W9-AMA-516

Pharmacology in Rehabilitation

4th Edition

Contemporary Perspectives in Rehabilitation

Steven L. Wolf, PT, PhD, FAPTA, Editor-in-Chief

Pharmacology in Rehabilitation, 4th Edition
Charles D. Ciccone, PT, PhD

Vestibular Rehabilitation, 3rd Edition
Susan J. Herdman, PT, PhD, FAPTA

Modalities for Therapeutic Intervention, 4th Edition
Susan L. Michlovitz, PT, PhD, CHT and **Thomas P. Nolan, Jr.**, PT, MS, OCS

Fundamentals of Musculoskeletal Imaging, 2nd Edition
Lynn N. McKinnis, PT, OCS

Wound Healing: Alternatives in Management, 3rd Edition
Luther C. Kloth, PT, MS, CWS, FAPTA, and
Joseph M. McCulloch, PT, PhD, CWS, FAPTA

Evaluation and Treatment of the Shoulder:
An Integration of the Guide to Physical Therapist Practice
Brian J. Tovin, PT, MMSc, SCS, ATC, FAAOMPT and
Bruce H. Greenfield, PT, MMSc, OCS

Cardiopulmonary Rehabilitation: Basic Theory and Application, 3rd Edition
Frances J. Brannon, PhD, **Margaret W. Foley**, RN, MN,
Julie Ann Starr, PT, MS, CCS, and **Lauren M. Saul**, MSN, CCRN

For more information on each title in the *Contemporary Perspectives in Rehabilitation* series, go to www.fadavis.com.

Pharmacology in Rehabilitation

4th Edition

Charles D. Ciccone, PT, PhD
Professor
Department of Physical Therapy
School of Health Sciences
and Human Performance
Ithaca College
Ithaca, New York

F. A. DAVIS COMPANY • Philadelphia

F. A. Davis Company
1915 Arch Street
Philadelphia, PA 19103
www.fadavis.com

Copyright © 2007 by F. A. Davis Company

Copyright © 1990 and 1996 by F. A. Davis Company. All rights reserved. This book is protected by copyright. No part of it may be reproduced, stored in a retrieval system, or transmitted in any from or by any means, electronic, mechanical, photocopying, recording, or otherwise, without written permission from the publisher.

Printed in the United States of America

Last digit indicates print number: 10 9 8 7 6

Publisher: Margaret Biblis
Acquisitions Editor/Developmental Editor: Melissa Duffield
Manager Art and Design: Carolyn O'Brien

As new scientific information becomes available through basic and clinical research, recommended treatments and drug threrapies undergo changes. The author and publisher have done everything possible to make this book accurate, up to date, and in accord with accepted standards at the time of publication. The author, editors, and publisher are not responsible for errors or omissions or for consequences from application of the book, and make no warranty, expressed or implied, in regard to the contents of the book. Any practice described in this book should be applied by the reader in accordance with professional standards of care used in regard to the unique circumstances that may apply in each situation. The reader is advised always to check product information (package inserts) for changes and new information regarding dose and contraindications before administering any drug. Caution is especially urged when using new or infrequently ordered drugs.

Library of Congress Cataloging-in-Publication Data

Ciccone, Charles D., 1953–
    Pharmacology in rehabilitation / Charles D. Ciccone. — 4th ed.
        p. ; cm.
    Includes bibliographical references and index.
    ISBN-13: 978-0-8036-1377-5
    ISBN-10: 0-8036-1377-6
1.   Pharmacology. 2.   Medical rehabilitation. I.   Title.
    [DNLM: 1.   Drug Therapy. 2.   Pharmacokinetics. 3.   Pharmacology. 4.   Rehabilitation.
WB 330 C568p 2007]
    RM301.C515 2007
    615′.1—dc22

                                                                                    2006101581

Authorization to photocopy items for internal or personal use, or the internal or personal use of specific clients, is granted by F. A. Davis Company for users registered with the Copyright Clearance Center (CCC) Transactional Reporting Service, provided that the fee of $.25 per copy is paid directly to CCC, 222 Rosewood Drive, Danvers, MA 01923. For those organizations that have been granted a photocopy license by CCC, a separate system of payment has been arranged. The fee code for users of the Transactional Reporting Service is: 8036–1377/07 0 + $.25.

Dedicated to Penny, Kate, and Alex for providing constant faith, support, and inspiration.

Foreword

There are very peculiar ways in which one can mark time. We often do so by observing the rate at which our siblings, children, or grandchildren grow, especially when we are not in daily contact, or by how we inevitably underestimate the length of time transpired since we last encountered an old friend. In this context, it seems remarkable that over 13 years have transpired since I first discussed with Chuck Ciccone the prospects for a text on pharmacology for our *Contemporary Perspectives in Rehabilitation*. The realization that the first edition of *Pharmacology in Rehabilitation* appeared more than a decade ago is even more astounding. The basis for the genesis of such a book was founded on the belief that rehabilitation specialists received little formal training about drug interactions and how any single pharmacological agent could impact either treatment plans or outcomes. Chuck took it upon himself to generate a text that would address this educational and clinical shortcoming. The result is very clear. *Pharmacology in Rehabilitation* **is** the "gold standard" among all texts addressing this content for nonphysician rehabilitation specialists.

So why is it important to create a fourth edition within one decade? Why is a more superficial compendium of information about drugs and their actions inadequate? The answer to these questions is directly related to the rapidly emerging responsibilities incumbent upon rehabilitation specialists. During the past 5 years, the advent of clinical doctoral programs in physical and occupational therapy has heralded a rapid transformation in these educational arenas. Several attributes now take on a meaning that previously might have been underappreciated. First, the label of "doctor" implies an *expectation* on the part of the consumer that the practitioner is the penultimate expert on providing an analysis and treatment plan for improving upon the pathology of any system's movement, whether muscle, joint, pulmonary, etc. Second, given the status associated with the professional label, there is an associated *obligation* on the part of the practitioner to address all aspects of the patients' signs and symptoms. This obligation requires that the clinician differentiate patient responses to treatment from patient responses to pharmacy. As one physical therapist so astutely told me, her recognition that a patient was not responding to pain medication taken well above the specified dosage, in the absence of any evidence for malingering behavior, resulted in the subsequent detection and successful removal of a renal tumor. Third, as practitioners, the DPT or DOT now assumes a greater *responsibility* for keeping a contemporary knowledge base about the interface between treatment plan and concurrent synergies or exacerbations that might result from single or multiple medications taken by the patient.

This collection of attributes can be best appreciated if the student is first informed and the clinician is educated about the most recent medications, their pharmokinetics, and the interactions they have with patients with specific diagnoses. Since the drug industry is arguably one of the most dynamic corporate structures in the world, changes in pharmacy occur at an alarmingly fast rate, one that will increase even more dramatically as transplants and the sequelae resulting from genetic engineering (as two examples) take on greater roles in medicine. Such rapid changes, then, call for contemporary and comprehensive updates in available information. Such updates must be presented in a manner that is compelling, yet easy to understand.

Inclusive in this perception is the absolute requirement that the student or clinician be able to relate to the text meaningfully. Toward this important goal, the 4th edition of *Pharmacology in Rehabilitation* is designed to address rehabilitation relevance in every clinical chapter as well as to present important case histories to reinforce this relevance. New materials on agents used in or even as complementary and alternative medicines have been added. Moreover, we have made efforts to add to the appeal of the book through the addition of colorization, use of double columns, and encasing the text within a newly designed hard cover. These changes are in contradistinction to one standard that remains immutable—Dr. Ciccone's remarkable gift for taking complex material and making it easy to understand.

For those clinicians who have in their possession early editions of this book, I invite you to compare your copy to the 4th edition as validation for the assertions made in this Foreword. We have not compromised the comprehensive nature of this volume in favor of a "simpler" approach to understanding pharmacology. We believe that the topic, by its very nature and from the implications inherent in its knowledge base, requires a comprehensive, yet user-friendly, delivery. This belief system remains unhindered in this latest edition; yet the problem-solving and evidence-based nature of the content is preserved and enhanced.

The thought of having a reference text for rehabilitation specialists was considered by us to be a unique concept 13 years ago. Today, many doctoral programs include pharmacology as a separate course or as an important component in teaching the rationale for treatment approaches and their assessment. There is much gratification to be gained from recognizing this transformation and in knowing that the content of this book contributes to the evolving maturation of our educational programs and our clinical services.

Steven L. Wolf, PT, PhD, FAPTA
Series Editor

Preface

In one sense, pharmacology can be considered a "good news, bad news" scenario. The good news is that exciting and innovative changes in drug therapy continue to occur at lightning speed. The bad news is that it is often difficult for health care practitioners to stay abreast of this rapidly changing field. Oftentimes, drug therapies that were considered state-of-the-art only a few years ago are now outdated and replaced by more contemporary treatments.

Hence, the fourth edition of this text has been revised extensively to reflect the science and practice of pharmacology, with particular emphasis on how drug therapy impacts patients receiving physical rehabilitation. Efforts were made to use the peer-reviewed literature to obtain the most recent information on pharmacotherapeutics. This information has become incredibly accessible because of computerized databases such as PubMed and resources such as the FDA website. The volume of this information, however, is so extensive that I was often astounded by the number of articles on a given topic. It was certainly a challenge to condense this information into a meaningful format for busy students and clinicians. Nonetheless, I believe this edition is successful in presenting the most recent and pertinent details of pharmacotherapeutics and that it underscores the relevance of this topic to physical therapy and occupational therapy.

As in previous editions, basic pharmacology concepts are addressed in the first section (Chapters 1 through 4), with subsequent chapters dealing with drug applications in specific diseases and pathological conditions. Chapters that deal with specific diseases begin with background information on each system or disorder, followed by detailed descriptions of the physiologic and pharmacologic actions of these drugs, their primary beneficial and adverse effect, and how drug therapy can impact physical rehabilitation. A new chapter on complementary and alternative medications (Chapter 38) has been added to this edition. This chapter complements the other chapters that deal with more traditional and conventional medications. This edition also has a new "look," with many features added to help students and clinicians access this information more easily.

Once again, I am pleased to present students and clinicians with a resource that might ultimately improve their ability to provide therapeutic interventions. Pharmacology continues to expand both in terms of the number of medications available to our patients, and in our understanding of how drugs can be used most effectively as part of a comprehensive health care regimen. It is essential that we understand the beneficial and adverse affects of medications commonly taken by our patients, and consider how we can capitalize on the beneficial effects while dealing with drug side effects. I hope this book will continue to serve as a primary resource on this topic, and that readers find this fourth edition interesting and useful.

Charles D. Ciccone

Acknowledgments

This edition is the culmination of the invaluable assistance and input from some very talented people. In particular, I want to thank Barbara MacDermott Costa, Linda D. Crane, John F. Decker, Mark Greve, Sandra B. Levine, Donald L. Merrill, Grace Minerbo, Peter Panus, and Jeffrey Rothman. I am deeply indebted to these individuals for their suggestions on previous editions. Without their help, it is unlikely that the fourth edition of this text would have ever become a reality.

I would also like to thank Bonnie DeSombre, Fred Estabrook, and Cheryl Tarbell for their help in preparing various tables and figures appearing in this text.

Finally, Steve Wolf, editor of the CPR series, has been a strong and consistent advocate for this book, and I thank him for his steadfast support and encouragement over the years. I also want to thank the staff at F. A. Davis Company for their help and proficiency in developing this text. In particular, Margaret Biblis and Melissa Duffield were instrumental in developing the fourth edition of this text, and for implementing most of the obvious changes in the design and presentation of this material. I cannot thank them enough for all their insight and expertise, and I am sure their efforts will be appreciated by everyone who uses this text.

Reviewer List

Susan Sullivan Glenney, PT, MS
Former Assistant Professor
Department of Physical Therapy
University of Hartford
West Hartford, Connecticut

Gary Gorniak, PT, PhD
Director and Associate Professor
Physical Therapy Program
University of St. Augustine for Health Sciences
St. Augustine, Florida

Ellen Wruble Hakim, PT, DScPT, MS, CWS
Assistant Professor
Department of Physical Therapy and Rehabilitation
Science
University of Maryland School of Medicine
Baltimore, Maryland

Steven Raymond Tippett, PT, PhD, SCS, ATC
Associate Professor
Department of Physical Therapy and Health Science
Bradley University
Peoria, Illinois

Contents

Chapter 34. Treatment of Infections II: Antiviral Drugs, 523

Chapter 35. Treatment of Infections III: Antifungal and Antiparasitic Drugs, 545

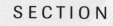

General Principles of Pharmacology

Chapter 1

Basic Principles of Pharmacology

Pharmacology is the study of drugs. In its broadest definition, a drug can be described as "any substance that, when taken into a living organism, may modify one or more of its functions."[28] In this sense, a drug includes any substance that alters physiologic function in the organism, regardless of whether the effect is beneficial or harmful. In terms of clinical pharmacology, it has traditionally been the beneficial or therapeutic effects that have been of special interest. Throughout history, certain naturally occurring chemicals have been used to relieve pain or treat disease in humans. Within the past century, the use of natural, semisynthetic, and synthetic chemical agents has expanded to the point where many diseases can be prevented or cured, and the general health and well-being of many individuals has dramatically improved through therapeutic drug use.

Because of the extensive clinical use of therapeutic medications, members of the medical community must have some knowledge of the basic types of drugs and the mechanisms of their actions. Although this has always been true for individuals who prescribe and administer drugs (i.e., physicians and nurses), it is now recognized that members of other health-related professions must have a fundamental knowledge of pharmacology.

An understanding of basic drug mechanisms can help practitioners such as physical therapists, occupational therapists, and other rehabilitation specialists better understand a patient's response to the drug. In addition, the knowledge of how certain rehabilitative procedures may interact with medications is helpful in getting an optimal response in the patient's drug and therapy treatment. For instance, scheduling the patient for therapy when certain drugs reach their peak effect may improve the therapy session dramatically. This may be true for drugs that decrease pain (analgesics) or improve the patient's motor skills (anti-Parkinson drugs). Conversely, some therapy sessions that require the patient's active participation may be rendered useless if scheduled when medications such as sedatives reach their peak effect. Also, any adverse responses occurring due to direct interaction between the therapy treatment and certain medications may be avoided or controlled by understanding a drug's pharmacologic aspects. For example, a patient who is taking a peripheral vasodilator may experience a profound decrease in blood pressure when he or she is placed in a hot whirlpool. By understanding the implications of such an interaction, the therapist can be especially alert for any detrimental effects on the patient, or they may institute a different therapy treatment for them.

In order to help the reader have a more focused approach to the study of drugs, pharmacology is often divided into several areas of interest (Fig. 1–1). **Pharmacotherapeutics** is the area of pharmacology that refers to the use of specific drugs to prevent, treat, or diagnose a disease. For the purposes of this text, the effects of drugs on humans will be of primary concern, with animal pharmacology mentioned only in reference to drug testing and research in animals.

When drugs are used therapeutically in humans, the way that the body interacts with the drug and what specific effect it has on an individual must be known. Consequently, pharmacotherapeutics is divided into two functional areas: pharmacokinetics and pharmacodynamics (see Fig. 1–1). **Pharmacokinetics** is the study of how the body deals with the drug in terms of the way it is absorbed, distributed, and eliminated.

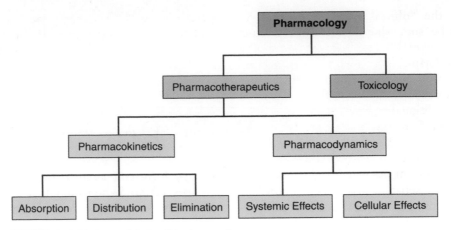

FIGURE 1–1 ▼ Areas of study within pharmacology.

Pharmacodynamics is the analysis of what the drug does to the body, including the mechanism by which the drug exerts its effect. In this text, the basic principles of pharmacokinetics will be outlined in Chapters 2 and 3, and the pharmacodynamics and pharmacokinetics of specific drugs will be discussed in their respective chapters.

Toxicology is the study of the harmful effects of chemicals. Although it can be viewed as a subdivision of pharmacology, toxicology has evolved into a separate area of study because of the scope of all the therapeutic agents' adverse effects as well as environmental toxins and poisons. However, because virtually every medication can produce adverse effects, a discussion of toxicology must be included in pharmacotherapeutics. For the purposes of this text, discussions of drug toxicity are limited to the unwanted effects that occur when therapeutic drugs reach excessively high (toxic) levels. The toxic side effects of individual drugs are covered in the chapters describing the therapeutic effects of that drug.

Pharmacy deals with the preparation and dispensing of medications. Although pharmacy is also frequently considered a subdivision of pharmacology, this area has evolved into a distinct professional discipline. Care must be taken not to use the terms "pharmacy" and "pharmacology" interchangeably, because these are quite different areas of study.

Drug Nomenclature

One of the most potentially confusing aspects of pharmacology is the variety of names given to different drugs or even to the same compound. Students of pharmacology, as well as clinicians, are often faced with myriad terms representing the same drug.[14,17] Many problems in drug terminology arise from the fact that each drug can be identified according to its *chemical*, *generic*, or *trade* name[12] (Table 1–1). **Chemical names** refer to the specific compound's structure and are usually fairly long and cumbersome. The **generic name**

Table 1–1	EXAMPLES OF DRUG NOMENCLATURE	
Chemical	**Generic (Nonproprietary)**	**Trade/Brand-Name (Proprietary)**
N-Acetyl-p-aminophenol	Acetaminophen	Tylenol, Panadol, many others
3,4-Dihydroxyphenyl-L-alanine	Levodopa	Larodopa
5,5-Phenylethylbarbituric acid	Phenobarbital	Luminal, Eskabarb
7-Chloro-1,3-dihydro-1-methyl-5-phenyl-2H-1,4-benzodiazepin-2-one	Diazepam	Valium

(also known as the "official" or "nonproprietary" name) tends to be somewhat shorter and is often derived from the chemical name. A **trade name** (also known as the brand name) is assigned to the compound by the pharmaceutical company and may or may not bear any reference at all to the chemical and generic terminology. An additional problem with trade names is that several manufacturers may be marketing the same compound under different names, thus adding to the confusion. If there is no existing patent for that compound or if the patent has expired, the same drug may be marketed by separate drug companies.[24] For practical purposes, the generic name is often the easiest and most effective way to refer to a drug, and this terminology will be used frequently in this text.

Drug nomenclature is also a source of confusion and potential errors in medication use, especially when different drugs have names that look or sound alike.[14] It has been estimated, for example, that up to 25 percent of all medication errors are caused by name confusion.[2,13] This fact seems especially true for drugs with similar brand names.[14] Consider, for example, the confusion that could occur when trying to differentiate between the following three brand-name products: Celebrex, Cerebryx, and Celexa.[14] These three brand names correspond with an analgesic (see Chapter 15), an antiseizure drug (see Chapter 9) and an antidepressant (see Chapter 7), respectively. Despite their similar brand names, these three products represent three distinct pharmacologic classes that are used in very different clinical situations. Hence, practitioners need to be especially careful when documenting the use of specific medications, and make sure that the correct drug name is used to identify each product.

Substitution of Generic Drugs for Brand-Name Products

A common question among practitioners and patients is whether the generic form of a drug can be substituted for the brand-name product. Generic forms are typically less expensive than their brand-name counterparts, and substitution of a generic drug can help reduce health care costs.[16] The generic form of the drug should be as safe and effective as the original brand-name product, provided that the generic form satisfies certain criteria.[10,29] Specifically, the generic form should undergo testing to establish that it has the same type and amount of the active ingredient(s), the same administration route, the same pharmacokinetic

profile (drug absorption, plasma levels, and so forth), and the same therapeutic effects as the brand-name drug.[3] If such testing is done, the two drugs are said to be "bioequivalent."[7]

Unless bioequivalence is established, however, it can only be assumed that substituting a generic drug will produce therapeutic effects that are similar to the brand-name drug. Likewise, establishing bioequivalence of a generic form does not guarantee that a given patient will not experience different effects from the generic form compared to the brand-name product. That is, certain patients might simply respond differently to a the generic form of a drug because of individual differences in their ability to absorb and metabolize certain generic products, even if these products have been shown to be similar to their brand-name counterpart during bioequivalence testing. This fact seems especially true for drugs that tend to produce a wider range of therapeutic and adverse effects when tested in a specific patient, or within a group of patients (i.e., drugs with more intrasubject and intersubject variability).[20] Hence, there are a number of issues that should be considered before a generic drug is substituted, and practitioners may want to prescribe a specific brand-name drug based on the pharmacologic profile of that drug and the specific way that the drug may affect a given patient.

What Constitutes a Drug: Development and Approval of Therapeutic Agents

In the United States, the **Food and Drug Administration (FDA)** is responsible for monitoring the use of existing drugs as well as developing and approving of new ones.[9,19,21] The analogous body in Canada is the Health Products and Food Branch of the Department of National Health and Welfare. The two primary concerns of these agencies are (1) whether or not the drug is effective in treating a certain condition and (2) whether the drug is reasonably safe for human use.

Drug Approval Process

The development of a new drug involves extensive preclinical (animal) and clinical (human) studies.[19,21] The basic procedure for testing a new drug is outlined here and is summarized in Table 1–2. Details about the phases of drug testing can also be found on the FDA website (http://www.fda.gov/cder/handbook).

Table 1–2	DRUG DEVELOPMENT AND APPROVAL		
Testing Phase	**Purpose**	**Subjects**	**Usual Time Period**
Preclinical testing	Initial laboratory tests to determine drug effects and safety	Laboratory animals	1–2 yrs
Investigational New Drug (IND) Application			
Human (clinical) testing: Phase I	Determine effects, safe dosage, pharmacokinetics	Small number (< 100) of healthy volunteers	<1 yr
Phase II	Assess drug's effectiveness in treating a specific disease/disorder	Limited number (200–300) patients with target disorder	2 yrs
Phase III	Assess safety and effectiveness in a larger patient population	Large number (1000–3000) patients targeted	3 yrs
New Drug Application (NDA) Approval			
Phase IV (postmarketing surveillance)	Monitor any problems that occur after NDA approval	General patient population	Indefinite

Animal (Preclinical) Studies

Drugs are typically tested in animals initially, often using several different species. Initial information on the basic pharmacokinetic and pharmacodynamic properties of the compound is obtained. Information on dosage and toxicity is also obtained from these animal trials.

Human (Clinical) Studies

If the results from animal trials are favorable, the drug sponsor files an investigational new drug (IND) application with the FDA. If approved as an IND, the sponsor may begin testing the drug in humans. Human, or "clinical" testing, is divided into three primary phases.

Phase I. The drug is usually tested in a relatively small number of healthy volunteers. The purpose of this phase is to obtain some initial information about the pharmacologic actions, and the drug's possible toxic effects in humans. In general, between 20 to 80 subjects are studied in phase 1, but the actual number of subjects will vary according to the drug,

Phase II. The drug is tested in a relatively small sample (200 to 300 people) with a specific dis-

ease or pathologic condition. The primary goal of phase 2 is to evaluate the effectiveness of the drug, and to assess the side effects and other risks.

Phase III. Clinical evaluation is expanded to include more patients (several hundred to several thousand) as well as more evaluators. Additional information is obtained regarding the drug's safety and effectiveness in a large patient population.

At the end of phase III, the drug sponsor applies for a new drug application (NDA). Results from clinical testing are reviewed extensively by the FDA, and if found favorable, the NDA is approved. At this point, the drug can be marketed and prescribed for use in the general population.

A fourth phase known as "postmarketing surveillance" should be instituted after the NDA is approved. Postmarketing surveillance refers to all of the methods used to continue monitoring drug safety and effectiveness after approval for public use.[19,21] These methods often consist of reports from health care providers that describe specific rare adverse effects that were not discovered during clinical testing.[24] A certain drug, for example, could cause a specific adverse effect in only 1 in 10,000 patients taking the drug.[1] It is very likely that such an adverse effect could be missed during phase I through phase III of the clinical trials because the drug is typically tested only in a few thousand subjects (e.g., 1000 to 3000 people). In addition to monitoring adverse effects, postmarketing surveillance can use more formal research methods to obtain information about how a specific drug is used in clinical practice and how that drug compares to similar drugs on the market.[24] Hence, postmarketing surveillance has been advocated as being critical in ensuring that the safety and efficacy of the drug continues to be monitored when it is used by the general patient population.[18,24]

The development of a new drug in the United States is an extremely expensive and time-consuming process.[11] The time course for the entire testing process from the beginning of animal trials to the end of phase III human testing may be as long as 7 to 9 years. The FDA has made provisions, however, to shorten the development and review process for drugs designed to treat serious and life-threatening conditions, especially if the drug shows substantial benefits over existing treatments, or no drugs are currently available for these conditions.[25] This type of accelerated development/review (also known as "fast track" drug development) is typically used for drugs that show promise in treating conditions such as cancer or acquired immunodeficiency syndrome (AIDS). Hence, these fast tract drugs may be made available for patient use even before formal clinical testing is completed.[27] The FDA will, however, require that drug testing be continued even after the drug is approved, and efforts must be made to ensure that it actually provides the therapeutic benefits that were initially promised.[27] The approval process can also be expedited if a drug has already received approval for treating one condition, but is now being considered for use in other "supplemental" conditions.[24]

The process of drug testing and approval does seem to be fairly rigorous in its ability to screen out ineffective or potentially harmful drugs. Out of thousands of newly synthesized compounds, only one will ever be released as a prescription drug.[1]

Prescription Versus Over-the-Counter Medication

In the United States, pharmacotherapeutic agents are divided into drugs requiring a prescription for use and drugs available as nonprescription, or **over-the-counter (OTC)**.[8] Nonprescription drugs can be pur-

chased directly by the consumer, whereas prescription medications may be ordered or dispensed only by an authorized practitioner (i.e., physician, dentist, or other appropriate health care provider). Prescription or nonprescription drug classification falls under the jurisdiction of the FDA.[8] In general, OTC medications are used to treat relatively minor problems and to make the consumer more comfortable until the condition is resolved. These medications have been judged to be safe for use by the consumer without direct medical supervision, and the chances of toxic effects are usually small when the medications are taken in the recommended amounts.[8] Of course, the patient may ingest more than the recommended amount, and in the case of an overdose, the danger always exists for potentially harmful effects, even if the drug is nonprescription in nature.[6,15,22]

The role of OTC products in the health care market has expanded dramatically in recent years.[4,23] Many drugs that were formerly available only by prescription are now available in a nonprescription form. Transition of a prescription drug to an OTC product usually occurs when the drug's marketing company applies to the FDA and receives approval to develop and market it in a nonprescription form. FDA approval is based on the drug having an adequate safety profile, and the FDA may require other stipulations such as lowering the drug dosage in the OTC product.

The fact that more and more prescription drugs are now available in a nonprescription form offers some obvious benefits. Increased availability of OTC products can make it easier for consumers to gain access to these medications.[4,5] In addition, OTC products are typically less expensive than prescription drugs, and the purported savings might help contain overall medication costs. The actual cost to the patient, however, might be greater for an OTC product because the patient must pay directly "out of pocket."[4] That is, health care programs with prescription drug plans may cover the majority of a prescription drug's cost, whereas the patient often must pay directly for the entire cost of an OTC product. The actual money spent by patients (i.e., the out-of-pocket cost) might therefore be greater for OTC products compared to prescription drugs. Hence the overall benefits of OTC products on health care costs remains complex.[4]

Despite the potential benefits of OTC products, there are some obvious concerns about their increased use and emphasis on self-care that permeates today's health care market. Consumers must realize that these products are important therapeutic medications and must be used appropriately.[23,26] There is also the chance that inappropriate OTC use can cause serious interactions with a patient's prescription medications, or that OTC products can delay the use of more effective medications.[4] The impact of such OTC compounds is discussed in this text in the appropriate chapters.

It is therefore clear that consumers need to be educated about the use of such medications and reminded that OTC products can produce substantial benefits and adverse effects. All health care providers, including physical therapists and occupational therapists, need to be in a position to help educate and counsel their patients about the benefits and drawbacks of such medications. While therapists should not directly prescribe or administer OTC products, therapists can provide information about the proper use and potential benefits of these medications.

Controlled Substances

In 1970, federal legislation was enacted to help control the abuse of legal and illegal drugs. The Comprehensive Drug Abuse Prevention and Control Act (or Controlled Substances Act) placed drugs into specific categories, or "schedules," according to their potential for abuse.[12] Descriptions of the schedules for controlled drugs can be found on the FDA website (http://www.fda.goc/opacom/laws/cntrlsbb.htm), and these schedules are described briefly below.

Schedule I. These drugs are regarded as having the highest potential for abuse, and are not typically used as an acceptable medical treatment in the United States. Legal use of agents in this category is restricted to approved research studies or therapeutic use in a very limited number of patients (e.g., use of marijuana as an antiemetic). Examples of schedule I drugs include heroin, lysergic acid diethylamide (LSD), psilocybin, mescaline, peyote, marijuana, tetrahydrocannabinols, and several other hallucinogens.

Schedule II. Drugs in this category are approved for specific therapeutic purposes but still have a high potential for abuse and possible addiction. Examples include opioids such as morphine and fentanyl, and drugs containing methamphetamine.

Schedule III. Although these drugs have a lower abuse potential than those in schedules I and II, there is still the possibility of developing mild to moderate physical dependence, strong psychologic dependence, or both. Drugs in schedule III include certain opioids (e.g., codeine) that are combined in a limited dosage with other nonopioid drugs. Other drugs in this category are anabolic steroids, certain barbiturates, and amphetamines that are not included in schedule II.

Schedule IV. These drugs supposedly have a lower potential for abuse than schedule III drugs, with only a limited possibility of physical dependence, psychologic dependence, or both. Examples include certain antianxiety drugs (meprobamate), certain barbiturates (barbital, phenobarbital), and a variety of other depressants and stimulants.

Schedule V. These drugs have the lowest relative abuse potential. Drugs in this category consist primarily of low doses of opioids that are used in cough medications and antidiarrheal preparations.

Several other criteria relate to the different controlled substance schedules, such as restrictions on prescription renewal and penalties for illegal possession of drugs in different schedules. For a further discussion of controlled substances, the reader is referred to another source.[12]

Basic Concepts in Drug Therapy

All drugs exert their beneficial effects by reaching some specific target cell or tissue. On the cellular level, the drug in some way changes the function of the cell either to help restore normal physiologic function or to prevent a disease process from occurring. In general, the **dose** of a drug must be large enough to allow an adequate concentration to reach the target site, thus producing a beneficial response. However, the administered **dosage** must not be so excessive that toxicologic effects are produced. Some aspects of the relationship between dose and response are discussed here.

Dose-Response Curves and Maximal Efficacy

The relationship between the dose of a drug and a specific response to the drug is illustrated in Figure 1–2. Typically, very low doses do not produce any observable effect. At some threshold dose, the response

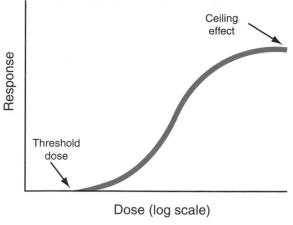

FIGURE 1–2 ▼ Dose-response curve.

begins to occur and continues to increase in magnitude before reaching a plateau. The plateau in the response indicates that there will be no further increment in the response even if the dosage continues to be increased. The point at which there is no further increase in the response is known as **ceiling effect,** or **maximal efficacy,** of the drug.[24]

  Dose-response curves are used to provide information about the dosage range over which the drug is effective, as well as the peak response that can be expected from the drug. In addition, the characteristic shape of the dose-response curve and the pres-

ence of the plateau associated with maximal efficacy can be used to indicate specific information about the binding of the drug to cellular receptors. The relevance of dose-response curves to drug-receptor interactions is discussed further in Chapter 4.

Potency

One criterion used frequently when comparing drugs is the concept of **potency**. Potency is related to the dose that produces a given response in a specific amplitude.[24] When two drugs are compared, the more potent drug requires a lower dose to produce the same effect as a higher dose of the second drug. For instance, in Figure 1–3, a dose of 10 mg of drug A would lower blood pressure by 25 percent, whereas 80 mg of drug B would be required to produce the same response. Consequently, drug A would be described as being more potent. It should be noted that potency is not synonymous with maximal efficacy. Drug B is clearly able to exert a greater maximal effect than drug A. Consequently, the term "potency" is often taken to be much more significant than it really is.[24] The potency of a drug is often misinterpreted by the layperson as an indication of the drug's overall therapeutic benefits, whereas potency really just refers to the fact that less of the compound is required to produce a given response. In fact, neither potency nor maximal efficacy fully indicates a drug's therapeutic

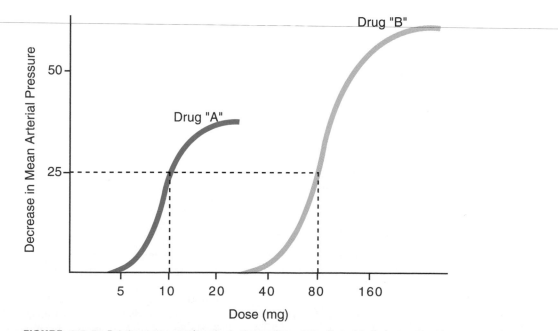

FIGURE 1–3 ▼ Relative potency and maximal efficacy of two drugs. Drug A is more potent, and drug B has a greater maximal efficacy.

potential. Other factors such as the therapeutic index (described further on) and drug selectivity (see Chapter 4) are also important in comparing and ultimately choosing the best medication for a given problem.

Elements of Drug Safety

Quantal Dose-Response Curves and the Median Effective Dose

The dose-response curves shown in Figures 1–2 and 1–3 represent the graded response to a drug as it would occur in a single individual or in a homogeneous population. In reality, variations in drug responses that are caused by individual differences in the clinical population need to be considered when trying to assess whether a drug is safe as well as effective. Consequently, the relationship between the dose of the drug and the occurrence of a certain response is measured in a large group of people (or animals if the drug is being tested preclinically). When plotted, this relationship yields a cumulative, or *quantal*, dose-response curve (Fig. 1–4).[24] This curve differs from the dose-response curve discussed previously in that it is not the magnitude of the response that increases with increasing the dosage, but the percentage of the population who

exhibit a specific response as the dosage is increased. The response is not graded; it is either present or it is absent in each member of the population. For example, a headache medication is administered in an increasing dosage to 1000 people. At some dose, some of the individuals will begin to respond to the drug by reporting the absence of their headache. As the dosage is increased, more and more individuals will experience pain relief because of the medication, until finally 100 percent of the population report that their headaches are gone. Again, it is the percentage of the population who respond in a specific way (e.g., reporting loss of their headaches) that is measured relative to the dose of the drug. An important reference point in this type of cumulative dose-response curve is the **median effective dose** (ED_{50}).[24] This is the dose at which 50 percent of the population respond to the drug in a specified manner.

Median Toxic Dose

In the aforementioned example, relief from pain was the desired response, which is often termed the "beneficial" effect. As dosages of the drug continue to be increased, however, adverse or toxic effects may become apparent. To continue the earlier example, higher doses of the same medication may be associated

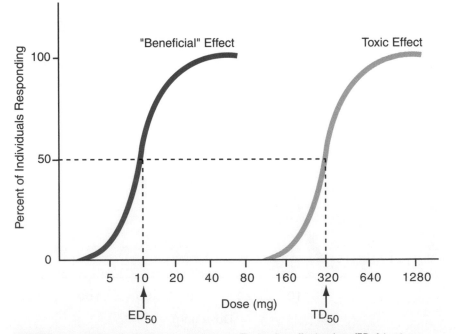

FIGURE 1–4 ▼ Cumulative dose-response curve. The median effective dose (ED_{50}) is 10 mg, and the median toxic dose (TD_{50}) is 320 mg. The therapeutic index (TI) for this drug is 32.

with the appearance of a specific toxic effect such as acute gastric hemorrhage. As the dosage is increased, more and more individuals will then begin to exhibit that particular adverse effect. The dose at which 50 percent of the group exhibits the adverse effect is termed the **median toxic dose** (TD_{50}). In animal studies, the toxic effect studied is often the death of the animal. In these cases, high doses of the drug are used to determine the **median lethal dose** (LD_{50})—the dose that causes death in 50 percent of the animals studied.[24] Of course, the LD_{50} is not a relevant term in clinical use of the drug in humans, but it does serve to provide some indication of the drug's safety in preclinical animal trials.

Therapeutic Index

The median effective and toxic doses are used to determine the **therapeutic index** (TI).[24] The TI is calculated as the ratio of the TD_{50} to the ED_{50}:

$$TI = \frac{TD_{50}}{ED_{50}}$$

In animal studies in which the median lethal dose is known, the TI is often calculated using the LD_{50} in place of the TD_{50}. In either human or animal studies, the TI is used as an indicator of the drug's safety.[24] The greater the value of the TI, the safer the drug is considered to be. In essence, a large TI indicates that it takes a much larger dose to evoke a toxic response than it does to cause a beneficial effect.

It should be noted, however, that the TI is a relative term. Acetaminophen, a nonprescription analgesic, has a TI of approximately 27 (i.e., the ratio of the median toxic dose to the median effective dose equals 27). Prescription agents tend to have lower TIs. For instance, the narcotic analgesic meperidine (Demerol)

has a TI of 8, and the sedative-hypnotic diazepam (Valium) has a TI equal to 3. Other prescription agents such as cancer chemotherapeutics (methotrexate, vincristine, and so on) may have very low TIs, some close to 1. However, a low TI is often acceptable in these agents, considering the critical nature of cancer and similar serious conditions. The consequences of not using the drug outweighs the risks of some of the toxic effects.

To help keep the risk of toxicity to a minimum with low-TI drugs, it is generally advisable to periodically monitor blood levels. This helps prevent concentrations from quickly reaching toxic levels. This precaution is usually not necessary with high-TI drugs, because there is a greater margin of error (i.e., blood levels can rise quite a lot above the therapeutic concentration before becoming dangerous).

SUMMARY

In its broadest sense, pharmacology is the study of the effects of chemicals on living organisms. Most discussions of clinical pharmacology deal primarily with the beneficial effects of specific drugs on humans, and the manner in which these drugs exert their therapeutic effects. Since all drugs have the potential to produce unwanted or toxic responses, some discussion of a drug's adverse effects is also essential in pharmacology. Drugs used therapeutically are subjected to extensive testing prior to approval for use in humans and are classified as either prescription or over-the-counter, depending on their dosage, effectiveness, and safety profile. Finally, certain characteristic relationships exist between the dose of a drug and the response or effect it produces. Such relationships can provide useful information about drug efficacy and potency and about the relative safety of different compounds.

References

1. Berkowitz BA. Basic and clinical evaluation of new drugs. In: Katzung BG, ed. *Basic and Clinical Pharmacology*. 9th ed. New York: Lange Medical Books/McGraw Hill; 2004.
2. Berman A. Reducing medication errors through naming, labeling, and packaging. *J Med Syst*. 2004; 28:9–29.
3. Borgheini G. The bioequivalence and therapeutic efficacy of generic versus brand-name psychoactive drugs. *Clin Ther*. 2003;25:1578–1592.
4. Brass EP. Changing the status of drugs from prescription to over-the-counter availability. *N Engl J Med*. 2001;345:810–816.
5. Brass EP. Implications of a switch from prescription to over-the-counter status for allergy drugs. *Curr Allergy Asthma Rep*. 2004;4:245–250.
6. Bromer MQ, Black M. Acetaminophen hepatotoxicity. *Clin Liver Dis*. 2003;7:351–367.
7. Chen ML, Shah V, Patnaik R, et al. Bioavailability and bioequivalence: an FDA regulatory overview. *Pharm Res*. 2001;18:1645–1650.
8. Corelli RL. Therapeutic and toxic potential of over-the-counter agents. In: Katzung BG, ed. *Basic and Clinical Pharmacology*. 9th ed. New York: Lange Medical Books/McGraw Hill; 2004.
9. Cowan CC. The process of evaluating and regulating a new drug: phases of a drug study. *AANA J*. 2002;70: 385–390.

10. Dighe SV. A review of the safety of generic drugs. *Transplant Proc.* 1999;31(suppl 3A):23S–24S.

11. DiMasi JA, Hansen RW, Grabowski HG. The price of innovation: new estimates of drug development costs. *J Health Econ.* 2003;22:151–185.

12. Edwards L. Appendix I. Principles of prescription order writing and patient compliance. In: Hardman JG, et al, eds. *The Pharmacological Basis of Therapeutics.* 10th ed. New York: McGraw Hill; 2001.

13. Gremillion L, Hogan DJ. Dermatologic look- or sound-alike medications. *J Drugs Dermatol.* 2004;3: 61–64.

14. Hoffman JM, Proulx SM. Medication errors caused by confusion of drug names. *Drug Saf.* 2003;26: 445–452.

15. Jones A. Over-the-counter analgesics: a toxicology perspective. *Am J Ther.* 2002;9:245–257.

16. Kirking DM, Ascione FJ, Gaither CA, Welage LS. Economics and structure of the generic pharmaceutical industry. *J Am Pharm Assoc.* 2001;41: 578–584.

17. Lambert BL, Chang KY, Lin SJ. Immediate free recall of drug names: effects of similarity and availability. *Am J Health Syst Pharm.* 2003;60:156–168.

18. Lasser KE, Allen PD, Woolhandler SJ, et al. Timing of new black box warnings and withdrawals for prescription medications. *JAMA.* 2002;287:2215–2120.

19. Lipsky MS, Sharp LK. From idea to market: the drug approval process. *J Am Board Fam Pract.* 2001;14: 362–367.

20. Meredith P. Bioequivalence and other unresolved issues in generic drug substitution. *Clin Ther.* 2003; 25:2875–2890.

21. Moore SW. An overview of drug development in the United States and current challenges. *South Med J.* 2003;96:1244–1256.

22. Motola G, Mazzeo F, Rinaldi B, et al. Self-prescribed laxative use: a drug-utilization review. *Adv Ther.* 2002; 19:203–238.

23. Newton GD, Pray WS, Popovich NG. New OTC drugs and devices 2003: a selective review. *J Am Pharm Assoc (Wash DC).* 2004;44:211–225.

24. Nies AS. Principles of therapeutics. In: Hardman JG, et al, eds. *The Pharmacological Basis of Therapeutics.* 10th ed. New York: McGraw Hill; 2001.

25. Reichert JM. Trends in development and approval times for new therapeutics in the United States. *Nat Rev Drug Discov.* 2003;2:695–702.

26. Roumie CL, Griffin MR0. Over-the-counter analgesics in older adults: a call for improved labelling and consumer education. *Drugs Aging.* 2004;21:485–498.

27. Shih WJ, Ouyang P, Quan H, Lin Y, Michiels B, Bijnens L. Controlling type I error rate for fast track drug development programmes. *Stat Med.* 2003;22: 665–675.

28. Venes D, Thomas CL (eds). *Taber's Cyclopedic Medical Dictionary.* 19th ed. Philadelphia: FA Davis;2004.

29. Welage LS, Kirking DM, Ascione FJ, Gaither CA. Understanding the scientific issues embedded in the generic drug approval process. *J Am Pharm Assoc (Wash DC).* 2001;41:856–867.

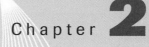

Chapter 2

Pharmacokinetics I: Drug Administration, Absorption, and Distribution

Pharmacokinetics is the study of the way that the body deals with pharmacologic compounds. In other words, what does the body do to the drug? This includes the manner in which the drug is administered, absorbed, distributed, and eventually eliminated from the body. These topics are discussed in this chapter and the next.

Routes of Administration

In general, drugs can be administered via two primary routes: through the alimentary canal **(enteral administration)** or through nonalimentary routes **(parenteral administration).** Each major route has several variations, and each offers distinct advantages and disadvantages. The primary features of some of the major routes are discussed here. For a more detailed description of the specific methodology involved in drug administration, the reader is referred to several excellent discussions of this topic.[10,34,86]

Enteral

Oral

The primary way that drugs are given enterally is through the oral route. This is the most common method of administering medications and offers several distinct advantages. Oral administration is the easiest method of taking medications, especially when self-administration is necessary or desired. The oral route is also relatively safe because drugs enter the system in a fairly controlled manner. This avoids the large, sudden increase in plasma drug levels, which can occur when the drug is administered by other methods such as through intravenous injection. Most medications that are administered orally are absorbed from the small intestine, thus utilizing the large surface area of the intestinal microvilli to enhance its entry into the body.

Several disadvantages may preclude drugs from being given orally. Drugs that are administered by mouth must have a relatively high degree of lipid solubility in order to pass through the gastrointestinal mucosa and into the bloodstream. Large, nonlipid-soluble compounds are absorbed very poorly from the alimentary canal and will eventually be lost from the body in the feces. Absorption of some nonlipid-soluble substances (peptides, small proteins) can be enhanced to some extent by encapsulating these agents in lipid vesicles (liposomes); this technique was recently developed to enable the oral administration of drugs that were formerly administered only through injection or some other parenteral route.[82] Other drawbacks to the oral route include the fact that certain medications may irritate the stomach and cause discomfort, vomiting, or even damage to the gastric mucosa. The acidic environment and presence of digestive proteases in the stomach may also cause various compounds to be degraded and destroyed prior to absorption from the gastrointestinal tract.[49]

Drugs that are given orally are subject to a phenomenon known as the **first-pass effect.**[10,86] After

Table 2–1	ROUTES OF DRUG ADMINISTRATION		
Route	**Advantages**	**Disadvantages**	**Examples**
Enteral			
Oral	Easy, safe, convenient	Limited or erratic absorption of some drugs; chance of first-pass inactivation in liver	Analgesics; sedative-hypnotics; many others
Sublingual	Rapid onset; not subject to first-pass inactivation	Drug must be easily absorbed from oral mucosa	Nitroglycerin
Rectal	Alternative to oral route; local effect on rectal tissues	Poor or incomplete absorption; chance of rectal irritation	Laxatives; suppository forms of other drugs
Parenteral			
Inhalation	Rapid onset; direct application for respiratory disorders; large surface area for systemic absorption	Chance of tissue irritation; patient compliance sometimes a problem	General anesthetics; anti-asthmatic agents
Injection	Provides more direct administration to target tissues; rapid onset	Chance of infection if sterility is not maintained	Insulin; antibiotics; anti-cancer drugs; narcotic analgesics
Topical	Local effects on surface of skin	Only effective in treating outer layers of skin	Antibiotic ointments; creams used to treat minor skin irritation and injury
Transdermal	Introduces drug into body without breaking the skin; can provide steady, prolonged delivery via medicated patch	Drug must be able to pass through dermal layers intact	Nitroglycerin; motion sickness medications; drugs used with phonophoresis and iontophoresis

absorption from the alimentary canal, the drug is transported directly into the liver via the portal vein, where a significant amount of the drug may be metabolized and destroyed prior to reaching its site of action. The dosage of the orally administered drug must be sufficient enough to allow an adequate amount of the compound to survive hepatic degradation and to eventually reach the target tissue.[10] Some drugs—such as nitroglycerin—undergo such extensive inactivation from the first-pass effect that it is usually preferable to administer them through nonoral routes.[86]

A final limitation of the oral route is that the amount and rate at which the drug eventually reaches the bloodstream tends to be somewhat less predictable with oral administration compared with more direct routes, such as injection. Factors that affect intestinal absorption (intestinal infection, presence of food, rate of gastric emptying, amount of visceral blood flow, and so on) can alter the usual manner in which a drug is absorbed into the body from the gastrointestinal tract.[6,21,39,86]

Sublingual and Buccal

Drugs are administered sublingually by placing the drug under the tongue. Buccal administration occurs when the drug is placed between the cheek and gums. A drug that is administered sublingually or buccally is then absorbed through the oral mucosa into the venous system that is draining the mouth region. These veins eventually carry blood to the superior vena cava, which in turn carries blood to the heart. Consequently, a drug administered sublingually or buccally can reach the systemic circulation without being subjected to first-pass inactivation in the liver.[70,90] This provides an obvious advantage for drugs such as nitroglycerin that would be destroyed in the liver when absorbed from the stomach or intestines. These routes also offer a means of enteral administration to people who have difficulty swallowing or to patients who cannot be given drugs rectally.[54] The restrictions of the sublingual and buccal routes are that the amount of drug that can be administered is somewhat limited, and the drug must be able to pass easily through the oral mucosa in order to reach the venous drainage of the mouth.

Rectal

A final method of enteral administration is via the rectum. Many drugs are available as rectal suppositories to allow administration through this route. This method is less favorable because many drugs are absorbed poorly or incompletely, and irritation of the rectal mucosa may occur.[86] Rectal administration does offer the advantage of allowing drugs to be given to a patient who is unconscious, or when vomiting prevents drugs from being taken orally. However, the rectal route is used most often for treating local conditions such as hemorrhoids.

Parenteral

All methods of drug administration that do not use the gastrointestinal tract are termed *parenteral*. Parenteral administration generally allows the drug to be delivered to the target site more directly, and the quantity of the drug that actually reaches the target site is often more predictable.[86] Also, drugs given parenterally are not usually subject to first-pass inactivation in the liver. Other advantages and disadvantages of various parenteral routes are discussed further on in this section.

Inhalation

Drugs that exist in a gaseous or volatile state, or that can be suspended as tiny droplets in an aerosol form, may be given via inhalation. Pulmonary administration is advantageous because of the large (alveolar) surface area for diffusion of the drug into the pulmonary circulation and it is generally associated with rapid entry of the drug into the bloodstream.[43] This method is used extensively in administering the volatile general anesthetics (e.g., halothane) and it is also advantageous when applying medications directly

to the bronchial and alveolar tissues for the treatment of specific pulmonary pathologies.[42] The pulmonary route may also be a potential way to administer larger nonlipid-soluble agents such as peptides, small proteins (including insulin), and DNA.[3,30,69]

One limitation of the inhalation route is that the drug must not irritate the alveoli or other areas of the respiratory tract. Also, some patients have trouble administering drugs by this route, and drug particles tend to be trapped by cilia and mucus in the respiratory tract. Both of these factors tend to limit the ability to predict exactly how much of the drug eventually reaches the lungs. Efforts continue to advance the use of inhaled drugs by improving the physicochemical properties of these drugs, and also by improving the devices used to deliver these drugs (i.e., inhalers).[20] Technological advancements in inhaled drugs will be addressed in more detail when respiratory medications are addressed later in this text (see Chapter 26).

Injection

Various types of injection can be used to introduce the drug either systemically or locally. If sterility is not maintained, all types of injection have the disadvantage of possible infection, and certain types of injection are more difficult, if not impossible, for the patient to self-administer. Specific types of injection include the following routes.

Intravenous. The bolus injection of a medication into a peripheral vein allows an accurate, known quantity of the drug to be introduced into the bloodstream over a short period of time, frequently resulting in peak levels of the drug appearing almost instantaneously in the peripheral circulation and thus reaching the target site rapidly. This occurrence is advantageous in emergency situations when it is necessary for the medication to exert an immediate effect. Of course, adverse reactions may also occur because of the sudden appearance of large titers of the drug in the plasma. Any unexpected side effects or miscalculations in the amount of the administered drug are often difficult to deal with after the full dose has been injected. In certain situations, an indwelling intravenous cannula (IV "line") can be used to allow the prolonged, steady infusion of a drug into the venous system. This method prevents large fluctuations in the plasma concentration of the drug and allows the dosage of drug to be maintained at a specific level for as long as desired.

Intra-arterial. The injection of a drug directly into an artery is understandably a difficult and dangerous procedure. This method permits a large dose of the medication to reach a given site, such as a specific organ, and may be used to focus the administration of drugs into certain tissues. Intra-arterial injections are used occasionally in cancer chemotherapy to administer the anticancer drug directly to the tumor site with minimal exposure of the drug to other healthy tissues. This route may also be used to focus the administration of other substances such as radiopaque dyes for various diagnostic procedures.

Subcutaneous. Injecting medications directly beneath the skin is used when a local response is desired, such as in certain situations requiring local anesthesia. Also, a slower, more prolonged release of the medication into the systemic circulation can be achieved in situations where this is the desired effect. A primary example is insulin injection in a patient with diabetes mellitus. Subcutaneous administration provides a relatively easy route of parenteral injection that can be performed by patients themselves, providing they are properly trained.

Some limitations are that the amount of drug that can be injected in this fashion is fairly small and that the injected drug must not irritate or inflame the subcutaneous tissues. The subcutaneous route can also be used when certain types of drug preparations are implanted surgically beneath the skin, so that the drug is slowly dispersed from the implanted preparation and then absorbed into the bloodstream for prolonged periods of time.[62,86] A common example of this form of subcutaneous administration is the use of implanted hormonal contraceptive products (e.g., Norplant).[9,53] The use of these implantable contraceptives is discussed in more detail in Chapter 30.

Intramuscular. The large quantity of skeletal muscle in the body allows this route to be an easily accessible site for parenteral administration. Intramuscular injections can be used to treat a problem located directly in the injected muscle. For example, botulinum toxin and other substances can be injected directly into hyperexcitable muscles to control certain types of muscle spasms or spasticity (see Chapter 13).[7,78] Alternatively, intramuscular injection can be used as a method for a relatively steady, prolonged release of the drug into the systemic circulation to control conditions such as psychosis,[2] or to administer certain vaccines.

Intramuscular injection offers the advantage of providing a relatively rapid effect (i.e., within a few minutes), while avoiding the sudden, large increase in plasma levels seen with intravenous injection. The major problem with intramuscular administration is that many drugs injected directly into a muscle cause significant amounts of local pain and prolonged soreness, tending to limit the use of this route for repeated injections.

Intrathecal. Intrathecal injections are given by injecting the medication within a sheath, and frequently refer to injections within the spinal subarachnoid space (i.e., the space between the arachnoid membrane and the pia mater that help form the meninges surrounding the spinal cord). This particular type of intrathecal route allows drugs such as narcotic analgesics, local anesthetics, and antispasticity drugs to be applied directly to an area adjacent to the spinal cord, thereby allowing these drugs to gain better access to the cord.[55,60,79] Also, intrathecal injections allow certain drugs—such as antibiotics and anticancer drugs—to bypass the blood-brain barrier and reach the central nervous system (see Chapter 5).[86] Other intrathecal injections include administration of the drug within a tendon sheath or bursa, which may be used to treat a local condition such as an inflammation within those structures.

Topical

Drugs given topically are applied to the surface of the skin or mucous membranes. Most medications applied directly to the skin are absorbed fairly poorly through the epidermis and into the systemic circulation and are used primarily to treat problems that exist on the skin itself. Common examples of topical administration include the use of antibiotics to treat cutaneous infections, application of anti-inflammatory steroids to reduce skin inflammation, and the use of various topical products to promote wound healing.[11,59,74,85] Topical application to mucous membranes is also used frequently to treat problems on the membrane itself.[86] Significant amounts of the drug, however, can be readily absorbed through the mucous membrane and into the bloodstream. Topical application of drugs to mucous membranes can therefore provide a fairly easy and convenient way to administer drugs systemically. Certain medications, for example, can be administered to the nasal mucosa (via nasal spray),[22,36] to the occular membranes (via eye drops),[87] or to other mucous membranes to facilitate systemic absorption and treat disorders throughout the body.[86] Nonetheless, the potential for adverse systemic effects must also be considered if large amounts of topically administered drugs are absorbed inadvertently into the body.[86]

Transdermal

Unlike topical administration, transdermal application consists of applying drugs directly to the surface of the skin with the intent that they *will* be absorbed through the dermal layers and into either the subcutaneous tissues or the peripheral circulation. A transdermally administered drug must possess two basic properties: (1) it must be able to penetrate the skin, and (2) it must not be degraded to any major extent by drug-metabolizing enzymes located in the dermis.[44] Absorption may be enhanced by mixing the drug in an oily base or in some other chemical enhancer, thus increasing solubility and permeability through the dermis.[4,80]

Transdermal administration provides a slow, controlled release of the drug into the body that is effective in maintaining plasma levels of the drug at a relatively constant level for prolonged periods of time.[65] Drugs that can be administered transdermally are often delivered through medicated "patches" that can be adhered to the skin much like a small adhesive bandage. This method has been used for some time to allow the prolonged administration of drugs such as nitroglycerin and some antimotion sickness medications such as scopolamine. The use of transdermal patches has been expanded recently to include other medications such as hormonal agents (estrogen, testosterone) and opioid analgesics (fentanyl).[58] Likewise, transdermal nicotine patches have received a great deal of attention for their use in helping people to quit smoking cigarettes.[58] Researchers continue to explore the use of the transdermal route, and the use of transdermal patches continues to gain acceptance as a safe and effective method of administering many medications.

The transdermal route also includes the use of iontophoresis and phonophoresis to administer the drug. In iontophoresis, electric current is used to "drive" the ionized form of the medication through the skin.[4,18,19,56] Phonophoresis uses ultrasound waves to enhance transmission of the medication through the dermis.[4,12,56] Both phonophoresis and iontophoresis are often used to treat pain and inflammation by transmitting specific medications to a subcutaneous tissue such as a muscle, tendon, or bursa. These forms of transdermal administration are important in a rehabilitation setting since they are often administered by a physical therapist following a prescription written by a physician. Specific medications that can be administered via iontophoresis or phonophoresis are listed in Appendix A. For a more detailed description of how

these transdermal routes are employed, the reader is referred to several additional sources.[12,18,19]

Drug Absorption and Distribution: Bioavailability

Although several routes exist for the administration of drugs, merely introducing the drug into the body does not ensure that the compound will reach all tissues uniformly or that the drug will even reach the appropriate target site. For instance, oral administration of a drug that affects the myocardium will not have any pharmacologic effect unless the drug is absorbed from the gastrointestinal tract into the bloodstream. The extent to which the drug reaches the systemic circulation is referred to as **bioavailability,** which is a parameter expressed as the percentage of the drug administered that reaches the bloodstream.[17,86] For instance, if 100 g of a drug is given orally, and 50 g eventually make it into the systemic circulation, the drug is said to be 50 percent bioavailable. If 100 g of the same compound were injected intravenously, the drug would be 100 percent bioavailable by that route.

Consequently, bioavailability depends on the route of administration as well as the drug's ability to cross membrane barriers. Once in the systemic circulation, further distribution into peripheral tissues may also be important in allowing the drug to reach the target site. Many drugs must eventually leave the systemic capillaries and enter other cells. Thus, drugs have to move across cell membranes and tissue barriers to get into the body and be distributed within the body. In this section, the ability of these membranes to affect absorption and distribution of drugs is discussed.

Membrane Structure and Function

Throughout the body, biologic membranes act as barriers that permit some substances to pass freely, while others pass through with difficulty or not at all. This differential separation serves an obvious protective effect by not allowing certain substances to enter the body or by limiting the distribution of the substance within the body. In effect, the body is separated into various "compartments" by these membranes. In the case of pharmacotherapeutics, there is often the need for the drug to cross one or more of these membrane barriers to reach the target site.

The ability of the membrane to act as a selective barrier is related to the membrane's normal structure and physiologic function. The cell membrane is composed primarily of lipids and proteins. Membrane lipids are actually *phospholipids*, which are composed of a polar, hydrophilic "head" (which contains a phosphate group) and a lipid, hydrophobic "tail" (Fig. 2–1). The phospholipids appear to be arranged in a bilayer, with the hydrophobic tails of the molecule oriented toward the membrane's center and the hydrophilic heads facing away from the center of the membrane. Interspersed throughout the lipid bilayer are membrane proteins, which can exist primarily in the outer or inner portion of the membrane or can span the entire width of the cell membrane (see Fig. 2–1).

Recent evidence also suggests that the distribution of phospholipids and proteins within the cell membrane is not random, but that certain areas of the cell membrane are organized into special regions or "domains."[35,52,63] In particular, certain domains appear to consist primarily of lipids such as cholesterol and sphingolipids.[27,50] These lipid domains are often described as lipid "rafts" that move freely about the cell membrane and these lipid rafts appear to be important in controlling various cell functions including cell signaling, endocytosis, and ion channel function.[27,50] Future research will help further define the role of the lipid rafts and other specific domains within the cell membrane.

The lipid bilayer that composes the basic structure of the cell membrane acts as a water barrier. The lipid portion of the membrane is essentially impermeable to water and other nonlipid-soluble substances (electrolytes, glucose). Lipid-soluble compounds (including most drugs) are able to pass directly through the membrane by becoming dissolved in the lipid bilayer. Nonlipid-soluble substances, including water, may be able to pass through the membrane because of the presence of membrane pores.[5] Small holes or channels appear to exist in the membrane, thereby allowing certain substances to pass from one side of the membrane to the other. These channels are believed to be formed by some of the membrane proteins that span the width of the membrane.[41] The ability a substance has to pass through a specific pore depends primarily on the size, shape, and electrical charge of the molecule. Also, in excitable membranes (nerve, muscle) some of these pores are dynamic in nature and appear to have the ability to "open" and "close," thus regulating the flow of certain ions in and out of the cell.[73,91] These dynamic ion channels are especially important in pharmacology because many drugs can affect their ability to open and close, thus altering cell excitability by regulating the movement of ions across the cell membrane.[45,81,84]

Movement Across Membrane Barriers

Drugs and other substances that pass through biologic membranes usually do so via passive diffusion, active transport, facilitated diffusion, or some "special" process such as endocytosis (Fig. 2–2). Each of these mechanisms is discussed here.

Passive Diffusion

Drugs and other substances will pass through a membrane by way of diffusion providing two essential criteria are met. First, there must be some type of difference or "gradient" on one side of the membrane

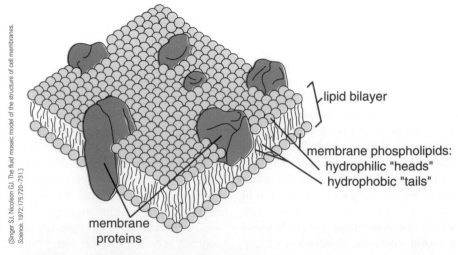

(Singer SJ, Nicolson GJ. The fluid mosaic model of the structure of cell membranes. *Science.* 1972;175:720–731.)

lipid bilayer

membrane phospholipids:
hydrophilic "heads"
hydrophobic "tails"

membrane proteins

FIGURE 2–1 ▼ Schematic diagram of the cell membrane.

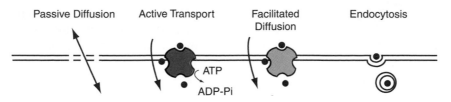

Passive Diffusion   Active Transport   Facilitated   Endocytosis
                                         Diffusion

ATP

ADP-Pi

FIGURE 2–2 ▼ Schematic diagram summarizing the ways in which substances may cross the cell membrane. Energy is expended during active transport by hydrolyzing adenosine triphosphate (ATP) into adenosine diphosphate (ADP) and inorganic phosphate (Pi). The three other mechanisms do not require any net energy expenditure. See text for further discussion of how and when each mechanism is utilized.

compared to the other. A concentration gradient, for example, occurs when the concentration of the substance differs on one side of the membrane compared to that on the other side. When this gradient occurs, the diffusing substance can move "downhill" from the area of high concentration to that of low concentration. In addition to a concentration difference, diffusion can also occur because of the presence of a pressure gradient or, in the case of charged particles, an electrical potential gradient. The rate of the diffusion is dependent on several factors, including the magnitude of the gradient, the size of the diffusing substance, the distance over which diffusion occurs, and the temperature at which diffusion occurs.[41] The term *passive diffusion* is often used to emphasize the fact that this movement occurs without expending any energy. The driving forces in passive diffusion are the electrical, chemical, and pressure differences on the two sides of the membrane.

For passive diffusion through a membrane to occur, the second essential factor is that the membrane must be permeable to the diffusing substance. As mentioned earlier, nonlipid-soluble compounds can diffuse through the membrane via specific pores. Some nonlipid-soluble drugs such as lithium are small enough to diffuse through these pores. Many drugs, however, are able to diffuse directly through the lipid bilayer; hence, they must be fairly lipid soluble. Passive lipid diffusion is nonselective, and a drug with a high degree of lipid solubility can gain access to many tissues because of its ability to pass directly through the lipid portion of the cell membrane. As indicated earlier, certain nonlipid-soluble substances—including some proteins—can be encapsulated in lipid vesicles, thereby enhancing their lipid solubility and increasing their ability to cross lipid membranes by passive diffusion.

Effect of Ionization on Lipid Diffusion. Passive lipid diffusion of certain drugs is also dependent on whether or not the drug is ionized. Drugs will diffuse more readily through the lipid layer if they are in their neutral, nonionized form. Most drugs are weak acids or weak bases,[86] meaning that they have the potential to become positively charged or negatively charged, depending on the pH of certain body fluids. In the plasma and in most other fluids, most drugs remain in their neutral, nonionized form because of the relatively neutral pH of these fluids. In specific fluids, however, a drug may exist in an ionized state, and the absorption of the drug will be affected because of the decreased lipid solubility associated with ionization. For instance, when a weak acid is in an acidic environment (e.g., gastric secretions of the stomach), it tends to be in its neutral, nonionized form. The same drug will become positively charged if the pH of the solution increases and becomes more basic (e.g., the digestive fluids in the duodenum). A weak acid such as aspirin will be nonionized and will therefore be absorbed fairly easily from the stomach because of its lipid solubility (Fig. 2–3). This same drug will be poorly absorbed if it reaches the basic pH of the duodenum and becomes ionized. Conversely, a drug that is a weak base will be ionized and poorly absorbed from the acidic environment of the stomach. The same drug will be nonionized and will therefore be lipid soluble when it reaches the duodenum, allowing it to be absorbed from the proximal small intestine.

Diffusion Trapping. Changes in lipid solubility caused by ionization can also be important when the body attempts to excrete a drug in the urine. Here the situation becomes slightly more complex because the urine can sometimes be acidic and at other times basic in nature. In either situation, it is often desirable for the drug to remain ionized while in the urine so that the drug will be excreted from the body. If the drug becomes nonionized while in the nephron, it may be reabsorbed back into the body because of its increased lipid solubility. An ionized form of the drug will remain "trapped" in the nephron and will eventually be excreted in the urine.[66] Thus, if the urine is basic, weak acids will become trapped in the nephron

(From Clark JB, Queener SF, and Karb VB. *Pharmacological Basis of Nursing Practice* 4th ed. St. Louis, MO: CV Mosby; 1993:p. 8, with permission.)

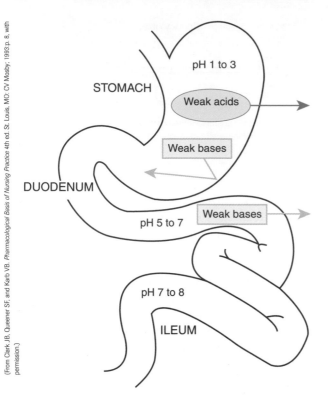

FIGURE 2–3 ▼ Effect of pH and ionization on absorption of drugs from the gastrointestinal tract. Weak acids and bases are absorbed from the stomach and duodenum, respectively, when they are in their neutral, nonionized form.

and will be excreted more readily. Weak bases will be excreted better if the urine is acidic. The importance of the kidneys in excreting drugs from the body is discussed further in Chapter 3.

Diffusion Between Cell Junctions. So far, the diffusion of drugs and other substances through individual cell membranes has been discussed. Often, groups of cells will join together to form a barrier that separates one body compartment from another. In some locations, cells form "tight junctions" with each other and do not allow any appreciable space to exist between adjacent cells. In these cases, the primary way that a drug may diffuse across the barrier is by diffusing first into and then out of the other side of the cells comprising the barrier. Such locations include the epithelial lining of the gastrointestinal tract and the capillary endothelium of the brain (one of the reasons for the blood-brain barrier). In other tissues such as peripheral capillaries, there may be relatively large gaps between adjacent cells. Here, relatively large substances with molecular weights as high as 30,000 may be able to diffuse across the barrier by diffusing between adjacent cells.

Osmosis. Osmosis refers to the special case of diffusion where the diffusing substance is water. In this situation, water moves from an area where it is highly concentrated to an area of low concentration. Of course, permeability is still a factor when osmosis occurs across a membrane or tissue barrier. During osmosis, certain drugs may simply travel with the diffusing water, thus crossing the membrane by the process of "bulk flow." This is usually limited to osmosis through the gaps between adjacent cells because membrane pores are often too small to allow the passage of the drug molecule along with the diffusing water.

Active Transport

Active or carrier-mediated transport involves using membrane proteins to transport substances across the cell membrane (see Fig. 2–2). Membrane proteins that span the entire membrane may serve as some sort of carrier that shuttles substances from one side of the membrane to the other.[41] Characteristics of active transport include the following:

Carrier specificity. The protein carrier exhibits some degree of specificity for certain substances, usually discriminating among different compounds according to their shape and electrical charge. This specificity is not absolute, and some compounds that resemble one another will be transported by the same group of carriers.

Expenditure of energy. The term *active* transport implies that some energy must be used to fuel the carrier system. This energy is usually in the form of adenosine triphosphate (ATP) hydrolysis.

Ability to transport substances against a concentration gradient. Carrier-mediated active transport may be able to carry substances "uphill"—that is, from areas of low concentration to areas of high concentration.

The role of active transport in moving drugs across cell membranes has some important implications. Essentially, the drug can use one of the body's active transport systems if the drug resembles some endogenous substance that is routinely carried by the transport system. Thus, drugs that resemble amino acids and small peptides can be absorbed from the gastrointestinal (GI) tract via active transport proteins that normally absorb these substances into the body. Active transport systems in the kidneys, liver, brain, intestines, and placenta are likewise responsible for the movement of organic ions, peptides, and other substances across cell membranes, and these transport systems play an important role in the disposition of certain drugs within these tissues.[23,40,83,89] Conversely, some drugs may exert their effect by either facilitating or inhibiting endogenous transport systems that affect cellular homeostasis. For example, some of the drugs used to treat excess gastric acid secretion (e.g., famotidine, ranitidine; see Chapter 27) inhibit the active transport of hydrogen ions into the stomach, thus reducing the formation of hydrochloric acid within the stomach.[67] Hence, medications can interact with the body's active transport systems in several ways and researchers continue to develop new methods to enhance a drug's effects by using or modifying active transport pathways.

Facilitated Diffusion

Facilitated diffusion, as the name implies, bears some features of both active transport and passive diffusion. A protein carrier is present in facilitated diffusion, but no net energy is expended in transporting the substance across the cell membrane.[41] As a result, in most cases of facilitated diffusion there is an inability to transport substances uphill against a concentration gradient. The entry of glucose into skeletal muscle cells via facilitated diffusion is probably the best example of this type of transport in the body.[61] As in active transport, the movement of drugs across membranes through facilitated diffusion is fairly infrequent, but certain medications may affect the rate at which endogenous facilitated diffusion occurs.

Special Processes

Certain cells have the ability to transport substances across their membranes through processes such as endocytosis. Here the drug is engulfed by the cell via an invagination of the cell membrane. Although limited in scope, this method does allow certain large, nonlipid-soluble drugs to enter the cell.

Distribution of Drugs Within the Body

Factors Affecting Distribution

Following administration, the extent to which a drug is uniformly distributed throughout the body or sequestered in a specific body compartment depends on several factors:

1. *Tissue permeability.* As discussed earlier, the ability to pass through membranes radically affects the extent to which a drug moves around within the body. A highly lipid-soluble drug can potentially reach all of the different body compartments and enter virtually every cell it reaches.[88] A large nonlipid-soluble compound will remain primarily in the compartment or tissue to which it is administered. Also, certain tissues such as the brain capillary endothelium have special characteristics that limit the passage of drugs. This so-called blood-brain barrier limits the movement of drugs out of the bloodstream and into the central nervous system tissue.

2. *Blood flow.* If a drug is circulating in the bloodstream, it will gain greater access to tissues that are highly perfused. More of the drug will reach organs that receive a great deal of blood flow—such as the brain, kidneys, and exercising skeletal muscle—than will other, less active tissues such as adipose stores.[86] Similarly, diseases that reduce blood flow to specific tissues and organs will result in less drug being delivered to those tissues.[25]

3. *Binding to plasma proteins.* Certain drugs will form reversible bonds to circulating proteins in the bloodstream such as albumin.[86] This fact is significant because only the unbound or "free" drug is able to reach the target tissue and exert a pharmacologic effect. Basically, the fraction of the drug that remains bound to the circulating proteins is sequestered within the vascular system and not available for therapeutic purposes in other tissues and organs.

4. *Binding to subcellular components.* In a situation similar to plasma protein binding, drugs that are bound within specific cells are unable to leave the cell and be distributed throughout other fluid compartments. Several drugs, for example, bind to subcellular organelles such as the lysosome, thus trapping the drug within the cell. Examples of this type of subcellular binding include certain antidepressants, antipsychotics, and other drugs with a relatively high pH that are attracted by the acidic environment found inside the lysosome.[24,88]

Volume of Distribution

The distribution of a given drug within the body is often described by calculating the **volume of distribution (V_d)** for that drug.[8,86] V_d is the ratio of the amount of drug administered to the concentration of drug in the plasma:

V_d = amount of drug administered ÷ concentration of drug in plasma.

V_d is used to estimate a drug's distribution by comparing the calculated V_d with the total amount of body water in a normal person. A normal 70 kg man has a total body fluid content of approximately 42 L (5.5 L blood, 12.0 L extracellular fluid, 24.5 L intracellular fluid). If the calculated V_d of a drug is approximately equal to the total amount of body water, then the drug is distributed uniformly throughout all of the body's fluids. If the V_d of the drug is far less than 42 L, then the drug is being retained in the bloodstream due to factors such as plasma protein binding. A V_d much greater than 42 L indicates that the drug is being concentrated in the tissues. It should be noted that V_d is not a "real" value; that is, it does not indicate the actual amount of fluid in the body, but is merely an arbitrary figure that reflects the apparent distribution of a drug using total body water as a reference point. Table 2–2 gives some examples of the calculation of the V_d for three different types of drugs.

Drug Storage

Storage Sites

Following administration and absorption, many drugs are "stored" to some extent at certain locations in the body[86]; that is, prior to drug elimination, the drug may be sequestered in its active form in a relatively inert tissue that may be different from the target site of the drug. Some storage sites include the following:

1. *Adipose.* The primary site for drug storage in the body is adipose tissue. Because many drugs are lipid soluble, fat deposits throughout the body can serve as a considerable reservoir for these compounds. In some individuals, the amount of fat in the body can reach as high as 40 to 50 percent of body weight, thus creating an extensive storage compartment. Once drugs have been stored in adipose tissue, they tend to remain there for long periods of time because of the low metabolic rate and poor blood perfusion of these tissues. Examples of drugs that tend to be stored in fat include highly lipid-soluble anesthetics such as the barbiturates (thiopental) and inhalation anesthetics (halothane).
2. *Bone.* Bone acts as a storage site for several toxic agents, especially heavy metals like lead. Also, drugs such as the tetracyclines, which bind to and form molecular complexes with the crystal components within the skeletal matrix, are stored within bone.
3. *Muscle.* Binding of drugs to components within the muscle may create the long-term storage of these compounds. Various agents may be actively transported into the muscle cell and may form reversible bonds to intracellular structures such as proteins, nucleoproteins, or phospholipids. An example is the antimalarial drug quinacrine.

Table 2–2	EXAMPLES OF VOLUME OF DISTRIBUTION				
Drug	Amount Administered	Plasma Concentration	Volume of Distribution	Indication	Examples
A	420 mg	0.01 mg/mL	420 mg ÷ 0.01 mg/mL = 42,000 mL = 42 L	Uniform distribution	Erythromycin; lithium
B	420 mg	0.05 mg/mL	420 mg ÷ 0.05 mg/mL = 8400 mL = 8.4 L	Retained in plasma	Aspirin; valproic acid
C	420 mg	0.001 mg/mL	420 mg ÷ 0.001 mg/mL = 420,000 mL = 420 L	Sequestered in tissues	Morphine; quinidine

4. *Organs.* Drugs are often stored within certain organs such as the liver and kidneys. As in muscle cells, the drug may enter the cell passively or by active transport and then form bonds to subcellular components. Examples include antimicrobial aminoglycoside agents (such as gentamicin and streptomycin), which accumulate in renal proximal tubular cells.

Adverse Consequences of Drug Storage

High concentrations of drugs, drug metabolites, and toxic compounds within tissues can cause local damage to the tissues in which they are stored. This event is particularly true for toxic compounds that are incorporated and stored in the matrix of bone or that are highly concentrated within specific organs. Lead poisoning, for example, causes several well-known and potentially devastating effects when this metal accumulates, in the CNS, bone, GI tract, and several other tissues.

Exposing various organs to high concentrations of therapeutic drugs can also result in myriad problems. Actaminophen, for example, is normally metabolized in the liver to form several highly reactive by-products or metabolites (see Chapter 15). When normal doses of acetaminophen are metabolized in a reasonably healthy liver, these metabolites are rapidly inactivated in the liver and subsequently excreted by the kidneys. Very high doses of acetaminophen, however, result in the formation of excessive amounts of a toxic metabolite that can react with hepatic proteins and cause severe liver damage.[64] Hence, organs such as the liver and the kidneys are often subjected to local damage when these organs must deal with high concentrations of therapeutic and toxic agents.

Another problem with drug storage occurs when the storage site acts as a reservoir that "soaks up" the drug and prevents it from reaching the target site. For instance, a highly lipid-soluble drug such as a general anesthetic must be administered at a sufficient dose to ensure that there will be enough drug available to reach the CNS, despite the tendency for much of the drug to be sequestered in the body's fat stores. Storage sites may also be responsible for the redistribution of drugs. This occurrence is seen when the drug begins to leak out of the storage reservoir after plasma levels of the drug have begun to diminish. In this way, the drug may be reintroduced to the target site long after the original dose should have been eliminated. This redistribution may explain why certain individuals experience prolonged effects of the drug or extended adverse side effects.

Newer Techniques for Drug Delivery

Controlled-Release Preparations

Controlled-release preparations, also known as *timed-release*, *sustained-release*, *extended-release*, or *prolonged-action preparations*, are generally designed to permit a slower and more prolonged absorption of the drug from the gastrointestinal tract and other routes of administration.[86] This technique may offer several advantages such as decreasing the number of doses needed each day, preventing large fluctuations in the amount of drug appearing in the plasma, and sustaining plasma levels throughout the night.[13,37] This type of preparation has been used successfully with several types of drugs, including cardiovascular medications (beta blockers, calcium channel blockers),[26,77] narcotic analgesics such as morphine,[13,28] and anti-Parkinson medications that contain L-dopa.[46,75] Controlled-release preparations will probably continue to gain popularity as a means for administering these and other medications in the future.[86]

Implanted Drug Delivery Systems

Several techniques have been developed whereby a type of drug "reservoir" is implanted surgically within the body and is then released in a controlled fashion from the implanted reservoir.[38,76] These drug reservoirs typically consist of a small container placed under the skin in the abdomen. The containers are often programmed to allow a small, measured dose of the drug to be released periodically from the reservoir. Alternatively, the reservoir can be controlled electronically from outside of the body through the use of small, remote-controlled devices, thus allowing the patient to regulate release of the drug as needed. In some cases, the drug reservoir may be connected by a small cannula to a specific body compartment—such as the subarachnoid space or epidural space—so that the drug can be delivered directly into that space. This type of system appears to be very helpful in applying certain drugs such as analgesics, anesthetics, and muscle relaxants into the spinal cord.[29,38,76]

Another type of implantable system has been developed recently that incorporates the drug into some type of biodegradable or nonbiodegradable substance such as a polymer matrix or gel.[53,57,71] The drug-polymer complex is then implanted in the body and the drug is slowly released into surrounding tissues (nonbiodegradable), or is released as the matrix gradually dissolves (biodegradable). This type of system is probably best known for administering contraceptive hormones such as progesterone (Norplant; see Chapter 30); these implants have also shown promise in delivering other medications such as local anesthetics, insulin, and vaccines.[71]

Hence, implantable drug delivery systems are being considered as a potential means of administering several drugs including analgesics, muscle relaxants, and hormones. Improvements in the technology of this type of drug delivery will hopefully permit increased clinical applications of these systems in the near future. The use of implantable drug delivery systems with specific types of medications will be discussed in more detail when these medications are addressed in subsequent chapters in this book.

Targeting Drug Delivery to Specific Cells and Tissues

Some very innovative approaches have been attempted on a molecular level to try to target the drug specifically to the cells that require treatment. For instance, specific types of antibodies (monoclonal antibodies) can be synthesized and attached to certain drugs such as the cytotoxic agents often used in cancer chemotherapy.[1,32] The antibodies are then attracted to antigens located on the surface of the tumor cells. This offers the distinct advantage of focusing the drug more directly on the cancerous cells rather than on healthy human tissues. Other cellular techniques have been investigated that could also help direct the drug to the affected tissues. It may be possible, for example, to link a drug to a modified virus so that the virus transports and helps insert the drug directly into specific cells;[47,51] the virus, of course, must be modified so that it will not cause viral infection. Other nonviral techniques include encapsulating the drug in a certain type of fat particle (liposome) or attaching the drug to certain proteins that will be attracted to the surface receptors of specific cells.[14,48] These viral and nonviral techniques have been particularly important in helping deliver DNA to specific cells in order to modify the genetic regulation of those cells (gene-based therapy).[47,48,51]

Drugs can also be targeted to specific sites by capitalizing on unique physiologic properties of various tissues and organs. Certain drugs, for example, might be activated by enzymes that are found only in the kidneys, thereby targeting these drugs specifically to the kidneys.[31] Abnormal tissues, including some tumors, might also have specialized enzymes that could be used to activate certain drugs only after the drugs reach these tissues.[68] Various techniques can also be used to modify a drug so that it is activated only after reaching the colon.[15,16] This action will allow the drug to be administered orally, but remain inactive as a "prodrug" until it reaches the colon, where it will then become activated to treat local problems or be absorbed into the systemic circulation.[33,72]

The idea of targeting drugs to specific tissues through various cellular and chemical mechanisms is still relatively new. These techniques have shown considerable promise, however, and may ultimately be extremely useful in increasing the effectiveness of certain drugs while decreasing side effects.

SUMMARY

In order for any drug to be effective, it must be able to reach specific target tissues. The goal of drug administration is to deliver the drug in the least complicated manner while still allowing sufficient concentrations of the active form of the drug to arrive at the desired site. Each route of administration has certain advantages and disadvantages that will determine how much and how fast the drug is delivered to specific tissues. In addition to the route of administration, the distribution of the drug within the body must be taken into account. Simply introducing the drug into certain body fluids such as the bloodstream does not ensure its entry into the desired tissues. Factors such as tissue permeability and protein binding may influence how the drug is dispersed within the various fluid compartments within the body. Finally, some drugs have a tendency to be stored in certain tissues for prolonged periods of time. This storage may produce serious toxic effects if high concentrations of the compound damage the cells in which it is stored.

References

1. Abou-Jawde R, Choueiri T, Alemany C, Mekhail T. An overview of targeted treatments in cancer. *Clin Ther.* 2003;25:2121–2137.
2. Altamura AC, Sassella F, Santini A, et al. Intramuscular preparations of antipsychotics: uses and relevance in clinical practice. *Drugs.* 2003;63:493–512.
3. Barnett AH. Exubera inhaled insulin: a review. *Int J Clin Pract.* 2004;58:394–401.
4. Barry BW. Novel mechanisms and devices to enable successful transdermal drug delivery. *Eur J Pharm Sci.* 2001;14:101–114.
5. Benga G. Birth of water channel proteins—the aquaporins. *Cell Biol Int.* 2003;27:701–709.
6. Berkes J, Viswanathan VK, Savkovic SD, Hecht G. Intestinal epithelial responses to enteric pathogens: effects on the tight junction barrier, ion transport, and inflammation. *Gut.* 2003;52:439–451.
7. Berweck S, Heinen F. Use of botulinum toxin in pediatric spasticity (cerebral palsy). *Mov Disord.* 2004; (Suppl 8)19:S162–S167.
8. Bjorkman S. Prediction of the volume of distribution of a drug: which tissue-plasma partition coefficients are needed? *J Pharm Pharmacol.* 2002;54:1237–1245.
9. Brache V, Faundes A, Alvarez F. Risk-benefit effects of implantable contraceptives in women. *Expert Opin Drug Saf.* 2003;2:321–332.
10. Bracht S. Methods in drug delivery. In: Sirtori CR, et al, eds. *Clinical Pharmacology.* London: McGraw-Hill International Ltd; 2000.
11. Briggs M, Nelson EA. Topical agents or dressings for pain in venous leg ulcers. *Cochrane Database Syst Rev.* 2003;CD001177.
12. Byl NN. The use of ultrasound as an enhancer for transcutaneous drug delivery: phonophoresis. *Phys Ther.* 1995;75:539–553.
13. Caldwell JR. Avinza—24-h sustained-release oral morphine therapy. *Expert Opin Pharmacother.* 2004; 5:469–472.
14. Cattel L, Ceruti M, Dosio F. From conventional to stealth liposomes: a new frontier in cancer chemotherapy. *Tumori.* 2003;89:237–249.
15. Chourasia MK, Jain SK. Polysaccharides for colon targeted drug delivery. *Drug Deliv.* 2004;11:129–148.
16. Chourasia MK, Jain SK. Pharmaceutical approaches to colon targeted drug delivery systems. *J Pharm Pharm Sci.* 2003;6:33–66.
17. Ciccone CD. Basic pharmacokinetics and the potential effect of physical therapy interventions on pharmacokinetic variables. *Phys Ther.* 1995;75:343–351.
18. Ciccone CD. Iontophoresis. In: Robinson AJ, Snyder-Mackler L, eds. *Clinical Electrophysiology* 2nd ed. Baltimore: Lippincott Williams & Wilkins; 1994.
19. Costello CT, Jeske AH. Iontophoresis: applications in transdermal medication delivery. *Phys Ther.* 1995; 75:554–563.
20. Courrier HM, Butz N, Vandamme TF. Pulmonary drug delivery systems: recent developments and prospects. *Crit Rev Ther Drug Carrier Syst.* 2002; 19:425–498.
21. Dahan A, Altman H. Food-drug interaction: grapefruit juice augments drug bioavailability—mechanism, extent and relevance. *Eur J Clin Nutr.* 2004;58:1–9.
22. Dahlof C. Clinical applications of new therapeutic deliveries in migraine. *Neurology.* 2003;61(suppl 4): S31–S34.
23. Daniel H. Molecular and integrative physiology of intestinal peptide transport. *Annu Rev Physiol.* 2004;66:361–384.
24. Daniel WA. Mechanisms of cellular distribution of psychotropic drugs. Significance for drug action and interactions. *Prog Neuropsychopharmacol Biol Psychiatry.* 2003;27:65–73.
25. De Paepe P, Belpaire FM, Buylaert WA. Pharmacokinetic and pharmacodynamic considerations when treating patients with sepsis and septic shock. *Clin Pharmacokinet.* 2002;41:1135–1151.
26. Eisenberg MJ, Brox A, Bestawros AN. Calcium channel blockers: an update. *Am J Med.* 2004;116:35–43.
27. Fullekrug J, Simons K. Lipid rafts and apical membrane traffic. *Ann N Y Acad Sci.* 2004;1014:164–169.
28. Gabrail NY, Dvergsten C, Ahdieh H. Establishing the dosage equivalency of oxymorphone extended release and oxycodone controlled release in patients with cancer pain: a randomized controlled study. *Curr Med Res Opin.* 2004;20:911–918.
29. Gerber HR. Intrathecal morphine for chronic benign pain. *Best Pract Res Clin Anaesthesiol.* 2003;17:429–442.
30. Groneberg DA, Witt C, Wagner U, et al. Fundamentals of pulmonary drug delivery. *Respir Med.* 2003; 97:382–387.
31. Haas M, Moolenaar F, Meijer DK, de Zeeuw D. Specific drug delivery to the kidney. *Cardiovasc Drugs Ther.* 2002;16:489–496.
32. Harris M. Monoclonal antibodies as therapeutic agents for cancer. *Lancet Oncol.* 2004;5:292–302.
33. Haupt S, Rubinstein A. The colon as a possible target for orally administered peptide and protein drugs. *Crit Rev Ther Drug Carrier Syst.* 2002;19:499–551.
34. Holland N, Adams MO. *Core Concepts in Pharmacology.* Upper Saddle River, NJ: Prentice-Hall; 2003.
35. Holthuis JC, van Meer G, Huitema K. Lipid microdomains, lipid translocation and the organization of intracellular membrane transport (Review). *Mol Membr Biol.* 2003;20:231–241.
36. Illum L. Is nose-to-brain transport of drugs in man a reality? *J Pharm Pharmacol.* 2004;56:3–17.
37. Kilts CD. Potential new drug delivery systems for antidepressants: an overview. *J Clin Psychiatry.* 2003; 64(suppl 18):31–33.
38. Korenkov AI, Niendorf WR, Darwish N, et al. Continuous intrathecal infusion of baclofen in patients with spasticity caused by spinal cord injuries. *Neurosurg Rev.* 2002;25:228–230.
39. Kunta JR, Sinko PJ. Intestinal drug transporters: in vivo function and clinical importance. *Curr Drug Metab.* 2004;5:109–124.
40. Kusuhara H, Sugiyama Y. Role of transporters in the tissue-selective distribution and elimination of drugs: transporters in the liver, small intestine, brain and kidney. *J Control Release.* 2002;78:43–54.

41. Kutchai HC. Cellular membranes and transmembrane transport of solutes and water. In: Berne RM, Levy MN, eds. *Principles of Physiology*. 3rd ed. St Louis, MO: CV Mosby; 2000.

42. Labiris NR, Dolovich MB. Pulmonary drug delivery. Part II: the role of inhalant delivery devices and drug formulations in therapeutic effectiveness of aerosolized medications. *Br J Clin Pharmacol*. 2003;56:600–612.

43. Labiris NR, Dolovich MB. Pulmonary drug delivery. Part I: physiological factors affecting therapeutic effectiveness of aerosolized medications. *Br J Clin Pharmacol*. 2003;56:588–599.

44. Langer R. Transdermal drug delivery: past progress, current status, and future prospects. *Adv Drug Deliv Rev*. 2004;56:557–558.

45. Lesage F. Pharmacology of neuronal background potassium channels. *Neuropharmacology*. 2003;44:1–7.

46. LeWitt PA, Nyholm D. New developments in levodopa therapy. *Neurology*. 2004;62(suppl 1):S9–S16.

47. Lundstrom K. Latest development in viral vectors for gene therapy. *Trends Biotechnol*. 2003;21:117–122.

48. Lundstrom K, Boulikas T. Viral and non-viral vectors in gene therapy: technology development and clinical trials. *Technol Cancer Res Treat*. 2003;2:471–486.

49. Mahato RI, Narang AS, Thoma L, Miller DD. Emerging trends in oral delivery of peptide and protein drugs. *Crit Rev Ther Drug Carrier Syst*. 2003;20:153–214.

50. Martens JR, O'Connell K, Tamkun M. Targeting of ion channels to membrane microdomains: localization of KV channels to lipid rafts. *Trends Pharmacol Sci*. 2004;25:16–21.

51. Mata M, Glorioso JC, Fink DJ. Targeted gene delivery to the nervous system using herpes simplex virus vectors. *Physiol Behav*. 2002;77:483–488.

52. Maxfield FR. Plasma membrane microdomains. *Curr Opin Cell Biol*. 2002;14:483–487.

53. Meirik O, Fraser IS, d'Arcangues C. WHO Consultation on Implantable Contraceptives for Women. Implantable contraceptives for women. *Hum Reprod Update*. 2003;9:49–59.

54. Mercadante S, Fulfaro F. Alternatives to oral opioids for cancer pain. *Oncology*. 1999;13:215–229.

55. Miles J. Intrathecal treatment for spasticity. *Stereotact Funct Neurosurg*. 2001;76:246–248.

56. Mitragotri S. Synergistic effect of enhancers for transdermal drug delivery. *Pharm Res*. 2000;17:1354–1359.

57. Moses MA, Brem H, Langer R. Advancing the field of drug delivery: taking aim at cancer. *Cancer Cell*. 2003;4:337–341.

58. Murphy M, Carmichael AJ. Transdermal drug delivery systems and skin sensitivity reactions. Incidence and management. *Am J Clin Dermatol*. 2000;1:361–368.

59. Nelson EA, Bradley MD. Dressings and topical agents for arterial leg ulcers. *Cochrane Database Syst Rev*. 2003; CD001836.

60. Penn RD. Intrathecal medication delivery. *Neurosurg Clin N Am*. 2003;14:381–387.

61. Pereira LO, Lancha AH Jr. Effect of insulin and contraction up on glucose transport in skeletal muscle. *Prog Biophys Mol Biol*. 2004;84:1–27.

62. Perez-Marrero R, Tyler RC. A subcutaneous delivery system for the extended release of leuprolide acetate for the treatment of prostate cancer. *Expert Opin Pharmacother*. 2004;5:447–457.

63. Pike LJ. Lipid rafts: heterogeneity on the high seas. *Biochem J* 2004;378(Pt 2):281–292.

64. Pineiro-Carrero VM, Pineiro EO. Liver. *Pediatrics*. 2004;113(suppl):1097–1106.

65. Prausnitz MR, Mitragotri S, Langer R. Current status and future potential of transdermal drug delivery. *Nat Rev Drug Discov*. 2004;3:115–124.

66. Proudfoot AT, Krenzelok EP, Vale JA. Position Paper on urine alkalinization. *J Toxicol Clin Toxicol*. 2004; 42:1–26.

67. Robinson M, Horn J. Clinical pharmacology of proton pump inhibitors: what the practising physician needs to know. *Drugs*. 2003;63:2739–2754.

68. Rooney PH, Telfer C, McFadyen MC, et al. The role of cytochrome P450 in cytotoxic bioactivation: future therapeutic directions. *Curr Cancer Drug Targets* 2004; 4:257–265.

69. Royle P, Waugh N, McAuley L, et al. Inhaled insulin in diabetes mellitus. *Cochrane Database Syst Rev*. 2004; CD003890.

70. Senel S, Kremer M, Nagy K, Squier C. Delivery of bioactive peptides and proteins across oral (buccal) mucosa. *Curr Pharm Biotechnol*. 2001;2: 175–186.

71. Sershen S, West J. Implantable, polymeric systems for modulated drug delivery. *Adv Drug Deliv Rev*. 2002; 54:1225–1235.

72. Shareef MA, Khar RK, Ahuja A, et al. Colonic drug delivery: an updated review. *AAPS PharmSci*. 2003; 5:E17.

73. Shoshan-Barmatz V, Gincel D. The voltage-dependent anion channel: characterization, modulation, and role in mitochondrial function in cell life and death. *Cell Biochem Biophys*. 2003;39:279–292.

74. Spann CT, Tutrone WD, Weinberg JM, et al. Topical antibacterial agents for wound care: a primer. *Dermatol Surg*. 2003;29:620–626.

75. Stocchi F, Barbato L, Nordera G, et al. Entacapone improves the pharmacokinetic and therapeutic response of controlled release levodopa/carbidopa in Parkinson's patients. *J Neural Transm*. 2004;111: 173–180.

76. Taira T, Hori T. Clinical application of drug pump for spasticity, pain, and restorative neurosurgery: other clinical applications of intrathecal baclofen. *Acta Neurochir Suppl*. 2003;87:37–38.

77. Tangeman HJ, Patterson JH. Extended-release metoprolol succinate in chronic heart failure. *Ann Pharmacother*. 2003;37:701–710.

78. Tilton AH. Injectable neuromuscular blockade in the treatment of spasticity and movement disorders. *J Child Neurol*. 2003;18(suppl 1):S50–S66.

79. Tobias JD. A review of intrathecal and epidural analgesia after spinal surgery in children. *Anesth Analg*. 2004;98:956–965.

80. Touitou E. Drug delivery across the skin. *Expert Opin Biol Ther*. 2002;2:723–733.

81. Triggle DJ. Drug targets in the voltage-gated calcium channel family: why some are and some are not. *Assay Drug Dev Technol.* 2003;1:719–733.
82. Ulrich AS. Biophysical aspects of using liposomes as delivery vehicles. *Biosci Rep.* 2002;22:129–150.
83. van Montfoort JE, Hagenbuch B, Groothuis GM, et al. Drug uptake systems in liver and kidney. *Curr Drug Metab.* 2003;4:185–211.
84. Wang SY, Wang GK. Voltage-gated sodium channels as primary targets of diverse lipid-soluble neurotoxins. *Cell Signal.* 2003;15:151–159.
85. Webster GF. Topical medications: a focus on antifungals and topical steroids. *Clin Cornerstone.* 2001;4: 33–38.
86. Wilkinson GR. Pharmacokinetics: the dynamics of drug absorption, distribution, and elimination. In: Hardman JG, et al eds. *The Pharmacological Basis of Therapeutics.* 10th ed. New York: McGraw Hill; 2001.
87. Wilson CG. Topical drug delivery in the eye. *Exp Eye Res.* 2004;78:737–743.
88. Yokogawa K, Ishizaki J, Ohkuma S, Miyamoto K. Influence of lipophilicity and lysosomal accumulation on tissue distribution kinetics of basic drugs: a physiologically based pharmacokinetic model. *Methods Find Exp Clin Pharmacol.* 2002; 24:81–93.
89. You G. The role of organic ion transporters in drug disposition: an update. *Curr Drug Metab.* 2004;5: 55–62.
90. Zhang H, Zhang J, Streisand JB. Oral mucosal drug delivery: clinical pharmacokinetics and therapeutic applications. *Clin Pharmacokinet.* 2002;41: 661–680.
91. Zhorov BS, Tikhonov DB. Potassium, sodium, calcium and glutamate-gated channels: pore architecture and ligand action. *J Neurochem.* 2004;88:782–799.

Chapter 3

Pharmacokinetics II: Drug Elimination

All drugs must be eliminated from the body eventually to terminate their effect and to prevent excessive accumulation of the drug. Drugs are usually eliminated by chemically altering the original compound while it is still in the body so that it is no longer active (*biotransformation*), by excreting the active form of the drug from the body (*excretion*), or by a combination of biotransformation and excretion. These methods of drug elimination will be discussed here.

Biotransformation

Drug metabolism, or **biotransformation**, refers to chemical changes that take place in the drug following administration. Enzymes that are located within specific tissues are responsible for catalyzing changes in the drug's structure and subsequently altering the pharmacologic properties of the drug. The location of these enzymes and the reactions involved in biotransformation are discussed later in this chapter.

Biotransformation usually results in an altered version of the original compound known as a **metabolite,** which is usually inactive or has a greatly reduced level of pharmacologic activity. Occasionally, the metabolite has a higher level of activity than the original compound. In these cases, the drug may be given in an inactive, or "prodrug," form that will activate via biotransformation following administration. However, after it has exerted its pharmacologic effect, drug termination is the primary function of biotransformation.[53]

Inactivating a drug and terminating its effects after it is no longer needed are often essential. For instance, the effects of general and local anesthetics must eventually wear off, allowing the patient to resume normal functioning. Although termination of drug activity can occur when the active form of the drug is excreted from the body via organs such as the kidneys, excretory mechanisms are often too slow to effectively terminate any activity within a reasonable time period. If excretion were the only way to terminate drug activity, some compounds would continue to exert their effects for several days or even weeks. Drug biotransformation into an inactive form usually occurs within a matter of minutes or hours, thus reducing the chance for toxic effects caused by drug accumulation or prolonged drug activity.

Cellular Mechanisms of Drug Biotransformation

The chemical changes that occur during drug metabolism are usually caused by oxidation, reduction, hydrolysis, or conjugation of the original compound.[28,52,60] Examples of each type of reaction are listed in Table 3–1. Each type of reaction and the location of the enzymes catalyzing the reaction are also discussed here.

1. *Oxidation.* Oxidation occurs when either oxygen is added or hydrogen is removed from the original compound. Oxidation reactions comprise the predominant method of drug biotransformation in the body, and the primary enzymes that catalyze these reactions are known collectively as the cytochrome P450 monooxygenases.[27,28,52] These enzymes are primarily located on the smooth endoplasmic reticulum of specific cells and are sometimes referred to as the **drug**

Table 3–1	EXAMPLES OF DRUG BIOTRANSFORMATION REACTIONS	

I. Oxidation — Examples

A. Side chain (aliphatic) hydroxylation

$$RCH_2CH_3 \xrightarrow{[O]} RCHCH_3 \;(OH)$$

Ibuprofen

B. N-oxidation

$$(R)_2NH \xrightarrow{[O]} (R)_2NOH$$

Acetaminophen

C. Deamination

$$RCH_2NH_2 \xrightarrow{[O]} RCHO + NH_3$$

Diazepam

II. Reduction

A. Nitro reductions

$$RNO_2 \rightarrow RNH_2$$

Dantrolene

B. Carbonyl reductions

$$RCR' \;(O) \rightarrow RCHR' \;(OH)$$

Methadone

III. Hydrolysis

A. Esters

$$RCOR' \;(O) \rightarrow RCOOH + R'OH$$

Aspirin

B. Amides

$$RCNR' \;(O) \rightarrow RCOOH + R'NH2$$

Lidocaine

IV. Conjugation

A. Acetylation

$$RNH_2 + AcetylCoA \rightarrow RNHCCH_3 \;(O) + CoA\text{-}SH$$

Clonazepam

B. Glycine conjugation

$$RCOOH \rightarrow RCSCoA \;(O) + NH_2CH_2COOH \rightarrow$$

$$RCNHCH_2COOH \;(O) + CoA\text{-}SH$$

Benzoic acid

Parent drug compounds are represented by the letter "R." Examples are types of drugs that undergo biotransformation via the respective type of chemical reaction.

microsomal metabolizing system (DMMS). The general scheme of drug oxidation as catalyzed by the DMMS is shown in Figure 3–1.

2. *Reduction.* Reduction reactions consist of removing oxygen or adding hydrogen to the original compound. Enzymes that are located in the cell cytoplasm are usually responsible for drug reduction.

3. *Hydrolysis.* The original compound is broken into separate parts. The enzymes responsible

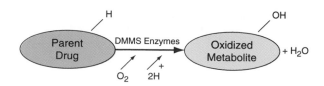

FIGURE 3–1 ▼ Drug oxidation catalyzed by drug microsomal metabolizing system (DMMS) enzymes.

for the hydrolysis of the drug are located at several sites within the cell (i.e., the endoplasmic reticulum and cytoplasm) as well as extracellularly (e.g., circulating in the plasma).

4. *Conjugation.* In conjugation reactions, the intact drug or the metabolite of one of the reactions described earlier, is coupled to an endogenous substance such as acetyl coenzyme A (acetyl CoA), glucuronic acid, or an amino acid. Enzymes catalyzing drug conjugations are found in the cytoplasm and on the endoplasmic reticulum.

The chemical reactions involved in drug biotransformation are also classified as either phase I or phase II reactions.[27,28,52,60] Phase I reactions consist of those using oxidation, reduction, or hydrolysis. Phase II reactions involve conjugation of the parent drug or the metabolite of a drug that was already metabolized using a phase I reaction.

Regardless of the type of chemical reaction used, biotransformation also helps in metabolite excretion from the body by creating a more polar compound.[18,53,60] After one or more of the reactions just described occurs, the remaining drug metabolite usually has a greater tendency to be ionized in the body's fluids. The ionized metabolite is more water soluble, thus becoming transported more easily in the bloodstream to the kidneys. Upon reaching the kidneys, the polar metabolite can be excreted from the body in the urine. The contribution of biotransformation toward renal excretion is discussed in a later section.

Organs Responsible for Drug Biotransformation

The primary location for drug metabolism is the liver.[5,60] Enzymes responsible for drug metabolism, such as the cytochrome P450 enzymes, are abundant on hepatic smooth endoplasmic reticulum; liver cells also contain other cytoplasmic enzymes responsible for drug reduction and hydrolysis. Other organs that contain metabolizing enzymes and exhibit considerable drug transformation abilities include the lungs, kid-

neys, gastrointestinal epithelium, and skin. Drug metabolism can be radically altered in conditions where these tissues are damaged. For instance, inactivation of certain drugs may be significantly delayed in the patient with hepatitis or cirrhosis of the liver.[47,61] As expected, dosages in these patients must be adjusted accordingly to prevent drug accumulation and toxicity.

Enzyme Induction

A frequent problem in drug metabolism is the phenomenon of **enzyme induction**.[9,13,62] Prolonged use of certain drugs "induces" the body to be able to enzymatically destroy the drug more rapidly, usually because either more metabolizing enzymes are being manufactured or less are being degraded. Enzyme induction may cause drugs to be metabolized more rapidly than expected, thus decreasing their therapeutic effect. This may be one reason why **tolerance** to some drugs occurs when it is used for extended periods (tolerance is the need for increased drug dosages to produce the same effect). Long-term ingestion or inhalation of other exogenous compounds such as alcohol, cigarette smoke, or environmental toxins may also cause enzyme induction.[9,39,49] When this occurs, medicinal drugs may be more rapidly metabolized even when they are first administered because of the preexisting enzyme induction.

Drug Excretion

The kidneys are the primary sites for drug excretion.[33,56] The functional unit of the kidney is the nephron (Fig. 3–2), and each kidney is composed of approximately 1 million nephrons. Usually, the metabolized or conjugated version of the original drug reaches the nephron and is then filtered at the glomerulus. Following filtration, the compound traverses the proximal convoluted tubule, loop of Henle, and distal convoluted tubule before reaching the collecting ducts. If a compound is not reabsorbed while moving through the nephron, it will ultimately leave the body in the urine. As discussed earlier, biotransformation plays a significant role in creating a polar, water-soluble metabolite that is able to reach the kidneys through the bloodstream. Only relatively polar drugs or their metabolites will be excreted in significant amounts by the kidneys because the ionized metabolite has a greater tendency to remain in the nephron and not be reabsorbed into the body.[60] Nonpolar compounds that are filtered by the kidneys are

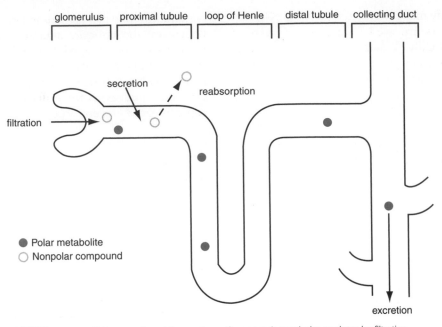

FIGURE 3–2 ▼ Drug excretion at the nephron. Compounds reach the nephron by filtration and/or secretion. Polar metabolites remain trapped in the nephron and are eventually excreted. Nonpolar compounds are able to diffuse back into the body (reabsorption).

relatively lipophilic and can easily be reabsorbed back into the body passively by diffusing through the wall of the nephron. However, the polar metabolite is relatively impermeable to the epithelium lining, and the metabolite tends to remain "trapped" in the nephron following filtration, where it will eventually be excreted in the urine (see Fig. 3–2).

In addition to filtration, some drugs may be secreted into the nephron by active transport mechanisms located in the proximal convoluted tubule. Several distinct types of transport proteins have been identified that secrete substances such as organic cations (e.g., uric acid), organic anions (e.g., choline, histamine), prostaglandins, conjugated drug metabolites, and a variety of other compounds.[25,42,33] Certain drugs can also be transported by one of these carrier systems so that they are actively secreted into the nephron. For example, penicillin G is actively secreted via the transport system for organic acids, and morphine is secreted by the organic base transport system. In these cases, elimination of the drug is enhanced by the combined effects of tubular secretion and filtration in delivering the drug to the urine.

Other routes for drug excretion include the lungs and gastrointestinal tract. The lungs play a significant role in excreting volatile drugs, that is, drugs that are usually administered by inhalation. Consequently, the lungs serve as the route of both administration and excretion for drugs such as gaseous anesthetics. The gastrointestinal tract usually plays only a minor role in drug excretion. Certain drugs can be excreted by the liver into the bile and subsequently reach the duodenum via the bile duct. If the drug remains in the gastrointestinal tract, it will eventually be excreted in the feces. However, most of the secreted bile is reabsorbed, and drugs contained in it are often reabsorbed simultaneously.

Other minor routes for drug excretion include the sweat, saliva, and breast milk of lactating mothers. Although drugs excreted via lactation are considered a relatively minor route with regard to loss from the mother, the possibility that the infant may imbibe substantial concentrations of the drug does exist. Careful consideration for the welfare of the nursing infant must always be a factor when administering medications to the lactating mother.[10,21]

Drug Elimination Rates

The rate at which a drug is eliminated is significant in determining the amount and frequency of the dosage of the drug. If a drug is administered much faster than it is eliminated, the drug will accumulate excessively in the body and reach toxic levels. Conversely, if elimination greatly exceeds the rate of delivery, the concentration in the body may never reach therapeutic levels. Several parameters are used to indicate the rate at which a drug is usually eliminated so that dosages may be adjusted accordingly. Two of the primary measurements are *clearance* and *half-life*.[58,60]

Clearance

Clearance of a drug (CL) can be described either in terms of all organ's and tissue's ability to eliminate the drug (systemic clearance) or in terms of a single organ or tissue's ability to eliminate the drug.[7,38,60] To calculate clearance from a specific organ, two primary factors must be considered. First, the blood flow to the organ (Q) determines how much drug will be delivered to the organ for elimination. Second, the fraction of drug removed from the plasma as it passes through the organ must be known. This fraction, termed the *extraction ratio*, is equal to the difference in the concentration of drug entering (Ci) and exiting (Co) the organ, divided by the entering concentration (Ci). Clearance by an individual organ is summarized by the following equation:

$$CL = Q \times [(Ci - Co) \div Ci].$$

The calculation of clearance using this equation is illustrated by the following example. Aspirin is metabolized primarily in the liver. Normal hepatic blood flow (Q) equals 1500 mL/min. If the blood entering the liver contains 200 μg/mL of aspirin (Ci) and the blood leaving the liver contains 134 μg/mL (Co), hepatic clearance of aspirin is calculated as follows:

$$CL_{hepatic} = Q \times [(Ci - Co) \div Ci]$$

$$= 1500 \text{ mL/min} \times [(200 \ \mu g/mL - 134$$
$$\mu g/mL) \div 200 \ \mu g/mL]$$

$$= 495 \text{ mL/min}.$$

This example illustrates that clearance is actually the amount of plasma that the drug can be totally removed from per unit time. As calculated here, the liver would be able to completely remove aspirin from 495 mL of blood each minute. Tetracycline, a common antibacterial drug, has a clearance equal to 130 mL/min, indicating that this drug would be completely removed from approximately 130 mL of plasma each minute.

Clearance is dependent on the organ or tissue's ability to extract the drug from the plasma as well as the perfusion of the organ. Some tissues may have an excellent ability to remove the drug from the bloodstream, but clearance is limited because only a small amount of blood reaches the organ. Conversely, highly perfused organs may be ineffective in removing the drug, thus prolonging its activity.

In terms of drug elimination from the entire body, systemic clearance is calculated as the sum of all individual clearances from all organs and tissues (i.e., systemic CL = hepatic CL + renal CL + lung CL, and so on). Note that the elimination of the drug includes the combined processes of drug loss from the body (excretion) as well as inactivation of the drug through biotransformation.[7,58,60]

Half-Life

In addition to clearance, the **half-life** of the drug is important in describing the duration of activity of the compound. Half-life is defined as the amount of time required for 50 percent of the drug remaining in the body to be eliminated.[59,60] Most drugs are eliminated in a manner such that a fixed portion of the drug is eliminated in a given time period. For example, a drug such as acetaminophen with a half-life of 2 hours indicates that in each 2-hour period, 50 percent of the acetaminophen still in the body will be eliminated (Fig. 3–3).

Half-life is a function of both clearance and volume of distribution (V_d);[38] that is, the time it takes to eliminate 50 percent of the drug depends not only on the ability of the organ(s) to remove the drug from the plasma, but also on the distribution or presence

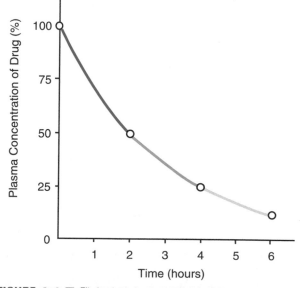

FIGURE 3–3 ▼ Elimination of a drug with a half-life of 2 hours. Fifty percent of the drug remaining in the bloodstream is eliminated in each 2-hour period.

of the drug in the plasma (see Chapter 2 for a description of V_d). A drug that undergoes extensive inactivation in the liver may have a long half-life if it is sequestered intracellularly in skeletal muscle. Also, disease states that affect either clearance or V_d will affect the half-life of the drug, so dosages must be altered accordingly.

Dosing Schedules and Plasma Concentration

With most medications, it is desirable to bring plasma concentrations of the drug up to a certain level and maintain it at that level. If the drug is administered by continuous intravenous administration, this can be done fairly easily by matching the rate of administration with the rate of drug elimination (clearance) once the desired plasma concentration is achieved (Fig. 3–4). In situations where the drug is given at specific intervals, the dosage must be adjusted to provide an average plasma concentration over the dosing period. Figure 3–4 illustrates that if the dosing interval is relatively long (e.g., 12 hours), the dose must be considerably large to provide the same relative plasma concentration that would exist in a shorter dosing interval (e.g., 8 hours). Note also that larger doses given further apart result in greater plasma fluctuations; that is, greater maximum and minimum plasma levels over the dosing period. Giving smaller doses

more frequently provides an equivalent average concentration without the extreme peaks and valleys associated with longer intervals.

Variations in Drug Response and Metabolism

The fact that different people react differently to the same relative drug dosage is an important and often critical aspect of pharmacology. Two patients who are given the same drug may exhibit different magnitudes of a beneficial response as well as different adverse effects. Several primary factors that are responsible for variations in the response to drugs are discussed below.

1. *Genetic factors.* Genetic variability can result in altered drug pharmacokinetics in certain individuals. In extreme cases, genetic variations may result in abnormal or absent drug-metabolizing enzymes.[60] This deficiency can be harmful or even fatal if the drug is not metabolized and begins exerting toxic effects due to accumulation or prolonged pharmacologic activity. For example, some individuals lack the appropriate plasma cholinesterase to break down circulating acetylcholine and acetylcholine-like compounds.[55] Succinylcholine is a neuromuscular blocking agent that is usually administered during general anesthesia to ensure muscular relax-

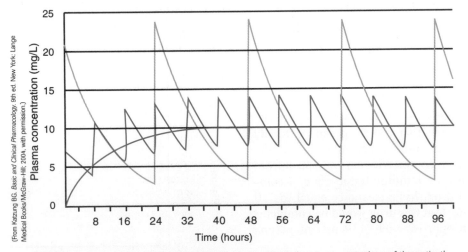

(From Katzung BG. *Basic and Clinical Pharmacology*, 9th ed. New York: Lange Medical Books/McGraw-Hill; 2004, with permission.)

FIGURE 3–4 ▼ Relationship between dosing interval and plasma concentrations of the antiasthmatic drug theophylline. A constant intravenous infusion (shown by the smoothly rising line) yields a desired plasma level of 10 mg/L. The same *average* plasma concentration is achieved when a dose of 224 mg is taken every 8 hours, or a dose of 672 mg every 24 hours. However, note the fluctuations in plasma concentration seen when doses are taken at specific hourly intervals.

ation during surgery. Normally, the succinylcholine is quickly degraded by plasma
cholinesterase; however, individuals lacking the
appropriate form of cholinesterase may suffer
respiratory paralysis because the succinylcholine
exerts its effect much longer than the expected
period of time.

In addition to the extreme case described
above, we now realize that many people have
subtle but important differences in the genes
controlling the synthesis of many drug-related
proteins. These differences—know as genetic
polymorphisms—will result in the production of
proteins that are somewhat different in structure
and function.[32,40,45] From this, various aspects of
drug disposition and response will be affected.[3,23,29] For example, differences in proteins
that transport drugs across membranes will
result in altered absorption, distribution, and
excretion of drugs using these transport systems.
Differences in the genetic control of drug
metabolizing proteins (enzymes) will likewise
result in altered metabolism and biotransformation of specific drugs. Finally, differences in the
proteins that function as drug receptors on
specific cells and target tissues (see Chapter 4)
might cause variability in the tissues' responses.

The potential influence of genetic variability
on drug responses and metabolism has actually
evolved into a branch of genetics known as
pharmacogenetics, or pharmacogenomics.[15]
Research in pharmacogenetics will continue to
expand as more details emerge about human
genetic make-up (i.e., the human genome project). We can tailor drug therapy more specifically for patients by realizing how specific genetic
differences might influence drug responses.[15,20,29,40] That is, doses can be adjusted to
account for genetic differences in drug disposition, and certain drugs can be avoided altogeth-
er in people who lack the appropriate enzymes
for these drugs. Drug regimens that take into
account genetic variability will ultimately result
in better drug effects with fewer side effects.

2. *Disease.* Structural or functional damage to an
organ or tissue responsible for drug metabolism
or excretion presents an obvious problem in
pharmacology. Diseases initiating change in tissue function or blood flow to specific organs like
the liver and kidneys can dramatically affect the
elimination of various drugs.[44,47,60] Certain dis-

eases may also impair the absorption and distribution of the drug, further complicating the
problem of individualized response. The significance of disease in affecting the patient's
response is crucial since response to a medication may be affected by the very same pathology that the drug is being used to treat. For
instance, renal excretion of antibiotics, such as
the aminoglycosides, is altered radically in many
types of bacterial infection, but these drugs are
typically administered to treat the same infections altering their own excretion.[60] Consequently, great care must be taken to adjust the
dosage accordingly when administering medications in conditions where drug disposition
might be altered by various diseases.[24,47,60]

3. *Drug interactions.* When two or more drugs are
present in the body at the same time, the
chance exists that they may interact and alter
each other's effects and metabolism.[3,19] The
majority of drug-drug interactions are insignificant and do not result in any clinically meaningful adverse effects.[11,46] Likewise, certain drug
combinations and interactions can be beneficial
because two or more compounds might act synergistically to produce a cumulative effect that
is greater than each drug would produce alone.
Several drugs, for example, are often administered simultaneously so that they augment each
other when treating conditions such as hypertension, cancer, and human immunodeficiency
virus infection. However, certain combinations
can lead to serious adverse effects and interactions. For example, two or more drugs can have
additive effects that cause an adverse response,
even if each drug is given in a nontoxic dose.
For instance, taking two central nervous system
(CNS) depressants simultaneously (e.g., barbiturates and alcohol) may cause such severe CNS
inhibition that the additive effects are lethal.

In contrast to an additive effect, drugs with
opposite actions may essentially cancel each
other out, thus negating or reducing the beneficial effects of one or both medications. A drug
that causes bronchodilation (i.e., for the treatment of asthma) will be negated by an agent
that constricts the bronchioles.

Some of the most serious problems occur
during drug interactions because one drug
delays the biotransformation of the other. If
a second compound inhibits the enzymes that

normally metabolize a drug, the original drug will exert its effect for prolonged periods, possibly leading to toxic effects.[60] For instance, the antiulcer drug cimetidine (Tagamet) inhibits the hepatic metabolism of oral anticoagulants such as warfarin (Coumadin). Taking these two drugs together tends to cause elevated plasma levels of the anticoagulant, which may prolong blood clotting and lead to a possible hemorrhage. Another type of interaction occurs when two or more drugs alter each other's absorption and distribution, and can occur when they compete for the same active transport carrier or bind to the same plasma proteins. An example is the interaction between aspirin and methotrexate, a drug used to treat cancer and rheumatoid arthritis. Aspirin can displace methotrexate from its binding site on plasma proteins, thus allowing relatively high amounts of unbound or "free" methotrexate to exist in the bloodstream. The increased levels of free methotrexate may lead to toxic effects.

Considering the large number of drugs on the market, it is well beyond the scope of this text to discuss all of the clinically relevant drug interactions. The prescribing physician and pharmacist, however, must carefully evaluate the potential for drug interactions. Likewise, physical therapists, occupational therapists, and other individuals dealing with patients taking medications must be alert for any abnormal symptoms or untoward effects because they may indicate a possible drug interaction.

4. *Age.* In general, older patients are more sensitive to drugs.[8,37] Drugs are usually not metabolized as quickly in the elderly, primarily because of decreases in liver and kidney function that typically accompany the aging process.[31,48,57] Decreased drug elimination therefore results in higher plasma levels in older adults than those occurring in younger adults given equivalent doses.[31,63] Older adults also suffer more illnesses, and consequently receive more drugs than younger adults; this fact further increases their vulnerability to altered drug responses.[4] Various other age-related changes in physiology (increased body fat, decreased cardiovascular function, and so forth) can affect pharmacokinetics and pharmacodynamics in older adults.[8,57]

Children are also subject to problems and variability in drug metabolism.[54] Because liver

and kidney function is immature, newborns may be deficient in specific drug-metabolizing enzymes, thus prolonging the effects of drugs.[1,16,22] Infants also differ from adults in several other key factors affecting drug disposition including differences in membrane function, plasma proteins, regional blood flow, and body composition (i.e., percentage of body fat and total body water).[54] Hence, drug absorption, distribution, and elimination will be altered in infants, and these alterations will be especially problematic in infants who are born prematurely.

5. *Diet.* Diet is shown to affect the absorption, metabolism, and response to many drugs.[12,30] Animal and human studies indicated that the total caloric input as well as the percentage of calories obtained from different sources (carbohydrates, proteins, and fats) influence drug pharmacokinetics.[17,26] Specific dietary constituents such as cruciferous vegetables and charcoal-broiled beef can also alter drug metabolism.[17]

Fortunately, most food-drug interactions are not serious and will not alter the clinical effects of the drug. There are, however, a few well-known food-drug combinations that should be avoided because of their potentially serious interaction. For example, it was recently discovered that grapefruit juice inhibits the enzymes that metabolize certain drugs as they are absorbed from the gastrointestinal (GI) tract. As a result, taking these drugs orally with grapefruit juice will result in *increased* drug bioavailability because more of the drug's active form will reach the bloodstream.[12,19] This increased bioavailability will result in plasma levels that are higher than expected, thereby increasing the risk of side effects and adverse reactions.

Another important food-drug interaction involves certain foods such as fermented cheese and wine. These foods contain high amounts of tyramine, which stimulates the release of catecholamines (norepinephrine, epinephrine) within the body. Hence, these foods should not be ingested with drugs that inhibit the monoamine oxidase enzyme (MAO inhibitors). MAO-inhibiting drugs work by suppressing the destruction of catecholamines, thus allowing higher levels of norepinephrine and epinephrine to occur. (MAO inhibitors are frequently used in the treatment of depression; see Chapter 7.) Consequently, when MAO inhibitors are taken with tyramine-containing foods, excessive levels of catecholamines may develop, leading to a dangerous increase in blood pressure (hypertensive crisis).

A number of other potential food-drug interactions occur, but it is beyond the scope of this text to discuss all of them. These interactions are addressed in more detail elsewhere.[19,30,34] Clinicians should therefore be aware of these well-known interactions and be on the alert for others as new drugs arrive on the market.

6. *Sex* Men and women may have distinct differences in the way that certain drugs are absorbed, distributed, and metabolized.[14,35,50] This idea makes sense when one considers that sex-related differences in body composition, gastrointestinal function, enzyme activity, and various other systems can potentially affect pharmacokinetic variables.[14,35,50] Drug disposition may also be influenced in women by the cyclic hormonal variations occurring during the menstrual cycle, whereas men do not typically undergo such routine hormonal fluctuations.[14] Pharmacokinetics can clearly differ between men and women, and future research is needed to determine how sex-related differences affect the therapeutic outcomes of specific drugs.[14,50]

7. *Other factors.* A number of additional factors may alter the predicted response of the patient to a drug. As discussed earlier, environmental and occupational hazards may produce certain toxins that alter drug absorption and metabolism.[9,62] Factors such as cigarette smoking and alcohol consumption have been shown to influence the metabolism of specific compounds.[39,49] Drug distribution and metabolism may be altered in the obese patient,[6] or in response to chronic and acute exercise.[7,43] Individuals with spinal cord injuries have a decreased ability to absorb certain drugs from their gastrointestinal tract, presumably because of a general decrease in gastrointestinal motility.[51] Conversely, patients with extensive burn injuries may have increased gastrointestinal absorption and therefore increased bioavailability of certain drugs, although the reason for this effect is not clear.[36,41]

There are many factors that influence the way each individual responds to a medication, and these factors must be taken into account whenever possible. Clinicians should also realize that these factors are not mutually exclusive. For example, a premature infant with genetic polymorphisms might present an extremely complex pharmacologic dilemma because of the combination of very young age and genetic variability.[23] In older adults, the combined effects of old age *and* disease can likewise increase the complexity of pharmacokinetic variability. Hence, special care must be taken in prescribing appropriate dosages in any situation where the predicted responses to drug therapy might be altered by one or more of the factors described.

SUMMARY

Drug elimination occurs because of the combined effects of drug metabolism and excretion. Elimination is essential in terminating drug activity within a reasonable and predictable time frame. Various tissues and organs (especially the liver and kidneys) are involved in drug elimination, and injury or disease of these tissues can markedly alter the response to certain drugs. In cases of disease or injury, dosages must frequently be adjusted to prevent adverse side effects from altered elimination rates. Many other environmental, behavioral, and genetic factors may also alter drug metabolism and disposition, and possible variability in the patient's response should always be a matter of concern when selecting the type and amount of the drug.

References

1. Alcorn J, McNamara PJ. Ontogeny of hepatic and renal systemic clearance pathways in infants: part II. *Clin Pharmacokinet.* 2002;41:1077–1094.
2. Ament PW, Bertolino JG, Liszewski JL. Clinically significant drug interactions. *Am Fam Physician.* 2000;61:1745–1754.
3. Attar M, Lee VH. Pharmacogenomic considerations in drug delivery. *Pharmacogenomics.* 2003;4:443–461.
4. Bressler R, Bahl JJ. Principles of drug therapy for the elderly patient. *Mayo Clin Proc.* 2003;78:1564–1577.
5. Buratti S, Lavine JE. Drugs and the liver: advances in metabolism, toxicity, and therapeutics. *Curr Opin Pediatr.* 2002;14:601–607.

6. Cheymol G. Effects of obesity on pharmacokinetics implications for drug therapy. *Clin Pharmacokinet.* 2000;39:215–231.

7. Ciccone CD. Basic pharmacokinetics and the potential effect of physical therapy interventions on pharmacokinetic variables. *Phys Ther.* 1995;75:343–351.

8. Ciccone, CD. Geriatric pharmacology. In: Guccione AA, ed. *Geriatric Physical Therapy.* 2nd ed. St. Louis: CV Mosby; 2000.

9. Conney AH. Induction of drug-metabolizing enzymes: a path to the discovery of multiple cytochromes P450. *Annu Rev Pharmacol Toxicol.* 2003;43:1–30.

10. Della-Giustina K, Chow G. Medications in pregnancy and lactation. *Emerg Med Clin North Am.* 2003;21:585–613.

11. Egger SS, Drewe J, Schlienger RG. Potential drug–drug interactions in the medication of medical patients at hospital discharge. *Eur J Clin Pharmacol.* 2003;58:773–778.

12. Evans AM. Influence of dietary components on the gastrointestinal metabolism and transport of drugs. *Ther Drug Monit.* 2000;22:131–136.

13. Fuhr U. Induction of drug metabolising enzymes: pharmacokinetic and toxicological consequences in humans. *Clin Pharmacokinet.* 2000;38:493–504.

14. Gandhi M, Aweeka F, Greenblatt RM, Blaschke TF. Sex differences in pharmacokinetics and pharmacodynamics. *Annu Rev Pharmacol Toxicol.* 2004;44:499–523.

15. Goldstein DB, Tate SK, Sisodiya SM. Pharmacogenetics goes genomic. *Nat Rev Genet.* 2003;4:937–947.

16. Gow PJ, Ghabrial H, Smallwood RA, et al. Neonatal hepatic drug elimination. *Pharmacol Toxicol.* 2001;88:3–15.

17. Harris RZ, Jang GR, Tsunoda S. Dietary effects on drug metabolism and transport. *Clin Pharmacokinet.* 2003;42:1071–1088.

18. Hlavica P. N-oxidative transformation of free and N-substituted amine functions by cytochrome P450 as means of bioactivation and detoxication.*Drug Metab Rev.* 2002;34:451–477.

19. Huang SM, Lesko LJ. Drug-drug, drug-dietary supplement, and drug-citrus fruit and other food interactions: what have we learned? *J Clin Pharmacol.* 2004;44:559–569.

20. Ingelman-Sundberg M. Pharmacogenetics of cytochrome P450 and its applications in drug therapy: the past, present and future. *Trends Pharmacol Sci.* 2004;25:193–200.

21. Ito S, Lee A. Drug excretion into breast milk—overview. *Adv Drug Deliv Rev.* 2003;55:617–627.

22. Johnson TN. The development of drug metabolising enzymes and their influence on the susceptibility to adverse drug reactions in children. *Toxicology.* 2003;192:37–48.

23. Kapur G, Mattoo T, Aranda JV. Pharmacogenomics and renal drug disposition in the newborn. *Semin Perinatol.* 2004;28:132–140.

24. Krishnan V, Murray P. Pharmacologic issues in the critically ill. *Clin Chest Med.* 2003;24:671–688.

25. Lee W, Kim RB. Transporters and renal drug elimination. *Annu Rev Pharmacol Toxicol.* 2004;44:137–166.

26. Leibovitch ER, Deamer RL, Sanderson LA. Food-drug interactions: careful drug selection and patient counseling can reduce the risk in older patients. *Geriatrics.* 2004;59:19–22, 32–33.

27. Lewis DF. 57 varieties: the human cytochromes P450. *Pharmacogenomics.* 2004;5:305–318.

28. Long A, Walker JD. Quantitative structure–activity relationships for predicting metabolism and modeling cytochrome p450 enzyme activities. *Environ Toxicol Chem.* 2003;22:1894–1899.

29. Ma MK, Woo MH, McLeod HL. Genetic basis of drug metabolism. *Am J Health Syst Pharm.* 2002;59:2061–2069.

30. Maka DA, Murphy LK. Drug–nutrient interactions: a review. *AACN Clin Issues.* 2000;11:580–589.

31. Mangoni AA, Jackson SH. Age-related changes in pharmacokinetics and pharmacodynamics: basic principles and practical applications. *Br J Clin Pharmacol.* 2004;57:6–14.

32. Marzolini C, Tirona RG, Kim RB. Pharmacogenomics of the OATP and OAT families. *Pharmacogenomics.* 2004;5:273–282.

33. Masereeuw R, Russel FG. Mechanisms and clinical implications of renal drug excretion. *Drug Metab Rev.* 2001;33:299–351.

34. McCabe BJ. Prevention of food-drug interactions with special emphasis on older adults. *Curr Opin Clin Nutr Metab Care.* 2004;7:21–26.

35. Meibohm B, Beierle I, Derendorf H. How important are gender differences in pharmacokinetics? *Clin Pharmacokinet.* 2002;41:329–342.

36. Neudeck BL, Foster DR, Li LY, et al. The effects of thermal injury on transcellular permeability and intestinal P glycoprotein in rats. *Burns.* 2003;29:803–809.

37. Noble RE. Drug therapy in the elderly. *Metabolism.* 2003;52(suppl 2):27–30.

38. Obach RS. The prediction of human clearance from hepatic microsomal metabolism data. *Curr Opin Drug Discov Devel.* 2001;4:36–44.

39. Oneta CM, Lieber CS, Li J, et al. Dynamics of cytochrome P4502E1 activity in man: induction by ethanol and disappearance during withdrawal phase. *J Hepatol.* 2002;36:47–52.

40. Oscarson M. Pharmacogenetics of drug metabolising enzymes: importance for personalized medicine. *Clin Chem Lab Med.* 2003;41:573–580.

41. Peng X, Yan H, You Z, et al. Effects of enteral supplementation with glutamine granules on intestinal mucosal barrier function in severe burned patients. *Burns.* 2004;30:135–139.

42. Perri D, Ito S, Rowsell V, Shear NH. The kidney—the body's playground for drugs: an overview of renal drug handling with selected clinical correlates. *Can J Clin Pharmacol.* 2003;10:17–23.

43. Persky AM, Eddington ND, Derendorf H. A review of the effects of chronic exercise and physical fitness level on resting pharmacokinetics. *Int J Clin Pharmacol Ther.* 2003;41:504–516.

44. Pichette V, Leblond FA. Drug metabolism in chronic renal failure. *Curr Drug Metab.* 2003;4:91–103.

45. Pirmohamed M, Park BK. Cytochrome P450 enzyme polymorphisms and adverse drug reactions. *Toxicology.* 2003;192:23–32.

46. Piscitelli S. Preventing dangerous drug interactions. *J Am Pharm Assoc.* 2000;40(suppl 1):S44–S45.

47. Rodighiero V. Effects of liver disease on pharmacokinetics. An update. *Clin Pharmacokinet.* 1999;37:399–431.

48. Schmucker DL. Liver function and phase I drug metabolism in the elderly: a paradox. *Drugs Aging.* 2001;18:837–851.

49. Schoedel KA, Tyndale RF. Induction of nicotine-metabolizing CYP2B1 by ethanol and ethanol-metabolizing CYP2E1 by nicotine: summary and implications. *Biochim Biophys Acta.* 2003;1619:283–290.

50. Schwartz JB. The influence of sex on pharmacokinetics. *Clin Pharmacokinet.* 2003;42:107–121.

51. Segal JL, Hayes KC, Brunnemann SR, et al. Absorption characteristics of sustained-release 4 aminopyridine (fampridine SR) in patients with chronic spinal cord injury. *J Clin Pharmacol.* 2000;40:402–409.

52. Sheweita SA. Drug-metabolizing enzymes: mechanisms and functions. *Curr Drug Metab.* 2000;1:107–132.

53. Srivastava P. Drug metabolism and individualized medicine. *Curr Drug Metab.* 2003;4:33–44.

54. Strolin Benedetti M, Baltes EL. Drug metabolism and disposition in children. *Fundam Clin Pharmacol.* 2003;17:281–299.

55. Taylor P. Agents acting at the neuromuscular junction and autonomic ganglia. In: Hardman JG, et al, eds. *The Pharmacological Basis of Therapeutics.* 10th ed. New York: McGraw Hill; 2001.

56. Tett SE, Kirkpatrick CM, Gross AS, McLachlan AJ. Principles and clinical application of assessing alterations in renal elimination pathways. *Clin Pharmacokinet.* 2003;42:1193–1211.

57. Turnheim K. When drug therapy gets old: pharmacokinetics and pharmacodynamics in the elderly. *Exp Gerontol.* 2003;38:843–853.

58. Urso R, Blardi P, Giorgi G. A short introduction to pharmacokinetics. *Eur Rev Med Pharmacol Sci.* 2002;6:33–44.

59. Wright JG, Boddy AV. All half-lives are wrong, but some half-lives are useful. *Clin Pharmacokinet.* 2001;40:237–244.

60. Wilkinson GR. Pharmacokinetics: the dynamics of drug absorption, distribution, and elimination. In: Hardman JG, et al, eds. *The Pharmacological Basis of Therapeutics.* 10th ed. New York: McGraw Hill; 2001.

61. Yang LQ, Li SJ, Cao YF, et al. Different alterations of cytochrome P450 3A4 isoform and its gene expression in livers of patients with chronic liver disease. *World J Gastroenterol.* 2003;9:359–363.

62. You L. Steroid hormone biotransformation and xenobiotic induction of hepatic steroid metabolizing enzymes. *Chem Biol Interact.* 2004;147:233–246.

63. Zeeh J, Platt D. The aging liver: structural and functional changes and their consequences for drug treatment in old age. *Gerontology.* 2002;48:121–127.

Chapter 4

Drug Receptors

A receptor is a component of the cell where a drug binds and initiates a chain of biochemical events.[2] Most drugs exert their effect by binding to and activating such a receptor, which brings about some change in the physiologic function of the cell. These receptors can be any cellular macromolecule, but many receptors have been identified as proteins or protein complexes that are located on or within the cell.[45,57] The general mechanisms of receptor function, in conjunction with their cellular location, are discussed here.

Receptors Located on the Cell's Surface

The principle site for receptors that recognize endogenous and exogenous compounds is the outer surface of the cell membrane.[2] By placing receptors on its outer surface, the cell is able to differentiate and respond to specific substances that approach the cell, without actually allowing these substances to enter. These surface receptors are primarily responsive to specific amino acid, peptide, or amine compounds. Surface receptors can affect cell function (1) by acting as an ion channel and directly altering membrane permeability, (2) by acting enzymatically to directly influence function within the cell, or (3) by being linked to regulatory proteins that control other chemical and enzymatic processes within the cell. Each of the three basic ways that surface receptors can affect cell function is addressed here.

Surface Receptors Linked Directly to Ion Channels

Membrane receptors may be involved directly in the cellular response to the drug by acting as an ion pore and thus changing the membrane permeability.[61]

Perhaps the most well-known example is the acetylcholine receptor located on the postsynaptic membrane of the neuromuscular junction[49,56] (Fig. 4–1). When bound by acetylcholine molecules, the receptor activates and opens a pore through the cell membrane, thereby increasing the permeability of the muscle cell to sodium.[38,56] This action results in depolarization and excitation of the cell because of sodium influx. Another important example of a receptor–ion channel system is the **gamma-aminobutyric acid (GABA)-benzodiazepine–chloride ion channel complex** found on neuronal membranes in the central nervous sys-

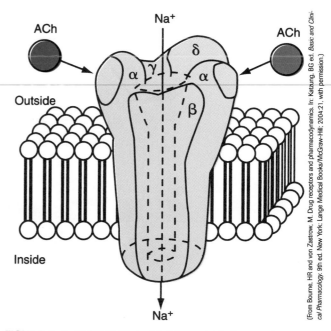

(From Bourne, HR and von Zastrow, M. Drug receptors and pharmacodynamics. In: Katzung, BG ed. *Basic and Clinical Pharmacology*: 9th ed. New York: Lange Medical Books/McGraw-Hill; 2004:21, with permission.)

FIGURE 4–1 ▼ Schematic model of the acetylcholine receptor, an example of a surface receptor that is linked directly to an ion channel. Binding of two acetylcholine (ACh) molecules to the outer surface of the receptor protein induces the opening of a central ion channel, thus allowing sodium to enter the cell.

tem.[46,51] In this situation, the membrane's permeability to chloride is increased by the binding of both the neurotransmitter GABA and benzodiazepine drugs such as diazepam (Valium) and chlordiazepoxide (Librium). The function of this chloride ion channel complex is discussed in more detail in Chapter 6. Surface receptors for other substances—such as ions (sodium, potassium, calcium) and amino acids (glutamate)—have been identified, and are likewise linked directly to ion channels that control permeability of the cell membrane.[37,61]

Surface Receptors Linked Directly to Enzymes

Some proteins that span the entire width of the cell membrane may have an extracellular receptor site (binding domain) as well as an intracellular enzymatic component (catalytic domain)[21,44] (Fig. 4–2). Drugs and endogenous chemicals that bind to the receptor site can change the enzyme activity of the intracellular catalytic component, thus altering the biochemical function within the cell.[43] Receptor-enzyme systems in this category are often referred to as *protein tyrosine kinases* because binding of an appropriate substance to the outer (receptor) component initiates the phosphorylation of certain tyrosine amino acids on the inner (catalytic) component of the protein, which in turn increases the enzyme activity of the intracellular component (see Fig. 4–2).[22,43] The activated enzymatic component of the receptor then catalyzes the activation of other substrates within the cell.

It appears that insulin and certain growth factors may exert their effects by acting through this type of tyrosine kinase receptor-enzyme system.[21,44] Insulin, for example, binds to the extracellular component of a protein located on skeletal muscle cells, thereby initiating activation of this protein's enzymatic activity on the inner surface of the cell membrane. This change in enzyme function causes further changes in cell activity, which ultimately result in increased glucose uptake in the muscle cell. The function of insulin receptors and their role in the cause and treatment of diabetes mellitus are discussed in more detail in Chapter 32.

Surface Receptors Linked to Regulatory (G) Proteins: Role of the Second Messenger

Rather than directly affecting membrane permeability or directly influencing enzyme activity, other membrane receptors affect cell function by linking to an intermediate regulatory protein that is located on the inner surface of the cell's membrane.[2,23,45] These regulatory proteins are activated by binding guanine

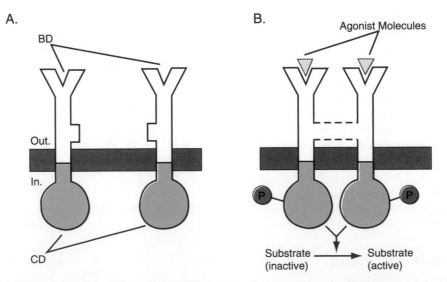

FIGURE 4–2 ▼ Example of a surface receptor that is linked directly to intracellular enzyme activity. (*A*) The receptor exists in an inactive state as two subunits: each subunit has a binding domain (BD) on the outer surface and a catalytic domain (CD) on the inner surface. (*B*) Binding of agonist molecules to the BDs causes the subunits to join together and induces phosphorylation (P) of tyrosine receptors on the CD. Tyrosine phosphorylation initiates enzymatic activity of the catalytic units, which then causes substrate activation within the cell.

nucleotides; hence they are often termed **G proteins**.[2] When an appropriate substance binds to the surface receptor, the receptor moves laterally in the cell membrane, and attaches to the regulatory G protein.[24] This attachment activates the G protein, which in turn alters the activity of a type of intracellular effector (such as an enzyme or ion channel), ultimately leading to a change in cell function.[27,59]

Receptors that are linked to G proteins (also called G protein–coupled receptors) represent the primary way that signals from the surface receptor are transduced into the appropriate response within the cell.[2,23] There appear to be two types of regulatory G proteins: a stimulatory protein (G_s), which increases the cellular response, and an inhibitory protein (G_i), which decreases that response (Fig. 4–3). The two types of G proteins are linked to two different receptors that are responsive to different drugs.

Certain drugs affect the cell by binding to a receptor that is linked to a G_s protein. The activated receptor activates the G_s protein, which in turn activates the effector system that opens an ion channel or activates a specific enzyme. Conversely, a drug that binds to a receptor that is linked to a G_i protein, inhibits channel opening or intracellular enzyme activity.

Hence, regulatory G proteins help account for how drugs can bind to one type of receptor and stimulate cell function, whereas drugs that bind to a different receptor on the same cell can inhibit cell activity. G proteins also seem to be important in mediating the other cell responses to stimulation or inhibition. For instance, cell function may continue to be

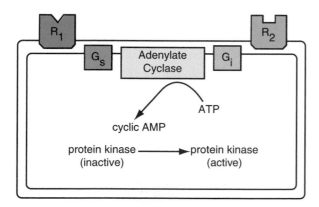

FIGURE 4–3 ▼ Schematic diagram of a surface receptor–second messenger system. In this example, the second messenger is cAMP, which is synthesized from ATP by the adenylate cyclase enzyme. The enzyme is linked to surface receptors (R_1 and R_2) by regulatory G proteins. G_s stimulates the enzyme and G_i inhibits enzyme activity. Thus, a drug binding to R_1 will increase production of cAMP, while a different drug binding to R_2 will inhibit cAMP production.

affected through the action of G proteins even after the drug has left the binding site on the cell's surface[2]; that is, the drug may bind to the cell for only a short period, but this binding is sufficient to initiate the interaction of the G protein with the intracellular effector system. Sustained influence of the G protein on the effector system helps explain why the cell may continue to exhibit a response even after the drug has dissociated from it, or even after the drug has been eliminated from the body completely.

As indicated earlier, many G protein–coupled receptors are linked directly to an intracellular enzyme. Drugs and other substances that exert their effects through receptor–G protein–enzyme systems often form (or inhibit the formation of) an intracellular compound known as a **second messenger**. In effect, the drug acts as the first messenger, which triggers a biochemical change in the cell, but the drug itself does not enter. The second messenger, which is the substance produced inside the cell, actually mediates the change in function.

The primary example of this type of second messenger strategy is the **adenylate cyclase–cyclic adenosine monophosphate (cAMP)** system present in many cells (see Fig. 4–3).[50,53] Adenylate cyclase, an enzyme that is located on the inner surface of the cell membrane, is responsible for hydrolyzing adenosine triphosphate (ATP) into cAMP. Cyclic AMP acts as the second messenger in this system by activating other enzymes (i.e., protein kinases) throughout the cell. Thus, drugs that bind to a surface receptor that is linked to a G_s protein will increase adenylate cyclase activity, resulting in increased production of cAMP within the cell. Other drugs bound to a different receptor that is linked to a G_i protein will inhibit adenylate cyclase activity, resulting in decreased production of cAMP.

The adenylate cyclase–cAMP system is associated with specific membrane receptors such as the beta-adrenergic receptors.[20] Other surface receptors may also be linked to this particular effector–second messenger system, or they may be linked to other intracellular processes that use different second messengers including: cyclic guanine monophosphate (cGMP), cyclic adenosine diphosphoribose (cADPR), diacylglycerol, phosphoinositides, nicotinic acid adenine dinucleotide phosphate (NAADP), and calcium ions.[11,17,28,34,39,42,47,48]

Finally, alterations in the synthesis, function, and regulation of G proteins have been identified in certain pathologic conditions, including alcoholism, diabetes mellitus, heart failure, and certain tumors.[20,26,35,41,52,60]

This illustrates the fact that G proteins seem to play an integral role in mediating the cell's response to various substances in both normal and disease states. The importance of these regulatory proteins will almost certainly continue to emerge as additional information about their structure and function becomes available.

Intracellular Receptors

Receptors have been identified at intracellular locations such as the cytoplasm and the nucleus.[1,4,10] These intracellular receptors are specific for certain endogenous hormones, and the drugs that affect them. For instance, steroid and steroidlike compounds exert some of their effects by initially interacting with a receptor that is located in the cytoplasm.[4,6,31] Specifically, these hormones form a complex with the receptor in the cytoplasm, and the hormone-receptor complex then moves to the cell's nucleus, where it affects the function of specific genes. Thyroid hormones (thyroxin, triiodothyronine) appear to bind directly to a receptor located on the chromatin in the cell's nucleus.[18] In either case, cell function is altered because the hormone-receptor complex affects specific genes in the DNA and causes changes in gene expression and messenger RNA transcription. Altered transcription of specific genes results in altered cellular protein synthesis, which ultimately results in altered cell function.[1]

Hence, certain endogenous hormones and hormone-like drugs exert some of their effects by acting on receptors located within the cell. It has become clear, however, that these substances might also exert some of their effects by binding to a second set of receptors located on the cell surface.[10,18] That is, surface receptors have been identified for steroid and thyroid hormones, and stimulation of these surface receptors might compliment or exaggerate the effects of the intracellular receptors.[1,31] The role of intracellular receptors, and their analogous surface receptors, is discussed further in this text in the chapters that deal with specific drugs that bind to these cellular components.

Drug-Receptor Interactions

The ability a drug has to bind to any receptor is dictated by factors such as the drug's size and shape relative to the configuration of the binding site on the receptor. The electrostatic attraction between the drug and the receptor may also be important in determining the extent to which the drug binds to the receptor. This drug-receptor interaction is somewhat analogous to a key fitting into a lock. The drug acts as a "key" that will only fit into certain receptors. Once inserted into a suitable receptor, the drug activates the receptor, much like a key turning and "activating" the appropriate lock. To carry this analogy one step further, unlocking a door to a room would increase the "permeability" of the room in a manner similar to the direct effect of certain activated membrane receptors (e.g., the acetylcholine receptor on the neuromuscular junction). Other types of key-lock interactions would be "linked" to some other event, such as using a key to start an automobile engine. This situation is analogous to linking a surface receptor to some intracellular enzymatic process that would affect the internal "machinery" of the cell.

Although key-lock analogy serves as a crude example of drug-receptor interactions, the attraction between a drug and any receptor is much more complex. Binding a drug to a receptor is not an all-or-none phenomenon, but is graded depending on the drug in question. Some drugs will bind readily to the receptor, some moderately, some very little, or some not at all. The term **affinity** is used to describe the amount of attraction between a drug and a receptor.[45] Affinity is actually related to the drug amount that is required to bind to the unoccupied receptors.[25] A drug with a high affinity binds readily to the open receptors, even if the concentration of the drug is relatively low. Drugs with moderate or low affinity require a higher concentration in the body before the receptors become occupied.

In addition to the relative degree of affinity of different drugs for a receptor, apparently the status of the receptor may also vary under specific conditions. Receptors may exist in variable affinity states (super-high, high, low) depending on the influence of local regulators such as guanine nucleotides, ammonium ions, and divalent cations.[45] These local regulators are also known as **allosteric modulators**, which can bind to specific sites on the receptor that are distinct from the primary (drug) binding site, and thereby increase or decrease the affinity for the drug.[23,36] Membrane receptors may also be influenced by the local environment of the lipid bilayer. The amount of flexibility or "fluidity" of the cell membrane is recognized as being critical in providing a suitable environment in which membrane constituents such as receptors can optimally function. Physical and chemical factors (including other drugs) may change the fluidity and organization of the membrane, thereby disrupting the normal orientation of the receptor and subsequently altering its affinity state and ability to interact with a drug.[9,29]

The exact way in which a drug activates a receptor has been the subject of considerable debate. Binding a drug to the receptor is hypothesized to cause the receptor to undergo some sort of temporary change in its shape or conformation. The change in structure of the activated receptor then mediates a change in cell function, either directly or by linking to some effector system. Studies have suggested that certain receptor proteins, such as the acetylcholine receptor, undergo a specific change in structure after binding with specific chemicals.[38, 55, 56] This event certainly seems plausible because most receptors have been identified as protein molecules, and proteins are known to be able to reversibly change their shape and conformation as part of normal physiologic function.[45] This fact should not, however, rule out other possible ways in which an activated receptor may mediate changes in cell function. Future research will continue to clarify the role of conformational changes as well as other possible mechanisms of receptor activation.

Functional Aspects of Drug-Receptor Interactions

The interaction between the drug and the receptor dictates several important aspects of pharmacology, including those discussed here.

Drug Selectivity and Receptor Subtypes

A drug is said to be *selective* if it affects only one type of cell or tissue and produces a specific physiologic response. For instance, a drug that is cardioselective will affect heart function without affecting other tissues such as the gastrointestinal tract or respiratory system. The selectivity of a particular drug is a function of the drug's ability to interact with specific receptors on the target tissue, and not with other receptors on the target tissue or on other tissues (Fig. 4–4). In reality, drug selectivity is a relative term because no drug produces only one effect. Drugs can be compared with one another, however, with the more selective drug being able to affect one type of tissue or organ with only a minimum of other responses.

The issue of drug selectivity is related closely to the fact that many receptor populations can be divided into various subtypes according to specific structural and functional differences between subgroups of the receptor. A primary example is the cholinergic (acetylcholine) receptor found on various tissues throughout the body. These receptors can be classified into two primary subtypes: muscarinic and nicotinic. Acetylcholine will bind to either subtype, but drugs such as nicotine will bind preferentially to the nicotinic subtype, and muscarine (a toxin found in certain mushrooms) will bind preferentially to the muscarinic subtype.

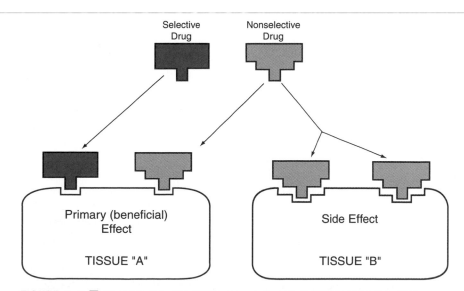

FIGURE 4–4 ▼ Drug selectivity. The diagram represents an ideal situation where the selective drug produces only beneficial effects and the nonselective drug exerts both beneficial and non-beneficial effects. Drug selectivity is actually a relative term, because all drugs produce some side effects; however, a selective drug produces fewer side effects than a nonselective agent.

Other types of receptors can be divided and subdivided in a similar manner. For example, the adrenergic receptor (i.e., the receptor for epinephrine or "adrenaline") is divided into two primary subtypes (alpha and beta), with each subtype having two primary divisions (alpha-1 and alpha-2; beta-1 and beta-2). Epinephrine will stimulate all adrenergic receptor subtypes, but certain drugs will only affect one of the primary divisions (e.g., a beta-selective drug), or even one subtype within each division (e.g., a beta-1 selective drug). The functional significance of adrenergic and cholinergic receptors is discussed in more detail in Chapter 18. Receptor subtypes also exist for other substances (opioids, dopamine, GABA, hormones, and so forth); the significance of these will be addressed in their respective chapters in this text.

The fact that many receptors can be classified into subtypes presents the opportunity to develop drugs that will produce fairly selective effects because they affect only one receptor subtype.[5,16] A beta-1 selective drug, for example, will primarily affect the heart because the heart basically contains the beta-1 subtype of adrenergic receptor, while other tissues (lungs, arterioles) contain other subtypes of adrenergic receptors. Research is ongoing to learn more about the structure and function of receptor populations and their subtypes. By knowing the characteristics of a specific receptor subtype, drugs can be designed to affect only that subtype and therefore will produce more selective effects with fewer side effects.[5,13]

Dose-Response

The shape of the typical dose-response curve discussed in Chapter 1 is related to the number of receptors that are bound by the drug (see Fig. 1–2), because within certain limits of the drug concentration, the response is essentially proportional to the number of receptors occupied by the drug.[2,25] At low dosages, for example, only a few receptors are bound by the drug; hence, the effect is relatively small. As the dosage (and drug concentration) increases, more receptors become occupied and the response increases. Finally, at a certain dosage, all available receptors will be occupied, and the response will be maximal. Increasing the dosage beyond the point at which the maximal effect is reached will not produce any further increase in response because all the receptors are bound by the drug. It should be noted, however, that the relationship between drug receptors and drug response is not a simple linear relationship for many drugs. A drug that

occupies half the available receptors, for example, may produce a response that is greater than 50 percent of the maximal response.[25] Clearly, other factors influence the absolute magnitude of the response, including factors that influence the relative affinity for the drug, and how well the occupied receptor can transmit the signal to the cell's effector mechanisms. It is, nonetheless, essentially true that increasing or decreasing the amount of drug available to the appropriate receptors will bring about a concomitant increase or decrease in the response to that drug.[45]

Classification of Drugs: Agonist Versus Antagonist

So far, drug-receptor interactions have been used to describe the process by which a drug occupies a receptor and in some way activates it. The activated receptor then brings about a change in cell function. A drug that can bind to a receptor and initiate a change in the function of the cell is referred to as an **agonist**. An agonist is identified as having affinity and efficacy.[2,45] As discussed earlier, *affinity* refers to the fact that there is an attraction, or desire, for the drug to bind to a given receptor. The second characteristic, *efficacy*, indicates that the drug will activate the receptor and will subsequently lead to a change in the function of the cell. Whereas an agonist has both affinity and efficacy, an **antagonist** has only affinity. This means that the drug will bind to the receptor, but it will not cause any direct change in the function of the receptor or cell (Fig. 4–5). Antagonists are significant because, by occupying the receptor, they prevent the agonistic compound from having any effect on the cell. Antagonists are often referred to as *blockers* because of their ability to block the effect of another chemical. The primary pharmacologic significance of these antagonists has been their use in blocking the effects of certain endogenous compounds. A classic example of this is the use of the so-called beta blockers, which occupy specific receptors on the myocardium, thus preventing circulating catecholamines from increasing heart rate and contractility. Other examples of antagonistic drugs are discussed in their appropriate chapters.

Competitive Versus Noncompetitive Antagonists

Pharmacologic antagonists are generally divided into two categories depending on whether they are com-

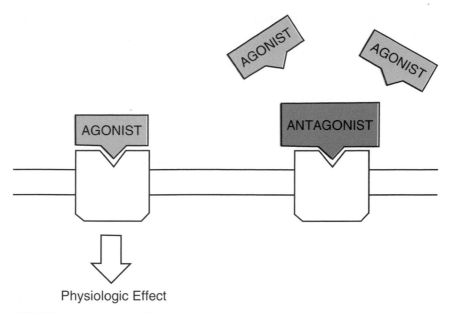

FIGURE 4–5 ▼ Drug classification: agonist versus antagonist. The antagonist (blocker) prevents the agonist from binding to the receptor and exerting a physiologic effect.

peting with the agonist for the receptor.[2,45] *Competitive antagonists* are so classified because they seem to be vying for the same receptor as the agonist. In other words, both the agonist and antagonist have an equal opportunity to occupy the receptor. For practical purposes, whichever drug concentration is greater tends to have the predominant effect. If the number of competitive antagonist molecules far exceeds the number of agonist molecules, the antagonists will occupy most of the receptors and the overall effect will be inhibition of the particular response. Conversely, a high concentration of an agonist relative to an antagonist will produce a pharmacologic effect, because the agonist will occupy most of the receptors. In fact, raising the concentration of the agonist with a competitive antagonist present can actually overcome the original inhibition, because the competitive antagonists form rather weak bonds with the receptor and can be displaced from it by a sufficient concentration of agonist molecules.[2,45] This is an important advantage of competitive antagonists because, if necessary, the inhibition caused by the antagonist can be overcome simply by administering high concentrations of the agonist.

In contrast to competitive antagonists, *noncompetitive antagonists* form strong, essentially permanent, bonds to the receptor. Noncompetitive antagonists either have an extremely high affinity for the receptor or actually form irreversible covalent bonds to the receptor.[2,45] Once bound to the receptor, the noncompetitive antagonist cannot be displaced by the agonist, regardless of how much agonist is present. Thus the term *noncompetitive* refers to the inability of the agonist to compete with the antagonist for the receptor site. The obvious disadvantage to this type of receptor blocker is that the inhibition cannot be overcome in cases of an overdose of the antagonist. Also, noncompetitive antagonists often remain bound for the receptor's lifespan, and their effect is terminated only after the receptor has been replaced as part of the normal protein turnover within the cell. Consequently, the inhibition produced by a noncompetitive blocker tends to remain in effect for long periods (i.e., several days).

Partial Agonists

Drugs are classified as *partial agonists* when they do not evoke a maximal response compared to a strong agonist. This classification is used even though the partial agonist occupies all available receptors.[3,32] In fact, partial agonists can be thought of as having an efficacy that lies somewhere between that of a full agonist and a full noncompetitive antagonist. The lack of a maximal response is not caused by decreased drug-receptor affinity. On the contrary, partial agonists often have a high affinity for the receptor. The decreased efficacy may be caused by the fact that the partial agonist does not completely activate the receptor after it binds, and that binding results in a lower level of any postreceptor events (e.g., less activation of G proteins, smaller changes in enzyme function).

Hence, the realization that certain drugs act as partial agonists has led to the idea that a range of efficacy can exist, depending on how specific drugs interact with their respective receptors.[3] At one end of this range are the drugs that bind strongly and produce a high degree of efficacy (strong agonists), while the other end of the spectrum contains drugs that bind strongly and produce no effect (strong antagonists). Agents that fall between these two extremes (partial agonists) can have varying degrees of agonistic activity. These partial agonists can also have certain clinical advantages. For instance, certain antipsychotic drugs that function as partial agonists may reduce psychotic episodes without excessive side effects.[15,32] Other examples of how partial agonists can be used clinically are discussed elsewhere in this text.

Mixed Agonist–Antagonists and Inverse Agonists

Some agents will stimulate certain receptor subtypes, while simultaneously blocking the effects of endogenous substances on other receptor subtypes (the concept of receptor subtypes was addressed earlier in this chapter). These agents are known as mixed agonist–antagonists, and they are especially useful in certain clinical situations.[2] In some women, for example, it is often beneficial to stimulate estrogen receptors on bone to prevent osteoporosis, while simultaneously blocking the effects of estrogen on breast tissues to prevent cancer. Hence, certain drugs known as selective estrogen receptor modulators (SERMs; see Chapters 30, 31, and 36) can differentiate between the subtypes of estrogen receptors on these two tissues, and act as an agonist on bone and an antagonist on breast tissues.[19] These agents are a good example of drugs with mixed agonist–antagonist activity, and other drugs with this type of mixed activity will be discussed in their respective chapters throughout this text.

Finally, it has been proposed that some drugs could function as inverse agonists.[3,25] As this classification implies, these drugs would bind to the same receptor as the agonist, but have the *opposite* effect on cellular function compared to the agonist. This effect is different from a traditional, or neutral, antagonist that binds to the tissue and simply prevents an increase in the agonist's effect. By creating the opposite effect, inverse agonists could bring about a decrease in activ-

ity in situations where the receptor is too active or overstimulated.[25] Future studies will be needed to determine to what extent inverse agonists might be useful as therapeutic agents.

Receptor Regulation

Receptor responses are not static but are regulated by endogenous and exogenous factors. In general, a prolonged increase in the stimulation of various receptors will lead to a *decrease* in receptor function, and decreased stimulation will lead to an *increase* in receptor numbers or sensitivity (Fig. 4–6). The mechanisms and significance of these receptor changes are described here.

Receptor Desensitization and Down-Regulation

As presented in Figure 4–6, overstimulation of postsynaptic receptors by endogenous substances (neurotransmitters, hormones) or by exogenous agonists (drugs) may lead to a functional decrease in the appropriate receptor population.[54,58] In effect, the cell becomes less responsive to the prolonged stimulation by decreasing the number of active receptors. The term desensitization is used to describe a fairly brief and transient decrease in responsiveness.[2,8] Desensitization is believed to occur because of the addition of phosphate residues (phosphorylation) or some other chemical modification to the receptor protein.[25,33] Adding a phosphate molecule seems to cause some membrane receptors to be uncoupled from their intermediate regulatory proteins and consequently from the rest of the cell's biochemical machinery.[40] Receptor desensitization helps account for the decrease in response that may be seen even though the agonist remains present in high concentration in the body. The decrease in responsiveness caused by desensitization is fairly brief, however, and a return to normal response may occur within a few minutes after the agonist is removed.

Receptor **down-regulation** describes a slower, more prolonged process in which the actual number of available receptors is diminished.[30,33] Although the exact mechanisms responsible for down-regulation are not fully understood, it appears that prolonged exposure of the agonist causes increased receptor removal, decreased receptor synthesis, or a combination of

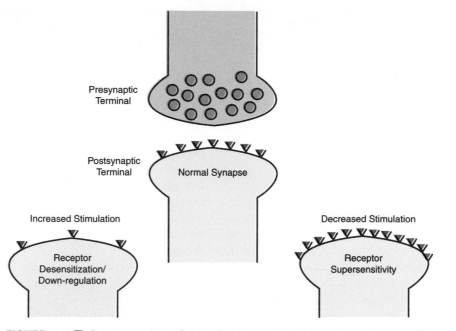

FIGURE 4–6 ▼ Receptor regulation. Functionally active receptor sites are represented by an "X." Increased stimulation results in a decrease in receptor numbers (desensitization/down-regulation), while decreased stimulation causes increased receptor numbers (supersensitivity).

increased removal and decreased synthesis.[40] In any event, the cell undergoes a decrease in responsiveness that remains in effect long after the agonist is removed (i.e., several days). Normal sensitivity to the agonist will be reestablished only when the cell has had the chance to replace and restore the receptors that were eliminated during downregulation.

Receptor desensitization and down-regulation appear to be examples of a negative feedback system used by the cell to prevent overstimulation by an agonist. The cell appears to selectively decrease its responsiveness to a particular stimulus in order to protect itself from excessive perturbation. Receptor down-regulation is important pharmacologically because it may be one of the primary reasons that a decrease in drug responsiveness occurs when certain drugs are used for prolonged periods.[33] Likewise, receptor desensitization and downregulation have been linked to several pathological situations, and drugs that prevent these decreases in receptor function could prove useful in conditions such as acute CNS injury, cardiac disease, or HIV infection.[8,12,30] Conversely, some drugs, such as the antidepressants, may exert their beneficial effects by intentionally causing receptor down-regulation and desensitization in certain neural pathways that cause

clinical depression. These drugs are discussed in detail in Chapter 7.

Receptor Supersensitivity

A prolonged decrease in the stimulation of the postsynaptic receptors can result in a functional increase in receptor sensitivity. The best example of this is the denervation supersensitivity seen when a peripheral nerve is severed.[7] In this situation, the lack of presynaptic neurotransmitter release results in a compensatory increase in postsynaptic receptor numbers on the muscle cell. Similarly, the loss of the endogenous neurotransmitter dopamine in neurodegenerative conditions such as Parkinson disease can result in supersensitivity of receptors for that neurotransmitter.[14] This increased receptor sensitivity becomes problematic because administration of dopaminelike drugs can cause excessive or untoward responses (see Chapter 10).[14]

A somewhat different type of denervation supersensitivity can also occur when receptor antagonist drugs are used for prolonged periods. Here the postsynaptic receptors are blocked by the antagonistic drug, and are unavailable for stimulation by the appropriate agonist. The postsynaptic neuron interprets this as if the synapse were denervated and responds by manufacturing more receptors, resulting in a compensatory *increase* in function at the synapse that was supposed to be blocked by the antagonist. Again, drug therapy could be affected in this situation because the dose of the blocker will need to be altered to cope with the new, larger population of receptors.

Nonreceptor Drug Mechanisms

Certain drugs do not appear to exert their effects by binding to a specific cellular component.[45] For example, certain cancer chemotherapeutic agents act as "antimetabolites" by becoming incorporated into the manufacture of specific cellular components. The drug acts as an improper ingredient in the biosynthesis of the component, so that the cell does not manufacture harmful or unwanted materials. In addition, many common antacids work by directly neutralizing stomach acid; that is, these drugs act via a chemical reaction rather than through a specific receptor molecule. Other drugs may affect cell function without first binding to a receptor by directly altering enzyme function or by acting as "chelating agents," which bind to harmful compounds such as heavy metals and prevent them from exerting toxic effects. Additional nonreceptor-mediated mechanisms of specific compounds are discussed when those drugs are examined in their respective chapters.

SUMMARY

Many drugs and endogenous chemicals exert their effects by first binding to and activating a cellular receptor. Cellular receptors seem to be proteins located on the cell surface or at specific locations within the cell. The primary role of the receptor is to recognize specific chemicals from the vast number of compounds that are introduced to the cell and to initiate a change in cell function by interacting with a specific agent. Activated receptors mediate a change in function by altering cell permeability or modifying the biochemical function within the cell, or both. The exact mechanism by which a receptor affects cell function depends on the type and location of the receptor.

Drug-receptor interactions are significant pharmacologically because they account for some of the basic pharmacodynamic principles such as drug selectivity and the relationship between drug dose and response. Also, the development of chemical agents that block specific receptors (antagonists) has been useful in moderating the effects of endogenous compounds on specific physiologic processes. Finally, changes in receptor number and sensitivity have been implicated as being important in the altered response seen in certain drugs with prolonged use. Information about the relationship between drugs and cellular receptors has been, and will continue to be, critical to our understanding of how drugs work, as well as to helping researchers develop new compounds.

References

1. Bassett JH, Harvey CB, Williams GR. Mechanisms of thyroid hormone receptor–specific nuclear and extra nuclear actions. *Mol Cell Endocrinol.* 2003;213:1–11.
2. Bourne HR, von Zastrow M. Drug receptors and pharmacodynamics. In: Katzung, BG, ed. *Basic and Clinical Pharmacology.*, 9th ed. New York: Lange Medical Books/McGraw-Hill; 2004.
3. Brink CB, Harvey BH, Bodenstein J, et al. Recent advances in drug action and therapeutics: relevance of novel concepts in G-protein–coupled receptor and signal transduction pharmacology. *Br J Clin Pharmacol.* 2004;57:373–387.
4. Buckbinder L, Robinson RP. The glucocorticoid receptor: molecular mechanism and new therapeutic opportunities. *Curr Drug Targets Inflamm Allergy.* 2002;1:127–136.
5. Bunnelle WH, Dart MJ, Schrimpf MR. Design of ligands for the nicotinic acetylcholine receptors: the quest for selectivity. *Curr Top Med hem.* 2004; 4:299–334.
6. Carlberg C. Current understanding of the function of the nuclear vitamin D receptor in response to its natural and synthetic ligands. *Recent Results Cancer Res.* 2003;164:29–42.
7. Csillik B, Nemcsok J, Chase B, et al. Infraterminal spreading and extrajunctional expression of nicotinic acetylcholine receptors in denervated rat skeletal muscle. *Exp Brain Res.* 1999;125:426–434.
8. El-Armouche A, Zolk O, Rau T, Eschenhagen T. Inhibitory G-proteins and their role in desensitization of the adenylyl cyclase pathway in heart failure. *Cardiovasc Res.* 2003;60:478–487.
9. Elmendorf JS. Fluidity of insulin action. *Mol Biotechnol.* 2004;27:127–138.
10. Farach-Carson MC, Davis PJ. Steroid hormone interactions with target cells: cross talk between membrane and nuclear pathways. *J Pharmacol Exp Ther.* 2003; 307:839–845.

11. Feil R, Lohmann SM, de Jonge H, et al. Cyclic GMP dependent protein kinases and the cardiovascular system: insights from genetically modified mice. *Circ Res.* 2003;93:907–916.

12. Frandsen A, Schousboe A. AMPA receptor–mediated neurotoxicity: role of Ca2 + and desensitization. *Neurochem Res.* 2003;28:1495–1499.

13. Gentilucci L. New trends in the development of opioid peptide analogues as advanced remedies for pain relief. *Curr Top Med Chem.* 2004;4:19–38.

14. Gerfen CR. D1 dopamine receptor supersensitivity in the dopamine depleted striatum animal model of Parkinson's disease. *Neuroscientist.* 2003;9:455–462.

15. Grunder G, Carlsson A, Wong DF. Mechanism of new antipsychotic medications: occupancy is not just antagonism. *Arch Gen Psychiatry.* 2003;60: 974–977.

16. Grutter T, Le Novere N, Changeux JP. Rational understanding of nicotinic receptors drug binding. *Curr Top Med Chem.* 2004;4:645–650.

17. Guse AH. Regulation of calcium signaling by the second messenger cyclic adenosine diphosphoribose (cADPR). *Curr Mol Med.* 2004;4:239–248.

18. Harvey CB, Williams GR. Mechanism of thyroid hormone action. *Thyroid.* 2002;12:441–446.

19. Haskell SG. Selective estrogen receptor modulators. *South Med J.* 2003;96:469–476.

20. Hata JA, Koch WJ. Phosphorylation of G protein–coupled receptors: GPCR kinases in heart disease. *Mol Interv.* 2003;3:264–272.

21. Hawkes C, Kar S. The insulin-like growth factor-II/mannose-6-phosphate receptor: structure, distribution and function in the central nervous system. *Brain Res Brain Res Rev.* 2004;44:117–140.

22. Hubbard SR, Till JH. Protein tyrosine kinase structure and function. *Annu Rev Biochem.* 2000; 69:373–398.

23. Jensen AA, Spalding TA. Allosteric modulation of G-protein coupled receptors. *Eur J Pharm Sci.* 2004; 21:407–420.

24. Kenakin T. Drug efficacy at G protein–coupled receptors. *Annu Rev Pharmacol Toxicol.* 2002;42:349–379.

25. Kenakin T. Principles: receptor theory in pharmacology. *Trends Pharmacol Sci.* 2004;25:186–192.

26. Kowluru A, Morgan NG. GTP-binding proteins in cell survival and demise: the emerging picture in the pancreatic beta-cell. *Biochem Pharmacol.* 2002;63: 1027–1035.

27. Kowluru A. Regulatory roles for small G proteins in the pancreatic beta cell: lessons from models of impaired insulin secretion. *Am J Physiol Endocrinol Metab.* 2003;285:E669–E684.

28. Kuhn M. Structure, regulation, and function of mammalian membrane guanylyl cyclase receptors, with a focus on guanylyl cyclase-A. *Circ Res.* 2003; 93:700–709.

29. Leifert WR, Jahangiri A, McMurchie EJ. Membrane fluidity changes are associated with the antiarrhythmic effects of docosahexaenoic acid in adult rat cardiomyocytes. *J Nutr Biochem.* 2000;11:38–44.

30. Levesque K, Finzi A, Binette J, Cohen EA. Role of CD4 receptor down regulation during HIV-1 infection. *Curr HIV Res.* 2004;2:51–59.

31. Levin ER. Cell localization, physiology, and nongenomic actions of estrogen receptors. *J Appl Physiol.* 2001;91:1860–1867.

32. Lieberman JA. Dopamine partial agonists: a new class of antipsychotic. *CNS Drugs.* 2004;18:251–267.

33. Liu-Chen LY. Agonist-induced regulation and trafficking of kappa opioid receptors. *Life Sci.* 2004;75: 511–536.

34. Macrez N, Mironneau J. Local Ca2 + signals in cellular signalling. *Curr Mol Med.* 2004;4:263–275.

35. Mailliard WS, Diamond I. Recent advances in the neurobiology of alcoholism: the role of adenosine. *Pharmacol Ther.* 2004;101:39–46.

36. May LT, Christopoulos A. Allosteric modulators of G-protein–coupled receptors. *Curr Opin Pharmacol.* 2003;3:551–556.

37. McFeeters RL, Oswald RE. Emerging structural explanations of ionotropic glutamate receptor function. *FASEB J.* 2004;18:428–438.

38. Miyazawa A, Fujiyoshi Y, Unwin N. Structure and gating mechanism of the acetylcholine receptor pore. *Nature.* 2003;423:949–955.

39. Newton AC. Diacylglycerol's affair with protein kinase C turns 25. *Trends Pharmacol Sci.* 2004;25:175–177.

40. Ossovskaya VS, Bunnett NW. Protease-activated receptors: contribution to physiology and disease. *Physiol Rev.* 2004;84:579–621.

41. Petrofski JA, Koch WJ. The beta-adrenergic receptor kinase in heart failure. *J Mol Cell Cardiol.* 2003;35: 1167–1174.

42. Pilz RB, Casteel DE. Regulation of gene expression by cyclic GMP. *Circ Res.* 2003;93:1034–1046.

43. Romano G. The complex biology of the receptor for the insulin-like growth factor-1. *Drug News Perspect.* 2003;16:525–531.

44. Roskoski R Jr. The ErbB/HER receptor protein–tyrosine kinases and cancer. *Biochem Biophys Res Commun.* 2004;319:1–11.

45. Ross EM, Kenakin,TP. Pharmacodynamics: mechanisms of drug action and the relationship between drug concentration and effect. In: Hardman, JG, et al, eds. *The Pharmacological Basis of Therapeutics.* 10th ed. New York: McGraw-Hill; 2001.

46. Rudolph U, Mohler H. Analysis of GABA$_A$ receptor function and dissection of the pharmacology of benzodiazepines and general anesthetics through mouse genetics. *Annu Rev Pharmacol Toxicol.* 2004;44:475–498.

47. Schulz I, Krause E. Inositol 1,4,5-trisphosphate and its co-players in the concert of Ca2 + signalling—new faces in the line up. *Curr Mol Med.* 2004;4:313–322.

48. Shisheva A. Regulating Glut4 vesicle dynamics by phosphoinositide kinases and phosphoinositide phosphatases. *Front Biosci.* 2003;8:s945–946.

49. Sine SM. The nicotinic receptor ligand binding domain. *J Neurobiol.* 2002;53:431–446.

50. Skalhegg BS, Tasken K. Specificity in the cAMP/PKA signaling pathway. Differential expression,

52 SECTION 1 General Principles of Pharmacology

regulation, and subcellular localization of subunits of PKA. *Front Biosci.* 2000;5:D678–D693.

51. Steiger JL, Russek SJ. GABA$_A$ receptors: building the bridge between subunit mRNAs, their promoters, and cognate transcription factors. *Pharmacol Ther.* 2004; 101:259–281.

52. Tan CM, Brady AE, Nickols HH, et al. Membrane trafficking of G protein–coupled receptors. *Annu Rev Pharmacol Toxicol.* 2004;44:559–609.

53. Tasken K, Aandahl EM. Localized effects of cAMP mediated by distinct routes of protein kinase A. *Physiol Rev.* 2004;84:137–167.

54. Toews ML, Prinster SC, Schulte NA. Regulation of alpha-1B adrenergic receptor localization, trafficking, function, and stability. *Life Sci.* 2003;74:379–389.

55. Unwin N. Structure and action of the nicotinic acetylcholine receptor explored by electron microscopy. *FEBS Lett.* 2003;555:91–95.

56. Unwin N, Miyazawa A, Li J, Fujiyoshi Y. Activation of the nicotinic acetylcholine receptor involves a switch in conformation of the alpha subunits. *J Mol Biol.* 2002;319:1165–1176.

57. Watson CS, Gametchu B. Proteins of multiple classes may participate in nongenomic steroid actions. *Exp Biol Med (Maywood).* 2003;228:1272–1281.

58. Woolf PJ, Linderman JJ. Untangling ligand induced activation and desensitization of G-protein–coupled receptors. *Biophys J.* 2003;84:3–13.

59. Yin D, Gavi S, Wang HY, Malbon CC. Probing receptor structure/function with chimeric G-protein–coupled receptors. *Mol Pharmacol.* 2004;65:1323–1332.

60. Yowell CW, Daaka Y. G protein–coupled receptors provide survival signals in prostate cancer. *Clin Prostate Cancer.* 2002;1:177–181.

61. Zhorov BS, Tikhonov DB. Potassium, sodium, calcium and glutamate-gated channels: pore architecture and ligand action. *J Neurochem.* 2004;88:782–799.

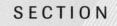

Pharmacology of the Central Nervous System

Chapter 5

General Principles of Central Nervous System Pharmacology

The central nervous system (CNS) is responsible for controlling bodily functions as well as being the center for behavioral and intellectual abilities. Neurons within the CNS are organized into highly complex patterns that mediate information through synaptic interactions. CNS drugs often attempt to modify the activity of these neurons in order to treat specific disorders or to alter the general level of arousal of the CNS. This chapter presents a simplified introduction to the organization of the CNS and the general strategies that can be used with drugs to alter activity within the brain and spinal cord.

CNS Organization

The CNS can be grossly divided into the brain and spinal cord (Fig. 5–1). The brain is subdivided according to anatomic or functional criteria. The following is a brief overview of the general organization of the brain and spinal cord, with some indication of where particular CNS drugs tend to exert their effects. This chapter is not intended to be an extensive review of neuroanatomy—a more elaborate discussion of CNS structure and function can be found in several excellent sources.[25,28,40,41]

Cerebrum

The largest and most rostral aspect of the brain is the *cerebrum* (see Fig. 5–1). The cerebrum consists of bilateral hemispheres, with each hemisphere anatomically divided into several lobes (frontal, temporal, parietal, and occipital). The outer cerebrum, or cerebral cortex, is the highest order of conscious function and integration in the CNS. Specific cortical areas are responsible for sensory and motor functions as well as intellectual and cognitive abilities. Other cortical areas are involved in short-term memory and speech. The cortex also operates in a somewhat supervisory capacity regarding lower brain functioning and may influence the control of other activities such as the autonomic nervous system. With regard to CNS drugs, most therapeutic medications tend to affect cortical function indirectly by first altering the function of lower brain and spinal cord structures. An exception is the group of drugs used to treat epilepsy; these drugs are often targeted directly for hyperexcitable neurons in the cerebral cortex. In addition, drugs that attempt to enhance cognitive function in conditions such as Alzheimer disease (cholinergic stimulants; see Chapter 19) might also exert their primary effects in the cerebrum.

Basal Ganglia

A group of specific areas located deep within the cerebral hemispheres is collectively termed the *basal ganglia*. Components of the basal ganglia include the caudate nucleus, putamen, globus pallidus, lentiform nucleus, and substantia nigra. The basal ganglia are primarily involved in the control of motor activities; deficits in this area are significant in movement disorders such as Parkinson disease and Huntington chorea. Certain medications used to treat these movement disorders exert their effects by interacting with basal ganglia structures.

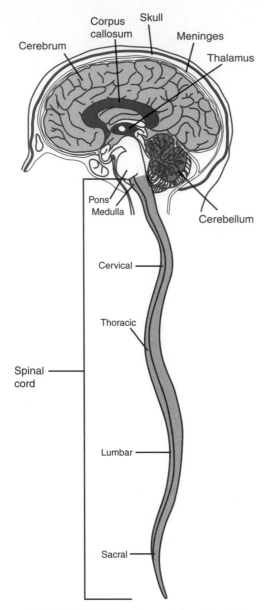

FIGURE 5–1 ▼ General organization of the CNS.

Diencephalon

The area of the brain enclosing the third ventricle is the *diencephalon*. This area consists of several important structures, including the thalamus and hypothalamus. The thalamus contains distinct nuclei that are crucial in the integration of certain types of sensations and their relay to other areas of the brain (such as the somatosensory cortex). The hypothalamus is involved in the control of diverse body functions including temperature control, appetite, water balance, and certain emotional reactions. The hypothalamus is also significant in its control over the function of hormonal release from the pituitary gland. Several CNS drugs affecting sensation and control of the body functions listed, manifest their effects by interacting with the thalamus and hypothalamus.

Mesencephalon and Brainstem

The *mesencephalon*, or *midbrain*, serves as a bridge between the higher areas of the brain (cerebrum and diencephalon) and the *brainstem*. The brainstem consists of the pons and the medulla oblongata. In addition to serving as a pathway between the higher brain and spinal cord, the midbrain and brainstem are the locations of centers responsible for controlling respiration and cardiovascular function (vasomotor center).

The reticular formation is also located in the midbrain and brainstem. The reticular formation is comprised of a collection of neurons that extend from the reticular substance of the upper spinal cord through the midbrain and the thalamus. The reticular formation monitors and controls consciousness and is also important in regulating the amount of arousal or alertness in the cerebral cortex. Consequently, CNS drugs that affect the arousal state of the individual tend to exert their effects on the reticular formation. Sedative-hypnotics and general anesthetics tend to decrease activity in the reticular formation, whereas certain CNS stimulants (caffeine, amphetamines) may increase arousal through a stimulatory effect on reticular formation neurons.

Cerebellum

The *cerebellum* lies posterior to the brainstem and is separated from it by the fourth ventricle. Anatomically it is divided into two hemispheres, each consisting of three lobes (anterior, posterior, and flocculonodular). The function of the cerebellum is to help plan and coordinate motor activity and to assume responsibility for comparing the actual movement with the intended motor pattern. The cerebellum interprets various sensory input and helps modulate motor output so that the actual movement closely resembles the intended motor program. The cerebellum is also concerned with the vestibular mechanisms responsible for maintaining balance and posture. Therapeutic medications are not usually targeted directly for the cerebellum, but incoordination and other movement disorders may result if a drug exerts a toxic side effect on the cerebellum.

Limbic System

So far, all of the structures described have been grouped primarily by their anatomic relationships with the brain. The *limbic system* is comprised of several structures that are dispersed throughout the brain but are often considered as a functional unit or system within the CNS. Major components of the limbic system include cortical structures (such as the amygdala, hippocampus, and cingulate gyrus), the hypothalamus, certain thalamic nuclei, mamillary bodies, septum pellucidum, and several other structures and tracts. These structures are involved in the control of emotional and behavioral activity. Certain aspects of motivation, aggression, sexual activity, and instinctive responses may be influenced by activity within the limbic system. CNS drugs affecting these aspects of behavior, including some antianxiety and antipsychotic medications, are believed to exert their beneficial effects primarily by altering activity in the limbic structures.

Spinal Cord

At the caudal end of the brainstem, the CNS continues distally as the *spinal cord.* The spinal cord is cylindrically shaped and consists of centrally located gray matter that is surrounded by white matter. The gray matter serves as an area for synaptic connections between various neurons. The white matter consists of the myelinated axons of neurons, which are grouped into tracts ascending or descending between the brain and specific levels of the cord. Certain CNS drugs exert some or all of their effects by modifying synaptic transmission in specific areas of gray matter, while other CNS drugs, such as narcotic analgesics, may exert an effect on synaptic transmission in the gray matter of the cord as well as on synapses in other areas of the brain. Some drugs may be specifically directed toward the white matter of the cord. Drugs such as local anesthetics can be used to block action potential propagation in the white matter so that ascending or descending information is interrupted (i.e., a spinal block).

The Blood-Brain Barrier

The *blood-brain barrier* refers to the unique structure and function of CNS capillaries.[15,43] Certain substances are not able to pass from the bloodstream into the CNS, despite the fact that these substances are able to pass from the systemic circulation into other peripheral tissues. This fact suggests the existence of some sort of unique structure and function of the CNS capillaries that prevents many substances from entering the brain and spinal cord—hence, the term **blood-brain barrier**. This barrier effect is caused primarily by the tight junctions that occur between capillary endothelial cells; in fact, CNS capillaries lack the gaps and fenestrations that are seen in peripheral capillaries. Also, nonneuronal cells in the CNS (e.g., astrocytes) and the capillary basement membrane seem to contribute to the relative impermeability of this barrier. Functionally, the blood-brain barrier acts as a selective filter and seems to protect the CNS by limiting the harmful substances that enter into the brain and spinal cord.

The blood-brain barrier obviously plays an important role in clinical pharmacotherapeutics. To exert their effects, drugs targeted for the CNS must be able to pass from the bloodstream into the brain and spinal cord. In general, nonpolar, lipid-soluble drugs are able to cross the blood-brain barrier by passive diffusion.[6,13] Polar and lipophobic compounds are usually unable to enter the brain. Some exceptions occur because of the presence of carrier-mediated transport systems in the blood-brain barrier.[23] Some substances (such as glucose) are transported via facilitated diffusion, while other compounds (including some drugs) may be able to enter the brain by active transport. However, the transport processes that carry drugs into the brain are limited to certain specific compounds, and the typical manner by which most drugs enter the brain is by passive lipid diffusion.[20]

Several active transport systems also exist on the blood-brain barrier that are responsible for *removing* drugs and toxins from the brain.[6,11] That is, certain drugs can enter the brain easily via diffusion or another process, but these drugs are then rapidly and efficiently transported out of the brain and back into the systemic circulation.[6,13] This effect creates an obvious problem because these drugs will not reach therapeutic levels within the CNS, and won't be beneficial. Hence, the blood-brain barrier has many structural and functional characteristics that influence CNS drugs, and researchers continue to explore ways that these characteristics can be modified to ensure adequate drug delivery to the brain and spinal cord.[15,23]

CNS Neurotransmitters

The majority of neural connections in the human brain and spinal cord are characterized as chemical

Table 5–1	CENTRAL NEUROTRANSMITTERS	
Transmitter	**Primary CNS Location**	**General Effect**
Acetylcholine	Cerebral cortex (many areas); basal ganglia; limbic and thalamic regions; spinal interneurons	Excitation
Norepinephrine	Neurons originating in brainstem and hypothalamus that project throughout other areas of brain	Inhibition
Dopamine	Basal ganglia; limbic system	Inhibition
Serotonin	Neurons originating in brainstem that project upward (to hypothalamus) and downward (to spinal cord)	Inhibition
GABA (gamma-aminobutyric acid)	Interneurons throughout the spinal cord, cerebellum, basal ganglia, cerebral cortex	Inhibition
Glycine	Interneurons in spinal cord and brainstem	Inhibition
Glutamate, aspartate	Interneurons throughout brain and spinal cord	Excitation
Substance P	Pathways in spinal cord and brain that mediate painful stimuli	Excitation
Enkephalins	Pain suppression pathways in spinal cord and brain	Excitation

synapses. The term *chemical synapse* indicates that a chemical neurotransmitter is used to propagate the nervous impulse across the gap that exists between two neurons. Several distinct chemicals have been identified as neurotransmitters within the brain and spinal cord (Table 5–1). Groups of neurons within the CNS tend to use one of these neurotransmitters to produce either excitation or inhibition of the other neurons. Although each neurotransmitter can be generally described as either excitatory or inhibitory within the CNS, some transmitters may have different effects depending on the nature of the postsynaptic receptor involved. As discussed in Chapter 4, the interaction of the transmitter and the receptor dictates the effect on the postsynaptic neuron.

The fact that several distinct neurotransmitters exist and that neurons using specific transmitters are organized functionally within the CNS has important pharmacologic implications. Certain drugs may alter the transmission in pathways using a specific neurotransmitter while having little or no effect on other transmitter pathways. This allows the drug to exert a rather specific effect on the CNS, so many disorders may be rectified without radically altering other CNS functions. Other drugs may have a much more general effect and may alter transmission in many CNS regions. To provide an indication of neurotransmitter function, the major categories of CNS neurotransmitters and their general locations and effects are discussed subsequently.

Acetylcholine

Acetylcholine is the neurotransmitter found in many areas of the brain as well as in the periphery (skeletal neuromuscular junction, some autonomic synapses). In the brain, acetylcholine is abundant in the cerebral cortex, and seems to play a critical role in cognition and memory.[22,32] Neurons originating in the large pyramidal cells of the motor cortex and many neurons originating in the basal ganglia also secrete acetylcholine from their terminal axons. In general, acetylcholine synapses in the CNS are excitatory in nature.

Monoamines

Monoamines are a group of structurally similar CNS neurotransmitters that include the **catecholamines** (dopamine, norepinephrine) and 5-hydroxytryptamine (serotonin).[36] **Dopamine** exerts different effects at various locations within the brain.[29,37] Within the basal ganglia, dopamine is secreted by neurons that originate in the substantia nigra and project to the corpus striatum. As such, it is important in regulating motor control, and the loss of these dopaminergic neurons results in symptoms commonly associated with Parkinson disease (see Chapter 10). Dopamine also influences mood and emotions, primarily via its presence in the hypothalamus and other structures within the limbic system. Although its effects within the brain are very complex, dopamine generally inhibits the neurons onto which it is released.

Norepinephrine is secreted by neurons that originate in the locus caeruleus of the pons and projects throughout the reticular formation. Norepinephrine is generally regarded as an inhibitory transmitter within the CNS, but the overall effect following activity of norepinephrine synapses is often general excitation of the brain, probably because norepinephrine directly inhibits other neurons that produce inhibition. This phenomenon of *disinhibition* causes excitation by removing the influence of inhibitory neurons.

Serotonin (also known as 5-hydroxytryptamine) is released by cells originating in the midline of the pons and brainstem and is projected to many different areas, including the dorsal horns of the spinal cord and the hypothalamus. Serotonin is considered to be a strong inhibitor in most areas of the CNS and is believed to be important in mediating the inhibition of painful stimuli. It is also involved in controlling many aspects of mood and behavior, and problems with serotonergic activity have been implicated in several psychiatric disorders, including depression and anxiety.[12,17] The roles of serotonin and the other monoamines in psychiatric disorders are discussed in Chapters 6–8.

Amino Acids

Several amino acids, such as glycine and gamma-aminobutyric acid (GABA), are important inhibitory transmitters in the brain and spinal cord. Glycine seems to be the inhibitory transmitter used by certain interneurons located throughout the spinal cord, and this amino acid also causes inhibition in certain areas of the brain.[4,8] Likewise, GABA is found throughout the CNS, and is believed to be the primary neurotransmitter used to cause inhibition at presynaptic and postsynaptic neurons in the brain and spinal cord.[5,10,26,30] Other amino acids such as aspartate and glutamate have been found in high concentrations throughout the brain and spinal cord; these substances cause excitation of CNS neurons.[2,3,42] These excitatory amino acids have received a great deal of attention lately because they may also produce neurotoxic effects when released in large amounts during CNS injury and certain neurologic disorders (epilepsy, amyotrophic lateral sclerosis, and so forth).[1,2,3,16]

Peptides

Many peptides have already been established as CNS neurotransmitters.[25] One peptide that is important from a pharmacologic standpoint is substance P, which is an excitatory transmitter that is involved in spinal cord pathways transmitting pain impulses.[14,19,38] Increased activity at substance P synapses in the cord serves to mediate the transmission of painful sensations, and certain drugs such as the opioid analgesics may decrease activity at these synapses. Other peptides that have important pharmacologic implications include three families of compounds: the endorphins, enkephalins, and dynorphins.[21] These peptides, also known as the endogenous opioids, are excitatory transmitters in certain brain synapses that inhibit painful sensations. Hence, endogenous opioids in the brain are able to decrease the central perception of pain. The interaction of these compounds with exogenous opioid drugs is discussed in Chapter 14.

Finally, peptides such as galanin, leptin, neuropeptide Y, vasoactive intestinal polypeptide (VIP), and pituitary adenylate cyclase–activating polypeptide (PACAP) have been identified in various areas of the CNS. These and other peptides may affect various CNS functions, either by acting directly as neurotransmitters or by acting as cotransmitters moderating the effects of other neurotransmitters.[7,24,27,34]

Other Transmitters

In addition to the well-known substances, other chemicals are continually being identified as potential CNS neurotransmitters. Recent evidence has implicated substances such as adenosine and adenosine triphosphate (ATP) as transmitters or modulators of neural transmission in specific areas of the brain and in the autonomic nervous system.[31,39] Many other chemicals that are traditionally associated with functions outside the CNS are being identified as possible CNS transmitters, including histamine, nitric oxide, and certain hormones (vasopressin, oxytocin).[9,33] As the function of these chemicals and other new transmitters becomes clearer, the pharmacologic significance of drugs that affect these synapses will undoubtedly be considered.

CNS Drugs: General Mechanisms

The majority of CNS drugs work by modifying synaptic transmission in some way. Figure 5–2 shows a typical chemical synapse that is found in the CNS. Most drugs that attempt to rectify CNS-related disorders do so by either increasing or decreasing transmission at specific synapses. For instance, psychotic behavior has been associated with overactivity in central synapses that use dopamine as a neurotransmitter (see Chapter 8). Drug therapy in this situation consists of agents that decrease activity at central dopamine synapses. Conversely, Parkinson disease results from a decrease in activity at specific dopamine synapses (see Chapter 10). Antiparkinsonian drugs attempt to increase dopaminergic transmission at these synapses and bring synaptic activity back to normal levels.

A drug that modifies synaptic transmission must somehow alter the quantity of the neurotransmitter that is released from the presynaptic terminal or affect the stimulation of postsynaptic receptors, or both. When considering a typical synapse, such as the one shown in Figure 5–2, there are several distinct sites at which a drug may alter activity in the synapse. Specific ways a drug may modify synaptic transmission are presented here.

1. *Presynaptic action potential.* The arrival of an action potential at the presynaptic terminal initiates neurotransmitter release. Certain drugs, such as local anesthetics, block propagation along neural axons so that the action potential fails to reach the presynaptic terminal, which effectively eliminates activity at that particular synapse. Also, the amount of depolarization or the height of the action potential arriving at the presynaptic terminal is directly related to the amount of transmitter released. Any drug or endogenous chemical that limits the amount of depolarization occurring in the presynaptic terminal will inhibit the synapse because less neurotransmitter is released. In certain situations, this is referred to as *presynaptic inhibition*, because the site of this effect is at the presynaptic terminal. The endogenous neurotransmitter GABA is believed to exert some of its inhibitory effects via this mechanism.

2. *Synthesis of neurotransmitter.* Drugs that block the synthesis of neurotransmitter will eventually deplete the presynaptic terminal and impair transmission. For example, metyrosine (Demser)

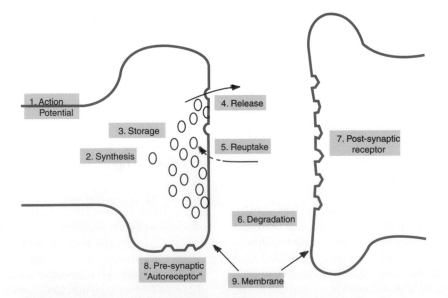

FIGURE 5–2 ▼ Sites at which drugs can alter transmission at a CNS synapse.

inhibits an enzyme that is essential for catecholamine biosynthesis in the presynaptic terminal. Treatment with metyrosine results in decreased synthesis of transmitters such as dopamine and norepinephrine.

3. *Storage of neurotransmitter.* A certain amount of chemical transmitter is stored in presynaptic vesicles. Drugs that impair this storage will decrease the ability of the synapse to continue to transmit information for extended periods. An example of this is the antihypertensive drug reserpine (Serpalan, Serpasil), which impairs the ability of adrenergic terminals to sequester and store norepinephrine in presynaptic vesicles.

4. *Release.* Certain drugs will increase synaptic activity by directly increasing the release of neurotransmitter from the presynaptic terminal. Amphetamines appear to exert their effects on the CNS primarily by increasing the presynaptic release of catecholamine neurotransmitters (e.g., norepinephrine). Conversely, other compounds may inhibit the synapse by directly decreasing the amount of transmitter released during each action potential. An example is botulinum toxin (Botox), which can be used as a skeletal muscle relaxant because of its ability to impair the release of acetylcholine from the skeletal neuromuscular junction (see Chapter 13).

5. *Reuptake.* After the neurotransmitter is released, some chemical synapses terminate activity primarily by transmitter reuptake. Reuptake involves the movement of the transmitter molecule back into the presynaptic terminal. A drug that impairs the reuptake of transmitter allows more of it to remain in the synaptic cleft and continue to exert an effect. Consequently, blocking reuptake actually increases activity at the synapse. For instance, tricyclic antidepressants (see Chapter 7) impair the reuptake mechanism that pumps amine neurotransmitters back into the presynaptic terminal, which allows the transmitter to continue to exert its effect and prolong activity at the synapse.

6. *Degradation.* Some synapses rely primarily on the enzymatic breakdown of the released transmitter to terminate synaptic activity. Inhibition of the enzyme responsible for terminating the transmitter allows more of the active transmitter to remain in the synaptic cleft, thereby increasing activity at the synapse. An example is using a drug that inhibits the **cholinesterase**

enzyme as a method of treating myasthenia gravis. In myasthenia gravis, there is a functional decrease in activity at the skeletal neuromuscular junction. Anticholinesterase drugs such as neostigmine (Prostigmin) and pyridostigmine (Mestinon) inhibit acetylcholine breakdown, allowing more of the released neurotransmitter to continue to exert an effect at the neuromuscular synapse.

7. *Postsynaptic receptor.* As discussed in Chapter 4, chemical antagonists can be used to block the postsynaptic receptor, thus decreasing synaptic transmission. The best-known example of this is the use of beta blockers. These agents are antagonists that are specific for the beta-adrenergic receptors on the myocardium, and they are frequently used to treat hypertension, cardiac arrhythmias, and angina pectoris. Other drugs may improve synaptic transmission by affecting the receptor directly so there is a tendency for increased neurotransmitter binding or improved receptor–effector coupling, or both. For instance, benzodiazepines (e.g., diazepam [Valium], chlordiazepoxide [Librium, others]) appear to enhance the postsynaptic effects of the inhibitory neurotransmitter GABA.

8. *Presynaptic autoreceptors.* In addition to postsynaptic receptors, there are also receptors on the presynaptic terminal of some types of chemical synapses. These presynaptic receptors seem to serve as a method of negative feedback in controlling neurotransmitter release.[18,35] During high levels of synaptic activity, the accumulation of neurotransmitter in the synaptic cleft may allow binding to the presynaptic receptors and limit further release of chemical transmitter. Certain drugs may also be able to attenuate synaptic activity through presynaptic autoreceptors. For instance, clonidine (Catapres), may exert some of its antihypertensive effects by binding to presynaptic receptors on sympathetic postganglionic neurons and impairing the release of norepinephrine onto the peripheral vasculature. The use of drugs that alter synaptic activity by binding to these autoreceptors is still somewhat new, however, and the full potential for this area of pharmacology remains to be determined.

9. *Membrane effects.* Drugs may alter synaptic transmission by affecting membrane organization and fluidity. Membrane fluidity is basically

the amount of flexibility or mobility of the lipid bilayer. Drugs that alter the fluidity of the presynaptic membrane could affect the way that presynaptic vesicles fuse with and release their neurotransmitter. Drug-induced changes in the postsynaptic membrane would affect the receptor environment and thereby alter receptor function. Membrane modification will result in either increased or decreased synaptic transmission, depending on the drug in question and the type and magnitude of membrane change. Alcohol (ethanol) and general anesthetics were originally thought to exert their effects by producing reversible changes in the fluidity and organization of the cell membranes of central neurons. Although this idea has been challenged somewhat, these drugs may still exert some of their effects via neuronal membranes.

A CNS drug does not have to adhere specifically to only one of these methods of synaptic modification. Some drugs may affect the synapse in two or more ways. For example, the antihypertensive agent guanethidine (Ismelin) impairs both presynaptic storage and release of norepinephrine. Other drugs such as barbiturates may affect both the presynaptic terminal and the postsynaptic receptor in CNS synapses.

SUMMARY

Drugs affecting the brain and spinal cord usually exert their effects by somehow modifying synaptic transmission. In some instances, drugs may be targeted for specific synapses in an attempt to rectify some problem with transmission at that particular synapse. Other drugs may increase or decrease the excitability of CNS neurons in an attempt to have a more general effect on the overall level of consciousness of the individual. Specific categories of CNS drugs and their pharmacodynamic mechanisms are discussed in succeeding chapters.

References

1. Aarts MM, Tymianski M. Novel treatment of excitotoxicity: targeted disruption of intracellular signaling from glutamate receptors. *Biochem Pharmacol.* 2003;66:877–886.
2. Arundine M, Tymianski M. Molecular mechanisms of calcium-dependent neurodegeneration in excitotoxicity. *Cell Calcium.* 2003;34:325–337.
3. Arundine M, Tymianski M. Molecular mechanisms of glutamate-dependent neurodegeneration in ischemia and traumatic brain injury. *Cell Mol Life Sci.* 2004; 61:657–668.
4. Awatramani GB, Turecek R, Trussell LO. Inhibitory control at a synaptic relay. *J Neurosci.* 2004;24: 2643–2647.
5. Barral J, Toro S, Galarraga E, Bargas J. GABAergic presynaptic inhibition of rat neostriatal afferents is mediated by Q-type Ca(2+) channels. *Neurosci Lett.* 2000;283:33–36.
6. Begley DJ. ABC transporters and the blood-brain barrier. *Curr Pharm Des.* 2004;10:1295–1312.
7. Bjorbaek C, Kahn BB. Leptin signaling in the central nervous system and the periphery. *Recent Prog Horm Res.* 2004;59:305–331.
8. Breustedt J, Schmitz D, Heinemann U, Schmieden V. Characterization of the inhibitory glycine receptor on entorhinal cortex neurons. *Eur J Neurosci.* 2004; 19:1987–1991.
9. Cherian L, Hlatky R, Robertson CS. Nitric oxide in traumatic brain injury. *Brain Pathol.* 2004;14:195–201.
10. Ciranna L, Licata F, Li Volsi G, Santangelo F. Role of GABA A and GABA B receptors in GABA-induced inhibition of rat red nucleus neurons. *Neurosci Lett.* 2003;341:221–224.
11. de Boer AG, van der Sandt IC, Gaillard PJ. The role of drug transporters at the blood-brain barrier. *Annu Rev Pharmacol Toxicol.* 2003;43:629–656.
12. Elhwuegi AS. Central monoamines and their role in major depression. *Prog Neuropsychopharmacol Biol Psychiatry.* 2004;28:435–451.
13. Elsinga PH, Hendrikse NH, Bart J, Vaalburg W, van Waarde A. PET Studies on P-glycoprotein function in the blood-brain barrier: how it affects uptake and binding of drugs within the CNS. *Curr Pharm Des.* 2004;10:1493–1503.
14. Fras C, Kravetz P, Mody DR, Heggeness MH. Substance P-containing nerves within the human vertebral body. An immunohistochemical study of the basivertebral nerve. *Spine J.* 2003;3:63–67.
15. Fricker G, Miller DS. Modulation of drug transporters at the blood-brain barrier. *Pharmacology.* 2004;70: 169–176.
16. Gillessen T, Budd SL, Lipton SA. Excitatory amino acid neurotoxicity. *Adv Exp Med Biol.* 2002;513: 3–40.
17. Gingrich JA, Ansorge MS, Merker R, Weisstaub N, Zhou M. New lessons from knockout mice: the role of serotonin during development and its possible contribution to the origins of neuropsychiatric disorders. *CNS Spectr.* 2003;8:572–577.
18. Gothert M. Modulation of noradrenaline release in human cardiovascular tissues. *Pharmacol Toxicol.* 2003;92:156–159.
19. Guo TZ, Offley SC, Boyd EA, Jacobs CR, Kingery WS. Substance P signaling contributes to the vascular

and nociceptive abnormalities observed in a tibial fracture rat model of complex regional pain syndrome type I. *Pain.* 2004;108:95–107.

20. Habgood MD, Begley DJ, Abbott NJ. Determinants of passive drug entry into the central nervous system. *Cell Mol Neurobiol.* 2000;20:231–253.

21. Janecka A, Fichna J, Janecki T. Opioid receptors and their ligands. *Curr Top Med Chem.* 2004;4:1–17.

22. Jones BE. Activity, modulation and role of basal forebrain cholinergic neurons innervating the cerebral cortex. *Prog Brain Res.* 2004;145:157–169.

23. Kabanov AV, Batrakova EV. New technologies for drug delivery across the blood brain barrier. *Curr Pharm Des.* 2004;10:1355–1363.

24. Kalra SP, Kalra PS. Neuropeptide Y. A physiological orexigen modulated by the feedback action of ghrelin and leptin. *Endocrine.* 2003;22:49–56.

25. Kandel ER, Schwartz JH, Jessell TM. *Principles of Neural Science.* 4th ed. New York: McGraw-Hill; 2000.

26. Ma CL, Kelly JB, Wu SH. Presynaptic modulation of GABAergic inhibition by GABA(B) receptors in the rat's inferior colliculus. *Neuroscience.* 2002;114:207–215.

27. Morilak DA, Cecchi M, Khoshbouei H. Interactions of norepinephrine and galanin in the central amygdala and lateral bed nucleus of the stria terminalis modulate the behavioral response to acute stress. *Life Sci.* 2003;73:715–726.

28. Nicholls JG, Martin AR, Wallace BG, Fuchs PA. *From Neuron to Brain.* 4th ed. Sunderland, MA: Sinauer Associates; 2001.

29. Nieoullon A, Coquerel A. Dopamine: a key regulator to adapt action, emotion, motivation and cognition. *Curr Opin Neurol.* 2003;(suppl 2):S3–S9.

30. Parnas I, Rashkovan G, Ravin R, Fischer Y. Novel mechanism for presynaptic inhibition: GABA(A) receptors affect the release machinery. *J Neurophysiol.* 2000;84:1240–1246.

31. Pearson T, Currie AJ, Etherington LA, et al. Plasticity of purine release during cerebral ischemia: clinical implications? *J Cell Mol Med.* 2003;7:362–375.

32. Pepeu G, Giovannini MG. Changes in acetylcholine extracellular levels during cognitive processes. *Learn Mem.* 2004;11:21–27.

33. Philippu A, Prast H. Importance of histamine in modulatory processes, locomotion and memory. *Behav Brain Res.* 2001;124:151–159.

34. Pozo D. VIP- and PACAP-mediated immunomodulation as prospective therapeutic tools. *Trends Mol Med.* 2003;9:211–217.

35. Raiteri M. Presynaptic autoreceptors. *J Neurochem.* 2001;78:673–675.

36. Schweighofer N, Doya K, Kuroda S. Cerebellar aminergic neuromodulation: towards a functional understanding. *Brain Res Brain Res Rev.* 2004; 44:103–116.

37. Smidt MP, Smits SM, Burbach JP. Molecular mechanisms underlying midbrain dopamine neuro development and function. *Eur J Pharmacol.* 2003; 480:75–88.

38. Vachon P, Masse R, Gibbs BF. Substance P and neurotensin are up regulated in the lumbar spinal cord of animals with neuropathic pain. *Can J Vet Res.* 2004; 68:86–92.

39. Volonte C, Amadio S, Cavaliere F, D'Ambrosi N, Vacca F, Bernardi G. Extracellular ATP and neurodegeneration. *Curr Drug Targets CNS Neurol Disord.* 2003;2:403–412.

40. Waxman SG. *Clinical Neuroanatomy.* 25th ed. New York: McGraw-Hill; 2003.

41. Webster RA , ed. *Neurotransmitters, Drugs, and Brain Function.* New York: John Wiley and Sons; 2001.

42. Willis C, Lybrand S, Bellamy N. Excitatory amino acid inhibitors for traumatic brain injury. *Cochrane Database Syst Rev.* 2004;CD003986.

43. Wolburg H, Lippoldt A. Tight junctions of the blood-brain barrier: development, composition and regulation. *Vascul Pharmacol.* 2002;38:323–337.

Chapter 6

Sedative-Hypnotic and Antianxiety Agents

Drugs that are classified as sedative-hypnotics are used both to relax the patient and to promote sleep.[59] As the name "sedative" implies, these drugs exert a calming effect and serve to pacify the patient. At higher doses, the same drug can produce drowsiness and initiate a relatively normal state of sleep (hypnosis). At still higher doses, some sedative-hypnotics (especially barbiturates) will eventually bring on a state of general anesthesia. Because of their general central nervous system (CNS)-depressant effects, some sedative-hypnotic drugs are also used for other functions such as treating epilepsy or producing muscle relaxation. However, the sleep-enhancing effects will be of concern in this chapter.

By producing sedation, many drugs will also decrease the level of anxiety in a patient. Of course, these anxiolytic properties often cause a decrease in the level of alertness in the individual. However, certain agents are available that can reduce anxiety without an overt sedative effect. Those medications that selectively produce antianxiety effects are discussed later in this chapter.

Sedative-hypnotic and antianxiety drugs are among the most commonly used drugs worldwide. For example, it is estimated that insomnia affects between 10 to 15 percent of the general population, and that pharmacological management can be helpful in promoting normal sleep.[18,42] Moreover, people who are ill, or who have recently been relocated to a new environment (hospital, nursing home), will often have difficulty sleeping and might need some form of sedative-hypnotic agent.[8,35,41] Likewise, a person who sustains an injury or illness will certainly have some apprehension concerning his or her welfare.[33] If necessary, this apprehension can be controlled to some extent by using antianxiety drugs during the course of rehabilitation. Consequently, many patients receiving physical therapy and occupational therapy take sedative-hypnotic and antianxiety agents to help promote sleep and decrease anxiety; rehabilitation specialists should understand the basic pharmacology of these agents.

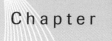 Sedative-Hypnotic Agents

Sedative-hypnotics fall into two general categories: benzodiazepines and nonbenzodiazepines (Table 6–1). At present, benzodiazepines are typically used to promote normal sedation and sleep, especially in relatively acute or short-term situations. These agents will be addressed first, followed by a description of the nonbenzodiazepine hypnotics.

Benzodiazepines

Benzodiazepines are a family of compounds that share the same basic chemical structure and pharmacological effects. Although the more famous members of this family are associated with treating anxiety (e.g., diazepam [Valium]; see later in this chapter), several benzodiazepines are indicated specifically to promote sleep (Table 6–1). These agents exert hypnotic effects similar to those of nonbenzodiazepines—such as the barbiturates—but benzodiazepines are generally regarded as safer because there is less of a chance for lethal overdose.[22] Benzodiazepines, however, are not without their drawbacks, and they can cause resid-

Table 6–1	COMMON SEDATIVE-HYPNOTIC DRUGS			

Oral Adult Dose (mg)

Generic Name	Trade Name	Sedative	Hypnotic*
Barbiturates			
Amobarbital	Amytal	25–100 BID or TID	65–200
Aprobarbital	Alurate	40 TID	40–160
Butabarbital	Busodium, Butisol, others	15–30 TID or QID	50–100
Pentobarbital	Nembutal	20 TID or QID	100
Phenobarbital	Solfoton	15–40 BID or TID	100–320
Secobarbital	Seconal	30–50 TID or QID	100
Benzodiazepines**			
Estazolam	ProSom	——	1–2
Flurazepam	Dalmane	——	15–30
Quazepam	Doral	——	7.5–15
Temazepam	Restoril	——	7.5–30
Triazolam	Halcion	——	0.125–0.25
Others			
Chloral hydrate	Noctec	250 TID	500–1000
Ethchlorvynol	Placidyl	——	500–1000
Glutethimide	(generic)	——	250–500
Promethazine	Phenergan, others	——	25–50
Zaleplon	Sonata	——	10
Zolpidem	Ambien	——	10

*Hypnotic doses are typically administered as a single dose at bedtime.
**Benzodiazepines listed here are indicated specifically as hypnotic agents and are not approved for other uses (antianxiety, anticonvulsant, and so forth). Virtually all benzodiazepines have sedative-hypnotic effects, and other benzodiazepines may be administered to produce sedation or sleep, depending on the dosage and the patient.

ual effects the day after they are administered; prolonged use can also cause tolerance and physical dependence (see "Problems and Adverse Effects," later in this chapter).[39,60]

Mechanism of Benzodiazepine Effects

The benzodiazepines exert their effects by increasing the inhibitory effects at CNS synapses that use the neurotransmitter gamma-aminobutyric acid (GABA).[48,49] These inhibitory synapses are associated with a membrane protein complex containing three primary components: (1) a binding site for GABA, (2) a binding site for benzodiazepines, and (3) an ion channel that is specific for chloride ions (Fig. 6–1).[48,55] GABA typically exerts its inhibitory effects by binding to its receptor site on this complex and by initiating an increase in chloride conductance through the channel. Increased chloride conductance facilitates chloride entry into the neuron and results in hyperpolarization, or a decreased ability to raise the neuron to its firing threshold. By binding to their own respective site on the complex, benzodiazepines potentiate the effects of GABA and increase the inhibition at these synapses.

Consequently, the presence of the GABA-benzodiazepine–chloride ion channel complex accounts for the specific mechanism of action of this class of sedative-hypnotics. By increasing the inhibitory effects at GABAergic synapses located in the reticular formation, benzodiazepines can decrease the level of arousal in the individual. In other words, the general excitation level in the reticular activating system decreases, and relaxation and sleep are enhanced.

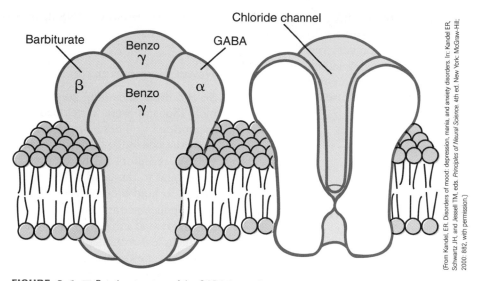

FIGURE 6–1 ▼ Putative structure of the GABA-benzodiazepine-chloride ion channel complex. The centrally located chloride ion channel is modulated by the binding of GABA to the alpha subunit of the receptor. The binding and effects of GABA are enhanced by the binding of benzodiazepines to the gamma subunits or barbiturates to the beta subunit.

(From Kandel, ER, Schwartz JH, and Jessell TM, eds. *Principles of Neural Science.* 4th ed. New York: McGraw-Hill; 2000: 882, with permission.)

Research has also indicated that there are at least three primary types of GABA receptors, and these receptors are classified as GABA A, B, and C according to their structural and functional characteristics.[5,28,49] $GABA_A$ and $GABA_C$ receptors, for example, cause inhibition by increasing chloride entry, whereas $GABA_B$ receptors may cause inhibition by increasing potassium *exit* (efflux) from CNS neurons.[14] At the present time, it appears that benzodiazepines act primarily on the $GABA_A$ subtype and that the therapeutic effects of these drugs (sedation, hypnosis, decreased anxiety) are mediated through the $GABA_A$ receptor, which is found in the brain.[3,48,49] Hence, clinically used benzodiazepines are basically $GABA_A$ receptor agonists.

Furthermore, the $GABA_A$ receptor is composed of several subunits (alpha, beta, gamma); it appears that individual subunits on this receptor mediate specific effects.[3,11] Sedation, for example, seems to be mediated by the alpha 1 subunit, whereas other beneficial effects such as decreased anxiety might be mediated by the alpha 2 and alpha 3 subunits. Benzodiazepines seem to affect all of these subunits, hence their ability to produce sedative and antianxiety effects.[3]

These drugs, however, might also exert certain side effects (tolerance, dependence) by affecting other subunits on the $GABA_A$ receptor. A drug that is selective for only the alpha 1 subunit might exert sedative effects without producing as many side effects. Some of the newer nonbenzodiazepine drugs such as zolpidem (Ambien) and zaleplon (Sonata) appear to be more specific for the alpha 1 subunit, and might therefore produce sedative effects with fewer side effects.[51] These newer drugs are addressed later in this chapter.

Because of these new advances, scientists continue to study the molecular biology of the $GABA_A$ receptor, and clarify how benzodiazepines affect these receptors. Likewise, differences between the principal GABA receptors (A, B, C) has encouraged the development of drugs that are more selective to GABA receptors located in certain areas of the CNS. The muscle relaxant baclofen (Lioresal), for example, may be somewhat more selective for $GABA_B$ receptors in the spinal cord than for other $GABA_A$ or $GABA_C$ receptors that are found in the brain (see Chapter 13). Future drug development will continue to exploit the differences between the GABA receptor subtypes so that drugs are more selective and can produce more specific beneficial effects with fewer side effects.

Finally, the discovery of a CNS receptor that is specific for benzodiazepines has led to some interesting speculation as to the possible existence of some type of endogenous sedative-like agent. The presence of a certain type of receptor to indicate that the body produces an appropriate agonist for that receptor makes sense. For instance, the discovery of opiate receptors initiated the search for endogenous opiate-like substances, which culminated in the discovery of the enkephalins. It has been surmised that certain endogenous steroids such as allopregnanolone (a metabolic byproduct of progesterone) can bind to the GABA receptors in the CNS and produce sedative-hypnotic effects. Continued research in this area may someday reveal the exact role of steroids and other endogenous substances, and the focus of pharmacologic treatment can then be directed toward stimulating the release of endogenous sedative-hypnotic agents

Nonbenzodiazepines

Barbiturates

The barbiturates are a group of CNS depressants that share a common chemical origin: barbituric acid. The potent sedative-hypnotic properties of these drugs have been recognized for some time, and their status as the premier medication used to promote sleep went unchallenged for many years. However, barbiturates are associated with a relatively small therapeutic index; approximately 10 times the therapeutic dose can often be fatal. These drugs are also very addictive, and their prolonged use is often a problem in terms of drug abuse. Consequently, the lack of safety of the barbiturates and their strong potential for addiction and abuse necessitated the development of alternative nonbarbiturate drugs such as the benzodiazepines. Still, some barbiturates are occasionally used for their **hypnotic** properties; these drugs are listed in Table 6–1.

Despite their extensive use in the past, the exact mechanism of the barbiturates remains somewhat unclear. When used in sedative-hypnotic doses, barbiturates may function in a similar fashion to the benzodiazepines in that they also potentiate the inhibitory effects of GABA.[21] This idea suggests that barbiturates may affect the GABA-benzodiazepine–chloride ion channel complex described above.[21] Indeed, considerable evidence exists that barbiturates bind directly to the $GABA_A$ receptor at a site that is different from the binding site for GABA or benzodiazepines (see Fig. 6–1).[21] Barbiturates may, however, also exert effects that are not mediated through an effect on the GABA-benzodiazepine–chloride ion channel. At higher doses, for instance, barbiturates may also directly increase the release of inhibitory transmitters such as glycine, and increase the release of excitatory transmitters such as glutamate.[21,30] Regardless of their exact mechanism, barbiturates are effective sedative-hypnotics because of their specificity for neurons in the midbrain portion of the reticular formation as well as some limbic system structures. At higher doses, barbiturates also depress neuronal excitability in other areas of the brain and spinal cord. Their role in producing general anesthesia

by this more extensive CNS depression is discussed in Chapter 11.

Newer, Nonbenzodiazepine Sedative-Hypnotics

Several drugs including zolpidem (Ambien) and zaleplon (Sonata) were developed recently as sedative-hypnotics.[19,25] These drugs are chemically different from the benzodiazepines, but still seem to affect the $GABA_A$ receptors in the brain. That is, these newer drugs bind to the $GABA_A$ receptor, which then causes GABA to bind more effectively, thus increasing chloride conductance and the level of inhibition in the neuron. Increased inhibition in certain areas of the brain results in less arousal and the promotion of sleep.

These newer drugs appear to be as effective as the benzodiazepines in promoting sleep. The drugs also seem to have a lower risk of producing certain side effects and causing problems when discontinued (see "Problems and Adverse Effects," below).[20,25,62] This difference might be explained by the fact that newer, nonbenzodiazepine drugs bind preferentially to the alpha 1 subunit of the $GABA_A$ receptor.[19,51,52] As discussed earlier, stimulation of this particular subunit seems to mediate sedation without producing other side effects. Hence, drugs like zolpidem and zaleplon are gaining acceptance for the treatment of sleep disorders, and efforts continue to develop other nonbenzodiazepine drugs that selectively affect this receptor.

Other Nonbenzodiazepines

Several other nonbenzodiazepine compounds can be prescribed for their sedative-hypnotic properties (see Table 6–1). These compounds are chemically dissimilar from one another, but share the ability to promote relaxation and sleep via depressing the CNS. Cyclic ethers and alcohols (including ethanol) can be included in this category, but their use specifically as sedative-hypnotics is fairly limited at present. The recreational use of ethanol in alcoholic beverages is an important topic in terms of abuse and long-term effects. However, since this area is much too extensive to be addressed here, only their effects as sedative-hypnotics is considered.

Alcohol (ethanol) and other sedative-hypnotics—neither benzodiazepine nor barbiturate in nature—work through mechanisms that are poorly understood. In the past, it was thought that alcohols exerted their CNS-depressant effects directly on neuronal membrane composition and fluidity. These and other highly lipid-soluble substances could simply dissolve in the lipid bilayer and inhibit neuronal excitability by temporarily disrupting membrane structures in the presynaptic and postsynaptic regions of CNS neurons.[17] Recent evidence, however, suggests that alcohol may act on protein receptors much in the same way as the benzodiazepines and barbiturates. That is, alcohol may exert most of its effects by activating GABA$_A$ receptors and increasing GABA-mediated inhibition in the CNS.[17,31] In any event, alcohol and similar agents bring about a decrease in neuronal transmission, which causes fairly widespread CNS depression which accounts for the subsequent sedative effects of such compounds.

Pharmacokinetics

Benzodiazepine and nonbenzodiazepine sedative-hypnotics are usually highly lipid soluble. They are typically administered orally and are absorbed easily and completely from the gastrointestinal tract. Distribution is fairly uniform throughout the body, and these drugs reach the CNS readily because of their high degree of lipid solubility. Sedative-hypnotics are metabolized primarily by the oxidative enzymes of the drug-metabolizing system in liver cells. Termination of their activity is accomplished either by hepatic enzymes or by storage of these drugs in non-CNS tissues; that is, by sequestering the drugs in adipose and other peripheral tissues, their CNS-depressant effects are not exhibited. However, when the drugs slowly leak out of their peripheral storage sites, they can be redistributed to the brain and can cause low levels of sedation. This occurrence may help explain the "hangoverlike" feelings that are frequently reported the day after taking sedative-hypnotic drugs. Finally, excretion of these drugs takes place through the kidney after their metabolism in the liver. As with most drug biotransformations, metabolism of sedative-hypnotics is essential in creating a polar metabolite that is readily excreted by the kidney.

Problems and Adverse Effects

Residual Effects

The primary problem associated with sedative-hypnotic use is the residual effects that can occur the day after administration. Individuals who take a sedative-hypnotic to sleep at night sometimes complain of drowsiness and decreased motor perf day.[39,60,62] These hangoverlike effe by the drug being redistributed to peripheral storage sites or may simply occu the drug has not been fully metabolized.

Anterograde amnesia is another problem sometimes associated with sedative-hypnotic use.[39] The patient may have trouble recalling details of events that occurred for a certain period of time before the drug was taken. Although usually a minor problem, this can become serious if the drug-induced amnesia exacerbates an already existing memory problem, as might occur in some elderly patients.

These residual problems can be resolved somewhat by taking a smaller dose or by using a drug with a shorter half-life (see Table 6–2).[60,63] Also, newer nonbenzodiazepine agents such as zolpidem and zaleplon appear to have milder effects, perhaps because of their relatively short half-life and the limited duration of action.[32,58] These newer drugs have therefore been advocated in people who are prone to residual effects (e.g., older adults), and people who need to use these drugs for an extended period of time.

Tolerance and Physical Dependence

Another potential problem with long-term sedative-hypnotic drug use is that prolonged administration may cause tolerance and physical dependence. *Drug tolerance* is the need to take more of a drug to exert the same effect. *Dependence* is described as the onset of withdrawal symptoms if drug administration is ceased. Although these problems were originally thought to be limited to barbiturates, benzodiazepines and other sedative-hypnotics are now recognized as also causing tolerance and dependence when taken continually for several weeks.[36]

The manner and severity of withdrawal symptoms varies according to the type of drug and the extent of physical dependence.[50] Withdrawal after short-term benzodiazepine use may be associated with problems such as sleep disturbances (i.e., so-called rebound insomnia).[34,62] As discussed earlier, withdrawal effects seem to be milder with the newer nonbenzodiazepine agents (zolpidem and zaleplon).[34,62] Newer agents, however, are not devoid of these problems and care should be taken with prolonged use, especially in people with psychiatric disorders or a history of substance abuse.[26]

Consequently, the long-term use of these drugs should be avoided, and other nonpharmacologic meth-

| Table 6–2 | PHARMACOKINETIC PROPERTIES OF BENZODIAZEPINE SEDATIVE-HYPNOTICS | | |

Drug	Time to Peak Plasma Concentration (hr)*	Relative Half-Life	Comments
Estazolam (ProSom)	2.0	Intermediate	Rapid oral absorption
Flurazepam (Dalmane)	0.5–1.0	Long	Long elimination half-life because of active metabolites
Quazepam (Doral)	2.0	Long	Daytime drowsiness more likely than with other benzodiazepines
Temazepam (Restoril)	1–2	Short-intermediate	Slow oral absorption
Triazolam (Halcion)	Within 2	Short	Rapid oral absorption

*Adult oral hypnotic dose.

ods of reducing stress and promoting relaxation (e.g., mental imagery, biofeedback) should be instituted before tolerance and physical dependence.[40,56] If the sedative-hypnotic drug has been used for an extended period, tapering off the dosage rather than abruptly stopping it has been recommended as a safer way to terminate administration.[25]

Other Side Effects

Other *side effects* such as gastrointestinal discomfort (nausea and vomiting), dry mouth, sore throat, and muscular incoordination have been reported, but these occur fairly infrequently and vary according to the exact drug used. Cardiovascular and respiratory depression may also occur, but these problems are dose-related and are usually not significant, except in cases of overdose.

Antianxiety Drugs

Anxiety can be described as a fear or apprehension over a situation or event that an individual feels is threatening. These events can range from a change in employment or family life to somewhat irrational phobias concerning everyday occurrences. Anxiety disorders can also be classified in several clinical categories including generalized anxiety disorder, social anxiety disorder, panic disorder, obsessive-compulsive disorder, and posttraumatic stress syndrome.[54] Antianxiety drugs can help decrease the tension and nervousness

associated with many of these syndromes until the situation is resolved or until the individual is counseled effectively in other methods of dealing with his or her anxiety.

Many drugs—including sedative-hypnotics—have the ability to decrease anxiety levels, but this is usually at the expense of an increase in sedation. Frequently, alleviating anxiety without producing excessive sedation is desirable so that the individual can function at home, on the job, and so on. Consequently, certain drugs are available that have significant anxiolytic properties at doses that produce minimal sedation. Benzodiazepine drugs and other nonbenzodiazepine strategies for dealing with anxiety are discussed here.

Benzodiazepines

As discussed previously, because of their relative safety, the benzodiazepines are typically the front-line drugs used to treat many forms of anxiety.[13,16] In terms of anxiolytic properties, diazepam (Valium) is the prototypical antianxiety benzodiazepine (Fig. 6–2). The extensive use of this drug in treating nervousness and apprehension has made the trade name of this compound virtually synonymous with a decrease in tension and anxiety. When prescribed in anxiolytic dosages, diazepam and certain other benzodiazepines (Table 6–3) will decrease anxiety without major sedative effects. Some sedation, however, may occur even at anxiolytic dosages; these drugs can be used as sedative-hypnotics simply by increasing the dosage.

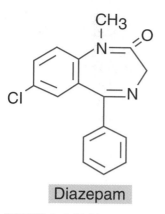

Diazepam

FIGURE 6–2 ▼ Diazepam (Valium).

The mechanism of action of the benzodiazepines was discussed previously in this chapter. The antianxiety properties of these drugs involve a mechanism similar or identical to their sedative-hypnotic effects (i.e., potentiating GABAergic transmission).[37] Benzodiazepines also seem to increase inhibition in the spinal cord, which produces some degree of skeletal muscle relaxation, which may contribute to their antianxiety effects by making the individual feel more relaxed. The use of these drugs as skeletal muscle relaxants is further discussed in Chapter 13.

Buspirone

Buspirone (BuSpar) is an antianxiety agent that was approved in 1986 for treating general anxiety disorder.[2] This agent is not a benzodiazepine. It belongs instead to a drug class known as the azapirones.[2] Therefore, buspirone does not act on the GABA receptor, but exerts its antianxiety effects by increasing the effects of 5-hydroxytryptamine (serotonin) in certain areas of the brain.[12] Buspirone is basically a serotonin agonist that stimulates certain serotonin receptors, especially the 5-HT1A serotonin receptor subtype.[6,10] This increase in serotonergic influence is beneficial in treating general anxiety disorder and possibly in panic disorder, obsessive-compulsive disorder, posttraumatic stress syndrome, and various other disorders that are influenced by CNS serotonin levels.[7]

More importantly, buspirone has a much better side-effect profile than traditional antianxiety drugs. Buspirone seems to produce less sedation and psychomotor impairment than benzodiazepine agents.[2] There is a much smaller risk of developing tolerance and dependence to buspirone and the potential for abuse is much lower than with other anxiolytics.[57] Buspirone has only moderate efficacy, however, and this drug may not take effect as quickly in patients with severe anxiety.[57] Nonetheless, buspirone offers a

Table **6–3**	BENZODIAZEPINE ANTIANXIETY DRUGS		
Generic Name	**Trade Name**	**Antianxiety Dose (mg)***	**Relative Half-Life**
Alprazolam	Xanax	0.25–0.5 TID	Short–intermediate
Chlordiazepoxide	Librium, others	5–25 TID or QID	Long
Clonazepam	Klonopin	0.25–0.50 BID	Intermediate
Clorazepate	Tranxene, others	7.5–15 BID to QID	Long
Diazepam	Valium, others	2–10 BID to QID	Long
Halazepam	Paxipam	20–40 TID or QID	Long
Lorazepam	Ativan	1–3 BID or TID	Short–intermediate
Oxazepam	Serax	10–30 TID or QID	Short–intermediate

*Dose refers to initial adult oral dose. Dosage is adjusted depending on the patient's response. Doses are likewise often lower in elderly or debilitated patients.

safer alternative to traditional antianxiety drugs such as benzodiazepines, especially if patients need to receive treatment for an extended period of time. Development of additional azapirones and other drugs that influence serotonin activity may continue to provide better and safer antianxiety agents in the future.

Use of Antidepressants in Anxiety

Many patients with anxiety also have symptoms of depression.[47] It therefore seems reasonable to include antidepressant drugs as part of the pharmacological regimen in these patients. Hence, patients with a combination of anxiety and depression often take a traditional antianxiety agent such as a benzodiazepine along with an antidepressant.[44] The pharmacology of the antidepressants is addressed in Chapter 7.

Antidepressant drugs, however, might have direct anxiolytic effects. That is, certain antidepressants such as paroxetine (Paxil) or venlafaxine (Effexor) can help reduce anxiety independent of their effects on depression.[1,47] These antidepressants have therefore been advocated as an alternative treatment for anxiety, especially for people who cannot tolerate the side effects of traditional anxiolytics, or who might be especially susceptible to the addictive properties of drugs like the benzodiazepines.[1,9,46] Moreover, antidepressants such as paroxetine or venlafaxine are now considered effective as the primary treatment for several forms of anxiety, including generalized anxiety disorder, social phobia, and panic disorder.[4,29,53] Antidepressants, either used alone or in combination with antianxiety drugs, have become an important component in the treatment of anxiety.

Other Antianxiety Drugs

The ideal antianxiety agent is nonaddictive, safe (i.e., relatively free from harmful side effects and potential for lethal overdose), and not associated with any sedative properties. Drugs such as meprobamate (Miltown) and barbiturates are not currently used to any great extent because they do not meet any of these criteria and are no more effective in reducing anxiety than benzodiazepines. As indicated earlier, buspirone and certain antidepressants currently offer an effective and somewhat safer method of treating anxiety, and the use of these agents has increased dramatically in recent years. Another option includes the beta-adrenergic antagonists (beta blockers, see Chapter 20) because

these drugs can decrease situational anxiety without producing sedation.[27] In particular, beta blockers such as propranolol (Inderal) have been used by musicians and other performing artists to decrease cardiac palpitations, muscle tremors, hyperventilation, and other manifestations of anxiety that tend to occur before an important performance.[43] Beta blockers probably exert their antianxiety effects through their ability to decrease activity in the sympathetic nervous system, that is, through their sympatholytic effects. These drugs may exert both peripheral sympatholytic effects (e.g., blockade of myocardial beta-1 receptors) as well as decreasing central sympathetic tone. In any event, beta blockers may offer a suitable alternative to decrease the effects of nervousness without a concomitant decrease in levels of alertness or motivation.[43] Again, these drugs have gained popularity with performing artists as a way to blunt the symptoms of performance anxiety without actually diminishing the anticipation and excitement that is requisite for a strong performance.

Problems and Adverse Effects

Most of the problems that occur with benzodiazepine anxiolytic drugs are similar to those mentioned regarding the use of these agents as sedative-hypnotics. Sedation is still the most common side effect of anxiolytic benzodiazepines, even though this effect is not as pronounced as with their sedative-hypnotic counterparts.[61] Still, even short-term use of these drugs can produce psychomotor impairment, especially during activities that require people to remain especially alert, such as driving a car.[60,61] Addiction and abuse are problems with chronic benzodiazepine use, and withdrawal from these drugs can be a serious problem.[36] Also, anxiety can return to, or exceed, pretreatment levels when benzodiazepines are suddenly discontinued, a problem known as rebound anxiety.[1,13] The fact that chronic benzodiazepine use can cause these problems reinforces the idea that these drugs are not curative and should be used only for limited periods of time as an adjunct to other nonpharmacologic procedures such as psychologic counseling.[24,45]

Problems and side effects associated with buspirone include dizziness, headache, nausea, and restlessness. Antidepressants such as paroxetine and venlafaxine also produce a number of side effects (described in Chapter 7) depending on the specific agent. Nonetheless, these newer, nonbenzodiazepine anxiolytics tend to produce less sedation, and their potential for addiction is lower compared to benzodiazepines. Hence, nonbenzodiazepine drugs might be an attractive alternative, especially in patients who are prone to sedation (e.g., older adults), patients with a history of substance abuse, or people who need chronic anxiolytic treatment.

Special Consideration of Sedative-Hypnotic and Antianxiety Agents in Rehabilitation

Although these drugs are not used to directly influence the rehabilitation of musculoskeletal or other somatic disorders, the prevalence of their use in patient populations is high. Any time a patient is hospitalized for treatment of a disorder, a substantial amount of apprehension and concern exists. The foreign environment of the institution as well as a change in the individual's daily routine can understandably result in sleep disturbances.[23] Likewise, older adults often have trouble sleeping, and the use of sedative-hypnotic agents is common, especially in patients living in nursing homes or other facilities.[8,35,41] Individuals who are involved in rehabilitation programs, both as inpatients and as outpatients, may also have a fairly high level of anxiety because of concern about their health and ability to resume normal functioning.[33] Acute and chronic illnesses can create uncertainty about a patient's future family and job obligations as well as doubts about his or her self-image. The tension and anxiety produced may necessitate pharmacologic management.

The administration of sedative-hypnotic and antianxiety drugs has several direct implications for the rehabilitation session. Obviously the patient will be much calmer and more relaxed after taking an antianxiety drug, thus offering the potential benefit of gaining the patient's full cooperation during a physical or occupational therapy treatment. Anxiolytic benzodiazepines, for example, reach peak blood levels 2 to 4 hours after oral administration, so scheduling the rehabilitation session during that time may improve the patient's participation in treatment. Of course, this rationale will backfire if the drug produces significant hypnotic effects. Therapy sessions that require the patient to actively participate in activities such as gait training or therapeutic exercise will be essentially useless and even hazardous if the patient is extremely drowsy. Consequently, scheduling patients for certain types of rehabilitation within several hours after administration of sedative-hypnotics or sedative-like anxiolytics is counterproductive and should be avoided.

Finally, benzodiazepines and other drugs used to treat sleep disorders and anxiety are often associated with falls and subsequent trauma including hip fractures, especially in older adults.[15,45,60] The risk of falls is greater in people who have a history of doing so or who have other problems that would predispose them to falling (vestibular disorders, impaired vision, and so forth). Therapists can identify such people and intervene to help prevent this through balance training, environmental modifications (removing cluttered furniture, throw rugs, and so forth), and similar activities. Therapists can help plan and implement nonpharmacological interventions to help decrease anxiety and improve sleep. Interventions such as regular physical activity, massage, and various relaxation techniques may be very helpful in reducing stress levels and promoting normal sleep.[38,40,56] Therapists can therefore help substitute nonpharmacological methods for traditional sedative-hypnotic and antianxiety drugs, thus improving the patient's quality of life by avoiding drug-related side effects.

SUMMARY

Sedative-hypnotic and antianxiety drugs play a prominent role in today's society. The normal pressures of daily life often result in tension and stress, which affects an individual's ability to relax or cope with stress. These problems are compounded when there is some type of illness or injury present. As would be expected, a number of patients seen in a rehabilitation setting are taking these drugs. Benzodiazepines have long been the premier agents used to treat sleep disorders and anxiety; they all share a common mechanism of action, and they potentiate the inhibitory effects of GABA in the CNS. With regard to their sedative-hypnotic effects, benzodiazepines such as flurazepam and triazolam are commonly used to promote sleep. Although these drugs are generally safer than their forerunners, they are not without their problems. Newer nonbenzodiazepine sedative-hypnotics such as zolpidem and zaleplon may also be effective in treating sleep disorders, and these newer agents may be somewhat safer than their benzodiazepine counterparts. Benzodiazepines such as diazepam (Valium)

CASE STUDY

Sedative-Hypnotic Drugs

Brief History. R.S. is a 34-year-old construction worker who sustained a fracture-dislocation of the vertebral column in an automobile accident. He was admitted to an acute care facility, where a diagnosis of complete paraplegia was made at the T-12 spinal level. Surgery was performed to stabilize the vertebral column. During the next 3 weeks, his medical condition improved. At the end of 1 month, he was transferred to a rehabilitation facility to begin an intensive program of physical and occupational therapy. Rehabilitation included strengthening and range-of-motion (ROM) exercises, as well as training in wheelchair mobility, transfers, and activities of daily living (ADLs). However, upon arriving at the new institution, R.S. complained of difficulty sleeping. Flurazepam (Dalmane) was prescribed at a dosage of 20 mg administered orally each night at bedtime.

Problem/Influence of Medication. During his daily rehabilitation regimen, the therapists noted that R.S.'s performance and level of attentiveness were markedly poor during the morning sessions. He was excessively lethargic and drowsy, and his speech was slurred. These symptoms were present to a much greater extent than the normal slow start that occurs in some patients on wakening in the morning. The therapists also found that when ADL or mobility training was taught during the morning sessions, there was poor carryover from day to day regarding these activities.

Decision/Solution. The benzodiazepine drug appeared to be producing a hangoverlike effect, which limited the patient's cognitive skills during the early daily activities. Initially this problem was dealt with by reserving the early morning session for stretching and ROM activities, and then gradually moving into upper-body strengthening. Activities that required more patient learning and comprehension were done later in the morning or in the afternoon. Also, this hangoverlike problem was brought to the attention of the physician, and the hypnotic drug was ultimately switched to zolpidem (Ambien) because this is a relatively short-acting nonbenzodiazepine with a half-life of 2.6 hours (range 1.4–4.5 hours), compared to flurazepam (Dalmane), which is a long-acting benzodiazepine that can have a half-life of up to 74 hours (range 47–100 hours) because of its active metabolites. Switching to zolpidem might also result in fewer problems (i.e., rebound insomnia) when it is time to discontinue the drug.

---

leave as are also used frequently to reduce anxiety, but the introduction of newer drugs such as buspirone and specific antidepressants (paroxetine, venlafaxine) have provided an effective but somewhat safer alternative for treating anxiety. Because of the potential for physical and psychologic dependence, sedative-hypnotic and antianxiety drugs should not be used indefinitely. These drugs should be prescribed judiciously as an adjunct to helping patients deal with the source of their problems.

References

1. Allgulander C, Bandelow B, Hollander E, et al. WCA recommendations for the long-term treatment of generalized anxiety disorder. *CNS Spectr.* 2003;8(suppl 1): 53–61.
2. Apter JT, Allen LA. Buspirone: future directions. *J Clin Psychopharmacol.* 1999;19:86—93.
3. Atack JR. Anxioselective compounds acting at the GABA (A) receptor benzodiazepine binding site. *Curr Drug Targets CNS Neurol Disord.* 2003;2:213–232.
4. Bandelow B, Zohar J, Hollander E, et al. World Federation of Societies of Biological Psychiatry (WFSBP) guidelines for the pharmacological treatment of anxiety, obsessive-compulsive and posttraumatic stress disorders. *World J Biol Psychiatry.* 2002;3:171–199.
5. Bettler B, Kaupmann K, Mosbacher J, Gassmann M. Molecular structure and physiological functions of GABA (B) receptors. *Physiol Rev.* 2004;84:835–867.
6. Bond AJ, Wingrove J, Baylis M, Dalton J. Buspirone decreases physiological reactivity to unconditioned and conditioned aversive stimuli. *Psychopharmacology.* 2003;165:291–295.
7. Bond AJ, Wingrove J, Valerie Curran H, Lader MH. Treatment of generalised anxiety disorder with a short course of psychological therapy combined with buspirone or placebo. *J Affect Disord.* 2002;72: 267–271.
8. Bourne RS, Mills GH. Sleep disruption in critically ill patients pharmacological considerations. *Anaesthesia.* 2004;59:374–384.
9. Brawman-Mintzer O. Pharmacologic treatment of generalized anxiety disorder. *Psychiatr Clin North Am.* 2001;24:119–137.
10. Bronowska A, Les A, Chilmonczyk Z, et al. Molecular dynamics of buspirone analogues interacting with the 5-HT1A and 5-HT2A serotonin receptors. *Bioorg Med Chem.* 2001;9:881–895.

11. Burt DR. Reducing GABA receptors. *Life Sci*. 2003; 73:1741–1717.

12. Chilmonnczyk Z, Cybulski J, Bronowska A, Les A. Molecular modeling of buspirone–serotonin receptor interactions. *Acta Pol Pharm*. 2000;57:281–288.

13. Chouinard G. Issues in the clinical use of benzodiazepines: potency, withdrawal, and rebound. *J Clin Psychiatry*. 2004;65(suppl 5):7–12.

14. Costa E. From GABA$_A$ receptor diversity emerges a unified vision of GABAergic inhibition. *Annu Rev Pharmacol Toxicol*. 1998;38:321–350.

15. Cumming RG, Le Couteur DG. Benzodiazepines and risk of hip fractures in older people: a review of the evidence. *CNS Drugs*. 2003;17:825–837.

16. Davidson JR. Use of benzodiazepines in social anxiety disorder, generalized anxiety disorder, and posttraumatic stress disorder. *J Clin Psychiatry*. 2004;65(suppl 5):29–33.

17. Davies M. The role of GABA$_A$ receptors in mediating the effects of alcohol in the central nervous system. *J Psychiatry Neurosci*. 2003;28:263–274.

18. Drake CL, Roehrs T, Roth T. Insomnia causes, consequences, and therapeutics: an overview. *Depress Anxiety*. 2003;18:163–176.

19. Drover DR. Comparative pharmacokinetics and pharmacodynamics of short acting hypnosedatives: zaleplon, zolpidem and zopiclone. *Clin Pharmacokinet*. 2004;43:227–238.

20. Dundar Y, Dodd S, Strobl J, et al. Comparative efficacy of newer hypnotic drugs for the short-term management of insomnia: a systematic review and meta-analysis. *Hum Psychopharmacol*. 2004;19:305–322.

21. Evers AS, Crowder CM. General anesthetics. In: Hardman JG, et al., eds. *The Pharmacological Basis of Therapeutics*. 10th ed. New York: McGraw-Hill; 2001.

22. Fraser AD. Use and abuse of the benzodiazepines. *Ther Drug Monit*. 1998;20:481–489.

23. Frighetto L, Marra C, Bandali S, et al. An assessment of quality of sleep and the use of drugs with sedating properties in hospitalized adult patients. *Health Qual Life Outcomes*. 2004;2:17.

24. Gorman JM. Treating generalized anxiety disorder. *J Clin Psychiatry*. 2003;64(suppl 2):24–29.

25. Grunstein R. Insomnia. Diagnosis and management. *Aust Fam Physician*. 2002;31:995–1000.

26. Hajak G, Muller WE, Wittchen HU, et al. Abuse and dependence potential for the non-benzodiazepine hypnotics zolpidem and zopiclone: a review of case reports and epidemiological data. *Addiction*. 2003;98:1371–1378.

27. James IM. Practical aspects of the use of beta-blockers in anxiety states: situational anxiety. *Postgrad Med J*. 1984;60(suppl 2):19–25.

28. Johnston GA. Medicinal chemistry and molecular pharmacology of GABA(C) receptors. *Curr Top Med Chem*. 2002;2:903–913.

29. Kapczinski F, Lima MS, Souza JS, Schmitt R. Antidepressants for generalized anxiety disorder. *Cochrane Database Syst Rev*. 2003;CD003592.

30. Kitayama M, Hirota K, Kudo M, Kudo T, Ishihara H, Matsuki A. Inhibitory effects of intravenous anaesthetic agents on K (+)-evoked glutamate release from rat cerebrocortical slices. Involvement of voltage sensitive Ca (2+) channels and GABA (A) receptors. *Naunyn Schmiedebergs Arch Pharmacol*. 2002;366:246–253.

31. Kumar S, Fleming RL, Morrow AL. Ethanol regulation of gamma–aminobutyric acid A receptors: genomic and nongenomic mechanisms. *Pharmacol Ther*. 2004; 101:211–226.

32. Lader MH. Implications of hypnotic flexibility on patterns of clinical use. *Int J Clin Pract Suppl*. 2001;116: 14–19.

33. Lecrubier Y. Posttraumatic stress disorder in primary care: a hidden diagnosis. *J Clin Psychiatry*. 2004;65 (suppl 1):49–54.

34. Lee YJ. Overview of the therapeutic management of insomnia with zolpidem. *CNS Drugs*. 2004; 18(suppl 1):17–23; discussion 41, 43–45.

35. Lenhart SE, Buysse DJ. Treatment of insomnia in hospitalized patients. *Ann Pharmacother*. 2001;35: 1449–1457.

36. Longo LP, Johnson B. Addiction: part I. Benzodiazepines—side effects, abuse risk and alternatives. *Am Fam Physician*. 2000;61:2121–2128.

37. Lydiard RB. The role of GABA in anxiety disorders. *J Clin Psychiatry*. 2003;64(Suppl 3):21–27.

38. Mamtani R, Cimino A. A primer of complementary and alternative medicine and its relevance in the treatment of mental health problems. *Psychiatr Q*. 2002;73: 367–381.

39. Mitler MM. Nonselective and selective benzodiazepine receptor agonists—where are we today? *Sleep*. 2000;23 (suppl 1):S39–S47.

40. Morgan K, Dixon S, Mathers N, et al. Psychological treatment for insomnia in the regulation of long-term hypnotic drug use. *Health Technol Assess*. 2004;8: 1–68.

41. Nagel CL, Markie MB, Richards KC, Taylor JL. Sleep promotion in hospitalized elders. *Medsurg Nurs*. 2003; 12:279–289.

42. Neubauer DN. Pharmacologic approaches for the treatment of chronic insomnia. *Clin Cornerstone*. 2003;5:16–27.

43. Nies AS. Clinical pharmacology of the beta-adrenergic blockers. *Med Probl Perform Art*. 1986;1:25–31.

44. Pary R, Matuschka PR, Lewis S, et al. Generalized anxiety disorder. *South Med J*. 2003;96:581–586.

45. Petrovic M, Mariman A, Warie H, et al. Is there a rationale for prescription of benzodiazepines in the elderly? Review of the literature. *Acta Clin Belg*. 2003;58:27–36.

46. Rickels K, Rynn M. Pharmacotherapy of generalized anxiety disorder. *J Clin Psychiatry*. 2002; 63(Suppl 14):9–16.

47. Rouillon F. Long term therapy of generalized anxiety disorder. *Eur Psychiatry*. 2004;19:96–101.

48. Rudolph U. Identification of molecular substrate for the attenuation of anxiety: a step toward the development of better anti-anxiety drugs. *ScientificWorld Journal*. 2001;1:192–193.

49. Rudolph U, Mohler H. Analysis of GABA$_A$ receptor function and dissection of the pharmacology of benzodiazepines and general anesthetics through mouse genetics. *Annu Rev Pharmacol Toxicol.* 2004;44:475–498.

50. Salzman C. Addiction to benzodiazepines. *Psychiatr Q.* 1998;69:251–261.

51. Sanger DJ. The pharmacology and mechanisms of action of new generation, non-benzodiazepine hypnotic agents. *CNS Drugs.* 2004; 18(suppl 1):9–15; discussion 41, 43–45.

52. Sanna E, Busonero F, Talani G, et al. Comparison of the effects of zaleplon, zolpidem, and triazolam at various GABA (A) receptor subtypes. *Eur J Pharmacol.* 2002;451:103–110.

53. Sheehan DV, Mao CG. Paroxetine treatment of generalized anxiety disorder. *Psychopharmacol Bull.* 2003;37 (suppl 1):64–75.

54. Shelton CI. Diagnosis and management of anxiety disorders. *J Am Osteopath Assoc.* 2004; 104(suppl 3):S2–S5.

55. Sigel E. Mapping of the benzodiazepine recognition site on GABA (A) receptors. *Curr Top Med Chem.* 2002;2:833–839.

56. Smith MT, Perlis ML, Park A, et al. Comparative meta-analysis of pharmacotherapy and behavior therapy for persistent insomnia. *Am J Psychiatry.* 2002;159:5–11.

57. Sramek JJ, Zarotsky V, Cutler NR. Generalised anxiety disorder: treatment options. *Drugs.* 2002;62: 1635–1648.

58. Terzano MG, Rossi M, Palomba V, Smerieri A, Parrino L. New drugs for insomnia: comparative tolerability of zopiclone, zolpidem and zaleplon. *Drug Saf.* 2003;26:261–282.

59. Trevor AJ, Way WL. Sedative-hypnotic drugs. In: Katzung BG, ed. *Basic and Clinical Pharmacology.* 9th ed. New York: Lange Medical Books/McGraw Hill; 2004.

60. Vermeeren A. Residual effects of hypnotics: epidemiology and clinical implications. *CNS Drugs.* 2004;18:297–328.

61. Verster JC, Volkerts ER. Clinical pharmacology, clinical efficacy, and behavioral toxicity of alprazolam: a review of the literature. *CNS Drug Rev.* 2004;10:45–76.

62. Wagner J, Wagner ML. Non-benzodiazepines for the treatment of insomnia. *Sleep Med Rev.* 2000;4:551–581.

63. Wang JS, DeVane CL. Pharmacokinetics and drug interactions of the sedative hypnotics. *Psychopharmacol Bull.* 2003;37:10–29.

Chapter 7

Drugs Used to Treat Affective Disorders: Depression and Bipolar Syndrome

Affective disorders comprise the group of mental conditions that includes depression, bipolar syndrome (manic-depression), and several others that are characterized by a marked disturbance in a patient's mood.[41] Patients with an affective disorder typically present with an inappropriate disposition, feeling unreasonably sad and discouraged (major depressive disorder) or fluctuating between periods of depression and excessive excitation and elation (bipolar disorder).

Because these forms of mental illness are relatively common, many rehabilitation specialists will work with patients who are receiving drug therapy for an affective disorder. Also, serious injury or illness may precipitate an episode of depression in the patient undergoing physical rehabilitation. Consequently, this chapter will discuss the pharmacologic management of affective disorders, as well as how antidepressant and antimanic drugs may influence the patient involved in physical therapy and occupational therapy.

Depression

Clinical Picture

Depression is considered to be the most prevalent mental illness in the United States, with approximately 15 percent of adults experiencing major depression at some point in their life.[73] Likewise, as many as 10 percent of Americans may experience major depression over a 1-year period.[43] In this sense, depression is a form of mental illness characterized by intense feelings of sadness and despair. While a certain amount of disappointment and sadness is part of everyday life, a diagnosis of clinical depression indicates that these feelings are increased in both intensity and duration to an incapacitating extent.

Depressive disorders are characterized by a general dysphoric mood (sadness, irritability, feeling "down in the dumps"), as well as by a general lack of interest in previously pleasurable activities. Other symptoms including anorexia, sleep disorders (either too much or too little), fatigue, lack of self-esteem, somatic complaints, and irrational guilt. Recurrent thoughts of death and suicide may also help lead to a diagnosis of depression. To initiate effective treatment, a proper diagnosis must be made; depression must not be confused with other mental disorders that also may influence mood and behavior (e.g., schizophrenia). To standardize the terminology and aid in recognizing depression, specific criteria for diagnosis has been outlined by the American Psychiatric Association.[2] Depressive disorders can also be subclassified according to the type, duration, and intensity of the patient's symptoms.[9,41,71] For the purpose of this chapter, the term *depression* will be used to indicate major depressive disorder, but readers should be aware that the exact type of depression may vary somewhat from person to person.

The causes of depression seem to be complex and unclear. Although a recent stressful incident, misfortune, or illness can certainly exacerbate an episode of depression, some patients may become depressed for no apparent reason. The role of genetic factors in depression has been explored but remains uncertain. Over the past few decades, it has been suggested that a central nervous system (CNS) neurochemical imbalance may be the underlying feature in depression, as well as in other forms of mental illness. The importance of these findings as related to pharmacologic treatment will be discussed later. However, factors responsible for initiating these changes in CNS function are unclear. Depression is undoubtedly caused by the complex interaction of a number of genetic, environmental, and biochemical factors.[18,38,46,57]

Treatment of depression is essential in minimizing the disruptive influence that this disease has on the patient's quality of life, and on his or her relationship with their family and job. Procedures ranging from psychotherapy to electroconvulsive treatment can be prescribed, depending on the severity and type. Drug treatment plays a major role in alleviating and preventing the occurrence of major depression, and this form of therapy is presented here.

Pathophysiology of Depression

It appears that depression is related to a disturbance in CNS neurotransmission involving certain chemicals know as amine neurotransmitters. These transmitters include 5-hydroxytryptamine (serotonin), norepi-

nephrine, and dopamine. Amine neurotransmitters are found in many areas of the brain, and are important in controlling many aspects of mood and behavior.

However, the exact problem in CNS amine neurotransmission remains a subject of much debate. One leading theory is that depression may be caused by an *increased* sensitivity of the presynaptic or postsynaptic receptors for these transmitters. That is, the neurochemistry of the brain has been changed in some way to make the amine receptors *more* sensitive to their respective amine neurotransmitters (norepinephrine, serotonin, and to a lesser extent, dopamine).[21] This theory is based primarily on the finding that antidepressant drugs prolong the activity of amine neurotransmission in the brain, thereby causing a compensatory decrease in the sensitivity of the amine receptors.[21,47]

The idea that depression is associated with changes in amine receptor sensitivity is summarized in Figure 7–1. For reasons that are still unclear, depression might occur because of an increase in postsynaptic receptor sensitivity to amine neurotransmitters, particularly norepinephrine and serotonin.[4] Antidepressant drugs increase amine transmission by a variety of methods, thereby bringing about overstimulation of the postsynaptic receptor. (The exact method by which these drugs increase amine stimulation is discussed later in this chapter.) Overstimulation

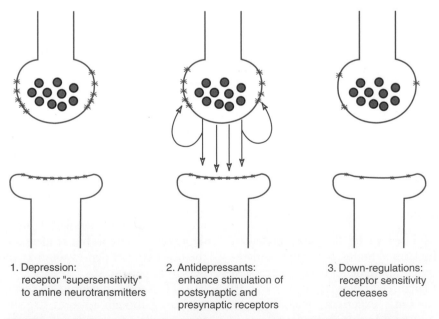

1. Depression:
   receptor "supersensitivity"
   to amine neurotransmitters

2. Antidepressants:
   enhance stimulation of
   postsynaptic and
   presynaptic receptors

3. Down-regulations:
   receptor sensitivity
   decreases

FIGURE 7–1 ▼ Theoretic basis for the mechanism and treatment of depression. Functionally active receptor sites are indicated by an "*." Depression is believed to be initiated by increased postsynaptic or presynaptic receptor sensitivity. Drugs that enhance stimulation of these receptors ultimately lead to receptor down-regulation, thus resolving the depression (see text for details).

of the postsynaptic receptor then leads to a compensatory down-regulation and decreased sensitivity of the receptor. As discussed in Chapter 4, this down-regulation is a normal response to overstimulation by either endogenous or exogenous agonists. As receptor sensitivity decreases, the clinical symptoms of depression might be resolved.

On the other hand, it has been suggested that the primary problem in depression is an increased sensitivity to receptors that are located on the *presynaptic* terminals of amine synapses.[54] These presynaptic "autoreceptors" normally regulate and limit the release of amine transmitters, such as norepinephrine or serotonin, from the presynaptic terminal. Increasing their sensitivity could result in a relative lack of adequate neurotransmitter release at these synapses. By causing overstimulation of these presynaptic receptors, antidepressant drugs could eventually normalize their sensitivity and help reestablish proper control and regulation of these amine synapses.[54]

It must be emphasized that it is difficult to prove the neurochemical changes that underlie depression, and the way that antidepressant drugs help resolve depression remains theoretical at present. Still, certain aspects of drug therapy tend to support the amine hypothesis and the putative changes in receptor sensitivity induced by drug therapy. For instance, there is usually a time lag of approximately 2 to 4 weeks before antidepressant drugs begin to work.[54] This latency period would be necessary for a compensatory change in receptor sensitivity to take place after drug therapy is initiated.[54]

Still, the exact neurochemical changes in depression are difficult to determine, and probably involve other neurotransmitters and receptors. For example, high levels of glucocorticoids, such as cortisol, are found in the bloodstream of certain people with depression.[15] This makes sense because cortisol is often released from the adrenal cortex in response to stress, and prolonged or severe stress can be a precipitating factor in certain forms of depression (see Chapter 28 for a description of cortisol production).[40,68] Apparently, excess glucocorticoid levels overstimulate glucocorticoid receptors in the brain, bringing about a compensatory *decrease* in the sensitivity and responsiveness of these receptors.[7] The decreased responsiveness of these glucocorticoid receptors is somehow related to the dysfunction in serotonin neurotransmission described above.[40] The relationship between glucocorticoid receptor sensitivity and dysfunctional serotonin activity is not completely understood, and the exact way that these systems interact has not been determined.[59] Nonetheless, it is apparent that stress hormones such as cortisol can play a role in the pathogenesis of depression, and research is currently underway to discover how antidepressant medications can help normalize glucocorticoid responsiveness in certain types of the disorder.[7]

Hence, complex neurochemical changes seem to occur in certain areas of the brain in people with depression, and these changes may vary depending on each person and the specific type of depression. Likewise, changes in other brain chemicals—such as brain-derived tropic factor, gamma-aminobutyric acid (GABA), substance P, glutamate, and cyclic adenosine monophosphate (cAMP) response element may also play a role in the pathophysiology of depression.[1,4,36,56] Changes in brain chemistry may be associated with altered neuronal structure and plasticity, and changes in cellular growth and hippocampus volume have been reported in people with depression.[42,50,66] Future research will continue to clarify the exact cellular and subcellular events that occur during depression, and how these events can be resolved pharmacologically. It is apparent, however, that current drug therapy is focused on modifying one or more receptor populations at brain synapses that use amine transmitters. These drugs are discussed here.

Antidepressant Drugs

The drugs that are currently used to treat depression are grouped into several categories, according to chemical or functional criteria. These categories consist of the tricyclics, monoamine oxidase (MAO) inhibitors, and second-generation drugs (Table 7–1). All three groups attempt to increase aminergic transmission, but by different mechanisms (Fig 7–2). Sympathomimetic stimulants such as the amphetamine drugs were also used on a limited basis to treat depression, but the powerful CNS excitation produced by amphetaminelike drugs and the potential for addiction and overdose have essentially eliminated their use as antidepressants. The pharmacologic effects of the primary antidepressant drug categories are discussed below.

Tricyclics. Drugs in this category share a common three-ring chemical structure (hence the name "tricyclic"). These drugs work by blocking the reuptake of amine neurotransmitters into the presynaptic terminal.[61,67] Actively transporting amine neurotransmitters back into the presynaptic terminal is the method by which most (50 to 80 percent) of the released transmitter is removed from the synaptic cleft. By blocking reuptake, tricyclics allow the released amines to

Table 7–1	COMMON ANTIDEPRESSANT DRUGS

Generic Name	Trade Name	Initial Adult Dose (mg/day)	Prescribing Limits* (mg/day)
Tricyclics			
Amitriptyline	Elavil, Endep, others	50–100	300
Amoxapine	Asendin	100–150	600
Clomipramine	Anafranil	75	300
Desipramine	Norpramin	100–200	300
Doxepin	Sinequan	75	300
Imipramine	Norfranil, Tofranil, others	75–200	300
Nortriptyline	Aventyl, Pamelor	75–100	150
Protriptyline	Vivactil	15–40	60
Trimipramine	Surmontil	75	300
Monoamine oxidase (MAO) inhibitors			
Isocarboxazid	Marplan	20	60
Phenelzine	Nardil	45	90
Tranylcypromine	Parnate	30	60
Second-generation agents			
Bupropion	Wellbutrin	150	400
Citalopram	Celexa	20	60
Escitalopram	Lexapro	10	20
Fluoxetine	Prozac	20	80
Fluvoxamine	Luvox	50	300
Maprotiline	Ludiomil	25–75	225
Mirtazapine	Remeron	15	45
Nefazodone	Serzone	200	600
Paroxetine	Paxil	20	50
Sertraline	Zoloft	50	200
Trazodone	Desyrel	150	600
Venlafaxine	Effexor	75	375

*Upper limits reflect dosages administered to patients with severe depression who are being treated as inpatients.

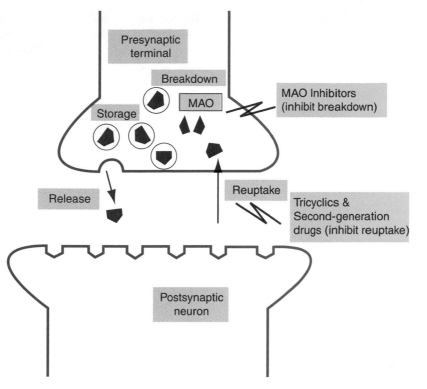

FIGURE 7–2 ▼ Effects of antidepressant drugs on amine synapses. All three types of drugs tend to increase the presence of amine transmitters (norepinephrine, dopamine, serotonin) in the synaptic cleft. Increased transmitter stimulation leads to postsynaptic receptor down-regulation/desensitization.

remain in the cleft and continue to exert their effects. The prolonged stimulation of these neurotransmitters (especially norepinephrine) leads to the compensatory decrease in receptor sensitivity, which ultimately leads to a decrease in depression.

In the past, tricyclic drugs such as amitriptyline and nortriptyline were the most commonly used antidepressants and were the standard against which other antidepressants were measured.[30] The use of tricyclic drugs as the initial treatment of depression has diminished somewhat in favor of some of the newer second-generation drugs, which may have more favorable side-effect profiles. Tricyclic agents, nonetheless, remain an important component in the management of depressive disorders, especially in more severe forms of depression that fail to respond to other antidepressants.[6,53]

Monoamine Oxidase Inhibitors. Monoamine oxidase (MAO) is an enzyme that is located at amine synapses and helps remove released transmitters through enzymatic destruction. Drugs that inhibit this enzyme allow more of the transmitter to remain in the synaptic cleft and continue to exert an effect.[74] As with

the tricyclics, MAO inhibitors directly increase activity at amine synapses, which can bring about changes in the activity and sensitivity of receptors at this synapse. MAO inhibitors are not usually the drugs of choice in depression, but they may be helpful if patients do not respond to other agents (tricyclics, second-generation drugs), or if other antidepressants produce intolerable side effects.

The MAO enzyme exists in two primary forms or subtypes: MAO type A and MAO type B.[4] These two subtypes are differentiated according to their ability to degrade specific amines and according to the ability of various drugs to inhibit one or both subtypes of the MAO enzyme. Preliminary evidence suggests that selective inhibition of MAO type A may be desirable in treating depression,[4] whereas inhibition of MAO type B may be more important in prolonging the effects of dopamine in Parkinson disease (see Chapter 10). Regardless, the MAO inhibitors currently used as antidepressants are relatively nonselective, meaning that they inhibit MAO A and MAO B fairly equally. Development of new MAO inhibitors may produce agents that are more selective for the MAO A subtype and may therefore produce better antidepressant effects with fewer side effects.[4]

Second-Generation Antidepressants. Because of the limitations of first-generation drugs such as the tricyclics and MAO inhibitors, a number of diverse compounds have been developed and continue to be evaluated for their antidepressant effects. There is some evidence that certain second-generation drugs are more effective in treating specific depressive symptoms in some patients, but the newer agents have not been proven to be categorically more effective than the older drugs.[12,48,70] The newer agents, however, tend to have a lower incidence of side effects such as cardiovascular problems, sedation, and so forth. Hence, these newer drugs may be better-tolerated and provide better long-term management of depression because of improved patient satisfaction and adherence to drug therapy.[58]

Newer antidepressants are chemically diverse, but most work by mechanisms similar to tricyclic drugs; that is, they block reuptake of norepinephrine and other monoamines. Hence, these drugs appear to exert their beneficial effects by bringing about a receptor sensitivity decrease, which seems to be the common denominator of antidepressant drugs' action. The second-generation drugs and their proposed mechanisms of action are summarized in Table 7–2. In addition, certain second-generation drugs are distinguished by their ability to selectively influence specific monoamines rather than all the amine transmitters simultaneously. Subcategories of these selective drugs are discussed below.

Selective serotonin reuptake inhibitors. Certain second-generation drugs have received attention because of their ability to selectively block the reuptake of 5-hydroxytryptamine (serotonin). Fluoxetine (Prozac) and similar agents (citalopram, escitalopram, fluvoxamine, paroxetine, sertraline, see Table 7–2) are functionally grouped together as selective serotonin reuptake inhibitors (SSRIs).[54,64] This distinguishes them from the tricyclics, MAO inhibitors, and other second-generation drugs because these other drugs tend to be nonselective in their effect on amine neurotransmitters and block the reuptake of norepinephrine and dopamine, as well as serotonin. The primary advantage of the SSRIs is that they produce fewer and less bothersome side effects than their nonselective counterparts. This improved side-effect profile can be very helpful in the long-term management of depression because patients may tolerate these drugs better and be more willing to take their medication on a

regular basis.[58] SSRIs may also be less toxic during overdose than more traditional antidepressants such as the tricyclics.[64,72] These serotonin selective drugs have therefore become the antidepressant drugs of choice for many patients, and are often prescribed as the initial method of treatment in people who are depressed.[64]

Other selective drugs. Drugs that are relatively selective for other types of monoamines are also administered as possible antidepressants. Reboxetine, for example, is a relatively new agent that selectively inhibits transmitter reuptake at norepinephrine synapses.[34,55] There is likewise an emerging group of drugs, such as venlafaxine, that selectively decrease serotonin and norepinephrine reuptake without an appreciable effect of dopamine synapses.[31] These drugs are known as serotonin/norepinephrine reuptake inhibitors (SNRIs), and they may be more effective than other agents in resolving depression, especially in resistant cases or in people with severe depression.[19,33,69] There is also some evidence that SNRIs such as venlafaxine and mirtazapine might take effect more quickly than traditional drugs such as the tricyclics and SSRIs.[11,19] The development of SNRIs and various other selective drugs—including SSRIs—has opened new opportunities for the optimal management of depression. Future studies will undoubtedly shed light on how these more selective agents can be best used to treat specific depressive symptoms and types of depression.

Pharmacokinetics

Antidepressants are usually administered orally. Dosages vary depending not only on each drug but also on the individual patient. Initial dosages generally start out relatively low and are increased slowly within the therapeutic range until beneficial effects are observed. Distribution within the body also varies with each type of antidepressant, but all eventually reach the brain to exert their effects. Metabolism takes place primarily in the liver, and metabolites of several drugs continue to show significant antidepressant activity. This fact may be responsible for prolonging the effects of the drug, even after it has undergone hepatic biotransformation. Elimination takes place by biotransformation and renal excretion.

Problems and Adverse Effects

Tricyclics. A major problem with the tricyclic antidepressants is sedation (Table 7–3). Although a

Table 7-2	SECOND-GENERATION ANTIDEPRESSANT DRUGS		
Drug	**Mechanism (Amine selectivity)**	**Advantages**	**Disadvantages**
	Selective serotonin reuptake inhibitors		
Citalopram (Celexa)	Strong, selective inhibition of serotonin reuptake	Low incidence of sedation and anticholinergic effects; does not cause orthostatic hypotension or cardiac arrhythmias	May cause sexual dysfunction (decreased libido, impotence)
Escitalopram (Lexapro)	Strong, selective inhibition of serotonin reuptake	Similar to citalopram	Similar to citalopram
Fluoxetine (Prozac)	Moderate, selective inhibition of serotonin reuptake	No sedative, anticholinergic, or cardiovascular side effects; helpful in obsessive-compulsive disorder	May cause anxiety, nausea, insomnia; long half-life can lead to accumulation
Fluvoxamine (Luvox)	Strong, selective inhibition of serotonin reuptake	Similar to fluoxetine	Similar to fluoxetine
Paroxetine (Paxil)	Strong, selective inhibition of serotonin reuptake	Similar to citalopram	Similar to citalopram
Sertraline (Zoloft)	Strong, selective inhibition of serotonin reuptake	Similar to fluoxetine	Similar to fluoxetine
	Other second-generation agents		
Bupropion (Wellbutrin, Zyban)	Primarily inhibits dopamine reuptake; little effect on norepinephrine or serotonin	Low sedative, anticholinergic, and cardiovascular side effects; also used as an intervention to quit cigarette smoking	May cause overstimulation (insomnia, tremor) and induce psychotic symptoms
Maprotiline (Ludiomil)	Moderate inhibition of norepinephrine reuptake	Sedating: useful in agitation	Possibility of seizures; overdoses lethal; long half-life
Mirtazapine (Remeron)	Exact mechanism unclear; may increase norepinephrine and serotonin activity by blocking inhibitory presynaptic autoreceptors	Low incidence of sedative, anticholinergic, and cardiovascular side effects	May cause agitation, anxiety, other mood changes
Nefazodone (Serzone)	Slight inhibition of serotonin and norepinephrine reuptake; may also block CNS serotonin receptors	Sedating: useful in agitation	May cause orthostatic hypotension because of antagonistic effect on vascular alpha-1 receptors

(Continued on following page)

Table 7–2	SECOND-GENERATION ANTIDEPRESSANT DRUGS *(Continued)*		
Drug	**Mechanism (Amineselectivity)**	**Advantages**	**Disadvantages**
Trazodone (Desyrel)	Slight inhibition of serotonin reuptake	Sedating: useful in agitation; lower relative risk of over-dose	May cause orthostatic hypotension (similar to nefazodone); serious problems related to pri-apism may also occur in men
Venlafaxine (Effexor)	Strong inhibition of norepi-nephrine and serotonin reuptake	Low risk of orthostatic hypotension, sedation, and anticholinergic side effects	May cause hypertension

certain degree of sedation may be desirable in some patients who are agitated and depressed, feelings of lethargy and sluggishness may impair patient adherence to drug therapy and result in a failure to take medication. A second major problem is that these drugs tend to have significant anticholinergic properties; that is, they act as if they are blocking certain central and peripheral acetylcholine receptors (see Table 7–3). Impairment of central acetylcholine transmission may cause confusion and delirium. The peripheral anticholinergic properties produce a variety of symptoms including dry mouth, constipation, urinary retention, and tachycardia. Other cardiovascular problems include arrhythmias and orthostatic hypotension, with the latter being particularly common in elderly patients. Finally, tricyclics have the highest potential for fatal overdose from an antidepressant.[62,72] This fact leads to a serious problem when one considers the risk of suicide among depressed patients. These drugs should be used cautiously in patients who have suicidal thoughts or a history of suicidal behaviors.

MAO Inhibitors. In contrast to the tricyclics, MAO inhibitors tend to produce CNS excitation, which can result in restlessness, irritability, agitation, and sleep loss. These drugs also produce some central and peripheral anticholinergic effects (e.g., tremor, confusion, dry mouth, urinary retention), but these effects tend to occur in a lesser extent than with the tricyclics (see Table 7–3). Because of the systemic MAO inhibition, excess activity at peripheral sympathetic adrenergic terminals may cause a profound increase in blood pressure, leading to a hypertensive crisis. This situation is exacerbated if other drugs that increase sympathetic nervous activity are being taken concurrently. Also, there is a distinct interaction between the MAO inhibitors and certain foods such as fermented cheese and wines.[76] These fermented foods contain tyramine, which stimulates the release of endogenous epinephrine and norepinephrine (the so-called cheese effect). The additive effect of increased catecholamine release (because of the ingested tyramine) and decreased catecholamine breakdown (because of MAO inhibition) can lead to excessive catecholamine levels and a hypertensive crisis.[76]

Second-Generation Drugs. The type and severity of side effects associated with newer antidepressants varies according to the specific drug in use. SSRIs and SNRIs, for example, generally produce less sedation, anticholinergic effects, and cardiovascular effects than the tricyclics, MAO inhibitors, and other second-generation drugs.[17] These newer drugs, however, are not devoid of side effects, and these agents often produce more gastrointestinal problems and insomnia than other antidepressants. Also, drugs that cause an excessive increase of serotonin activity in the brain may cause "serotonin syndrome," which is characterized by sweating, shivering, movement disorders (severe restlessness, dystonias, dyskinesias), muscle fasciculations, and other neuromuscular symptoms.[22,25] These symptoms typically disappear if the drug is discontinued, but they should be identified early or this syndrome could progress to seizures and coma.[25]

Advantages and disadvantages of common second-generation drugs are listed in Table 7–2, and comparison of these drugs to the tricyclics and MAO inhibitors is summarized in Table 7–3. Various factors, including potential side effects, are considered when selecting one of these drugs, and selection of the best drug must be done on a patient-by-patient basis.

Table 7–3	SIDE EFFECTS OF ANTIDEPRESSANT DRUGS*

Drug	Sedation	Anticholinergic Effects	Orthostatic Hypotension	Cardiac Arrhythmias	Seizures
Tricyclic drugs					
Amitriptyline	++++	++++	+++	+++	+++
Amoxapine	++	+++	++	++	+++
Clomipramine	++++	++++	++	+++	++++
Desipramine	++	++	++	++	++
Doxepin	++++	+++	++	++	+++
Imipramine	+++	+++	++++	+++	+++
Nortriptyline	++	++	+	++	++
Protriptyline	+	++	++	+++	++
Trimipramine	++++	++++	+++	+++	+++
Monoamine oxidase (MAO) inhibitors					
Phenelzine	++	+	++	+	+
Tranylcypromine	+	+	++	+	+
Second-generation drugs					
Bupropion	0	+	0	+	++++
Citalopram	+	0	0	0	++
Fluoxetine	0	0	0	0	++
Fluvoxamine	0	0	0	0	++
Maprotiline	+++	+++	++	++	++++
Mirtazapine	++	+	++	+	+
Nefazodone	+++	0	+++	+	++
Paroxetine	+	+	0	0	++
Sertraline	0	0	0	0	++
Trazodone	++++	0	+++	+	++
Venlafaxine	+	+	0	+	++

*Zero denotes no side effect, + a very low incidence, ++ a low incidence, +++ a moderate incidence, and ++++ a high incidence.

Adapted from Kando, et al. Depressive disorders. In: DiPiro JT, et al, eds. *Pharmacotherapy: A Pathophysiologic Approach.* 5th ed. New York: McGraw-Hill; 2002:1250, with permission.

Use of Antidepressants in Chronic Pain

Many chronic pain syndromes (neuropathic pain, fibromyalgia, chronic low back pain, and so forth) can be treated more effectively if antidepressants are included in the treatment regimen.[45,52,65] In particular, certain tricyclic agents such as amitriptyline, nortriptyline, doxepin, and desipramine: may help provide better pain relief when used along with traditional analgesic medications or, in some cases, when these tricyclic drugs are used alone.[45,60] Some studies attribute this effect to the fact that clinical depression is present in many patients with chronic pain; administering antidepressants will help provide optimal care by resolving the depressive symptoms.[3,14] There is considerable evidence, however, that antidepressants will help patients with chronic pain even if no symptoms of depression are present. That is, improvements in pain have been noted even when there has been no observed effect on the patient's mood. As indicated earlier, these drugs have the ability to modulate the influence of serotonin and other CNS monoamine neurotransmitters, and their effects on chronic pain may be related to the influence on monoamine transmission in critical pain pathways in the brain.[13,24,45] For the most part, however, the exact way that antidepressants affect pain perception remains unknown.

Hence, there is little doubt that antidepressants may be useful as an adjunct in the treatment of patients with chronic pain. Traditional tricyclic medications such as amitriptyline and nortriptyline are often considered the drugs of choice for chronic pain.[52] Newer drugs such as the SSRIs (e.g., paroxetine) and SNRIs (e.g., venlafaxine) might also be considered for some patients with fibromyalgia, neuropathies, and other forms of chronic pain.[29] Future research should help clarify how specific antidepressants can be used most effectively as part of a comprehensive regimen for treating various types of chronic pain.

Treatment of Bipolar Disorder: Antimanic Drugs

Bipolar Disorder

The form of depression discussed previously is often referred to as major depressive disorder or *unipolar depression*, in contrast to bipolar or "manic-depressive" disorder. As these terms imply, bipolar syndrome is associated with mood swings from one extreme (mania) to the other (depression).[10] Manic episodes are characterized by euphoria, hyperactivity, and talkativeness, and depressive episodes are similar to those described previously. Approximately 10 percent of all patients with depression are considered to exhibit bipolar syndrome.[10]

As in unipolar depression, the exact causes of bipolar disorder are unknown. One theory is that genetic and environmental factors conspire to increase norepinephrine and possibly serotonin influence in the brain.[23] This increase in neurotransmitter activity appears to be responsible for the manic episodes of this disorder. The subsequent depression may simply be a rebound from the general excitement of the manic episode. The exact cause of bipolar disorder is not clear; however, the manic episode of this condition may also be caused by neuroendocrine factors, an imbalance in cations such as sodium and calcium, or changes in the cellular and subcellular responses in specific brain neurons.[10,23] In any event, the treatment of bipolar disorder focuses on preventing the start of these pendulumlike mood swings by preventing the manic episodes. Hence, drugs used to treat manic-depression are really "antimanic drugs." The primary form of drug treatment consists of lithium salts (i.e., lithium carbonate, lithium citrate).[27,44] In addition, lithium is a useful adjunct to other antidepressant drugs in treatment-resistant unipolar depression.[16,28]

Lithium

Lithium (Li^+) is a monovalent cation included in the alkali metal group. Because of its small size (molecular weight 7) and single positive charge, lithium may influence neural excitability by competing with other cations including sodium, potassium, and calcium.[5] The exact way that lithium helps stabilize mood, however, is not known.[32] Several theories have been proposed, and lithium has been shown to produce several neurochemical effects that could contribute to its antimanic properties. In particular, lithium may stabilize neuronal excitability by decreasing the sensitivity of certain postsynaptic receptors and by uncoupling these receptors from their subcellular second-messenger systems.[5,10] For example, studies have shown that lithium can diminish the function of cAMP and other second-messenger systems that are normally stimulated by norepinephrine.[5,10] Lithium has also been shown to inhibit certain intracellular enzymes such as protein kinase C, glycogen synthetase kinase3-beta, and inositol monophosphatase, which may help account for decreased neuronal excitation and desensitization.[8,10,35] In addition, lithium has been shown to directly decrease the release of certain amine neurotransmitters (norepinephrine and dopamine) and to increase the effects of other transmitters (serotonin, acetylcholine, and GABA).[23] Obviously, lithium has the potential to influence synaptic function and neural excitability in many ways. Exactly how this drug is able to stabilize mood and prevent the manic episodes associated with bipolar disorder remains to be determined.[5,32]

Absorption and Distribution

Lithium is readily absorbed from the gastrointestinal tract and completely distributed throughout all the tissues in the body. During an acute manic episode, achieving blood serum concentrations between 1.0 and 1.4 mEq/L is desirable. Maintenance doses are somewhat lower, and serum concentrations that range from 0.5 to 1.3 mEq/L are optimal.

Problems and Adverse Effects of Lithium

A major problem with lithium use is the danger of accumulation within the body.[27] Lithium is not metabolized, and drug elimination takes place almost exclusively through excretion in the urine. Consequently, lithium has a tendency to accumulate in the body, and toxic levels can frequently be reached during administration.

Side effects are frequent with lithium, and the degree and type depends on the amount of lithium in the bloodstream. As Table 7–4 indicates, some side effects are present even when serum levels are within the therapeutic range.[23] However, toxic side effects become more apparent when serum concentrations reach 1.5 mEq/L, and become severe when serum levels exceed 3.0 mEq/L.[23] Progressive accumulation of lithium can lead to seizures, coma, and even death. Consequently, clinicians with patients receiving lithium should be aware of any changes in behavior that might indicate that this drug is reaching toxic levels. These changes can usually be resolved by adjusting the dosage or using a sustained-release form of lithium.[27] Also, serum titers of lithium should be monitored periodically to ensure that blood levels remain within the therapeutic range.[27]

Other Drugs Used in Bipolar Disorder

Although lithium remains the cornerstone of treatment for bipolar disorder, it is now recognized that other agents may be helpful, especially during manic episodes. In particular, antiseizure medications such as carbamazepine, valproic acid, gabapentin, and lamotrigine may help stabilize mood and limit manic symptoms.[20,26,49] Antipsychotic medications, including the newer agents such as clozapine and resperidone (see Chapter 8), may also be helpful as antimanic drugs.[63,75] Antiseizure and antipsychotic drugs are believed to be helpful because they act directly on CNS neurons to

Table 7–4	SIDE EFFECTS AND TOXICITY OF LITHIUM	
Mild (Below 1.5 mEq/L)	**Moderate (1.5–3.0 mEq/L)**	**Severe (Above 3.0 mEq/L)**
Fine hand tremor (resting)	Confusion	Choreoathetoid movements
Gastrointestinal upset	Lethargy	Seizures
Muscle weakness	Ataxia	Respiratory complications
Fatigue	Dysarthria	Coma
Problems with memory and concentration	Nystagmus Emesis Increased deep tendon reflexes Increased tremor Muscle fasciculations	Death

Adapted from: Fankhauser, pp 1280–1281,[23] with permission.

help prevent the neuronal excitation that seems to precipitate manic symptoms.[10] (Details about the pharmacology of antipsychotic and antiseizure drugs are addressed in Chapters 8 and 9, respectively.) Hence, these drugs can be used initially, along with lithium, to decrease manic mood swings, or to simply stabilize mood at baseline levels and to prevent the mood swings that characterize bipolar disorder. These additional drugs may be discontinued when the mood is stabilized, or they may be administered alone or with lithium treatment as maintenance therapy in the long-term treatment of bipolar disorder.[28,39,51]

Special Concerns in Rehabilitation Patients

■ ■ ■ Some amount of depression is certain to be present as a result of a catastrophic injury or illness. Patients receiving physical therapy and occupational therapy for any number of acute or chronic illnesses may be taking antidepressants in order to improve their mood and general well-being. Of course, therapists working in a psychiatric facility will deal with many patients taking antidepressant drugs, and severe depression may be the primary reason the patient is institutionalized in the first place. However, these drugs are also frequently prescribed to patients with a spinal cord injury, stroke, severe burn, multiple sclerosis, amputation, and so on. Therapists must realize that adequate treatment of depression is a very difficult clinical task. Even with optimal pharmacologic and psychologic intervention, it is estimated that up to one third of patients with depression may not adequately respond.[4] Depression is a very serious and complex psychological disorder, and the effects of drug treatment vary greatly from individual to individual. It is therefore imperative that the physician and other health care professionals work closely with the patient and the patient's family to find the drug that produces optimal results with a minimum of side effects. Again, this task is complicated by many issues including the complex interplay of factors causing depression in each patient and their rather unpredictable response to each type of antidepressant.

With regard to the impact of antidepressant and antimanic agents on the rehabilitation process, these drugs can be extremely beneficial in helping to improve a patient's outlook. The patient may become more optimistic regarding the future and may assume a more active role and interest in the rehabilitation process. This behavior can be invaluable in increasing patient cooperation and improving compliance with rehabilitation goals. However, certain side effects can be somewhat troublesome during rehabilitation treatments. Sedation, lethargy, and muscle weakness can occur with the tricyclics and lithium, which can present a problem if the patient's active cooperation is required. Other unpleasant side effects, such as nausea and vomiting, can also be disturbing during treatments. A more common and potentially more serious problem is the orthostatic hypotension that occurs predominantly with the tricyclics. This hypotension can cause syncope and subsequent injury if patients fall during gait training. Conversely, MAO inhibitors can increase blood pressure, and care should be taken to avoid a hypertensive crisis, especially during therapy sessions that tend to increase blood pressure (e.g., certain forms of exercise). Hence, patients should also be monitored regularly to detect an increase or decrease in blood pressure depending on the drug and the patient.

Finally, rehabilitation specialists should remember that some improvement in mood may occur within 2 weeks after beginning antidepressant drug treatment, but that these agents must often be administered for 1 month or more before an appreciable improvement in symptoms occurs.[4] During this period, drug therapy may actually precipitate an increase in depression, including increased thoughts of suicide.[37] Rehabilitation specialists should keep alert for any signs that a patient is becoming more depressed and possibly suicidal, especially during the first few weeks after antidepressant drug therapy is initiated.

CASE STUDY

Antidepressant Drugs

Brief History. J.G., a 71-year-old retired pharmacist, was admitted to the hospital with a chief complaint of an inability to move his right arm and leg. He was also unable to speak at the time of admission. The clinical impression was right hemiplegia caused by left-middle cerebral artery thrombosis. The patient also had a history of hypertension and had been taking cardiac beta blockers for several years. J.G.'s medical condition stabilized, and the third day after admission he was seen for the first time by a physical therapist. Speech and occupational therapy were also soon initiated. The patient's condition improved rapidly, and motor function began to return in the right side. Balance and gross motor skills increased until he could transfer from his wheelchair to his bed with minimal assistance, and gait training activities were being initiated. J.G. was able to comprehend verbal commands, but his speech remained markedly slurred and difficult to understand. During his first 2 weeks in the hospital, J.G. showed signs of severe depression. Symptoms increased until cooperation with the rehabilitation and nursing staff was being compromised. Imipramine (Tofranil) was prescribed at a dosage of 150 mg/day.

Problem/Influence of Medication. Imipramine is a tricyclic antidepressant, and these drugs are known to produce orthostatic hypotension during the initial stages of drug therapy. Since the patient is expressively aphasic, he will have trouble telling the therapist that he feels dizzy or faint. Also, the cardiac beta blockers will blunt any compensatory increase in cardiac output if blood pressure drops during postural changes.

Decision/Solution. The therapist decided to place the patient on the tilt table for the first day after imipramine was started and to monitor blood pressure regularly. While the patient was on the tilt table, weight shifting and upper-extremity facilitation activities were performed. The patient tolerated this well, so the therapist had him resume ambulation activities using the parallel bars on the following day. With the patient standing inside the bars, the therapist carefully watched for any subjective signs of dizziness or syncope in the patient (i.e., facial pallor, inability to follow instructions). Standing bouts were also limited in duration. By the third day, ambulation training continued with the patient outside the parallel bars, but the therapist made a point of having the patient's wheelchair close at hand in case the patient began to appear faint. These precautions of careful observation and short, controlled bouts of ambulation were continued throughout the remainder of the patient's hospital stay, and no incident of orthostatic hypotension was observed during physical therapy.

SUMMARY

Affective disorders such as depression and manic-depression are found frequently in the general population as well as in rehabilitation patients. Drugs commonly prescribed in the treatment of (unipolar) depression include the tricyclics and MAO inhibitors as well as the newer second-generation antidepressants. Lithium is the drug of choice for treating bipolar disorder, or manic-depression. All of these drugs seem to exert their effects by modifying CNS synaptic transmission and receptor sensitivity in amine pathways. The exact manner in which these drugs affect synaptic activity has shed some light on the possible neuronal changes that underlie these forms of mental illness. Antidepressant and antimanic drugs can improve the patient's attitude and compliance during rehabilitation, but therapists should be aware that certain side effects may alter the patient's physical and mental behavior.

References

1. Adell A. Antidepressant properties of substance P antagonists: relationship to monoaminergic mechanisms? *Curr Drug Targets CNS Neurol Disord.* 2004; 3:113–121.
2. American Psychiatric Association. *Diagnostic and Statistical Manual of Mental Disorders–Revised.* 4th ed. Washington, DC: American Psychiatric Association; 1994.
3. Bair MJ, Robinson RL, Katon W, Kroenke K. Depression and pain comorbidity: a literature review. *Arch Intern Med.* 2003;163:2433–2445.
4. Baldessarini RJ. Drugs and the treatment of psychiatric disorders: depression and anxiety disorders. In: Hardman JG, et al., eds. *The Pharmacological Basis of Therapeutics.* 10th ed. New York: McGraw-Hill; 2001.
5. Baldessarini RJ, Tarazi FI. Drugs and the treatment of psychiatric disorders: psychosis and mania. In: Hardman JG, et al., eds. *The Pharmacological Basis of Therapeutics.* 10th ed. New York: McGraw-Hill; 2001.
6. Barbui C, Guaiana G, Hotopf M. Amitriptyline for inpatients and SSRIs for outpatients with depression?

Systematic review and meta-regression analysis. *Pharmacopsychiatry*. 2004;37:93–97.

7. Barden N. Implication of the hypothalamic-pituitary–adrenal axis in the physiopathology of depression. *J Psychiatry Neurosci*. 2004;29:185–193.

8. Bauer M, Alda M, Priller J, Young LT; International Group for the Study of Lithium Treated Patients (IGSLI). Implications of the neuroprotective effects of lithium for the treatment of bipolar and neurodegenerative disorders. *Pharmacopsychiatry*. 2003;36(suppl 3):S250–S254.

9. Bauer M, Whybrow PC, Angst J, et al. World Federation of Societies of Biological Psychiatry (WFSBP) guidelines for biological treatment of unipolar depressive disorders, part 2: Maintenance treatment of major depressive disorder and treatment of chronic depressive disorders and subthreshold depressions. *World J Biol Psychiatry*. 2002;3:69–86.

10. Belmaker RH. Bipolar disorder. *N Engl J Med*. 2004;351:476–486.

11. Benkert O, Muller M, Szegedi A. An overview of the clinical efficacy of mirtazapine. *Hum Psychopharmacol*. 2002;17(suppl 1):S23–S26.

12. Blier P. The pharmacology of putative early-onset antidepressant strategies. *Eur Neuropsychopharmacol*. 2003;13:57–66.

13. Blier P, Abbott FV. Putative mechanisms of action of antidepressant drugs in affective and anxiety disorders and pain. *J Psychiatry Neurosci*. 2001;26:37–43.

14. Briley M. New hope in the treatment of painful symptoms in depression. *Curr Opin Investig Drugs*. 2003;4:42–45.

15. Brown ES, Varghese FP, McEwen BS. Association of depression with medical illness: does cortisol play a role? *Biol Psychiatry*. 2004;55:1–9.

16. Bschor T, Lewitzka U, Sasse J, et al. Lithium augmentation in treatment-resistant depression: clinical evidence, serotonergic and endocrine mechanisms. *Pharmacopsychiatry*. 2003;36(suppl 3):S230–S234.

17. Cassano P, Fava M. Tolerability issues during long-term treatment with antidepressants. *Ann Clin Psychiatry*. 2004;16:15–25.

18. Charney DS, Manji HK. Life stress, genes, and depression: multiple pathways lead to increased risk and new opportunities for intervention. *Sci STKE*. 2004;2004(225):re5.

19. Deakin B, Dursun S. Optimizing antidepressant treatment: efficacy and tolerability. *Int Clin Psychopharmacol*. 2002;17(suppl 1):S13–S24.

20. Dunner DL. Drug interactions of lithium and other antimanic/mood stabilizing medications. *J Clin Psychiatry*. 2003;64(suppl 5):38–43.

21. Elhwuegi AS. Central monoamines and their role in major depression. *Prog Neuropsychopharmacol Biol Psychiatry*. 2004;28:435–451.

22. Ener RA, Meglathery SB, Van Decker WA, Gallagher RM. Serotonin syndrome and other serotonergic disorders. *Pain Med*. 2003;4:63–74.

23. Fankhauser MP. Bipolar disorder. In: DiPiro JT, et al., eds. *Pharmacotherapy: A Pathophysiologic Approach*. 5th ed. New York: McGraw-Hill; 2002.

24. Fava M. The role of the serotonergic and noradrenergic neurotransmitter systems in the treatment of psychological and physical symptoms of depression. *J Clin Psychiatry*. 2003;64(suppl 13):26–29.

25. Finfgeld DL. Serotonin syndrome and the use of SSRIs. *J Psychosoc Nurs Ment Health Serv*. 2004;42:16–20.

26. Goldsmith DR, Wagstaff AJ, Ibbotson T, Perry CM. Lamotrigine: a review of its use in bipolar disorder. *Drugs*. 2003;63:2029–2050.

27. Goodwin FK. Rationale for long-term treatment of bipolar disorder and evidence for long-term lithium treatment. *J Clin Psychiatry*. 2002;63(suppl 10):5–12.

28. Goodwin FK. Rationale for using lithium in combination with other mood stabilizers in the management of bipolar disorder. *J Clin Psychiatry*. 2003;64(suppl 5):18–24.

29. Grothe DR, Scheckner B, Albano D. Treatment of pain syndromes with venlafaxine. *Pharmacotherapy*. 2004;24:621–629.

30. Guaiana G, Barbui C, Hotopf M. Amitriptyline versus other types of pharmacotherapy for depression. *Cochrane Database Syst Rev*. 2003;CD004186.

31. Gupta RK, Tiller JW, Burrows GD. Dual action antidepressants and some important considerations. *Aust N Z J Psychiatry*. 2003;37:190–195.

32. Gurvich N, Klein PS. Lithium and valproic acid: parallels and contrasts in diverse signaling contexts. *Pharmacol Ther*. 2002;96:45–66.

33. Gutierrez MA, Stimmel GL, Aiso JY. Venlafaxine: a 2003 update. *Clin Ther*. 2003;25:2138–2154.

34. Hajos M, Fleishaker JC, Filipiak-Reisner JK, et al. The selective norepinephrine reuptake inhibitor antidepressant reboxetine: pharmacological and clinical profile. *CNS Drug Rev*. 2004;10:23–44.

35. Harwood AJ, Agam G. Search for a common mechanism of mood stabilizers. *Biochem Pharmacol*. 2003;66:179–189.

36. Hashimoto K, Shimizu E, Iyo M. Critical role of brain-derived neurotrophic factor in mood disorders. *Brain Res Brain Res Rev*. 2004;45:104–114.

37. Healy D, Whitaker C. Antidepressants and suicide: risk–benefit conundrums. *J Psychiatry Neurosci*. 2003;28:331–337.

38. Heim C, Plotsky PM, Nemeroff CB. Importance of studying the contributions of early adverse experience to neurobiological findings in depression. *Neuropsychopharmacology*. 2004;29:641–648.

39. Herman E. Lamotrigine: a depression mood stabiliser. *Eur Neuropsychopharmacol*. 2004;14(suppl 2):S89–S93.

40. Joels M, Verkuyl JM, Van Riel E. Hippocampal and hypothalamic function after chronic stress. *Ann N Y Acad Sci*. 2003;1007:367–378.

41. Jonas BS, Brody D, Roper M, Narrow WE. Prevalence of mood disorders in a national sample of young American adults. *Soc Psychiatry Psychiatr Epidemiol*. 2003;38:618–624.

42. Kempermann G, Kronenberg G. Depressed new neurons—adult hippocampal neurogenesis and a cellular plasticity hypothesis of major depression. *Biol Psychiatry*. 2003;54:499–503.

43. Kessler RC, McGonagle KA, Zhao S, et al. Lifetime and 12-month prevalence of DSM-III-R psychiatric disorders in the United States. Results from the national comorbidity survey. *Arch Gen Psychiatry.* 1994;51:8–19.

44. Kleindienst N, Greil W. Lithium in the long-term treatment of bipolar disorders. *Eur Arch Psychiatry Clin Neurosci.* 2003;253:120–125.

45. Lawson K. Tricyclic antidepressants and fibromyalgia: what is the mechanism of action? *Expert Opin Investig Drugs.* 2002;11:1437–1445.

46. Lesch KP. Gene-environment interaction and the genetics of depression. *J Psychiatry Neurosci.* 2004;29:174–184.

47. Lucki I, O'Leary OF. Distinguishing roles for norepinephrine and serotonin in the behavioral effects of antidepressant drugs. *J Clin Psychiatry.* 2004;65(suppl 4):11–24.

48. MacGillivray S, Arroll B, Hatcher S, et al. Efficacy and tolerability of selective serotonin reuptake inhibitors compared with tricyclic antidepressants in depression treated in primary care: systematic review and meta-analysis. *BMJ.* 2003;326:1014.

49. Macritchie K, Geddes JR, Scott J, et al. Valproate for acute mood episodes in bipolar disorder. *Cochrane Database Syst Rev.* 2003;CD004052.

50. Malberg JE. Implications of adult hippocampal neurogenesis in antidepressant action. *J Psychiatry Neurosci.* 2004;29:196–205.

51. Malhi GS, Mitchell PB, Salim S. Bipolar depression: management options. *CNS Drugs.* 2003;17:9–25.

52. Mattia C, Coluzzi F. Antidepressants in chronic neuropathic pain. *Mini Rev Med Chem.* 2003;3:773–784.

53. Nierenberg AA, Papakostas GI, Petersen T, et al. Nortriptyline for treatment-resistant depression. *J Clin Psychiatry.* 2003;64:35–39.

54. Nutt DJ. The neuropharmacology of serotonin and noradrenaline in depression. *Int Clin Psychopharmacol.* 2002;17(suppl 1):S1–S12.

55. Page ME. The promises and pitfalls of reboxetine. *CNS Drug Rev.* 2003;9:327–342.

56. Paul IA, Skolnick P. Glutamate and depression: clinical and preclinical studies. *Ann N Y Acad Sci.* 2003;1003:250–272.

57. Paykel ES. Life events and affective disorders. *Acta Psychiatr Scand Suppl.* 2003;418:61–66.

58. Peretti S, Judge R, Hindmarch I. Safety and tolerability considerations: tricyclic antidepressants vs. selective serotonin reuptake inhibitors. *Acta Psychiatr Scand Suppl.* 2000;403:17–25.

59. Porter RJ, Gallagher P, Watson S, Young AH. Corticosteroid-serotonin interactions in depression: a review of the human evidence. *Psychopharmacology (Berl).* 2004;173:1–17.

60. Reisner L. Antidepressants for chronic neuropathic pain. *Curr Pain Headache Rep.* 2003;7:24–33.

61. Richelson E. Interactions of antidepressants with neurotransmitter transporters and receptors and their clinical relevance. *J Clin Psychiatry.* 2003;64(suppl 13):5–12.

62. Roose SP. Compliance: the impact of adverse events and tolerability on the physician's treatment decisions. *Eur Neuropsychopharmacol.* 2003;13(suppl 3):S85–S92.

63. Sachs GS. Unmet clinical needs in bipolar disorder. *J Clin Psychopharmacol.* 2003;23(suppl 1):S2–S8.

64. Sampson SM. Treating depression with selective serotonin reuptake inhibitors: a practical approach. *Mayo Clin Proc.* 2001;76:739–744.

65. Schnitzer TJ, Ferraro A, Hunsche E, Kong SX. A comprehensive review of clinical trials on the efficacy and safety of drugs for the treatment of low back pain. *J Pain Symptom Manage.* 2004;28:72–95.

66. Sheline YI, Mittler BL, Mintun MA. The hippocampus and depression. *Eur Psychiatry.* 2002;17(suppl 3):300–305.

67. Stahl SM, Grady MM. Differences in mechanism of action between current and future antidepressants. *J Clin Psychiatry.* 2003;64(suppl 13):13–17.

68. Tafet GE, Bernardini R. Psychoneuroendocrinological links between chronic stress and depression. *Prog Neuropsychopharmacol Biol Psychiatry.* 2003;27:893–903.

69. Thase ME. Effectiveness of antidepressants: comparative remission rates. *J Clin Psychiatry.* 2003;64(suppl 2):3–7.

70. Vaswani M, Linda FK, Ramesh S. Role of selective serotonin reuptake inhibitors in psychiatric disorders: a comprehensive review. *Prog Neuropsychopharmacol Biol Psychiatry.* 2003;27:85–102.

71. Waraich P, Goldner EM, Somers JM, Hsu L. Prevalence and incidence studies of mood disorders: a systematic review of the literature. *Can J Psychiatry.* 2004;49:124–138.

72. Whyte IM, Dawson AH, Buckley NA. Relative toxicity of venlafaxine and selective serotonin reuptake inhibitors in overdose compared to tricyclic antidepressants. *QJM.* 2003;96:369–374.

73. Wong ML, Licinio J. From monoamines to genomic targets: a paradigm shift for drug discovery in depression. *Nat Rev Drug Discov.* 2004;3:136–151.

74. Yamada M, Yasuhara H. Clinical pharmacology of MAO inhibitors: safety and future. *Neurotoxicology.* 2004;25:215–221.

75. Yatham LN. Acute and maintenance treatment of bipolar mania: the role of atypical antipsychotics. *Bipolar Disord.* 2003;5(suppl 2):7–19.

76. Youdim MB, Weinstock M. Therapeutic applications of selective and non selective inhibitors of monoamine oxidase A and B that do not cause significant tyramine potentiation. *Neurotoxicology.* 2004;25:243–250.

Antipsychotic Drugs

Psychosis is the term used to describe the more severe forms of mental illness. Psychoses are actually a group of mental disorders characterized by marked thought disturbance and an impaired perception of reality. The most common form of psychosis by far is schizophrenia; it is estimated that 1 percent of the world population has the disorder.[23,47] Other psychotic disorders include psychotic depression and severe paranoid disorders. In the past, strong, sedativelike drugs were the primary method of treating patients with psychosis. The goal was to pacify these patients so that they were no longer combative and abusive to themselves and others. These drugs were commonly referred to as "major tranquilizers" and had the obvious disadvantage of sedating a patient so that his or her cognitive and motor skills were compromised.

As researchers learned more about the neurologic changes involved in psychosis, drugs were developed to specifically treat disorders rather than simply sedate the patient. These antipsychotic drugs, or **neuroleptics,** as some clinicians refer to them, represent a major breakthrough in the treatment of schizophrenia and other psychotic disorders.

Physical and occupational therapists frequently encounter patients taking antipsychotics. Therapists employed in a psychiatric facility will routinely treat patients taking these medications. Therapists who practice in nonpsychiatric settings may still encounter these patients for various reasons. For instance, a patient on an antipsychotic medication who sustains a fractured hip may be seen at an orthopedic facility. Consequently, knowledge of antipsychotic pharmacology will be useful to all rehabilitation specialists.

Because of the prevalence of schizophrenia, this chapter concentrates on the treatment of this psychotic disorder. Also, the pathogenesis and subsequent treatment of other forms of psychosis are similar to those of schizophrenia, and this specific condition will be used as an example of the broader range of psychotic conditions.

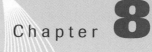

Schizophrenia

The *Diagnostic and Statistical Manual of Mental Disorders* lists several distinct criteria necessary for a diagnosis of schizophrenia.[5] These criteria include a marked disturbance in the thought process, which may include bizarre delusions and auditory hallucinations (i.e., "hearing voices"). Also, a decreased level of function in work, social relations, and self-care may be present. Other factors include the duration of these and additional symptoms (at least 6 months) and a differential diagnosis from other forms of mental illness (such as affective disorders and organic brain syndrome).

The exact cause of schizophrenia has been the subject of extensive research. It appears that genetic factors (i.e., chromosomal abnormalities that cause deviations in brain structure and function) are the primary risk factors in the majority of people with schizophrenia (70% to 80%).[15,23] Environmental factors (social stresses, prenatal or childhood brain injury, and so forth) seem to be the underlying cause in the remaining 20% to 30% of people with schizophrenia.[23] The precise role of these factors, and the interplay between genetic and environmental factors, continues to be elucidated.[28,50, 61]

The advent of antipsychotic drugs represents one of the most significant developments in the treatment of schizophrenia and similar disorders. These drugs are believed to be the single most important reason for the abrupt decrease in the number of mental patients admitted to public hospitals during the 1950s and 1960s.[22] This observation does not imply that these drugs cure schizophrenia. Schizophrenia and other psychoses are believed to be incurable, and psychotic episodes can recur throughout a patient's lifetime. However, these drugs can normalize the patient's behavior and thinking during an acute psychotic episode, and maintenance dosages are believed to help prevent the recurrence of psychosis. Consequently, the ability of people with psychosis to take care of themselves and cooperate with others is greatly improved.

Neurotransmitter Changes in Schizophrenia

Schizophrenia appears to be caused by an overactivity of dopamine pathways in certain parts of the brain such as the limbic system.[2,23] This idea is based primarily on the fact that most antipsychotics block dopamine receptors, thereby reducing dopaminergic hyperactivity in mesolimbic pathways and other limbic structures (see the next section of this chapter). The increased dopamine influence underlying psychosis could be caused by excessive dopamine synthesis and release by the presynaptic neuron, decreased dopamine breakdown at the synapse, increased postsynaptic dopamine receptor sensitivity, or a combination of these and other factors.

Consequently, increased dopamine transmission in areas such as the limbic system seems to be the primary neurochemical change associated with schizophrenia and other psychotic syndromes. However, given the complexity of central neurotransmitter interaction, changes in dopamine activity in the limbic system will almost certainly result in changes in other neurotransmitters in other parts of the brain. Indeed, there is substantial evidence that individuals with psychosis might also have decreased activity in cortical pathways that use glutamate as a neurotransmitter,[15,37,41] and it seems likely that other transmitters such as gamma-aminobutyric acid (GABA) and 5-hydroxytriptamine (serotonin) may also be affected during the pathogenesis and treatment.[16,23] Moreover, the increased dopamine activity in subcortical structures may result in an *decreased* activity in cortical dopamine activity.[2] This imbalance in dopamine activity in different brain regions might explain the different symptoms associated with psychosis. That is, positive symptoms such as agitation and hallucinations might be caused by excess dopamine influence in subcortical regions, whereas negative symptoms such as withdrawn behavior and cognitive

impairment might result from diminished cortical dopamine activity.[1]

Hence, it appears that the primary neurochemical change in schizophrenia is increased dopamine activity in certain limbic structures, but that this dopamine hyperactivity brings about subsequent changes in neurotransmitter activity in other areas of the brain as well. Resolving all these neurochemical changes might ultimately provide optimal treatment for people with schizophrenia and other forms of psychosis. For now, however, antipsychotic drugs are mainly focused on resolving the increased dopaminergic activity that seems to initiate psychosis. These drugs are discussed in more detail in the next sections of this chapter.

Antipsychotic Mechanism of Action

Antipsychotic drugs used to successfully treat schizophrenia block central dopamine receptors to some extent (Fig. 8–1).[19,23] These drugs share some structural similarity to dopamine, which allows them to bind to the postsynaptic receptor, but they do not activate it. This action effectively blocks the receptor from the effects of the released endogenous neurotransmitter (see Fig. 8–1). Any increased activity at central dopamine synapses is therefore negated by a postsynaptic receptor blockade.

It has become evident, however, that there are several subcategories of dopamine receptors, and these receptor subtypes are identified as D1, D2, D3,

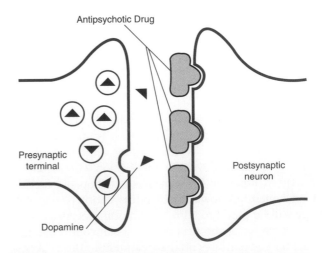

FIGURE 8–1 ▼ Effects of antipsychotic drugs on dopamine synapses. Antipsychotics act as postsynaptic receptor antagonists to block the effects of overactive dopamine transmission.

and so on.[18] The clinical effects and side effects of specific antipsychotic medications are therefore related to their ability to affect certain dopamine receptor populations. The receptor that appears to be most important in mediating antipsychotic effects is the D2 receptor subtype.[32,51] Most antipsychotic medications therefore have some ability to block the D2 subtype. It is also clear, however, that other dopamine receptor subtypes play a role in the pathogenesis of psychosis, and that certain antipsychotic drugs may produce specific effects because of their affinity for specific receptor subtypes. For example, newer antipsychotics such as clozapine block D4 receptors, and this action may help explain differences in the effects and side effects of these drugs.[62]

Consequently, antipsychotic drugs all share a basic mechanism of action that involves dopamine receptor blockade. It is apparent, however, that they are not all equal in their ability to affect specific subtypes of dopamine receptors, and that their effectiveness and side effects are related to their affinity and preference for certain receptors. As indicated earlier, other neurotransmitters may also be involved in the pathogenesis of psychosis, and differences in specific antipsychotic medications may be related to their ability to directly or indirectly affect these other transmitters as well as block dopamine influence. Future studies will continue to clarify how current antipsychotics exert their beneficial effects and how new agents can be developed to be more selective in their effects on dopamine and other neurotransmitter pathways.

Antipsychotic Medications

Antipsychotic medications are listed in Tables 8–1 and 8–2. These agents comprise a somewhat diverse group in terms of their chemical background and potency—that is, the dosage range typically needed to achieve antipsychotic effects. As indicated earlier, these agents all block dopamine receptors to some extent, despite their chemical diversity. In addition to their chemical differences, antipsychotics can be classified as either traditional agents or newer "atypical" antipsychotics according to their efficacy and side effects. Differences between these two classes are described here.

Traditional Antipsychotics

Traditional antipsychotics are associated with more side effects than newer counterparts, including an in-creased incidence of extrapyramidal (motor) side effects. This increased risk may be due to the traditional agents' tendencies to bind to several types of CNS dopamine receptors, including the receptors that influence motor function. This fact seems especially true for high-potency traditional agents such as haloperidol (Haldol) and fluphenazine (Prolixin). These agents have a strong affinity for CNS dopamine receptors and can exert beneficial effects when used in low dosages (see Table 8–1). Other traditional agents such as chlorpromazine (Thorazine) and thioridazine (Mellaril) have lower potency and must be used in high dosages to exert an antipsychotic effect. These low-potency agents tend to cause fewer extrapyramidal (motor) side effects but are associated with an increased incidence of other problems, such as sedative and anticholinergic side effects (e.g., dry mouth, constipation, urinary retention). These side effects and their possible long-term implications are discussed further in this chapter.

Traditional agents are also somewhat less predictable, and there tends to be more patient-to-patient variability in the beneficial (antipsychotic) effects of these medications.[18] Newer atypical drugs may be somewhat safer and more predictable, and these agents are described next.

Atypical Antipsychotics

Several newer antipsychotic medications have been developed that seem different or "atypical," compared with their predecessors. These agents include clozapine (Clozaril), risperidone (Risperdal), and several others listed in Tables 8–1 and 8–2. Although there is some debate about what exactly defines these drugs as "atypical," the most distinguishing feature is that they have a much better side-effect profile, including a decreased risk of producing extrapyramidal (motor) side effects.[17,45,57]

These newer, atypical agents seem to affect certain dopamine receptor subtypes differently than the older, more conventional drugs. In particular, the atypicals do not block the D2 receptors in the basal ganglia as strongly as conventional antipsychotics, hence their reduced risk of motor side effects.[52] There is also evidence that these drugs might have beneficial effects on other neurotransmitters, including glutamate, serotonin, and acetylcholine.[6,23,52] These additional effects might add to their antipsychotic benefits by improving cognition and reducing the incidence of other problems such as social withdrawal.[52]

Table 8-1	COMMON ANTIPSYCHOTIC DRUGS		
Generic Name	**Trade Name**	**Usual Dosage Range (mg/d)***	**Maximum recommended dosage (mg/d)****
Aripiprazole***	Abilify	10–30	30
Chlorpromazine	Thorazine	100–800	1000
Clozapine***	Clozaril	50–600	900
Fluphenazine	Permitil, Prolixin	2–20	40
Haloperidol	Haldol	2–20	100
Loxapine	Loxitane	10–80	250
Molindone	Moban	10–100	225
Mesoridazine	Serentil	50–400	500
Olanzapine***	Zyprexa	10–20	20
Perphenazine	Trilafon, Triavil	10–64	64
Prochlorperazine	Comazol, Compazine	15–150	150
Quetiapine***	Seroquel	250–600	800
Risperidone***	Risperdal	2–6	16
Thioridazine	Mellaril	100–800	800
Thiothixene	Navane	4–40	60
Trifluoperazine	Stelazine	5–40	80
Triflupromazine	Vesprin	6–150	150
Ziprasidone***	Geodon	40–160	200

*Dosage range represents usual adult oral dose. Lower dosages may be indicated for older or debilitated patients.
**Maximum recommended dosage represents the upper limit that can be administered each day to control severe psychotic symptoms, usually in hospitalized patients.
***Atypical antipsychotics. See text for details.

Regarding efficacy, the newer atypical agents seem to be at least as effective as the conventional drugs, but the atypical drugs can reduce the incidence of relapse compared to conventional agents.[23,46] Given the therapeutic benefits and reduced risk of side effects, these atypical drugs are usually considered first when treating psychosis.[23] If these atypical drugs are not effective, the more conventional or traditional agents are administered.[23,45]

Pharmacokinetics

Antipsychotics are usually administered orally. During the acute stage of a psychotic episode, the daily dosage is often divided into three or four equal amounts. Maintenance doses are usually lower and can often be administered once each day. Under certain conditions, antipsychotics can be given intramuscularly.

Table 8–2	SIDE EFFECTS OF TRADITIONAL AND ATYPICAL ANTIPSYCHOTIC DRUGS*		
Drug	**Sedation**	**Extrapyramidal Effects**	**Anticholinergic Effects**
		Traditional antipsychotics	
Chlorpromazine	++++	+++	+++
Fluphenazine	+	++++	+
Haloperidol	+	++++	+
Loxapine	+++	+++	++
Mesoridazine	+++	+	++
Molindone	+	+++	++
Perphenazine	++	+++	++
Prochlorperazine	++	++++	+
Thioridazine	++++	+++	++++
Thiothixene	+	++++	+
Trifluoperazine	++	+++	++
Triflupromazine	+++	+++	++++
		Atypical antipsychotics	
Aripiprazole	++	+	+
Clozapine	++++	+	++++
Olanzapine	++	++	++
Quetiapine	++	+	+
Risperidone	+	++	+
Ziprasidone	++	++	+

*Incidence of side effects are classified as follows: + a very low incidence, ++ a low incidence, +++ a moderate incidence, and ++++ a high incidence.

During acute episodes, intramuscular injections tend to reach the bloodstream faster than an orally administered drug and may be used if the patient is especially agitated.

Conversely, certain forms of intramuscular antipsychotics that enter the bloodstream slowly have been developed. This method of "depot administration" may prove helpful if the patient has poor self-adherence to drug therapy and neglects to take his or her medication regularly.[10,34] For example, depot preparations of conventional antipsychotics such as fluphenazine decanoate and haloperidol decanoate, can be injected every 2 to 4 weeks, respectively, and serve as a method of slow, continual release during the maintenance phase of psychosis.[4] More recently, an injectable form of risperidone, an atypical antipsychotic, has been developed, and this product might provide beneficial long-term effects with fewer side effects.[10,26]

Metabolism of antipsychotics is through two mechanisms: conjugation with glucuronic acid and oxidation by hepatic microsomal enzymes. Both mechanisms of metabolism and subsequent inactivation take place in the liver. Some degree of enzyme induction may occur because of prolonged use of antipsychotics, which may be responsible for increasing the rate of metabolism of these drugs.

Other Uses of Antipsychotics

Occasionally, antipsychotics are prescribed for conditions other than classic psychosis. As discussed in Chapter 7, an antipsychotic can be used alone or combined with lithium during an acute manic phase of bipolar disorder.[9,43] These drugs are also effective in decreasing nausea and vomiting occurring when dopamine agonists and precursors are administered to treat Parkinson disease. The antiemetic effect of antipsychotics is probably caused by their ability to block dopamine receptors located on the brainstem that cause vomiting when stimulated by the exogenous dopamine.

Antipsychotics are often used in Alzheimer disease and other cases of dementia to help control aggression and agitation.[7,38,58] There is concern, however, that these agents should be used carefully in patients with Alzheimer disease, and that these drugs should not be overused just to sedate these patients. Likewise, side effects should be minimized by considering one of the newer atypical agents, and by using the lowest effective dose.[33,38,40] Still, additional research is needed to determine how these drugs can be used most effectively to improve quality of life in people with various forms of dementia.[27,30,56]

Problems and Adverse Effects

Extrapyramidal Symptoms

One of the more serious problems occurring from the use of antipsychotics is the production of abnormal movement patterns.[36,44] Many of these aberrant movements are similar to those seen in patients with lesions of the extrapyramidal system and are often referred to as extrapyramidal side effects. The basic reason that these motor problems occur is because dopamine is an important neurotransmitter in motor pathways, especially in the integration of motor function that takes place in the basal ganglia. Because antipsychotic drugs block CNS dopamine receptors, it makes sense that

motor side effects are a potential complication. The unintentional antagonism of dopamine receptors in areas of motor integration (as opposed to the beneficial blockade of behaviorally related receptors) results in a neurotransmitter imbalance that creates several distinct types of movement problems.

Thus, most antipsychotics are associated with some type of motor side effect because these drugs are relatively nonselective in their ability to block CNS dopamine receptors. As noted earlier, the newer (atypical) agents such as clozapine and resperidone are not associated with as high an incidence of extrapyramidal side effects. Several hypotheses exist to explain the lower incidence, including the idea that the atypical antipsychotics block serotonin receptors more than the dopamine type 2 (D2) receptors associated with motor side effects.[13] Alternatively, it has been proposed that atypical agents block dopamine receptors long enough to cause a therapeutic effect, but not long enough to cause receptor supersensitivity and other changes that result in motor side effects.[13] The exact reasons for their lower incidence of extrapyramidal side effects, however, is not known.

At present, however, extrapyramidal side effects continue to be one of the major drawbacks of antipsychotic medications. The primary types of extrapyramidal side effects, the manifestations of each type, and the relative time of their onset are shown in Figure 8–2. Some factors involved in patient susceptibility and possible treatment of these side effects are discussed here.

Tardive Dyskinesia. The disorder of **tardive dyskinesia** is characterized by a number of involuntary and fragmented movements.[21] In particular, rhythmic movements of the mouth, tongue, and jaw are present, and the patient often produces involuntary sucking and smacking noises. Because this condition often involves the tongue and orofacial musculature, serious swallowing disorders (dysphagia) may also occur.[55] Other symptoms include choreoathetoid movements of the extremities and dystonias of the neck and trunk. As indicated in Table 8–2, certain antipsychotics, such as the traditional high-potency drugs, are associated with a greater incidence of tardive dyskinesia. Other risk factors include advanced patient age, affective mood disorders, diabetes mellitus, history of alcohol abuse, and continual use of the drug for 6 months or longer.[18,29,49] On the other hand, use of newer, atypical antipsychotics is associated with a much lower risk of tardive dyskinesia, even in high-risk patients.[20,31] Still, tardive dyskinesia is relatively common, with an estimated prevalence of 24% of people with chronic psychosis.[36]

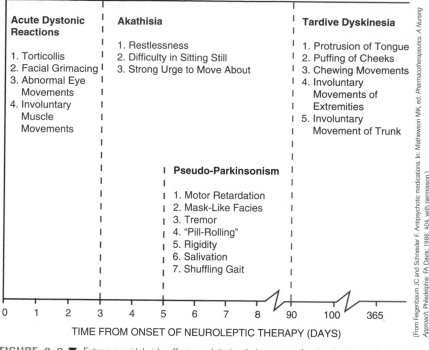

Acute Dystonic Reactions	Akathisia	Tardive Dyskinesia
1. Torticollis 2. Facial Grimacing 3. Abnormal Eye Movements 4. Involuntary Muscle Movements	1. Restlessness 2. Difficulty in Sitting Still 3. Strong Urge to Move About	1. Protrusion of Tongue 2. Puffing of Cheeks 3. Chewing Movements 4. Involuntary Movements of Extremities 5. Involuntary Movement of Trunk

Pseudo-Parkinsonism

1. Motor Retardation
2. Mask-Like Facies
3. Tremor
4. "Pill-Rolling"
5. Rigidity
6. Salivation
7. Shuffling Gait

0 1 2 3 4 5 6 7 8   90 100 365

TIME FROM ONSET OF NEUROLEPTIC THERAPY (DAYS)

(From Feigenbaum JC and Schneider F. Antipsychotic medications. In: Mathewson MK, ed. *Pharmacotherapeutics: A Nursing Approach.* Philadelphia: FA Davis; 1986: 404, with permission.)

FIGURE 8–2 ▼ Extrapyramidal side effects and their relative onset after beginning antipsychotic drug therapy.

Tardive dyskinesia induced by antipsychotic drugs may be caused by "disuse supersensitivity" of the dopamine receptor.[12,36] Although the presynaptic neurons are still intact, drug blockade of the postsynaptic receptor induces the postsynaptic neuron to respond by "up-regulating" the number or sensitivity of the receptors. This increase in receptor sensitivity causes a functional increase in dopaminergic influence, leading to a neurotransmitter imbalance between dopamine and other central neurotransmitters such as acetylcholine and GABA. In addition, changes in the structure of striatonigral neurons and other brain structures appear to accompany the functional changes in neurotransmitter sensitivity.[12,36] These functional and structural changes result in the symptoms of tardive dyskinesia.

Tardive dyskinesia is the most feared side effect of antipsychotic drugs.[24] In some patients, the symptoms will disappear if the drug is stopped or if the dosage is decreased, but this can take from several weeks to several years to occur. In other individuals, drug-induced tardive dyskinesia appears irreversible.[24] To prevent the occurrence of tardive dyskinesia, the lowest effective dose of the antipsychotic should be used, especially during the maintenance phase of drug therapy.[18] Also, patients taking these drugs for three months or more should undergo periodic reevaluation for any

symptoms of tardive dyskinesia.[18] The motor symptoms of tardive dyskinesia can be dealt with by lowering the drug dosage or by substituting an antipsychotic that produces fewer extrapyramidal side effects (see Table 8–2). Early intervention is generally believed to be the most effective way of preventing the permanent changes associated with antipsychotic-induced tardive dyskinesia.[21]

Other drugs have been used to try to alleviate the symptoms of drug-induced tardive dyskinesia.[53,54] Agents such as anticholinergic drugs (e.g., atropinelike drugs), GABA-enhancing drugs (e.g., benzodiazepines), and calcium channel blockers have been used to attempt to rectify the transmitter imbalance or the cellular changes created by the increased dopamine sensitivity. Reserpine has also been used in some patients because of its ability to deplete presynaptic stores of dopamine, thus limiting the influence of this neurotransmitter. However, these additional agents tend to be only marginally successful in reducing the dyskinesia symptoms, and their use tends to add complexity to the drug management of patients with psychoses. Thus, the best course of action continues to be judicious administration of these drugs, using the lowest effective dose, and early recognition and intervention if extrapyramidal symptoms appear.[18]

Pseudoparkinsonism. The motor symptoms seen in Parkinson disease (see Chapter 10) are caused by a deficiency in dopamine transmission in the basal ganglia. Because antipsychotic drugs block dopamine receptors, some patients may understandably experience symptoms similar to those seen in Parkinson disease. These symptoms include resting tremor, bradykinesia, and rigidity. Elderly patients are more susceptible to these drug-induced parkinsonian-like symptoms, probably because dopamine content (and therefore dopaminergic influence) tends to be lower in older individuals.[22] The outcome of antipsychotic-induced parkinsonism is usually favorable, and these symptoms normally disappear when the dosage is adjusted or the drug is withdrawn. Drugs used as adjuncts in treating Parkinson disease (e.g., amantadine, benztropine mesylate) may also be administered to deal with parkinsonianlike side effects.[11] However, primary antiparkinsonian drugs such as levodopa and dopamine agonists are not typically used to treat these side effects because they tend to exacerbate the psychotic symptoms.

Akathisia. Patients taking antipsychotics may experience sensations of motor restlessness and may complain of an inability to sit or lie still. This condition is known as **akathisia**.[25,35] Patients may also appear agitated, may "pace the floor," and may have problems with insomnia. Akathisia can usually be dealt with by altering the dosage or type of medication. If this is unsuccessful, beta-2 adrenergic receptor blockers (propranolol) may help decrease the restlessness associated with akathisia by a mechanism involving central adrenergic receptors.[25] Anticholinergic drugs may also be used to treat akathisia, but it is not clear if these drugs actually reduce symptoms associated with akathisia.[42]

Dyskinesia and Dystonias. Patients may exhibit a broad range of movements in the arms, legs, neck, and face including torticollis, oculogyric crisis, and opisthotonos.[8] These movements are involuntary and uncoordinated, and may begin fairly soon after initiating antipsychotic therapy (i.e., even after a single dose).[8] If they persist during therapy, other drugs such as antiparkinsonian adjuncts or benzodiazepines (e.g., diazepam) may be used to try to combat the aberrant motor symptoms.

Neuroleptic Malignant Syndrome. Patients taking relatively high doses of the more potent antipsychotics may experience a serious disorder known as neuroleptic malignant syndrome (NMS).[48] Symptoms of NMS include catatonia, stupor, rigidity, tremors, and fever.[14] These symptoms are rather severe, and can lead to death if left untreated.[48] Treatment typically consists of stopping the antipsychotic drug and providing supportive care. The exact causes of NMS are unclear, but the risk of developing this syndrome is increased in patients who are mentally retarded, who are agitated, or when traditional antipsychotics are administered at high doses or via intramuscular injection.[60]

Nonmotor Effects

Sedation

Antipsychotics have varying degrees of sedative properties. Contrary to previous beliefs, sedative properties do not enhance the antipsychotic efficacy of these drugs. Consequently, sedative side effects offer no benefit and can be detrimental in withdrawn psychotic patients.

Anticholinergic Effects

Some antipsychotics also produce significant anticholinergic effects, manifested by a variety of symptoms such as blurred vision, dry mouth, constipation, and urinary retention. Fortunately, these problems are usually self-limiting as many patients become tolerant to the anticholinergic side effects while remaining responsive to the antipsychotic properties.

Other Side Effects

Orthostatic hypotension is a frequent problem during the initial stages of antipsychotic therapy. This problem usually disappears after a few days. Certain antipsychotic drugs such as chlorpromazine are associated with photosensitivity, and care should be taken when exposing these patients to ultraviolet irradiation. The newer, atypical drugs can produce metabolic side effects that result in substantial weight gain, increased plasma lipids, and diabetes mellitus.[3,39] Thus, these newer drugs pose less risk of motor symptoms, but can cause side effects that ultimately produce serious cardiovascular and endocrine problems.[3,59] Finally, abrupt withdrawal of antipsychotic drugs after prolonged use often results in nausea and vomiting, so it is advisable to decrease dosage gradually rather than to suddenly stop administration.

Special Concerns in Rehabilitation Patients

■ ■ ■ Antipsychotic drugs have been a great benefit to patients seen in various rehabilitation facilities. Regardless of the reason these individuals are referred to physical therapy and occupational therapy, the improved behavior and reality perception usually provided by drug therapy will surely enhance the patient's cooperation during rehabilitation. Because these drugs tend to normalize patient behavior, the withdrawn patient often becomes more active and amiable, while the agitated patient becomes calmer and more relaxed. Also, remission of some confusion and impaired thinking will enable the patient to follow instructions more easily. Patients with paranoid symptoms may have fewer delusions of persecution and will feel less threatened by the entire therapy environment.

The benefits of antipsychotic drugs must be weighed against their side effect risks. The less serious side effects such as sedation and some of the anticholinergic effects (blurred vision, dry mouth, constipation) can be bothersome during the treatment session. Orthostatic hypotension should be guarded against, especially during the first few days after drug therapy is initiated. However, the major problems have to do with the antipsychotic drug's extrapyramidal motor effects. Therapists treating patients on antipsychotic medications should remain alert for early signs of motor involvement. Chances are good that the therapist may be the first person to notice a change in posture, balance, or involuntary movements. Even subtle problems in motor function should be brought to the attention of the medical staff immediately. This early intervention may diminish the risk of long-term or even permanent motor dysfunction.

CASE STUDY

Antipsychotic Drugs

Brief History. R.F., a 63-year-old woman, has been receiving treatment for schizophrenia intermittently for many years. She was last hospitalized for an acute episode 7 months ago and has since been on a maintenance dosage of haloperidol (Haldol), 25 mg/d. She is also being seen as an outpatient for treatment of rheumatoid arthritis in both hands. Her current treatment consists of gentle heat and active range-of-motion exercises, three times each week. She is being considered for possible metacarpophalangeal joint replacement.

Problem/Influence of Medication. During the course of physical therapy, the therapist noticed the onset and slow, progressive increase in writhing gestures of both upper extremities. Extraneous movements of her mouth and face were also observed, including chewinglike jaw movements and tongue protrusion.

Decision/Solution. These initial extrapyramidal symptoms suggested the onset of tardive dyskinesia. The therapist notified the patient's physician, and drug therapy was progressively shifted from haloperidol to the atypical agent clozapine (Clozaril), 450 mg/d. The extrapyramidal symptoms gradually diminished over the next 8 weeks and ultimately disappeared.

SUMMARY

Antipsychotic drugs represent one of the major advances in the management of mental illness. Drugs are currently available that diminish the symptoms of psychosis and improve a patient's ability to cooperate with others and to administer self-care. Despite their chemical diversity, antipsychotics all seem to exert beneficial effects by blocking central dopamine receptors. Therefore, psychoses such as schizophrenia may be caused by an overactivity of CNS dopaminergic pathways.

Because of the rather nonspecific blockade of dopaminergic receptors, antipsychotics are associated with several adverse side effects. The most serious of these are abnormal movement patterns that resemble tardive dyskinesia, Parkinson disease, and other lesions associated with the extrapyramidal system. In some cases, these aberrant motor activities may become irreversible and persist even after drug therapy is terminated. Rehabilitation specialists may play a critical role in recognizing the early onset of these motor abnormalities. When identified early, potentially serious motor problems can be dealt with by altering the dosage or type of antipsychotic agent.

References

1. Abi-Dargham A. Do we still believe in the dopamine hypothesis? New data bring new evidence. *Int J Neuropsychopharmacol.* 2004;7(suppl 1): S1–S5.
2. Abi-Dargham A, Moore H. Prefrontal DA transmission at D1 receptors and the pathology of schizophrenia. *Neuroscientist.* 2003;9:404–416.
3. Abidi S, Bhaskara SM. From chlorpromazine to clozapine—antipsychotic adverse effects and the clinician's dilemma. *Can J Psychiatry.* 2003;48:749–755.
4. Altamura AC, Sassella F, Santini A, et al. Intramuscular preparations of antipsychotics: uses and relevance in clinical practice. *Drugs.* 2003;63:493–512.
5. American Psychiatric Association. *Diagnostic and Statistical Manual of Mental Disorders.* Revised 4th ed. Washington, DC: American Psychiatric Association; 1994.
6. Ananth J, Parameswaran S, Hara B. Drug therapy in schizophrenia. *Curr Pharm Des.* 2004;10:2205–2217.
7. Ballard CG, Margallo-Lana ML. The relationship between antipsychotic treatment and quality of life for patients with dementia living in residential and nursing home care facilities. *J Clin Psychiatry.* 2004;65(suppl 11):23–28.
8. Ballerini M, Bellini S, Niccolai C, et al. Neuroleptic-induced dystonia: incidence and risk factors. *Eur Psychiatry.* 2002;17:366–368.
9. Belmaker RH. Bipolar disorder. *N Engl J Med.* 2004;351:476–486.
10. Bhanji NH, Chouinard G, Margolese HC. A review of compliance, depot intramuscular antipsychotics and the new long-acting injectable atypical antipsychotic risperidone in schizophrenia. *Eur Neuropsychopharmacol.* 2004;14:87–92.
11. Burgyone K, Aduri K, Ananth J, Parameswaran S. The use of antiparkinsonian agents in the management of drug-induced extrapyramidal symptoms. *Curr Pharm Des.* 2004;10:2239–2248.
12. Casey DE. Tardive dyskinesia: pathophysiology and animal models. *J Clin Psychiatry.* 2000;61(suppl 4):5–9.
13. Casey DE. Pathophysiology of antipsychotic drug-induced movement disorders. *J Clin Psychiatry.* 2004;65(suppl 9):25–28.
14. Chandran GJ, Mikler JR, Keegan DL. Neuroleptic malignant syndrome: case report and discussion. *CMAJ.* 2003;169:439–442.
15. Collier DA, Li T. The genetics of schizophrenia: glutamate not dopamine? *Eur J Pharmacol.* 2003;480: 177–184.
16. Conley RR, Kelly DL. Current status of antipsychotic treatment. *Curr Drug Targets CNS Neurol Disord.* 2002;1:123–128.
17. Correll CU, Leucht S, Kane JM. Lower risk for tardive dyskinesia associated with second-generation antipsychotics: a systematic review of 1-year studies. *Am J Psychiatry.* 2004;161:414–425.
18. Crismon ML, Dorson PG. Schizophrenia. In: DiPiro JT, et al, eds. *Pharmacotherapy: A Pathophysiologic Approach.* 5th ed. New York: McGraw-Hill; 2002.
19. Dean B, Scarr E. Antipsychotic drugs: evolving mechanisms of action with improved therapeutic benefits. *Curr Drug Targets CNS Neurol Disord.* 2004;3:217–225.
20. Dolder CR, Jeste DV. Incidence of tardive dyskinesia with typical versus atypical antipsychotics in very high risk patients. *Biol Psychiatry.* 2003;53:1142–1145.
21. Fernandez HH, Friedman JH. Classification and treatment of tardive syndromes. *Neurologist.* 2003;9:16–27.
22. Finkel SI. Psychotherapeutic agents in older adults. Antipsychotics: old and new. *Clin Geriatr Med.* 1998; 14:87–100.
23. Freedman R. Schizophrenia. *N Engl J Med.* 2003;349: 1738–1749.
24. Friedman JH. Historical perspective on movement disorders. *J Clin Psychiatry.* 2004;65(suppl 9):3–8.
25. Gogtay N, Sporn A, Alfaro CL, et al. Clozapine-induced akathisia in children with schizophrenia. *J Child Adolesc Psychopharmacol.* 2002;12:347–349.
26. Harrison TS, Goa KL. Long-acting risperidone: a review of its use in schizophrenia. *CNS Drugs.* 2004;18:113–132.
27. Hoeh N, Gyulai L, Weintraub D, Streim J. Pharmacologic management of psychosis in the elderly: a critical review. *J Geriatr Psychiatry Neurol.* 2003;16: 213–218.
28. Howes OD, McDonald C, Cannon M, et al. Pathways to schizophrenia: the impact of environmental factors. *Int J Neuropsychopharmacol.* 2004;(suppl 1):S7–S13.
29. Jeste DV. Tardive dyskinesia in older patients. *J Clin Psychiatry.* 2000;61(suppl 4):27–32.
30. Jeste DV, Dolder CR. Treatment of non-schizophrenic disorders: focus on atypical antipsychotics. *J Psychiatr Res.* 2004;38:73–103.
31. Kane JM. Tardive dyskinesia rates with atypical antipsychotics in adults: prevalence and incidence. *J Clin Psychiatry.* 2004;65(suppl 9):16–20.
32. Kapur S, Mamo D. Half a century of antipsychotics and still a central role for dopamine D2 receptors. *Prog Neuropsychopharmacol Biol Psychiatry.* 2003;27: 1081–1090.

33. Kasckow JW, Mulchahey JJ, Mohamed S. The use of novel antipsychotics in the older patient with neurodegenerative disorders in the long-term care setting. *J Am Med Dir Assoc.* 2004;5:242–248.

34. Keith SJ, Kane JM. Partial compliance and patient consequences in schizophrenia: our patients can do better. *J Clin Psychiatry.* 2003;64:1308–1315.

35. Kim JH, Byun HJ. Prevalence and characteristics of subjective akathisia, objective akathisia, and mixed akathisia in chronic schizophrenic subjects. *Clin Neuropharmacol.* 2003;26:312–316.

36. Kulkarni SK, Naidu PS. Pathophysiology and drug therapy of tardive dyskinesia: current concepts and future perspectives. *Drugs Today.* 2003;39:19–49.

37. Laruelle M, Kegeles LS, Abi-Dargham A. Glutamate, dopamine, and schizophrenia: from pathophysiology to treatment. *Ann N Y Acad Sci.* 2003;1003:138–158.

38. Lawlor BA. Behavioral and psychological symptoms in dementia: the role of atypical antipsychotics. *J Clin Psychiatry.* 2004;65(suppl 11):5–10.

39. Lebovitz HE. Metabolic consequences of atypical antipsychotic drugs. *Psychiatr Q.* 2003;74:277–290.

40. Lee PE, Gill SS, Freedman M, et al. Atypical antipsychotic drugs in the treatment of behavioural and psychological symptoms of dementia: systematic review. *BMJ.* 2004;329:75.

41. Leriche L, Diaz J, Sokoloff P. Dopamine and glutamate dysfunctions in schizophrenia: role of the dopamine D3 receptor. *Neurotox Res.* 2004;6:63–71.

42. Lima AR, Weiser KV, Bacaltchuk J, Barnes TR. Anticholinergics for neuroleptic-induced acute akathisia. *Cochrane Database Syst Rev.* 2004;CD003727.

43. Masan PS. Atypical antipsychotics in the treatment of affective symptoms: a review. *Ann Clin Psychiatry.* 2004;16:3–13.

44. Masand PS. Side effects of antipsychotics in the elderly. *J Clin Psychiatry.* 2000;61(suppl 8):43–49; discussion 50–51.

45. Meltzer HY. What's atypical about atypical antipsychotic drugs? *Curr Opin Pharmacol.* 2004;4:53–57.

46. Mortimer AM. Novel antipsychotics in schizophrenia. *Expert Opin Investig Drugs.* 2004;13:315–329.

47. Mueser KT, McGurk SR. Schizophrenia. *Lancet.* 2004;363:2063–2072.

48. Nicholson D, Chiu W. Neuroleptic malignant syndrome. *Geriatrics.* 2004;59:36, 38–40.

49. Oosthuizen PP, Emsley RA, Maritz JS, et al. Incidence of tardive dyskinesia in first-episode psychosis patients treated with low-dose haloperidol. *J Clin Psychiatry.* 2003;64:1075–1080.

50. Palomo T, Archer T, Kostrzewa RM, Beninger RJ. Gene-environment interplay in schizopsychotic disorders. *Neurotox Res.* 2004;6:1–9.

51. Remington G. Understanding antipsychotic "atypicality": a clinical and pharmacological moving target. *J Psychiatry Neurosci.* 2003;28:275–284.

52. Serretti A, De Ronchi D, Lorenzi C, Berardi D. New antipsychotics and schizophrenia: a review on efficacy and side effects. *Curr Med Chem.* 2004;11:343–358.

53. Soares-Weiser KV, Joy C. Miscellaneous treatments for neuroleptic-induced tardive dyskinesia. *Cochrane Database Syst Rev.* 2003;CD000208.

54. Soares-Weiser K, Rathbone J. Calcium channel blockers for neuroleptic induced tardive dyskinesia. *Cochrane Database Syst Rev.* 2004;CD000206.

55. Stewart JT. Dysphagia associated with risperidone therapy. *Dysphagia.* 2003;18:274–275.

56. Sultzer DL. Psychosis and antipsychotic medications in Alzheimer's disease: clinical management and research perspectives. *Dement Geriatr Cogn Disord.* 2004;17:78–90.

57. Sussman N. Choosing an atypical antipsychotic. *Int Clin Psychopharmacol.* 2002;17(suppl 3):S29–S33.

58. Tariot PN, Profenno LA, Ismail MS. Efficacy of atypical antipsychotics in elderly patients with dementia. *J Clin Psychiatry.* 2004;65(suppl 11):11–15.

59. Trenton A, Currier G, Zwemer F. Fatalities associated with therapeutic use and overdose of atypical antipsychotics. *CNS Drugs.* 2003;17:307–324.

60. Viejo LF, Morales V, Punal P, et al. Risk factors in neuroleptic malignant syndrome. A case-control study. *Acta Psychiatr Scand.* 2003;107:45–49.

61. Walker E, Kestler L, Bollini A, Hochman KM. Schizophrenia: etiology and course. *Annu Rev Psychol.* 2004;55:401–430.

62. Wong AH, Van Tol HH. The dopamine D4 receptors and mechanisms of antipsychotic atypicality. *Prog Neuropsychopharmacol Biol Psychiatry.* 2003;27:1091–1099.

Chapter 9

Antiepileptic Drugs

Epilepsy is a chronic neurologic disorder characterized by recurrent seizures.[33] Seizures are episodes of sudden, transient disturbances in cerebral excitation that occur when a sufficient number of cerebral neurons begin to fire rapidly and in synchronized bursts.[42] Depending on the type of seizure, neuronal activity may remain localized in a specific area of the brain, or it may spread to other areas of the brain. In some seizures, neurons in the motor cortex are activated, leading to skeletal muscle contraction via descending neuronal pathways. These involuntary, paroxysmal skeletal muscle contractions seen during certain seizures are referred to as *convulsions*. However, convulsions are not associated with all types of epilepsy, and other types of seizures are characterized by a wide variety of sensory or behavioral symptoms.

Epilepsy is associated with the presence of a group or focus of cerebral neurons that are hyperexcitable, or "irritable." The spontaneous discharge of these irritable neurons initiates the epileptic seizure. The reason for the altered excitability of these focal neurons, and thus the cause of epilepsy, varies depending on the patient.[20,42] In some patients, a specific incident such as a stroke, tumor, encephalopathy, head trauma, or other CNS injury probably caused damage to certain neurons, resulting in their altered threshold. In other patients, the reason for seizures may be less distinct or unknown, perhaps relating to a congenital abnormality, birth trauma, or genetic factor. A systemic metabolic disorder such as infection, hypoglycemia, hypoxia, or uremia may precipitate seizure activity. Once the cause of the seizures is identified in this last group of individuals, the epilepsy can be treated by resolving the metabolic disorder. Epilepsy resulting from these combined causes affects approximately 5 to 10 people per 1000 in the general population, making this one of the most common neurologic disorders.[30]

Although some innovative approaches using surgery, neural stimulation, and dietary control have been reported,[8,9,32,45] drug therapy remains the primary method for treating epilepsy. In general, antiepileptic medications are successful in eliminating seizures in 50 percent of the patient population, and can reduce seizure activity substantially in an additional 25 percent of patients with epilepsy.[20] Some of the newer antiepileptic medications such as gabapentin (Neurontin) have also been used to treat certain types of pain, including neuropathic pain and migraine headaches.[25,37] This chapter, however, will focus on the use of these medications in resolving seizure disorders.

Several types of drugs are currently available, and certain compounds work best in specific types of epilepsy. Consequently, the type of epilepsy must be determined by observing the patient and using diagnostic tests such as electroencephalography (EEG).[21] The classification system most commonly used in characterizing epilepsy is discussed here.

Classification of Epileptic Seizures

In an attempt to standardize the terminology used in describing various forms of epilepsy, the International League Against Epilepsy[10] proposed the classification scheme outlined in Table 9–1. Seizures are divided into two major categories: partial and generalized. A third category of "unclassified" seizures is sometimes included to encompass additional seizure types not fitting into the two major groups. Originally devised in the 1980s, this classification system has been revised periodically, and it will undoubtedly continue to be revised as more is learned about the cause and symptoms of specific seizures.[29,34]

Table 9–1	CLASSIFICATION OF SEIZURES

Seizure Type	Classification
I. Partial seizures	
A. Simple partial seizures	Limited (focal) motor or sensory signs (e.g., convulsions confined to one limb, specific sensory hallucinations); consciousness remains intact
B. Complex partial seizures (needed to differentiate this from absence seizures)	Consciousness impaired; bizarre behavior; wide variety of other manifestations; specific electroencephalography (EEG) abnormality
C. Partial becoming generalized	Symptoms progressively increase until seizure resembles a generalized (tonic-clonic) seizure
II. Generalized seizures	
A. Absence (petit mal) seizures	Sudden, brief loss of consciousness; motor signs may be absent or may range from rapid eye-blinking to symmetrical jerking movements of entire body
B. Myoclonic seizures	Sudden, brief, "shocklike" contractions of muscles in the face and trunk, or in one or more extremities; contractions may be single or multiple; consciousness may be impaired
C. Clonic seizures	Rhythmic, synchronized contractions throughout the body; loss of consciousness
D. Tonic seizures	Generalized sustained muscle contractions throughout body; loss of consciousness
E. Tonic-clonic (grand mal) seizures	Major convulsions of entire body; sustained contraction of all muscles (tonic phase) followed by powerful rhythmic contractions (clonic phase); loss of consciousness
F. Atonic seizures	Sudden loss of muscle tone in the head and neck, one limb, or throughout the entire body; consciousness may be maintained or lost briefly
III. Unclassified seizures	
All other seizures that do not fit into one of the aforementioned categories.	

Source: Modified from Commission on Classification and Terminology of the International League Against Epilepsy, pp 493–495,[10] with permission.

In partial seizures only part of the brain (i.e., one cerebral hemisphere) is involved, whereas in generalized seizures the whole brain is involved. Partial seizures that spread throughout the entire brain are referred to as "partial becoming generalized" or "secondarily generalized" seizures.

Partial and generalized seizures are subdivided depending on the specific symptoms that occur during the epileptic seizure (see Table 9–1). As a rule, the outward manifestations of the seizure depend on the area of the brain involved. Simple partial seizures that remain localized within the motor cortex for the right hand may cause involuntary, spasm like movements of only the right hand. Other partial seizures produce motor and sensory symptoms, and affect consciousness and memory as well. These usually fall into the category of complex partial seizures.

Generalized seizures are subclassified depending on the type and degree of motor involvement, as well as other factors such as EEG recordings. The most well-known and dramatic seizure of the generalized group is the tonic-clonic, or "grand mal," seizure. Absence, or "petit mal," seizures also fall into the generalized seizure category. Drug therapy for generalized and partial seizures is discussed later in "Drugs Used to Treat Epilepsy."

Rationale for Drug Treatment

Even in the absence of drug therapy, individual seizures are usually self-limiting. Brain neurons are unable to sustain a high level of synaptic activity for more than a few minutes, and the seizure ends spontaneously. However, the uncontrolled recurrence of seizures is believed to cause further damage to the already injured neurons, and can be potentially harmful to healthy cells.[15,36] In particular, seizures can cause structural and functional changes in neuronal pathways, resulting in impaired cerebral activity and increased susceptibility to additional seizures.[22,36]

Certain types of seizures will also be harmful if the patient loses consciousness or goes into convulsions and injures himself or herself during a fall. Certain types of convulsions are potentially fatal if cardiac irregularities result and the individual goes into cardiac arrest. Even relatively minor seizures may be embarrassing to a person, and social interaction may be compromised if the individual is afraid of having a seizure in public. Consequently, a strong effort is made to find an effective way to control or eliminate the incidence of seizures.

Drugs Used to Treat Epilepsy

Table 9–2 lists the drugs commonly used to treat epilepsy according to their chemical classes and mechanisms of action. These drugs generally try to inhibit firing of certain cerebral neurons, usually by increasing the inhibitory effects of gamma-aminobutyric acid (GABA), by decreasing the effects of excitatory amino acids (glutamate, aspartate), or by altering the movement of ions (sodium, calcium) across the neuronal membrane.[20,39,42] In some cases, however, the exact way that antiepileptic drugs exert their beneficial effects is obscure or unknown.[20] Specific details of each chemical class of drugs are discussed here. Because these drugs tend to have many adverse side effects, only the frequently occurring or more serious problems are listed for each category.

Barbiturates

Phenobarbital (various trade names) and other barbiturates such as mephobarbital (Mebaral) are prescribed in virtually all types of adult seizures, but seem to be especially effective in generalized tonic-clonic and simple and complex partial seizures. These agents are considered to be very safe and effective in the treatment of seizures, but their use is often limited because of their strong tendency to produce sedation. Primidone (Mysoline) is another barbituratelike drug that is recommended in several types of epilepsy but is particularly useful in generalized tonic-clonic seizures not responding to other drugs.

Mechanism of Action. Barbiturates are known to increase the inhibitory effects of GABA (see Chapter 6), and this effect is probably the primary way that these drugs decrease seizure activity. Barbiturates may also produce some of their antiseizure effects by inhibiting calcium entry into excitatory presynaptic nerve terminals and thereby decreasing the release of excitatory neurotransmitters such as glutamate.[20]

Adverse Side Effects. Sedation (primary problem), nystagmus, ataxia, folate deficiency, vitamin K deficiency, and skin problems are typical side effects. A paradoxical increase in seizures and an increase in hyperactivity may occur in some children.

Benzodiazepines

Several members of the benzodiazepine group are effective in treating epilepsy, but most are limited because of problems with sedation and tolerance. Some agents such as diazepam (Valium) and lorazepam (Ativan) are used in the acute treatment of status epilepticus (see "Treatment of Status Epilepticus"), but only a few are used in the long-term treatment of epilepsy. Clonazepam (Klonopin) is recommended in specific forms of absence seizures (e.g., the Lennox-Gastaut variant) and may also be useful in minor generalized seizures such as akinetic spells and myoclonic jerks. Clorazepate (Tranxene) is another benzodiazepine that is occasionally used as an adjunct in certain partial seizures.

Table 9–2	CHEMICAL CLASSIFICATION AND ACTIONS OF ANTIEPILEPTIC AGENTS

Chemical Class	Possible Mechanism of Action
Barbiturates Amobarbital (Amytal)* Mephobarbital (Mebaral) Pentobarbital (Nembutal)* Phenobarbital (Solfoton, others) Primidone (Mysoline) Secobarbital (Seconal)*	Potentiate inhibitory effects of GABA**; may also decrease excitatory effects of glutamate
Benzodiazepines Clonazepam (Klonopin) Clorazepate (Tranxene) Diazepam (Valium) Lorazepam (Ativan)	Potentiate inhibitory effects of GABA
Carboxylic acids Valproic acid (Depakene, Depakote, others)	Unclear; may hyperpolarize membrane through an effect on potassium channels; higher concentrations increase CNS GABA concentrations
Hydantoins Ethotoin (Peganone) Fosphenytoin (Cerebyx)* Mephenytoin (Mesantoin) Phenytoin (Dilantin)	Primary effect is to stabilize membrane by blocking sodium channels in repetitive-firing neurons; higher concentrations may also influence concentrations of other neurotransmitters (GABA, norepinephrine, others)
Iminostilbenes Carbamazepine (Tegretol) Oxcarbazepine (Trileptal)	Similar to hydantoins
Succinimides Ethosuximide (Zarontin) Methsuximide (Celontin)	Affect calcium channels; appear to inhibit spontaneous firing in thalamic neurons by limiting calcium entry

*Parental use only (IV injection).
**GABA = gamma-aminobutyric acid.

Mechanism of Action. These drugs are known to potentiate the inhibitory effects of GABA in the brain (see Chapter 6), and their antiepileptic properties are probably exerted through this mechanism.

Adverse Side Effects. Sedation, ataxia, and behavioral changes can be observed.

Hydantoins

This category includes phenytoin (Dilantin), mephenytoin (Mesantoin), ethotoin (Peganone), and fosphenytoin (Cerebyx). Phenytoin is often the first drug considered in treating many types of epilepsy, and it is especially effective in treating partial seizures and generalized tonic-clonic seizures. Mephenytoin has similar properties but is somewhat more toxic, and ethotoin has been effective in treating absence seizures. The latter two drugs are usually reserved for use if the patient has not responded to other, less toxic drugs. Finally, fosphenytoin can be administered intravenously in emergency situations to treat continuous, uncontrolled seizures (status epilepticus, a condition addressed later in this chapter).

Mechanism of Action. Phenytoin stabilizes neural membranes and decreases neuronal excitability by decreasing sodium entry into rapidly firing neurons. This drug basically inhibits the ability of sodium channels to reset from an inactive to active state after the neuron has fired an action potential. By inhibiting the reactivation of sodium channels, phenytoin prolongs the time between action potentials (absolute refractory period) so that neurons must slow their firing rate to a normal level. At higher doses, phenytoin may also decrease neuronal excitability by increasing the effects of GABA and by influencing the movement of potassium and calcium across the nerve membrane, but these effects generally occur at higher drug concentrations than those used therapeutically to control seizures. Less is known about the molecular mechanisms of the other drugs in this category, but they probably work by a similar effect on the sodium channels.

Adverse Side Effects. Gastric irritation, confusion, sedation, dizziness, headache, cerebellar signs (nystagmus, ataxia, dysarthria), gingival hyperplasia, increased body and facial hair (hirsutism), and skin disorders are typical adverse effects.

Iminostilbenes

The primary drugs in this category are carbamazepine (Tegretol) and oxcarbazepine (Trileptal). Carbamazepine has been shown to be effective in treating all types of epilepsy except absence seizures, and it is often considered the primary agent for treating partial and tonic-clonic seizures. Carbamazepine is regarded as equivalent to phenytoin in efficacy and side effects, and may be substituted for that drug, depending on patient response. Alternatively, oxcarbazepine can be used alone or with other antiepileptics to treat partial seizures in adults, and it is a treatment adjunct in partial seizures in children between ages 4 to 16.

Mechanism of Action. These drugs are believed to exert their primary antiepileptic effects in a manner similar to phenytoin—that is, they stabilize the neuronal membrane by slowing the recovery of sodium channels firing too rapidly. Carbamazepine may also inhibit the presynaptic uptake and release of norepinephrine, and this effect may contribute to its antiseizure activity.

Adverse Side Effects. Dizziness, drowsiness, ataxia, blurred vision, anemia, water retention (because of abnormal antidiuretic hormone [ADH] release), cardiac arrhythmias, and congestive heart failure can occur with use of these drugs.

Succinimides

Drugs in this category include ethosuximide (Zarontin), methsuximide (Celontin), and phensuximide (Milontin). All three drugs are primary agents in the treatment of absence (petit mal) seizures, but ethosuximide is the most commonly prescribed.

Mechanism of Action. These drugs are known to increase the seizure threshold and limit the spread of electrical activity in the brain, but their exact cellular mechanism is unknown. They may exert their beneficial effects by decreasing calcium influx in certain thalamic neurons. The spontaneous, rhythmic entry of calcium into thalamic neurons may be responsible for initiating partial seizures, and the succinimides prevent their onset by blunting calcium influx. Additional research is needed to elaborate on this theory.

Adverse Side Effects. Gastrointestinal distress (nausea, vomiting), headache, dizziness, fatigue, lethargy, movement disorders (dyskinesia, bradykinesia), and skin rashes and itching are common side effects.

Valproic Acid

Valproic acid (Depakene, Depakote, other trade names) is classified as a carboxylic acid, and is used primarily to treat absence seizures or as a secondary agent in generalized tonic-clonic forms of epilepsy. This drug is also used to treat bipolar disorder (manic-depression), especially during the acute manic phase (see Chapter 7).

Mechanism of Action. High concentrations of valproic acid are associated with increased levels of GABA in the brain, and this increase in GABAergic inhibition may be responsible for this drug's antiepileptic action. However, lower concentrations are still effective in limiting seizures and do not increase CNS GABA, indicating that some other mechanism must occur. This drug may, for example, increase potassium conductance and efflux from certain neurons, thereby hyperpolarizing the neuron and decreasing its excitability. Valproic acid also exerts some of its effects in a manner similar to phenytoin; that is, it limits sodium entry into rapidly firing neurons. Hence, the exact way in which this drug is effective against partial seizures remains to be determined, and valproic acid may actually work through a combination of several different molecular mechanisms.

Adverse Side Effects. Gastrointestinal distress, temporary hair loss, weight gain or loss, and impaired platelet function are documented adverse reactions.

Newer "Second-Generation" Agents

The medications described earlier have been on the market for many years and have been used routinely for decreasing seizure activity. Beginning with the introduction of felbamate in 1993, several new or "second-generation" drugs have also been approved by the FDA and are currently in use (Table 9–3). In most cases, these newer drugs are not more effective than their predecessors.[24] These newer agents, however, generally have favorable pharmacokinetic characteristics (absorption, distribution, metabolism, and so forth) and have relatively mild side effects that allow their use along with the more traditional antiseizure medications.[5,16]

Hence, these newer drugs are often used as adjuncts or "add-on" therapy to other drugs.[11,13] The combinations often allow adequate seizure control in patients who did not respond to a single traditional antiseizure agent. Likewise, as more is learned about these newer drugs, some are being used alone as the initial treatment, or in certain types of seizures that are resistant to other drugs.[11,14,12] Second-generation antiseizure medications currently available are described here.

Felbamate (Felbatol). Felbamate is indicated for treatment of partial seizures in adults and children as well as generalized absence seizures (Lennox-Gastaut syndrome) in children. Felbamate appears to bind to specific receptors in the brain (the *N*-methyl-D-aspartate receptor) and block the effects of excitatory amino acids such as glutamate. Reduced influence of these excitatory amino acids results in decreased seizure activity. As indicated, this drug first appeared on the market in 1993, and represented the first "new generation" antiseizure agent. It was soon recognized, however, that felbamate may cause severe toxic effects such as aplastic anemia and liver failure.[20] Felbamate is therefore not widely prescribed and its use is typically limited to patients with severe epilepsy who fail to respond to other antiseizure drugs. Other common side effects include insomnia, headache, dizziness, and gastrointestinal problems (anorexia, nausea, and vomiting).

Gabapentin (Neurontin). Gabapentin is used primarily to treat partial seizures in adults and partial seizures in children that have not responded to other treatments. As the name implies, gabapentin was designed to act as a GABA agonist. However, the exact antiseizure mechanism of this drug is unclear.[20] Gabapentin appears to work by increasing GABA release or by acting at a receptor that is different from the GABA receptor.[3,17] The primary side effects of this drug are sedation, fatigue, dizziness, and ataxia.

Lamotrigine (Lamictal). Lamotrigine is used primarily as an adjunct to other medications in adults with partial seizures, although it has also been used

Table 9–3	SECOND-GENERATION ANTIEPILEPTICS	
Generic Name	**Trade Name**	**Primary Indication(s)**
Felbamate	Felbatol	Used alone or as an adjunct in partial seizures in adults; treatment adjunct in partial and generalized seizures associated with Lennox-Gastaut syndrome in children
Gabapentin	Neurontin	Treatment adjunct in partial seizures in adults and children over age 3
Lamotrigine	Lamictal	Use alone or as a treatment adjunct in partial seizures in adults over age 16; treatment adjunct in generalized seizures associated with Lennox-Gastaut syndrome in adults and children over age 2
Levetiracetam	Keppra	Treatment adjunct in partial onset seizures in adults
Tiagabine	Gabitril	Treatment adjunct in partial seizures in adults and children over age 12
Topiramate	Topamax	Treatment adjunct in partial onset seizures
Zonisamide	Zonegran	Treatment adjunct in partial seizures in adults

alone to treat partial and generalized seizures in adults and children. This drug exerts some of its effects by a stabilizing sodium channels in a manner similar to carbamazepine and phenytoin. Lamotrigine may also inhibit the release of excitatory amino acids by inhibiting sodium entry into the presynaptic terminals of neurons firing too rapidly.[20] The primary side effects include dizziness, headache, ataxia, vision problems, and skin rash.

Levetiracetam (Keppra). Levetiracetam has been successful in treating partial seizures in adults when used in conjunction with traditional antiseizure drugs. This drug does not appear to decrease seizure activity via one of the common antiseizure mechanisms (stabilize sodium channels, increase GABA inhibition, and so forth), and the mechanism of this drug is therefore unknown. Levetiracetam is usually well tolerated, although some patients may experience sedation, dizziness, and generalized weakness.

Tiagabine (Gabitril). Tiagabine is used primarily as an adjunct to other drugs in adults with partial seizures that are poorly controlled by traditional drug therapy. This drug inhibits the reuptake of GABA after it is released from presynaptic terminals, thereby inhibiting seizure activity by enabling GABA to remain active in the synaptic cleft for longer periods.[2] The primary side effects of this drug are dizziness,

weakness, and a slight tendency for psychiatric disturbances (anxiety, depression).

Topiramate (Topamax). Topiramate is used primarily as an adjunct to other medications in adults with partial seizures. This drug appears to limit seizure activity through several complimentary mechanisms including inhibition of sodium channel opening, blockade of excitatory amino acid receptors, and stimulation of GABA receptors.[2,41] Primary side effects include sedation, dizziness, fatigue, and ataxia.

Zonisamide (Zonegran). Zonisamide is used primarily as an adjunct to other medications in adults with partial seizures. This drug stabilizes sodium channels in a manner similar to carbamazepine and phenytoin, and may also exert some of its antiseizure effects by inhibiting calcium entry into rapidly firing neurons. Zonisamide is fairly well tolerated, although side effects may include sedation, ataxia, loss of appetite, and fatigue.

Selection of a Specific Antiepileptic Agent

It is apparent from the preceding discussion that certain drugs are often preferred when treating certain types of seizures. Table 9–4 lists some of the more

Table 9–4	COMMON METHODS OF TREATING SPECIFIC SEIZURES	
Seizure Type	**First-line Drugs**	**Alternative Agents**
Partial seizures	Carbamazepine Phenytoin Lamotrigine Valproic acid Oxcarbazepine	Gabapentin Topiramate Levetiracetam Zonisamide Tiagabine Primidone, phenobarbital Felbamate
Generalized seizures		
Absence	Valproic acid, ethosuximide	Lamotrigine
Myoclonic	Valproic acid, clonazepam	Lamotrigine, topiramate, felbamate
Tonic-clonic	Phenytoin, carbamazepine, valproic acid	Lamotrigine, topiramate, phenobarbital, primidone, oxcarbazepine

Source: Gidal BE, et al. Epilepsy. In: DiPiro JT, et al, eds. *Pharmacotherapy: A Pathophysiologic Approach.* 5th ed. New York: McGraw-Hill; 2002:1036.

common types of seizures and the primary and alternative agents used to treat each seizure type. It is important to note, however, that while Table 9–4 indicates general guidelines for drug selection, selection of the best agent must be done on a patient-by-patient basis. Some patients will understandably exhibit a better response to agents that are not typically used as the first or second choice for a specific type of seizure. Hence, some trial and error may occur before the best drug is found, and drug selection may need to be altered periodically throughout the patient's lifetime to achieve optimal results.[31]

Thus, a fairly large number of drugs can be used to treat epileptic seizures (see Tables 9–2 and 9–3), but certain agents are usually considered first when attempting to treat the most common types. These agents comprise a fairly small group that tend to be used most often; the drugs and their relevant dosing parameters are listed in Table 9–5. Again, alternative antiseizure drugs can be used if commonly used drugs are ineffective or poorly tolerated. As indicated earlier, one of the newer agents can also be added to traditional drugs if patients do not respond to single-drug therapy.

Table 9–5   DOSAGES OF COMMON ANTIEPILEPTIC DRUGS*

	Adult			Child	
Drug	Initial Dose (mg)	Increment** (mg)	Maintenance (mg/d)	Initial Dose (mg/kg/d)	Maintenance (mg/kg/d)
Carbamazepine	200 BID	200 q wk	600–1800	10 qd	10–35 (<6 years)
Ethosuximide	250 qd	250 q 3–7d	750	15	15–40
Felbamate	600–1200 qd	600–1200 q 1–2 wk	2400–3600	15	15–45
Gabapentin	300 qd	300 q 3–7 d	1200–3600	10	25–50
Lamotrigine	25 qd	25 q 2 wk	400	0.15–0.5	5
Levetiracetam	500 BID	500 q wk	2000–4000	20	40–100
Oxcarbazepine	300 qd	300 q wk	900–2400	8–10	30–46
Phenobarbital	30–60 qd	30 q 1–2 wk	60–120	3	3–6
Phenytoin	200 qd	100 q 5–7 d	200–300	4	4–8
Primidone	125–250 qd	250 q 1–2 wk	500–750	10	10–25
Tiagabine	4 qd	4–8 q wk	16–32	0.1	0.4
Topiramate	25 qd	25 q 1–2 wk	100–400	3	3–9
Valproic acid	250 qd	250 q 3–7 d	750–3000	15	15–45
Zonisamide	100 qd	100 q 2 wk	200–400	4	4–12

Abbreviations: BID = twice a day; qd = every day.
*Dosages reflect monotherapy. Dosages may vary if combining the drug with other antiseizure agents, or other drugs that affect liver enzyme function.
**Increments reflect the rate that dosage can typically be increased when trying to find the appropriate therapeutic dose.
Source: Ranta A, Fountain NB. Seizures and epilepsy in adolescents and adults. In: Rakel RE, Bope ET, eds. Conn's Current Therapy 2005. New York: Elsevier/Saunders; 2005: 1026.

Single-Drug Therapy Versus Drug Combinations in Epilepsy

In the past, an effort was made to use only one drug (primary agent), with an additional drug (secondary agent) being added only if the epilepsy is especially resistant to management with the primary medication.[6] The use of a single drug (monotherapy) offers several advantages, including fewer side effects, a lack of drug interactions, better ability of the patient to adhere to the drug regimen, lower cost, and better seizure control because the patient was able to tolerate a higher dose of a single agent.[31] Likewise, management of adverse side effects in single-drug therapy is easier because there is no question about which drug is producing the adverse effect.

As indicated earlier, the development of the newer antiseizure medications has advanced the strategy of using two drugs rather than a single agent. Because these newer drugs have relatively predictable pharmacokinetic and side-effect profiles, they can be added to traditional medications without excessive complications and risk to the patient.[4,31] Combination therapy is therefore a more common approach to treating seizure disorders than it was in the past.

Pharmacokinetics

When given for the long-term control of epilepsy, these drugs are normally administered orally. Daily oral doses are usually divided into three or four equal quantities, and the amount of each dose varies widely depending on the specific drug and the severity of patient seizures. Distribution within the body is fairly extensive, with all antiepileptic drugs eventually reaching the brain to exert their beneficial effects. Drug biotransformation usually occurs via liver microsomal oxidases, and this is the primary method of drug termination.

Special Precautions During Pregnancy

Most women with epilepsy continue to take their antiseizure medications when they become pregnant, and eventually give birth to normal, healthy babies.[44] Nonetheless, the incidence of birth defects is increased somewhat in children of mothers with epilepsy compared with children of mothers who are not epilep-

tic.[23,26,44] Problems such as stillbirth, microencephaly, mental retardation, infant seizures, and congenital malformations (cleft palate, cardiac defects, neural tube defects) occur more frequently in children of women with seizure disorders. There is considerable debate as to whether this is a side effect of antiepileptic drug therapy or a sequela of the epilepsy itself. Because there is at least some concern that fetal malformations may be a drug side effect, some mothers may choose to discontinue drug therapy during their pregnancies.[44] This action obviously places the mother at risk for uncontrolled seizures, which may be even more harmful to the mother and unborn child.

Hence, women taking antiepileptic drugs should discuss the potential risks with their family members and physician, and consider whether they will continue taking their medication(s).[38] If an expectant mother continues to take her medication(s), using one drug (monotherapy) at the lowest effective dose will help reduce the risk of harmful effects on the fetus.[1,43] In addition, mothers should receive optimal prenatal care (folic acid supplementation, proper amounts of exercise, rest, and so forth) to help ensure the baby's health.[27,43] After delivery, the baby should be monitored initially for drug-related effects such as withdrawal symptoms, and should be subsequently evaluated for developmental delays that might become apparent later in childhood.[27]

Treatment of Status Epilepticus

Status epilepticus is a series of seizures occurring without any appreciable period of recovery between individual seizures.[19,28] Essentially the patient experiences one long, extended seizure. This may be brought on by a number of factors such as sudden withdrawal from antiepileptic drugs, cerebral infarct, systemic or intracranial infection, or withdrawal from addictive drugs including alcohol.[19,28] If untreated, status epilepticus will result in permanent damage or death, especially if the seizures are generalized tonic-clonic in nature.[18] Consequently, this event is regarded as a medical emergency that should be resolved as rapidly as possible.

Treatment begins with standard emergency procedures such as maintaining an airway, starting an IV line for blood sampling and drug administration, and so on.[28] The first drugs administered are usually benzodiazepines: lorazepam (Ativan) or diazepam (Valium) given intravenously. This approach is followed by phenytoin, which is also administered intravenously. The phenytoin is given concurrently with or immediately after the benzodiazepine so that seizures are controlled when the relatively short-acting benzodiazepine is metabolized. If seizures continue despite these drugs, phenobarbital is given intravenously. If all other attempts fail, general anesthesia (e.g., halothane) may be used as a last resort. When the status epilepticus is eventually controlled, an attempt is made to begin or reinstitute chronic antiepileptic therapy.

Withdrawal of Antiseizure Medications

Many people with seizure disorders will need to adhere to a regimen of antiseizure medications throughout their lifetime. There appears, however, to be a certain percentage of patients who can discontinue their medications once their seizures are under control. It is estimated, for example, that as many as 60 to 70 percent of people who have epilepsy can remain seizure-free after their medication is withdrawn.[7] Factors associated with successful medication withdrawal include being free of seizures for at least 2 years while on medication(s), having a normal neurologic examination prior to withdrawal, and being young when the seizures started.[35,40]

Withdrawal of medications must, of course, be done under close medical supervision. Likewise, medications are usually tapered-off over an extended period of time (6 months) rather than being suddenly discontinued.[7] Nonetheless, it appears that a large proportion of people with epilepsy may be able to maintain seizure-free status once their seizures are controlled by the appropriate medications.

Special Concerns in Rehabilitation Patients

■ ■ ■ Rehabilitation specialists must always be cognizant of their patients who have a history of seizures and who are taking antiepileptic drugs. Patients being treated for conditions unrelated to epilepsy (e.g., the outpatient with low back pain) should be identified as potentially at risk for a seizure during the therapy session. This knowledge will better prepare the therapist to recognize and deal with such an episode. This approach emphasizes the need for a thorough medical history of all patients. Also, therapists may help determine the efficacy of antiepileptic drug therapy. The primary goal in any patient taking antiepileptic drugs is maintaining the drug dosage within a therapeutic window. Dosage must be high enough to adequately control seizure activity, but not so high as to invoke serious side effects. By constantly observing and monitoring patient progress, rehabilitation specialists may help determine if this goal is being met. By noting changes in either seizure frequency or side effects, physical therapists, occupational therapists, and other rehabilitation personnel may help the medical staff arrive at an effective dosing regimen. This information can be invaluable in helping achieve optimal patient care with a minimum of adverse side effects.

Some of the more frequent side effects may affect physical therapy and other rehabilitation procedures. Headache, dizziness, sedation, and gastric disturbances (nausea, vomiting) may be bothersome during the therapy session. Often, these reactions can be addressed by scheduling therapy at a time of day when these problems are relatively mild. The optimal treatment time will vary from patient to patient, depending on the particular drug, dosing schedule, and age of the patient. Cerebellar side effects such as ataxia also occur frequently and may impair the patient's ability to participate in various functional activities. If ataxia persists despite efforts to alter drug dosage or substitute another agent, coordination exercises may be instituted to help resolve this problem. Skin conditions (dermatitis, rashes, etc.) are another frequent problem in long-term antiepileptic therapy. Any therapeutic modalities that might exacerbate these conditions should be discontinued.

Finally, in some patients, seizures tend to be exacerbated by environmental stimuli such as lights and sound. In such patients, conducting the therapy session in a busy, noisy clinic may be sufficient to precipitate a seizure, especially if the epilepsy is poorly controlled by drug therapy. Also, certain patients may have a history of increased seizure activity at certain times of the day, which may be related to when the antiepileptic drug is administered. Consequently, certain patients may benefit if the therapy session is held in a relatively quiet setting at a time when the chance of a seizure is minimal.

CASE STUDY

Antiepileptic Drugs

Brief History. F.B. is a 43-year-old man who works in the mail room of a large company. He was diagnosed in childhood as having generalized tonic-clonic epilepsy, and his seizures have been managed successfully with various drugs over the years. Most recently, he has been taking carbamazepine (Tegretol), 800 mg/d (i.e., one 200-mg tablet, QID). One month ago, he began complaining of dizziness and blurred vision, so the dosage was reduced to 600 mg/d (one 200 mg tablet TID). He usually took the medication after meals. Two weeks ago, he injured his back while lifting a large box at work. He was evaluated in physical therapy as having an acute lumbosacral strain. He began to attend physical therapy daily as an outpatient. Treatment included heat, ultrasound, and manual therapy, and the patient was also being instructed in proper body mechanics and lifting technique. F.B. continued to work at his normal job, but he avoided heavy lifting. He would attend therapy on his way home from work, at about 5 PM.

Problem/Influence of Medication. F.B. arrived at physical therapy the first afternoon stating that he had had a particularly long day. He was positioned prone on a treatment

table, and hot packs were placed over his low back. As the heat was applied, he began to drift off to sleep. Five minutes into the treatment, he had a seizure. Because of a thorough initial evaluation, the therapist was aware of his epileptic condition and protected him from injury during the seizure. The patient regained consciousness and rested quietly until he felt able to go home. No long-term effects were noted from the seizure.

Decision/Solution. The seizure may have been precipitated by a number of factors, including the recent decrease in drug dosage and the fact that he was nearing the end of a dosing interval. (He had taken his last dose at lunch and would take his next dose after he went home and had dinner.) The fact that he was tired and fell asleep during the treatment probably played a role. He reported later that when seizures do occur, they tend to be when he is asleep. To prevent the recurrence of seizures, the therapy session was rescheduled to earlier in the day, at 8 AM (his schedule was flexible enough that he could attend therapy before going to work). Also, he took his first dose of the day approximately 1 hour before arriving at physical therapy. No further seizures occurred during the course of rehabilitation, and F.B.'s lumbosacral strain was resolved after 2 weeks of physical therapy.

SUMMARY

Epilepsy is a chronic condition characterized by recurrent seizures. Causes of this disorder range from a distinct traumatic episode to obscure or unknown origins. Seizures are categorized according to the clinical and electrophysiologic manifestations that occur during the seizure. Fortunately, most individuals with epilepsy (up to 75 percent) can be treated successfully with antiepileptic drugs. Although these drugs do

not cure this disorder, reduction or elimination of seizures will prevent further CNS damage. Currently, a wide variety of drugs are used, with certain agents being the most successful in specific types of epilepsy. As in any area of pharmacotherapeutics, these drugs are not without adverse side effects. Some of these side effects may become a problem in rehabilitation patients, so therapists should be ready to alter the time and type of treatment as needed to accommodate these side effects. Physical therapists and other rehabilitation personnel should also be alert for any behavioral or functional changes in the patient that might indicate a problem in drug therapy. Insufficient drug therapy (as evidenced by

increased seizures) or possible drug toxicity (as evidenced by increased side effects) should be brought to the physician's attention so that these problems can be rectified.

References

1. Adab N, Tudur SC, Vinten J, et al. Common antiepileptic drugs in pregnancy in women with epilepsy. *Cochrane Database Syst Rev.* 2004;CD004848.
2. Angehagen M, Ben-Menachem E, Ronnback L, Hansson E. Novel mechanisms of action of three antiepileptic drugs, vigabatrin, tiagabine, and topiramate. *Neurochem Res.* 2003;28:333–340.
3. Ashton H, Young AH. GABA-ergic drugs: exit stage left, enter stage right. *J Psychopharmacol.* 2003;17:174–178.
4. Baulac M. Rational conversion from antiepileptic polytherapy to monotherapy. *Epileptic Disord.* 2003;5:125–132.
5. Beghi E. Efficacy and tolerability of the new antiepileptic drugs: comparison of two recent guidelines. *Lancet Neurol.* 2004;3:618–621.
6. Ben-Menachem E, Scheepers B, Stodieck S. Epilepsy: from consensus to daily practice. *Acta Neurol Scand Suppl.* 2003;180:5–15.
7. Britton JW. Antiepileptic drug withdrawal: literature review. *Mayo Clin Proc.* 2002;77:1378–1388.
8. Buchhalter JR, Jarrar RG. Therapeutics in pediatric epilepsy, part 2: epilepsy surgery and vagus nerve stimulation. *Mayo Clin Proc.* 2003;78:371–378.
9. Cohen-Gadol AA, Britton JW, Wetjen NM, et al. Neurostimulation therapy for epilepsy: current modalities and future directions. *Mayo Clin Proc.* 2003;78:238–248.
10. Commission on Classification and Terminology of the International League Against Epilepsy. Proposal for revised clinical and electroencephalographic classification of epileptic seizures. *Epilepsia.* 1989;30:389–399.
11. Deckers CL, Knoester PD, de Haan GJ, et al. Selection criteria for the clinical use of the newer antiepileptic drugs. *CNS Drugs.* 2003;17:405–421.
12. French JA, Kanner AM, Bautista J, et al. Efficacy and tolerability of the new antiepileptic drugs I: treatment of new onset epilepsy: report of the Therapeutics and Technology Assessment Subcommittee and Quality Standards Subcommittee of the American Academy of Neurology and the American Epilepsy Society. *Neurology.* 2004;62:1252–1260.
13. French JA, Kanner AM, Bautista J, et al. Efficacy and tolerability of the new antiepileptic drugs II: treatment of refractory epilepsy: report of the Therapeutics and Technology Assessment Subcommittee and Quality Standards Subcommittee of the American Academy of Neurology and the American Epilepsy Society. *Neurology.* 2004;62:1261–1273.
14. Gil-Nagel A. Review of new antiepileptic drugs as initial therapy. *Epilepsia.* 2003;44(suppl 4):3–10.
15. Haut SR, Veliskova J, Moshe SL. Susceptibility of immature and adult brains to seizure effects. *Lancet Neurol.* 2004;3:608–617.
16. LaRoche SM, Helmers SL. The new antiepileptic drugs: scientific review. *JAMA.* 2004;291:605–614.
17. Maneuf YP, Gonzalez MI, Sutton KS, et al. Cellular and molecular action of the putative GABA-mimetic, gabapentin. *Cell Mol Life Sci.* 2003;60:742–750.
18. Manno EM. New management strategies in the treatment of status epilepticus. *Mayo Clin Proc.* 2003;78:508–518.
19. Marik PE, Varon J. The management of status epilepticus. *Chest.* 2004;126:582–591.
20. McNamara JO. Drugs effective in the therapy of the epilepsies. In: Hardman JG, et al, eds. *The Pharmacological Basic of Therapeutics.* 10th ed. New York: McGraw-Hill; 2001.
21. Mendiratta A. Clinical neurophysiology of epilepsy. *Curr Neurol Neurosci Rep.* 2003;3:332–340.
22. Morimoto K, Fahnestock M, Racine RJ. Kindling and status epilepticus models of epilepsy: rewiring the brain. *Prog Neurobiol.* 2004;73:1–60.
23. Morrow JI, Craig JJ. Anti-epileptic drugs in pregnancy: current safety and other issues. *Expert Opin Pharmacother.* 2003;4:445–456.
24. Onat F, Ozkara C. Adverse effects of new antiepileptic drugs. *Drugs Today (Barc).* 2004;40:325–342.
25. Pappagallo M. Newer antiepileptic drugs: possible uses in the treatment of neuropathic pain and migraine. *Clin Ther.* 2003;25:2506–2538.
26. Pennell PB. The importance of monotherapy in pregnancy. *Neurology.* 2003;60(suppl 4):S31–S38.
27. Penovich PE, Eck KE, Economou VV. Recommendations for the care of women with epilepsy. *Cleve Clin J Med.* 2004;71(suppl 2):S49–S57.
28. Phelps SJ, Hovinga CA, Boucher BA. Status epilepticus. In: DiPiro JT, et al, eds. *Pharmacotherapy: A Pathophysiologic Approach.* 5th ed. New York: McGraw-Hill; 2002.
29. Riviello JJ. Classification of seizures and epilepsy. *Curr Neurol Neurosci Rep.* 2003;3:325–331.
30. Sander JW. The epidemiology of epilepsy revisited. *Curr Opin Neurol.* 2003;16:165–170.
31. Sander JW. The use of antiepileptic drugs—principles and practice. *Epilepsia.* 2004;45(suppl 6):28–34.
32. Shaefi S, Harkness W. Current status of surgery in the management of epilepsy. *Epilepsia.* 2003;44(suppl 1):43–47.
33. Shneker BF, Fountain NB. Epilepsy. *Dis Mon.* 2003;49:426–478.

34. Sirven JI. Classifying seizures and epilepsy: a synopsis. *Semin Neurol.* 2002;22:237–246.

35. Specchio LM, Beghi E. Should antiepileptic drugs be withdrawn in seizure-free patients? *CNS Drugs.* 2004; 18:201–212.

36. Sperling MR. The consequences of uncontrolled epilepsy. *CNS Spectr.* 2004;9:98–101, 106–109.

37. Spina E, Perugi G. Antiepileptic drugs: indications other than epilepsy. *Epileptic Disord.* 2004; 6: 57–75.

38. Tatum WO, 4th, Liporace J, Benbadis SR, Kaplan PW. Updates on the treatment of epilepsy in women. *Arch Intern Med.* 2004;164:137–145.

39. Tidwell A, Swims M. Review of the newer antiepileptic drugs. *Am J Manag Care.* 2003;9: 253–276.

40. Verrotti A, Trotta D, Salladini C, et al. Risk factors for recurrence of epilepsy and withdrawal of antiepileptic therapy: a practical approach. *Ann Med.* 2003;35: 207–215.

41. Waugh J, Goa KL. Topiramate: as monotherapy in newly diagnosed epilepsy. *CNS Drugs.* 2003;17: 985–992.

42. Webster RA. The epilepsies. In: Webster RA, ed. *Neurotransmitters, Drugs and Brain Function.* New York: John Wiley and Sons; 2001.

43. Yerby MS. Clinical care of pregnant women with epilepsy: neural tube defects and folic acid supplementation. *Epilepsia.* 2003;44(suppl 3):33–40.

44. Yerby MS, Kaplan P, Tran T. Risks and management of pregnancy in women with epilepsy. *Cleve Clin J Med.* 2004;71(suppl 2):S25–S37.

45. Yudkoff M, Daikhin Y, Nissim I, et al. Ketogenic diet, brain glutamate metabolism and seizure control. *Prostaglandins Leukot Essent Fatty Acids.* 2004;70: 277–285.

Chapter 10

Pharmacological Management of Parkinson Disease

Parkinson disease is a movement disorder character-ized by resting tremor, bradykinesia, rigidity, and pos-tural instability.[3,29,32] In Parkinson disease, there is a slow, progressive degeneration of certain dopamine-secreting neurons in the basal ganglia.[29,59,66] Several theories have been proposed to explain this sponta-neous neuronal degeneration, including the possibili-ty that the disease may be caused by a combination of genetic and environmental factors (see "Etiology of Parkinson Disease: Potential Role of Toxic Sub-stances").[22,83] However, the precise initiating factor in Parkinson disease is still unknown.

The clinical syndrome of parkinsonism (i.e., rigidity, bradykinesia) may be caused by other factors such as trauma, infectious agents, antipsychotic drugs, cerebrovascular disease, and various forms of cortical degeneration (including Alzheimer disease).[46,48,54,63] However, the most frequent cause of parkinsonism is the spontaneous slow, selective neuronal degeneration characteristic of Parkinson disease itself.[59,66] Also, the drug management of parkinsonism caused by these other factors closely resembles the management of Parkinson disease.[48] Consequently, this chapter will address the idiopathic onset and pharmacologic treat-ment of Parkinson disease per se.

Parkinson disease usually begins in the fifth or sixth decade, and symptoms progressively worsen over a period of 10 to 20 years. It is estimated that more than 1 percent of the U.S. population older than 60 years is afflicted with Parkinson disease, making it one of the most prevalent neurologic disorders affecting elderly individuals.[59] In addition to the symptoms of bradykinesia and rigidity, a patient with advanced Parkinson disease maintains a flexed posture and speaks in a low, soft voice (microphonia). If left untreated, the motor problems associated with this ill-ness eventually lead to total incapacitation. Rehabilita-tion specialists are often involved in treating patients with this illness due to its prevalence and its associated motor problems.

Fortunately, the pharmacologic management of Parkinson disease has evolved to where the symptoms associated with this disorder can be greatly diminished in many patients. The use of levodopa (L-dopa) alone or in combination with other drugs can improve motor function and general mobility well into the advanced stages of this disease. Drugs used in treating Parkinson disease do not cure this condition, and motor function often tends to slowly deteriorate regardless of when drug therapy is initiated.[51,57,79] However, by alleviating the motor symptoms (i.e., bradykinesia and rigidity), drug therapy can allow patients with Parkinson disease to continue to lead relatively active lifestyles, thus improving their overall physiologic and psychologic well-being.

Pathophysiology of Parkinson Disease

During the past 40 years, the specific neuronal changes associated with the onset and progression of Parkinson disease have been established. Specific alterations in neurotransmitter balance in the basal ganglia are responsible for the symptoms associated with this disorder.[59,66] The basal ganglia are groups of nuclei located in the brain that are involved in the coordination and regulation of motor function. One such nucleus, the substantia nigra, contains the cell bodies of neurons that project to other areas such as the putamen and caudate nucleus (known col-lectively as the "corpus striatum"). The neurotrans-mitter used in this nigrostriatal pathway is dopamine. The primary neural abnormality in Parkinson disease is that dopamine-producing cells in the substantia nigra begin to degenerate, resulting in the eventual loss of dopaminergic input into the corpus striatum.[48,59]

Consequently, the decrease in striatal dopamine seems to be the initiating factor in the symptom onset associated with Parkinson disease. However, it also appears that the lack of dopamine results in an activity increase in basal ganglia cholinergic pathways.[3] Illustrated in Figure 10–1, there is a balance between dopaminergic and cholinergic influence in the basal ganglia under normal conditions. However, the loss of dopaminergic influence in Parkinson disease appears to allow cholinergic influence to dominate.

The relationship between these two neurotransmitters suggests that the role of striatal dopamine may be to modulate acetylcholine release; that is, the lack of

inhibitory dopaminergic influence allows excitatory acetylcholine pathways to run wild. Thus, the symptoms associated with Parkinson disease may be directly caused by increased cholinergic influence occurring secondary to dopamine loss. Current research also suggests that other imbalances involving transmitters such as gamma-aminobutyric acid (GABA), 5-hydroxytryptamine (serotonin), endogenous opioids, and excitatory amino acids (glutamate) may also be present in the basal ganglia subsequent to the loss of dopamine.[3,66] In any event, drug therapy focuses on resolving the dopamine-acetylcholine imbalance to restore normal motor function in Parkinson disease.

Etiology of Parkinson Disease: Genetic and Environmental Factors

As stated previously, the exact factors that initiate the loss of striatal dopamine are unknown in most patients with Parkinson disease. However, recent evidence suggests that genetic factors may interact with environmental factors to make certain individuals susceptible to the destruction of dopaminergic neurons in the substantia nigra.[22,35,83]

Regarding the genetic factors, mutations of several genes have been identified that might play a causative role in Parkinson disease.[22,35] These genes are responsible for controlling the production of alpha-synuclein (a small presynaptic protein) and other neuronal proteins.[6,14,45] Defects in the genes regulating the production of these proteins appear to lead to the overproduction and abnormal accumulation of proteins in neuronal tissues, especially in people with certain forms of Parkinson disease such as early onset parkinsonism and other familial forms.[11,34] As proteins accumulate, they can cause damage to specific cellular components such as the mitochondria and cell membrane.[33,42] Indeed, Parkinson disease and several other neurodegenerative disorders are associated with the formation of Lewy bodies, which are clumps of proteins found in the neuronal tissues.[48,78]

Abnormal protein accumulation therefore seems to play a role in the degenerative changes seen in Parkinson disease. The actual neuronal death, however, may be caused by the formation of harmful byproducts of oxygen metabolism, better known as oxygen "free radicals."[38,75] A free radical is a chemical species that has an unpaired electron in its outer shell.[15] In order to become more stable, the free radical steals an electron from some other cellular component such as a

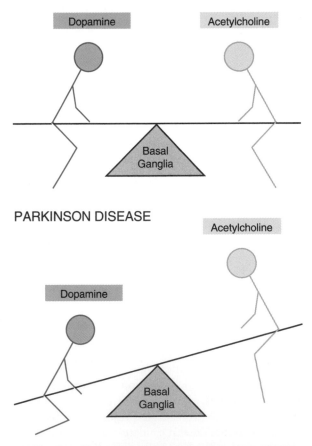

NORMAL

Dopamine   Acetylcholine

Basal Ganglia

PARKINSON DISEASE

Acetylcholine

Dopamine

Basal Ganglia

FIGURE 10–1 ▼ Schematic representation of the neurotransmitter imbalance in Parkinson disease. Normally, a balance exists between dopamine and acetylcholine in the basal ganglia. In Parkinson disease, decreased dopaminergic influence results in increased acetylcholine influence.

protein, DNA molecule, or membrane phospholipid. In this process, the free radical damages the cellular component, subsequently damaging the cell. Free radicals, for example, might initiate or accelerate the abnormal accumulation and aggregation of alpha-synuclein and other proteins within the neuron.[20] Consequently, cells subjected to this free radical-induced damage are said to undergo oxidative stress because loss of electrons (oxidation) of proteins and other cellular components leads to harmful effects on the cell.[15,33]

Hence, oxygen free radicals might ultimately be responsible for causing the degeneration and death of substantia nigra neurons. Production of these free radicals appears to be increased in people with Parkinson disease, either in response to protein accumulation, or because of a primary defect in mitochondrial function.[8,14,21] Regardless of the initiating factor, excess production of free radicals in the basal ganglia could lead to a vicious cycle whereby the free radicals accelerate protein accumulation and damage the mitochondria, which in turn causes more free radical production, and so on.[30,38]

It therefore appears that neurons in the substantia nigra might ultimately be destroyed because genetic factors lead to neuronal protein accumulation and free radical-induced oxidative stress that causes the degeneration and death of these neurons. As indicated earlier, however, the influence of environmental factors should be considered.[49,64] It has been theorized, for example, that environmental toxins (e.g., herbicides, insecticides, fungicides) accelerate the neuronal destruction in people with Parkinson disease.[14] Much of this evidence is based on the finding that a compound known as 1-methyl-4-phenyl-1,2,3,6-tetrahydropyridine (MPTP) appears to be selectively toxic to these neurons and can invoke parkinsonism in primates.[84]

The theory that a toxin like MPTP might cause Parkinson disease was formulated in a rather interesting fashion. In 1982, several young adults in their 20s and 30s developed permanent, severe parkinsonism.[5] Since the onset of Parkinson disease before age 40 is extremely rare, these individuals aroused a great deal of interest. Upon close investigation, all of these individuals were found to have experimented with synthetic heroin-like drugs. These so-called designer drugs were manufactured by drug dealers in an attempt to create an illicit supply of narcotics for sale to heroin addicts. However, the illicit narcotics contained the toxin MPTP, which was discovered to cause selective destruction of substantia nigra neurons.[5]

The discovery of toxin-induced parkinsonism in drug addicts led to the idea that idiopathic Parkinson disease may occur when susceptible individuals are exposed to some environmental toxin.[14] Exposure to such a toxin through industrial waste or certain herbicides may begin the neuronal changes that ultimately result in Parkinson disease. A specific environmental factor, however, has not been identified yet.

Nonetheless, it seems possible that environmental factors might interact with genetic factors to bring about the neuronal destruction associated with Parkinson disease. Environmental toxins, for example, might serve as the trigger for neuronal death in people who have genetic variations that make them vulnerable to these toxins. The exact cause of Parkinson disease remains unknown, however, and future research will hopefully clarify the link between genetic factors, environmental factors, and the mechanism of cell death in the substantia nigra.

The idea that toxins and free radicals may cause neuronal damage in Parkinson disease has also led to research in ways to delay or prevent the destructive effects of these chemicals.[49,60] For example, it has been suggested that certain medications might have neuroprotective effects if they control the production and harmful effects of endogenous toxins such as free radicals. Such medications are often referred to as "antioxidants" because they may help control oxidative stress caused by free radicals. This idea has encouraged the development and use of agents that might delay the neurodegenerative changes seen in Parkinson disease. In particular, drugs used to decrease the symptoms of Parkinson disease (dopamine agonists, selegiline, see later) as well as antioxidants such as vitamin E, have been investigated for any possible neuroprotective effects.[15,30,66] To date, no agent has been identified that is overwhelmingly successful in delaying the neuronal changes occurring in Parkinson disease. Nonetheless, future research may continue to clarify the exact reason for the degeneration of substantia nigra neurons, and drugs that help prevent this degeneration could conceivably be developed to decrease or even eliminate the neuronal death that underlies the disease.

Therapeutic Agents in Parkinsonism

An overview of the drugs used to treat Parkinson disease is shown in Table 10–1. The primary drug used is levodopa. Other agents such as amantadine, anticholinergic drugs, catechol-O-methyltransferase

Table 10–1	OVERVIEW OF DRUG THERAPY IN PARKINSON DISEASE	
Drug	**Mechanism of Action**	**Special Comments**
Levodopa	Resolves dopamine deficiency by being converted to dopamine after crossing blood-brain barrier.	Still the best drug for resolving parkinsonian symptoms; long-term use limited by side effects and decreased efficacy.
Dopamine agonists Bromocriptine Cabergoline Pergolide Pramipexole Ropinirole	Directly stimulates dopamine receptors in basal ganglia.	May produce fewer side effects (dyskinesias, fluctuations in response) than levodopa; preliminary evidence suggests that early use may also delay the progression of Parkinson disease.
Anticholinergics (see Table 10–2)	Inhibit excessive acetylcholine influence caused by dopamine deficiency.	Use in Parkinson disease limited by frequent side effects.
Amantadine	Unclear; may inhibit the effects of excitatory amino acids in the basal ganglia.	May be used alone during early/mild stages or added to drug regimen when levodopa loses effectiveness.
Selegiline	Inhibits the enzyme that breaks down dopamine in the basal ganglia; enables dopamine to remain active for longer periods of time.	May improve symptoms, especially in early stages of Parkinson disease; ability to produce long-term benefits unclear.
COMT* inhibitors Entacapone Tolcapone	Help prevent breakdown of dopamine in peripheral tissues; allows more levodopa to reach the brain.	Useful as an adjunct to levodopa/carbidopa administration; may improve and prolong effects of levodopa.

*COMT: catechol-O-methyltransferase

inhibitors, and direct-acting dopamine agonists can be used alone or in conjunction with levodopa, depending on the needs of the patient. Each of these agents is discussed below.

Levodopa

Because the underlying problem in Parkinson disease is a deficiency of dopamine in the basal ganglia, simple substitution of this chemical would seem to be a logical course of action. However, dopamine does not cross the blood-brain barrier. Administration of dopamine either orally or parenterally will therefore be ineffective because it will be unable to cross from the systemic circulation into the brain where it is needed. Fortunately, the immediate precursor to dopamine, dihydroxyphenylalanine (dopa; Fig. 10–2), crosses the blood-brain barrier quite readily. Dopa, or more specifically levodopa (the L-isomer of dopa), is able to cross the brain capillary endothelium through an active transport process that is specific for this molecule and other large amino acids.[66,71] Upon entering the brain, levodopa is then transformed into dopamine by decarboxylation from the enzyme **dopa decarboxylase** (Fig. 10–3).

Administration of levodopa often dramatically improves all symptoms of parkinsonism, especially bradykinesia and rigidity. The decrease in symptoms and increase in function are remarkable in patients who respond well to the drug. As with any medication, there is a portion of the population who—for unknown reasons—do not respond well or simply cannot tolerate the drug. Also, prolonged use of levodopa is associated with some rather troublesome and frustrating side effects (see "Problems and Adverse Effects of Levodopa Therapy"). However, the use of levodopa has been the most significant advancement in the management of Parkinson disease, and it remains the most effective single drug in the treatment of most patients with this disorder.[32,41,52]

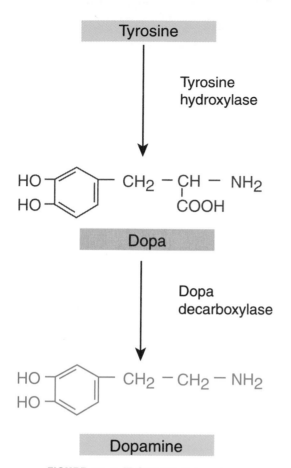

FIGURE 10-2 ▼ Synthesis of dopamine.

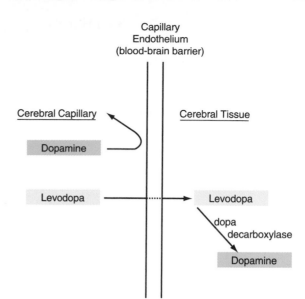

FIGURE 10-3 ▼ Selective permeability of the blood-brain barrier to levodopa.

Levodopa Administration and Metabolism: Use of Peripheral Decarboxylase Inhibitors

Levodopa is usually administered orally; the daily dose is determined according to each patient's needs. Dosages of levodopa are also minimized by administering it with a companion drug that inhibits premature levodopa breakdown (i.e., a peripheral decarboxylase inhibitor such as carbidopa, discussed later in this section). Levodopa dosages are progressively increased until a noticeable reduction in symptoms occurs, or until side effects begin to be a problem. Daily titers are usually divided into two to three doses per day, and individual doses are often given with meals to decrease gastrointestinal irritation.

Following absorption from the gastrointestinal tract, levodopa is rapidly converted to dopamine by the enzyme dopa decarboxylase. This enzyme is distributed extensively throughout the body and can be found in locations such as the liver, intestinal mucosa, kidneys, and skeletal muscle. Conversion of levodopa to dopamine in the periphery is rather extensive—less than 1 percent of the levodopa that is administered reaches the brain in that form.[66] This fact is significant because only levodopa will be able to cross the blood-brain barrier to be subsequently transformed into dopamine. Any levodopa that is converted prematurely to dopamine in the periphery must remain there, becoming essentially useless in alleviating parkinsonism symptoms.

Consequently, when given alone, rather large quantities of levodopa must be administered to ensure that enough levodopa reaches the brain in that form. This is often undesirable because the majority of the levodopa ends up as dopamine in the peripheral circulation, and these high levels of circulating dopamine can cause some unpleasant gastrointestinal and cardiovascular side effects (see the next section). An alternative method is to give levodopa in conjunction with a peripheral decarboxylase inhibitor (Fig. 10–4). The simultaneous use of a drug that selectively inhibits the dopa decarboxylase enzyme outside of the CNS enables more levodopa to reach the brain before being converted to dopamine.

Carbidopa is a peripheral decarboxylase inhibitor that is given in conjunction with levodopa to prevent peripheral decarboxylation (see Fig. 10–4).[48,66] Use of carbidopa with levodopa dramatically decreases the amount of levodopa needed to achieve a desired effect.[48] Another decarboxylase inhibitor known as benserazide is available outside of the United States;

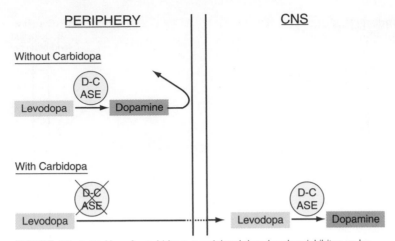

FIGURE 10–4 ▼ Use of a carbidopa, a peripheral decarboxylase inhibitor, on levodopa absorption. Without carbidopa, most of the levodopa is converted to dopamine in the periphery, rendering it unable to cross the blood-brain barrier. Carbidopa inhibits the peripheral decarboxylase (D-C ase) enzyme so that levodopa can cross the blood-brain barrier intact. Carbidopa does not cross the blood-brain barrier so that conversion of levodopa to dopamine still occurs within the CNS.

this drug can also be used to prevent peripheral conversion of levodopa to dopamine.[62]

Since levodopa is almost always administered along with a decarboxylase inhibitor such as carbidopa, these two drugs are often combined in the same pill and marketed under the trade name Sinemet. (Preparations of levodopa with benserazide are marketed as Madopar.) When prepared together as Sinemet, levodopa and carbidopa are combined in specific proportions, usually a fixed carbidopa-to-levodopa ratio of either 1:4 or 1:10.[48] The Sinemet preparation that is typically used to initiate therapy consists of tablets containing 25 mg of carbidopa and 100 mg of levodopa. This ratio is used to achieve a rapid and effective inhibition of the dopa decarboxylase enzyme. A 10:100- or 25:250-mg preparation of carbidopa to levodopa is usually instituted as the parkinsonism symptoms become more pronounced and there is a need for larger relative amounts of levodopa. When administered with carbidopa, levodopa dosages typically begin at 200–300 mg/d, and are increased periodically according to the needs of the patient. Average maintenance dosages of levodopa range between 600–700 mg/d, and the maximum dosage is often 800 mg/d; however, these are highly variable from patient to patient.

Levodopa-carbidopa is also available in a controlled-release preparation (Sinemet CR) that is absorbed more slowly and is intended to provide prolonged effects.[48] The use of this controlled-release preparation may be helpful in patients who respond well to levodopa initially but experience dyskinesias

and fluctuations in response, such as end-of-dose akinesia and the on-off phenomenon.[48] Problems related to levodopa therapy are described in the next section of this chapter.

Problems and Adverse Effects of Levodopa Therapy

Gastrointestinal Problems. Levodopa administration is often associated with nausea and vomiting. These symptoms can be quite severe, especially during the first few days of drug use. However, the incidence of this problem is greatly reduced if levodopa is given in conjunction with a peripheral decarboxylase inhibitor such as carbidopa. The reduction in nausea and vomiting when levodopa peripheral decarboxylation to dopamine is inhibited suggests that these symptoms may be caused by excessive levels of peripherally circulating dopamine.

Cardiovascular Problems. Some problems with cardiac arrhythmias may arise in a patient taking levodopa. However, these problems are usually fairly minor unless the patient has a history of cardiac irregularity. Caution should be used in cardiac patients undergoing levodopa therapy, especially during exercise.

Postural hypotension can also be an extremely troublesome problem in a patient taking levodopa. Again, this side effect is usually diminished when peripheral decarboxylation is inhibited and peripheral dopamine levels are not allowed to increase excessively. Still, patients undergoing physical therapy or similar regimens should be carefully observed during changes in posture and should be instructed to avoid sudden postural adjustments. This factor is especially true in patients beginning or resuming levodopa therapy.

Dyskinesias. A more persistent and challenging problem is the appearance of various movement disorders in patients taking levodopa for prolonged periods. Approximately 80 percent of patients receiving chronic levodopa therapy begin to exhibit various dyskinesias such as choreoathetoid movements, ballismus, dystonia, myoclonus, and various tics and tremors.[3] The specific type of movement disorder can vary from patient to patient, but tends to remain constant within the individual patient. The onset of dyskinetic side effects is particularly frustrating since levodopa ameliorates one form of the movement disorder only to institute a different motor problem.

The onset of dyskinesias usually occurs after the patient has been receiving levodopa therapy for periods ranging from 3 months to several years. In some patients, these abnormal movements may simply be caused by drug-induced overstimulation of dopaminergic pathways in the basal ganglia, and decreasing the daily dosage of levodopa should help. Because levodopa has a short half-life and erratic absorption, the drug may also cause dyskinesias due to its intermittent or pulsatile stimulation of dopamine receptors.[43,68] That is, the sudden rapid influx of levodopa into the brain may combine with endogenous neuronal dopamine release to cause excessive stimulation resulting in various dyskinesias.[52]

The reason for dyskinesias in some patients, however, may be far more complex. Certain patients, for example, may exhibit dyskinesias when plasma levodopa levels are rising or falling, or even when plasma levels are at a minimum.[66] There is evidently an intricate relationship between the basal ganglia neurons that continue to release or respond to dopamine and the pharmacologic replacement of dopamine through levodopa therapy. Dyskinesias may actually be the result of functional and structural adaptations of these neurons caused by periodic fluctuations in dopamine influence supplied from exogenous sources (levodopa).[7,68]

Regardless of the exact neural mechanism that underlies these dyskinesias, the goal of levodopa therapy is to find a regimen that diminishes the incapacitating parkinsonism symptoms without causing other movement disorders.[73] Strategies for minimizing dyskinesias include adjusting the dose of levodopa, using a controlled-release form of this drug, and incorporating other anti-Parkinson medications into the patient's drug regimen.[7,68] In some patients, dyskinesias may be somewhat difficult to control because the optimal dosage of levodopa may fall into a fairly narrow range, and some of the parkinsonism symptoms may appear quite similar to the dyskinetic side effects. The physician, physical therapist, patient, and other individuals dealing with the patient should make careful observations to determine if adjustments in levodopa therapy are resulting in the desired effect.

Behavioral Changes. A variety of mental side effects have been reported in patients taking levodopa. Psychotic symptoms seem especially prevalent, although depression, anxiety, and other changes in behavior have also been noted.[29,57] These problems are especially prevalent in older patients or individuals who have some preexisting psychologic disturbance.[48] Unlike the gastrointestinal and vascular problems described earlier, psychotic symptoms appear to be exacerbated if levodopa is used in conjunction with carbidopa. This event may be caused by greater quantities of levodopa crossing the blood-brain barrier before being converted to dopamine, thus generating higher quantities of dopamine within the brain. This idea seems logical considering that increased activity in certain dopamine pathways seems to be the underlying cause of psychosis (see Chapter 8). Treatment of these symptoms is often difficult because traditional antipsychotic medications tend to increase the symptoms of Parkinson disease. However, some of the newer "atypical" antipsychotics such as clozapine (Chapter 8) may help decrease psychotic symptoms without causing an increase in parkinsonism.[48,77]

Diminished Response to Levodopa. One of the most serious problems in levodopa therapy is that the drug seems to become less effective in many patients when it is administered for prolonged periods. When used continually for periods of 3 to 4 years, the ability of levodopa to relieve parkinsonism symptoms often progressively diminishes to the point where the drug is no longer effective.[57,79] One explanation for this occurrence is that the patient develops a tolerance to the drug. A second theory is that the decreased effectiveness of levodopa may be caused by a progressive increase in the severity of the underlying disease rather than a decrease in drug's efficacy. These two theories on the decreased effectiveness of levodopa have initiated a controversy as to whether or not levodopa therapy should be started early or late in the course of Parkinson disease (see "Clinical Course of Parkinson Disease: When to Use Specific Drugs").

Regardless of why this occurs, the loss of levodopa efficacy can be a devastating blow to the patient who had previously experienced excellent therapeutic results from this drug.

Fluctuations in Response to Levodopa. Several distinct fluctuations in the response to levodopa are fairly common in most patients.[67,69,80] **End-of-dose akinesia** describes the phenomenon where the effectiveness of the drug simply seems to wear off prior to the next dose. This condition, known also as "wearing off," is usually resolved by adjusting the quantity and timing of levodopa administration (i.e., smaller doses may be given more frequently), or by using a sustained release form of the drug.

A more bizarre and less understood fluctuation in response is the **on-off phenomenon**. Here, the effectiveness of levodopa may suddenly and spontaneously decrease, resulting in the abrupt worsening of parkinsonism symptoms (the "off" period). Remission of symptoms may then occur spontaneously or after taking a dose of levodopa (the "on" period). This on-off pattern may repeat itself several times during the day. Although the exact reasons for this phenomenon are unclear, the off periods are directly related to diminishing plasma levels of levodopa.[66] These low levels may occur when the absorption of orally administered levodopa is delayed by poor gastrointestinal motility or if levodopa must compete with large amino acids for transport across the intestinal mucosa.[24] The off periods can be eliminated by administering levodopa continuously by intravenous infusion, thus preventing the fall in plasma levels. However, this is not a long-term solution, and alterations in the oral dosage schedule may have to be made in an attempt to maintain plasma levels at a relatively constant level. Specifically, the drug can be taken with smaller amounts of food and meals that are relatively low in protein so that levodopa absorption is not overwhelmed by dietary amino acid absorption. As indicated earlier, use of a controlled-release formulation such as Sinemet CR can also help alleviate various fluctuations by allowing a more steady, controlled release of levodopa into the bloodstream, thus preventing the fluctuations in plasma levodopa that seem to be responsible for the on-off phenomenon and similar problems.

Drug Holidays from Levodopa

Drug holidays are sometimes used in the patient who has become refractory to the beneficial effects of levodopa or has had a sudden increase in adverse side effects.[3] During this period, the patient is gradually removed from all anti-Parkinson medication for 3 days to 3 weeks while under close medical supervision. The purpose of the holiday is to allow the body to recover from any toxicity or tolerance that may have developed because of prolonged use of levodopa at relatively high dosages. Drug holidays are done with the hope that levodopa can eventually be resumed at a lower dosage and with better results. Drug holidays do appear to be successful in some patients with Parkinson disease. Beneficial effects may be achieved at only half of the preholiday dosage, and the incidence of side effects (such as dyskinesias, confusion, and the on-off phenomenon) may be markedly reduced.[3]

Despite these potential benefits, drug holidays are no longer used routinely because of their potential risk to the patient. Considering that these patients are in the advanced stages of Parkinson disease, discontinuing the anti-Parkinson medications even temporarily results in severe immobility, which can lead to problems such as venous thrombosis, pulmonary embolism, pneumonia, and other impairments that could increase morbidity and mortality.[3] Hence, drug holidays may still be used on a limited basis in a few select patients with Parkinson disease, but this intervention is not used routinely at the present time.

Other Drugs Used to Treat Parkinson Disease

Dopamine Agonists

Because the basic problem in Parkinson disease is a deficiency of striatal dopamine, it would seem logical that drugs similar in function to dopamine would be effective in treating this problem. However, many dopamine agonists have serious side effects that prevent their clinical use. A few dopamine agonists such as bromocriptine (Parlodel), pergolide (Permax), and newer agents such as pramipexole (Mirapex), ropinirole (Requip), and cabergoline (Dostinex) (see Table 10–1) have been developed to treat Parkinson disease without causing excessive adverse effects.[37,61] These dopamine agonists have traditionally been used in conjunction with levodopa, especially in patients who have begun to experience a decrease in levodopa effects, or in those who experience problems such as end-of-dose akinesia and the on-off effect.[48] Simultaneous administration of levodopa with a dopamine agonist permits optimal results with relatively smaller doses of each drug.

Dopamine agonists can also be used alone in the early stages of mild-to-moderate parkinsonism, thus providing an alternative if other anti-Parkinson drugs (including levodopa) are poorly tolerated.[61,76] When used alone, dopamine agonists do not usually cause the dyskinesias and fluctuations in motor responses occurring with levodopa therapy.[36,76] Several of these drugs tend to have a longer half-life than levodopa, and therefore produce a steadier and more prolonged effect on dopamine receptors.[9,19] Dopamine agonists may also be more selective than levodopa in stimulating certain dopamine receptor subtypes such as the D2 receptor, thus resulting in fewer abnormal motor responses.[37] Hence, these drugs continue to gain acceptance as initial treatment for patients with Parkinson disease.

There is also evidence that dopamine agonists may help normalize endogenous dopamine activity, thus having a neuroprotective effect on substantia nigra neurons.[61] As indicated earlier, certain medications are being investigated for their potential to delay or prevent the degeneration of dopamine-producing neurons in the basal ganglia. Dopamine agonists could produce such a neuroprotective effect by providing continuous stimulation of dopamine receptors and preventing the free radical-induced damage that is associated with abnormal dopamine synthesis and breakdown.[12,86] Long-term studies should help clarify if early use of dopamine agonists is successful in slowing the progression of Parkinson disease.

Dopamine agonists may produce adverse side effects such as nausea and vomiting. Postural hypotension is also a problem in some patients. With prolonged use, these drugs may cause CNS-related side effects such as confusion and hallucinations.

Anticholinergic Drugs

As mentioned previously, the deficiency of striatal dopamine results in excessive activity in certain cholinergic pathways in the basal ganglia. Consequently, drugs that limit acetylcholine transmission are used to help alleviate the symptoms of Parkinson disease, especially tremors and rigidity. Various **anticholinergic** agents are available for this purpose, (Table 10–2), and these drugs work by blocking acetylcholine receptors in the basal ganglia.[66] These drugs are fairly nonselective, however, and they tend to produce a wide variety of side effects because they block acetylcholine receptors in various tissues throughout the body (see below). When used alone, anticholinergics are usually only mildly to moderately successful in reducing symptoms and they are typically used in conjunction with levodopa or other anti-Parkinson drugs to obtain optimal results.

Anticholinergics are associated with many side effects including mood change, confusion, hallucinations, drowsiness, and cardiac irregularity.[13,39] In addition, blurred vision, dryness of the mouth, nausea/vomiting, constipation, and urinary retention are fairly common. Antihistamine drugs with anticholinergic properties are also used occasionally (Table 10–2).

Table 10–2	ANTICHOLINERGIC DRUGS USED IN TREATING PARKINSONISM		
Generic Name	**Trade Name**	**Daily Dosage (mg/d)**	**Prescribing Limit (mg/d)**
Benztropine mesylate	Cogentin	1.0–2.0	6
Biperiden	Akineton	6.0–8.0	16
Diphenhydramine*	Benadryl	75–200	300
Ethopropazine	Parsidol	50–100	600
Procyclidine	Kemadrin	7.5–15.0	20
Trihexyphenidyl	Artane	6.0–10.0	15

*Antihistamine drug with anticholinergic properties.

These drugs tend to be somewhat less effective in treating parkinsonism, but appear to have milder side effects than their anticholinergic counterparts.

Amantadine

Amantadine (Symmetrel) was originally developed as an antiviral drug, and its ability to reduce parkinsonian symptoms was discovered by chance.[18] Amantadine was being used to treat influenza in a patient with Parkinson disease, and a noticeable improvement in the patient's tremor and rigidity was also observed. Since that time, amantadine has been approved for use in patients with Parkinson disease and is usually given along with levodopa. Preliminary evidence suggests that this drug may help reduce dyskinesias and other motor complications associated with levodopa therapy in people with advanced Parkinson disease.[23,55,65,74] Additional research, however, is needed to confirm this effect.[18]

Amantadine appears to work by blocking the N-methyl-D-aspartate (NMDA) receptor in the brain, thereby inhibiting the effects of excitatory amino acids such as glutamate.[18,47] This suggests that excitatory neurotransmitters play a role in motor complications associated with advanced Parkinson disease.[23,65] Future research may discover other ways of controlling these excitatory neurotransmitters, thus providing additional treatments for people with advanced Parkinson disease.

The primary adverse effects associated with amantadine are orthostatic hypotension, CNS disturbance (e.g., depression, confusion, hallucinations), and patches of skin discoloration on the lower extremities (livedo reticularis). However, these side effects are relatively mild compared to those of other anti-Parkinson drugs and are usually reversed by altering the drug dosage.

Selegiline

Selegiline (Deprenyl, Eldepryl) is a drug that potently and selectively inhibits the monoamine oxidase type B (MAO$_B$) enzyme. This enzyme is responsible for breaking down dopamine. By inhibiting this enzyme, selegiline prolongs the local effects of dopamine at CNS synapses. Thus, selegiline can be used alone in the early stages of Parkinson disease to prolong the effects of endogenous dopamine produced within the basal ganglia. Early administration of selegiline may alleviate motor symptoms so that patients do not need to begin taking levodopa until later in the course of this disease.[48] Selegiline may also be combined with levodopa therapy because selegiline prolongs the action of dopamine and allows the reduction of parkinsonism symptoms using a relatively low dose of levodopa.[48] Another MAO$_B$ inhibitor, rasagiline (Azilect), has also been developed recently, and exerts effects similar to selegiline.[2,85]

It has been suggested that selegiline may actually slow the progression of Parkinson disease.[70] Theoretically, selegiline could have neuroprotective effects because this drug inhibits dopamine oxidation, thus preventing excessive production of harmful free radicals during dopamine breakdown.[15,28] Selegiline, however, may actually have neuroprotective effects that are unrelated to its effects on dopamine metabolism.[70] It has been suggested, for example, that selegiline may decrease the synthesis of proteins that ultimately lead to cell death (apoptosis) in neurons that have undergone some sort of injury.[27,72] Thus, administration of selegiline early in the course of Parkinson disease may help delay its progression. Nonetheless, the actual effects of this drug on disease progression remain unclear, and future studies will hopefully clarify whether early use produces long-term benefits in people with Parkinson disease.

Selegiline is relatively safe in terms of short-term adverse side effects. With some MAO inhibitors, there is frequently a sudden, large increase in blood pressure if the patient ingests foods containing tyramine (see Chapter 7). However, selegiline does not appear to cause a hypertensive crisis even when such tyramine-containing foods are eaten.[48] Other side effects include dizziness, sedation, gastrointestinal distress, and headache.

Catechol-O-Methyltransferase Inhibitors

A relatively new group of drugs including entacapone (Comtan) and tolcapone (Tasmar) were developed to enhance the effects of levodopa. These drugs inhibit an enzyme known as catechol-O-methyltransferase (COMT). This enzyme converts levodopa to an inactive metabolite known as 3-O-methyldopa; hence, these drugs are referred to as COMT inhibitors.[10] By preventing levodopa conversion in peripheral tissues, more levodopa is available to reach the brain and exert beneficial effects. Hence, these drugs are used as an adjunct to levodopa therapy to provide better therapeutic effects using smaller doses of levodopa.[53] Evidence suggests that adding a COMT inhibitor to levodopa therapy may also reduce fluctuations in the response to levodopa, and prolong the periods of levodopa effectiveness ("on" time) with shorter periods of unresponsiveness ("off" time).[53,56]

The primary problem associated with COMT inhibitors is an initial increase in dyskinesias.[10] This problem may be due to the fact that the COMT inhibitor is allowing more levodopa to reach the brain, and that the levodopa dosage needs to be lowered accordingly. Other side effects include nausea, diarrhea, dizziness, and muscle pain/cramps.

Clinical Course of Parkinson Disease: When to Use Specific Drugs

Controversy exists as to when specific anti-Parkinson drugs should be employed.[1,16] Much of the debate focuses on when levodopa therapy should be initiated. Without question, levodopa is the most effective pharmacological treatment for reducing the motor symptoms of Parkinson disease. As mentioned previously, however, long-term use of levodopa poses several risks, and the effectiveness of this drug seems to diminish after several years of use. Consequently, some practitioners question whether levodopa therapy should be withheld until the parkinsonian symptoms become severe enough to truly impair motor function. In theory, this saves the levodopa for more advanced stages of this disease, when it would be needed the most.[48]

Recently, some sources suggested that dopamine agonists might be a suitable alternative to levodopa as the initial treatment of Parkinson disease.[1,16] Dopamine agonists can help resolve parkinsonian symptoms, sparing the use of levodopa until later in the course of the disease. As indicated, dopamine agonists may also have a reduced incidence of dyskinesias, and may slow the degeneration of substantia nigra neurons (neuroprotective effect). Thus, early use of these medications could potentially slow the progression of Parkinson disease. Levodopa can also be incorporated into the drug regimen as disability increases, along with other medications such as amantadine, anticholinergics, COMT inhibitors, and selegiline.[48]

There is no clear consensus of which drugs should be used in the initial and subsequent treatment of Parkinson disease. Future research should help clarify whether it is better to begin treatment with dopamine agonists, and to save levodopa and other medications until later in the disease course. Ultimately, the physi-

cian should select specific medications based on a patient's individual characteristics at each stage of the disease.[48]

Neurosurgical Interventions in Parkinson Disease

Several innovative approaches have been studied to try to achieve a more permanent resolution to the dopamine imbalance in Parkinson disease. One approach is to surgically implant dopamine-producing cells into the substantia nigra to replace the cells that have been destroyed by the disease process.[26,58] This strategy, however, is limited by several issues, including how to get a supply of viable cells. A potential source of these cells has been from fetal mesenchymal tissues. Embryonically derived stem cells have the potential to differentiate into virtually any type of human cell, thus providing a source that could be used to repair damaged tissues in many degenerative conditions including Parkinson disease.[25,40]

This approach, however, has generated considerable concern about the ethical use of fetal tissues for medical research and treatment. Alternative sources such as stem cells from adult bone marrow or human chromaffin cells have also been considered, but these sources might not be as effective as cells from embryonic tissues.[26] Regardless of their source, there are some practical limitations associated with implanting a sufficient number of these cells into a small area deep in the brain and then keeping these cells alive and producing dopamine. Patients who would benefit from such transplants are typically older and somewhat debilitated with a possible reduction in blood flow and oxygenation of tissues deep in the brain. These facts, combined with the presence of the original pathologic process that caused Parkinson disease, may limit the transplanted tissues chances for survival.

Hence, tissue transplants have not shown overwhelming clinical success, and the future of this technique as an effective and widely used method of treating Parkinson disease remains doubtful at present.[58] It may be possible that new developments, including the use of cell cultures as a source of dopamine-producing cells and the use of drugs to prolong the survival of transplanted tissues, may improve the clinical outcome of this technique. Still, it remains to be seen whether tissue transplants will ever be a practical and routine method of treating the rather large number of patients with the disease.

An alternative nonpharmacological treatment involves the use of specific surgeries (pallidotomy, thalotomy) to produce lesions in specific neuronal pathways in patients with advanced Parkinson disease.[82] These surgical lesions, however, are associated with many risks and side effects.[50] An alternative strategy consists of surgically implanting electrodes into deep brain structures such as the globus pallidus, thalamus, and subthalamic nucleus.[44,82] High-frequency stimulation of these structures may help normalize neuronal circuitry within the basal ganglia, and help resolve the motor symptoms of advanced Parkinson disease.[4,44] It is beyond the scope of this chapter to review these newer surgical and electrical stimulation techniques. Nonetheless, these nonpharmacologic interventions continue to be developed and will hopefully provide an alternative treatment for patients who have become refractory to drug therapy during the advanced stages of the disease.[82]

SUMMARY

The cause of Parkinson disease remains unknown. However, the neuronal changes that produce the symptoms associated with this movement disorder

Special Considerations for Rehabilitation

■ ■ ■ Therapists who are treating patients with Parkinson disease usually wish to coordinate the therapy session with the peak effects of drug therapy. In patients receiving levodopa, this usually occurs approximately 1 hour after a dose of the medication has been taken. If possible, scheduling the primary therapy session in elderly patients after the breakfast dose of levodopa often yields optimal effects from the standpoint of both maximal drug efficacy and low fatigue levels.

Therapists working in hospitals and other institutions are sometimes faced with the responsibility of treating patients who are on a drug holiday. As discussed previously, the patient is placed in the hospital for several days and all anti-Parkinson medication is withdrawn so that the patient may recover from the adverse effects of prolonged levodopa administration. During the drug holiday, the goal of physical therapy is to maintain patient mobility as much as possible. Obviously, without anti-Parkinson drugs, this task is often quite difficult. Many patients are well into the advanced stages of the disease, and even a few days without medication can produce profound debilitating effects. Consequently, any efforts to maintain joint range of motion and cardiovascular fitness during the drug holiday are crucial in helping the patient resume activity when medications are reinstated.

Therapists should also be aware of the need to monitor blood pressure in patients receiving anti-Parkinson drugs. Most of these drugs cause orthostatic hypotension, especially during the first few days treatment. Dizziness and syncope often occur because of a sudden drop in blood pressure when the patient stands up. Because patients with Parkinson disease are susceptible to falls, this problem is only increased by the chance of orthostatic hypotension. Consequently, therapists must be especially careful to guard against falls by the patient taking anti-Parkinson drugs.

Finally, rehabilitation specialists should recognize that they can have a direct and positive influence on the patient's health and need for drug treatment. There is consensus that an aggressive program of gait training, balance activities, and other appropriate exercises can be extremely helpful in promoting optimal health and function in patients with Parkinson disease.[17,31,81] Using physical therapy and occupational therapy interventions to maintain motor function can diminish the patient's need for anti-Parkinson drugs. The synergistic effects of physical rehabilitation and the judicious use of drugs will ultimately provide better results than either intervention used alone.

CASE STUDY

Anti-Parkinson Drugs

Brief History. M.M. is a 67-year-old woman who was diagnosed with Parkinson disease 6 years ago, at which time she was treated with anticholinergic drugs (i.e., benztropine mesylate, diphenhydramine). After approximately 2 years, bradykinesia and the rigidity associated with this disease began to be more pronounced, so she was started on a combination of levodopa-carbidopa. The initial levodopa dosage was 400 mg/d. She was successfully maintained on levodopa for the next 3 years, with minor adjustments in the dosage. During that time, M.M. had been living at home with her husband. During the past 12 months, her husband noted that her ability to get around seemed to be declining, so the levodopa dosage was progressively increased to 600 mg/d. The patient was also referred to physical therapy on an outpatient basis in an attempt to maintain mobility and activities of daily living (ADL). She began attending physical therapy three times per week, and a regimen designed to maintain musculoskeletal flexibility, posture, and balance was initiated.

Problem/Influence of Medication. The patient was seen by the therapist three mornings each week. After a few sessions, the therapist observed that there were certain days when the patient was able to actively and vigorously participate in the therapy program. On other days, the patient was essentially akinetic, and her active participation in exer-cise and gait activities was virtually impossible. There was no pattern to her good and bad days, and the beneficial effects of the rehabilitation program seemed limited by the rather random effects of her medication. The patient stated that these akinetic episodes sometimes occurred even on nontherapy days.

Decision/Solution. After discussions with the patient and her husband, the therapist realized that the morning dose of levodopa was sometimes taken with a rather large breakfast. On other days, the patient consumed only a light breakfast. In retrospect, the akinetic episodes usually occurred on days when a large morning meal was consumed. The therapist surmised that this probably occurred because the large breakfast was impairing absorption of levodopa from the gastrointestinal tract. The patient was probably exhibiting the on-off phenomenon sometimes seen in patients receiving long-term levodopa therapy, which was brought on by the impaired absorption of the drug. This problem was resolved by having the patient consistently take the morning dose with a light breakfast. On mornings when the patient was still hungry, she waited 1 hour before consuming additional food to allow complete absorption of the medication. The problem was also brought to the physician's attention, and the physician prescribed a sustained release form of levodopa/carbidopa (Sinemet CR) to help provide a more continuous and prolonged absorption.

---

have been identified. Degeneration of dopaminergic neurons in the substantia nigra results in a deficiency of dopamine and subsequent overactivity of acetylcholine in the basal ganglia. Pharmacologic treatment attempts to rectify this dopamine-acetylcholine imbalance. Although no cure is currently available, drug therapy can dramatically improve the clinical picture in many patients by reducing the incapacitating symptoms of parkinsonism.

The use of levodopa and several other medications has allowed many patients with Parkinson disease to remain active despite the disease's steadily degenerative nature. Levodopa, currently the drug of choice in treating parkinsonism, often produces remarkable improvements in motor function. However, levodopa is associated with several troublesome side effects, and the effectiveness of this drug tends to diminish with time. Other agents, such as dopamine agonists, amantadine, selegiline, anticholinergic drugs, and COMT inhibitors, can be used alone, in combination with levodopa, or with each other to prolong the functional status of the patient. Physical therapists and other rehabilitation specialists can maximize the effectiveness of their treatments by coordinating therapy sessions with drug administration. Therapists also play a vital role in maintaining function in the patient with Parkinson disease when the efficacy of these drugs begins to diminish.

References

1. Ahlskog JE. Parkinson's disease: is the initial treatment established? *Curr Neurol Neurosci Rep.* 2003;3:289–295.

2. Am OB, Amit T, Youdim MB. Contrasting neuroprotective and neurotoxic actions of respective metabolites of anti-Parkinson drugs rasagiline and selegiline. *Neurosci Lett.* 2004;355:169–172.

3. Aminoff MJ. Pharmacologic management of parkinsonism and other movement disorders. In: Katzung, BG, ed. *Basic and Clinical Pharmacology*, 9th ed. New York: Lange Medical Books/McGraw Hill; 2004.

4. Ashkan K, Wallace B, Bell BA, Benabid AL. Deep brain stimulation of the subthalamic nucleus in Parkinson's disease 1993–2003: where are we 10 years on? *Br J Neurosurg.* 2004;18:19–34.

5. Ballard PA, Tetrud JW, Langston JW. Permanent human parkinsonism due to 1-methyl-4-phenyl-1,2,3,6-tetrahydropyridine (MPTP): seven cases. *Neurology.* 1985;35:949–956.

6. Baptista MJ, Cookson MR, Miller DW. Parkin and alpha-synuclein: opponent actions in the pathogenesis of Parkinson's disease. *Neuroscientist.* 2004;10:63–72.

7. Barone P. Clinical strategies to prevent and delay motor complications. *Neurology.* 2003;61(suppl 3): S12–S16.

8. Beal MF. Mitochondria, oxidative damage, and inflammation in Parkinson's disease. *Ann N Y Acad Sci.* 2003; 991:120–131.

9. Bracco F, Battaglia A, Chouza C, et al. The long-acting dopamine receptor agonist cabergoline in early Parkinson's disease: final results of a 5-year, double-blind, levodopa-controlled study. *CNS Drugs.* 2004; 18:733–746.

10. Brooks DJ. Safety and tolerability of COMT inhibitors. *Neurology.* 2004;62(suppl 1):S39–S46.

11. Burke RE. Recent advances in research on Parkinson disease: synuclein and parkin. *Neurologist.* 2004;10: 75–81.

12. Chalimoniuk M, Stepien A, Strosznajder JB. Pergolide mesylate, a dopaminergic receptor agonist, applied with L-DOPA enhances serum antioxidant enzyme activity in Parkinson disease. *Clin Neuropharmacol.* 2004;27:223–229.

13. Chan DK. The art of treating Parkinson disease in the older patient. *Aust Fam Physician.* 2003;32:927–931.

14. Chung KK, Dawson VL, Dawson TM. New insights into Parkinson's disease. *J Neurol.* 2003;250(suppl 3): III15–III24.

15. Ciccone CD. Free-radical toxicity and antioxidant medications in Parkinson disease. *Phys Ther.* 1998;78: 313–319.

16. Clarke CE. Neuroprotection and pharmacotherapy for motor symptoms in Parkinson's disease. *Lancet Neurol.* 2004;3:466–474.

17. Comella CL, Stebbins GT, Brown-Toms N, Goetz CG. Physical therapy and Parkinson disease: a controlled clinical trial. *Neurology.* 1994;44:376–378.

18. Crosby NJ, Deane KH, Clarke CE. Amantadine for dyskinesia in Parkinson's disease. *Cochrane Database Syst Rev.* 2003;CD003467.

19. Curran MP, Perry CM. Cabergoline: a review of its use in the treatment of Parkinson's disease. *Drugs.* 2004;64:2125–2141.

20. Dauer W, Przedborski S. Parkinson's disease: mechanisms and models. *Neuron.* 2003;39:889–909.

21. Dawson TM, Dawson VL. Molecular pathways of neurodegeneration in Parkinson's disease. *Science.* 2003;302:819–822.

22. Dekker MC, Bonifati V, van Duijn CM. Parkinson's disease: piecing together a genetic jigsaw. *Brain.* 2003;126:1722–1733.

23. Del Dotto P, Pavese N, Gambaccini G, et al. Intravenous amantadine improves levadopa induced dyskinesias: an acute double-blind placebo-controlled study. *Mov Disord.* 2001; 16:515–520.

24. Djaldetti R, Melamed, E. Management of response fluctuations: practical guidelines. *Neurology.* 1998;51 (suppl 2):S36–S40.

25. Doss MX, Koehler CI, Gissel C, et al. Embryonic stem cells: a promising tool for cell replacement therapy. *J Cell Mol Med.* 2004;8:465–473.

26. Drucker-Colin R, Verdugo-Diaz L. Cell transplantation for Parkinson's disease: present status. *Cell Mol Neurobiol.* 2004;24:301–316.

27. Ebadi M, Sharma SK. Peroxynitrite and mitochondrial dysfunction in the pathogenesis of Parkinson's disease. *Antioxid Redox Signal.* 2003;5:319–335.

28. Ebadi M, Sharma S, Shavali S, El Refaey H. Neuroprotective actions of selegiline. *J Neurosci Res.* 2002; 67:285–289.

29. Fahn S. Description of Parkinson's disease as a clinical syndrome. *Ann N Y Acad Sci.* 2003;991:1–14.

30. Fernandez-Espejo E. Pathogenesis of Parkinson's disease: prospects of neuroprotective and restorative therapies. *Mol Neurobiol.* 2004;29:15–30.

31. Formisano R, Pratesi L, Modarelli FT, et al. Rehabilitation and Parkinson disease. *Scand J Rehabil Med.* 1992;24:157–160.

32. Guttman M, Kish SJ, Furukawa Y. Current concepts in the diagnosis and management of Parkinson's disease. *CMAJ.* 2003;168:293–301.

33. Hashimoto M, Rockenstein E, Crews L, Masliah E. Role of protein aggregation in mitochondrial dysfunction and neurodegeneration in Alzheimer's and Parkinson's diseases. *Neuromolecular Med.* 2003; 4:21–36.

34. Hattori N, Mizuno Y. Pathogenetic mechanisms of parkin in Parkinson's disease. *Lancet.* 2004;364: 722–724.

35. Huang Y, Cheung L, Rowe D, Halliday G. Genetic contributions to Parkinson's disease. *Brain Res Brain Res Rev.* 2004;46:44–70.

36. Inzelberg R, Schechtman E, Nisipeanu P. Cabergoline, pramipexole and ropinirole used as monotherapy in early Parkinson's disease: an evidence-based comparison. *Drugs Aging.* 2003;20:847–855.

37. Jenner P. Dopamine agonists, receptor selectivity and dyskinesia induction in Parkinson's disease. *Curr Opin Neurol.* 2003;16(suppl 1):S3–S7.

38. Jenner P. Oxidative stress in Parkinson's disease. *Ann Neurol.* 2003;53(suppl 3):S26–S38.

39. Katzenschlager R, Sampaio C, Costa J, Lees A. Anticholinergics for symptomatic management of Parkinson's disease. *Cochrane Database Syst Rev.* 2003; CD003735.

40. Kim SU. Human neural stem cells genetically modified for brain repair in neurological disorders. *Neuropathology.* 2004;24:159–171.

41. Lang AE, Obeso JA. Challenges in Parkinson's disease: restoration of the nigrostriatal dopamine system is not enough. *Lancet Neurol.* 2004;3:309–316.

42. Lee SJ. Alpha-synuclein aggregation: a link between mitochondrial defects and Parkinson's disease? *Antioxid Redox Signal.* 2003;5:337–348.

43. LeWitt PA, Nyholm D. New developments in levodopa therapy. *Neurology.* 2004;62(suppl 1): S9–S16.

44. Lozano AM, Mahant N. Deep brain stimulation surgery for Parkinson's disease: mechanisms and consequences. *Parkinsonism Relat Disord.* 2004;10(suppl 1): S49–S57.

45. Marin I, Lucas JI, Gradilla AC, Ferrus A. Parkin and relatives: the RBR family of ubiquitin ligases. *Physiol Genomics.* 2004;17:253–263.

46. Mattson MP. Infectious agents and age-related neurodegenerative disorders. *Ageing Res Rev.* 2004;3: 105–120.

47. Moresco RM, Volonte MA, Messa C, et al. New perspectives on neurochemical effects of amantadine in the brain of parkinsonian patients: a PET-[(11)C] raclopride study. *J Neural Transm.* 2002;109: 1265–1274.

48. Nelson MV, Berchou RC, LeWitt PA. Parkinson disease. In: DiPiro, JT, et al, eds. *Pharmacotherapy: A Pathophysiologic Approach.* 5th ed. New York: McGraw-Hill, NY; 2002.

49. Nomoto M. Clinical pharmacology and neuroprotection in Parkinson's disease. *Parkinsonism Relat Disord.* 2003;9(suppl 2):S55–S58.

50. Okun MS, Vitek JL. Lesion therapy for Parkinson's disease and other movement disorders: update and controversies. *Mov Disord.* 2004;19:375–389.

51. Olanow CW. The scientific basis for the current treatment of Parkinson's disease. *Annu Rev Med.* 2004;55: 41–60.

52. Olanow CW, Agid Y, Mizuno Y, et al. Levodopa in the treatment of Parkinson's disease: current controversies. *Mov Disord.* 2004;19:997–1005.

53. Olanow CW, Stocchi F. COMT inhibitors in Parkinson's disease: can they prevent and/or reverse levodopa-induced motor complications? *Neurology.* 2004;62(suppl 1):S72–S81.

54. O'Suilleabhain P, Dewey RB, Jr. Movement disorders after head injury: diagnosis and management. *J Head Trauma Rehabil.* 2004;19:305–313.

55. Paci C, Thomas A, Onofrj M. Amantadine for dyskinesia in patients affected by severe Parkinson's disease. *Neurol Sci.* 2001;22:75–76.

56. Poewe W. The role of COMT inhibition in the treatment of Parkinson's disease. *Neurology.* 2004;62 (suppl 1):S31–S38.

57. Rascol O, Payoux P, Ory F, et al. Limitations of current Parkinson's disease therapy. *Ann Neurol.* 2003; 53(suppl 3):S3–S15.

58. Roitberg B, Urbaniak K, Emborg M. Cell transplantation for Parkinson's disease. *Neurol Res.* 2004;26: 355–362.

59. Samii A, Nutt JG, Ransom BR. Parkinson's disease. *Lancet.* 2004;363:1783–1793.

60. Schapira AH, Olanow CW. Neuroprotection in Parkinson disease: mysteries, myths, and misconceptions. *JAMA.* 2004;291:358–364.

61. Schwarz J. Rationale for dopamine agonist use as monotherapy in Parkinson's disease. *Curr Opin Neurol.* 2003;16(suppl 1):S27–S33.

62. Shen H, Kannari K, Yamato H, et al. Effects of benserazide on L-DOPA-derived extracellular dopamine levels and aromatic L-amino acid decarboxylase activity in the striatum of 6-hydroxydopamine-lesioned rats. *Tohoku J Exp Med.* 2003;199:149–159.

63. Sibon I, Tison F. Vascular parkinsonism. *Curr Opin Neurol.* 2004;17:49–54.

64. Siderowf A, Stern M. Update on Parkinson disease. *Ann Intern Med.* 2003;138:651–658.

65. Snow BJ, Macdonald L, Mcauley D, Wallis W. The effect of amantadine on levodopa induced dyskinesias in Parkinson's disease: a double-blind, placebo-controlled study. *Clin Neuropharmacol.* 2000; 23:82–85.

66. Standaert DG, Young AB. Treatment of central nervous system degnerative disorders. In: Hardman, JG, et al, eds. *The Pharmacological Basis of Therapeutics.* 10th ed. New York: McGraw-Hill; 2001.

67. Stocchi F. Prevention and treatment of motor fluctuations. *Parkinsonism Relat Disord.* 2003;9(suppl 2): S73–S81.

68. Stocchi F, Olanow CW. Continuous dopaminergic stimulation in early and advanced Parkinson's disease. *Neurology.* 2004;62(suppl 1):S56–S63.

69. Swope DM. Rapid treatment of "wearing off" in Parkinson's disease. *Neurology.* 2004;62(suppl 4): S27–S31.

70. Tabakman R, Lecht S, Lazarovici P. Neuroprotection by monoamine oxidase B inhibitors: a therapeutic strategy for Parkinson's disease? *Bioessays.* 2004;26: 80–90.

71. Tamai I, Tsuji A. Transporter-mediated permeation of drugs across the blood-brain barrier. *J Pharm Sci.* 2000;89:1371–1388.

72. Tatton W, Chalmers-Redman R, Tatton N. Neuroprotection by deprenyl and other propargylamines: glyceraldehyde-3-phosphate dehydrogenase rather than monoamine oxidase B. *J Neural Transm.* 2003;110:509–515.

73. Thanvi BR, Lo TC. Long term motor complications of levodopa: clinical features, mechanisms, and management strategies. *Postgrad Med J.* 2004;80:452–458.

74. Thomas A, Iacono D, Luciano AL, et al. Duration of amantadine benefit on dyskinesia of severe Parkinson's disease. *J Neurol Neurosurg Psychiatry.* 2004;75: 141–143.

75. Tieu K, Ischiropoulos H, Przedborski S. Nitric oxide and reactive oxygen species in Parkinson's disease. *IUBMB Life.* 2003;55:329–335.

76. Tintner R, Jankovic J. Dopamine agonists in Parkinson's disease. *Expert Opin Investig Drugs.* 2003;12: 1803–1820.

77. Tolosa E. Advances in the pharmacological management of Parkinson disease. *J Neural Transm Suppl.* 2003;64:65–78.

78. Trzesniewska K, Brzyska M, Elbaum D. Neurodegenerative aspects of protein aggregation. *Acta Neurobiol Exp.* 2004;64:41–52.

79. Tuite P, Riss J. Recent developments in the pharmacological treatment of Parkinson's disease. *Expert Opin Investig Drugs.* 2003;12:1335–1352.

80. van Laar T. Levodopa-induced response fluctuations in patients with Parkinson's disease: strategies for management. *CNS Drugs.*2003;17:475–489.

81. Wade DT, Gage H, Owen C, et al. Multidisciplinary rehabilitation for people with Parkinson's disease: a randomised controlled study. *J Neurol Neurosurg Psychiatry.* 2003;74:158–162.

82. Walter BL, Vitek JL. Surgical treatment for Parkinson's disease. *Lancet Neurol.* 2004;3:719–728.

83. Warner TT, Schapira AH. Genetic and environmental factors in the cause of Parkinson's disease. *Ann Neurol.* 2003;53(suppl 3):S16–S25.

84. Wichmann T, DeLong MR. Pathophysiology of Parkinson's disease: the MPTP primate model of the human disorder. *Ann N Y Acad Sci.* 2003;991: 199–213.

85. Youdim MB, Bar Am O, Yogev-Falach M, et al. Rasagiline: neurodegeneration, neuroprotection, and mitochondrial permeability transition. *J Neurosci Res.* 2005;79:172–179.

86. Yuan H, Sarre S, Ebinger G, Michotte Y. Neuroprotective and neurotrophic effect of apomorphine in the striatal 6-OHDA-lesion rat model of Parkinson's disease. *Brain Res.* 2004;1026:95–107.

Chapter 11

General Anesthetics

The discovery and development of anesthetic agents has been one of the most significant contributions in the advancement of surgical technique. Before the use of anesthesia, surgery was used only as a last resort and was often performed with the patient conscious, but physically restrained by several large "assistants." During the past century, general and local anesthetic drugs have been used to allow surgery to be performed in a manner that is safer, that is much less traumatic to the patient, and that permits lengthier and more sophisticated surgical procedures.

Anesthetics are categorized as general or local, depending on whether or not the patient remains conscious when the anesthetic is administered. General anesthetics are usually administered during the more extensive surgical procedures. Local anesthetics are given when analgesia is needed in a relatively small, well-defined area, or when the patient needs to remain conscious during surgery. The use of general anesthesia and general anesthetic agents is presented in this chapter; local anesthetics are dealt with in Chapter 12.

Most physical therapists and other rehabilitation specialists are usually not involved in working with patients while general anesthesia is actually being administered. However, knowledge of how these agents work will help the therapist understand some of the residual effects that may occur when the patient is recovering from the anesthesia. This knowledge will help the therapist understand how these effects may directly influence the therapy sessions that take place during the first few days after procedures in which general anesthesia was used.

General Anesthesia: Requirements

During major surgery (such as laparotomy, thoracotomy, joint replacement, amputation), the patient should be unconscious throughout the procedure and, upon awakening, have no recollection of what occurred during the surgery. An ideal anesthetic agent must be able to produce each of the following conditions:

1. Loss of consciousness and sensation.
2. Amnesia (i.e., no recollection of what occurred during the surgery).
3. Skeletal muscle relaxation (this requirement is currently met with the aid of skeletal muscle blockers used in conjunction with the anesthetic [see "Neuromuscular Blockers," later]).
4. Inhibition of sensory and autonomic reflexes.
5. A minimum of toxic side effects (i.e., be relatively safe).
6. Rapid onset of anesthesia; easy adjustment of the anesthetic dosage during the procedure; and rapid, uneventful recovery after administration is terminated.

Current general anesthetics meet these criteria quite well, providing that the dose is high enough to produce an adequate level of anesthesia but not so high that problems occur. The relationship between dosage and level or plane of anesthesia is discussed in the next section, "Stages of General Anesthesia."

Stages of General Anesthesia

During general anesthesia, the patient goes through a series of stages as the anesthetic dosage and amount of anesthesia reaching the brain progressively increase. Four stages of anesthesia are commonly identified.[39]

Stage I. Analgesia. The patient begins to lose somatic sensation but is still conscious and somewhat aware of what is happening.

Stage II. Excitement (Delirium). The patient is unconscious and amnesiac but appears agitated and restless. This paradoxical increase in the level of excitation is highly undesirable because patients may injure themselves while thrashing about. Thus, an effort is made to move as quickly as possible through this stage and on to stage III.

Stage III. Surgical Anesthesia. As the name implies, this level is desirable for the surgical procedure and begins with the onset of regular, deep respiration. Some sources subdivide this stage into several planes, according to respiration rate and reflex activity. [39]

Stage IV. Medullary Paralysis. This stage is marked by the cessation of spontaneous respiration because respiratory control centers located in the medulla oblongata are inhibited by excessive anesthesia. The ability of the medullary vasomotor center to regulate blood pressure is also affected, and cardiovascular collapse ensues. If this stage is inadvertently reached during anesthesia, respiratory and circulatory support must be provided or the patient will die.[39]

Consequently, the goal of the anesthetist is to bring the patient to stage III as rapidly as possible and to maintain the patient at that stage for the duration of the surgical procedure. This goal is often accomplished by using both an intravenous and an inhaled anesthetic agent (see next section, "General Anesthetic Agents: Classification and Use According to Route of Administration"). Finally, the anesthetic should not be administered any longer than necessary, or recovery will be delayed. This state is often accomplished by beginning to taper off the dosage toward the end of the surgical procedure so that the patient is already recovering as surgery is completed.

General Anesthetics: Classification and Use According to Route of Administration

Specific agents are classified according to the two primary routes of administration—intravenous or inhaled.[11,39] Intravenously injected anesthetics offer the advantage of a rapid onset, thus allowing the patient to pass through the first two stages of anesthesia very quickly. The primary disadvantage is that there is a relative lack of control over the level of anesthesia if too much of the drug is injected. Inhaled anesthetics provide an easier method of making adjustments in the dosage during the procedure, but it takes a relatively long time for the onset of the appropriate level of anesthesia. Consequently, a combination of injected and inhaled agents is often used sequentially during lengthier surgical procedures.[10] The intravenous drug is injected first to quickly get the patient to stage III, and an inhaled agent is then administered to maintain the patient in a stage of surgical anesthesia. Ultimately, the selection of exactly which agents will be used depends on the type and length of the surgical procedure and any possible interactions with other anesthetics or medical problems of the patient. Specific injected and inhaled anesthetics are presented here.

General Anesthetics: Specific Agents

Inhalation Anesthetics

Anesthetics administered by this route exist either as gases or as volatile liquids that can be easily mixed with air or oxygen and then inhaled by a patient. When administered, a system of tubing and valves is usually employed to deliver the anesthetic drug directly to the patient through an endotracheal tube or a mask over the face (Figure 11–1). This delivery system offers the obvious benefit of focusing the drug on the patient without anesthetizing everyone else in the room. These systems also allow for easy adjustment of the rate of delivery and concentration of the inhaled drug.

Inhaled anesthetics currently in use include halogenated volatile liquids such as desflurane, enflurane, halothane, isoflurane, methoxyflurane, and sevoflurane (Table 11–1). These volatile liquids are all chemically similar, but newer agents such as desflurane and sevoflurane are often used preferentially because they permit a more rapid onset, a faster recovery, and better control during anesthesia compared to older agents such as halothane.[9,15] These volatile liquids likewise represent the primary form of inhaled anesthetics. The only gaseous anesthetic currently in widespread use is nitrous oxide, which is usually reserved for relatively short-term procedures (e.g., tooth extractions). Earlier inhaled anesthetics, such as ether, chloroform, and cyclopropane, are not currently used because they are explosive in nature or produce toxic effects that do not occur with the more modern anesthetic agents.

Intravenous Anesthetics

When given in appropriate doses, several categories of central nervous system (CNS) depressants can serve as

Text continued on page 139

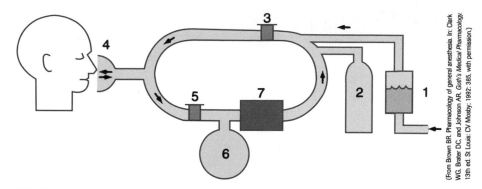

(From Brown BR. Pharmacology of general anesthesia. In: Clark WG, Brater DC, and Johnson AR. *Goth's Medical Pharmacology.* 13th ed. St Louis: CV Mosby; 1992: 385, with permission.)

FIGURE 11–1 ▼ Schematic diagram of a closed anesthesia system. (*1*) Vaporizer for volatile liquid anesthetics. (*2*) Compressed gas source. (*3*) Inhalation unidirectional valve. (*4*) Mask. (*5*) Unidirectional exhalation valve. (*6*) Rebreathing bag. (*7*) Carbon dioxide absorption chamber.

Table 11–1	GENERAL ANESTHETICS

Anesthetic	**Representative Structure**

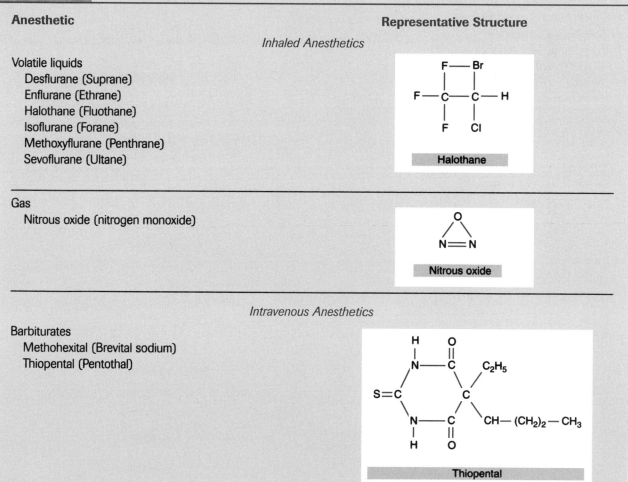

Inhaled Anesthetics

Volatile liquids
   Desflurane (Suprane)
   Enflurane (Ethrane)
   Halothane (Fluothane)
   Isoflurane (Forane)
   Methoxyflurane (Penthrane)
   Sevoflurane (Ultane)

Gas
   Nitrous oxide (nitrogen monoxide)

Intravenous Anesthetics

Barbiturates
   Methohexital (Brevital sodium)
   Thiopental (Pentothal)

(Continued on following page)

Table 11–1   GENERAL ANESTHETICS *(Continued)*

Anesthetic	Representative Structure

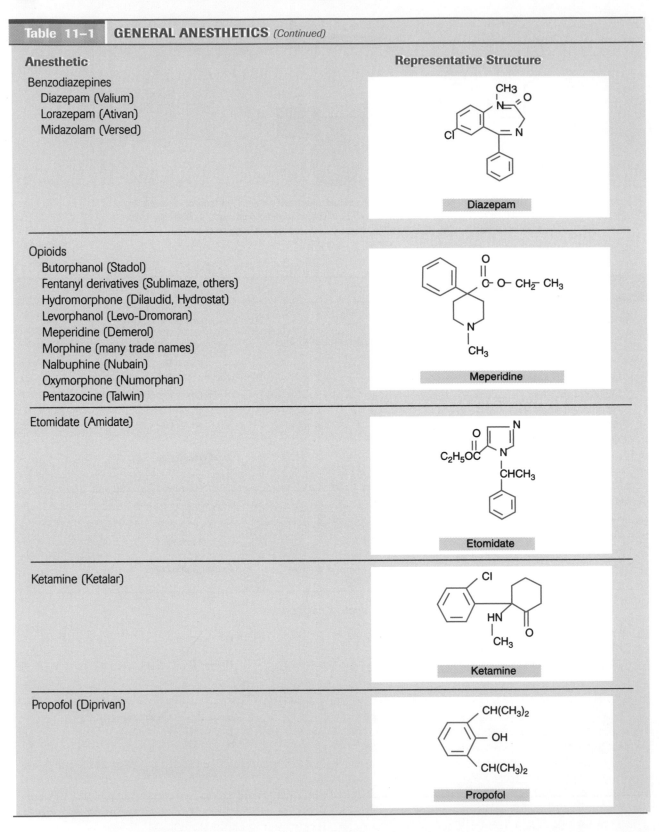

Benzodiazepines
  Diazepam (Valium)
  Lorazepam (Ativan)
  Midazolam (Versed)

Diazepam

Opioids
  Butorphanol (Stadol)
  Fentanyl derivatives (Sublimaze, others)
  Hydromorphone (Dilaudid, Hydrostat)
  Levorphanol (Levo-Dromoran)
  Meperidine (Demerol)
  Morphine (many trade names)
  Nalbuphine (Nubain)
  Oxymorphone (Numorphan)
  Pentazocine (Talwin)

Meperidine

Etomidate (Amidate)

Etomidate

Ketamine (Ketalar)

Ketamine

Propofol (Diprivan)

Propofol

general anesthetics (see Table 11–1).[38,39] Barbiturate drugs such as thiopental, thiamylal, and methohexital have been used commonly to induce anesthesia in many situations. Barbiturates are noted for their fast onset (when administered intravenously) and relative safety when used appropriately. Several other types of drugs including benzodiazepines (diazepam, lorazepam, midazolam) and opioid analgesics (fentanyl, morphine, meperidine) have also been used to induce or help maintain general anesthesia. Although these other agents are often used as preoperative sedatives, larger doses can be used alone or in combination with other general anesthetics to produce anesthesia in short surgical or diagnostic procedures, or where other general anesthetics may be contraindicated (e.g., cardiovascular disease).

Another intravenous general anesthetic is ketamine (Ketalar). This agent produces a somewhat different type of condition known as *dissociative anesthesia*.[16,39] This term is used because of the clinical observation that the patient appears detached or dissociated from the surrounding environment. The patient appears awake but is sedated and usually unable to recall events that occurred when the ketamine was in effect. Dissociative anesthesia is useful during relatively short diagnostic or surgical procedures (e.g., endoscopy) or during invasive procedures in children or certain high-risk patients (e.g., some older adults or people with low blood pressure or bronchospastic disease).[11,16]

A similar type of anesthesia is produced by combining the opioid fentanyl with the antipsychotic drug droperidol. The combination of these two agents produces a condition known as *neuroleptanalgesia*, which is also characterized by a dissociation from what is happening around the patient, with or without loss of consciousness.[39] An inhaled anesthetic such as nitrous oxide can also be added to convert neuroleptanalgesia to neuroleptanesthesia.[39] Neuroleptanalgesia and neuroleptanesthesia are typically used for short surgical procedures, including endoscopy or burn dressings, or for patients who are seriously ill and may not tolerate general anesthesia using more conventional methods.

Finally, newer intravenous anesthetics such as etomidate (Amidate) and propofol (Diprivan) are available. Etomidate is a hypnoticlike drug that causes a rapid onset of general anesthesia with a minimum of cardiopulmonary side effects. Hence, this drug may be useful in patients with compromised cardiovascular or respiratory function. Propofol is a short-acting hypnotic that is useful as a general anesthetic in some short invasive procedures, or to maintain anesthesia in longer procedures.[22] Recovery from propofol may also be more rapid than with other anesthetics, making this drug useful when early mobilization of the patient is desirable.[38]

Pharmacokinetics

Following either injection or inhalation administration, general anesthetics become widely and uniformly distributed throughout the body, largely because of their high degree of lipid solubility. As a result, a great deal of the anesthetic may become temporarily stored in adipose tissues and slowly washed out when the patient is recovering from surgery. If the person was anesthetized for an extended period of time and has large deposits of fat, this washout may take quite some time.[11,17] During this period, symptoms such as confusion, disorientation, and lethargy may occur, presumably because the drug is being redistributed to the CNS. The patient's age also influences anesthetic requirements and distribution, with older individuals usually requiring less anesthetic for a given procedure.[29] Since older people need smaller concentrations of anesthetic, the chance that more anesthetic may be administered during surgery than is needed is increased and recovery will be somewhat delayed.

Depending on the individual drug, elimination occurs primarily through excretion from the lungs, biotransformation in the liver, or a combination of these two methods.[39] If the patient has any pulmonary or hepatic dysfunction, elimination of the anesthetic will be further delayed.

Mechanisms of Action

Although general anesthetics have been used extensively for over 150 years, debate still exists as to exactly how these drugs work. Clearly these drugs are able to inhibit the neuronal activity throughout the CNS. It appears that they can decrease activity of neurons in the reticular activating system in the brain, and this action explains their ability to produce unconsciousness and lack of memory (amnesia) during surgery.[7] General anesthetics likewise inhibit neuronal function in the spinal cord, and this action explains their ability to produce immobility and inhibit motor responses to painful stimuli.[7]

The exact way in which these drugs affect these neurons remains somewhat speculative. In the past, it was believed that general anesthetics primarily affected the lipid bilayer of CNS neurons. This so-called general perturbation theory was based on the premise that general anesthetic molecules become dissolved directly in the nerve membrane's lipid bilayer and serve to generally perturb membrane function by increasing membrane fluidity and disrupting the phospholipid environment that surrounds the protein channel.[7] Membrane excitability would be decreased because ion channels, including sodium channels, are unable to open and allow the influx of sodium needed to initiate an action potential (Fig. 11–2). The primary support for the membrane perturbation theory was the direct correlation between anesthetic potency and lipid solubility,[39] meaning that the more easily the drug dissolves in the bilayer, the less is needed to achieve a given level of anesthesia. This theory was further supported by the fact that general anesthetics all produce a similar effect, even though they have quite diverse chemical structures (see Table 11–1). Presumably, if drugs bind to a certain type of receptor, they should share some structural similarities.

More recent evidence, however, suggests that general anesthetics bind to specific receptors located on the outer surface of CNS neurons.[7,14] In particular, many general anesthetics bind to CNS receptors that are specific for gamma-aminobutyric acid (GABA). As discussed in Chapter 6, GABA receptors contain a chloride ion channel that, when activated by GABA, increases influx of chloride ions into the neuron, thereby inhibiting that neuron. By binding to specific GABA receptors (the $GABA_A$ subtype), general anesthetics increase the effects of GABA, thus enhancing CNS inhibition throughout the CNS.[27,28] This widespread CNS inhibition ultimately leads to a state of general anesthesia.

Hence, many general anesthetics exert their primary effects by binding to inhibitory $GABA_A$ receptors in the brain and cord. This fact seems true for both the commonly used intravenous anesthetics (barbiturates, benzodiazepines, propofol, etomidate) as well as the typical inhaled forms (halothane, enflurane, sevoflurane).[19] Some of their anesthetic effects, however, might also be mediated by other receptors. Many general anesthetics, for example, also bind to excitatory acetylcholine receptors on CNS neurons, and inhibit the function of these receptors. This combination of increased inhibition (through GABA receptors) and decreased excitation (through acetylcholine receptors) would certainly explain why

No Drug
(Na⁺ channel shown open)

Anesthetized
(Na⁺ channel closed)

A. General Perturbation Theory

B. Specific Receptor Theory

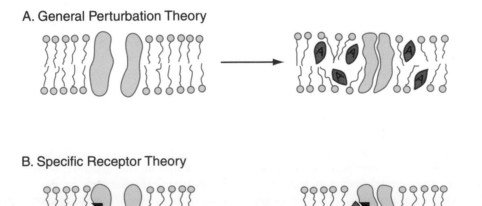

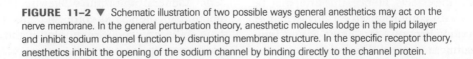

FIGURE 11–2 ▼ Schematic illustration of two possible ways general anesthetics may act on the nerve membrane. In the general perturbation theory, anesthetic molecules lodge in the lipid bilayer and inhibit sodium channel function by disrupting membrane structure. In the specific receptor theory, anesthetics inhibit the opening of the sodium channel by binding directly to the channel protein.

these drugs are so effective in reducing the level of consciousness and excitability throughout the brain and cord.[34,41]

In addition to GABA and acetylcholine receptors, other CNS receptors have been implicated in mediating the effects of specific general anesthetics. Opioids, for example, decrease transmission in nociceptive pathways by binding to specific presynaptic and postsynaptic opioid receptors in the brain and spinal cord (see Chapter 14). Injected anesthetics such as ketamine, and certain inhaled agents (nitrous oxide), bind to the *N*-methyl-D-aspartate (NMDA) receptor in the brain, thus inhibiting the excitatory effects of glutamate.[34,41] Other proteins that might be affected by anesthetics include serotonin receptors and ion channels that are specific for sodium, potassium, or calcium.[7,35].

Hence, it is believed that general anesthetics exert most, if not all, of their effects by binding to one or more neuronal receptors in the CNS. This idea is a departure from the general perturbation theory described earlier; that is, that the inhaled anesthetics affected the lipid bilayer rather than a specific protein. Continued research will continue to clarify the mechanism of these drugs, and future studies may lead to more agents that produce selective anesthetic effects by acting at specific receptor sites in the brain and spinal cord.

Adjuvants in General Anesthesia

Preoperative Medications

Frequently, a preoperative sedative is given to a patient 1 to 2 hours before the administration of general anesthesia.[2,36] Sedatives are usually administered orally or by intramuscular injection, and are given while the patient is still in his or her room. This approach serves to relax the patient and reduce anxiety when arriving at the operating room. Commonly used preoperative sedatives include barbiturates (secobarbital, pentobarbital), opioids (butorphanol, meperidine), and benzodiazepines (diazepam, lorazepam) (Table 11–2). Different sedatives are selected depending on the patient, the type of general anesthesia used, and the preference of the physician.

A number of other medications may be used preoperatively to achieve various goals (see Table 11–2).[5,40] Antihistamines (promethazine, hydroxyzine) offer the dual advantage of producing sedation and reducing vomiting (antiemesis). Antacids and other drugs that increase gastric pH are sometimes used to decrease stomach acidity and thus reduce the risk of serious lung damage if gastric fluid is aspirated during general surgery. Preoperative administration of an anti-inflammatory steroid (dexamethasone) can likewise help control postoperative symptoms such as pain and vomiting.[4,12] In the past, anticholinergics (atropine, scopolamine) were administered to help reduce bronchial secretions and aid in airway intubation. However, anesthetics currently in use do not produce excessive airway secretions (as did prior agents), so the preoperative use of anticholinergics is no longer critical.[11]

Neuromuscular Blockers

Skeletal muscle paralysis is essential during surgical procedures. The patient must be relaxed to allow proper positioning on the operating table and to prevent spontaneous muscle contractions from hampering the surgery.[23,24] Imagine the disastrous effects that a muscular spasm in the arm would have on a delicate procedure such as nerve repair or limb reattachment. Neuromuscular paralysis also makes it easier for the patient to be ventilated mechanically because the thoracic wall is more compliant and does not offer as much resistance to mechanical inflation and deflation of the chest cavity. Hence, these drugs are used as an adjunct to general anesthesia as well as in other situations that require mechanical ventilation (intensive care units).

Most currently used general anesthetics also produce skeletal muscle relaxation, but it takes a larger dose of the anesthetic to produce adequate muscular relaxation than is needed to produce unconsciousness and amnesia; that is, the patient must be well into stage III and almost into stage IV of anesthesia before muscle paralysis is complete. Consequently, a drug that blocks the skeletal neuromuscular junction is given in conjunction with a general anesthetic to allow the use of a lower dose of anesthetic while still ensuring skeletal muscle paralysis. These drugs work by blocking the postsynaptic acetylcholine receptor located at the skeletal neuromuscular junction.

Several different neuromuscular blockers are currently available, and the choice of a specific agent depends primarily on the desired length of action and the agent's potential side effects (Table 11–3).[21,23] Possible side effects include cardiovascular problems (tachycardia), increased histamine release, increased

Table 11–2	PREOPERATIVE PREMEDICATION: DRUGS AND DOSES USED		
Classification	**Preoperative Indication**	**Drug**	**Method of Administration***
Barbiturates	Decrease anxiety; facilitate induction of anesthesia	Amobarbital	Oral: 200 mg 1 to 2 hours before surgery
		Butabarbital	Oral: 50–100 mg 60 to 90 minutes before surgery
		Pentobarbital	Oral: 100 mg IM: 150–200 mg
		Phenobarbital	IM: 130–200 mg 60 to 90 minutes before surgery
		Secobarbital	Oral: 200–300 mg 1 to 2 hours before surgery
Opioids**	Provide analgesic, antianxiety, and sedative effects	Butorphanol	IV: 2 mg 60–90 minutes before surgery
		Meperidine	IM: 1–2.2 mg/kg body weight (100 mg maximum) 30 to 90 minutes before surgery
Benzodiazepines	Decrease anxiety and tension; provide sedation and amnesia	Chlordiazepoxide	IM: 50–100 mg 1 hour before surgery
		Diazepam	IM or IV: 5–10 mg prior to surgery
		Lorazepam	IM: 0.05 mg/kg body weight (4 mg maximum) 2 hours before surgery IV: 0.044–0.05 mg/kg body weight (4 mg maximum) 15 to 20 minutes before surgery
Antihistamines	Provide sedative-hypnotic effects	Diphenhydramine	Oral: 50 mg 20 to 30 minutes before surgery
		Hydroxyzine	Oral: 50–100 mg
Anticholinergics	Prevent excessive salivation and respiratory tract secretions	Atropine	Oral: 2 mg IM: 0.2–0.6 mg 30 to 60 minutes before surgery
		Glycopyrrolate	IM: 0.0044 mg/kg body weight 30 to 60 minutes before induction of anesthesia
		Scopolamine	IM: 0.2–0.6 mg 30 to 60 minutes before induction of anesthesia

*Typical adult doses. IV, intravenous; IM, intramuscular.
**Virtually all opioids can be used as a preoperative medication. Selection of a specific type and dose can be individualized based on the needs of each patient.

Classification	Preoperative Indication	Drug	Method of Administration*
Antacids (H2 receptor blockers)	Reduce gastric acidity; help prevent aspiration pneumonitis	Cimetidine	IM: 300 mg 1 hour before induction of anesthesia; 300 mg every 4 hours until patient responds to commands
		Ranitidine	IM: 50 mg 45 to 60 minutes before induction of anesthesia

plasma potassium levels (hyperkalemia), residual muscle pain and weakness, and immunologic reactions (anaphylaxis).[13,25] Selection of a specific agent is therefore designed to minimize the risk of a certain side effect in a specific patient; for example, a drug that produces relatively little cardiovascular effects would be selected for a patient with cardiovascular disease.

Efforts are also made to use small doses of relatively short-acting agents so that the length of muscle paralysis is kept to a minimum.[6] The paralytic effects of these agents should disappear by the end of the surgical procedure. If necessary, drugs such as neostigmine or edrophonium can also be administered to help reverse the effects of neuromuscular blockade.[24,30] These drugs inhibit the enzyme that breaks down acetylcholine (the acetylcholinesterase), thereby prolonging its effects and hastening recovery of motor function. The pharmacology of acetylcholinesterase inhibitors is addressed in more detail in Chapter 19.

Nonetheless, residual effects of the neuromuscular blocker can persist in some patients long after surgery is complete.[6,13] The most serious complication is residual paralysis; that is, skeletal muscle contraction remains depressed for several hours after the drug should have worn off.[8,18] In extreme cases, this residual paralysis necessitates that the patient remain in intensive care with a mechanical ventilator to provide respiratory support.

It is not always clear why certain patients do not recover adequately from neuromuscular blockade. In

Table 11–3   NEUROMUSCULAR JUNCTION BLOCKERS

Generic Name	Trade Name	Time of Onset (min)*	Clinical Duration (min)	Relative Duration
Nondepolarizing blockers				
Tubocurarine	–	4–6	80–120	Long
Atracurium	Tracrium	2–4	30–60	Intermediate
Doxacurium	Nuromax	4–6	90–120	Long
Mivacurium	Mivacron	2–4	12–18	Short
Pancuronium	Pavulon	4–6	120–180	Long
Pipecuronium	Arduan	2–4	80–100	Long
Rapacuronium	Raplon	1–2	15–30	Intermediate
Rocuronium	Zemuron	1–2	30–60	Intermediate
Vecuronium	Norcuron	2–4	60–90	Intermediate
Depolarizing blockers				
Succinylcholine	Anectine, others	1–1.5	5–8	Ultrashort

*Reflects usual adult intravenous dose.
Source: Adapted from Taylor.[37]

some cases, the residual effects are attributed to genetic differences in the enzymes responsible for metabolizing the neuromuscular blocker.[37] If these enzymes are deficient or absent, the patient cannot adequately metabolize the blocker, hence paralysis continues for days or even weeks. In other patients, residual effects may occur if the patient has a concurrent neuromuscular condition such as a spinal cord injury, peripheral neuropathies, intracranial lesions, or muscle pathologies.[26,32]

Efforts should be made to use these drugs sparingly, and to check that their effects have worn off before the patient leaves the operating room. In fact, electric stimulation of a peripheral nerve (e.g., ulnar nerve) can be used to objectively determine if there is residual muscle paralysis.[1] The muscles supplied by the nerve must show an appropriate twitch response to a given electric stimulus to insure that the patient has recovered adequately from the neuromuscular blocking drug.[20,31]

It should also be realized that neuromuscular junction blockers are an adjunct to general anesthesia but that these blockers do not cause anesthesia or analgesia when used alone.[26,33] The patient must receive an adequate amount of the general anesthetic throughout the surgery when a neuromuscular junction blocker is used. This idea is critical considering that the patient will be paralyzed by the neuromuscular junction blocker and unable to respond to painful stimuli if the anesthesia is inadequate. Failure to provide adequate anesthesia has resulted in some harrowing reports from patients who were apparently fully awake during surgery but unable to move or cry out.[26,33]

Two general types of neuromuscular blockers are discussed here. They are classified according to those that depolarize the skeletal muscle cell when binding to the cholinergic receptor and those that do not.[37]

Nondepolarizing Blockers. These drugs act as competitive antagonists of the postsynaptic receptor; that is, they bind to the receptor but do not activate it (see Chapter 4). This binding prevents the agonist (acetylcholine) from binding to the receptor; the result is paralysis of the muscle cell. These drugs all share a structural similarity to curare (the first neuromuscular blocker), which explains their affinity and relative selectivity for the cholinergic receptor at the skeletal neuromuscular junction. Specific agents, their onset, and duration of action are listed in Table 11–3.

Depolarizing Blockers. Although these drugs also inhibit transmission at the skeletal neuromuscular junction, their mechanism is different from that of the nondepolarizing agents. These drugs initially act like acetylcholine by binding to and stimulating the receptor, resulting in depolarization of the muscle cell. However, the enzymatic degradation of the drug is not as rapid as the destruction of acetylcholine, so the muscle cell remains depolarized for a prolonged period. While depolarized, the muscle is unresponsive to further stimulation. The cell must become repolarized, or reprimed, before the cell will respond to a second stimulus. This event is often referred to as phase I blockade.[37] If the depolarizing blocker remains at the synapse, the muscle cell eventually repolarizes, but it will remain unresponsive to stimulation by acetylcholine. This occurrence is referred to as phase II blockade and is believed to occur because the drug exerts some sort of modification on the receptor. This modification could be in the form of a temporary change in the receptor's shape. Clinically, when these drugs are first administered, they are often associated with a variable amount of muscle tremor and fasciculation (because of the initial depolarization), but this is followed by a period of flaccid paralysis. Although several drugs that act as depolarizing blockers are available, the only agent currently in clinical use is succinylcholine (see Table 11–3).[37]

SUMMARY

General anesthesia has been used for some time to permit surgical procedures of various types and durations. Several different effective agents are currently available and are relatively safe in producing a suitable anesthetic condition in the patient. General anesthetics are classified according to their two primary routes of administration: inhalation and intravenous infusion. Specific anesthetic agents and anesthetic adjuvants (preoperative sedatives, neuromuscular blockers, etc.) are primarily selected according to the type of surgical procedure being performed and the overall condition of the patient. Health professionals should be cognizant of the fact that their patients may take some time to fully recover from the effects of general anesthesia and should adjust their postoperative care accordingly.

Special Concerns in Rehabilitation

■ ■ ■ A rehabilitation specialist is most likely to encounter major problems when the patient is not quite over the effects of the anesthesia. Dealing with a patient the day after surgery or even on the same day might be difficult because he or she is woozy. Some anesthetics may produce confusion or psychoticlike behavior (delirium) during the recovery period, especially in older adults.[3] Muscle weakness may also occur for a variable amount of time, especially if a neuromuscular blocker was used during the surgical procedure. Of course, patients who are in relatively good health and who have had relatively short or minor surgeries will have minimal residual effects. However, patients who are debilitated or who have other medical problems impairing drug elimination may continue to show some anesthesia aftereffects for several days.[3] These problems should disappear with time, so the therapist must plan activities accordingly until recovery from the anesthetic is complete.

Another problem that therapists frequently deal with is the tendency for bronchial secretions to accumulate in the lungs of patients recovering from general anesthesia. General anesthetics depress mucociliary clearance in the airway, leading to a pooling of mucus, which may produce respiratory infections and atelectasis. Therapists play an important role in preventing this accumulation by encouraging the patient's early mobilization and by implementing respiratory hygiene protocols (i.e., breathing exercises and postural drainage).

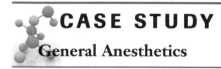

CASE STUDY

General Anesthetics

Brief History. B.W., a 75-year-old woman, fell at home and experienced a sudden sharp pain in her left hip. She was unable to walk and was taken to a nearby hospital where x-ray examination showed an impacted fracture of the left hip. The patient was alert and oriented at the time of admission. She had a history of arteriosclerotic cardiovascular disease and diabetes mellitus, but her medical condition was stable. The patient was relatively obese, and a considerable amount of osteoarthritis was present in both hips. Two days after admission, a total hip arthroplasty was performed under general anesthesia. Meperidine (Demerol) was given intramuscularly as a preoperative sedative. General anesthesia was induced by intravenous administration of thiopental (Pentothal) and sustained by inhalation of halothane (Fluothane). The surgery was completed successfully, and physical therapy was initiated at the patient's bedside on the subsequent day.

Problem/Influence of Medication. At the initial therapy session, the therapist found the patient to be extremely lethargic and disoriented. She appeared confused about recent events and was unable to follow most commands. Apparently, she was experiencing some residual effects of the general anesthesia.

Decision/Solution. The patient's confusion and disorientation precluded any activities that required her cooperation, including any initial attempts at weight-bearing exercises. The therapist limited the initial session to passive- and active-assisted exercises of both lower extremities. Active upper-extremity exercises were encouraged within the limitations of the patient's ability to follow instructions. These exercises were instituted to help increase metabolism and excretion of the remaining anesthesia. The patient was also placed on a program of breathing exercises in an effort to facilitate excretion of the anesthesia, as well as to maintain respiratory function and prevent the accumulation of mucus in the airways. As the patient's mental disposition gradually improved, the therapist initiated partial weight bearing in the parallel bars. From there, the patient progressed to a walker and was soon able to ambulate independently using the device. Within 1 week after the surgery, no overt residual effects of the anesthesia were noted, and the remainder of the hospital stay was uneventful.

References

1. Baykara N, Solak M, Toker K. Predicting recovery from deep neuromuscular block by rocuronium in the elderly. *J Clin Anesth.* 2003;15:328–333.
2. Bauer KP, Dom PM, Ramirez AM, O'Flaherty JE. Preoperative intravenous midazolam: benefits beyond anxiolysis. *J Clin Anesth.* 2004;16:177–183.
3. Bekker AY, Weeks EJ. Cognitive function after anaesthesia in the elderly. *Best Pract Res Clin Anaesthesiol.* 2003;17:259–272.
4. Bisgaard T, Klarskov B, Kehlet H, Rosenberg J. Preoperative dexamethasone improves surgical outcome after laparoscopic cholecystectomy: a randomized double-blind placebo-controlled trial. *Ann Surg.* 2003;238:651–660.
5. Chia YY, Lo Y, Liu K, et al. The effect of promethazine on postoperative pain: a comparison of preoperative, postoperative, and placebo administration in patients following total abdominal hysterectomy. *Acta Anaesthesiol Scand.* 2004;48:625–630.
6. Cammu G. Postoperative residual curarisation: complication or malpractice? *Acta Anaesthesiol Belg.* 2004;55:245–249.
7. Campagna JA, Miller KW, Forman SA. Mechanisms of actions of inhaled anesthetics. *N Engl J Med.* 2003;348:2110–2124.
8. Debaene B, Plaud B, Dilly MP, Donati F. Residual paralysis in the PACU after a single intubating dose of nondepolarizing muscle relaxant with an intermediate duration of action. *Anesthesiology.* 2003;98:1042–1048.
9. Eger EI, 2nd. Characteristics of anesthetic agents used for induction and maintenance of general anesthesia. *Am J Health Syst Pharm.* 2004;61(suppl 4):S3–S10.
10. Eger EI, White PF, Bogetz MS. Clinical and economic factors important to anaesthetic choice for day-case surgery. *Pharmacoeconomics.* 2000;17:245–262.
11. Elhakim M, Ali NM, Rashed I, et al. Dexamethasone reduces postoperative vomiting and pain after pediatric tonsillectomy. *Can J Anaesth.* 2003;50:392–397.
12. Eriksson LI. Residual neuromuscular blockade. Incidence and relevance. *Anaesthesist.* 2000;49(suppl 1):S18–S19.
13. Evers AS, Crowder CM. General anesthetics. In: Hardman JG, et al, eds. *The Pharmacological Basis of Therapeutics.* 10th ed. New York: McGraw-Hill; 2001.
14. Friederich P. Basic concepts of ion channel physiology and anaesthetic drug effects. *Eur J Anaesthesiol.* 2003;20:343–353.
15. Golembiewski J. Considerations in selecting an inhaled anesthetic agent: case studies. *Am J Health Syst Pharm.* 2004;61(suppl 4):S10–S17.
16. Ivani G, Vercellino C, Tonetti F. Ketamine: a new look to an old drug. *Minerva Anestesiol.* 2003;69:468–471.
17. Joshi GP. Inhalational techniques in ambulatory anesthesia. *Anesthesiol Clin North America.* 2003;21:263–272.
18. Kim KS, Lew SH, Cho HY, Cheong MA. Residual paralysis induced by either vecuronium or rocuronium after reversal with pyridostigmine. *Anesth Analg.* 2002;95:1656–1660.
19. Kitamura A, Sato R, Marszalec W, et al. Halothane and propofol modulation of gamma-aminobutyric acid A receptor single-channel currents. *Anesth Analg.* 2004;99:409–415.
20. Kopman AF, Kopman DJ, Ng J, Zank LM. Antagonism of profound cisatracurium and rocuronium block: the role of objective assessment of neuromuscular function. *J Clin Anesth.* 2005;17:30–35.
21. Lee C. Conformation, action, and mechanism of action of neuromuscular blocking muscle relaxants. *Pharmacol Ther.* 2003;98:143–169.
22. Marik PE. Propofol: therapeutic indications and side-effects. *Curr Pharm Des.* 2004;10:3639–3649.
23. McManus MC. Neuromuscular blockers in surgery and intensive care, part 1. *Am J Health Syst Pharm.* 2001;58:2287–2299.
24. McManus MC. Neuromuscular blockers in surgery and intensive care, part 2. *Am J Health Syst Pharm.* 2001;58:2381–2395.
25. Mertes PM, Laxenaire MC. Adverse reactions to neuromuscular blocking agents. *Curr Allergy Asthma Rep.* 2004;4:7–16.
26. Messahel FM, Al-Qahtani AS. Awareness during surgery. *Saudi Med J.* 2003;24:967–970.
27. Rudolph U, Antkowiak B. Molecular and neuronal substrates for general anaesthetics. *Nat Rev Neurosci.* 2004;5:709–720.
28. Rudolph U, Mohler H. Analysis of GABA A receptor function and dissection of the pharmacology of benzodiazepines and general anesthetics through mouse genetics. *Annu Rev Pharmacol Toxicol.* 2004;44:475–498.
29. Sadean MR, Glass PS. Pharmacokinetics in the elderly. *Best Pract Res Clin Anaesthesiol.* 2003;17:191–205.
30. Saitoh Y, Hattori H, Sanbe N, et al. Reversal of vecuronium with neostigmine in patients with diabetes mellitus. *Anaesthesia.* 2004;59:750–754.
31. Samet A, Capron F, Alla F, et al. Single acceleromyographic train-of-four, 100 Hertz tetanus or double-burst stimulation: which test performs better to detect residual paralysis? *Anesthesiology.* 2005;102:51–56.
32. Schreiber JU, Mencke T, Biedler A, et al. Postoperative myalgia after succinylcholine: no evidence for an inflammatory origin. *Anesth Analg.* 2003;96:1640–1644.
33. Sigalovsky N. Awareness under general anesthesia. *AANA J.* 2003;71:373–379.
34. Sloan TB. Anesthetics and the brain. *Anesthesiol Clin North America.* 2002;20:265–292.
35. Sonner JM, Antognini JF, Dutton RC, et al. Inhaled anesthetics and immobility: mechanisms, mysteries, and minimum alveolar anesthetic concentration. *Anesth Analg.* 2003;97:718–740.
36. Tamura M, Nakamura K, Kitamura R, et al. Oral premedication with fentanyl may be a safe and effective alternative to oral midazolam. *Eur J Anaesthesiol.* 2003;20:482–486.

37. Taylor P. Agents acting at the neuromuscular junction and autonomic ganglia. In: Hardman JG, et al, eds. *The Pharmacological Basis of Therapeutics.* 10th ed. New York: McGraw Hill; 2001.

38. Tesniere A, Servin F. Intravenous techniques in ambulatory anesthesia. *Anesthesiol Clin North America.* 2003;21:273–288.

39. Trevor AJ, White PF. General anesthetics. In: Katzung BG, ed. *Basic and Clinical Pharmacology.* 9th ed. New York: Lange Medical Books/McGraw-Hill; 2004.

40. Turner KE, Parlow JL, Avery ND, et al. Prophylaxis of postoperative nausea and vomiting with oral, long-acting dimenhydrinate in gynecologic outpatient laparoscopy. *Anesth Analg.* 2004;98:1660–1664.

41. Villars PS, Kanusky JT, Dougherty TB. Stunning the neural nexus: mechanisms of general anesthesia. *AANA J.* 2004;72:197–205.

Chapter 12

Local Anesthetics

Local anesthesia produces a loss of sensation in a specific body part or region. Frequently this application occurs before performing a relatively minor surgical procedure. This approach involves introducing an anesthetic drug near the peripheral nerve that innervates the desired area. The basic goal is to block afferent neural transmission along the peripheral nerve so that the procedure is painless. When a local anesthetic is introduced in the vicinity of the spinal cord, transmission of impulses may be effectively blocked at a specific level of the cord, allowing more extensive surgical procedures to be performed (e.g., caesarean delivery) because a larger region of the body is being anesthetized. This approach, however, is still considered a local anesthetic because the drug acts locally at the spinal cord and the patient remains conscious during the surgical procedure.

Using a local anesthetic during a surgical procedure offers several advantages over the use of general anesthesia, including a relatively rapid recovery and lack of residual effects.[13,15] There is a virtual absence of the postoperative confusion and lethargy often seen after general anesthesia. In most cases of minor surgery, patients are able to leave the practitioner's office or hospital almost as soon as the procedure is completed. In more extensive procedures, local anesthesia offers the advantage of not interfering with cardiovascular, respiratory, and renal functioning. This fact can be important in patients with problems in these physiological systems. During childbirth, local (spinal) anesthesia imposes a lesser risk to the neonate than general anesthesia.[14,41] The primary disadvantages of local anesthesia are the length of time required to establish an anesthetic effect and the risk that analgesia will be incomplete or insufficient for the respective procedure.[47] The latter problem can usually be resolved by administering more local anesthesia if the procedure is relatively minor, or by switching to a general anesthetic during a major procedure in the event of an emergency arising during surgery.

In nonsurgical situations, local anesthetics are sometimes used to provide analgesia. These drugs may be used for short-term pain relief in conditions such as musculoskeletal and joint pain (e.g., bursitis, tendinitis), or in more long-term situations such as pain relief in cancer or treatment of chronic pain. In addition, local anesthetics may be used to block efferent sympathetic activity in conditions such as reflex sympathetic dystrophy syndrome. During these nonsurgical applications, physical therapists and other rehabilitation personnel will often be directly involved in treating the patient while the local anesthetic is in effect. If prescribed by a physician, the local anesthetic may actually be administered by the physical therapist via phonophoresis or iontophoresis. Consequently, these individuals should have adequate knowledge of the pharmacology of local anesthetics.

Types of Local Anesthetics

Commonly used local anesthetics are listed in Table 12–1. These drugs share a common chemical strategy consisting of both a lipophilic and hydrophilic group connected by an intermediate chain (Fig. 12–1). A local anesthetic is chosen depending on factors such as: (1) the operative site and nature of the procedure; (2) the type of regional anesthesia desired (such as single peripheral nerve block or spinal anesthesia); (3) the patient's size and general health; and (4) the duration of action of the anesthetic.[3]

The "caine" suffix (lidocaine, procaine, and so on) usually identifies local anesthetics.. The first clinically useful local anesthetic identified was cocaine in

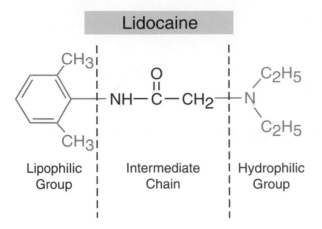

FIGURE 12–1 ▼ Structure of lidocaine. The basic structure of a lipophilic and hydrophilic group connected by an intermediate chain is common to most local anesthetics.

1884. However, its tendency for abuse and its high incidence of addiction and systemic toxicity initiated the search for safer local anesthetics such as those in Table 12–1. One should note that cocaine abuse grew because of its effects on the brain, not for its local anesthetic effects. Cocaine produces intense feelings of euphoria and excitement through increased synaptic transmission in the brain. This fact explains why cocaine abusers inject or apply this drug to the nasal mucous membranes (i.e., "snorting," so that it absorbs through those membranes and into systemic circulation where it ultimately reaches the brain).

Pharmacokinetics

Local anesthetics are administered through a variety of routes and techniques depending on the specific clinical situation (see "Clinical Use of Local Anesthetics," below). In local anesthesia, the drug should remain at the site of administration. For instance, injecting procaine (Novocain) into the trigeminal nerve area during a dental procedure will be more effective if it is not washed away from the administration site by blood flow through that region. Likewise, injection of a local anesthetic into the area surrounding the spinal cord (e.g., epidural or spinal injection, see next section) will be more effective if the drug remains near the administration site.[31,32] Consequently, a vasoconstricting agent (e.g., epinephrine) is often administered simultaneously to help prevent washout from the desired site.[42,46] Preventing the anesthetic from reaching the bloodstream is also beneficial because local anes-

thetics can cause toxic side effects when sufficient amounts reach the systemic circulation (see "Systemic Effects of Local Anesthetics," later). This occurrence is usually not a problem in most single, small doses of regional anesthesia, but the build-up of the drug in the bloodstream should be monitored if these drugs are administered repeatedly or continuously to treat chronic pain.[51,59]

Local anesthetics are usually eliminated by hydrolyzing or breaking apart the drug molecule. This metabolic hydrolysis is catalyzed by hepatic enzymes or enzymes circulating in the plasma (e.g., the plasma cholinesterase). Once metabolized, the kidneys excrete the polar drug metabolites.

Clinical Use of Local Anesthetics

The primary clinical uses of local anesthetics according to their method of administration and specific indications are presented here.

1. *Topical administration.* Local anesthetics can be applied directly to the surface of the skin, mucous membranes, cornea, and other regions to produce analgesia. This is usually done for the symptomatic relief of minor surface irritation and injury (minor burns, abrasions, inflammation). Local anesthetics can also be applied topically to reduce pain prior to minor surgical procedures such as wound cleansing, myringotomy, circumcision, and cataract surgery.[7,52,57] A topical anesthesia can be made by applying a single agent or a mixture of two or more local anesthetics (e.g., lidocaine and prilocaine).[4,49,52]

   Topical anesthesia has also been used to improve motor function in some patients with skeletal muscle hypertonicity resulting from a cerebrovascular accident (CVA) or head trauma.[53] In this situation, a local anesthetic (e.g., 20% benzocaine) can be sprayed on the skin overlying hypertonic muscles, and then various exercises and facilitation techniques can be performed to increase and improve mobility in the affected limbs. The rationale of this treatment is that it temporarily decreases abnormal or excessive excitatory feedback of cutaneous receptors on efferent motor pathways so that normal integration and control of motor function can be reestablished. Preliminary evidence has suggested that repeated application of this

Table 12–1	COMMON LOCAL ANESTHETICS			
Generic Name	**Trade Name(s)**	**Onset of Action**	**Duration of Action**	**Principle Use(s)**
Articane	Septocaine	Rapid	Intermediate	Peripheral nerve block
Benzocaine	Americaine, others	–	–	Topical
Bupivacaine	Marcaine, Sensor-caine	Slow to Intermediate	Long	Infiltration; Peripheral nerve block; Epidural; Spinal; Sympathetic block
Butamben	Butesin Picrate	–	–	Topical
Chloroprocaine	Nesacaine	Rapid	Short	Infiltration; Peripheral nerve block; Epidural; Intravenous regional block
Dibucaine	Nupercainal	–	–	Topical
Etidocaine	Duranest	Rapid	Long	Infiltration; Peripheral nerve block; Epidural
Levobupivacaine	Chirocaine	Slow to Intermediate	Short to Long	Infiltration; Peripheral nerve block; Epidural
Lidocaine	Xylocaine	Rapid	Intermediate	Infiltration; Peripheral Nerve Block; Epidural; Spinal; Transdermal; Topical; Sympathetic block; Intravenous regional block
Mepivacaine	Carbocaine, Polo-caine	Intermediate to Rapid	Intermediate	Infiltration; Peripheral nerve block; Epidural; Intravenous regional block
Pramoxine	Prax, Tronolane	–	–	Topical
Prilocaine	Citanest	Rapid	Intermediate	Infiltration; Peripheral nerve block

(Continued on following page)

Table 12–1	COMMON LOCAL ANESTHETICS *(Continued)*			
Generic Name	**Trade Name(s)**	**Onset of Action**[*]	**Duration of Action**[*]	**Principle Use(s)**
Procaine	Novocain	Intermediate	Short	Infiltration; Peripheral nerve block; Spinal
Tetracaine	Pontocaine	Rapid	Intermediate to Long	Topical; Spinal

*Values for onset and duration of action refer to use during injection. Relative durations of action are as follows: short = 30–60 min; intermediate = 1–3 hr; and long = 3–10 hr of action.
Source: USP DI, 25th Edition. Copyright 2005. Thomson MICROMEDEX. Permission granted.

technique may produce long-lasting improvements in joint mobility and gait characteristics in patients with hypertonicity caused by various central nervous system (CNS) disorders.[53]

2. *Transdermal administration.* The drug is applied to the surface of the skin or other tissues with the intent that the drug will absorb into underlying tissues. Transdermal administration of some local anesthetics may be enhanced by the use of electrical current (iontophoresis) or ultrasound (phonophoresis; see Appendix A).[18,50,66] Moreover, iontophoresis and phonophoresis offer the advantage of anesthetizing a region of the skin before treating painful subcutaneous structures (bursae, tendons, other soft tissues) without breaking the skin. Physical therapists can therefore use iontophoresis and phonophoresis to administer local anesthetics, such as lidocaine, for treating certain musculoskeletal injuries. However, a comprehensive discussion of the efficacy of these techniques in physical therapy practice is beyond the scope of this chapter. Readers are directed to several references at the end of this chapter that address this topic in more detail.[12,18,20]

Administration of local anesthetics via iontophoresis can also be used to produce topical anesthesia prior to certain dermatologic procedures. For example, lidocaine iontophoresis can adequately anesthetize a small patch of skin for performing a minor surgical procedure (placement of an intravenous catheter, laser treatment of port-wine stains, and so forth).[18,50,66] Iontophoretic application of local anesthetics offers

a noninvasive alternative to subcutaneous injection of these drugs, and use of iontophoresis seems to be gaining popularity as a method for producing local anesthesia before specific dermatologic surgeries.[29]

Finally, local anesthetics can be administered via a transdermal patch.[1] In particular, transdermal patches containing 5% lidocaine have been used to treat localized pain in musculoskeletal conditions (osteoarthritis, low back pain, myofascial pain)[22,25,26] and various types of neuropathic pain (postherpetic neuralgia, diabetic neuropathy).[2,24,58] As indicated in Chapter 2, transdermal patches provide a convenient and predictable method for administering drugs to a given anatomical site, and lidocaine patches are now being used to provide symptomatic relief in many conditions involving fairly localized pain.

3. *Infiltration anesthesia.* The drug is injected directly into the selected tissue, allowing it to diffuse to sensory nerve endings within that tissue. This technique saturates an area such as a skin laceration for performing surgical repair (suturing).

4. *Peripheral nerve block.* The anesthetic is injected close to the nerve trunk so that transmission along the peripheral nerve is interrupted.[61] This type of local anesthesia is common in dental procedures (restorations, tooth extractions, and so on) and can also be used to block other peripheral nerves to allow certain surgical procedures of the hand, foot, shoulder, and so forth.[11,56,65] Injection near larger nerves (femoral, sciatic) or around a nerve plexus (brachial plexus)

can also be used to anesthetize larger areas of an upper or lower extremity.[23,37,39] Nerve blocks can be classified as minor when only one distinct nerve (e.g., ulnar, median) is blocked, or major, when several peripheral nerves or a nerve plexus (brachial, lumbosacral) is involved.

Nerve blocks can also be continued after the completion of the surgery to provide optimal pain management.[28,55] In this situation, a small catheter is left implanted near the nerve(s) so that small dosages of the local anesthetic are administered for the first 24 hours or so after surgery. Continuous peripheral nerve blocks have therefore been used to control postsurgical pain in several clinical situations, and these techniques should continue to gain acceptance as technical improvements are made in this form of drug delivery.[39,55] Prolonged administration of local anesthetics within skeletal muscle, however, can produce localized muscle pain and necrosis.[67,68] Hence, therapists should be aware of this possibility if patients report muscle pain and weakness following the use of continuous peripheral nerve blocks.

5. *Central neural blockade.* The anesthetic is injected within the spaces surrounding the spinal cord[10] (Fig.12–2). Specifically, the term **epidural nerve blockade** refers to injection of the drug into the epidural space—that is, the space between the bony vertebral column and the dura mater. A variation of epidural administration known as a "caudal block" is sometimes performed by injecting the local anesthetic into the lumbar epidural space via the sacral hiatus (see Fig. 12–2). **Spinal nerve blockade** refers to injection within the subarachnoid space—that is, the space between the arachnoid membrane and the pia mater. Spinal blockade is also referred to as "intrathecal anesthesia" because the drug is injected within the tissue sheaths surrounding the spinal cord (*intrathecal* means within a sheath; see Chapter 2).

In theory, epidural and spinal blocks can be done at any level of the cord, but they are usually administered at the L3-4 or L4-5 vertebral interspace (i.e., caudal to the L-2 vertebral body, which is the point where the spinal cord ends). Epidural anesthesia is somewhat easier to perform than spinal blockade because the epidural space is larger and more accessible than the subarachnoid space. However, spinal anesthesia is

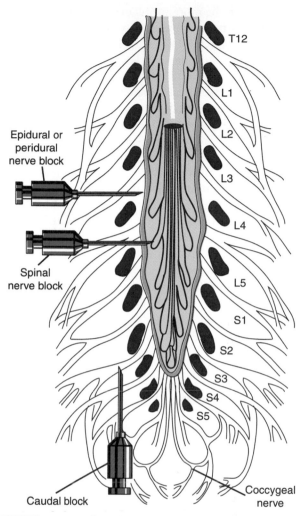

FIGURE 12–2 ▼ Sites of epidural and spinal administration of a local anesthetic. Caudal block represents epidural administration via the sacral hiatus. (From Clark JB, Queener SF, Karb VB. *Pharmacological Basis of Nursing Practice.* 4th ed. St Louis: CV Mosby; 1993: 688. Reproduced with permission.)

more rapid and usually creates a more effective or solid block using a smaller amount of the local anesthetic.[10,44] The drawback, of course, is that higher concentrations of the drug are administered in close proximity to neural structures during spinal anesthesia. Local anesthetics are neurotoxic when administered in high concentrations.[62,63] Spinal anesthesia therefore carries a somewhat higher risk for neurotoxicity because a relatively large amount of the local anesthetic is being introduced fairly close to the spinal cord and related neural structures (cauda equina). Any physical damage from the injection technique or neurotoxicity from the drugs will therefore be more problematic during spinal administration compared to the epidural route.

Central neural blockade is used whenever analgesia is needed in a large region, and epidural and spinal routes are used frequently to administer local anesthetics during obstetric procedures (including caesarean delivery).[30,44] These routes can also be used as an alternative to general anesthesia for other surgical procedures including lumbar spine surgery and hip and knee arthroplasty.[23,45] The epidural and intrathecal routes have also been used to administer anesthetics and narcotic analgesics for relief of acute and chronic pain.[6,19] In these instances, an indwelling catheter is often left implanted in the epidural or subarachnoid space to allow repeated or continuous delivery of the anesthetic to the patient. The use of implanted drug delivery systems in managing chronic and severe pain is discussed further in Chapters 14 and 17.

6. *Sympathetic block.* Although blockade of sympathetic function usually occurs during peripheral and central nerve blocks, sometimes the selective interruption of sympathetic efferent discharge is desirable. This intervention is especially useful in cases of complex regional pain syndrome (CRPS). This syndrome, also known as reflex sympathetic dystrophy syndrome (RSDS) and causalgia, involves increased sympathetic discharge to an upper or lower extremity, often causing severe pain and dysfunction in the distal part of the extremity. As part of the treatment, a local anesthetic can be administered to interrupt sympathetic discharge to the affected extremity.[33,64] One approach is to inject the local anesthetic into the area surrounding the sympathetic chain ganglion that innervates the affected limb. For example, injection near the stellate ganglion is performed when the upper extremity is involved, and injections around the sympathetic ganglion at the L-2 vertebral level are used for lower-extremity CRPS.[33] Usually a series of five injections on alternate days is necessary to attenuate the sympathetic discharge and to provide remission from the CRPS episode. Alternatively, the local anesthetic can be administered subcutaneously to an affected area,[38] or injected intravenously into the affected limb using regional intravenous block techniques (see next section).[35] Hence, several techniques are currently being used to promote sympathetic blockade using local anesthetic drugs. With these techniques, the goal is not to provide analgesia, but rather to impair efferent sympathetic outflow to the affected extremity.

7. *Intravenous Regional Anesthesia (Bier block).* During intravenous regional anesthesia (also known as Bier block), the anesthetic is injected into a peripheral vein located in a selected limb (arm or leg).[9] The local vasculature can then carry the anesthetic to the nerves in that extremity, thereby producing anesthesia in the limb. A tourniquet is also applied proximally on the limb to localize the drug temporarily within the extremity, and to prevent the anesthetic from reaching the systemic circulation where it would cause toxic effects on the heart and CNS. This technique is somewhat difficult to use because the tourniquet can cause pain or increase the risk of ischemic neuropathy if left in place for more than 2 hours.[48] Intravenous regional block, however, can be used to anesthetize the forearm-hand or distal leg-ankle-foot for short periods to allow certain surgical procedures or to treat conditions such as CRPS.[34,35]

Mechanism of Action

Local anesthetics work by blocking action potential propagation along neuronal axons, which is believed to occur from the anesthetic molecule inhibiting the opening of membrane sodium channels.[44,60] The sudden influx of sodium into the neuron through open (activated) ion channels depolarizes the neuron during impulse propagation. If the sodium ion channels are inhibited from opening along a portion of the axon, the action potential will not be propagated past that point. If the neuron is sensory in nature, this information will not reach the brain and will result in anesthesia of the area innervated by that neuron.

Exactly how local anesthetics inhibit the sodium channel from opening has been the subject of much debate. Although several theories exist, the current consensus is that local anesthetics temporarily attach to a binding site or receptor located on or within the sodium channel.[16,36,60] These receptors probably control the opening of the channel, and when bound by the anesthetic molecule, the sodium channel is maintained in a closed, inactivated position. Several sites have been proposed to explain exactly where the local

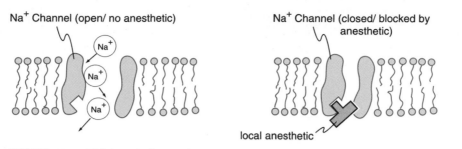

FIGURE 12–3 ▼ Schematic diagram showing mechanism of action of local anesthetics on the nerve membrane. Local anesthetics appear to bind directly to a site within the sodium channel, thereby locking the channel in a closed position, thus preventing sodium entry and action potential propagation.

anesthetic binds on the sodium channel protein (Fig. 12–3).[36,43,60] The most likely binding site is within the lumen or pore of the channel itself, possibly at the inner, cytoplasmic opening of the channel.[16,60] When bound by the anesthetic molecule, this site may effectively lock the sodium channel shut (much in the same way that the appropriate key fitting into a door keyhole is able to lock a door).

Consequently, local anesthetics appear to bind directly to sodium channels on the nerve axon. By keeping these channels in a closed, inactivated state, the anesthetic prevents action potential propogation along the affected portion of the axon. Likewise, only a relatively short portion of the axon (e.g., the length of 3 nodes of Ranvier in a myelinated neuron) needs to be affected by the anesthetic to block action potential propogation.[62] That is, the anesthetic does not need to affect the entire length of the axon, but block only one specific segment of the axon to completely prevent sensory or motor information from being transmitted past the point of the blockade.

Differential Nerve Block

Differential nerve block refers to the ability of a given local anesthetic dose to block specific nerve fiber groups depending on the size (diameter) of the fibers.[54, 62] In general, smaller diameter fibers seem to be the most sensitive to anesthetic effects, with progressively larger fibers being affected as anesthetic concentration increases.[62] This point is significant because different diameter fibers transmit different types of information (Table 12–2). Thus, information transmitted by the smallest fibers will be lost first, with other types of transmission being successively lost as the local anesthetic effect increases. The smallest diameter (type C) fibers that transmit pain are usually the first sensory information blocked as the anesthetic takes effect. Type C fibers also transmit postganglionic autonomic information, including sympathetic vasomotor control of the peripheral vasculature, and are most susceptible to block by local anesthetics. Other sensory information—such as temperature, touch, and proprioception—is successively lost as the concentration and effect of the anesthetic increases. Finally, skeletal motor function is usually last to disappear because efferent impulses to the skeletal muscle are transmitted over the large type A-alpha fibers.

The exact reason for the differential susceptibility of nerve fibers based on their axonal diameter is not known. One possible explanation is that the anesthetic is able to affect a critical length of the axon more quickly in unmyelinated fibers, or small myelinated neurons with nodes of Ranvier that are spaced closely together compared to larger fibers where the nodes are farther apart.[17] As indicated earlier, a specific length of the axon must be affected by the anesthetic so that action potentials cannot be transmitted past the point of blockade. Other factors such as the firing rate of each axon or the position of the axon in the nerve bundle (e.g., in the outer part of the bundle versus buried toward the center of the nerve) may also affect susceptibility to local anesthesia.[62] In any event, from a clinical perspective the smaller-diameter fibers appear to be affected first, although the exact reasons for this phenomenon remain to be determined.

The clinical importance of a differential nerve block is that certain sensory modalities may be blocked without the loss of motor function. Fortuitously, the most susceptible modality is pain because analgesia is usually the desired effect. If the dosage and administration of the anesthetic is optimal, it will produce analgesia without any significant loss of skeletal muscle function. This fact may be advantageous if motor function is required, such as during labor and delivery.[14] If

Table 12-2	RELATIVE SIZE AND SUSCEPTIBILITY TO BLOCK OF TYPES OF NERVE FIBERS				
Fiber Type*	Function	Diameter (μm)	Myelination	Conduction Velocity (m/s)	Sensitivity to Block
Type A					
Alpha	Proprioception, motor	12–20	Heavy	70–120	+
Beta	Touch, pressure	5–12	Heavy	30–70	++
Gamma	Muscle spindles	3–6	Heavy	15–30	++
Delta	Pain, temperature	2–5	Heavy	12–30	+++
Type B	Preganglionic, auto- nomic	< 3	Light	3–15	++++
Type C					
Dorsal Root	Pain	0.4–1.2	None	0.5–2.3	++++
Sympathetic	Postganglionic	0.3–1.3	None	0.7–2.3	++++

*Fiber types are classified according to the system established by Gasser and Erlanger. *Am J Physiol.* 1929; 88:581. Reproduced with permission from Katzung BG. *Basic and Clinical Pharmacology.* 9th ed. New York: Lange Medical Books/McGraw Hill; 2004.

local anesthetics are used to produce sympathetic blockade, postganglionic type C fibers are the first to be blocked, thus producing the desired effect at the lowest anesthetic concentration.

Systemic Effects of Local Anesthetics

The intent of administering a local anesthetic is to produce a regional effect on specific neurons. However, these drugs may occasionally be absorbed into the general circulation and exert various effects on other organs and tissues. Because local anesthetics inhibit action potential initiation and propogation, the most important systemic effects involve the CNS and cardiovascular system.[8,21,27] That is, local anesthetics can inadvertently disrupt the excitability of the CNS and cardiac tissues if meaningful amounts of these drugs reach the systemic circulation.

Regarding CNS effects, virtually all local anesthetics stimulate the brain initially, and symptoms such as somnolence, confusion, agitation, excitation, and seizures can occur if sufficient amounts reach the brain via the bloodstream.[8,17] Central excitation is usually followed by a period of CNS depression. This depression may result in impaired respiratory function, and death may occur due to respiratory depression.[17] The primary cardiovascular effects associated with local anesthetics include decreased cardiac excitation, heart rate, and force of contraction.[5,17] Again, this general inhibitory effect on the myocardium may produce serious consequences if sufficient amounts of the local anesthetic reach the general circulation.[17]

Systemic effects are more likely to occur with long-acting anesthetics if an excessive dose is used, if absorption into the blood stream is accelerated for some reason, or if the drug is accidentally injected into the systemic circulation rather than into extravascular tissues.[17,40] Other factors that can predispose a patient to systemic effects include the type of local anesthetic administered, as well as the route and method of administration.[3] Therapists and other health care professionals should always be alert for signs of the systemic effects of local anesthetics in patients. Early symptoms of CNS toxicity include ringing/buzzing in the ears (tinnitus), agitation, restlessness, and decreased cutaneous sensation around the mouth or other areas of the skin.[59] Changes in heart rate (bradycardia), electrocardiogram (ECG) abnormalities, or clinical signs of cardiac depression (fatigue, dizziness) may indicate cardiotoxicity. Again, early recognition of these CNS and cardiac abnormalities is essential to help avert fatalities due to the drug's systemic effects.

Significance in Rehabilitation

Physical therapists may encounter the use of local anesthetics in several patient situations because of their various clinical applications. For example, therapists may be directly involved in the topical or transdermal administration of local anesthetics. As discussed earlier, repeated topical application of local anesthetics may help produce long-term improvements in motor function in patients with skeletal muscle hypertonicity, so therapists may want to consider incorporating topical anesthetics into the treatment of certain patients with CNS dysfunction. Therapists may also administer local anesthetics transdermally, using the techniques of iontophoresis and phonophoresis. Agents such as lidocaine can be administered through this method for the treatment of acute inflammation in bursitis, tendinitis, and so on.

Therapists may also be working with patients who are receiving local anesthetic injections for the treatment of CRPS/RSDS. Since these patients often receive a series of anesthetic injections, therapists may want to schedule the rehabilitation session immediately after each injection so that
cises and other rehabilitatic
anesthetic is still in effect.
reestablish normal sympath
flow to the affected extremit
are obtained from the sympa

Finally, therapists may
are receiving central neural b..........
epidural or spinal injection. These procedures are common during natural and caesarean childbirth and in some other surgical procedures. Administration of local anesthetics into the spaces around the spinal cord are also used to treat individuals with severe and chronic pain—that is, patients recovering from extensive surgery, patients who have cancer, or patients with other types of intractable pain. In these situations, therapists may notice that an indwelling catheter has been placed in the patient's epidural or subarachnoid space to allow repeated or sustained administration of the spinal anesthesia.

In situations where central neural blockade is used, therapists should be especially aware that sensation might be diminished below the level of epidural or spinal administration. Decreased sensation to thermal agents and electrical stimulation will occur when the central block is in effect.[10] Likewise, motor function may be affected in the lower extremities when local anesthetics are administered spinally or epidurally.[10] Hence, therapists should test sensation and motor strength before applying any physical agents or attempting ambulation with patients who have received some type of central neural blockade using a local anesthetic.

CASE STUDY

Local Anesthetics

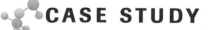

Brief History. R.D. is a 35-year-old man who developed pain in his right shoulder after spending the weekend chopping firewood. He was examined by a physical therapist and evaluated as having supraspinatus tendinitis. Apparently, this tendinitis recurred intermittently, usually after extensive use of the right shoulder. During past episodes, the tendinitis was resistant to treatment and usually took several months to resolve.

Decision/Solution. The therapist began an aggressive rehabilitation program consisting of daily heat, ultra-
sound, soft-tissue massage, and exercise. Soft-tissue massage consisted of transverse-friction techniques applied to the supraspinatus tendon. In order to improve the patient's tolerance to this technique, 5 percent lidocaine (Xylocaine) solution was administered via iontophoresis prior to the transverse-friction massage. This approach allowed R.D. and the therapist to perform both the massage technique and subsequent exercises more aggressively. Under this regimen, the supraspinatus tendinitis was resolved and the patient had full, pain-free use of the right shoulder within 3 weeks.

‍IARY

‍l anesthetics are used frequently when a limited, well-defined area of anesthesia is required, as is the case for most minor surgical procedures. Depending on the method of administration, local anesthetics can be used to temporarily block transmission in the area of peripheral nerve endings, along the trunk of a single peripheral nerve, along several peripheral nerves or plexuses, or at the level of the spinal cord. Local anesthetics may also be used to block efferent sympathetic activity. These drugs appear to block transmission along nerve axons by binding to membrane sodium channels and by preventing the channels from opening during neuronal excitation. Physical therapists may frequently encounter the use of these agents in their patients for both short-term and long-term control of pain, as well as in the management of sympathetic hyperactivity.

References

1. Argoff CE, Galer BS, Jensen MP, et al. Effectiveness of the lidocaine patch 5% on pain qualities in three chronic pain states: assessment with the Neuropathic Pain Scale. *Curr Med Res Opin.* 2004;20(suppl 2):S21–S28.
2. Barbano RL, Herrmann DN, Hart-Gouleau S, et al. Effectiveness, tolerability, and impact on quality of life of the 5% lidocaine patch in diabetic polyneuropathy. *Arch Neurol.* 2004;61:914–918.
3. Berde CB, Strichartz GR. Local anesthetics. In: Miller RD, ed. *Anesthesia. Volume 1.* 5th ed. Philadelphia: Churchill Livingstone; 2000.
4. Bloch Y, Levkovitz Y, Atshuler A, et al. Use of topical application of lidocaine-prilocaine cream to reduce injection-site pain of depot antipsychotics. *Psychiatr Serv.* 2004;55:940–941.
5. Borgeat A, Ekatodramis G, Blumenthal S. Interscalene brachial plexus anesthesia with ropivacaine 5 mg/mL and bupivacaine 5 mg/mL: effects on electrocardiogram. *Reg Anesth Pain Med.* 2004;29:557–563.
6. Bourne MH. Analgesics for orthopedic postoperative pain. *Am J Orthop.* 2004;33:128–135.
7. Brady-Fryer B, Wiebe N, Lander JA. Pain relief for neonatal circumcision. *Cochrane Database Syst Rev.* 2004;CD004217.
8. Breslin DS, Martin G, Macleod DB, et al. Central nervous system toxicity following the administration of levobupivacaine for lumbar plexus block: a report of two cases. *Reg Anesth Pain Med.* 2003;28:144–147.
9. Brill S, Middleton W, Brill G, Fisher A. Bier's block: 100 years old and still going strong! *Acta Anaesthesiol Scand.* 2004;48:117–122.
10. Brown DL. Spinal, epidural, and caudal anesthesia. In: Miller RD, ed. *Anesthesia. Volume 1* 5th ed. Philadelphia: Churchill Livingstone; 2000.
11. Budenz AW. Local anesthetics in dentistry: then and now. *J Calif Dent Assoc.* 2003;31:388–396.
12. Byl NN. The use of ultrasound as an enhancer for transcutaneous drug delivery: phonophoresis. *Phys Ther.* 1995;75:539–553.
13. Capdevila X, Dadure C. Perioperative management for one day hospital admission: regional anesthesia is better than general anesthesia. *Acta Anaesthesiol Belg.* 2004;(suppl 55):33–36.
14. Capogna G, Camorcia M. Epidural analgesia for childbirth: effects of newer techniques on neonatal outcome. *Paediatr Drugs.* 2004;6:375–386.
15. Casati A, Cappelleri G, Aldegheri G, et al. Total intravenous anesthesia, spinal anesthesia or combined sciatic-femoral nerve block for outpatient knee arthroscopy. *Minerva Anestesiol.* 2004;70:493–502.
16. Catterall WA. Molecular mechanisms of gating and drug block of sodium channels. *Novartis Found Symp.* 2002;241:206–218.
17. Catterall WA, Mackie K. Local anesthetics. In: Hardman JG, et al, eds. *The Pharmacological Basis of Therapeutics.* 10th ed. New York: McGraw-Hill; 2001.
18. Ciccone CD. Iontophoresis. In: Robinson AJ, Snyder-Mackler L, eds. *Clinical Electrophysiology.* 3rd ed. Baltimore: Williams and Wilkins; In press.
19. Colwell CW, Jr. The use of the pain pump and patient-controlled analgesia in joint reconstruction. *Am J Orthop.* 2004;33(suppl 5):10–12.
20. Costello CT, Jeske AH. Iontophoresis: applications in transdermal medication delivery. *Phys Ther.* 1995;75:554–563.
21. Crews JC, Rothman TE. Seizure after levobupivacaine for interscalene brachial plexus block. *Anesth Analg.* 2003;96:1188–1190.
22. Dalpiaz AS, Lordon SP, Lipman AG. Topical lidocaine patch therapy for myofascial pain. *J Pain Palliat Care Pharmacother.* 2004;18:15–34.
23. Davies AF, Segar EP, Murdoch J, et al. Epidural infusion or combined femoral and sciatic nerve blocks as perioperative analgesia for knee arthroplasty. *Br J Anaesth.* 2004;93:368–374.
24. Davies PS, Galer BS. Review of lidocaine patch 5% studies in the treatment of postherpetic neuralgia. *Drugs.* 2004;64:937–947.
25. Galer BS, Gammaitoni AR, Oleka N, et al. Use of the lidocaine patch 5% in reducing intensity of various pain qualities reported by patients with low-back pain. *Curr Med Res Opin.* 2004;20(suppl 2):S5–S12.
26. Gammaitoni AR, Galer BS, Onawola R, et al. Lidocaine patch 5% and its positive impact on pain qualities in osteoarthritis: results of a pilot 2-week, open-label study using the Neuropathic Pain Scale. *Curr Med Res Opin.* 2004;20(suppl 2):S13–S19.

27. Graf BM. The cardiotoxicity of local anesthetics: the place of ropivacaine. *Curr Top Med Chem.* 2001; 1:207–214.

28. Grant SA, Nielsen KC, Greengrass RA, et al. Continuous peripheral nerve block for ambulatory surgery. *Reg Anesth Pain Med.* 2001;26:209–214.

29. Greenbaum SS. Iontophoresis as a tool for anesthesia in dermatologic surgery: an overview. *Dermatol Surg.* 2001;27:1027–1030.

30. Gogarten W. Spinal anaesthesia for obstetrics. *Best Pract Res Clin Anaesthesiol.* 2003;17:377–392.

31. Hocking G, Wildsmith JA. Intrathecal drug spread. *Br J Anaesth.* 2004;93:568–578.

32. Inoue S, Kawaraguchi Y, Kitaguchi K, Furuya H. Inclusion of epinephrine to hyperbaric tetracaine and the supine position enhance the cephalad spread of spinal anaesthesia compared with hyperbaric tetracaine alone in the lithotomy position. *Acta Anaesthesiol Scand.* 2004;48:342–346.

33. Karakurum G, Pirbudak L, Oner U, et al. Sympathetic blockade and amitriptyline in the treatment of reflex sympathetic dystrophy. *Int J Clin Pract.* 2003;57: 585–587.

34. Karalezli N, Karalezli K, Iltar S, et al. Results of intravenous regional anaesthesia with distal forearm application. *Acta Orthop Belg.* 2004;70:401–405.

35. Lake AP. Intravenous regional sympathetic block: past, present and future? *Pain Res Manag.* 2004;9:35–37.

36. Leuwer M, Haeseler G, Hecker H, et al. An improved model for the binding of lidocaine and structurally related local anaesthetics to fast-inactivated voltage-operated sodium channels, showing evidence of cooperativity. *Br J Pharmacol.* 2004;141:47–54.

37. Liisanantti O, Luukkonen J, Rosenberg PH. High-dose bupivacaine, levobupivacaine and ropivacaine in axillary brachial plexus block. *Acta Anaesthesiol Scand.* 2004;48:601–606.

38. Linchitz RM, Raheb JC. Subcutaneous infusion of lidocaine provides effective pain relief for CRPS patients. *Clin J Pain.* 1999;15:67–72.

39. Long TR, Wass CT, Burkle CM. Perioperative interscalene blockade: an overview of its history and current clinical use. *J Clin Anesth.* 2002;14:546–556.

40. Mather LE, Chang DH. Cardiotoxicity with modern local anaesthetics: is there a safer choice? *Drugs.* 2001; 61:333–342.

41. Mattingly JE, D'Alessio J, Ramanathan J. Effects of obstetric analgesics and anesthetics on the neonate: a review. *Paediatr Drugs.* 2003;5:615–627.

42. Naftalin LW, Yagiela JA. Vasoconstrictors: indications and precautions. *Dent Clin North Am.* 2002;46: 733–746.

43. Nau C, Wang GK. Interactions of local anesthetics with voltage-gated Na+ channels. *J Membr Biol.* 2004; 201:1–8.

44. Ng K, Parsons J, Cyna AM, Middleton P. Spinal versus epidural anaesthesia for caesarean section. *Cochrane Database Syst Rev.* 2004;CD003765.

45. Parker MJ, Handoll HH, Griffiths R. Anaesthesia for hip fracture surgery in adults. *Cochrane Database Syst Rev.* 2004;CD000521.

46. Pitkanen M, Rosenberg PH. Local anaesthetics and additives for spinal anaesthesia—characteristics and factors influencing the spread and duration of the block. *Best Pract Res Clin Anaesthesiol.* 2003;17: 305–322.

47. Portnoy D, Vadhera RB. Mechanisms and management of an incomplete epidural block for cesarean section. *Anesthesiol Clin North America.* 2003;21:39–57.

48. Rodola F, Vagnoni S, Ingletti S. An update on Intravenous Regional Anaesthesia of the arm. *Eur Rev Med Pharmacol Sci.* 2003;7:131–138.

49. Rogers TL, Ostrow CL. The use of EMLA cream to decrease venipuncture pain in children. *J Pediatr Nurs.* 2004;19:33–39.

50. Rose JB, Galinkin JL, Jantzen EC, Chiavacci RM. A study of lidocaine iontophoresis for pediatric venipuncture. *Anesth Analg.* 2002;94:867–871.

51. Rosenberg PH, Veering BT, Urmey WF. Maximum recommended doses of local anesthetics: a multifactorial concept. *Reg Anesth Pain Med.* 2004; 29:564–575.

52. Rosenthal D, Murphy F, Gottschalk R, et al. Using a topical anaesthetic cream to reduce pain during sharp debridement of chronic leg ulcers. *J Wound Care.* 2001;10:503–505.

53. Sabbahi MA, De Luca CJ: Topical anesthetic-induced improvements in the mobility of patients with muscular hypertonicity: preliminary results. *J Electromyogr Kinesiol.* 1991;1:41–46.

54. Sakai T, Tomiyasu S, Yamada H, et al. Quantitative and selective evaluation of differential sensory nerve block after transdermal lidocaine. *Anesth Analg.* 2004; 98:248–251.

55. Shinaman RC, Mackey S. Continuous peripheral nerve blocks. *Curr Pain Headache Rep.* 2005;9:24–29.

56. Singelyn FJ, Lhotel L, Fabre B. Pain relief after arthroscopic shoulder surgery: a comparison of intraarticular analgesia, suprascapular nerve block, and interscalene brachial plexus block. *Anesth Analg.* 2004; 99:589–592.

57. Soliman MM, Macky TA, Samir MK. Comparative clinical trial of topical anesthetic agents in cataract surgery: lidocaine 2% gel, bupivacaine 0.5% drops, and benoxinate 0.4% drops. *J Cataract Refract Surg.* 2004; 30:1716–1720.

58. Stacey BR. Management of peripheral neuropathic pain. *Am J Phys Med Rehabil.* 2005;84(suppl):S4–S16.

59. Stewart J, Kellett N, Castro D. The central nervous system and cardiovascular effects of levobupivacaine and ropivacaine in healthy volunteers. *Anesth Analg.* 2003;97:412–416.

60. Tsang SY, Tsushima RG, Tomaselli GF, et al. A multifunctional aromatic residue in the external pore vestibule of Na+ channels contributes to the local anesthetic receptor. *Mol Pharmacol.* 2005;67:424–434.

61. Wedel DJ. Nerve blocks. In: Miller RD, ed. *Anesthesia. Volume 1.* 5th ed. Philadelphia: Churchill Livingstone; 2000.

62. White PF, Katzung BG. Local anesthetics. In: Katzung BG, ed. *Basic and Clinical Pharmacology.* 9th ed. New York: Lange Medical Books/McGraw-Hill; 2004.

63. Yamashita A, Matsumoto M, Matsumoto S, et al. A comparison of the neurotoxic effects on the spinal cord of tetracaine, lidocaine, bupivacaine, and ropivacaine administered intrathecally in rabbits. *Anesth Analg.* 2003;97:512–519.

64. Yung Chung O, Bruehl SP. Complex Regional Pain Syndrome. *Curr Treat Options Neurol.* 2003;5:499–511.

65. Zaric D, Boysen K, Christiansen J, Haastrup U, Kofoed H, Rawal N. Continuous popliteal sciatic nerve block for outpatient foot surgery—a randomized, controlled trial. *Acta Anaesthesiol Scand.* 2004;48:337–341.

66. Zempsky WT, Sullivan J, Paulson DM, Hoath SB. Evaluation of a low-dose lidocaine iontophoresis system for topical anesthesia in adults and children: a randomized, controlled trial. *Clin Ther.* 2004;26:1110–1119.

67. Zink W, Graf BM. Local anesthetic myotoxicity. *Reg Anesth Pain Med.* 2004;29:333–340.

68. Zink W, Seif C, Bohl JR, et al. The acute myotoxic effects of bupivacaine and ropivacaine after continuous peripheral nerve blockades. *Anesth Analg.* 2003;97:1173–1179.

Drugs Affecting Skeletal Muscle

Chapter 13

Skeletal Muscle Relaxants

Skeletal muscle relaxants are used to treat conditions associated with hyperexcitable skeletal muscle—specifically, spasticity and muscle spasms. Although these two terms are often used interchangeably, spasticity and muscle spasms represent two distinct abnormalities. The use of relaxant drugs, however, is similar in each condition because the ultimate goal is to normalize muscle excitability without a profound decrease in muscle function. Considering the number of rehabilitation patients with muscle hyperexcitability that is associated with either spasm or spasticity, skeletal muscle relaxants represent an important class of drugs to the rehabilitation specialist.

Drugs discussed in this chapter are used to decrease muscle excitability and contraction via an effect at the spinal cord level, at the neuromuscular junction, or within the muscle cell itself. Some texts also classify neuromuscular junction blockers such as curare and succinylcholine as skeletal muscle relaxants. However, these drugs are more appropriately classified as skeletal muscle *paralytics* because they eliminate muscle contraction by blocking transmission at the myoneural synapse. This type of skeletal muscle paralysis is used primarily during general anesthesia; using neuromuscular blockers as an adjunct in surgery was discussed in Chapter 11. Skeletal muscle relaxants do not typically prevent muscle contraction; they only attempt to normalize muscle excitability to decrease pain and improve motor function.

Increased Muscle Tone: Spasticity Versus Muscle Spasms

Much confusion and consternation often arise from the erroneous use of the terms "spasticity" and "spasm." For the purpose of this text, these terms will be used to describe two different types of increased excitability, which result from different underlying pathologies. *Spasticity* occurs in many patients following an injury to the central nervous system (CNS), including cord-related problems (multiple sclerosis, spinal cord transection) and injuries to the brain (CVA, cerebral palsy, acquired brain injury). Although there is considerable controversy about the exact changes in motor control, most clinicians agree that spasticity is characterized primarily by an exaggerated muscle stretch reflex (Fig. 13–1).[40,52,79] This abnormal reflex activity is velocity-dependent, with a rapid lengthening of the muscle invoking a strong contraction in the

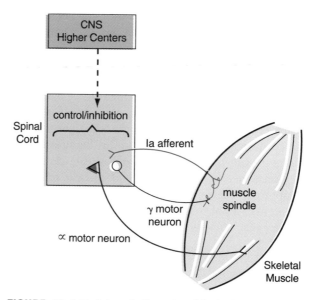

FIGURE 13–1 ▼ Schematic illustration of the basic components of the stretch reflex. Normally, higher CNS centers control the sensitivity of this reflex by inhibiting synaptic connections within the spinal cord. Spasticity is thought to occur when this higher center influence is lost because of cerebral trauma or damage to descending pathways in the spinal cord.

stretched muscle. The neurophysiologic mechanisms underlying spasticity are complex, but this phenomenon occurs when supraspinal inhibition or control is lost because of a lesion in the spinal cord or brain.[40,52,54] Presumably, specific upper motor neuron lesions interrupt the cortical control of stretch reflex and alpha motor neuron excitability. Spasticity, therefore, is not in itself a disease but rather the motor sequela to pathologies such as cerebral vascular accident (CVA), cerebral palsy, multiple sclerosis (MS), and traumatic lesions to the brain and spinal cord (including quadriplegia and paraplegia).

Skeletal muscle *spasms* are used to describe the increased tension often seen in skeletal muscle after certain musculoskeletal injuries and inflammation (muscle strains, nerve root impingements, etc.) occur.[20,96] This tension is involuntary, so the patient is unable to relax the muscle. Spasms differ from spasticity because spasms typically arise from an orthopedic injury to a musculoskeletal structure or peripheral nerve root rather than an injury to the CNS. Likewise, muscle spasms are often a continuous, tonic contraction of specific muscles rather than the velocity-dependent increase in stretch reflex activity commonly associated with spasticity. The exact reasons for muscle spasms are poorly understood. According to some authorities, muscle spasms occur because a vicious cycle is created when the initial injury causes muscular pain and spasm, which increases afferent nociceptive input to the spinal cord, further exciting the alpha motor neuron to cause more spasms, and so on.[61,96] Other experts believe that muscle spasms occur because of a complex protective mechanism, whereby muscular contractions are intended to support an injured vertebral structure or peripheral joint.[96] Regardless of the exact reason, tonic contraction of the affected muscle is often quite painful because of the buildup of pain-mediating metabolites (e.g., lactate).

Consequently, various skeletal muscle relaxants attempt to decrease skeletal muscle excitation and contraction in cases of spasticity and spasm. Specific drugs and their mechanisms of action are discussed here.

Specific Agents Used to Produce Skeletal Muscle Relaxation

Skeletal muscle relaxants are categorized in this chapter according to their primary clinical application: agents used to decrease spasms and agents used to

decrease spasticity. One agent, diazepam (Valium), is indicated for both conditions and will appear in both categories. Finally, the use of botulinum toxin (Botox) as an alternative strategy for reducing focal spasms or spasticity will be addressed.

Agents Used to Treat Muscle Spasms

Diazepam

The effects of diazepam (Valium) on the CNS and its use as an antianxiety drug are discussed in Chapter 6. Basically, diazepam and other benzodiazepines work by increasing the central inhibitory effects of gamma-aminobutyric acid (GABA); that is, diazepam binds to receptors located at GABAergic synapses and increases the GABA-induced inhibition at that synapse. Diazepam appears to work as a muscle relaxant through this mechanism, potentiating the inhibitory effect of GABA on alpha motor neuron activity in the spinal cord.[40,102] The drug also exerts some supraspinal sedative effects; in fact, some of its muscle relaxant properties may derive from the drug's ability to produce a more generalized state of sedation.[101]

Uses. Diazepam is one of the oldest medications for treating muscle spasms, and has been used extensively in treating spasms associated with musculoskeletal injuries such as acute low-back strains. Diazepam has also been used to control muscle spasms associated with tetanus toxin; the use of valium in this situation can be life-saving as well by inhibiting spasms of the larynx and other muscles.[51,65]

Adverse Effects. The primary side effect with diazepam is that dosages successful in relaxing skeletal muscle also produce sedation and a general reduction in psychomotor ability.[40,101] However, this effect may not be a problem and may actually be advantageous for the patient recovering from an acute musculoskeletal injury. For example, a patient with an acute lumbosacral strain may benefit from the sedative properties because he or she will remain fairly inactive, thereby allowing better healing during the first few days after the injury. Continued use, however, may be problematic because of diazepam's sedative effects. The drug can also produce tolerance and physical dependence, and sudden withdrawal after prolonged use can cause seizures, anxiety, agitation, tachycardia, and even death.[102] Likewise, an overdose with diazepam can result in coma or death as well.[102] Hence, this drug might be beneficial for the short-term management of acute muscle spasms, but long-term use should be discouraged.

Polysynaptic Inhibitors

A variety of centrally acting compounds have been used in an attempt to enhance muscle relaxation and decrease muscle spasms (see Table 13–1). Some examples are carisoprodol (Soma, Vanadom), chlorphenesin carbamate (Maolate), chlorzoxazone (Paraflex, Parafon Forte, others), cyclobenzaprine (Flexeril), metaxalone (Skelaxin), methocarbamol (Carbacot, Robaxin, Skelex), and orphenadrine citrate (Antiflex, Norflex, others). The mechanism of action of these drugs is not well defined.[8] Research in animals has suggested that these drugs may decrease polysynaptic reflex activity in the spinal cord, hence the term "polysynaptic inhibitors." A polysynaptic reflex arc in the spinal cord is comprised of several small interneurons that link incoming (afferent) input into the dorsal horn with outgoing (efferent) outflow onto the alpha motor neuron. By inhibiting the neurons in the polysynaptic pathways, these drugs could decrease alpha motor neuron excitability and therefore cause relaxation of skeletal muscle.

It is not clear, however, exactly how these drugs inhibit neurons involved in the polysynaptic pathways. There is preliminary evidence that one of these compounds (cyclobenzaprine) might block serotonin receptors on spinal interneurons, thereby decreasing the excitatory influence of serotonin on alpha motor neuron activity.[50,55] Although this effect has been attributed to cyclobenzaprine in animals (rats), the effect of this drug and other muscle relaxants in humans remains to be determined.

On the other hand, these compounds have a general depressant effect on the CNS; that is, they cause a global decrease in CNS excitability that results in generalized sedation. It therefore seems possible that some of their muscle relaxant effects are caused by their sedative powers rather than a selective effect on specific neuronal reflex pathways.[11,92] This observation is not to say that they are ineffective, because clinical research has shown that these drugs can be superior to a placebo in producing subjective muscle relaxation.[8,20,80,97] However, the specific ability of these drugs to relax skeletal muscle remains doubtful, and it is generally believed that their muscle relaxant properties are secondary to a nonspecific CNS sedation.

Uses. These drugs are typically used as adjuncts to rest and physical therapy for the short-term relief of

Table 13–1	DRUGS COMMONLY USED TO TREAT SKELETAL MUSCLE SPASMS		
Drug	Usual Adult Oral Dosage (mg)	Onset of Action (min)	Duration of Action (hr)
Carisoprodol (Soma, Vanadom)	350 TID and bedtime	30	4–6
Chlorphenesin carbamate (Maolate)	Initially: 800 TID; reduce to 400 QID or less	–	–
Chlorzoxazone (Paraflex, Parafon Forte, others)	250–750 TID or QID	Within 60	3–4
Cyclobenzaprine (Flexeril)	10 TID	Within 60	12–24
Diazepam (Valium)	2–10 TID or QID	15–45	Variable
Metaxalone (Skelaxin)	800 TID or QID	60	4–6
Methocarbamol (Carbacot, Robaxin, Skelex)	1000 QID or 1500 TID	Within 30	24
Orphenadrine citrate (Antiflex, Norflex, others)	100 BID	Within 60	12

muscle spasms associated with acute, painful muscu-loskeletal injuries.[9,14,97] When used to treat spasms, these compounds are often given with a nonsteroidal anti-inflammatory agent (NSAIDs; see Chapter 15), or sometimes incorporated into the same tablet with an analgesic such as acetaminophen or aspirin. For instance, Norgesic is one of the brand names for orphenadrine combined with aspirin (and caffeine). Such combinations have been reported to be more effective than the individual components given sepa-rately.[8]

Adverse Effects. Because of their sedative proper-ties, the primary side effects of these drugs are drowsi-ness and dizziness (see Table 13–2). A variety of additional adverse effects, including nausea, light-headedness, vertigo, ataxia, and headache, may occur depending on the patient and the specific drug admin-istered (Table 13–2). Cases of fatal overdose have also been documented for several of these drugs, including cyclobenzaprine and metaxolone.[70,86]

Long term or excessive use of these medica-tions may also cause tolerance and physical depend-ence.[14,31] In particular, carisoprodol should be used cautiously because this drug is metabolized in the body to form meprobamate, which is a controlled sub-stance (see Chapter 1) that has sedative/anxiolytic properties but is not used extensively because it has strong potential for abuse.[13,73] Hence, use of cariso-prodol represents a rather unique situation where the drug itself or its metabolic byproduct (meprobamate) can produce effects and side effects that lead to addic-tion and abuse, especially in people with a history of substance abuse.[13,73] Likewise, discontinuing cariso-prodol suddenly after long term use can lead to with-drawal symptoms such as anxiety, tremors, muscle twitching, and hallucinations.[72]

Consequently, polysynaptic inhibitors can help provide short-term relief for muscle spasms associ-ated with certain musculoskeletal conditions, and they may work synergistically with physical therapy and other interventions during acute episodes of back pain, neck pain, and so forth. Nonetheless, they have some rather serious side effects and potential for abuse, and the long-term use of these drugs should be discouraged.

Agents Used to Treat Spasticity

The three agents traditionally used in the treatment of spasticity are baclofen, diazepam, and dantrolene sodi-um (see Table 13–3, Fig. 13–2). Two newer agents, gabapentin and tizanidine, are also available for treat-ing spasticity in various conditions. All of these agents are addressed below.

Table 13–2 RELATIVE SIDE EFFECTS OF POLYSYNAPTIC INHIBITORS USED AS ANTISPASM AGENTS

Drug	Drowsiness	Dizziness or Lightheadedness	Headache	Nausea and Vomiting
Carisoprodol	M	L	L	L
Chlorphenesin carbamate	L	L	R	R
Chlorzoxazone	M	M	L	L
Cyclobenzaprine	M	M	L	L
Metaxalone	M	M	M	M
Methocarbamol	M	M	L	L
Orphenadrine citrate	L	L	L	L

Relative incidence of side effects: M = more frequent; L = less frequent; R = rare.
Taken from *USP DI, 25th Edition.* Copyright 2005.Thompson MICROMEDEX.

Table 13-3	ANTISPASTICITY DRUGS	
Drug	**Oral Dosage**	**Comments**
Baclofen (Lioresal)	Adult: 5 mg TID initially; increase by 5 mg at 3-day intervals as required; maximum recommended dosage is 80 mg/day. Children: No specific pediatric dosage is listed; the adult dose must be decreased according to the size and age of the child.	More effective in treating spasticity resulting from spinal cord lesions (versus cerebral lesions).
Dantrolene sodium (Dantrium)	Adult: 25 mg/d initially; increase up to 100 mg 2, 3, or 4 times per day as needed; maximum recommended dose is 400 mg/day. Children (older than 5 yr of age): initially, 0.5 mg/kg body weight BID; increase total daily dosage by 0.5 mg/kg every 4–7 days as needed, and give total daily amount in 4 divided dosages; maximum recommended dose is 400 mg/d.	Exerts an effect directly on the muscle cell; may cause generalized weakness in all skeletal musculature.
Diazepam (Valium)	Adult: 2–10 mg TID or QID. Children (older than 6 mo of age): 1.0–2.5 mg TID or QID (in both adults and children, begin at lower end of dosage range and increase gradually as tolerated and needed).	Produces sedation at dosages that decrease spasticity.
Gabapentin (Neurontin)	Adult:* initially, 300 mg TID. Can be gradually increased up to 3600 mg/d based on desired response. Children* (3–12 years of age): Initially, 10–15 mg/kg body weight in 3 divided dosages; increase over 3 days until desired effect or a maximum of 50 mg/kg/d.	Developed originally as an anticonvulsant; may also be helpful as an adjunct to other drugs in treating spasticity associated with spinal cord injury and multiple sclerosis.
Tizanidine (Zanaflex)	Adult: 8 mg every 6–8 hours as needed. Children: The safety and effficacy of this drug in treating spasticity in children have not been established.	May reduce a in spinal cord disorders while producing fewer side effects and less generalized muscle weakness than other agents (oral baclofen, diazepam).

*Anticonvulsant dose

Baclofen

The chemical name of baclofen is beta (*p*-chlorophenyl)-GABA. As this name suggests, baclofen is a derivative of the central inhibitory neurotransmitter GABA. However, there appear to be some differences between baclofen and GABA. Baclofen seems to bind preferentially to certain GABA receptors, which have been classified as $GABA_b$ receptors (as opposed to $GABA_a$ receptors).[64,95] Preferential binding to $GABA_b$ receptors enables baclofen to act as a GABA agonist, inhibiting transmission within the spinal cord at specific synapses.[40,64] To put this in the context of its use as a muscle relaxant, baclofen appears to have an

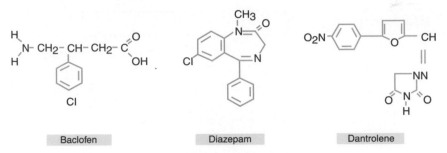

FIGURE 13–2 ▼ Structure of three primary antispasticity drugs.

inhibitory effect on alpha motor neuron activity within the spinal cord. This inhibition apparently occurs via inhibiting excitatory neurons that synapse with the alpha motor neuron (presynaptic inhibition), as well as directly affecting the alpha motor neuron itself (postsynaptic inhibition).[40,102] The result is decreased firing of the alpha motor neuron, with a subsequent relaxation of the skeletal muscle.

Uses. Baclofen is administered orally to treat spasticity associated with lesions of the spinal cord, including traumatic injuries resulting in paraplegia or quadriplegia and spinal cord demyelination resulting in MS.[30,102] Baclofen is often the drug of choice in reducing the muscle spasticity associated with MS because it produces beneficial effects with a remarkable lack of adverse side effects when used in patients with MS.[4] The drug also does not cause as much generalized muscle weakness as direct-acting relaxants such as dantrolene, which can be a major advantage of baclofen treatment in many patients with MS.[101] Baclofen also appears to produce fewer side effects when used appropriately to reduce spasticity secondary to traumatic spinal cord lesions, thus providing a relatively safe and effective form of treatment.[102] When administered systemically, baclofen is less effective in treating spasticity associated with supraspinal lesions (stroke, cerebral palsy), because these patients are more prone to the adverse side effects of this drug and because baclofen does not readily penetrate the blood-brain barrier.[40,102]

Oral baclofen has also been used to reduce alcohol consumption in people who are chronic alcohol abusers.[21,22] Apparently, relatively low doses of baclofen can reduce the cravings and desire for alcohol consumption via the effects of this drug on CNS GABA receptors.[21] Future studies will help clarify the role of this drug in treating chronic alcoholism.

Adverse Effects. When initiating baclofen therapy, the most common side effect is transient drowsiness, which usually disappears within a few days.[30] When given to patients with spinal cord lesions, there are usually few other adverse effects. When given to patients who have had a CVA or to elderly individuals, there is sometimes a problem with confusion and hallucinations. Other side effects, occurring on an individual basis, include fatigue, nausea, dizziness, muscle weakness, and headache. Abrupt discontinuation of baclofen may also cause withdrawal symptoms such as hyperthermia, hallucinations, and seizures.[30] Increased seizure activity has also been reported following baclofen overdose, and in selected patient populations such as certain children with cerebral palsy and certain adults with multiple sclerosis.[48,81]

Intrathecal Baclofen

Although baclofen is administered orally in most patients (Table 13–3) it can also be administered intrathecally in patients with severe, intractable spasticity.[71,103] Intrathecal administration is the delivery of a drug directly into the subarachnoid space surrounding a specific level of the spinal cord. This places the drug very close to the spinal cord, thus allowing increased drug effectiveness with much smaller drug doses. Likewise, fewer systemic side effects occur because the drug tends to remain in the area of the cord rather than circulating in the bloodstream and causing adverse effects on other tissues.

When baclofen is administered intrathecally for the long-term treatment of spasticity, a small catheter is usually implanted surgically so that the open end of the catheter is located in the subarachnoid space and the other end is attached to some type of programmable pump. The pump is implanted subcutaneously in the abdominal wall and is adjusted to deliver the drug at a slow, continuous rate. The rate of infusion is adjusted over time to achieve the best clinical reduction in spasticity.

Intrathecal baclofen delivery using implantable pumps has been used in patients with spasticity of spinal origin (spinal cord injury, multiple sclerosis),[57,103] and in patients with spasticity resulting from supraspinal (cerebral) injury, including cerebral palsy, CVA, and traumatic brain injury.[1,40,94] Studies involving these patients have typically noted a substantial decrease in rigidity (as indicated by decreased Ashworth scores, decreased reflex activity, and so forth).[57,103] Patient satisfaction is generally favorable, and caregivers for younger children report ease of care following implantation of intrathecal baclofen pumps.[17,43] There is growing evidence that intrathecal baclofen can also reduce pain of central origin in people with spasticity; that is, continuous baclofen administration to the subarachnoid space may inhibit the neural circuitry that induces chronic pain in people with stroke and other CNS injuries.[85,90]

Uses. Intrathecal baclofen can result in decreased spasticity and increased comfort in many people with severe spasticity. This intervention can also result in functional improvements, especially in cases where voluntary motor control was being masked by spasticity.[16] Ambulatory patients with spasticity resulting from a CVA, for example, may be able to increase their walking speed and increase their functional mobility after intrathecal baclofen therapy.[37,74]

These functional improvements, however, may not occur in all types of spasticity. Patients with severe spasticity of spinal origin, for example, may not experience improvements in mobility or decreased disability.[103] If these patients do not have adequate voluntary motor function there is simply not enough residual motor ability to perform functional tasks after spasticity is reduced. Nonetheless, these patients may still benefit from intrathecal baclofen because of decreased rigidity and pain, which can result in improved self-care and the ability to perform daily living activities.[37,74,76]

Adverse effects. Despite these benefits, intrathecal baclofen is associated with a number of potential complications. Primary among these is the possibility of a disruption in the delivery system; that is, a pump malfunction or a problem with the delivery catheter can occur.[42,60,67,69] In particular, the catheter can become obstructed, or the tip of the catheter can become displaced so that baclofen is not delivered into the correct area of the subarachnoid space. Increased drug delivery due to a pump malfunction could cause overdose and lead to respiratory depression, decreased cardiac function, and coma.[40] Conversely, abruptly

stopping the drug due to pump failure, pump removal, or delivery catheter displacement/blockage may cause a withdrawal syndrome that includes fever, confusion, delirium, and seizures.[46,75,104]

A second major concern is the possibility that tolerance could develop with long-term, continuous baclofen administration. Tolerance is the need for more of a drug to achieve its beneficial effects when used for prolonged periods. Several studies have reported that dosage must indeed be increased progressively when intrathecal baclofen systems are used for periods of several months to several years.[40,63] Tolerance to intrathecal baclofen, however, can usually be dealt with by periodic adjustments in dosage, and tolerance does not usually develop to such an extent that intrathecal baclofen must be discontinued.

Hence, intrathecal baclofen offers a means of treating certain patients with severe spasticity who have not responded to more conventional means of treatment including oral baclofen. Additional research will help determine optimal ways that this intervention can be used to decrease spasticity. Further improvements in the technologic and mechanical aspects of intrathecal delivery, including better pumps and catheter systems, will also make this a safer and more practical method of treating these patients.

Dantrolene Sodium

The only muscle relaxant available that exerts its effect directly on the skeletal muscle cell is dantrolene sodium (Dantrium).[40,102] This drug works by impairing the release of calcium from the sarcoplasmic reticulum within the muscle cell during excitation (Fig. 13–3).[56,89] In response to an action potential, the release of calcium from sarcoplasmic storage sites initiates myofilament cross-bridging and subsequent muscle contraction. By inhibiting this release, dantrolene attenuates muscle contraction and therefore enhances relaxation.

Uses. Dantrolene is often effective in treating severe spasticity, regardless of the underlying pathology.[102] Patients with traumatic cord lesions, advanced MS, cerebral palsy, or CVAs will probably experience a reduction in spasticity with this drug. This drug is also invaluable in treating malignant hyperthermia, which is a potentially life-threatening reaction occurring in susceptible individuals following exposure to general anesthesia, muscle paralytics used during surgery, or certain antipsychotic medications (a condition also called neuroleptic malignant syndrome; see

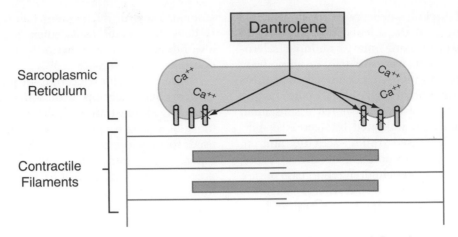

FIGURE 13-3 ▼ Possible mechanism of action of dantrolene sodium (Dantrium). Dantrolene blocks channels in the sarcoplasmic reticulum, thus interfering with calcium release onto the contractile (actin, myosin) filaments. Muscle contraction is reduced because less calcium is available to initiate cross-bridge formation between actin and myosin filaments.

Chapter 8).[2,58] In this situation, dantrolene inhibits skeletal muscle contraction throughout the body, thereby limiting the rise in body temperature generated by strong, repetitive skeletal muscle contractions.[58] Dantrolene is not prescribed to treat muscle spasms caused by musculoskeletal injury.

Adverse Effects. The most common side effect of dantrolene is generalized muscle weakness; this makes sense considering that dantrolene impairs sarcoplasmic calcium release in skeletal muscles throughout the body, not just in the hyperexcitable tissues. Thus, the use of dantrolene is sometimes counterproductive because the increased motor function that occurs when spasticity is reduced may be offset by generalized motor weakness. This drug may also cause severe hepatotoxicity, and cases of fatal hepatitis have been reported.[20,102] The risk of toxic effects on the liver seems to be greater in women over 40 years of age, and in individuals receiving higher doses of this drug (over 300 mg).[102] Other, less serious side effects that sometimes occur during the first few days of therapy include drowsiness, dizziness, nausea, and diarrhea, but these problems are usually transient.

Diazepam

As indicated earlier, diazepam is effective in reducing spasticity as well as muscle spasms because this drug increases the inhibitory effects of GABA in the CNS.

Uses. Diazepam is used in patients with spasticity resulting from cord lesions and is sometimes effective in patients with cerebral palsy.

Adverse effects. Use of diazepam as an antispasticity agent is limited by the sedative effects of this medication; that is, patients with spasticity who do not want a decrease in mental alertness will not tolerate diazepam therapy very well. Extended use of the drug can cause tolerance and physical dependence, and use of diazepam for the long-term treatment of spasticity should be avoided whenever possible.[102]

Gabapentin

Developed originally as an antiseizure drug (see Chapter 9), gabapentin (Neurontin) has also shown some promise in treating spasticity. This drug appears to cause inhibition in the spinal cord in a manner similar to GABA, but the exact mechanism of this drug remains to be determined. That is, gabapentin does not appear to bind to the same receptors as GABA, and this drug does not appear to directly increase the release or effects of endogenous GABA.[82,83] Nonetheless, gabapentin may decrease spasticity by raising the overall level of inhibition in the spinal cord, thereby decreasing excitation of the alpha motor neuron with subsequent skeletal muscle relaxation. The exact way that this drug exerts its antispasticity effects, however, remains to be determined.

Uses. Gabapentin is effective in decreasing the spasticity associated with spinal cord injury[102] and multiple sclerosis.[29] Additional research should clarify how this drug can be used alone or with other agents to provide optimal benefits in spasticity resulting from various spinal, and possibly cerebral, injuries.

Adverse effects. The primary side effects of this drug are sedation, fatigue, dizziness, and ataxia.

Tizanidine

Tizanidine (Zanaflex) is classified as an alpha-2 adrenergic agonist, meaning that this drug binds selectively to the alpha-2 receptors in the CNS and stimulates them. Alpha-2 receptors are found at various locations in the brain and spinal cord, including the presynaptic and postsynaptic membranes of spinal interneurons that control alpha motor neuron excitability. Stimulation of these alpha-2 receptors inhibits the firing of interneurons that relay information to the alpha motor neuron; that is, interneurons that comprise polysynaptic reflex arcs within the spinal cord.[27] Tizanidine appears to bind to receptors on spinal interneurons, decrease the release of excitatory neurotransmitters from their presynaptic terminals (presynaptic inhibition), and decrease the excitability of the postsynaptic neuron (postsynaptic inhibition).[40] Inhibition of spinal interneurons results in decreased excitatory input onto the alpha motor neuron, with a subsequent decrease in spasticity of the skeletal muscle supplied by that neuron.

Uses. Tizanidine has been used primarily to control spasticity resulting from spinal lesions (multiple sclerosis, spinal cord injury),[40] and this drug may also be effective in treating spasticity in people with cerebral lesions (CVA, acquired brain injury).[41,62] There is some concern, however, that tizanidine might slow neuronal recovery following brain injury, and some practitioners are therefore reluctant to use this drug during the acute phase of stroke or traumatic brain injury.[102] Because it may inhibit pain pathways in the spinal cord, tizanidine has also been used to treat chronic headaches and other types of chronic pain (fibromyalgia, chronic regional pain syndromes, and so forth).[77]

As an antispasticity drug, tizanidine appears to be as effective as orally administered baclofen or diazepam, but tizanidine generally has milder side effects and produces less generalized muscle weakness than these other agents.[40] Tizanidine is also superior to other alpha-2 agonists such as clonidine (Catapres) because tizanidine does not cause as much hypotension and other cardiovascular side effects. Clonidine exerts antispasticity as well as antihypertensive effects because this drug stimulates alpha-2 receptors in the cord and brainstem, respectively.[102] Use of clonidine in treating spasticity, however, is limited because of the cardiovascular side effects, and clonidine is used primarily for treating hypertension (see Chapter 21).

Adverse Effects. The most common side effects associated with tizanidine include sedation, dizziness, and dry mouth.[40] As indicated, however, tizanidine tends to have a more favorable side effect profile than other alpha-2 agonists, and this drug produces less generalized weakness than oral baclofen or diazepam. Tizanidine may therefore be a better alternative to these other agents in patients who need to reduce spasticity while maintaining adequate muscle strength for ambulation, transfers, and so forth.

Use of Botulinum Toxin as a Muscle Relaxant

Injection of botulinum toxin is a rather innovative way to control localized muscle hyperexcitability. Botulinum toxin is a purified version of the toxin that causes botulism. Systemic doses of this toxin can be extremely dangerous or fatal because botulinum toxin inhibits the release of acetylcholine from presynaptic terminals at the skeletal neuromuscular junction. Loss of presynaptic acetylcholine release results in paralysis of the muscle fiber supplied by that terminal. Systemic dissemination of botulinum toxin can therefore cause widespread paralysis, including loss of respiratory muscle function. Injection into specific muscles, however, can sequester the toxin within these muscles, thus producing localized effects that are beneficial in certain forms of muscle hyperexcitability.

Mechanism of action. The cellular actions of botulinum toxin at the neuromuscular junction have recently been clarified.[84] This toxin is attracted to glycoproteins located on the surface of the presynaptic terminal at the skeletal neuromuscular junction.[33] Once attached to the membrane, the toxin enters the presynaptic terminal and inhibits proteins that are needed for acetylcholine release (Figure 13–4).[84] Normally, certain proteins help fuse presynaptic vesicles with the inner surface of the presynaptic terminal, thereby allowing the vesicles to release acetylcholine via exocytosis. Botulinum toxin cleaves and destroys these fusion proteins, thus making it impossible for the neuron to release acetylcholine into the synaptic cleft.[32,84] Local injection of botulinum toxin into specific muscles will therefore decrease muscle excitation by disrupting synaptic transmission at the neuromuscular junction. The affected muscle will invariably undergo some degree of paresis and subsequent

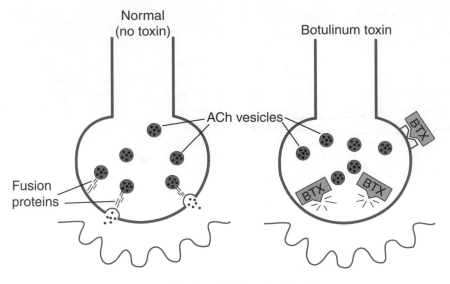

Skeletal Muscle Cell

FIGURE 13-4 ▼ Mechanism of action of botulinum toxin at the skeletal neuromuscular junction. At a normal synapse (shown on left), fusion proteins connect acetylcholine (ACh) vesicles with the presynaptic membrane, and ACh is released via exocytosis. Botulinum toxin (represented by "BTX" on the right) binds to the presynaptic terminal, and enters the terminal where it destroys the fusion proteins so that ACh cannot be released. See text for details.

relaxation because the toxin prevents the release of acetylcholine.

It has been suggested that botulinum toxin might have other effects on neuronal excitability. This toxin, for example, might also inhibit contraction of intrafusal muscle fibers that are located within skeletal muscle, and help control sensitivity of the stretch reflex.[33] Inhibiting these intrafusal fibers would diminish activity in the afferent limb of the stretch reflex, thereby contributing to the antispasticity effects of this intervention.[33]

Through its direct action on muscle excitability, botulinum toxin may also have other neurophysiological effects at the spinal cord level. That is, reducing spasticity might result in complex neurophysiologic changes at the spinal cord, ultimately resulting in more normal control of motor function in both the injected muscle and its antagonist.[45] In other words, reduction of excessive afferent discharge from the spastic muscle might help reestablish a more reasonable level of excitation at the cord level, thus improving efferent discharge to the injected muscle and its antagonist.[33,45] More research will be needed to help clarify how local administration of botulinum toxin can have direct effects on the injected muscle as well as reflex neurophysiological effects on the spinal cord.

Clinical use of botulinum toxin. Seven strains (serotypes) of botulinum toxin have been identified,

but only two types are currently available for clinical use: botulinum toxin types A and B.[15,23] These types differ somewhat in their chemistry, duration of action, and so forth. The most commonly used therapeutic type is botulinum toxin type A; this agent is marketed commercially under trade names such as Botox and Dysport. Botulinum toxin type B (Myobloc) is also available, and can be useful in patients who develop immunity to the type A form of this toxin (discussed later).

Botulinum toxin has been used for some time to control localized muscle dystonias, including conditions such as spasmodic torticollis, blepharospasm, laryngeal dystonia, strabismus, and several other types of focal dystonias.[6,25,26,87,93] When used therapeutically, small amounts of this toxin are injected directly into the dystonic muscles, which begin to relax within a few days to 1 week. This technique appears to be fairly safe and effective in many patients, but relief may only be temporary. Symptoms often return within 3 months after each injection, necessitating additional treatments.[40] Still, this technique represents a method for treating patients with severe, incapacitating conditions marked by focal dystonias and spasms.

More recently, there has been considerable interest in using botulinum toxin to reduce spasticity in specific muscles or muscle groups. This treatment has been used to treat spasticity resulting from various disorders including cerebral palsy,[10,68,78,99] traumatic brain injury,[36,66,98] CVA,[19,44,49] and spinal cord injury.[39] As with treatment of focal dystonias, the toxin is injected directly into selected muscles. If necessary, electromyography or ultrasonography can be used to identify specific muscles and guide the injection to the desired site within the muscle belly (e.g., the motor point of the muscle).[18,53,100] There is also some evidence that electrical stimulation of the nerve supplying the muscle for the first few days following injection may help increase the efficacy of the toxin, presumably by enhancing its uptake by the presynaptic nerve terminals.[38]

Botulinum toxin injection has been documented as a means to control severe spasticity in various clinical situations. This intervention, for example, can help remove spastic dominance in certain patients so that volitional motor function can be facilitated. For example, judicious administration of botulinum toxin can result in improved gait and other functional activities in selected patients with cerebral palsy, stroke, or traumatic brain injury.[7,36,49,78] Even if voluntary motor function is not improved dramatically, reducing spasticity in severely affected muscles may produce other musculoskeletal benefits. For example, injection of botulinum toxin can reduce spasticity so that muscles can be stretched or casted more effectively, thus helping to prevent joint contractures and decreasing the need for surgical procedures such as heel-cord lengthening and adductor release.[12,98]

These injections can likewise enable patients to wear and use orthotic devices more effectively. Injection into the triceps surae musculature can improve the fit and function of an ankle-foot orthosis by preventing excessive plantar flexor spasticity from "pistoning" the foot out of the orthosis.[49] Injections into severely spastic muscles can also increase patient comfort and ability to perform ADL and hygiene activities. Consider, for example, the patient with severe upper extremity flexor spasticity following a CVA. Local injection of botulinum toxin into the affected muscles may enable the patient to extend his or her elbow, wrist, and fingers, thereby allowing better hand cleansing, ability to dress, decreased pain, and so forth.[7]

Finally, local botulinum toxin administration has been advocated as a way to control muscle hyperexcitability in other clinical situations. There has, of course, been considerable interest in using this toxin for cosmetic reasons. Injection of botulinum toxin into specific facial muscles can paralyze these muscles, thereby reducing the appearance of wrinkles around the eyes, mouth, and so forth.[3,24] Nonetheless,

patients undergoing physical rehabilitation may also benefit from uses of this toxin. For example, patients with hyperactive (neurogenic) bladder following spinal cord injury can be treated by injecting botulinum toxin directly into the bladder detrusor muscle or external urethral sphincter.[28,59] This intervention may help normalize bladder function and promote more effective voiding.[28,47] Botulinum toxin has also been used to treat patients with chronic pain syndromes, including chronic headache, migraine, and various musculoskeletal disorders (back pain, whiplash injuries, and so forth).[24,88] Clearly, this intervention has many potential benefits in many different clinical situations, and additional research will be needed to document how botulinum toxin can be used to reduce muscle hyperexcitability and improve function in various patient populations.

Limitations and side effects. Botulinum toxin does not cure spasticity and there are a number of limitations to its use. In particular, only a limited number of muscles can be injected during a given treatment because only a limited amount of botulinum toxin can be administered during each set of injections. For example, the total amount of botulinum toxin type A injected during each treatment session is typically between 200–300 units in adults, with proportionally smaller amounts used in children depending on his or her size and age.[40] The typical dose of the type B form is 2500–5000 units. Exceeding these doses will cause an immune response whereby antibodies are synthesized against the toxin, making subsequent treatments ineffective because the patient's immune system will recognize and inactivate the toxin.[34,35,91] The number of muscles that can be injected is therefore often limited to one or two muscle groups; for example, the elbow and wrist flexors in one upper extremity of an adult, or the bilateral triceps surae musculature of a child.

As indicated earlier, the relaxant effects of the toxin are likewise temporary, and these effects typically diminish within 2 to 3 months after injection.[91] The effects apparently wear off because a new presynaptic terminal "sprouts" from the axon that contains the originally affected presynaptic terminal. This new terminal grows downward, reattaching to the skeletal muscle and creating a new motor end plate with a new source of acetylcholine. The effects of the previous injection are overcome when this new presynaptic terminal begins to function. Another injection will be needed to block the release from this new presynaptic terminal, thus allowing another 2 to 3 months of antispasticity effects. This fact raises the question of how many times the injection cycle can be repeated safely and effectively. At the present time, there is no clear limit to the number of times a muscle can be injected, providing, of course, that sufficient time has elapsed between each series of injections.[5] Longitudinal studies will be needed to determine if there are any detrimental effects of long-term use of this intervention.

Consequently, botulinum toxin represents a strategy for dealing with spasticity that is especially problematic in specific muscles or groups of muscles. Despite the rather ominous prospect of injecting a potentially lethal toxin into skeletal muscles, this intervention has a remarkably small incidence of severe adverse effects when administered at therapeutic doses.[5,44] Botulinum toxin can therefore be used as part of a comprehensive rehabilitation program to provide optimal benefits in certain patients with severe spasticity.

Pharmacokinetics

Most muscle relaxants are absorbed fairly easily from the gastrointestinal tract, and the oral route is the most frequent method of drug administration. In cases of severe spasms, certain drugs such as methocarbamol and orphenadrine can be injected intramuscularly or intravenously to permit a more rapid effect. Likewise, diazepam and dantrolene can be injected to treat spasticity if the situation warrants a faster onset. As discussed earlier, continuous intrathecal baclofen administration may be used in certain patients with severe spasticity, and local injection of botulinum toxin is a possible strategy for treating focal dystonias and spasticity. Metabolism of muscle relaxants is usually accomplished by hepatic microsomal enzymes; and the metabolite or intact drug is excreted through the kidneys.

Special Concerns in Rehabilitation Patients

■ ■ ■ Because of the very nature of their use, skeletal muscle relaxants are prescribed for many patients involved in rehabilitation programs. Physical therapists and other rehabilitation professionals will encounter these drugs applied as both antispasm and antispasticity agents. When used to reduce muscle spasms following nerve root impingements, muscle strains, and the like, these drugs will complement the physical therapy interventions. Concomitant use of muscle relaxants with thermal, electrotherapeutic, and manual techniques can produce optimal benefits during the acute phase of musculoskeletal injuries causing spasms. Of course, the long-term use of antispasm agents is not practical because these drugs often cause sedation, and they can have addictive properties that lead to tolerance and physical dependence. This fact further emphasizes the need for aggressive physical therapy so that the drugs can be discontinued as soon as possible. Physical therapists and occupational therapists can also help prevent reinjury and recurrence of spasms by improving the patient's muscle strength, flexibility, posture, and by teaching proper body mechanics and lifting techniques. These interventions may help decrease the incidence of spasms and the need for drugs used to treat them.

The pharmacologic reduction of spasticity is also an important goal in patients receiving physical therapy and occupational therapy. As indicated earlier, decreased spasticity can result in increased motor function, easier self-care or nursing care, and decreased painful and harmful effects of strong spastic contractions. Drug treatment is likewise synergistic with rehabilitation; that is, antispasticity agents can allow more effective passive range-of-motion and stretching activities, as well as permit more effective use of neuromuscular facilitation techniques, orthotic devices, and other interventions designed to reduce spasticity and improve function.

Rehabilitation specialists also play a critical role in helping patients adapt to sudden changes in muscle excitability caused by antispasticity drugs. Reducing spasticity may, in fact, adversely affect the individual relying on increased muscle tone to assist in functional activities such as ambulation. For example, patients who have had a CVA and use extensor spasticity in the lower extremity to support themselves when walking may begin to fall if this spasticity is reduced suddenly by drugs. This loss of support from the hypertonic muscles will hopefully be replaced by a more normal form of motor function.

Therapists can therefore play a vital role in facilitating the substitution of normal physiologic motor control for the previously used spastic tone. This idea seems especially true when one of the parenteral antispasticity techniques is used, such as intrathecal baclofen or botulinum toxin injections. For example, patients who receive intrathecal baclofen through programmable pump systems often require a period of intensive rehabilitation to enable the benefits from decreased spasticity and increased voluntary motor function to occur. Therapists must therefore be ready to use aggressive rehabilitation techniques to help patients adapt to the relatively rapid and dramatic decrease in muscle tone that is often associated with antispasticity drug therapy.

Rehabilitation specialists can also play a critical role in using certain antispasticity drugs effectively. In particular, therapists can help identify patients who are suitable candidates for botulinum toxin injections, and help evaluate these patients pre-injection and postinjection to determine if they achieved the desired outcomes. Rehabilitation specialists are, in fact, often in the best position to evaluate the effects of all antispasticity drugs. By working closely with the patient, the patient's family, and the physician, therapists can provide valuable feedback about the efficacy of antispasticity drugs and whether they are helping to produce improvements in the patient's function and well-being.

Finally, therapists may have to deal with the side effects of these drugs. Depending on the drug in question, problems with sedation, generalized muscle weakness, and hepatotoxicity can negate any beneficial effects from a reduction in muscle tone. Sedation, which may occur to a variable degree with all systemic skeletal muscle relaxants, must sometimes be accommodated in the rehabilitation program. If the patient needs to be awake and alert, treatments may have to be scheduled at a time of the day when the sedative effects are minimal.

In situations of generalized muscle weakness (i.e., during the use of dantrolene sodium or oral baclofen), there is often little that the physical therapist can do to resolve this problem. For instance, the patient with paraplegia who requires adequate upper extremity strength to perform transfers, wheelchair mobility, and ambulation with crutches and braces may find his or her ability to perform these activities compromised by the antispasticity drug. The role of the therapist in this situation may simply be to advise the patient that voluntary muscular power is limited and that some upper extremity strength deficits can be expected. The therapist may also work closely with the physician in trying to find the minimum acceptable dose for that patient or in attempting to find a better drug (e.g., switching from dantrolene to tizanidine).

CASE STUDY

Muscle Relaxants

Brief History. F.D. is a 28-year-old man who sustained complete paraplegia below the L-2 spinal level during an automobile accident. Through the course of rehabilitation he was becoming independent in self-care, and he had begun to ambulate in the parallel bars and with crutches while wearing temporary long leg braces. He was highly motivated to contin-

ue this progress and was eventually fitted with permanent leg orthoses. During this period, spasticity had increased in his lower extremities to the point where dressing and self-care were often difficult. Also, the ability of the patient to put his leg braces on was often compromised by lower extremity spasticity. The patient was started on oral baclofen (Lioresal) at an initial oral dosage of 15 mg/day. The daily dosage of baclofen was gradually increased until he was receiving 60 mg/day.

Problem/Influence of Medication. Although the baclofen was effective in controlling his spasticity, F.D. began to notice weakness in his arms and upper torso when he attempted to ambulate and transfer. This decrease in voluntary power in his upper extremities was caused by the generalized muscle weakness sometimes seen when this drug is used.

Decision/Solution. The therapist conferred with the patient's physician, and the decreased voluntary muscle power was noted. As an alternative, the patient was switched to tizanidine (Zanaflex). The dosage was adjusted until the spasticity was adequately reduced, and no further problems were noted.

SUMMARY

Skeletal muscle relaxants are used to treat the muscle spasms that result from musculoskeletal injuries or spasticity that occurs following lesions in the CNS. Depending on the specific agent, these drugs reduce muscle excitability by acting on the spinal cord, at the neuromuscular junction, or directly within the skeletal muscle fiber. Diazepam and polysynaptic inhibitors are used in the treatment of muscle spasms, but their effectiveness as muscle relaxants may be because of their nonspecific sedative properties. Agents used to treat spasticity include baclofen, dantrolene, diazepam, gabapentin, and tizanidine. Each drug works by a

somewhat different mechanism, and the selection of a specific antispasticity agent depends on the patient and the underlying CNS lesion (e.g., stroke, MS). Local injection of botulinum toxin can also be used to treat focal dystonias and spasticity, and this technique may help control spasms and spasticity in specific muscles or muscle groups. Physical therapists and other rehabilitation personnel will frequently work with patients taking these drugs for the treatment of either spasticity or spasms. Although there are some troublesome side effects, these drugs generally facilitate the rehabilitation program by directly providing benefits (muscle relaxation) that are congruent with the major rehabilitation goals.

References

1. Albright AL, Gilmartin R, Swift D, et al. Long-term intrathecal baclofen therapy for severe spasticity of cerebral origin. *J Neurosurg.* 2003;98:291–295.
2. Ali SZ, Taguchi A, Rosenberg H. Malignant hyperthermia. *Best Pract Res Clin Anaesthesiol.* 2003;17:519–533.
3. Aoki KR. Pharmacology and immunology of botulinum toxin type A. *Clin Dermatol.* 2003;21:476–480.
4. Bainbridge JL, Corboy JR, Gidal BE. Multiple sclerosis. In: DiPiro JT, et al, eds. *Pharmacotherapy: A Pathophysiologic Approach.* 5th ed. New York: McGraw-Hill; 2002.
5. Bakheit AM, Fedorova NV, Skoromets AA, et al. The beneficial antispasticity effect of botulinum toxin type A is maintained after repeated treatment cycles. *J Neurol Neurosurg Psychiatry.* 2004;75:1558–1561.
6. Balash Y, Giladi N. Efficacy of pharmacological treatment of dystonia: evidence-based review including meta-analysis of the effect of botulinum toxin and other cure options. *Eur J Neurol.* 2004;11:361–370.
7. Barnes M. Botulinum toxin—mechanisms of action and clinical use in spasticity. *J Rehabil Med.* 2003;41 (suppl):56–59.
8. Beebe FA, Barkin RL, Barkin S. A Clinical and Pharmacologic Review of Skeletal Muscle Relaxants for Musculoskeletal Conditions. *Am J Ther.* 2005;12:151–171.
9. Bernstein E, Carey TS, Garrett JM. The use of muscle relaxant medications in acute low back pain. *Spine.* 2004;29:1346–1351.
10. Berweck S, Heinen F. Use of botulinum toxin in pediatric spasticity (cerebral palsy). *Mov Disord.* 2004;19 (suppl 8):S162–S167.
11. Borenstein DG, Korn S. Efficacy of a low-dose regimen of cyclobenzaprine hydrochloride in acute skeletal muscle spasm: results of two placebo-controlled trials. *Clin Ther.* 2003;25:1056–1073.
12. Bottos M, Benedetti MG, Salucci P, et al. Botulinum toxin with and without casting in ambulant children with spastic diplegia: a clinical and functional assessment. *Dev Med Child Neurol.* 2003;45:758–762.
13. Bramness JG, Skurtveit S, Morland J. Impairment due to intake of carisoprodol. *Drug Alcohol Depend.* 2004;74:311–318.
14. Browning R, Jackson JL, O'Malley PG. Cyclobenzaprine and back pain: a meta-analysis. *Arch Intern Med.* 2001;161:1613–1620.
15. Callaway JE. Botulinum toxin type B (Myobloc): pharmacology and biochemistry. *Clin Dermatol.* 2004;22:23–28.
16. Campbell SK, Almeida GL, Penn RD, Corcos DM. The effects of intrathecally administered baclofen on function in patients with spasticity. *Phys Ther.* 1995;75:352–362.
17. Campbell WM, Ferrel A, McLaughlin JF, et al. Long-term safety and efficacy of continuous intrathecal baclofen. *Dev Med Child Neurol.* 2002;44:660–665.
18. Childers MK. Targeting the neuromuscular junction in skeletal muscles. *Am J Phys Med Rehabil.* 2004;83 (suppl):S38–S44.
19. Childers MK, Brashear A, Jozefczyk P, et al. Dose-dependent response to intramuscular botulinum toxin

type A for upper-limb spasticity in patients after a stroke. *Arch Phys Med Rehabil.* 2004;85:1063–1069.

20. Chou R, Peterson K, Helfand M. Comparative efficacy and safety of skeletal muscle relaxants for spasticity and musculoskeletal conditions: a systematic review. *J Pain Symptom Manage.* 2004;28:140–175.

21. Colombo G, Addolorato G, Agabio R, et al. Role of GABA(B) receptor in alcohol dependence: reducing effect of baclofen on alcohol intake and alcohol motivational properties in rats and amelioration of alcohol withdrawal syndrome and alcohol craving in human alcoholics. *Neurotox Res.* 2004;6:403–414.

22. Colombo G, Vacca G, Serra S, et al. Baclofen suppresses motivation to consume alcohol in rats. *Psychopharmacology.* 2003;167:221–224.

23. Comella CL, Pullman SL. Botulinum toxins in neurological disease. *Muscle Nerve.* 2004;29:628–644.

24. Cordivari C, Misra VP, Catania S, Lees AJ. New therapeutic indications for botulinum toxins. *Mov Disord.* 2004;19(suppl 8):S157–S161.

25. Costa J, Borges A, Espirito-Santo C, et al. Botulinum toxin type A versus botulinum toxin type B for cervical dystonia. *Cochrane Database Syst Rev.* 2005;CD004314.

26. Costa J, Espirito-Santo C, Borges A, et al. Botulinum toxin type A therapy for blepharospasm. *Cochrane Database Syst Rev.* 2005;CD004900.

27. Coward DM. Tizanidine: neuropharmacology and mechanism of action. *Neurology.* 1994;44(suppl 9):S6–S10.

28. Cruz F, Silva C. Botulinum toxin in the management of lower urinary tract dysfunction: contemporary update. *Curr Opin Urol.* 2004;14:329–334.

29. Cutter NC, Scott DD, Johnson JC, Whiteneck G. Gabapentin effect on spasticity in multiple sclerosis: a placebo-controlled, randomized trial. *Arch Phys Med Rehabil.* 2000;81:164–169.

30. Dario A, Tomei G. A benefit–risk assessment of baclofen in severe spinal spasticity. *Drug Saf.* 2004; 27:799–818.

31. Dillon C, Paulose-Ram R, Hirsch R, Gu Q. Skeletal muscle relaxant use in the United States: data from the Third National Health and Nutrition Examination Survey (NHANES III). *Spine.* 2004;29:892–896.

32. Dolly O. Synaptic transmission: inhibition of neurotransmitter release by botulinum toxins. *Headache.* 2003;43(suppl 1):S16–S24.

33. Dressler D, Adib Saberi F. Botulinum toxin: mechanisms of action. *Eur Neurol.* 2005;53:3–9.

34. Dressler D, Bigalke H. Botulinum toxin type B de novo therapy of cervical dystonia. Frequency of antibody induced therapy failure. *J Neurol.* 2005; 252:904–907.

35. Dressler D, Bigalke H. Antibody-induced failure of botulinum toxin type B therapy in de novo patients. *Eur Neurol.* 2004;52:132–135.

36. Fock J, Galea MP, Stillman BC, et al. Functional outcome following Botulinum toxin A injection to reduce spastic equinus in adults with traumatic brain injury. *Brain Inj.* 2004;18:57–63.

37. Francisco GE, Boake C. Improvement in walking speed in poststroke spastic hemiplegia after intrathecal baclofen therapy: a preliminary study. *Arch Phys Med Rehabil.* 2003;84:1194–1199.

38. Frasson E, Priori A, Ruzzante B, et al. Nerve stimulation boosts botulinum toxin action in spasticity. *Mov Disord.* 2005;20:624–629.

39. Fried GW, Fried KM. Spinal cord injury and use of botulinum toxin in reducing spasticity. *Phys Med Rehabil Clin N Am.* 2003;14:901–910.

40. Gallichio JE. Pharmacologic management of spasticity following stroke. *Phys Ther.* 2004;84:973–981.

41. Gelber DA, Good DC, Dromerick A, et al. Open-label dose-titration safety and efficacy study of tizanidine hydrochloride in the treatment of spasticity associated with chronic stroke. *Stroke.* 2001;32:1841–1846.

42. Gooch JL, Oberg WA, Grams B, et al. Complications of intrathecal baclofen pumps in children. *Pediatr Neurosurg.* 2003;39:1–6.

43. Gooch JL, Oberg WA, Grams B, et al. Care provider assessment of intrathecal baclofen in children. *Dev Med Child Neurol.* 2004;46:548–552.

44. Gordon MF, Brashear A, Elovic E, et al. Repeated dosing of botulinum toxin type A for upper limb spasticity following stroke. *Neurology.* 2004;63:1971–1973.

45. Gracies JM. Physiological effects of botulinum toxin in spasticity. *Mov Disord.* 2004;19(suppl 8):S120–S128.

46. Greenberg MI, Hendrickson RG. Baclofen withdrawal following removal of an intrathecal baclofen pump despite oral baclofen replacement. *J Toxicol Clin Toxicol.* 2003;41:83–85.

47. Hajebrahimi S, Altaweel W, Cadoret J, et al. Efficacy of botulinum-A toxin in adults with neurogenic overactive bladder: initial results. *Can J Urol.* 2005;12: 2543–2546.

48. Hansel DE, Hansel CR, Shindle MK, et al. Oral baclofen in cerebral palsy: possible seizure potentiation? *Pediatr Neurol.* 2003;29:203–206.

49. Hesse S. Recovery of gait and other motor functions after stroke: novel physical and pharmacological treatment strategies. *Restor Neurol Neurosci.* 2004;22: 359–369.

50. Honda M, Nishida T, Ono H. Tricyclic analogs cyclobenzaprine, amitriptyline and cyproheptadine inhibit the spinal reflex transmission through 5-HT(2) receptors. *Eur J Pharmacol.* 2003;458:91–99.

51. Ismoedijanto, Nassiruddin M, Prajitno BW. Case report: diazepam in severe tetanus treatment. *Southeast Asian J Trop Med Public Health.* 2004;35:175–180.

52. Ivanhoe CB, Reistetter TA. Spasticity: the misunderstood part of the upper motor neuron syndrome. *Am J Phys Med Rehabil.* 2004;83(suppl):S3–S9.

53. Kinnett D. Botulinum toxin A injections in children: technique and dosing issues. *Am J Phys Med Rehabil.* 2004;83(suppl):S59–S64.

54. Kita M, Goodkin DE. Drugs used to treat spasticity. *Drugs.* 2000;59:487–495.

55. Kobayashi H, Hasegawa Y, Ono H. Cyclobenzaprine, a centrally acting muscle relaxant, acts on descending serotonergic systems. *Eur J Pharmacol.* 1996;311: 29–35.

56. Kobayashi S, Bannister ML, Gangopadhyay JP, et al. Dantrolene stabilizes domain interactions within the ryanodine receptor. *J Biol Chem.* 2005;280:6580–6587.

57. Korenkov AI, Niendorf WR, Darwish N, et al. Continuous intrathecal infusion of baclofen in patients with spasticity caused by spinal cord injuries. *Neurosurg Rev.* 2002;25:228–230.

58. Krause T, Gerbershagen MU, Fiege M, et al. Dantrolene—a review of its pharmacology, therapeutic use and new developments. *Anaesthesia.* 2004;59:364–373.

59. Leippold T, Reitz A, Schurch B. Botulinum toxin as a new therapy option for voiding disorders: current state of the art. *Eur Urol.* 2003;44:165–174.

60. Lew SM, Psaty EL, Abbott R. An unusual cause of overdose after baclofen pump implantation: case report. *Neurosurgery.* 2005;56:E624.

61. Maigne JY, Vautravers P. Mechanism of action of spinal manipulative therapy. *Joint Bone Spine.* 2003; 70:336–341.

62. Meythaler JM, Guin-Renfroe S, Johnson A, Brunner RM. Prospective assessment of tizanidine for spasticity due to acquired brain injury. *Arch Phys Med Rehabil.* 2001;82:1155–1163.

63. Nielsen JF, Hansen HJ, Sunde N, Christensen JJ. Evidence of tolerance to baclofen in treatment of severe spasticity with intrathecal baclofen. *Clin Neurol Neurosurg.* 2002;104:142–145.

64. Ohliger-Frerking P, Wiebe SP, Staubli U, Frerking M. GABA(B) receptor-mediated presynaptic inhibition has history-dependent effects on synaptic transmission during physiologically relevant spike trains. *J Neurosci.* 2003;23:4809–4814.

65. Okoromah CN, Lesi FE. Diazepam for treating tetanus. *Cochrane Database Syst Rev.* 2004;CD003954.

66. O'Suilleabhain P, Dewey RB, Jr. Movement disorders after head injury: diagnosis and management. *J Head Trauma Rehabil.* 2004;19:305–313.

67. Pasquier Y, Cahana A, Schnider A. Subdural catheter migration may lead to baclofen pump dysfunction. *Spinal Cord.* 2003;41:700–702.

68. Pidcock FS. The emerging role of therapeutic botulinum toxin in the treatment of cerebral palsy. *J Pediatr.* 2004;145(suppl 2):S33–S35.

69. Plassat R, Perrouin Verbe B, Menei P, et al. Treatment of spasticity with intrathecal Baclofen administration: long-term follow-up, review of 40 patients. *Spinal Cord.* 2004;42:686–693.

70. Poklis JL, Ropero-Miller JD, Garside D, Winecker RE. Metaxalone (Skelaxin)-related death. *J Anal Toxicol.* 2004;28:537–541.

71. Rawlins PK. Intrathecal baclofen therapy over 10 years. *J Neurosci Nurs.* 2004;36:322–327.

72. Reeves RR, Beddingfield JJ, Mack JE. Carisoprodol withdrawal syndrome. *Pharmacotherapy.* 2004;24: 1804–1806.

73. Reeves RR, Carter OS, Pinkofsky HB, et al. Carisoprodol (soma): abuse potential and physician unawareness. *J Addict Dis.* 1999;18:51–56.

74. Remy-Neris O, Tiffreau V, Bouilland S, Bussel B. Intrathecal baclofen in subjects with spastic hemiplegia: assessment of the antispastic effect during gait. *Arch Phys Med Rehabil.* 2003;84:643–650.

75. Rigoli G, Terrini G, Cordioli Z. Intrathecal baclofen withdrawal syndrome caused by low residual volume in the pump reservoir: a report of 2 cases. *Arch Phys Med Rehabil.* 2004;85:2064–2066.

76. Sampson FC, Hayward A, Evans G, et al. Functional benefits and cost/benefit analysis of continuous intrathecal baclofen infusion for the management of severe spasticity. *J Neurosurg.* 2002;96:1052–1057.

77. Saper JR, Lake AE, 3rd, Cantrell DT, et al. Chronic daily headache prophylaxis with tizanidine: a double-blind, placebo-controlled, multicenter outcome study. *Headache.* 2002;42:470–482.

78. Sarioglu B, Serdaroglu G, Tutuncuoglu S, Ozer EA. The use of botulinum toxin type A treatment in children with spasticity. *Pediatr Neurol.* 2003;29: 299–301.

79. Satkunam LE. Rehabilitation medicine: 3. Management of adult spasticity. *CMAJ.* 2003;169:1173–1179.

80. Schnitzer TJ, Ferraro A, Hunsche E, Kong SX. A comprehensive review of clinical trials on the efficacy and safety of drugs for the treatment of low back pain. *J Pain Symptom Manage.* 2004;28:72–95.

81. Schuele SU, Kellinghaus C, Shook SJ, et al. Incidence of seizures in patients with multiple sclerosis treated with intrathecal baclofen. *Neurology.* 2005;64: 1086–1087.

82. Shimizu S, Honda M, Tanabe M, et al. Endogenous GABA does not mediate the inhibitory effects of gabapentin on spinal reflexes in rats. *J Pharmacol Sci.* 2004;94:137–143.

83. Shimizu S, Honda M, Tanabe M, Ono H. GABA B receptors do not mediate the inhibitory actions of gabapentin on the spinal reflex in rats. *J Pharmacol Sci.* 2004;96:444–449.

84. Simpson LL. Identification of the major steps in botulinum toxin action. *Annu Rev Pharmacol Toxicol.* 2004; 44:167–193.

85. Slonimski M, Abram SE, Zuniga RE. Intrathecal baclofen in pain management. *Reg Anesth Pain Med.* 2004;29:269–276.

86. Spiller HA, Cutino L. Fatal cyclobenzaprine overdose with postmortem values. *J Forensic Sci.* 2003;48: 883–884.

87. Sulica L. Contemporary management of spasmodic dysphonia. *Curr Opin Otolaryngol Head Neck Surg.* 2004;12:543–548.

88. Sycha T, Kranz G, Auff E, Schnider P. Botulinum toxin in the treatment of rare head and neck pain syndromes: a systematic review of the literature. *J Neurol.* 2004;251(suppl 1):I19–I30.

89. Szentesi P, Collet C, Sarkozi S, et al. Effects of dantrolene on steps of excitation-contraction coupling in mammalian skeletal muscle fibers. *J Gen Physiol.* 2001; 118:355–375.

90. Taira T, Hori T. Clinical application of drug pump for spasticity, pain, and restorative neurosurgery: other clinical applications of intrathecal baclofen. *Acta Neurochir Suppl.* 2003;87:37–38.

91. Tilton AH. Injectable neuromuscular blockade in the treatment of spasticity and movement disorders. *J Child Neurol.* 2003;18(suppl 1):S50–S66.

92. Toth PP, Urtis J. Commonly used muscle relaxant therapies for acute low back pain: a review of cariso-

prodol, cyclobenzaprine hydrochloride, and metaxalone. *Clin Ther.* 2004;26:1355–1367.

93. Truong D, Duane DD, Jankovic J, et al. Efficacy and safety of botulinum type A toxin (Dysport) in cervical dystonia: results of the first US randomized, double-blind, placebo-controlled study. *Mov Disord.* 2005; 20:783–791.

94. Turner MS. Early use of intrathecal baclofen in brain injury in pediatric patients. *Acta Neurochir Suppl.* 2003;87:81–83.

95. Vacher CM, Bettler B. GABA(B) receptors as potential therapeutic targets. *Curr Drug Targets CNS Neurol Disord.* 2003;2:248–259.

96. van Dieen JH, Selen LP, Cholewicki J. Trunk muscle activation in low-back pain patients, an analysis of the literature. *J Electromyogr Kinesiol.* 2003;13: 333–351.

97. van Tulder MW, Touray T, Furlan AD, et al. Muscle relaxants for non-specific low back pain. *Cochrane Database Syst Rev.* 2003;CD004252.

98. Verplancke D, Snape S, Salisbury CF, et al. A randomized controlled trial of botulinum toxin on lower limb spasticity following acute acquired severe brain injury. *Clin Rehabil.* 2005;19:117–125.

99. Wasiak J, Hoare B, Wallen M. Botulinum toxin A as an adjunct to treatment in the management of the upper limb in children with spastic cerebral palsy. *Cochrane Database Syst Rev.* 2004;CD003469.

100. Westhoff B, Seller K, Wild A, et al. Ultrasound-guided botulinum toxin injection technique for the iliopsoas muscle. *Dev Med Child Neurol.* 2003;45: 829–832.

101. White PF, Katzung BG. Skeletal muscle relaxants. In Katzung BG, ed. *Basic and Clinical Pharmacology.* 9th ed. New York: Lange Medical Books/McGraw Hill; 2004.

102. Zafonte R, Lombard L, Elovic E. Antispasticity medications: uses and limitations of enteral therapy. *Am J Phys Med Rehabil.* 2004;83(suppl):S50–S58.

103. Zahavi A, Geertzen JH, Middel B, et al. Long term effect (more than five years) of intrathecal baclofen on impairment, disability, and quality of life in patients with severe spasticity of spinal origin. *J Neurol Neurosurg Psychiatry.* 2004;75:1553–1557.

104. Zuckerbraun NS, Ferson SS, Albright AL, Vogeley E. Intrathecal baclofen withdrawal: emergent recognition and management. *Pediatr Emerg Care.* 2004;20: 759–764.

Drugs Used to Treat Pain and Inflammation

Chapter 14

Opioid Analgesics

Analgesic drug therapy and certain rehabilitation interventions share a common goal: pain relief. Consequently, analgesics are among the drugs most frequently taken by patients who are treated in a rehabilitation setting. The vast array of drugs that are used to treat pain can be roughly divided into two categories: opioid and nonopioid analgesics. Nonopioid analgesics are composed of drugs such as acetaminophen, aspirin, and similar agents. These drugs are discussed in Chapter 15.

Opioid analgesics are a group of naturally occurring, semisynthetic, and synthetic agents that are characterized by their ability to relieve moderate-to-severe pain. These drugs exert their effects by binding to specific neuronal receptors that are located primarily in the central nervous system (CNS). Opioid analgesics are also characterized by their potential ability to produce physical dependence, and these agents are classified as controlled substances in the United States because of their potential for abuse (see Chapter 1 for a description of controlled substance classification). Morphine (Fig. 14–1) is considered the prototypical opioid analgesic, and other drugs of this type are often compared to morphine in terms of efficacy and potency.[44,65]

In the past, the term "narcotic" was often applied to these compounds because—when taken—they tend to have sedative or sleep-inducing side effects and high doses can produce a state of unresponsiveness and stupor. Narcotic is a misleading name, however, because it describes a side effect rather than their principal therapeutic effect.

Likewise, these drugs are frequently referred to as "opiate" analgesics because some of these compounds are derived from opium (see the next section, "Source of Opioid Analgesics"). More recently, the term "opioid" has also been instituted to represent all types of narcotic analgesiclike agents, regardless of their origin.[27] Hence, most sources preferentially use the term "opioid" to describe these drugs, and clinicians should recognize that this term represents all of the morphinelike medications.

Source of Opioid Analgesics

As mentioned previously, opioid analgesics can be obtained from natural, synthetic, or semisynthetic sources. Synthetic agents, as the designation implies, are simply formulated from basic chemical components in the laboratory. The source of naturally occurring and semisynthetic narcotic analgesics is from the opium poppy.[27,65] When the extract from the seeds of this flower is allowed to dry and harden, the resulting substance is opium. Opium contains about 20 biologically active compounds, including morphine and codeine. Other derivatives from opium can also directly produce analgesia in varying degrees or can serve as precursors for analgesic drugs. The most notable of these precursors is thebaine, which can be modified chemically to yield compounds such as heroin. Likewise, semisynthetic narcotic analgesics are derived from these precursors. Semisynthetic opioids can also

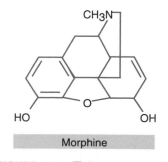

FIGURE 14–1 ▼ Structure of morphine.

be formulated by modifying one of the other naturally occurring narcotic drugs, such as morphine.

In addition to analgesic drugs and their precursors, opium also contains compounds that do not have any analgesic properties. These compounds can actually antagonize the analgesic effects of opioid agonists such as morphine. (As defined in Chapter 4, an *agonist* stimulates its respective receptor and exerts a physiologic response, whereas an *antagonist* blocks the receptor, thus preventing the response.) The role of these opioid antagonists is discussed in "Classification of Specific Agents," later in this chapter.

Endogenous Opioid Peptides and Opioid Receptors

Endogenous Opioids

Neurons at specific locations within the brain and spinal cord have been identified as having receptors that serve as binding sites for morphine and other similar exogenous substances.[27] Exogenous opioids exert their effects by binding to these receptors; the proposed mechanisms of these drug-receptor interactions are discussed later in "Mechanism of Action." The discovery of these opioid receptors also suggested the existence of an endogenous opioidlike substance. Rather than isolating one such compound, the search for an "endogenous morphine" has actually revealed several groups of peptides with analgesic and other pharmacologic properties. It is now recognized that three distinct families of endogenous opioids exist: the endorphins, enkephalins, and dynorphins.[27,72] These peptides are manufactured and released within the body to control pain under specific conditions.[29,65,81] Endogenous opioids are also released during other stressful situations, and these endogenous peptides interact with other neurochemicals (e.g., melatonin) and the immune system to help individuals deal with various types of physical and psychological stress.[23,66,67,85]

This chapter is not intended to elucidate all of the known details of the endogenous opioid peptide system or to illustrate how these endogenous compounds can be influenced by opioid drugs. The endogenous compounds described do exert their effects, however, via the same receptors as the exogenous opioid drugs. Obviously, there is the possibility for a great deal of interaction between the endogenous and exogenous opioids, and researchers continue to investigate how

exogenous drugs influence the function of the endogenous peptides, and vice versa.[25,63]

Opioid Receptors

Since their discovery, the opioid receptors have been examined in considerable detail. Studies in animals have suggested that rather than only one homogeneous opioid receptor, there are at least three primary classes known as mu, kappa, and delta receptors[69,82] (Table 14–1). Some sources also divide these primary classes into subcategories (i.e., mu_1, mu_2, $delta_1$, $delta_2$, $kappa_1$, $kappa_2$, $kappa_3$) based on how well various opioids affect these receptors.[65] The significance of these subcategories, however, has been questioned somewhat based on studies using opioid receptors that were cloned from rodent cell lines.[27] That is, it is not clear at the present time if the primary classes (mu, kappa, delta) can be subclassified based on structural or functional differences within each primary receptor class.[27] Nonetheless, mu opioid receptors are somewhat distinct from kappa receptors, and kappa receptors are distinct from delta receptors, and so forth. Hence, some specialization regarding both the location and the response of specific primary classes of opioid receptors does appear to exist (see Table 14–1).

Stimulation of all three classes of opioid receptors causes analgesia. The mu receptor, however, seems to be the most important in mediating the analgesic effects of many opioids, including morphine.[30,33] Mu receptors are located in specific locations in the brain and spinal cord, and opioids that are used clinically to reduce pain typically have a fairly high affinity for the mu class of opioid receptors.[27] Unfortunately, some of the more problematic side effects of opioid drugs may also be mediated by stimulation of mu receptors. For example, stimulation of mu receptors may also cause respiratory depression and constipation, and repeated stimulation of mu opioid receptors has been associated with the cellular changes that might lead to opioid abuse and addiction.[15,27]

The existence of several classes of opioid receptors has therefore lead to the development of drugs that are somewhat more selective in the receptor class or subclass that they stimulate. In particular, drugs that selectively stimulate kappa or delta receptors may still provide sufficient analgesia, but will be less likely to provoke problems like respiratory depression and opioid abuse if they avoid or even block (antagonize) the mu receptors. Certain opioid drugs, for example, stimulate kappa receptors while avoiding or blocking

Table 14–1	OPIOID RECEPTORS	
Receptor Class	**Primary Therapeutic Effect(s)**	**Other Effects**
Mu (μ)	Spinal and supraspinal analgesia	Sedation; respiratory depression; constipation; inhibits neurotransmitter release (acetylcholine, dopamine); increases hormonal release (prolactin; growth hormone)
Kappa (κ)	Spinal and supraspinal analgesia	Sedation; constipation; psychotic effects
Delta (δ)	Spinal and supraspinal analgesia	Increases hormonal release (growth hormone); inhibits neurotransmitter release (dopamine)

Adapted from Gutstein and Akil,[27] page 573.

the mu receptors. These agents are known as mixed agonist-antagonist opioids and their clinical significance is addressed in the next section, "Classification of Specific Agents."

The discovery of several classes of opioid receptors that cause different effects and side effects has important pharmacologic implications. Research in this area continues to expand our knowledge about the structural and functional aspects of these receptor classes. Drug developers will hopefully capitalize on the unique aspects of opioid receptor classes, and new agents will be produced that are even more specific in relieving pain without provoking excessive side effects.

Classification of Specific Agents

Opioid analgesics are classified as strong agonists, mild-to-moderate agonists, mixed agonist-antagonists, and antagonists according to their interaction with opioid receptors. Some of the opioids in these categories are listed in Table 14–2. The basic characteristics of each category and clinically relevant examples are also discussed here.

Strong Agonists. These agents are used to treat severe pain. As the name implies, these drugs have a high affinity for certain receptors and are believed to interact primarily with mu opioid receptors in the CNS. The best-known member of this group is morphine—the other strong agonists are pharmacologically similar. Examples of strong opioid agonists include the following:

- fentanyl (Actiq, Duragesic, Sublimaze)
- hydromorphone (Hydrostat, Dilaudid)

- levorphanol (Levo-Dromoran)
- meperidine (Demerol)
- methadone (Dolophine, Methadose)
- morphine (MS Contin, Roxanol, Statex, others)
- oxymorphone (Numorphan)

Mild-to-Moderate Agonists. These drugs are still considered agonists that stimulate opioid receptors, but they do not have as high an affinity or efficacy as the drugs listed previously. These drugs are more effective in treating pain of moderate intensity. Examples include the following:

- codeine
- hydrocodone (Hycodan)
- oxycodone (OxyContin, Roxicodone)
- propoxyphene (Darvon)

Mixed Agonist-Antagonists. These drugs exhibit some agonist and antagonistlike activity at the same time because the drugs have the ability to act differently at specific classes of opioid receptors. For instance, certain drugs in this category (butorphanol, nalbuphine, pentazocine) cause analgesia because they bind to and activate kappa receptors; that is, they are kappa receptor agonists. At the same time, these drugs block or only partially activate mu receptors, thus acting as mu receptor antagonists or partial agonists, respectively[27] (the effects of partial agonists are described in more detail in Chapter 4). Mixed agonist-antagonist opioids appear to have the advantage of producing adequate analgesia with less risk of the side effects associated with mu receptors, including respiratory depression. These drugs are therefore safer in terms of a reduced risk of fatal overdose.[27] These drugs may also have fewer addictive qualities than strong mu receptor agonists such as morphine.[27] Mixed agonist-

Table 14–2	OPIOID ANALGESICS			
Drug	**Route of Administration***	**Onset of Action (min)**	**Time to Peak Effect (min)**	**Duration of Action (hr)**
	Strong Agonists			
Fentanyl (Sublimaze)	IM	7–15	20–30	1–2
	IV	1–2	3–5	0.5–1
Hydromorphone (Hydrostat, Dilaudid)	Oral	30	90–120	4
	IM	15	30–60	4–5
	IV	10–15	15–30	2–3
	Sub-Q	15	30–90	4
Levorphanol (Levo-Dromoran)	Oral	10–60	90–120	4–5
	IM	—	60	4–5
	IV	—	Within 20	4–5
	Sub-Q	—	60–90	4–5
Meperidine (Demerol)	Oral	15	60–90	2–4
	IM	10–15	30–50	2–4
	IV	1	5–7	2–4
	Sub-Q	10–15	30–50	2–4
Methadone (Dolophine, Methadose)	Oral	30–60	90–120	4–6
	IM	10–20	60–120	4–5
	IV	—	15–30	3–4
Morphine (many trade names)	Oral	—	60–120	4–5
	IM	10–30	30–60	4–5
	IV	—	20	4–5
	Sub-Q	10–30	50–90	4–5
	Epidural	15–60	—	Up to 24
	Intrathecal	15–60	—	Up to 24
	Rectal	20–60	—	—
Oxymorphone (Numorphan)	IM	10–15	30–90	3–6
	IV	5–10	15–30	3–4
	Sub-Q	10–20	—	3–6
	Rectal	15–30	120	3–6
	Mild-to-Moderate Agonists			
Codeine (generic)	Oral	30–45	60–120	4
	IM	10–30	30–60	4
	Sub-Q	10–30	—	4
Hydrocodone (Hycodan)	Oral	10–30	30–60	4–6
Oxycodone (OxyContin, Roxicodone)	Oral	—	60	3–4
Propoxyphene (Darvon)	Oral	15–60	120	4–6

Drug	Route of Administration*	Onset of Action (min)	Time to Peak Effect (min)	Duration of Action (hr)
Mixed Agonist-Antagonist				
Butorphanol (Stadol)	IM	10–30	30–60	3–4
	IV	2–3	30	2–4
Nalbuphine (Nubain)	IM	Within 15	60	3–6
	IV	2–3	30	3–4
	Sub-Q	Within 15	–	3–6
Pentazocine (Talwin)	Oral	15–30	60–90	3
	IM	15–20	30–60	2–3
	IV	2–3	15–30	2–3
	Sub-Q	15–20	30–60	2–3

*IM = intramuscular; IV = intravenous; Sub-Q = subcutaneous.

antagonists, however, may produce more psychotropic effects (e.g., hallucinations, vivid dreams), and their maximal analgesic effect may not be as great as strong mu agonists.[65] Consequently, these drugs are not used extensively, but they do offer an alternative to strong-to-moderate opioid agonists in certain patients.

A new addition to this category is buprenorphine (Buprenex). This drug partially activates mu receptors but is an antagonist at kappa receptors. Because of these selective effects, buprenorphine has been advocated not only as an analgesic, but also as a treatment for opioid dependence and withdrawal.[26,84] The use of this drug in treating opioid addiction is discussed in more detail later in this chapter.

Examples of mixed agonist–antagonists include the following:

- butorphanol (Stadol)
- buprenorphine (Buprenex)
- nalbuphine (Nubain)
- pentazocine (Talwin)

Antagonists. These drugs block all opioid receptors, with a particular affinity for the mu variety. Because of their antagonistic properties, these agents will not produce analgesia but will displace opioid agonists from the opioid receptors and block any further effects of the agonist molecules. Consequently, these drugs are used primarily to treat opioid overdoses and addiction. Certain opioid antagonists (e.g., nalmefene, naloxone) can rapidly (within 1 to 2 minutes) and dramatically reverse the respiratory depression that is usually the cause of death in excessive opioid inges-

tion. Other antagonists (e.g., naltrexone) are used in conjunction with behavioral therapy to maintain an opioid-free state in individuals recovering from opioid addiction. Hence, the primary agents used clinically as opioid antagonists are the following:

- nalmefene (Revex)
- naloxone (Narcan)
- naltrexone (ReVia)

Pharmacokinetics

Some opioid analgesics can be given orally, a preferred route of administration in terms of convenience and safety. Several of these enteral drugs also come in suppository form, permitting rectal administration if nausea and vomiting prohibit the oral route. Some opioids—including morphine—are now available in sustained-release enteral preparations, thus allowing more prolonged effects and wider intervals between doses.[6,12,50] Because of poor intestinal absorption or significant first-pass inactivation, other agents must be administered parenterally, usually through subcutaneous or intramuscular injection. Intravenous administration is also used sometimes, but must be done slowly and with caution. When the intravenous route is used, the narcotic is frequently diluted and infusion pumps are used to allow the slow, controlled administration of the drug. The intravenous route or other parenteral routes (epidural and intrathecal infusion) can also be used to administer opioids during patient-controlled analgesia; this concept is addressed in Chapter 17.

The feasibility of using other relatively new methods for administering opioids has also been investigated. For instance, transdermal patches have been developed to administer morphine, and other opioids such as fentanyl (Duragesic Patch), a potent and fast-acting opioid.[12,68] The patch provides a convenient method for the steady, prolonged administration of these opioids into the systemic circulation. Transdermal opioid patches also avoid the direct administration of the drug to the gastrointestinal (GI) tract, and this fact may help reduce GI problems such as nausea and constipation.[39]

Iontophoresis techniques (i.e., the use of electric current to facilitate transdermal delivery) have also been advocated as a way to enhance transdermal opioid delivery to the systemic circulation.[11] By varying the amount of electric current, iontophoresis may ultimately allow the patient to control the rate of transdermal administration of the opioid.[10,76,78] Finally, certain opioids such as fentanyl can be administered systemically via lozenges or a "lollipop" that dissolves in the mouth (transmucosal delivery), or via nasal spray (intranasal administration).[21,54] It will be interesting to see if these newer methods of administration will gain widespread acceptance in the future.

Because of differing degrees of solubility, the distribution and subsequent onset of action of specific agents varies (see Table 14–2). Opioids are ultimately distributed throughout all tissues, and these agents probably exert their principal analgesic effects after they reach the CNS. Some opioid effects may also be mediated by peripheral receptors located at the site of painful inflammation (see "Mechanism of Action" below). Metabolic inactivation of these drugs takes place primarily in the liver, although some degree of metabolism also occurs in other tissues such as the kidneys, lungs, and CNS. The kidneys excrete the drug metabolite and—to a lesser extent—the intact drug in the urine.

Mechanism of Action

Effect of Opioids on the CNS

As discussed earlier, opioid receptors exist at specific locations throughout the CNS and possibly in peripheral nerve tissues as well. In the spinal cord, these receptors are concentrated on the neurons responsible for transmitting nociceptive input to higher (supraspinal) levels.[33] Opioid receptors have likewise been identified in several locations of the brain that are associated with pain transmission and interpretation.

These areas include the periaqueductal gray region of the spinoreticular tract, medial thalamic nuclei, hypothalamus, limbic system, and several other areas.[33,65,75]

It is well accepted that opioids exert analgesic effects by inhibiting afferent pain transmission in ascending pain pathways. By acting at the key CNS sites listed above, opioids can inhibit painful impulses from being sent from the periphery to the brain. It is also believed that opioids exert some of their analgesic effects by activating *descending* pain pathways.[27,33] That is, opioids can also affect efferent CNS pathways originating in higher centers (rostral medulla, locus ceruleus, midbrain periaqueductal gray area), and enhance the ability of these descending pathways to reduce painful sensations at the spinal cord level.[65] This effect probably occurs because opioids inhibit interneurons that normally inhibit the ability of these descending pathways to moderate pain. This effect, known as *disinhibition*, ultimately activates the descending pathways by removing the inhibitory effect of these interneurons.[33] By removing this inhibition, opioids allow these descending pathways to become more active and help control painful sensations. Hence, opioids seem to exert analgesic effects through their ability to decrease ascending (afferent) pain transmission, combined with their ability to activate descending (efferent) pathways that reduce pain.

Effect of Opioids on CNS Synapses

Opioids basically exert their analgesic effects by inhibiting synaptic transmission in key pain pathways in the spinal cord and brain. This inhibitory effect is mediated by opioid receptors that are located on both presynaptic and postsynaptic membranes of pain-mediating synapses (Fig. 14–2). In the spinal cord, for example, receptors are located on the presynaptic terminals of primary (first-order) nociceptive afferents, and when bound by opioids, they directly decrease the release of pain-mediating transmitters such as substance P.[35,38] Opioid drug-receptor interactions also take place on the postsynaptic membrane of the secondary afferent neuron—that is, the second-order nociceptive afferent neuron in the spinal cord.[19,33] When stimulated, these receptors also inhibit pain transmission by hyperpolarizing the postsynaptic neuron.[19]

Opioids therefore inhibit synaptic transmission by decreasing neurotransmitter release from the presynaptic terminal and by decreasing excitable (hyperpolarizing) postsynaptic neurons within key pain pathways in the spinal cord and brain. Again, these synaptic effects can either limit the transmission of painful stim-

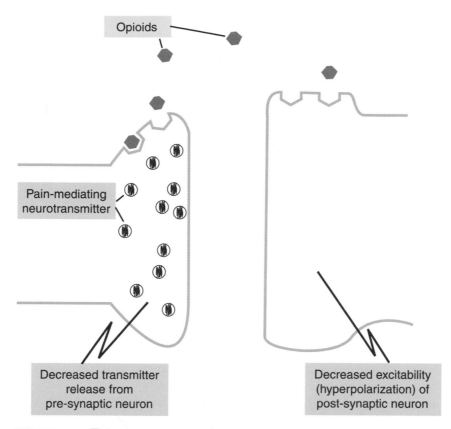

FIGURE 14–2 ▼ Schematic representation of how opioid analgesics may impair synaptic transmission in pain-mediating pathways. The drug binds to specific opioid receptors on the presynaptic and postsynaptic membranes.

uli in ascending pain pathways, or they can activate descending antinociceptive pathways by inhibiting interneurons that control these pathways. These effects are mediated through opioid receptors that are located on the membrane of these neurons, but are linked to the internal chemistry on the presynaptic and postsynaptic neurons through regulatory G proteins.[1,65]

As described in Chapter 4, regulatory G proteins act as an intermediate link between receptor activation and the intracellular effector mechanism that ultimately causes a change in cellular activity. In the case of opioid receptors, these G proteins interact with three primary cellular effectors: calcium channels, potassium channels, and the adenyl cyclase enzyme.[27] At the presynaptic terminal, stimulation of opioid receptors activates G proteins that in turn inhibit the opening of calcium channels on the nerve membrane.[65] Decreased calcium entry into the presynaptic terminal causes decreased neurotransmitter release because calcium influx mediates transmitter release at a chemical synapse. At the postsynaptic neuron, opioid receptors are linked via G proteins to potassium channels, and

activation of the receptor leads to an opening of these channels and a loss of potassium from the postsynaptic neuron.[46] A relative loss of potassium from the postsynaptic neuron causes hyperpolarization because efflux of potassium (a cation) results in a relative increase in the negative intracellular electric potential. The postsynaptic neuron is therefore more difficult to excite because the interior of the cell is more negative.

Finally, opioid receptors are linked via G proteins to the adenyl cyclase enzyme, and stimulation of the receptor leads to inhibition of this enzyme and decreased synthesis of cyclic adenosine monophosphate (cAMP). cAMP is an important second messenger that regulates neurotransmitter release from the presynaptic terminal and may also regulate the firing threshold of the postsynaptic neuron.[27] Opioid-mediated inhibition of this second messenger therefore helps to explain how these drugs alter pain transmission. Hence, opioid drugs exert their analgesic effects by interacting with receptors that are linked to several intracellular effector mechanisms that ultimately lead to decreased synaptic transmission in specific pain pathways.

Peripheral Effects of Opioids

Opioid receptors may exist outside the CNS, and some of the analgesic effects of opioid drugs may be mediated at peripheral sites.[34,64] Opioid receptors have been identified on the distal (peripheral) ends of primary afferent (sensory) neurons.[34,61] Binding opioid agents to these peripheral receptors will provide an analgesic effect by decreasing the excitability of these sensory neurons (Fig. 14–3). This idea is supported by the fact that endogenous opioids (endorphins, enkephalins) are often produced by leukocytes in peripheral tissues during certain types of painful inflammation, and that these endogenous substances seem to act locally on the peripheral sensory nerve terminals.[9,45,61] Likewise, results from some studies in animals and humans suggest that exogenous opioids can be administered directly into peripheral tissues (e.g., injected into an inflamed joint) and that these agents exert analgesic effects even though the drug never reaches the CNS.[27,65]

Hence, evidence suggests that opioid receptors exist outside the CNS and opioid drugs may help produce analgesia at these peripheral sites. However, the clinical significance of these peripheral opioid effects remains to be fully determined. For instance, these receptors may play a role in mediating only certain types of pain, such as the pain associated with inflammation.[59] Nonetheless, the fact that certain types of pain might be controlled by peripherally acting opioids has important pharmacologic implications. For instance, opioids that work exclusively in the periphery would not cause CNS-mediated side effects such as

sedation, respiratory depression, and tolerance. Peripheral-acting opioids could be developed by creating lipophobic compounds that are unable to cross the blood-brain barrier.[17,34] The use of these peripheral-acting drugs remains fairly experimental at the present time, and additional clinical trials are needed to determine whether this becomes a viable means of treating certain types of pain.

Clinical Applications

Treatment of Pain

Opioid analgesics are most effective in treating moderate-to-severe pain that is more or less constant in duration. These drugs are not as effective in treating sharp, intermittent pain—although higher dosages will relieve this type of pain as well. Some examples of the clinical usage of opioid analgesics include the treatment of acute pain following surgery, trauma, and myocardial infarction, as well as the treatment of chronic pain in patients with conditions such as cancer. Because of the potential for serious side effects (see "Problems and Adverse Effects" below), these drugs should be used only when necessary, and the dose should be titrated according to the patient's pain. Generally, oral administration of a mild-to-moderate opioid agonist should be used first, with stronger agonists being instituted orally and then parenterally if needed. In cases of chronic pain, pain control by nonopioid drugs should be attempted first. However, opioid analgesics should be instituted when the improvement in the quality of

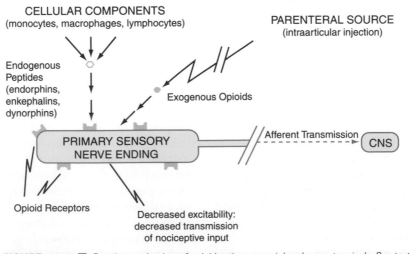

FIGURE 14–3 ▼ Putative mechanism of opioid action on peripheral nerve terminals. See text for discussion.

life offered to the patient with chronic pain clearly outweighs the potential risks of these drugs.[28,51]

Opioid analgesics often produce a rather unique form of analgesia as compared to the nonopioid agents. Opioids often alter the perception of pain rather than eliminating the painful sensation entirely. The patient may still be aware of the pain but it is no longer the primary focus of his or her attention. In a sense, the patient is no longer preoccupied by the pain. This type of analgesia is also often associated with euphoria and a sensation of floating. These sensations may be caused by the stimulation of specific types of opiate receptors within the limbic system (i.e., delta receptors).

The route of opioid administration appears to be important in providing effective pain relief.[2,7] Although the oral route is the easiest and most convenient, parenteral routes may be more effective in chronic or severe, intractable pain. In particular, administration directly into the epidural or intrathecal space has been suggested as being optimal in relieving pain following certain types of surgery, or in various types of acute or chronic pain.[7,13,24,31,57,71] Since it is impractical to reinsert a needle every time the drug is needed, indwelling catheters are often implanted surgically so that the tip of the catheter lies in the epidural or intrathecal space. The free end of the catheter can be brought out through the patient's skin and used to administer the opioid directly into the area surrounding the spinal cord. Alternatively, the catheter can be connected to some sort of a drug reservoir or pump that contains the opioid drug. Such devices can be located outside the patient's body or implanted surgically beneath the patient's skin (e.g., in the abdominal wall), and these pumps are programmed to deliver the drug at a fixed rate into the indwelling catheter.[2] Although these programmable drug delivery systems do have some risks, they appear to be an effective way of treating patients with severe, chronic pain from malignant and nonmalignant sources.[24]

The effectiveness of opioid analgesics also appears to be influenced by the dosing schedule. The current consensus is that orally administered opioids are more effective when given at regularly scheduled intervals rather than when the patient feels the need for the drug.[55,58] This may be because with regularly scheduled dosages, plasma concentrations may be maintained within a therapeutic range, rather than allowing the large plasma fluctuations that may occur if the drugs are given at sporadic intervals. On the other hand, it may simply be easier to control pain in its earlier stages before the pain can reach full intensity.[58]

Consistent with these hypotheses is the finding that continuous infusion of the opioid into the epidural or intrathecal space provides optimal pain relief postoperatively or in chronic, intractable pain.[2,40,83] Continuous infusion is associated with certain side effects, especially nausea and constipation, as well as the potential for disruption of the drug delivery system.[24,57,77] Problems with tolerance have also been reported during continuous administration,[27] but it is somewhat controversial whether tolerance really develops when these drugs are used appropriately in the clinical management of pain (see section on "Concepts of Addiction, Tolerance, and Physical Dependence"). Hence, the benefit-to-risk ratio for continuous epidural or intrathecal infusion is often acceptable in patients with severe pain. This method of opioid administration continues to gain acceptance.[24,57]

Use of Opioids in Patient-Controlled Analgesia

Finally, some rather innovative techniques have been employed whereby the patient is able to control the delivery of the analgesic.[5,20,60] These techniques are collectively known as patient-controlled analgesia (PCA) because the patient is able to periodically administer a specific dose of the drug (by pushing a button or some other device). PCA systems have some distinct advantages over conventional administration, and PCAs are often used following various types of surgery as well as in the treatment of certain types of chronic pain.[5,13,60] The use of opioids and other drugs in PCA systems is discussed in Chapter 17.

Other Opioid Uses

Opioids have several other clinical applications. These agents can be used as an anesthetic premedication or as an adjunct in general anesthesia. Opioids are effective in cough suppression, and the short-term use of codeine and codeinelike agents in this regard is quite common. Opioid agonists decrease gastrointestinal motility and can be used to control cases of severe diarrhea. This effect is probably mediated indirectly through an effect on the CNS, as well as through a direct effect on the intestine. Finally, opioid agonists are used as an adjunct in cases of acute pulmonary edema. These drugs probably do not directly improve ventilatory capacity, but they do serve to reduce feelings of intense panic and anxiety associated with the dyspnea inherent to this disorder. Patients feel they can breathe more easily following opioid administration.

Problems and Adverse Effects

Opioid analgesics produce a number of central and peripheral side effects.[32,48] Virtually all of these drugs have sedative properties and induce some degree of mental slowing and drowsiness. Patients taking opioids for the relief of pain may also become somewhat euphoric, although the manner and degree of such mood changes varies from individual to individual. One of the more potentially serious side effects is the respiratory depression often seen after narcotic administration.[56] Within a few minutes after administration, these drugs cause the breathing rate to slow down, which can last for several hours. Although not usually a major problem when therapeutic doses are given to relatively healthy individuals, respiratory depression can be severe or even fatal in seriously ill patients, in patients with pre-existing pulmonary problems, or in cases of overdose. Some cardiovascular problems such as orthostatic hypotension may also occur immediately after opioids are administered, especially when parenteral routes are used.

Finally, gastrointestinal distress in the form of nausea and vomiting is quite common with many of the narcotic analgesics. Because of their antiperistaltic action, these drugs can also cause constipation.[48] Because this constipating effect can be quite severe, laxatives and stool softeners (see Chapter 27) can be used to prevent opioid-induced constipation in certain people, such as with patients who are at risk for fecal impaction (e.g., people with spinal cord injuries), or with people who are taking opioids for an extended period of time (e.g., patients receiving opioids for treatment of cancer-related pain).[36,70]

Concepts of Addiction, Tolerance, and Physical Dependence

When used inappropriately, opioid drugs can produce addiction. The term *addiction* typically refers to situations in which an individual repeatedly seeks out and ingests certain substances for mood-altering and pleasurable experiences, such as the heroin addict who takes the drug illicitly to achieve an opioid "high." In this sense, addiction is a very complex phenomenon that has strong psychologic implications regarding why certain chemicals cause this behavior in certain people.

This concept of addiction is often separated from the physiologic changes that can accompany prolonged opioid use, namely tolerance and physical dependence. **Tolerance** is the need for more of a drug to achieve a given effect, and **physical dependence** is the onset of withdrawal symptoms if a drug is suddenly discontinued. Tolerance and physical dependence are also rather complex phenomena, and a complete discussion of the factors involved in producing these occurrences is not possible at this time. The primary characteristics of tolerance and physical dependence will be briefly discussed here as they relate to opioid usage.

Tolerance

Tolerance is defined as the need to progressively increase the dosage of a drug to achieve a therapeutic effect when the drug is used for prolonged periods.[53] When used for the treatment of pain in some patients, the dosage of the opioid may need to be increased periodically to continue to provide adequate relief. The physiologic reasons for tolerance are complex and probably involve changes in the intracellular response to repeated stimulation of opioid receptors. Prolonged exposure to opioids can also cause a decrease in the number and sensitivity of the opioid receptors—a phenomenon known as receptor downregulation and desensitization (see Chapter 4).[14,43,80] However, these changes in the quantity and sensitivity of opioid receptors do not seem to be the primary reasons for opioid tolerance.[62] It seems more likely that tolerance is caused by changes in the intracellular effectors that are coupled to the opioid receptor, namely the G proteins and intracellular effector mechanisms.[22,73] As described earlier, opioid receptors mediate their effects through regulatory G proteins that are linked to intracellular effectors, including the adenyl cyclase enzyme. Tolerance to opioid drugs, therefore, seems to be caused by long-term changes in G protein function and adenyl cyclase-induced synthesis of second messengers like cAMP.[42,79] In a sense, tolerance occurs because the internal biochemistry of the cell has been blunted by repeated stimulation of the G protein-effector mechanisms.

The physiologic changes that cause opioid tolerance typically follow a predictable time course. Tolerance begins after the first dose of the narcotic, but the need for increased amounts of the drug usually becomes obvious after 2 to 3 weeks of administration. Tolerance seems to last approximately 1 to 2 weeks after the drug is removed. This does not mean that the patient no longer has any desire for the drug, but that the patient will again respond to the initial dosage after 14 days or so. Other factors may influence the individual's desire for the drug long after any physiologic effects have disappeared (see "Physical Dependence").

Physical Dependence

Physical dependence is usually defined as the onset of withdrawal symptoms when the drug is abruptly removed. **Withdrawal syndrome** from opioid dependence is associated with a number of obvious and unpleasant symptoms (Table 14–3). In severe dependence, withdrawal symptoms become evident within 6 to 10 hours after the last dose of the drug, and symptoms reach their peak in the second or third day after the drug has been stopped. Withdrawal symptoms last approximately 5 days. This does not necessarily mean that the individual no longer desires the drug, only that the physical symptoms of withdrawal have ceased. Indeed, an addict may continue to crave the drug after months or years of abstinence.

Physical dependence must therefore be differentiated from the more intangible concepts of addiction and psychologic dependence. Psychologic dependence seems to be related to pleasurable changes in mood and behavior evoked by the drug. The individual is motivated to continually reproduce these pleasurable sensations because of the feelings of well-being, relaxation, and so on. Psychologic dependence seems to create the drug-seeking behavior that causes the addict to relapse into use of the drug long after the physiologic effects have disappeared.

Tolerance and Dependence During Therapeutic Opioid Use

Although tolerance and dependence can occur whenever opioid drugs are used indiscriminately for pro-

longed periods, there is some debate as to whether these phenomena must always accompany the therapeutic use of opioid drugs for the treatment of chronic pain. There is growing evidence that the risk of tolerance and dependence is actually very low when opioid drugs are used appropriately to treat chronic pain.[8,18] For example, there appear to be relatively few problems with long-term opioid use when these drugs are administered to treat pain in patients who do not have a history of substance abuse, who adhere to the prescribed opioid regimen, and who have pain from physiological rather than psychological causes.[18,52]

Some experts also feel that tolerance and physical dependence will not occur if the dosage is carefully adjusted to meet the patient's needs.[4,8] It is believed that when the opioid dose exactly matches the patient's need for pain control, there is no excess drug to stimulate the drug-seeking behavior commonly associated with opioid addiction. The opioid is essentially absorbed by the patient's pain. Of course, patients with chronic pain may still need to have the dosage increased periodically. This observation would be explained by the fact that the pain has increased because the patient's condition has worsened (e.g., the cancer has increased) rather than the idea that the patient developed pharmacologic tolerance to the drug.[28,51] Thus, many practitioners feel that problems with addiction, tolerance, and dependence are minimized when opioid drugs are used therapeutically. These agents are essentially being used for a specific reason—the treatment of pain—rather than for the pleasure-seeking purpose associated with the recreational use of these drugs. These drugs must, of course, be used carefully and with strict regard to using the lowest effective dose. Hence, there is consensus that opioids are very effective and important analgesic agents and should be used under appropriate therapeutic conditions without excessive fear of the patient developing addiction or becoming especially tolerant to the drug's effects.[4,18]

Pharmacological Treatment of Opioid Addiction

The inappropriate or illegal use and abuse of narcotics such as heroin is a major problem in many countries. Hence, various strategies have been employed to treat people who are addicted to heroin and other opioids. Methadone is the primary pharmacological intervention used to treat opioid addiction. Methadone is a strong opioid agonist, similar in potency and efficacy to morphine. While giving an opioid to treat an opi-

Table 14–3	ABSTINENCE SYNDROMES: SYMPTOMS OF NARCOTIC WITHDRAWAL	
Body aches	Runny nose
Diarrhea	Shivering
Fever	Sneezing
Gooseflesh	Stomach cramps
Insomnia	Sweating
Irritability	Tachycardia
Loss of appetite	Uncontrollable yawning
Nausea/vomiting	Weakness/fatigue

oid addiction may at first appear odd, methadone offers several advantages, such as milder withdrawal symptoms. Methadone is essentially substituted for the abused opioid (e.g., heroin), and is then slowly withdrawn as various methods of counseling are employed to discourage further drug abuse.[3,74] Use of methadone, however, remains controversial because of the rather low success rate of this intervention and the tendency for many subjects to relapse and return to opioid abuse.[37] Still, methadone maintenance programs are more successful than using no pharmacological intervention,[47] and methadone remains the primary drug strategy used to treat opioid addiction.[74]

Recently, buprenorphine has been advocated as an alternative pharmacological method for treating opioid addiction.[26,84] As indicated earlier, buprenorphine is a mixed agonist-antagonist that partially stimulates mu opioid receptors while acting as a strong antagonist at kappa opioid receptors. By weakly stimulating the mu receptors, this drug can sustain the opioid effects and prevent sudden withdrawal. At the same time, buprenorphine can block kappa receptors, thereby affecting some of the cellular changes that seem to promote opioid addiction. Hence, this drug offers another method of substituting a therapeutic agent for the abused opioid, with the ultimate goal being to eventually wean the patient from all opioid drugs.[16]

Hence, efforts continue to provide more effective pharmacological and nonpharmacological interventions for treating opioid addiction.[41] As more infor-

Special Concerns in Rehabilitation Patients

■ ■ ■ Physical therapists will encounter the use of opioid analgesics in patients requiring acute pain relief (following surgery, trauma, etc.) and chronic analgesia (for patients with terminal cancer and other types of severe chronic pain). The usual side effects of sedation and gastrointestinal discomfort may be bothersome during some of the therapy sessions. However, the relief of pain afforded by these drugs may be helpful in allowing a relatively more vigorous and comprehensive rehabilitation regimen. The benefits of pain relief usually outweigh side effects such as sedation. Scheduling therapy when these drugs reach their peak effects may be advantageous (see Table 14–2). One side effect that should be taken into account during therapy is the tendency of these drugs to produce respiratory depression. Opioids tend to make the medullary chemoreceptors less responsive to carbon dioxide, thus slowing down the respiratory rate and inducing a relative hypoxia and hypercapnia.[27] This fact should be considered if any exercise is instituted as part of the rehabilitation program. The respiratory response to this exercise may be blunted.

The tendency for these drugs to produce constipation is another side effect that could have important implications for patients receiving physical rehabilitation. Opioid-induced constipation is especially problematic in patients with spinal cord injuries or other conditions that decrease gastrointestinal motility. In such patients, opioids are often administered along with laxatives and GI stimulants (see Chapter 27) to minimize the constipating effects and risk of fecal impaction. Therapists should therefore be aware of these constipating effects and help educate patients and their families so that these effects do not result in serious problems.

Therapists may also be working with patients who are experiencing withdrawal symptoms from opioid drugs. Such patients may be in the process of being weaned off the therapeutic use of these agents, or they may be heroin addicts who have been hospitalized for other reasons (e.g., trauma, surgery). If not on some type of methadone maintenance, the addict may be experiencing a wide variety of physical symptoms including diffuse muscle aches. The therapist should be aware that these aches and pains may be caused by opioid withdrawal rather than an actual somatic disorder. Therapists may, however, help the patient cope with opioid withdrawal by using various physical agents (heat, electrotherapy) and manual techniques (massage, relaxation techniques) to alleviate these somatic symptoms.

CASE STUDY

Opioid Analgesics

Brief History. N.P., a 45-year-old woman, was involved in an automobile accident approximately 6 months ago. She received multiple contusions from the accident, but no major injuries were sustained. Two months later, she began to develop pain in the right shoulder. This pain progressively increased, and she was treated for bursitis using anti-inflammatory drugs. Her shoulder motion became progressively more limited; however, any movement of her glenohumeral joint caused rather severe pain. She was reevaluated and a diagnosis of adhesive capsulitis was made. The patient was admitted to the hospital, and while she was under general anesthesia, a closed manipulation of the shoulder was performed. When the patient recovered from the anesthesia, meperidine (Demerol) was prescribed for pain relief. This drug was given orally at a dosage of 75 mg every 4 hours. Physical therapy was also initiated the afternoon following the closed manipulation. Passive range-of-motion exercises were used to maintain the increased joint mobility achieved during the manipulative procedure.

Relevance to Therapy/Clinical Decision. The therapist arranged the treatment schedule so that the meperidine was reaching peak effects during the therapy session. The patient was seen approximately 1 hour following the oral administration of the drug. The initial session was scheduled at the patient's bedside because the patient was still woozy from the anesthesia. On the following day, therapy was continued in the physical therapy department. However, the patient was brought to the department on a stretcher to prevent an episode of dizziness brought on by orthostatic hypotension. On the third day, the patient's medication was changed to oxycodone (OxyContin), a mild-to-moderate opioid agonist. By this time, the patient was being transported to physical therapy in a wheelchair, and the therapy session also included active exercise. The patient was discharged on the fourth day after the manipulative procedure. She continued to attend therapy as an outpatient, and full function of her right shoulder was ultimately restored.

mation is gained about the cellular and subcellular mechanisms that cause addiction, we may see other agents being used to specifically treat these changes and thereby offer a more effective way to prevent and treat opioid abuse.

SUMMARY

Opioid analgesics represent some of the most effective methods of treating moderate-to-severe pain. When used properly, these agents can alleviate acute and chronic pain in a variety of situations. The use of these drugs is sometimes tempered with their tendency to produce tolerance and physical dependence, but their potential for abuse seems relatively low when these drugs are used appropriately to treat pain. Opioid drugs therefore represent the most effective pharmacologic means of helping patients deal with acute and chronic pain. The analgesic properties of these drugs often provide a substantial benefit in patients involved in rehabilitation. Physical therapists should be aware of some of the side effects, such as sedation and respiratory depression, and should be cognizant of the impact of these effects during the rehabilitation session.

References

1. Ahmad S, Dray A. Novel G protein-coupled receptors as pain targets. *Curr Opin Investig Drugs.* 2004; 5:67–70.
2. Alon E, Jaquenod M, Schaeppi B. Post-operative epidural versus intravenous patient-controlled analgesia. *Minerva Anestesiol.* 2003;69:443–446.
3. Amato L, Minozzi S, Davoli M, Vecchi S, Ferri M, Mayet S. Psychosocial combined with agonist maintenance treatments versus agonist maintenance treatments alone for treatment of opioid dependence. *Cochrane Database Syst Rev.* 2004;4:CD004147.
4. Antoin H, Beasley RD. Opioids for chronic noncancer pain. Tailoring therapy to fit the patient and the pain. *Postgrad Med.* 2004;116:37–40,43–44.
5. Aygun S, Kocoglu H, Goksu S, et al. Postoperative patient-controlled analgesia with intravenous tramadol, intravenous fentanyl, epidural tramadol and epidural ropivacaine + fentanyl combination. *Eur J Gynaecol Oncol.* 2004;25:498–501.
6. Bellissant E, Estebe JP, Sebille V, Ecoffey C. Effect of preoperative oral sustained-release morphine sulfate on postoperative morphine requirements in elective spine surgery. *Fundam Clin Pharmacol.* 2004;18: 709–714.

7. Block BM, Liu SS, Rowlingson AJ, et al. Efficacy of postoperative epidural analgesia: a meta-analysis. *JAMA*. 2003;290:2455–2463.

8. Bloodworth D. Issues in opioid management. *Am J Phys Med Rehabil*. 2005;84(suppl 3):S42–S55.

9. Brack A, Rittner HL, Machelska H, et al. Endogenous peripheral antinociception in early inflammation is not limited by the number of opioid-containing leukocytes but by opioid receptor expression. *Pain*. 2004;108:67–75.

10. Chelly JE, Grass J, Houseman TW, et al. The safety and efficacy of a fentanyl patient-controlled transdermal system for acute postoperative analgesia: a multicenter, placebo-controlled trial. *Anesth Analg*. 2004;98:427–433.

11. Ciccone CD. Iontophoresis. In: Robinson AJ, Snyder-Mackler L eds. *Clinical Electrophysiology* 2nd ed. Baltimore: Lippincott Williams & Wilkins, 1994.

12. Clark AJ, Ahmedzai SH, Allan LG, et al. Efficacy and safety of transdermal fentanyl and sustained-release oral morphine in patients with cancer and chronic non-cancer pain. *Curr Med Res Opin*. 2004;20:1419–1428.

13. Colwell CW, Jr. The use of the pain pump and patient-controlled analgesia in joint reconstruction. *Am J Orthop*. 2004;33(suppl 5):10–12.

14. Connor M, Osborne PB, Christie MJ. Mu-opioid receptor desensitization: is morphine different? *Br J Pharmacol*. 2004;143:685–696.

15. Contet C, Kieffer BL, Befort K. Mu opioid receptor: a gateway to drug addiction. *Curr Opin Neurobiol*. 2004;14:370–378.

16. Davids E, Gastpar M. Buprenorphine in the treatment of opioid dependence. *Eur Neuropsychopharmacol*. 2004;14:209–216.

17. DeHaven-Hudkins DL, Dolle RE. Peripherally restricted opioid agonists as novel analgesic agents. *Curr Pharm Des*. 2004;10:743–757.

18. Dews TE, Mekhail N. Safe use of opioids in chronic noncancer pain. *Cleve Clin J Med*. 2004;71:897–904.

19. Eckert WA 3rd, Light AR. Hyperpolarization of substantia gelatinosa neurons evoked by mu-, kappa-, delta 1-, and delta 2-selective opioids. *J Pain*. 2002;3:115–125.

20. Evans E, Turley N, Robinson N, Clancy M. Randomised controlled trial of patient controlled analgesia compared with nurse delivered analgesia in an emergency department. *Emerg Med J*. 2005;22:25–29.

21. Finn J, Wright J, Fong J, et al. A randomised crossover trial of patient controlled intranasal fentanyl and oral morphine for procedural wound care in adult patients with burns. *Burns*. 2004;30:262–268.

22. Gainetdinov RR, Premont RT, Bohn LM, et al. Desensitization of G protein-coupled receptors and neuronal functions. *Annu Rev Neurosci*. 2004;27:107–144.

23. Gein SV, Simonenko TA, Tendryakova SP. The effects of rotation stress on measures of immunity. The role of opiate receptors. *Neurosci Behav Physiol*. 2004;34:935–938.

24. Gerber HR. Intrathecal morphine for chronic benign pain. *Best Pract Res Clin Anaesthesiol*. 2003;17:429–442.

25. Gerrits MA, Lesscher HB, van Ree JM. Drug dependence and the endogenous opioid system. *Eur Neuropsychopharmacol*. 2003;13:424–434.

26. Gonzalez G, Oliveto A, Kosten TR. Combating opiate dependence: a comparison among the available pharmacological options. *Expert Opin Pharmacother*. 2004;5:713–725.

27. Gutstein HB, Akil H. Opioid analgesics. In: Hardman JG, et al, eds. *The Pharmacological Basis of Therapeutics*. 10th ed. New York: McGraw-Hill; 2001.

28. Hall EJ, Sykes NP. Analgesia for patients with advanced disease: 2. *Postgrad Med J*. 2004;80:190–195.

29. Han JS. Acupuncture and endorphins. *Neurosci Lett*. 2004;361:258–261.

30. Han W, Ide S, Sora I, et al. A possible genetic mechanism underlying individual and interstrain differences in opioid actions: focus on the mu opioid receptor gene. *Ann N Y Acad Sci*. 2004;1025:370–375.

31. Heitz JW, Viscusi ER. The evolving role of spinal agents in acute pain. *Curr Pain Headache Rep*. 2005;9:17–23.

32. Herndon CM, Kalauokalani DA, Cunningham AJ, et al. Anticipating and treating opioid-associated adverse effects. *Expert Opin Drug Saf*. 2003;2:305–319.

33. Inturrisi CE. Clinical pharmacology of opioids for pain. *Clin J Pain*. 2002;18(suppl 4):S3–S13.

34. Janson W, Stein C. Peripheral opioid analgesia. *Curr Pharm Biotechnol*. 2003;4:270–274.

35. Kerchner GA, Zhuo M. Presynaptic suppression of dorsal horn inhibitory transmission by mu-opioid receptors. *J Neurophysiol*. 2002;88:520–522.

36. Klaschik E, Nauck F, Ostgathe C. Constipation—modern laxative therapy. *Support Care Cancer*. 2003;11:679–685.

37. Kleber HD. Pharmacologic treatments for heroin and cocaine dependence. *Am J Addict*. 2003;12(suppl 2):S5–S18.

38. Kondo I, Marvizon JC, Song B, et al. Inhibition by spinal mu- and delta-opioid agonists of afferent-evoked substance P release. *J Neurosci*. 2005;25:3651–3660.

39. Kornick CA, Santiago-Palma J, Moryl N, et al. Benefit-risk assessment of transdermal fentanyl for the treatment of chronic pain. *Drug Saf*. 2003;26:951–973.

40. Kotake Y, Matsumoto M, Morisaki H, Takeda J. The effectiveness of continuous epidural infusion of low-dose fentanyl and mepivacaine in perioperative analgesia and hemodynamic control in mastectomy patients. *J Clin Anesth*. 2004;16:88–91.

41. Krantz MJ, Mehler PS. Treating opioid dependence. Growing implications for primary care. *Arch Intern Med*. 2004;164:277–288.

42. Law PY, Loh HH, Wei LN. Insights into the receptor transcription and signaling: implications in opioid tolerance and dependence. *Neuropharmacology*. 2004;47(suppl 1):300–311.

43. Liu-Chen LY. Agonist-induced regulation and trafficking of kappa opioid receptors. *Life Sci*. 2004;75:511–536.

44. Lugo RA, Kern SE. Clinical pharmacokinetics of morphine. *J Pain Palliat Care Pharmacother.* 2002; 16:5–18.

45. Machelska H, Schopohl JK, Mousa SA, et al. Different mechanisms of intrinsic pain inhibition in early and late inflammation. *J Neuroimmunol.* 2003;141:30–39.

46. Marker CL, Lujan R, Loh HH, Wickman K. Spinal G-protein-gated potassium channels contribute in a dose-dependent manner to the analgesic effect of mu- and delta- but not kappa-opioids. *J Neurosci.* 2005;25: 3551–3559.

47. Mattick RP, Breen C, Kimber J, Davoli M. Methadone maintenance therapy versus no opioid replacement therapy for opioid dependence. *Cochrane Database Syst Rev.* 2003;CD002209.

48. McNicol E, Horowicz-Mehler N, Fisk RA, et al. Management of opioid side effects in cancer-related and chronic noncancer pain: a systematic review. *J Pain.* 2003;4:231–256.

49. Molina PE. Endogenous opioid analgesia in hemorrhagic shock. *J Trauma.* 2003;54(suppl 5):S126–S132.

50. Morales ME, Gallardo Lara V, Calpena AC, et al. Comparative study of morphine diffusion from sustained release polymeric suspensions. *J Control Release.* 2004;95:75–81.

51. Moynihan TJ. Use of opioids in the treatment of severe pain in terminally ill patients—dying should not be painful. *Mayo Clin Proc.* 2003;78:1397–401. Review [erratum in *Mayo Clin Proc.* 2003;78:1579].

52. Olsen Y, Daumit GL. Opioid prescribing for chronic nonmalignant pain in primary care: challenges and solutions. *Adv Psychosom Med.* 2004;25:138–150.

53. Ossipov MH, Lai J, King T, et al. Antinociceptive and nociceptive actions of opioids. *J Neurobiol.* 2004;61: 126–148.

54. Paech MJ, Lim CB, Banks SL, Rucklidge MW, Doherty DA. A new formulation of nasal fentanyl spray for postoperative analgesia: a pilot study. *Anaesthesia.* 2003;58:740–744.

55. Patterson DR, Ptacek JT, Carrougher G, et al. The 2002 Lindberg Award. PRN vs regularly scheduled opioid analgesics in pediatric burn patients. *J Burn Care Rehabil.* 2002;23:424–430.

56. Pattinson KT, Bowes M, Wise RG, et al. Evaluation of a non-invasive method of assessing opioid induced respiratory depression. *Anaesthesia.* 2005;60:426–432.

57. Penn RD. Intrathecal medication delivery. *Neurosurg Clin N Am.* 2003;14:381–387.

58. Phero JC, Becker DE, Dionne RA. Contemporary trends in acute pain management. *Curr Opin Otolaryngol Head Neck Surg.* 2004;12:209–216.

59. Pol O, Puig MM. Expression of opioid receptors during peripheral inflammation. *Curr Top Med Chem.* 2004;4:51–61.

60. Prakash S, Fatima T, Pawar M. Patient-controlled analgesia with fentanyl for burn dressing changes. *Anesth Analg.* 2004;99:552–555.

61. Puehler W, Stein C. Controlling pain by influencing neurogenic pathways. *Rheum Dis Clin North Am.* 2005; 31:103–113, ix.

62. Raith K, Hochhaus G. Drugs used in the treatment of opioid tolerance and physical dependence: a review. *Int J Clin Pharmacol Ther.* 2004;42:191–203.

63. Rasmussen NA, Farr LA. Effects of morphine and time of day on pain and beta-endorphin. *Biol Res Nurs.* 2003;5:105–116.

64. Riviere PJ. Peripheral kappa-opioid agonists for visceral pain. *Br J Pharmacol.* 2004;141:1331–1334.

65. Schumacher MA, Basbaum AI, Way WL. Opioid analgesics and antagonists. In: Katzung BG ed. *Basic and Clinical Pharmacology.* 9th ed. New York: Lange Medical Books/McGraw Hill; 2004.

66. Shavali S, Ho B, Govitrapong P, et al. Melatonin exerts its analgesic actions not by binding to opioid receptor subtypes but by increasing the release of beta-endorphin an endogenous opioid. *Brain Res Bull.* 2005;64:471–479.

67. Sher L. The role of endogenous opioids in the placebo effect in post-traumatic stress disorder. *Forsch Komplementarmed Klass Naturheilkd.* 2004;11:354–359.

68. Skaer TL. Practice guidelines for transdermal opioids in malignant pain. *Drugs.* 2004;64:2629–2638.

69. Smith AP, Lee NM. Opioid receptor interactions: local and nonlocal, symmetric and asymmetric, physical and functional. *Life Sci.* 2003;73:1873–1893.

70. Tamayo AC, Diaz-Zuluaga PA. Management of opioid-induced bowel dysfunction in cancer patients. *Support Care Cancer.* 2004;12:613–618.

71. Tobias JD. A review of intrathecal and epidural analgesia after spinal surgery in children. *Anesth Analg.* 2004; 98:956–965.

72. Tordjman S, Carlier M, Cohen D, et al. Aggression and the three opioid families (endorphins, enkephalins, and dynorphins) in mice. *Behav Genet.* 2003;33: 529–536.

73. Tso PH, Wong YH. Molecular basis of opioid dependence: role of signal regulation by G-proteins. *Clin Exp Pharmacol Physiol.* 2003;30:307–316.

74. Uchtenhagen A. Substitution management in opioid dependence. *J Neural Transm Suppl.* 2003:33–60.

75. Vaughan CW, Bagley EE, Drew GM, et al. Cellular actions of opioids on periaqueductal grey neurons from C57B16/J mice and mutant mice lacking MOR-1. *Br J Pharmacol.* 2003;139:362–367.

76. Viscusi ER. Emerging techniques for postoperative analgesia in orthopedic surgery. *Am J Orthop.* 2004; 33(suppl 5):13–16.

77. Viscusi ER. Emerging techniques in the treatment of postoperative pain. *Am J Health Syst Pharm.* 2004;61 (suppl 1):S11–S14.

78. Viscusi ER, Reynolds L, Chung F, et al. Patient-controlled transdermal fentanyl hydrochloride vs intravenous morphine pump for postoperative pain: a randomized controlled trial. *JAMA.* 2004;291: 1333–1341.

79. von Zastrow M. A cell biologist's perspective on physiological adaptation to opiate drugs. *Neuropharmacology.* 2004;47(suppl 1):286–292.

80. von Zastrow M, Svingos A, Haberstock-Debic H, Evans C. Regulated endocytosis of opioid receptors:

cellular mechanisms and proposed roles in physiological adaptation to opiate drugs. *Curr Opin Neurobiol.* 2003;13:348–353.

81. Vrinten DH, Gispen WH, Kalkman CJ, Adan RA. Interaction between the spinal melanocortin and opioid systems in a rat model of neuropathic pain. *Anesthesiology.* 2003;99:449–454.

82. Wei LN, Law PY, Loh HH. Post-transcriptional regulation of opioid receptors in the nervous system. *Front Biosci.* 2004;9:1665–1679.

83. Werawatganon T, Charuluxanun S. Patient controlled intravenous opioid analgesia versus continuous epidural analgesia for pain after intra-abdominal surgery. *Cochrane Database Syst Rev.* 2005;CD004088.

84. Wesson DR. Buprenorphine in the treatment of opiate dependence: its pharmacology and social context of use in the U.S. *J Psychoactive Drugs.* 2004;suppl 2:119–128.

85. Zadina JE. Isolation and distribution of endomorphins in the central nervous system. *Jpn J Pharmacol.* 2002; 89:203–208.

Chapter 15

Nonsteroidal Anti-Inflammatory Drugs

This chapter discusses a chemically diverse group of substances that exert several distinct pharmacologic properties. These properties include (1) the ability to decrease inflammation, (2) the ability to relieve mild-to-moderate pain (analgesia), (3) the ability to decrease elevated body temperature associated with fever (antipyresis), and (4) the ability to decrease blood clotting by inhibiting platelet aggregation (anticoagulation). These drugs are commonly referred to as nonsteroidal anti-inflammatory drugs (NSAIDs) to distinguish them from the glucocorticoids (i.e., the other main group of drugs used to treat inflammation). Obviously, the term NSAID does not fully describe these agent's pharmacologic actions; a more inclusive terminology should also mention the analgesic, antipyretic, and anticoagulant effects. However, these drugs are typically referred to as NSAIDs, and this terminology is used throughout this chapter.

Because of their analgesic and anti-inflammatory effects, patients receiving physical therapy often take NSAIDs for any number of problems. These drugs are a mainstay in the treatment of many types of mild-to-moderate pain, and NSAIDs are especially useful in treating pain and inflammation occurring in acute and chronic musculoskeletal disorders. Other patients are given NSAIDs to treat fever or to prevent excessive blood clotting. Consequently, physical therapists and other rehabilitation specialists will notice that these drugs are used quite frequently in their patient population, with the specific therapeutic goal related to each patient's individual needs.

Aspirin and Other NSAIDs: General Aspects

The best representative of an NSAID is aspirin (acetylsalicylic acid; Fig. 15–1). Newer NSAIDs are usually compared to aspirin in terms of efficacy and safety. Acetaminophen is another agent that is similar to aspirin and other NSAIDs in its ability to decrease pain and fever. Acetaminophen, however, is not considered an NSAID because it lacks anti-inflammatory and anticoagulant properties. For a discussion of the comparative effects of aspirin, newer NSAIDs, and acetaminophen, see "Comparison of Aspirin with Other NSAIDs."

For years, it was a mystery how a drug like aspirin could exert such a diverse range of therapeutic effects;

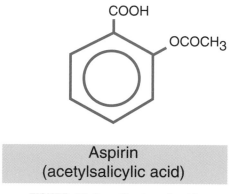

**Aspirin
(acetylsalicylic acid)**

FIGURE 15–1 ▼ Structure of aspirin.

that is, how could one drug influence so many different systems—effectively alleviating pain and inflammation, decreasing fever, and even affecting blood clotting? This issue was essentially resolved in the early 1970s, when aspirin was found to inhibit the synthesis of a group of endogenous compounds known collectively as the "prostaglandins." We now know that aspirin and the other NSAIDs exert most, if not all, of their therapeutic effects by interfering with the biosynthesis of prostaglandins and other related compounds.[37,91,103] To understand the way in which these drugs work, a brief discussion of prostaglandins and similar endogenously produced substances is presented.

Prostaglandins, Thromboxanes, and Leukotrienes

Prostaglandins are a group of lipidlike compounds that exhibit a wide range of physiologic activities.[37,48,68] With the exception of the red blood cell, virtually every type of living cell in the human body has been identified as being able to produce prostaglandins. These compounds appear to be hormones that act locally to help regulate cell function under normal and pathologic conditions. Other biologically active compounds known as the "thromboxanes" and "leukotrienes" are derived from the same precursor as the prostaglandins.[2,73,80] Together, the prostaglandins, thromboxanes, and leukotrienes are often referred to as eicosanoids because they all are derived from 20-carbon fatty acids that contain several double bonds.[66,73,88] (The term *eicosanoid* is derived from *eicosa*, meaning "20-carbon," and *enoic*, meaning "containing double bonds.")

Eicosanoid Biosynthesis

The biosynthetic pathway of prostaglandins and other eicosanoids is outlined in Figure 15–2. Basically, these compounds are derived from a 20-carbon essential fatty acid. In humans, this fatty acid is usually arachidonic acid,[68,73] which is ingested in the diet and stored as a phospholipid in the cell membrane. Thus, the cell has an abundant and easily accessible supply of this

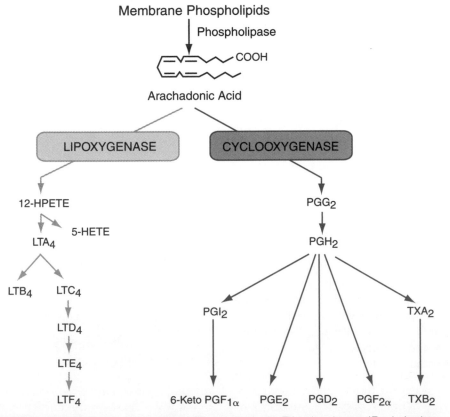

FIGURE 15–2 ▼ Eicosanoid biosynthesis. PG = prostaglandin; TX = thromboxane; LT = leukotriene.

precursor. When needed, arachidonic acid is cleaved from the cell membrane by a phospholipase enzyme (i.e., phospholipase A_2). The 20-carbon fatty acid can then be metabolized by several enzyme systems to generate a variety of biologically active compounds. One of the primary enzyme systems involves the cyclooxygenase (COX) enzyme, and a second system involves the lipoxygenase (LOX) enzyme. The prostaglandins and thromboxanes are ultimately synthesized from the cyclooxygenase pathway, and the leukotrienes come from the lipoxygenase system (see Fig. 15–2).[73]

Exactly which pathway is used in any particular cell depends on the type and quantity of enzymes in that cell, as well as its physiologic status. The end products within a given pathway (i.e., exactly which prostaglandins, thromboxanes, or leukotrienes will be formed) also depend on the individual cell. Any drug inhibiting one of these enzymes will also inhibit the formation of all of the subsequent products of that particular pathway. A drug that blocks the cyclooxygenase will essentially eliminate all prostaglandin and thromboxane synthesis in that cell. As this chapter will later discuss, aspirin and the other NSAIDs are cyclooxygenase inhibitors, which is the way that these drugs exert their therapeutic effects (see "Mechanism of NSAID Action: Inhibition of Prostaglandin and Thromboxane Synthesis").

Aspirin and other NSAIDs do not inhibit the lipoxygenase enzyme and thus do not appreciably decrease leukotriene synthesis.[73] Like the prostaglandins, leukotrienes are pro-inflammatory, but leukotrienes seem to be more important in mediating airway inflammation in conditions such as asthma and allergic rhinitis (see Chapter 26).[2,20] Drugs have therefore been developed to reduce leukotriene-mediated inflammation by either inhibiting the lipoxygenase enzyme (e.g., zileuton) or by blocking leukotriene receptors on respiratory tissues (e.g., montelukast and zafirlukast).[20,83] These antileukotriene drugs will be discussed in more detail in Chapter 26. The remainder of this chapter will focus on drugs that inhibit prostaglandin and thromboxane production by selectively inhibiting the cyclooxygenase enzyme.

Role of Eicosanoids in Health and Disease

The prostaglandins, thromboxanes, and leukotrienes have been shown to have a variety of effects on virtually every major physiologic system. Studies have indicated that these compounds can influence cardio-vascular, respiratory, renal, gastrointestinal, nervous, and reproductive function.[48,73] The biologic effects of the various eicosanoids cannot be generalized. Different classes of eicosanoids, and even different members within the same class, may exert various effects on the same system. For instance, certain prostaglandins such as the PGIs and PGEs tend to produce vasodilation in most vascular beds, whereas other prostaglandins (e.g., $PGF_{2\alpha}$) and the thromboxanes are often vasoconstrictors.[30,73,96] Some of the major effects of the eicosanoids are summarized in Table 15–1.

All of the effects of different prostaglandins, thromboxanes, and leukotrienes on various systems in the body cannot be reviewed in this chapter; this issue has been reviewed extensively elsewhere.[13,48,50,73,88] Of greater interest is the role of prostaglandins and related substances in pathologic conditions. In general, cells that are subjected to various types of trauma or disturbances in homeostasis tend to increase the production of prostaglandins.[50,73] This finding suggests that prostaglandins and other eicosanoids may be important in the protective response to cellular injury. In addition, prostaglandins are important in mediating some of the painful effects of injury and inflammation, as well as the symptoms of other pathologic conditions. Some of the better-documented conditions associated with excessive prostaglandin synthesis are listed here.

Inflammation. Increased prostaglandin synthesis is usually detected at the site of local inflammation.[21,66,73,101] Certain prostaglandins, such as PGE2, are thought to help mediate the local erythema and edema associated with inflammation by increasing local blood flow, increasing capillary permeability, and potentiating the permeability effects of histamine and bradykinin.[13,73] Leukotrienes, particularly LTB4, also contribute to the inflammatory response by increasing vascular permeability, and LTB4 has a potent chemotactic effect on polymorphonuclear leukocytes.[73,80]

Pain. Prostaglandins appear to help mediate painful stimuli in a variety of conditions (including inflammation). The compounds do not usually produce pain directly but are believed to increase the sensitivity of pain receptors to mechanical pressure and the effects of other pain-producing substances such as bradykinin.[73]

Fever. Prostaglandins appear to be pyretogenic; that is, they help produce the elevated body temperature during fever.[55] Although the details are somewhat unclear, prostaglandins produced in hypothalamic blood vessels may promote fever by altering the thermoregulatory set-point within the hypothalamus so

Table 15–1	PRIMARY PHYSIOLOGIC EFFECTS OF THE MAJOR CLASSES OF PROSTAGLANDINS, THROMBOXANES, AND LEUKOTRIENES					
Class	Vascular Smooth Muscle	Airway Smooth Muscle	Gastrointestinal Smooth Muscle	Gastrointestinal Secretions	Uterine Muscle (Nonpregnant)	Platelet Aggregation
PGAs	Vasodilation	—	—	Decrease	Relaxation	—
PGEs	Vasodilation	Bronchodilation	Contraction	Decrease	Relaxation	Variable
PGIs	Vasodilation	—	Relaxation	Decrease	—	Decrease
PGFs	Variable	Bronchoconstriction	Contraction	—	Contraction	—
TXA_2	Vasoconstriction	Bronchoconstriction	—	—	—	Increase
LTs	Vasoconstriction	Bronchoconstriction	Contraction	—	—	—

PGs = prostaglandins, TXs = thromboxanes, LTs = leukotrienes.

that body temperature is maintained at a higher level.[10] Alternatively, prostaglandin production may promote fever by stimulating vagal afferent neurons that originate peripherally near the diaphragm.[10] Regardless of their exact mechanism, prostaglandins clearly play a role in promoting fever associated with systemic infection and other pyretogenic disorders.[55]

Dysmenorrhea. The painful cramps that accompany menstruation in some women have been attributed at least in part to increased prostaglandin production in the endometrium of the uterus.[56,70]

Thrombus Formation. The thromboxanes, especially TXA_2, cause platelet aggregations that result in blood clot formation.[73] It is unclear whether excessive thrombus formation (as in deep vein thrombosis or coronary artery occlusion) is initiated by abnormal thromboxane production. Certainly, inhibition of thromboxane synthesis will help prevent platelet-induced thrombus formation in individuals who are prone to specific types of excessive blood clotting.[84]

Other Pathologies. Because of their many varied physiologic effects, the eicosanoids are involved in a number of other pathologic conditions. Prostaglandins have been implicated in cardiovascular disorders (hypertension), neoplasms (colon cancer), respiratory dysfunction (asthma), neurologic disorders (multiple sclerosis, allergic encephalomyelitis, affective disorders), endocrine dysfunction (Bartter syndrome, diabetes mellitus), and a variety of other problems.[7,17,40,77,93,110] The exact role of prostaglandins and the other eicosanoids in various diseases continues to be evaluated, and the role of these compounds in health and disease has become clearer with ongoing research.

Mechanism of NSAID Action: Inhibition of Prostaglandin and Thromboxane Synthesis

Aspirin and the other NSAIDs are all potent inhibitors of the cyclooxygenase enzyme.[37,84,91,103] Because cyclooxygenase represents the first step in the synthesis of prostaglandins and thromboxanes, drugs that inhibit this enzyme in any given cell will block the production of all prostaglandins and thromboxanes in that cell. Considering that prostaglandins and thromboxanes are implicated in producing pain, inflammation, fever, and excessive blood clotting, virtually all of the therapeutic effects of aspirin and similar drugs can be explained by their ability to inhibit the synthesis of these two eicosanoid classes.[103]

The cyclooxygenase or COX enzyme system is therefore the key site of NSAID action within the cell. It is now realized, however, that there are at least two primary subtypes (isozymes) of the COX enzyme: COX-1 and COX-2.[24,37,103] The COX-1 enzyme is a normal constituent in certain cells, and prostaglandins synthesized by COX-1 are typically responsible for mediating normal cell activity and maintaining homeostasis. For example, COX-1 enzymes located in the stomach mucosa synthesize prostaglandins that help protect the stomach lining from gastric acid, and COX-1 enzymes in the kidneys produce beneficial prostaglandins that help maintain renal function, especially when kidney function is compromised.[27,46,95] COX-1 is also the enzyme responsible for synthesizing prostaglandins and thromboxanes regulating normal platelet activity.[73]

The COX-2 enzyme, however, seems to be produced primarily in injured cells; that is, other chemical mediators (**cytokines**, growth factors) induce the injured cell to synthesize the COX-2 enzyme, and this enzyme then produces prostaglandins that mediate pain and other aspects of the inflammatory response.[19,61,84] There is also considerable evidence that the COX-2 form is responsible for producing prostaglandins in other pathological conditions such as colorectal cancer.[62,100]

The roles of COX-1 and COX-2 enzymes therefore seem quite different. The COX-1 enzyme is a "normal" cell component that synthesizes prostaglandins to help regulate and maintain cell activity. COX-2 represents an "emergency" enzyme that often synthesizes prostaglandins in response to cell injury (i.e., pain and inflammation). This difference has important implications for how NSAIDs exert their therapeutic effects and side effects. Aspirin and most of the traditional NSAIDs are nonselective—they inhibit both the COX-1 and COX-2 enzymes. These nonselective NSAIDs therefore cause primary beneficial effects (decreased pain and inflammation) by inhibiting the COX-2 enzyme. Because these drugs also inhibit the COX-1 enzyme, they also decrease the production of the beneficial and protective prostaglandins. It is the loss of these beneficial prostaglandins that accounts for the primary side effects of the NSAIDs; that is, loss of protective prostaglandins in the stomach and kidneys result in gastric damage and decreased renal function, respectively.

It follows that drugs selectively inhibiting the COX-2 enzyme offer certain advantages over aspirin and nonselective NSAIDs. Selective COX-2 inhibitors should decrease the production of prostaglandins that mediate pain and inflammation while sparing the synthesis of protective prostaglandins that are synthesized by COX-1. Such COX-2 selective drugs are currently available, and their pharmacology is addressed later in this chapter.

Aspirin: Prototypical NSAID

Acetylsalicylic acid, or aspirin, as it is commonly known (see Fig. 15–1), represents the major form of a group of drugs known as the salicylates. Other salicylates (sodium salicylate, choline salicylate) are used clinically, but aspirin is the most frequently used and appears to have the widest range of therapeutic effects. Because aspirin has been used clinically for more than 100 years, is inexpensive, and is readily available without prescription, many individuals may be under the impression that this drug is only a marginally effective therapeutic agent. On the contrary, aspirin is a very powerful and effective drug that should be considered a major medicine.[84] As discussed previously, aspirin is a potent inhibitor of all cyclooxygenase activity (COX-1 and COX-2), and thus it has the potential to affect a number of conditions involving excessive prostaglandin and thromboxane production.

Aspirin is the oldest and most widely used NSAID, and other NSAIDs are compared with aspirin in terms of efficacy and safety. Hence, this discussion focuses primarily on the clinical applications of aspirin and the problems typically associated with aspirin. For the most part, clinical use and problems can also be applied to most nonaspirin NSAIDs. The major similarities and differences between aspirin and the other NSAIDs are discussed in "Comparison of Aspirin with Other NSAIDs."

Clinical Applications of Aspirinlike Drugs

Treatment of Pain and Inflammation

Aspirin and other NSAIDs are effective in treating mild-to-moderate pain of various origins, including headache, toothache, and diffuse muscular aches and soreness. Aspirin appears to be especially useful in treating pain and inflammation in musculoskeletal and joint disorders.[71,87,89] The safe and effective use of aspirin in both rheumatoid arthritis and osteoarthritis is well documented (see Chapter 16).[53,66,84] Aspirin is also recommended for treating the pain and cramping associated with primary dysmenorrhea.[70]

Aspirin and aspirinlike drugs are also used to manage pain following certain types of surgery, including arthroscopic surgery.[15,16] These drugs can serve as the primary analgesic following other types of minor or intermediate surgeries, and they can be used after extensive surgery to decrease the need for high doses of other drugs such as opioids.[12,69] Ketorolac tromethamine (Toradol), for example, is a relatively new NSAID that has shown exceptional promise in treating postoperative pain. This drug can be given orally or by intramuscular injection, and it is reported to provide analgesic effects similar to opioid drugs (e.g., morphine) but without the associated side effects and risks.[26,69] Hence, ketorolac tromethamine provides a reasonable alternative for nonopioid management of postoperative pain and may be especially valuable when opioid side effects (sedation, respiratory depression) are harmful or undesirable.[12,26]

Treatment of Fever

Although the use of aspirin in treating fever in children is contraindicated (because of the association with Reye syndrome; see "Problems and Adverse Effects of Aspirinlike Drugs"), aspirin remains the primary NSAID used in treating fever in adults.[9] Ibuprofen is also used frequently as a nonprescription antipyretic NSAID in both adults and children.

Treatment of Vascular Disorders

As discussed previously, aspirin inhibits platelet-induced thrombus formation through its ability to inhibit thromboxane biosynthesis. Aspirin has therefore been used to help prevent the onset or recurrence of heart attacks in some individuals by inhibiting thrombus formation in the coronary arteries.[97,109] Similarly, daily aspirin use may help prevent transient ischemic attacks and stroke by preventing cerebral infarction in certain patients.[97,109] The role of aspirin in treating coagulation disorders is discussed in more detail in Chapter 25

Prevention of Cancer

There is now considerable evidence that regular aspirin use decreases the risk of colorectal cancer.[1,49,58] It has been estimated, for example, that people who use aspirin on a regular basis have a 40 to 50 percent lower risk of fatal colon cancer as compared with people who do not use aspirin.[78] Aspirin might also help prevent other types of cancers (e.g., skin, bladder, prostate can-

cers), but beneficial effects in these other cancers requires additional study.[3,74] It appears that certain prostaglandins help promote tumor growth and that aspirin and similar NSAIDs exert anticancer effects by inhibiting the synthesis of these prostaglandins.[17,78] Hence, aspirin continues to gain acceptance as an anticancer drug, especially in individuals who are at an increased risk for developing colon cancer.

Problems and Adverse Effects of Aspirinlike Drugs

Gastrointestinal Problems

The primary problem with all NSAIDs, including aspirin, is gastrointestinal damage. Problems ranging from minor stomach discomfort to variable amounts of upper gastrointestinal hemorrhage and ulceration are fairly common.[38,67] These effects are most likely caused by the loss of protective prostaglandins from the mucosal lining. Certain prostaglandins such as PGI_2 and PGE_2 are produced locally in the stomach, and these prostaglandins help protect the gastric mucosa by inhibiting gastric acid secretion, increasing the production of mucous in the stomach lining, and maintaining blood flow to the gastric mucosa.[84] By inhibiting the formation of these protective prostaglandins, aspirin and most traditional NSAIDs render the stomach more susceptible to damage from acidic gastric juices.[79]

Certain patients are likewise more susceptible to gastrointestinal injury from aspirinlike drugs. Factors such as advanced age, a history of ulcers, use of multiple NSAIDs, use of high doses of an NSAID, and use of other agents (anti-inflammatory steroids, anticoagulants) appear to increase the risk of serious gastrointestinal damage.[81] Helicobacter pylori, a bacterium that is sometimes present in the stomach (see Chapter 27), can also contribute to the increased risk of gastric irritation associated with NSAIDs.[4,23]

Several pharmacologic and nonpharmacologic strategies have been employed to manage gastrointestinal problems associated with aspirinlike drugs. One strategy has been to coat the aspirin tablet so that dissolution and release of the drug is delayed until it reaches the small intestine. These so-called enteric-coated forms of aspirin spare the stomach from irritation, but the duodenum and upper small intestine may still be subjected to damage.[38] Enteric-coated aspirin also has the disadvantage of delaying the onset of analgesic effects to relieve acute pain. Other methods such as buffering the aspirin tablet have also been used to help decrease stomach irritation. The rationale is that including a chemical buffer helps blunt the acidic effects of the aspirin molecule on the stomach mucosa. It is questionable, however, whether sufficient buffer is added to commercial aspirin preparations to actually make a difference in stomach irritation. During chronic aspirin therapy (e.g., treatment of arthritis), taking aspirin with meals may help decrease gastrointestinal irritation because the food in the stomach will offer some direct protection of the gastric mucosa. The presence of food, however, will also delay drug absorption, which may decrease the peak levels of drug that reach the bloodstream.

Recently, a great deal of attention has focused on other drugs that can prevent or treat the gastrointestinal side effects associated with aspirin and the other NSAIDs. Misoprostol (Cytotec) is a prostaglandin E_1 analog that inhibits gastric acid secretion and prevents gastric damage.[23,43] This drug has been beneficial in decreasing aspirin-induced irritation, but the clinical use of misoprostol is limited by side effects such as diarrhea.[43] Omeprazole (Prilosec), esomeprazole (Nexium), and lansoprazole (Prevacid) are drugs that inhibit the "proton pump" that is ultimately responsible for secreting gastric acid from mucosal cells into the lumen of the stomach (see Chapter 27). These proton pump inhibitors have therefore been used successfully to increase healing and decrease NSAID-induced ulcers.[34,43] Drugs that antagonize certain histamine receptors—that is, the H_2 receptor blockers—have also been used to decrease gastrointestinal damage.[43] As indicated in Chapter 27, histamine receptor (H_2) blockers such as cimetidine (Tagamet) and ranitidine (Zantac) inhibit gastric acid secretion by antagonizing histamine receptors in the gastric mucosa. These drugs are tolerated quite well but are generally not as effective in controlling NSAID-induced ulceration as other drugs such as misoprostol and proton pump inhibitors.[54]

Hence, currently available drugs such as misoprostol, proton pump inhibitors, and H_2 receptor blockers can be used to prevent or treat gastrointestinal damage in patients taking aspirin and other NSAIDs. These protective agents are not usually prescribed to every person taking aspirinlike drugs but are typically reserved for people who exhibit symptoms of gastrointestinal irritation or who are at risk for developing ulceration while undergoing NSAID therapy.[64]

COX-2 selective drugs comprise an alternative strategy for reducing the risk of gastric irritation. As indicated earlier, the COX-1 enzyme is responsible for synthesizing prostaglandins that help protect the stomach lining, whereas the COX-2 form synthesizes prostaglandins that promote pain, inflammation, and other pathological symptoms. A COX-2 drug is therefore more likely to inhibit production of the pathological prostaglandins, while sparing the production of beneficial prostaglandins in the stomach.[34,43] Indeed, COX-2 drugs are generally associated with a reduced incidence of gastric irritation.[4,25,54,57] Still, certain people can experience gastric problems with COX-2 drugs, and these drugs may produce other serious side effects. The risks and benefits of COX-2 drugs are addressed in more detail later in this chapter.

Other Side Effects

Aspirin and similar NSAIDs can cause other toxic side effects if used improperly or if taken by patients who have preexisting diseases. For instance, serious hepatotoxicity is rare with normal therapeutic use, but high doses of aspirinlike drugs can produce adverse changes in hepatic function in patients with liver disease.[85,99] Likewise, aspirin does not seem to cause renal disease in an individual with normal kidneys,[84] but problems such as nephrotic syndrome, acute interstitial nephritis, and even acute renal failure have been observed when aspirin is given to patients with impaired renal function, or people with decreased body water (volume depletion).[35,102]

Aspirinlike drugs appear to cause renal and hepatic problems by inhibiting the synthesis of prostaglandins that serve a protective role in maintaining blood flow and function in the liver and kidneys.[36,84] These protective prostaglandins appear to be important in sustaining adequate hepatic and renal function, especially when blood flow and perfusion pressure to these organs becomes compromised. Consequently, aspirin and aspirinlike drugs may create problems in other conditions such as hypovolemia, shock, hepatic cirrhosis, congestive heart failure, and hypertension.[36,84,102]

In cases of aspirin overdose, a condition known as aspirin intoxication or poisoning may occur. This event is usually identified by a number of symptoms, including headache, tinnitus, difficulty hearing, confusion, and gastrointestinal distress. More severe cases also result in metabolic acidosis and dehydration, which can be life-threatening. In adults, a dose of 10 to 30 g of aspirin is sometimes fatal, although much higher doses (130 g in one documented case) have been ingested without causing death.[84] Of course, much smaller doses can produce fatalities in children.

Evidence has suggested that aspirin may also be associated with a relatively rare condition known as Reye syndrome.[22] This condition occurs in children and teenagers, usually following a bout of influenza or chicken pox. Reye syndrome is marked by a high fever, vomiting, liver dysfunction, and increasing unresponsiveness, often progressing rapidly and leading to delirium, convulsions, coma, and possibly death. Because aspirin is one factor that may contribute to Reye syndrome, it is recommended that aspirin and other aspirinlike drugs not be used to treat fever in children and teenagers.[84] Nonaspirin antipyretics such as acetaminophen and ibuprofen are not associated with Reye syndrome, so products containing these drugs are preferred for treating fever in children and teenagers.[84]

A small number of individuals exhibit aspirin intolerance or supersensitivity.[84] These individuals comprise approximately 1 percent of the general population, but the incidence is considerably higher (10%–25%) in people with asthma or other hypersensitivity reactions.[84,94] People with aspirin intolerance will display allergiclike reactions, including acute bronchospasm, urticaria, and severe rhinitis, within a few hours after taking aspirin and aspirinlike NSAIDs.[45,76] These reactions may be quite severe, and cardiovascular shock may occur. Likewise, sensitivity to aspirin often indicates a concomitant sensitivity to other NSAIDs, including COX-2 selective drugs.[92] Consequently, the use of all NSAIDs is contraindicated in these individuals.[84]

Finally, there is preliminary evidence that aspirin and other commonly used NSAIDs may inhibit healing of certain tissues. In particular, it has been suggested that these drugs may inhibit bone healing after fracture and certain types of surgery (spinal fusion).[47,98] It seems that certain prostaglandins are important in stimulating the early stages of bone formation following fracture or bone surgery.[42] By inhibiting the synthesis of these prostaglandins, NSAIDS may retard bone healing and delay the formation of new bone.[47] Much of this evidence, however, is based on laboratory studies on animal models, and a definitive link between NSAIDs (including COX-2 drugs) and delayed bone healing in humans remains to be determined.[18,106] Still, some experts feel that it might be prudent to avoid the use of NSAIDs immediately following fracture or bone surgery.[31,98] More details are needed to determine if traditional NSAIDs and COX-2 selective agents are detrimental to bone heal-

ing in clinical situations, and whether these drugs should be avoided for a certain period following fracture or spinal surgery.

The effect of NSAIDs on healing of soft tissues is likewise uncertain. It was originally suggested that NSAIDs might inhibit the synthesis and transport of connective tissue components such as proteoglycans.[29,51] More recent findings indicate that NSAIDs may actually facilitate the incorporation of proteoglycans, hylauronan, and other components into soft tissues.[8] As such, NSAIDs may enhance the healing of soft tissues in certain conditions.[31] Once again, much of this evidence was obtained from animal and *in vitro* studies, and additional research will therefore be needed to determine if aspirin and other NSAIDs can affect the healing process of articular cartilage and other soft tissues.

Comparison of Aspirin with Other NSAIDs

A number of drugs that bear a functional similarity to aspirin have been developed during the past several decades, and a comprehensive list of currently available NSAIDs is shown in Table 15–2. Other NSAIDs are like aspirin in that they exert their therapeutic effects by inhibiting prostaglandin and thromboxane synthesis. Although specifically approved uses of individual members of this group vary, NSAIDs are used in much the same way as aspirin; that is, they are administered primarily for their analgesic and anti-inflammatory effects, with some members also used as antipyretic and anticoagulant agents. Dosages commonly used to achieve analgesic or anti-inflammatory effects with some of the more common NSAIDs are listed in Table 15–3.

With respect to therapeutic effects, there is no clear evidence that any of the commonly used NSAIDs are markedly better than aspirin as anti-inflammatory analgesics.[87] The primary differences between aspirin and other NSAIDs are related to the side effects and safety profile of each agent (see Table 15–2).[84] As a group, the nonaspirin NSAIDs tend to be associated with less gastrointestinal discomfort than plain aspirin, but most of these NSAIDs (with the possible exception of the COX-2 drugs; see later) are still associated with some degree of stomach irritation (Table 15–2).[72,87] Likewise, certain NSAIDs may offer an advantage over aspirin or other aspirinlike drugs because they are

Table 15–2	COMMON NONSTEROIDAL ANTI-INFLAMMATORY DRUGS	
Generic Name	**Trade Name(s)**	**Specific Comments—Comparison to Other NSAIDs**
Aspirin	Many trade names	Most widely used NSAID for analgesic and anti-inflammatory effects; also used frequently for antipyretic and anticoagulant effects.
Diclofenac	Voltaren	Substantially more potent than naproxen and several other NSAIDs; adverse side effects occur in 20% of patients.
Diflunisal	Dolobid	Has potency 3–4 times greater than aspirin in terms of analgesic and anti-inflammatory effects but lacks antipyretic activity.
Etodolac	Lodine	Effective as analgesic/anti-inflammatory agent with fewer side effects than most NSAIDs; may have gastric-sparing properties.
Fenoprofen	Nalfon	GI side effects fairly common but usually less intense than those occurring with similar doses of aspirin.
Flurbiprofen	Ansaid	Similar to aspirin's benefits and side effects; also available as topical ophthalmic preparation (Ocufen).
Ibuprofen	Motrin, many others	First nonaspirin NSAID also available in nonprescription form; fewer GI side effects than aspirin but GI effects still occur in 5%–15% of patients.
Indomethacin	Indocin	Relative high incidence of dose-related side effects; problems occur in 25%–50% of patients.
Ketoprofen	Orudis, Oruvail, others	Similar to aspirin's benefits and side effects but has relatively short half-life (1–2 hours).
Ketorolac	Toradol	Can be administered orally or by intramuscular injection; parenteral doses provide postoperative analgesia equivalent to opioids.
Meclofenamate	Meclomen	No apparent advantages or disadvantages compared to aspirin and other NSAIDs.
Mefanamic acid	Ponstel	No advantages; often less effective and more toxic than aspirin and other NSAIDs.
Nabumetone	Relafen	Effective as analgesic/anti-inflammatory agent with fewer side effects than most NSAIDs.
Naproxen	Anaprox, Naprosyn, others	Similar to ibuprofen in terms of benefits and adverse effects
Oxaprozin	Daypro	Analgesic and anti-inflammatory effects similar to aspirin; may produce fewer side effects than other NSAIDs.
Phenylbutazone	Cotylbutazone	Potent anti-inflammatory effects but long-term use limited by high incidence of side effects (10%–45% of patients).
Piroxicam	Feldene	Long half-life (45 hours) allows once-daily dosing; may be somewhat better tolerated than aspirin.

(Continued on following page)

Table 15–2	COMMON NONSTEROIDAL ANTI-INFLAMMATORY DRUGS *(Continued)*	
Generic Name	**Trade Name(s)**	**Specific Comments—Comparison to Other NSAIDs**
Sulindac	Clinoril	Relatively little effect on kidneys (renal-sparing), but may produce more GI side effects than aspirin.
Tolmetin	Tolectin	Similar to aspirin's benefits and side effects but must be given frequently (QID) because of short half-life (1 hour).

NSAID = nonsteroidal anti-inflammatory drugs, GI = gastrointestinal

Table 15–3	DOSAGES OF COMMON ORAL NSAIDs	
	Dosages (According to Desired Effect)	
Drug	**Analgesia**	**Anti-inflammation**
Aspirin (many trade names)	325–650 mg every 4 hr	3.6–5.4 g/d in divided doses
Diclofenac (Voltaren)	Up to 100 mg for the first dose; then up to 50 mg TID thereafter	Initially: 150–200 mg/d in 3–4 divided doses; try to reduce to 75–100 mg/d in 3 divided doses
Diflunisal (Dolobid)	1 g initially; 500 mg every 8–12 hr as needed	250–500 mg BID
Etodolac (Lodine)	400 mg initially; 200–400 mg every 6–8 hours as needed	400 mg BID or TID or 300 mg TID or QID; total daily dose is typically between 600–1200 mg/d
Fenoprofen (Nalfon)	200 mg every 4–6 hr	300–600 mg TID or QID
Flurbiprofen (Ansaid)	–	200–300 mg/d in 2–4 divided doses
Ibuprofen (Advil, Motrin, Nuprin, others)	200–400 mg every 4–6 hr as needed	1.2–3.2 g/d in 3–4 divided doses
Indomethacin (Indocin)	–	25–50 mg 2–4 times each day initially; can be increased up to 200 mg/d as tolerated
Ketoprofen (Orudis)	25–50 mg every 6–8 hr	150–300 mg/d in 3–4 divided doses
Meclofenamate (Meclomen)	50 mg every 4–6 hr	200–400 mg/d in 3–4 divided doses
Mefenamic acid (Ponstel)	500 mg initially; 250 mg every 6 hr as needed	–
Nabumetone (Relafen)	–	Initially: 1000 mg/d in a single dose or 2 divided doses. Can be increased to 1500–2000 mg/d in 2 divided doses if needed

Drug	Analgesia	Anti-inflammation
Naproxen (Naprosyn)	500 mg initially; 250 mg every 6–8 hr	250, 375, or 500 mg BID
Naproxen sodium (Aleve, Anaprox, others)	500–650 mg initially; 275 mg every 6–8 hr	275 or 550 mg BID
Oxaprozin (Daypro)	–	Initially: 1200 mg/d, then adjust to patient tolerance
Phenylbutazone (Butazolidin, Cotylbutazone)	–	300–600 mg/d in 3–4 divided doses initially; reduce as tolerated to lowest effective dose
Piroxicam (Feldene)	–	20 mg/d single dose; or 10 mg BID
Sulindac (Clinoril)	–	150 or 200 mg BID
Tolmetin (Tolectin)	–	400 mg TID initially; 600 mg–1.8 g/day in 3–4 divided doses

less toxic to other organs such as the liver and kidneys. The effect on these other organs, however, seems to be related more to the status of each patient rather than the drug. That is, all NSAIDs, including aspirin, are relatively safe in people with normal liver and kidney function when administered at moderate dosages for a short period of time.[84] A specific patient may also respond more favorably to a specific NSAID in terms of therapeutic effects (decreased pain, inflammation), but these responses are due to patient variability rather than a unique characteristic of the drug. Hence, it cannot be generalized that the non-aspirin NSAIDs are significantly better or worse than aspirin in terms of either therapeutic or adverse effects.[84]

The primary difference between aspirin and other NSAIDs is cost. Most of the NSAIDs still require a physician's prescription. The cost of prescription NSAIDs can be anywhere from 10 to 20 times more expensive than an equivalent supply of aspirin. NSAIDs that are available in nonprescription form (e.g., ibuprofen) can still cost up to five times as much as aspirin.

Consequently, the newer NSAIDs have not always been shown to be clinically superior to aspirin, but some agents may provide better effects in some patients. Considering the interpatient variability in drug response, there are surely cases in which another NSAID will produce better therapeutic effects with fewer side effects than aspirin.[108] If a patient responds equally well to a variety of NSAIDs, however, efforts should be made to use the NSAID that will produce adequate therapeutic effects at a minimal cost.[84]

COX-2 Selective Drugs

As discussed earlier, the cyclooxygenase enzyme that synthesizes prostaglandins exists in at least two forms: COX-1 and COX-2.[24,37,103] Aspirin and most other NSAIDs are nonselective cyclooxygenase inhibitors; that is, they inhibit both the COX-1 and COX-2 forms of the cyclooxygenase. This nonselective inhibition results in decreased synthesis of prostaglandins that cause pain and inflammation (COX-2 prostaglandins), as well as loss of prostaglandins that are protective and beneficial to tissues such as the stomach lining and kidneys (COX-1 prostaglandins). Recently, drugs have been developed that are selective for the COX-2 enzyme, hence the name COX-2 inhibitors. COX-2 selective drugs such as celecoxib (Celebrex) offer the obvious advantage of inhibiting synthesis of the inflammatory prostaglandins, while sparing synthesis of beneficial prostaglandins that help regulate normal physiologic function.[37,103]

It follows that use of COX-2 selective drugs should decrease pain and inflammation with minimal or no adverse effects on the stomach and other tissues. The burden of evidence indicates that this fact is indeed true; that is, COX-2 drugs have analgesic and anti-inflammatory effects similar to other NSAIDs, but have a much lower incidence of gastric irritation.[33,41] Likewise, COX-2 drugs do not inhibit platelet function because prostaglandins influencing normal platelet activity are under the control of the COX-1 isozyme.[73] Use of COX-2 drugs should therefore be beneficial in people who are at risk for prolonged bleeding and hemorrhage.

COX-2 drugs represent an important addition to the NSAID armamentarium. Although these drugs are not necessarily more effective in reducing pain and inflammation, they may avoid the gastritis associated with aspirin and other NSAIDs. The COX-2 drugs are not devoid of side effects, of course, and they may increase the risk of upper respiratory tract infections. Even though these drugs are purportedly easier on the stomach than traditional NSAIDs, certain patients may still experience **gastrointestinal (GI)** problems such as diarrhea, heartburn, stomach cramps, and upper GI bleeding. Nonetheless, COX-2 drugs offer an alternative to more traditional NSAIDs, and COX-2 agents may be especially useful to patients who cannot tolerate aspirin or other NSAIDs because of gastric irritation or other side effects with aspirin and the more traditional NSAIDs typically associated.[33]

COX-2 Drugs and the Risk of Heart Attack and Stroke

The primary concern about COX-2 drugs is that certain patients taking specific agents may have an increased risk of serious cardiovascular events such as heart attack and stroke.[14,75] By inhibiting the COX-2 form of the enzyme, these drugs inadvertently impair the production of prostacyclin, a prostaglandin that promotes vasodilation and prevents platelet-induced occlusion in the coronary and carotid arteries.[32,63] Simultaneously, these drugs do not inhibit the production of thromboxane from the COX-1 enzyme, and thromboxane is a prostaglandin that facilitates platelet aggregation and clot formation.[39] The balance of prostaglandin production is therefore shifted to favor increased platelet activity and an increased risk of clots in the coronary and carotid arteries in susceptible individuals.[6]

Thus, people who are prone to coronary ischemia or carotid occlusion may be at risk for heart attack or ischemic stroke when taking these COX-2 selective drugs. This finding was the primary reason that certain COX-2 drugs such as rofecoxib (Vioxx) and valdecoxib (Bextra) were taken off the market. On the other hand, there is growing evidence that the risk of heart attack and stroke may be acceptable if COX-2 drugs are used appropriately.[90,105,107] That is, patients must be screened carefully to determine individuals who are at risk for coronary or carotid ischemia.[28,60] Dosages must likewise be kept to a minimum to prevent untoward cardiovascular events.

At the time of this writing, celecoxib (Celebrex) is the only COX-2 selective drug that is still available. It will be interesting to see if new COX-2 drugs can be developed that have an acceptable cardiovascular risk profile. Likewise, efforts continue to clearly identify patients who should not take these drugs because of an increased risk for heart attack or ischemic stroke.

Acetaminophen

Acetaminophen (known also as paracetamol) has several distinct differences from aspirin and the other NSAIDs. Acetaminophen does appear to be equal to aspirin and NSAIDs in terms of analgesic and antipyretic effects, but it does not have any appreciable anti-inflammatory or anticoagulant effects.[44,84] One major advantage of acetaminophen is that this drug is not associated with upper gastrointestinal tract irritation.[82] Consequently, acetaminophen has been used widely in the treatment of noninflammatory conditions associated with mild-to-moderate pain and in patients who have a history of gastric damage (such as ulcers). Acetaminophen is, for example, often the first drug used to control pain in the early stages of osteoarthritis and other musculoskeletal conditions that do not have an inflammatory component.[5,104,111] In addition, Reye syndrome has not been implicated with acetaminophen use, so this drug is often used in treating fever in children and teenagers.[82]

The mechanism of action of acetaminophen is not fully understood. Acetaminophen does inhibit the cyclooxygenase enzyme, and its analgesic and antipyretic effects are probably mediated through prostaglandin inhibition. Why acetaminophen fails to exert anti-inflammatory and anticoagulant effects, however, is unclear. One explanation is that acetaminophen preferentially inhibits **central nervous system (CNS)** prostaglandin production but has little effect on peripheral cyclooxygenase activity.[10,44] This specific effect on central prostaglandins has generated the theory that a third subset of cyclooxygenase enzymes known as the COX-3 variant exists in the CNS, and that acetaminophen may be somewhat selective for this COX-3 subtype.[11] The existence and functional role of such a COX-3 enzyme, however, remains to be fully determined. Nonetheless, acetaminophen's analgesic and antipyretic effects are produced by specifically limiting prostaglandin production in central pain interpretation and thermoregulatory centers, respectively. Tissue inflammation and platelet aggregation would be peripheral events unaffected by acetaminophen, according to this theory.

Hence, acetaminophen is a very important and useful medication in the treatment of fever and mild to moderate pain. The fact that acetaminophen does not cause gastric irritation might also give users the false impression that it is a totally innocuous drug devoid of all adverse effects. On the contrary, high doses of acetaminophen (e.g., 15 g) can be especially toxic to the liver and may be fatal because of hepatic necrosis.[59,65,82] Normally, acetaminophen is metabolized in the liver via a series of reactions illustrated in Figure 15–3. In the liver, acetaminophen is converted initially into a highly reactive intermediate by-product known as **N-*acetyl-p*-benzoquinoneimine (NAPQI)**. This intermediate by-product is quickly detoxified by coupling it with **glutathione (GHS)** to create a final, nonreactive by-product (mercapturic acid) that is sent to the kidneys for excretion. At moderate doses, these reactions occur rapidly so that NAPQI does not accumulate within the liver. At high doses, however, the conversion of NAPQI to mercapturic acid is delayed, resulting in the accumulation of NAPQI. In sufficient amounts, this metabolite induces hepatic necrosis by binding to and inactivating certain liver proteins.[52] Likewise, previous damage to the liver may impair the ability of this organ to convert NAPQI to mercapturic acid, thus resulting in accumulation and damage even at relatively low doses. Hence, people with pre-existing liver disease or individuals who are chronic alcohol abusers may be particularly susceptible to liver damage caused by high doses of acetaminophen.[84,86]

Pharmacokinetics of NSAIDs and Acetaminophen

Aspirin is absorbed readily from the stomach and small intestine. Approximately 80 to 90 percent of aspirin remains bound to plasma proteins such as albumin. The remaining 10 to 20 percent is widely distributed throughout the body. The unbound or free drug exerts

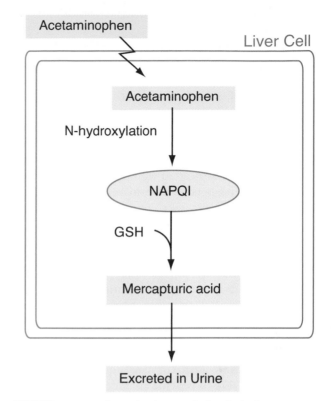

FIGURE 15–3 ▼ Acetaminophen metabolism. In the liver, acetaminophen is metabolized to a toxic intermediate **N-acetyl-p-benzoquinoneimine (NAPQI)**. NAPQI is quickly detoxified by conjugation with **glutathione (GSH)**, forming mercapturic acid, which is eliminated via the urine. High doses of acetaminophen or liver dysfunction can result in accumulation of NAPQI and subsequent toxicity to liver proteins.

the therapeutic effects. Aspirin itself (acetylsalicylic acid) is hydrolyzed to an active metabolite—salicylic acid. This biotransformation occurs primarily in the bloodstream, and the salicylic acid is further metabolized by oxidation or conjugation in the liver. Excretion of salicylic acid and its metabolites occurs through the kidneys. Although there is some pharmacokinetic variability within the nonaspirin NSAIDs, these drugs generally follow a pattern of absorption, protein binding, metabolism, and excretion similar to that of aspirin.

Acetaminophen is also absorbed rapidly and completely from the upper gastrointestinal tract. Plasma protein binding with acetaminophen is highly variable (20 to 50 percent) but is considerably less than with aspirin. As indicated earlier in this chapter, metabolism of acetaminophen occurs in the liver via conjugation with an endogenous substrate (glutathione), and the conjugated metabolites are excreted through the kidneys.

Special Concerns in Rehabilitation Patients

■ ■ ■ Aspirin and the other NSAIDs are among the most frequently used drugs in the rehabilitation population. Aside from the possibility of stomach discomfort, these drugs have a remarkable lack of adverse effects that could directly interfere with physical and occupational therapy. When used for various types of musculoskeletal pain and inflammation, these drugs can often provide analgesia without sedation and psychomimetic (hallucinogenic, etc.) effects that are associated with opioid (narcotic) analgesics. Thus, the therapy session can be conducted with the benefit of pain relief but without the loss of patient attentiveness and concentration. In inflammatory conditions, NSAIDs can be used for prolonged periods without the serious side effects associated with steroidal drugs (see Chapters 16 and 29). Of course, the limitation of NSAIDs is that they may not be as effective in moderate-to-severe pain or in severe, progressive inflammation. Still, these agents are a beneficial adjunct in many painful conditions and can usually help facilitate physical rehabilitation by relieving pain. The other clinical uses of these drugs (antipyresis, anticoagulation) may also be encountered in some patients, and these effects are also usually achieved with a minimum of adverse effects.

Acetaminophen is also frequently employed for pain relief in many physical rehabilitation patients. Remember that this drug is equal to an NSAID in analgesic properties, but lacks anti-inflammatory effects. Because both aspirin and acetaminophen are available without prescription, a patient may inquire about the differences between these two drugs. Clinicians should be able to provide an adequate explanation of the differential effects of aspirin and acetaminophen but should also remember that the suggested use of these agents should ultimately come from a physician.

CASE STUDY

Nonsteroidal Anti-Inflammatory Drugs

Brief History. D.B., a 38-year-old man, began to develop pain in his right shoulder. He was employed as a carpenter and had recently been working rather long hours building a new house. The increasing pain required medical attention. A physician evaluated the patient, and a diagnosis of subacromial bursitis was made. The patient was also referred to physical therapy, and a program of heat, ultrasound, and exercise was initiated to help resolve this condition.

Problem/Influence of Medication. During the initial physical therapy evaluation, the therapist asked if the patient was taking any medication for the bursitis. The patient responded that he had been advised by the physician to take aspirin as needed to help relieve the pain. When asked if he had done this, the patient said that he had taken some aspirin once or twice, especially when his shoulder pain kept him awake at night. When he was asked specifically what type of aspirin he had taken, he named a commercial acetaminophen preparation. Evidently the patient was unaware of the difference between acetaminophen and aspirin (acetylsalicylate).

Decision/Solution. The therapist explained the difference between aspirin and acetaminophen to the patient, pointing out that acetaminophen lacks any significant anti-inflammatory effects. After consulting with the physician to confirm that aspirin was recommended, the therapist suggested that the patient take the recommended dosage at regular intervals to help decrease the inflammation in the bursa, as well as to provide analgesia. The patient had used aspirin in the past without any problems, but the therapist cautioned the patient to contact his physician if any adverse effects were noted (e.g., gastrointestinal distress or tinnitus).

SUMMARY

Aspirin and similarly acting drugs comprise a group of therapeutic agents that are usually referred to as NSAIDs. In addition to their anti-inflammatory effects, these drugs are also known for their ability to decrease mild-to-moderate pain (analgesia), alleviate fever (antipyresis), and inhibit platelet aggregation (anticoagulation). These drugs seem to exert all of their therapeutic effects by inhibiting the function of the cellular cyclooxygenase enzyme, which results in decreased prostaglandin and thromboxane synthesis. Aspirin is the prototypical NSAID, and newer prescription and nonprescription drugs appear to be similar in terms of pharmacologic effects and therapeutic efficacy.

Newer drugs known as COX-2 inhibitors were also developed in an attempt to inhibit prostaglandins that cause pain and inflammation while sparing the production of beneficial prostaglandins that protect the stomach and other organs. These COX-2 drugs have the potential to produce therapeutic effects with less gastritis, but their status remains controversial because certain COX-2 agents may increase the risk of heart attack and stroke. Acetaminophen also seems to be similar to aspirin in analgesic and antipyretic effects, but acetaminophen lacks anti-inflammatory and anticoagulant properties. Patients requiring physical rehabilitation use aspirin, other NSAIDs, and COX-2 inhibitors frequently, which usually provides beneficial effects (analgesia, decreased inflammation, etc.) without producing cognitive side effects (sedation, mood changes) that can interfere with the rehabilitation program.

References

1. Arber N, Levin B. Chemoprevention of colorectal cancer: ready for routine use? *Recent Results Cancer Res.* 2005;166:213–230.
2. Arm JP. Leukotriene generation and clinical implications. *Allergy Asthma Proc.* 2004;25:37–42.
3. Asgari M, White E, Chren MM. Nonsteroidal anti-inflammatory drug use in the prevention and treatment of squamous cell carcinoma. *Dermatol Surg.* 2004;30: 1335–1342.
4. Becker JC, Domschke W, Pohle T. Current approaches to prevent NSAID-induced gastropathy—COX selectivity and beyond. *Br J Clin Pharmacol.* 2004;58: 587–600.
5. Bertin P, Keddad K, Jolivet-Landreau I. Acetaminophen as symptomatic treatment of pain from osteoarthritis. *Joint Bone Spine.* 2004;71:266–274.
6. Bing RJ, Lomnicka M. Why do cyclo-oxygenase-2 inhibitors cause cardiovascular events? *J Am Coll Cardiol.* 2002;39:521–522.
7. Birney Y, Redmond EM, Sitzmann JV, Cahill PA. Eicosanoids in cirrhosis and portal hypertension. *Prostaglandins Other Lipid Mediat.* 2003;72:3–18.
8. Blot L, Marcelis A, Devogelaer JP, Manicourt DH. Effects of diclofenac, aceclofenac and meloxicam on the metabolism of proteoglycans and hyaluronan in osteoarthritic human cartilage. *Br J Pharmacol.* 2000; 131:1413–1421.
9. Botting R. Antipyretic therapy. *Front Biosci.* 2004;9: 956–966.
10. Botting R. COX-1 and COX-3 inhibitors. *Thromb Res.* 2003;110:269–272.
11. Botting R, Ayoub SS. COX-3 and the mechanism of action of paracetamol/acetaminophen. *Prostaglandins Leukot Essent Fatty Acids.* 2005;72:85–87.
12. Bourne MH. Analgesics for orthopedic postoperative pain. *Am J Orthop.* 2004;33:128–135.
13. Boushel R, Langberg H, Risum N, Kjaer M. Regulation of blood flow by prostaglandins. *Curr Vasc Pharmacol.* 2004;2:191–197.
14. Bresalier RS, Sandler RS, Quan H, et al. Cardiovascular events associated with rofecoxib in a colorectal adenoma chemoprevention trial. *N Engl J Med.* 2005;352: 1092–1102.
15. Brill S, Plaza M. Non-narcotic adjuvants may improve the duration and quality of analgesia after knee arthroscopy: a brief review. *Can J Anaesth.* 2004;51: 975–978.
16. Brown AK, Christo PJ, Wu CL. Strategies for postoperative pain management. *Best Pract Res Clin Anaesthesiol.* 2004;18:703–717.
17. Brown JR, DuBois RN. COX-2: a molecular target for colorectal cancer prevention. *J Clin Oncol.* 2005;23: 2840–2855.
18. Brown KM, Saunders MM, Kirsch T, Donahue HJ, Reid JS. Effect of COX-2-specific inhibition on fracture-healing in the rat femur. *J Bone Joint Surg Am.* 2004;86–A:116–123.
19. Cannon GW, Breedveld FC. Efficacy of cyclooxygenase-2-specific inhibitors. *Am J Med.* 2001;110(suppl 3A):6S–12S.
20. Capra V, Rovati GE. Leukotriene modifiers in asthma management. *IDrugs.* 2004;7:659–666.
21. Carey MA, Germolec DR, Langenbach R, Zeldin DC. Cyclooxygenase enzymes in allergic inflammation and asthma. *Prostaglandins Leukot Essent Fatty Acids.* 2003; 69:157–162.
22. Casteels-Van Daele M, Van Geet C, Wouters C, Eggermont E. Reye syndrome revisited: a descriptive term covering a group of heterogeneous disorders. *Eur J Pediatr.* 2000;159:641–648.

23. Chan FK, Graham DY. Review article: prevention of non-steroidal anti-inflammatory drug gastrointestinal complications—review and recommendations based on risk assessment. *Aliment Pharmacol Ther.* 2004;19: 1051–1061.

24. Chandrasekharan NV, Simmons DL. The cyclooxygenases. *Genome Biol.* 2004;5:241.

25. Chang SY, Howden CW. Is no NSAID a good NSAID? Approaches to NSAID-associated upper gastrointestinal disease. *Curr Gastroenterol Rep.* 2004;6: 447–453.

26. Chen JY, Wu GJ, Mok MS, et al. Effect of adding ketorolac to intravenous morphine patient-controlled analgesia on bowel function in colorectal surgery patients—a prospective, randomized, double-blind study. *Acta Anaesthesiol Scand.* 2005;49:546–551.

27. Cheng HF, Harris RC. Cyclooxygenases, the kidney, and hypertension. *Hypertension.* 2004;43:525–530.

28. Clark DW, Layton D, Shakir SA. Do some inhibitors of COX-2 increase the risk of thromboembolic events? Linking pharmacology with pharmacoepidemiology. *Drug Saf.* 2004;27:427–456.

29. Collier S, Ghosh P. Comparison of the effects of NSAIDs on proteoglycan synthesis by articular cartilage explant and chondrocyte monolayer cultures. *Biochem Pharmacol.* 1991;41:1375–1384.

30. Creutzig A, Lehmacher W, Elze M. Meta-analysis of randomised controlled prostaglandin E1 studies in peripheral arterial occlusive disease stages III and IV. *Vasa.* 2004;33:137–144.

31. Dahners LE, Mullis BH. Effects of nonsteroidal anti-inflammatory drugs on bone formation and soft-tissue healing. *J Am Acad Orthop Surg.* 2004;12:139–143.

32. Dai W, Kloner RA. Relationship between cyclooxygenase-2 inhibition and thrombogenesis. *J Cardiovasc Pharmacol Ther.* 2004;9:51–59.

33. de Leval X, Julemont F, Benoit V, et al. First and second generations of COX-2 selective inhibitors. *Rev Med Chem.* 2004;4:597–601.

34. Dickman A, Ellershaw J. NSAIDs: gastroprotection or selective COX-2 inhibitor? *Palliat Med.* 2004;18: 275–286.

35. Ejaz P, Bhojani K, Joshi VR. NSAIDs and kidney. *J Assoc Physicians India.* 2004;52:632–640.

36. Epstein M. Non-steroidal anti-inflammatory drugs and the continuum of renal dysfunction. *J Hypertens Suppl.* 2002;20:S17–S23.

37. Fitzpatrick FA. Cyclooxygenase enzymes: regulation and function. *Curr Pharm Des.* 2004;10:577–588.

38. Fortun PJ, Hawkey CJ. Nonsteroidal antiinflammatory drugs and the small intestine. *Curr Opin Gastroenterol.* 2005;21:169–175.

39. Fowles RE. Potential cardiovascular effects of COX-2 selective nonsteroidal antiinflammatory drugs. *J Pain Palliat Care Pharmacother.* 2003;17:27–50.

40. Francois H, Coffman TM. Prostanoids and blood pressure: which way is up? *J Clin Invest.* 2004;114: 757–759.

41. Gajraj NM, Joshi GP. Role of cyclooxygenase-2 inhibitors in postoperative pain management. *Anesthesiol Clin North America.* 2005;23:49–72.

42. Gerstenfeld LC, Einhorn TA. COX inhibitors and their effects on bone healing. *Expert Opin Drug Saf.* 2004;3:131–136.

43. Goldstein JL. Challenges in managing NSAID-associated gastrointestinal tract injury. *Digestion.* 2004;69(suppl 1):25–33.

44. Graham GG, Scott KF. Mechanism of action of paracetamol. *Am J Ther.* 2005;12:46–55.

45. Grattan CE. Aspirin sensitivity and urticaria. *Clin Exp Dermatol.* 2003;28:123–127.

46. Gyires K. Gastric mucosal protection: from prostaglandins to gene-therapy. *Curr Med Chem.* 2005;12:203–215.

47. Harder AT, An YH. The mechanisms of the inhibitory effects of nonsteroidal anti-inflammatory drugs on bone healing: a concise review. *J Clin Pharmacol.* 2003; 43:807–815.

48. Hata AN, Breyer RM. Pharmacology and signaling of prostaglandin receptors: multiple roles in inflammation and immune modulation. *Pharmacol Ther.* 2004;103: 147–166.

49. Hawk ET, Levin B. Colorectal cancer prevention. *J Clin Oncol.* 2005;23:378–391.

50. Helliwell RJ, Adams LF, Mitchell MD. Prostaglandin synthases: recent developments and a novel hypothesis. *Prostaglandins Leukot Essent Fatty Acids.* 2004;70:101–113.

51. Henrotin Y, Bassleer C, Franchimont P. In vitro effects of etodolac and acetylsalicylic acid on human chondrocyte metabolism. *Agents Actions.* 1992;36:317–323.

52. Hinson JA, Reid AB, McCullough SS, James LP. Acetaminophen-induced hepatotoxicity: role of metabolic activation, reactive oxygen/nitrogen species, and mitochondrial permeability transition. *Drug Metab Rev.* 2004;36:805–822.

53. Hinz B, Brune K. Pain and osteoarthritis: new drugs and mechanisms. *Curr Opin Rheumatol.* 2004;16: 628–633.

54. Hooper L, Brown TJ, Elliott R, et al. The effectiveness of five strategies for the prevention of gastrointestinal toxicity induced by non-steroidal anti-inflammatory drugs: systematic review. *BMJ.* 2004; 329:948.

55. Ivanov AI, Romanovsky AA. Prostaglandin E2 as a mediator of fever: synthesis and catabolism. *Front Biosci.* 2004;9:1977–1993.

56. Jabbour HN, Sales KJ. Prostaglandin receptor signalling and function in human endometrial pathology. *Trends Endocrinol Metab.* 2004;15:398–404.

57. Jacobsen RB, Phillips BB. Reducing clinically significant gastrointestinal toxicity associated with nonsteroidal antiinflammatory drugs. *Ann Pharmacother.* 2004;38:1469–1481.

58. Jalving M, Koornstra JJ, De Jong S, et al. Review article: the potential of combinational regimen with non-steroidal anti-inflammatory drugs in the chemoprevention of colorectal cancer. *Aliment Pharmacol Ther.* 2005;21:321–339.

59. James LP, Mayeux PR, Hinson JA. Acetaminophen-induced hepatotoxicity. *Drug Metab Dispos.* 2003;31: 1499–1506.

60. Justice E, Carruthers DM. Cardiovascular risk and COX-2 inhibition in rheumatological practice. *J Hum Hypertens.* 2005;19:1–5.
61. Kiefer W, Dannhardt G. Novel insights and therapeutical applications in the field of inhibitors of COX-2. *Curr Med Chem.* 2004;11:3147–3161.
62. Koehne CH, Dubois RN. COX-2 inhibition and colorectal cancer. *Semin Oncol.* 2004;31(suppl 7):12–21.
63. Konstam MA, Weir MR. Current perspective on the cardiovascular effects of coxibs. *Cleve Clin J Med.* 2002; 69(suppl 1):SI47–SI52.
64. Lanas A. Economic analysis of strategies in the prevention of non-steroidal anti-inflammatory drug-induced complications in the gastrointestinal tract. *Aliment Pharmacol Ther.* 2004;20:321–331.
65. Lane JE, Belson MG, Brown DK, Scheetz A. Chronic acetaminophen toxicity: a case report and review of the literature. *J Emerg Med.* 2002;23:253–256.
66. Laufer S. Role of eicosanoids in structural degradation in osteoarthritis. *Curr Opin Rheumatol.* 2003;15: 623–627.
67. Lazzaroni M, Bianchi Porro G. Gastrointestinal side-effects of traditional non-steroidal anti-inflammatory drugs and new formulations. *Aliment Pharmacol Ther.* 2004;20 (suppl 2):48–58.
68. Leslie CC. Regulation of arachidonic acid availability for eicosanoid production. *Biochem Cell Biol.* 2004; 82:1–17.
69. Lowder JL, Shackelford DP, Holbert D, Beste TM. A randomized, controlled trial to compare ketorolac tromethamine versus placebo after cesarean section to reduce pain and narcotic usage. *Am J Obstet Gynecol.* 2003;189:1559–1562.
70. Marjoribanks J, Proctor ML, Farquhar C. Nonsteroidal anti-inflammatory drugs for primary dysmenorrhoea. *Cochrane Database Syst Rev.* 2003; CD001751.
71. Mason L, Moore RA, Edwards JE, et al. Topical NSAIDs for chronic musculoskeletal pain: systematic review and meta-analysis. *BMC Musculoskelet Disord.* 2004;5:28.
72. Moore N. Forty years of ibuprofen use. *Int J Clin Pract Suppl.* 2003;135:28–31.
73. Morrow JD, Roberts LJ. Lipid-derived autacoids: eicosanoids and platelet-activating factor. In: Hardman JG, et al, eds. *The Pharmacological Basis of Therapeutics.* 10th ed. New York: McGraw-Hill; 2001.
74. Moyad MA. An introduction to aspirin, NSAids, and COX-2 inhibitors for the primary prevention of cardiovascular events and cancer and their potential preventive role in bladder carcinogenesis: part II. *Semin Urol Oncol.* 2001;19:306–316.
75. Mukherjee D, Nissen SE, Topol EJ. Risk of cardiovascular events associated with selective COX-2 inhibitors. *JAMA.* 2001;286:954–959.
76. Nettis E, Colanardi MC, Ferrannini A, Tursi A. Update on sensitivity to nonsteroidal antiinflammatory drugs. *Curr Drug Targets Immune Endocr Metabol Disord.* 2001;1:233–240.
77. Nusing RM, Seyberth HW. The role of cyclooxygenases and prostanoid receptors in furosemide-like salt losing tubulopathy: the hyperprostaglandin E syndrome. *Acta Physiol Scand.* 2004;181:523–528.
78. Peek RM, Jr. Prevention of colorectal cancer through the use of COX-2 selective inhibitors. *Cancer Chemother Pharmacol.* 2004;54(suppl 1):S50–S56.
79. Perini R, Fiorucci S, Wallace JL. Mechanisms of nonsteroidal anti-inflammatory drug-induced gastrointestinal injury and repair: a window of opportunity for cyclooxygenase-inhibiting nitric oxide donors. *Can J Gastroenterol.* 2004;18:229–236.
80. Peters-Golden M, Canetti C, Mancuso P, Coffey MJ. Leukotrienes: underappreciated mediators of innate immune responses. *J Immunol.* 2005;174:589–594.
81. Peura DA. Prevention of nonsteroidal anti-inflammatory drug-associated gastrointestinal symptoms and ulcer complications. *Am J Med.* 2004;117(suppl 5A):63S–71S.
82. Prescott LF. Paracetamol: past, present, and future. *Am J Ther.* 2000;7:143–147.
83. Riccioni G, Di Ilio C, Conti P, et al. Advances in therapy with antileukotriene drugs. *Ann Clin Lab Sci.* 2004; 34:379–387.
84. Roberts LJ, Morrow JD. Analgesic-antipyretic and antiinflammatory agents and drugs employed in the treatment of gout. In: Hardman JG, et al, eds. *The Pharmacological Basis of Therapeutics.* 10th ed. New York: McGraw-Hill; 2001.
85. Rubenstein JH, Laine L. Systematic review: the hepatotoxicity of non-steroidal anti-inflammatory drugs. *Aliment Pharmacol Ther.* 2004;20:373–380.
86. Rumack BH. Acetaminophen misconceptions. *Hepatology.* 2004;40:10–15.
87. Sachs CJ. Oral analgesics for acute nonspecific pain. *Am Fam Physician.* 2005;71:913–918.
88. Sales KJ, Jabbour HN. Cyclooxygenase enzymes and prostaglandins in pathology of the endometrium. *Reproduction.* 2003;126:559–567.
89. Schnitzer TJ, Ferraro A, Hunsche E, Kong SX. A comprehensive review of clinical trials on the efficacy and safety of drugs for the treatment of low back pain. *J Pain Symptom Manage.* 2004;28:72–95.
90. Shaya FT, Blume SW, Blanchette CM, et al. Selective cyclooxygenase-2 inhibition and cardiovascular effects: an observational study of a Medicaid population. *Arch Intern Med.* 2005;165:181–186.
91. Simmons DL, Botting RM, Hla T. Cyclooxygenase isozymes: the biology of prostaglandin synthesis and inhibition. *Pharmacol Rev.* 2004;56:387–437.
92. Stevenson DD. Aspirin and NSAID sensitivity. *Immunol Allergy Clin North Am.* 2004;24:491–505.
93. Sublette ME, Russ MJ, Smith GS. Evidence for a role of the arachidonic acid cascade in affective disorders: a review. *Bipolar Disord.* 2004;6:95–105.
94. Szczeklik A, Sanak M, Nizankowska-Mogilnicka E, Kielbasa B. Aspirin intolerance and the cyclooxygenase-leukotriene pathways. *Curr Opin Pulm Med.* 2004;10: 51–56.
95. Takeeda M, Hayashi Y, Yamato M, et al. Roles of endogenous prostaglandins and cyclooxygenase izoenzymes in mucosal defense of inflamed rat stomach. *J Physiol Pharmacol.* 2004;55:193–205.

96. Tanaka Y, Yamaki F, Koike K, Toro L. New insights into the intracellular mechanisms by which PGI2 analogues elicit vascular relaxation: cyclic AMP-independent, Gs-protein mediated-activation of MaxiK channel. *Curr Med Chem Cardiovasc Hematol Agents.* 2004;2:257–265.

97. Tendera M, Wojakowski W. Role of antiplatelet drugs in the prevention of cardiovascular events. *Thromb Res.* 2003;110:355–359.

98. Thaller J, Walker M, Kline AJ, Anderson DG. The effect of nonsteroidal anti-inflammatory agents on spinal fusion. *Orthopedics.* 2005;28:299–303.

99. Traversa G, Bianchi C, Da Cas R, et al. Cohort study of hepatotoxicity associated with nimesulide and other non-steroidal anti-inflammatory drugs. *BMJ.* 2003;327:18–22.

100. Tuynman JB, Peppelenbosch MP, Richel DJ. COX-2 inhibition as a tool to treat and prevent colorectal cancer. *Crit Rev Oncol Hematol.* 2004;52:81–101.

101. Ueno A, Oh-ishi S. Critical roles for bradykinin and prostanoids in acute inflammatory reactions: a search using experimental animal models. *Curr Drug Targets Inflamm Allergy.* 2002;1:363–376.

102. Ulinski T, Guigonis V, Dunan O, Bensman A. Acute renal failure after treatment with non-steroidal anti-inflammatory drugs. *Eur J Pediatr.* 2004;163:148–150.

103. Vane JR, Botting RM. The mechanism of action of aspirin. *Thromb Res.* 2003;110:255–258.

104. Wegman A, van der Windt D, van Tulder M, Stalman W, de Vries T. Nonsteroidal antiinflammatory drugs or acetaminophen for osteoarthritis of the hip or knee? A systematic review of evidence and guidelines. *J Rheumatol.* 2004;31:344–354.

105. Weir MR, Sperling RS, Reicin A, Gertz BJ. Selective COX-2 inhibition and cardiovascular effects: a review of the rofecoxib development program. *Am Heart J.* 2003;146:591–604.

106. Wheeler P, Batt ME. Do non-steroidal anti-inflammatory drugs adversely affect stress fracture healing? A short review. *Br J Sports Med.* 2005;39:65–69.

107. White WB, Strand V, Roberts R, Whelton A. Effects of the cyclooxygenase-2 specific inhibitor valdecoxib versus nonsteroidal antiinflammatory agents and placebo on cardiovascular thrombotic events in patients with arthritis. *Am J Ther.* 2004;11:244–250.

108. Willkens RF. The selection of a nonsteroidal antiinflammatory drug: is there a difference? *J Rheumatol.* 1992;19(suppl 36):9–12.

109. Williams A, Hennekens CH. The role of aspirin in cardiovascular diseases—forgotten benefits? *Expert Opin Pharmacother.* 2004;5:109–115.

110. Zha S, Yegnasubramanian V, Nelson WG, et al. Cyclooxygenases in cancer: progress and perspective. *Cancer Lett.* 2004;215:1–20.

111. Zhang W, Jones A, Doherty M. Does paracetamol (acetaminophen) reduce the pain of osteoarthritis? A meta-analysis of randomised controlled trials. *Ann Rheum Dis.* 2004;63:901–907.

Chapter 16

Pharmacologic Management of Rheumatoid Arthritis and Osteoarthritis

Rheumatoid arthritis and osteoarthritis represent the two primary pathologic conditions that affect the joints and periarticular structures. Although the causes underlying these conditions are quite different from one another, both conditions can cause severe pain and deformity in various joints in the body. Likewise, pharmacologic management plays an important role in the treatment of each disorder. Because physical therapists and other rehabilitation specialists often work with patients who have rheumatoid arthritis or osteoarthritis, an understanding of the types of drugs used to treat these diseases is important.

This chapter will begin by describing the etiology of rheumatoid joint disease and the pharmacologic treatment of rheumatoid arthritis. An analogous discussion of osteoarthritis will follow. Hopefully, these descriptions will provide rehabilitation specialists with an understanding of drug therapy's role in arthritis, and the impact drugs can have on patients receiving physical therapy and occupational therapy.

Rheumatoid Arthritis

Rheumatoid arthritis is a chronic, systemic disorder that affects many different tissues in the body, but is primarily characterized by synovitis and the destruction of articular tissue.[49,90,100] This disease is associated with pain, stiffness, and inflammation in the small synovial joints of the hands and feet, as well as in larger joints such as the knee. Although marked by periods of exacerbation and remission, rheumatoid arthritis is often progressive in nature, with advanced stages leading to severe joint destruction and bone erosion.

Specific criteria for the diagnosis of rheumatoid arthritis in adults are listed in Table 16–1. In addition to the adult form of this disease, there is also a form of arthritis that occurs in children known commonly as juvenile rheumatoid arthritis, or by the more recent term juvenile idiopathic arthritis (JIA). Juvenile arthritis differs from the adult form of this disease—the age of onset (younger than 16 years) and other criteria help to differentiate these two types of rheumatoid joint disease.[69,109] Drug treatment of adult and juvenile rheumatoid arthritis is fairly similar, however, with the exception that children may not respond as well to certain medications (e.g., hydroxychloroquine, gold compounds, penicillamine) compared to adults.[79,80] Consequently, in this chapter most of the discussion of the management of rheumatoid arthritis is directed toward the adult form.

Rheumatoid arthritis affects about 0.5 to 1.0 percent of the population worldwide.[38,55] This disease occurs three times more often in women than in men, with women between the ages of 20 and 40 especially susceptible to the onset of rheumatoid joint disease.[90,101] Rheumatoid arthritis often causes severe pain and suffering, frequently devastating the patient's family and social life as well as his or her job situation.[5,55] The economic impact of this disease is also staggering; medical costs and loss of productivity exceed $1 billion annually in the United States.[5,55] Consequently, rheu-

Table 16–1	CRITERIA FOR THE CLASSIFICATION OF RHEUMATOID ARTHRITIS*
Criterion	**Definition**
1. Morning stiffness	Morning stiffness in and around the joints, lasting at least 1 hr before maximal improvement.
2. Arthritis of 3 or more joint areas	At least 3 joint areas simultaneously have had soft tissue swelling or fluid (not bony overgrowth alone) observed by a physician. The 14 possible areas are right or left PIP, MCP, wrist, elbow, knee, ankle, and MTP joints.†
3. Arthritis of hand joints	At least 1 area swollen (as defined above) in a wrist, MCP, or PIP joint.
4. Symmetric arthritis	Simultaneous involvement of the same joint areas (as defined in 2) on both sides of the body (bilateral involvement of PIPs, MCPs, or MTPs is acceptable without absolute symmetry).
5. Rheumatoid nodules	Subcutaneous nodules over bony prominences or extensor surfaces, or in juxtaarticular regions, observed by a physician.
6. Serum rheumatoid factor	Demonstration of abnormal amounts of serum rheumatoid factor by any method for which the result has been positive in <5% of normal control subjects.
7. Radiographic changes	Radiographic changes typical of rheumatoid arthritis on posteroanterior hand and wrist radiographs, which must include erosions or unequivocal bony decalcification localized in or most marked adjacent to the involved joints (osteoarthritis changes alone do not qualify).

*For classification purposes, a patient is diagnosed with rheumatoid arthritis if he or she has satisfied at least 4 of these 7 criteria. Criteria 1 through 4 must have been present for at least 6 weeks.

†PIP = proximal interphalangeal; MCP = metacarpophalangeal; MTP = metatarsophalangeal.

Source: Arnett, et al. The American Rheumatism Association 1987 Revised Criteria for the Classification of Rheumatoid Arthritis. Arthritis and Rheumatism.1988;31:315–324. Reprinted from *Arthritis and Rheumatism Journal*, copyright 1988. Used with permission from the American College of Rheumatology.

matoid arthritis is a formidable and serious problem in contemporary health care.

Immune Basis for Rheumatoid Arthritis

The initiating factor in rheumatoid arthritis is not known. It is apparent, however, that the underlying basis of this disease consists of some type of autoimmune response in genetically susceptible individuals.[29,32,94] Some precipitating factor (possibly a virus or other infectious agent) appears to initiate the formation of antibodies that are later recognized by the host as antigens.[29] Subsequent formation of new antibodies to these antigens then initiates a complex chain of events involving a variety of immune system components such as mononuclear phagocytes, T lymphocytes, and B lymphocytes.[38,100] These cells basically interact with each other to produce a number of arthritogenic mediators, including cytokines (interleukin-1, tumor necrosis factor-alpha), eicosanoids (prostaglandins, leukotrienes), and destructive enzymes (proteases, collagenases).[32,90,94] These substances act either directly or through other cellular components of the immune system to induce synovial cell proliferation and destruction of articular cartilage and bone.[29,100] Thus, the joint destruction in rheumatoid arthritis is the culmination of a series of events resulting from an inherent defect in the immune response in patients with this disease.[29,32]

Overview of Drug Therapy in Rheumatoid Arthritis

The drug treatment of rheumatoid arthritis has two goals: (1) to decrease joint inflammation and (2) to arrest the progression of this disease. Three general categories of drugs are available to accomplish these goals: (1) nonsteroidal anti-inflammatory drugs (NSAIDs), (2) glucocorticoids, and (3) a diverse group of agents known as *disease-modifying antirheumatic drugs (DMARDs)* (Table 16–2).[56,90] NSAIDs and glucocorticoids are used primarily to decrease joint inflammation, but these agents do not necessarily halt the progression of rheumatoid arthritis. DMARDs attempt to slow or halt the advancement of this disease, usually by interfering with the immune response that seems to be the underlying factor in rheumatoid arthritis.[56] Each of these major drug categories, as well as specific disease-modifying drugs, is discussed in the following sections.

Nonsteroidal Anti-Inflammatory Drugs

Aspirin and the other NSAIDs are usually considered the first line of defense in treating rheumatoid arthritis.[68,90] Although NSAIDs are not as powerful in reducing inflammation as glucocorticoids, they are associated with fewer side effects, and they offer the added advantage of analgesia. Consequently, NSAIDs such as aspirin are often the first drugs employed in treating rheumatoid arthritis; in fact, this disease can often be controlled for short periods in some patients

Table 16–2	DRUG CATEGORIES USED IN RHEUMATOID ARTHRITIS

I. Nonsteroidal Anti-Inflammatory Drugs

Aspirin (many trade names)	Ketoprofen (Orudis, others)
Celecoxib (Celebrex)*	Meclofenamate (Meclomen)
Diclofenac (Cataflam, Voltaren)	Nabumetone (Relafen)
Diflunisal (Dolobid)	Naproxen (Anaprox, Naprosyn)
Fenoprofen (Nalfon)	Oxaprozin (Daypro)
Flurbiprofen (Ansaid)	Piroxicam (Feldene)
Ibuprofen (many trade names)	Sulindac (Clinoril)
Indomethacin (Indocin)	Tolmetin (Tolectin)

II. Corticosteroids

Betamethasone (Celestone)	Methylprednisolone (Medrol, others)
Cortisone (Cortone acetate)	Prednisolone (Prelone, others)
Dexamethasone (Decadron, others)	Prednisone (Deltasone, others)
Hydrocortisone (Cortef, others)	Triamcinolone (Aristocort, others)

III. Disease-Modifying Antirheumatic Drugs

Adalimumab (Humira)	Etanercept (Enbrel)
Anakinra (Kineret)	Gold sodium thiomalate (Myochrysine)
Auranofin (Ridaura)	Hydroxychloroquine (Plaquenil)
Aurothioglucose (Solganal)	Infliximab (Remicade)
Azathioprine (Imuran)	Leflunomide (Arava)
Chloroquine (Aralen)	Methotrexate (Rheumatrex, others)
Cyclophosphamide (Cytoxan)	Penicillamine (Cuprimine, Depen)
Cyclosporine (Neoral, Sandimmune)	Sulfasalazine (Azulfidine)

*Subclassified as a cyclooxygenase type 2 (COX-2) inhibitor; see Chapter 15

by solely using an NSAID.[68] In patients who continue to experience progressive joint destruction despite NSAID therapy these drugs are often combined with disease-modifying agents (discussed later in this chapter). Usually, it is not advisable to use two different NSAIDs simultaneously because there is an increased risk of side effects without any appreciable increase in therapeutic benefits. Some amount of trial and error may be involved in selecting the best NSAID, and several agents may have to be given before an optimal drug is found. As discussed in Chapter 15, aspirin appears approximately equal to the newer, more expensive NSAIDs in terms of anti-inflammatory and analgesic effects, but some of the newer drugs may produce less gastrointestinal discomfort. In particular, the cyclooxygenase-2 (COX-2) selective drugs (see below) may be especially helpful in people with a history of peptic ulcers or other risk factors for gastrointestinal problems.[3] The choice of a specific NSAID ultimately depends on each patient's response to the therapeutic effects and side effects of any given agent.[84]

Finally, acetaminophen (paracetamol) products may provide some temporary analgesic effects in people with rheumatoid arthritis, but these products are not optimal because they lack anti-inflammatory effects. As discussed in Chapter 15, acetaminophen can be used to treat mild-to-moderate pain, but the lack of anti-inflammatory effects makes acetaminophen fall short of NSAIDs for conditions such as rheumatoid arthritis. Hence, patients with rheumatoid arthritis usually prefer the effects of NSAIDs to acetaminophen,[110] and acetaminophen products are not typically used for the routine treatment of this disease.

Mechanism of Action

The pharmacology of the NSAIDs was discussed in Chapter 15. Basically, aspirin and the other NSAIDs exert most or all of their anti-inflammatory and analgesic effects by inhibiting the synthesis of prostaglandins.[84,103] Certain prostaglandins (i.e., prostaglandin E_2 [PGE_2]) are believed to participate in the inflammatory response by increasing local blood flow and vascular permeability and by exerting a chemotactic effect on leukocytes.[61] Prostaglandins are also believed to sensitize pain receptors to the nociceptive effects of other pain mediators such as bradykinin.[84] Aspirin and other NSAIDs prevent the production of prostaglandins by inhibiting the COX enzyme that initiates prostaglandin synthesis. As discussed in Chapter 15, aspirin and most other NSAIDs inhibit all COX forms; that is,

these drugs inhibit the COX-1 form of the enzyme that produces beneficial and protective prostaglandins in certain tissues while also inhibiting the COX-2 form that synthesizes prostaglandins in painful and inflamed tissues.[84]

Newer NSAIDs, however, are known as COX-2 inhibitors because these drugs inhibit the specific form of COX-2 that synthesizes prostaglandins during pain and inflammation. COX-2 drugs such as celecoxib (Celebrex) spare the production of normal or protective prostaglandins produced by COX-1 in the stomach, kidneys, and platelets (see Chapter 15).[33,103] Hence, COX-2 selective drugs may be especially beneficial during long-term use in people with rheumatoid arthritis because they may be less toxic to the stomach and other tissues.[3] The effect of COX-2 selective drugs and other NSAIDs on prostaglandin biosynthesis is discussed in more detail in Chapter 15.

Adverse Side Effects

The problems and adverse effects of aspirin and other NSAIDs are discussed in Chapter 15. The most common problem with chronic use is stomach irritation, which can lead to gastric ulceration and hemorrhage. This can be resolved to some extent by taking aspirin in an enteric-coated form so that release is delayed until the drug reaches the small intestine. Other pharmacologic interventions such as prostaglandin analogs (misoprostol) and proton pump inhibitors (omeprazole [Prilosec], and so forth) can also be used if gastropathy continues to be a limiting factor during NSAID use (see Chapter 15). Chronic NSAID use can also produce bleeding problems (because of platelet inhibition) and impaired renal function, especially in an older or debilitated patient. Despite the potential for various side effects, aspirin and other NSAIDs continue to be used extensively by people with rheumatoid arthritis and are often used for extended periods without serious effects.

As indicated earlier, COX-2 selective drugs may reduce the risk of toxicity to the stomach, kidneys, and other tissues because these drugs spare the production of normal or protective prostaglandins in these tissues.[3] These drugs may cause other problems such as diarrhea, heartburn, gastrointestinal cramps, and an increased risk of upper respiratory tract infection. As indicated in Chapter 15, COX-2 drugs have also been associated with serious cardiovascular problems (heart attack, stroke), and these drugs should be avoided in people at risk for cardiac disease.

Glucocorticoids

Glucocorticoids such as prednisone are extremely effective anti-inflammatory agents, but they are associated with a number of serious side effects (see "Adverse Side Effects," below). Hence, these drugs (known also as corticosteroids) are commonly used to treat acute exacerbations in people with rheumatoid arthritis. In particular, the judicious short-term use of systemic (oral) glucocorticoids can serve as a bridge between an acute flare-up of rheumatoid joint disease and successful management by other drugs such as NSAIDs and disease-modifying agents.[43] Glucocorticoids can often be given systemically at high doses for short periods (a week or two) to provide anti-inflammatory effects. This so-called pulse treatment may be especially helpful in managing acute exacerbations of rheumatoid arthritis without producing the severe side effects associated with long-term use.[50]

Glucocorticoids can also be injected directly into the arthritic joint, a technique that can be invaluable in the management of acute exacerbations. There is, of course, considerable controversy about whether intra-articular glucocorticoids will produce harmful catabolic effects in joints that are already weakened by arthritic changes. At the very least, the number of injections into an arthritic joint should be limited, and a common rule of thumb is to not exceed more than four injections in one joint within one year.[77]

The long-term use of glucocorticoids, however, remains somewhat controversial.[52,96] While their short-term anti-inflammatory effects can be extremely helpful, high doses of glucocorticoids for prolonged periods can cause serious musculoskeletal problems and other adverse effects (see below). It was also believed that these drugs do not necessarily halt the progression of rheumatoid arthritis and that their short-term benefits are eventually lost during prolonged use.[102] More recent evidence, however, suggests that glucocorticoids such as prednisone may actually have some ability to retard disease progression.[11,24] That is, these drugs may have some beneficial disease-modifying properties similar to other DMARDs.[86] Furthermore, these beneficial effects may be achieved with fairly low doses, minimizing the risk of adverse effects.[11,24] Hence, the risks and benefits of long-term glucocorticoid administration continue to be investigated, and future research will help clarify how these drugs can be used most effectively alone or with other agents to manage rheumatoid arthritis.

Mechanism of Action

The details of the cellular effects of steroids are discussed in Chapter 29. Briefly, glucocorticoids bind to a receptor in the cytoplasm of certain cells (macrophages, leukocytes), thereby forming a glucocorticoid-receptor complex.[17,89] This complex then moves to the cell's nucleus where it binds to specific genes that regulate the inflammatory process. By binding to these genes, the glucocorticoid-receptor complex increases the production of several anti-inflammatory proteins while also inhibiting the production of many pro-inflammatory substances.[87]

These agents, for example, increase the production of proteins called annexins (previously known as lipocortins).[66] Annexins inhibit the phospholipase A_2 enzyme that normally liberates fatty acid precursors at the start of prostaglandin and leukotriene biosynthesis. Therefore, glucocorticoid-induced production of annexins blocks the first step in the synthesis of pro-inflammatory prostaglandins and leukotrienes.[66] Glucocorticoids likewise increase the production of proteins such as interleukin-10, interleukin-1 receptor antagonist, and neutral endopeptidase.[8] These other proteins contribute to anti-inflammatory effects by inhibiting, destroying, or blocking various other inflammatory chemicals, peptides, and proteins.[8]

In addition to direct effects on genes regulating inflammation, glucocorticoids also inhibit the transcription factors that initiate synthesis of pro-inflammatory cytokines (e.g., interleukin-1, tumor necrosis factor), enzymes (e.g., COX-2, nitric oxide synthase), and receptor proteins (e.g., natural killer receptors).[17,87,89] Glucocorticoids may also exert some of their effects via a membrane-bound receptor that regulates activity of macrophages, eosinophils, T lymphocytes, and several other types of cells involved in the inflammatory response.[89] Consequently, glucocorticoids affect many aspects of inflammation, and their powerful anti-inflammatory effects in rheumatoid arthritis result from their ability to blunt various cellular and chemical components of the inflammatory response.

Adverse Side Effects

The side effects of glucocorticoids are numerous (see Chapter 29). These drugs exert a general catabolic effect on all types of supportive tissue (i.e., muscle, tendon, bone). Osteoporosis is a particular a problem in the patient with arthritis because many of these patients have significant bone loss before even beginning steroid therapy. Glucocorticoids have been known to increase bone loss in patients with arthritis, especially when these drugs are used at higher doses for prolonged periods.[68,86] Glucocorticoids may also cause muscle wasting and weakness, as well as hypertension, aggravation of diabetes mellitus, glaucoma, and cataracts.[68,89] These side effects emphasize the need to limit glucocorticoid therapy as much as possible in patients with arthritis.

Disease-Modifying Antirheumatic Drugs

Disease-modifying antirheumatic drugs (DMARDs) are defined as "medications that retard or halt the progression of [rheumatoid] disease."[68] These drugs comprise an eclectic group of agents that are now recognized as essential in the early treatment of rheumatoid arthritis. That is, early and aggressive use of DMARDs can slow the progression of this disease before there is extensive damage to affected joints. When used in conjunction with NSAIDs and glucocorticoids, DMARDs can help improve the long-term outcomes of patients with rheumatoid arthritis, and can contribute to substantial improvements in quality-of-life.[12]

Hence, disease-modifying drugs are typically used to control synovitis and erosive changes during the active stages of rheumatoid joint disease.[68] There is still considerable concern, however, over DMARD's safety and efficacy. Older DMARDs, such as penicillamine and oral gold, were especially problematic, and many patients who started treatment on these drugs eventually discontinued drug therapy due to side effects or lack of therapeutic benefits.[68] Some of the newer DMARDs are substantially more effective, but these newer agents can still produce serious side effects such as hepatic and renal toxicity.[70] Despite these limitations, there has been a definite trend toward more frequent DMARD use, and to use these drugs earlier in the course of rheumatoid arthritis before excessive joint destruction has occurred.[4,68]

Disease-modifying agents currently used in treating rheumatoid arthritis are listed in Table 16–3. As the name implies, DMARDs attempt to induce remission by modifying the pathologic process inherent to rheumatoid arthritis. In general, DMARDs inhibit certain aspects of the immune response thought to be underlying rheumatoid disease. For example, these drugs can inhibit the function of monocytes and T and B lymphocytes, or affect specific inflammatory mediators (e.g., cytokines) that are responsible for perpetuating joint inflammation and destruction.[90] The pharmacology of specific DMARDs is discussed below.

Antimalarial Drugs

Originally used in the treatment of malaria, the drugs chloroquine (Aralen) and hydroxychloroquine (Plaquenil) have also been used to treat rheumatoid arthritis. In the past, these drugs have been used reluctantly because of the fear of retinal toxicity (see "Adverse Side Effects").[25] There is now evidence, however, that these agents can be used safely, but they are only marginally effective when compared to other DMARDs. These drugs are therefore not usually the first choice, but they can be used in patients who cannot tolerate other DMARDs, or in combination with another DMARD (e.g., methotrexate) for more comprehensive treatment.

Mechanism of Action. Antimalarials exert a number of effects, although it is unclear exactly which of these contributes to their ability to halt the progression in rheumatoid arthritis. These drugs are known to increase pH within certain intracellular vacuoles in macrophages and other immune-system cells.[35] This effect is believed to disrupt the ability of these cells to process antigenic proteins and present these antigens to T cells.[107] Decreased T-cell stimulation results in immunosuppression and attenuation of the arthritic response.[35] Antimalarials have also been shown to stabilize lysosomal membranes and impair DNA and RNA synthesis, although the significance of these effects in their role as antiarthritics remains unclear.[107]

Adverse Side Effects. Chloroquine and hydroxychloroquine are usually considered the safest DMARDs.[68] The major concern is that high doses of these drugs can produce irreversible retinal damage. Retinal toxicity is rare, however, when daily dosages are maintained below the levels typically used to treat rheumatoid arthritis (i.e., less than 3.5 to 4.0 mg/kg per day for chloroquine and less than 6.0 to 6.5 mg/kg per day for hydroxychloroquine).[60,63] Nonetheless, ocular exams should be scheduled periodically to ensure the safe and effective use of these drugs during prolonged administration.[16] Other side effects such as headache and gastrointestinal distress can occur, but these are relatively infrequent and usually transient.

Table 16-3   DISEASE-MODIFYING ANTIRHEUMATIC DRUGS

Drug	Trade Name	Usual Dosage	Special Considerations
Anakinra	Kineret	Subcutaneous injection: 100 mg/d.	Can be used alone or with other antiarthritic agents, but should not be used with tumor necrosis factor inhibitors.
Antimalarials			
Chloroquine	Aralen	Oral: Up to 4 mg/kg of lean body weight per day.	Periodic ophthalmic exams recommended to check for retinal toxicity.
Hydroxychloroquine	Plaquenil	Oral: Up to 6.5 mg/kg of lean body weight per day.	Similar to chloroquine.
Azathioprine	Imuran	Oral: 1 mg/kg body weight per day; can be increased after 6–8 wk up to maximum dose of 2.5 mg/kg body weight.	Relatively high toxicity; should be used cautiously in debilitated patients or patients with renal disease.
Cyclophosphamide	Cytoxan	Oral: 1.5–2 mg/kg body weight per day; can be increased to a maximum daily dose of 3 mg/kg body weight.	Long-term use is limited because of potential for carcinogenicity.
Cyclosporine	Neoral, Sandimmune	Oral: 2.5 mg/kg body weight per day; can be increased after 8 wk by 0.5–0.75 mg/kg body weight per day; dose can be increased after another 4 weeks to a maximum daily dose of 4 mg/kg body weight per day.	May cause nephrotoxicity and gastrointestinal problems.
Gold compounds			
Auranofin	Ridaura	Oral: 6 mg/once each day or 3 mg BID	May have a long latency (6–9 mo) before onset of benefits.
Aurothioglucose	Solganal	Intramuscular: 10 mg the 1st wk, 25 mg the 2nd and 3rd wk, then 25–50 mg each wk until total dose is 1 g. Maintenance doses of 25–50 mg every 2–4 wk can follow.	Effects occur somewhat sooner than oral gold, but still has long delay (4 mo).
Gold sodium thiomalate	Myochrysine	Similar to aurothioglucose.	Similar to aurothioglucose.

(Continued on following page)

Table 16–3	DISEASE-MODIFYING ANTIRHEUMATIC DRUGS *(Continued)*		
Drug	**Trade Name**	**Usual Dosage**	**Special Considerations**
Leflunomide	Arava	Oral: 100 mg/d for the first 3 days; continue with a maintenance dosage of 20 mg/d thereafter.	May decrease joint erosion/destruction with relatively few serious side effects; effects of long-term use remains to be determined.
Methotrexate	Rheumatrex, others	Oral: 2.5–5 mg every 12 hr for total of 3 doses/wk or 10 mg once each week. Can be increased up to a maximum of 20–25 mg/wk.	Often effective in halting joint destruction, but long-term use may be limited by toxicity.
Penicillamine	Cuprimine, Depen	Oral: 125 or 250 mg/d; can be increased to a maximum of 1.5 g/d.	Relatively high incidence of toxicity with long-term use.
Sulfasalazine	Azulfidine	Oral: 0.5–1.0 g/d for the first week; dose can be increased by 500 mg each week up to a maximum daily dose of 2–3 g/d.	Relatively high toxicity; may produce serious hypersensitivity reactions and blood dyscrasias.
Tumor Necrosis Factor Inhibitors			
Adalimumab	Humira	Subcutaneous injection: 40 mg every week if used alone; 40 mg every other week if used in combination with other antiarthritic agents such as methotrexate.	Relatively low incidence of serious side effects compared to other immunosuppressants.
Etanercept	Enbrel	Subcutaneous injection: 25 mg twice each week.	Similar to adalimumab.
Infliximab	Remicade	Slow intravenous infusion: 3 mg/ kg body weight. Additional doses at 2 and 6 weeks after first infusion, then every 8 weeks thereafter.	Should be administered in combination with methotrexate.

Azathioprine

Azathioprine (Imuran) is an immunosuppressant drug that is often used to prevent tissue rejection following organ transplants. Because of its immunosuppressant properties, this drug has been employed in treating cases of severe, active rheumatoid arthritis that have not responded to other agents.

Mechanism of Action. The mechanism of action of azathioprine in rheumatoid arthritis is not fully understood. This drug has been shown to impair the synthesis of DNA and RNA precursors, but it is unclear exactly how (or if) this is related to its immunosuppressant effects. Azathioprine can likewise inhibit lymphocyte proliferation, thereby impairing immune responses mediated by these cells.[54] This action accounts for the immunosuppressant effects of this drug and for its ability to blunt the autoimmune responses that govern rheumatoid disease.

Adverse Side Effects. Azathioprine is relatively toxic, with more frequent and more severe side effects than other DMARDs.[97] The primary side effects include fever, chills, sore throat, fatigue, loss of appetite, and nausea or vomiting; these effects often limit the use of this drug.

Gold Therapy

Compounds containing elemental gold were among the first drugs identified as DMARDs (Fig. 16–1). Specific compounds such as aurothioglucose (Solganal) and gold sodium thiomalate (Myochrysine) have been used in the past and are usually administered by intramuscular injection. An orally active gold compound, auranofin (Ridaura), has also been developed and offers the advantage of oral administration.[84] Auranofin is better tolerated than parenteral gold compounds in terms of adverse side effects.[84] In the past, gold therapy was often used to arrest further progression of rheumatoid joint disease. Because safer and more effective agents have been developed, gold compounds are no longer used routinely in the treatment of rheumatoid arthritis, but are reserved for patients who fail to respond to other DMARDs.[68]

Mechanism of Action. Although the exact mechanism is not fully understood, gold compounds probably induce remission in patients with rheumatoid arthritis by inhibiting the growth and function of T cells and mononuclear phagocytes.[27,84] These drugs accumulate in the lysosomes of macrophages and other synovial cells, thereby suppressing the action of key components in the cellular immune reaction inherent in this disease.[84] A number of additional cellular effects have been noted (decreased lysosomal enzyme release, decreased prostaglandin E_2 production), and these effects may also contribute to the effectiveness of gold compounds in treating rheumatoid arthritis.[84,111]

Adverse Side Effects. Adverse effects are relatively common with gold therapy, with approximately one third of patients experiencing some form of toxic effect.[84] The primary side effects caused by gold compounds are gastrointestinal distress (diarrhea, indigestion), irritation of the oral mucosa, and rashes and

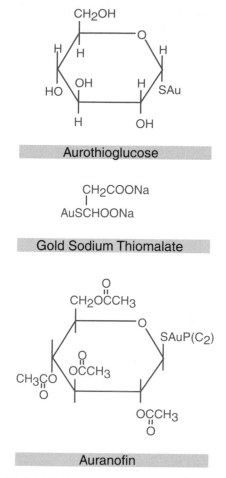

FIGURE 16–1 ▼ Gold compounds used to treat rheumatoid arthritis.

itching of the skin.[27,84] Other side effects include proteinuria, conjunctivitis, and blood dyscrasias (e.g., thrombocytopenia, leukopenia). As mentioned earlier, auranofin may be safer than parenteral gold compounds because it produces fewer cutaneous and potentially serious hematologic side effects, but auranofin tends to produce more gastrointestinal irritation than injected forms of gold.[84]

Leflunomide

Leflunomide (Arava) is a relative newcomer to the antirheumatic drug arsenal. This drug helps decrease pain and inflammation in rheumatoid joint disease, and leflunomide has been shown to slow the formation of bone erosions in arthritic joints.[19] Leflunomide is also fairly well tolerated by most patients and may produce beneficial effects fairly soon (1 month) after beginning treatment.[57,105] This drug is therefore a potential alternative in people who have failed to respond to other DMARDs such as methotrexate.[59,70]

Mechanism of Action. Leflunomide acts primarily by inhibiting the synthesis of RNA precursors in lymphocytes.[65,70] When stimulated, lymphocytes must radically increase their RNA synthesis to proliferate and become activated during the inflammatory response. Leflunomide blocks a key enzyme responsible for RNA synthesis, so that these lymphocytes cannot progress to a more activated state and cannot cause as much joint inflammation.[58,107]

Adverse Side Effects. Leflunomide's primary side effects include gastrointestinal distress, allergic reactions (skin rashes), and hair loss.[57] This drug can also affect the liver; liver function may need to be monitored periodically.[19,70]

Methotrexate

Methotrexate (Folex, Rheumatrex) is an antimetabolite used frequently in the treatment of cancer (see Chapter 36). There is considerable evidence that this drug is also one of the most effective DMARDs.[15,76] Methotrexate has been shown to slow the effects of rheumatoid arthritis as evidenced by decreased synovitis, decreased bone erosion, and less narrowing of the joint space.[37] The therapeutic effects of methotrexate have also been reported to be equal to, or better than, other DMARDs such as oral gold or azathioprine, and methotrexate may offer an advantage in terms of a rapid onset.[68,90] Hence, methotrexate's popularity as a DMARD has increased during the past few years, and this drug is often the first DMARD used to treat rheumatoid arthritis in both adults and children.[76]

Mechanism of Action. The ability of methotrexate and similar anticancer drugs to impair DNA and RNA synthesis is well known (see Chapter 36). Methotrexate inhibits the synthesis of folic acid, thus inhibiting the formation of nucleoproteins that serve as DNA precursors.[20] This action inhibits cellular replication by impairing the cell's ability to produce new genetic material, an effect that helps attenuate tumor cell replication in cancer. Nonetheless, methotrexate's effects on immune function and rheumatoid arthritis are somewhat unclear. This drug could affect immune function by inhibiting folic acid metabolism, thereby limiting the proliferation of lymphocytes and other cells that cause the autoimmune responses in rheumatoid disease. Methotrexate, however, also exerts other effects, including inhibition of inflammatory cytokines and stimulation of adenosine release.[90] The effects on adenosine release may be especially important because increased amounts of endogenous adenosine can inhibit various components of the immune response.[92] Regardless of the exact mechanism, methotrexate has become a mainstay in the management of rheumatoid arthritis.

Adverse Side Effects. Methotrexate is a relatively toxic drug, and a number of adverse side effects can occur.[15,90] The primary problems involve the gastrointestinal tract and include loss of appetite, nausea, and other forms of gastrointestinal distress (including intragastrointestinal hemorrhage).[90] Long-term methotrexate use in patients with rheumatoid arthritis has also been associated with pulmonary problems, hematologic disorders, liver dysfunction, and hair loss.[15] These side effects often limit the use of methotrexate with rheumatoid arthritis, and most patients who stop using this drug do so because of an adverse side effect rather than a loss of effectiveness.[104] Methotrexate does, however, offer a favorable benefit-to-risk ratio in many patients and has become one of the most commonly used DMARDs.

Penicillamine

Penicillamine (Cuprimine), a derivative of penicillin, is officially classified as a chelating agent that is often used in the treatment of heavy metal intoxication (e.g., lead poisoning). In addition, this drug has been used in patients with severe rheumatoid arthritis, and seems to be as effective as other DMARDs such as methotrexate, sulfasalazine, and gold therapy.[68,98] Penicillamine, however, tends to be substantially more toxic than other DMARDs, and is therefore used rarely in the treatment of specific patients with rheumatoid arthritis.[68]

Mechanism of Action. The basis for the antiarthritic effects of penicillamine is unknown. Reductions in serum immunoglobulin M-rheumatoid factor have been observed with penicillamine, and this drug has been shown to depress T-cell function.[53] These and similar findings suggest that penicillamine works by suppressing the immune response in rheumatoid arthritis, but the exact mechanisms remain to be determined.

Adverse Side Effects. Penicillamine is considered to be fairly toxic when compared with other DMARDs.[68] Side effects that have been reported as occurring more frequently include fever, joint pain, skin rashes and itching, and swelling of lymph glands. Other adverse effects that may occur less frequently are bloody or cloudy urine, swelling of feet and legs, unusual weight gain, sore throat, and excessive fatigue.

Tumor Necrosis Factor Inhibitors

Several agents are now available that inhibit the action of tumor necrosis factor-alpha (TNF-α). TNF-α is a small protein (cytokine) that is released from cells involved in the inflammatory response. TNF-α seems to be a key chemical mediator that promotes inflammation and joint erosion in rheumatoid arthritis.[83] Drugs that inhibit this chemical will therefore help delay the progression of this disease by decreasing TNF-α's destructive effects.[70]

Drugs in this group include etanercept (Enbrel), infliximab (Remicade), and adalimumab (Humira). These drugs are also referred to as "biologic" DMARDs because they affect the biologic response to a specific cytokine (TNF-α).[68] Etanercept was the first biologic DMARD— it was created by fusing human immunoglobulin (IgG) with an amino acid sequence that mimics the binding portion of the TNF receptor. TNF-α recognizes the binding portion on the drug, attaches to this portion, and therefore cannot bind to the real TNF receptor.

The two newer agents (infliximab and adalimumab) were developed using monoclonal antibody techniques. These techniques enable the drug to bind tightly to antigenic components on TNF-α, thereby forming a drug-cytokine molecule that is too large to bind to the real TNF receptor. In addition, infliximab and adalimumab can destroy cells that express TNF-α, thus further reducing the destructive effects of this cytokine.

There is substantial evidence that TNF-α inhibitors can retard the progression of inflammatory joint disease, and promote improvements in symptoms and quality-of-life with rheumatoid arthritis.[13,51] These drugs are not typically used as the initial treatment, but can be used alone or added to other agents (e.g., methotrexate) if patients do not have an adequate response to other DMARDs.[45,91] There is some concern about toxicity (see below), and these drugs must be given parenterally, usually by subcutaneous injection (twice each week for etanercept; every other week for adalimumab), or by slow intravenous infusion (every eight weeks for infliximab). Nonetheless, TNF-α inhibitors represent an important breakthrough in the drug treatment of rheumatoid arthritis.

Mechanism of Action. As indicated, these agents bind selectively to TNF-α (see Fig. 16–2).[7,70,91] This action prevents TNF-a from binding to surface receptors located on other inflammatory cells. TNF is therefore unable to activate other inflammatory cells that cause inflammation and joint destruction in rheumatoid arthritis.[70]

Adverse Side Effects. Patients taking TNF-α inhibitors may be prone to upper respiratory tract infections and other serious infections, including sepsis.[48,51,83] This increased risk of infection probably occurs because the drug inhibits a key component of the immune response—namely, TNF-α. These drugs

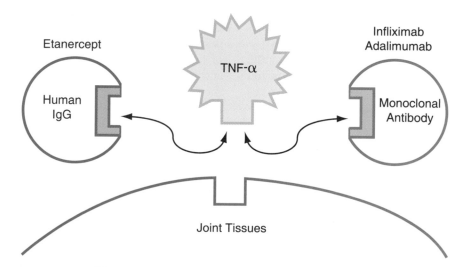

FIGURE 16–2 ▼ Schematic diagram illustrating the effects of tumor necrosis factor-alpha (TNF-α) inhibitors. Drugs such as etanercept, infliximab, and adalimumab attach directly to TNF-α, thereby preventing this destructive cytokine from reaching joint tissues. See text for more details.

are therefore contraindicated in people with infections, and administration should be discontinued if an infection develops.

Other potential adverse responses include malignancy (e.g., lymphoma), liver disease, heart failure, lupuslike disease, irritation around the injection site, and demyelinating disorders that mimic multiple sclerosis.[34,70,88] The incidence of these adverse effects, however, seems to be fairly low. For the most part, these drugs provide an acceptable risk-to-benefit ratio for most people with rheumatoid arthritis. Patients should, however, be screened carefully for any risk factors before beginning drug therapy, and should likewise be monitored periodically for any potential adverse reactions to these drugs.

Anakinra

Anakinra (Kineret) blocks the effects of interleukin-1 on joint tissues. Like TNF-α, interleukin-1 is a cytokine that promotes inflammation and joint destruction in rheumatoid arthritis.[23,36] By blocking interleukin-1 receptors on joint tissues, anakinra prevents the destructive events mediated by this cytokine. This drug appears to be moderately effective in limiting the progression of rheumatoid arthritis, and it is generally well tolerated.[36] Hence, anakinra is another option that can be used alone or in combination with other DMARDs such as methotrexate.[23]

Mechanism of Action. As indicated, anakinra is an antagonist (blocker) that is specific for the interleukin-1 receptor found on joint tissues, other tissues, and organs.[23] By blocking this receptor, the drug prevents interleukin-1 from binding to this receptor and exerting destructive effects on joint tissues.

Adverse Side Effects. Patients receiving anakinra may be more susceptible to bacterial infections and other infectious agents.[70] This drug is administered via subcutaneous injection, and irritation at the injection site is fairly common, but is usually not severe. More serious systemic allergic reactions may occur in a small number of patients.[70]

Other DMARDs

Because of the autoimmune basis of rheumatoid arthritis, various other drugs that affect the immune response are used on a limited basis. For instance, cyclosporine (Sandimmune), an immunosuppressant agent that is used to prevent rejection of organ transplants (see Chapter 37), is sometimes used to treat patients with rheumatoid arthritis who have not responded to other measures.[54] Sulfasalazine (Azulfidine), a drug that is typically used to treat inflammatory bowel disease, may also be helpful in treating rheumatoid arthritis because of its immunosuppressant effects.[68] Cyclophosphamide (Cytoxan) is used primarily to treat cancer, but this agent can be used to suppress the immune system in severe cases of rheumatoid arthritis.

In general, these drugs are more toxic and are usually reserved for patients who have not responded to more traditional DMARDs such as methotrexate. Drugs with immunosuppressant activity may also be used in combination with more traditional DMARDs to provide optimal benefits in certain patients. Combination drug therapy in rheumatoid arthritis is addressed in the next section.

DMARD Combinations Used in Rheumatoid Arthritis

There has been a great deal of interest in using several DMARDs simultaneously to achieve optimal effects in treating rheumatoid arthritis. The strategy of combination therapy is to attack the underlying disease process from several pharmacologic vantage points, much in the same way that combination therapies are used in other disorders such as hypertension (Chapter 21) and cancer (Chapter 36). Although the benefits of combining DMARDs have been questioned, most practitioners currently advocate a combination of two or more drugs so that optimal benefits can be achieved with a relatively low dose of each drug.[42,68] Likewise, the best way to combine specific DMARDs is still being investigated, with various combinations of new and old DMARDs being studied for efficacy and toxicity.[40,67] At present, methotrexate is typically the cornerstone of treatment, with other DMARDs added, depending on the needs of each patient.[76] For example, a triple combination of methotrexate with hydroxychloroquine and sulfasalazine has been advocated as an effective treatment for many patients.[39] In addition, some of the newer biologic agents such as the TNF-α inhibitors (etanercept, infliximab, adalamimab) and interleukin-1 inhibitors (anakinra) have been added to methotrexate to provide an effective combination in patients who have not responded to use of only one drug.[31,68]

The drawback of combination therapy is, of course, the potential for increased toxicity and drug interactions when several DMARDs are used simultaneously.[68] This fact is understandable, considering that many DMARDs have a relatively high risk of toxicity when used alone, and combining these drugs will certainly increase the risk of adverse drug reactions. There is, however, evidence that the incidence of side effects is not necessarily greater when DMARD combinations are used compared with a single drug such as methotrexate.[68,99] Hence, combination therapy continues to gain acceptance, and the use of two or three DMARDs early in the course of the disease may provide patients with the best hope for halting the progression of rheumatoid arthritis.[99] Continued research will hopefully lend additional insight to the best way that DMARDs can be combined to safely and effectively treat patients with rheumatoid arthritis.

Dietary Implications for Rheumatoid Arthritis

There is an ongoing search for other pharmacologic and nonpharmacologic interventions that can help arrest the progression of rheumatoid joint disease. There is some evidence, for example, that dietary manipulation can alleviate the symptoms of rheumatoid arthritis.[72] Diets that are high in fish oil and certain fatty acids (e.g., gammalinolenic acid) have been advocated for patients with rheumatoid arthritis because these diets may supply precursors that enhance the biosynthesis of certain endogenous anti-inflammatory and immunosuppressant compounds.[81,85] Foods that have antioxidant properties (e.g., fruits, vegetables) may also have beneficial effects in people with rheumatoid arthritis.[81] On the other hand, diets that are rich in meat and protein may exacerbate rheumatoid arthritis and similar inflammatory diseases.[21] Hence, dietary changes used in combination with drug therapy may provide additional benefits for some people with rheumatoid arthritis.

Osteoarthritis

Osteoarthritis far exceeds rheumatoid arthritis as the most common form of joint disease. The prevalence of osteoarthritis increases with age.[2] Approximately 50 to 80 percent of people aged 65 years have osteoarthritis to some extent, and virtually everyone over 75 years has some degree of osteoarthritic joint disease.[14] In contrast to rheumatoid joint disease, osteoarthritis does not seem to be caused by an immune response,

but rather an intrinsic defect in the joint cartilage. This defect causes a slow, progressive deterioration of articular cartilage that is accompanied by degenerative bony changes, including thickening of the subchondral bone, creation of subchondral bone cysts, and formation of large bony protrusions (osteophytes) at the joint margins.[14] Osteoarthritis typically occurs in large weight-bearing joints such as the knees and hips, as well as some of the smaller joints in the hands and feet.[18] Patients are described as having primary osteoarthritis when there is no apparent reason for the onset of joint destruction; in secondary osteoarthritis, a factor such as previous joint trauma, infection, or metabolic disease is responsible for triggering articular changes.[14] Obesity, genetic susceptibility, and joint vulnerability (malalignment, weakness, and so forth) have also been implicated as predisposing factors in osteoarthritis.[30]

Clearly, osteoarthritis is a different form of joint disease than rheumatoid arthritis. Hence, treatment of these conditions also differs somewhat. As discussed previously, rheumatoid arthritis is characterized by a severe inflammatory response that is perpetuated by a cellular immune reaction. Thus, drug therapy in rheumatoid disease consists of agents that are focused on directly relieving these inflammatory symptoms (i.e., NSAIDs or glucocorticoids) or drugs that attempt to arrest the cellular immune response that causes this inflammation (DMARDs). Treatment of joint inflammation is not a major focus of drug therapy in osteoarthritis, however. A mild inflammatory synovitis does occur in osteoarthritis, but this is secondary to the articular damage inherent to this disease.[14] Also, drug therapy represents one of the primary interventions in rheumatoid arthritis, whereas treatment of osteoarthritis should be focused more directly on nonpharmacologic measures such as physical therapy, weight loss, and joint replacement in the advanced stages of this disease.[93]

Hence, drug therapy in osteoarthritis is focused primarily on helping patients manage their pain and maintain an active lifestyle. When joint pain begins to be a problem, simple analgesics such as acetaminophen and NSAIDs have been the major form of drug therapy. Newer pharmacologic strategies are also emerging that attempt to slow or reverse the pathologic changes in osteoarthritis. These newer strategies use disease-modifying osteoarthritic drugs (DMOADs) rather than drugs that treat only the symptoms of osteoarthritis.[28,90] Two types of DMOADs will be addressed: drugs that attempt to directly improve the viscosity and function of synovial fluid (**viscosupplementation**) and agents that serve as precursors to the normal constituents of joint tissues (glucosamine and chondroitin sulfate).

Acetaminophen and NSAIDs

Acetaminophen is often the first drug used to treat osteoarthritis.[9,10] As indicated in Chapter 15, acetaminophen is as effective as NSAIDs in controlling pain, but acetaminophen does not have anti-inflammatory effects. The lack of anti-inflammatory effects is of less concern when acetaminophen is used in osteoarthritis because the inflammatory symptoms are milder. Acetaminophen is therefore successful in reducing pain, and because this drug does not cause gastric irritation, acetaminophen is often considered the drug of choice in mild-to-moderate osteoarthritis.[9,108] Hence, acetaminophen provides a relatively safe and effective form of analgesia for patients with osteoarthritis, especially when this drug needs to be administered for long periods of time.[9]

NSAIDs are also used for the symptomatic treatment of pain in osteoarthritis.[10,75] These drugs are used primarily for their analgesic properties, although the anti-inflammatory effects of NSAIDs can help control the mild synovitis that typically occurs in advanced osteoarthritis secondary to joint destruction.[75] If the primary goal is pain reduction, however, NSAIDs do not provide any advantage over acetaminophen. As indicated earlier, acetaminophen is often a better choice than traditional NSAIDs because most NSAIDs cause gastric irritation. The newer COX-2 selective NSAIDs (see Chapter 15) do not appear to cause as much gastric irritation as other NSAIDs, and these COX-2 drugs may be a valuable alternative to acetaminophen and traditional NSAIDs in the long-term treatment of osteoarthritis. COX-2 drugs, however, may increase the risk of serious cardiovascular problems (heart attack, stroke), and patients should be screened carefully for cardiovascular risk factors before beginning treatment with COX-2 drugs.[44]

Regardless of the exact drug used, there is no doubt that the analgesia produced by NSAIDs or acetaminophen plays a valuable role in the management of osteoarthritis. These drugs allow the patient to maintain a more active lifestyle and to participate in various activities, including exercise programs and other forms of physical therapy and occupational therapy. However, these drugs do not alter the progressive course of joint destruction and osteoarthritic changes. There is

preliminary evidence, in fact, that some of the NSAIDs may actually impair bone healing following fractures or surgery, but their effects on cartilage formation and soft tissue repair remain unclear (see Chapter 15).[26,46] At the present time, however, acetaminophen and NSAIDs remain the cornerstone of the pharmacologic treatment of joint pain in osteoarthritis.

Viscosupplementation

Viscosupplementation is a clinical procedure that is being used increasingly in the treatment of osteoarthritis. This technique uses a substance known as hyaluronan to restore the lubricating properties of synovial fluid in osteoarthritic joints.[6,41] Hyaluronan is a polysaccharide that can be injected into an arthritic joint to help restore the normal viscosity of the synovial fluid.[6] This treatment helps reduce joint stresses, thus limiting the progression of articular destruction seen in osteoarthritis.[106] Viscosupplementation has therefore been shown to reduce pain and improve function in osteoarthritis.[1,95]

When used to treat osteoarthritis, viscosupplementation typically consists of 2 to 10 weekly injections of hyaluronan Hyalgan, Synvisc, others. Patients often experience a decrease in pain within days after injection, and pain continues to diminish within the first weeks after treatment. Duration of relief is variable, but most patients who respond to viscosupplementation experience beneficial effects for 6 months to 1 year after a series of injections.[74]

Hence, viscosupplementation may temporarily attenuate the progressive changes in joint structure and function typically seen in osteoarthritis. Although these benefits are relatively transient, viscosupplementation can delay the need for more invasive surgical treatments such as joint replacement. This intervention is also tolerated fairly well, although a pseudoseptic reaction that produces local pain and swelling may occur.[41,106] Future clinical studies will be needed to determine how viscosupplementation can be used most effectively in the comprehensive treatment of people with osteoarthritis.

Glucosamine and Chondroitin Sulfate

It has been suggested that dietary supplements such as glucosamine and chondroitin sulfate may help protect articular cartilage and halt or reverse joint degeneration in osteoarthritis. These two compounds are key ingredients needed for the production of several components of articular cartilage and synovial fluid, including glycosaminoglycans, proteoglycans, and hyaluronic acid.[71,112] It seems reasonable that increased amounts of these ingredients should facilitate the repair of joint tissues, improve synovial fluid viscosity, and help restore joint function in conditions like osteoarthritis. Hence, several products containing glucosamine, or glucosamine combined with chondroitin sulfate, are currently available as nonprescription dietary supplements. These supplements typically contain oral dosages of 1500 mg/d glucosamine and 1200 mg/d chondroitin sulfate.[82]

Several recent studies suggest that chondroitin and glucosamine supplements can decrease pain and improve function in some patients with osteoarthritis.[47,62,64] Radiographic studies also indicate that these supplements can reduce joint space narrowing in knee osteoarthritis, thus providing some protective effects on joint structure.[78,82] These benefits may not occur in all patients—patients with a high rate of cartilage turnover may be more likely to experience positive effects because these supplements will provide the necessary substrates to sustain this turnover and maintain joint integrity.[22]

Consequently, it appears that glucosamine and chondroitin supplements are certainly worth a trial for many patients with osteoarthritis. Some gastrointestinal problems may occur, but these supplements are usually well tolerated. Although these supplements are available over-the-counter in the United States, people with osteoarthritis should consult their physician and pharmacist before self-administration. Likewise, patients should be educated on the proper dosage, and should be reminded that these products may need to be consumed for several weeks or months before beneficial effects become apparent. Long-term studies on the effects of these supplements are currently being conducted, and clinicians should try to stay abreast of any new information about the potential benefits of glucosamine and chondroitin.

Special Concerns for Antiarthritic Drug Therapy in Rehabilitation Patients

■ ■ ■ Drugs used to treat rheumatoid arthritis and osteoarthritis often play a vital role in permitting optimal rehabilitation of patients with joint disease. By decreasing pain and inflammation, these drugs help facilitate a more active and vigorous program of exercise and functional activity. Some drugs, such as the disease-modifying drugs used in rheumatoid arthritis and osteoarthritis, appear to be able to impair or even halt the progression of joint destruction. This may enable the therapist to help restore muscle strength and joint function rather than simply employ a program of maintenance therapy during a steady downward progression in patients with arthritis.

The influence of antiarthritic drugs on the rehabilitative process depends primarily on the type of drugs used. Beginning with the NSAIDs, there is little concern for adverse effects on physical therapy procedures. These drugs are relatively safe and are not usually associated with the type of side effects that will directly influence the physical rehabilitation of people with rheumatoid arthritis or osteoarthritis. If glucocorticoids are used, the therapist must be aware of adverse side effects; in particular, the catabolic effects of these agents on supporting tissues (muscle, tendon, bone, skin) must be considered. Range-of-motion and strengthening programs must be used judiciously to avoid fractures and soft-tissue injuries. Care must also be taken to prevent skin breakdown, especially when splints and other protective orthotic devices are employed.

The disease-modifying agents used in rheumatoid arthritis are associated with a number of side effects that could influence rehabilitation. Some of these drugs, such as the gold compounds and methotrexate, may cause headache and nausea, which may be bothersome during the therapy session. Joint pain and swelling may also occur with drugs such as methotrexate and peni-

Continued on following page

cillamine, and these effects may also become a problem during rehabilitation. A variety of other side effects can occur, depending on the particular DMARD being used and the sensitivity of the patient. Therapists should be aware of any changes in patient response, not only when a new drug is being started but also during the prolonged use of DMARDs.

Finally, the use of DMOADs (viscosupplementation, glucosamine, chondroitin) to restore joint function in osteoarthritis is fairly new, and it is not clear if these techniques will have any side effects that will have a direct impact on physical rehabilitation. Likewise, it remains to be seen if there are any rehabilitation techniques (exercise, physical agents) that could enhance the effectiveness of DMOADs. It is hoped that these techniques will work synergistically with physical therapy to improve function in patients with osteoarthritic joints.

CASE STUDY
Rheumatoid Arthritis

Brief History. A.T., a 75-year-old woman, was diagnosed with rheumatoid joint disease several years ago. She is currently being seen three times each week in physical therapy as an outpatient for a program of paraffin and active exercise to her wrists and hands. Resting splints were also fabricated for both hands, and these are worn at night to prevent joint deformity. The patient was also instructed in a home exercise program to maintain joint mobility in both upper extremities. Pharmacologic management in this patient originally consisted of NSAIDs, beginning with aspirin and later switching to ibuprofen. Six months ago, she was also placed on auranofin (Ridaura), which was instituted in an attempt to halt the progressive arthritic changes. This orally administered gold compound was given at a dosage of 3 mg twice each day.

Problem/Influence of Medication. The combination of an NSAID and a disease-modifying drug, along with the physical therapy program, seemed to be helping to decrease the patient's pain and joint stiffness. However, she began to develop skin rashes and itching on her arms and legs. The therapist noticed this while preparing the patient for her paraffin treatment. It seemed that these rashes might be occurring as a side effect of the auranofin. The therapist brought this to the attention of the physician, who concurred that this was probably a side effect of the gold therapy.

Decision/Solution. The patient was temporarily removed from auranofin therapy to see if this skin reaction would subside. In the interim, the therapist discontinued paraffin so that the rashes and itching would not be exacerbated. To continue to provide gentle heat, a warm whirlpool (100°F) was substituted for the paraffin bath. Also, the night splints were temporarily discontinued to prevent irritation to the affected areas. After 2 weeks, the skin rashes had virtually disappeared, and the original physical therapy program was resumed. After another week, the physician restarted DMARD therapy in the form of low dose methotrexate combined with etanercept (Enbrel). This combination was intended to provide a more comprehensive antiarthritic regimen, while reducing the chance of the allergic response that is common with gold compounds. No other adverse effects were noted, and the patient continued to notice improvements in her arthritic condition.

SUMMARY

Rheumatoid arthritis and osteoarthritis represent two distinct forms of joint disease that can produce devastating effects on the structure and function of synovial joints. Fortunately, management of these conditions has improved substantially through advancements in drug therapy. Rheumatoid arthritis can be treated pharmacologically with NSAIDs, glucocorticoids, and various DMARDs. NSAIDs, including aspirin, represent the primary form of drug therapy in the early stages of this disease, and these drugs are often used in conjunction with other drugs as the arthritic condition increases in severity. Glucocorticoids are often effective in decreasing the joint inflammation typically found in rheumatoid arthritis, but long-term use of these agents is limited because of their toxic effects. Disease-modifying drugs can slow or halt the progressive nature of rheumatoid arthritis by suppressing the immune response inherent in this disease. Although there is some concern about the efficacy and safety of these drugs, DMARDs have been a welcome addition to the rather limited arsenal of drugs used to treat rheumatoid arthritis.

Drug treatment of osteoarthritis differs somewhat from that of rheumatoid arthritis, with management of pain by using NSAIDs and acetaminophen constituting the major forms of drug therapy. A newer technique known as viscosupplementation has also been used to help restore the lubricating properties of the synovial fluid in osteoarthritic joints. Dietary supplements containing glucosamine and chondroitin sulfate may also help provide constituents that protect joint structure and function, and some people with osteoarthritis have benefited from their long-term use. In any event, drug therapy along with nonpharmacologic measures such as physical therapy can provide an effective way of dealing with the potentially devastating effects of rheumatoid arthritis and osteoarthritis.

References

1. Aggarwal A, Sempowski IP. Hyaluronic acid injections for knee osteoarthritis. Systematic review of the literature. *Can Fam Physician.* 2004;50:249–256.
2. Aigner T, Rose J, Martin J, Buckwalter J. Aging theories of primary osteoarthritis: from epidemiology to molecular biology. *Rejuvenation Res.* 2004; 7:134–145.
3. Akarca US. Gastrointestinal effects of selective and non-selective non-steroidal anti-inflammatory drugs. *Curr Pharm Des.* 2005;11:1779–1793.
4. Aletaha D, Smolen JS. DMARD use in early rheumatoid arthritis. Lessons from observations in patients with established disease. *Clin Exp Rheumatol.* 2003;21 (suppl 31):S169–S173.
5. Backman CL. Employment and work disability in rheumatoid arthritis. *Curr Opin Rheumatol.* 2004;16: 148–152.
6. Balazs EA. Viscosupplementation for treatment of osteoarthritis: from initial discovery to current status and results. *Surg Technol Int.* 2004;12:278–289.
7. Bang LM, Keating GM. Adalimumab: a review of its use in rheumatoid arthritis. *BioDrugs.* 2004;18: 121–139.
8. Barnes PJ. Anti-inflammatory actions of glucocorticoids: molecular mechanisms. *Clin Sci.* 1998;94: 557–572.
9. Bertin P, Keddad K, Jolivet-Landreau I. Acetaminophen as symptomatic treatment of pain from osteoarthritis. *Joint Bone Spine.* 2004;71:266–274.
10. Bijlsma JW. Analgesia and the patient with osteoarthritis. *Am J Ther.* 2002;9:189–197.
11. Bijlsma JW, Saag KG, Buttgereit F, da Silva JA. Developments in glucocorticoid therapy. *Rheum Dis Clin North Am.* 2005;31:1–17.
12. Blumenauer B, Cranney A, Clinch J, Tugwell P. Quality of life in patients with rheumatoid arthritis: which drugs might make a difference? *Pharmacoeconomics.* 2003;21:927–940.
13. Blumenauer B, Judd M, Cranney A, et al. Etanercept for the treatment of rheumatoid arthritis. *Cochrane Database Syst Rev.* 2003;CD004525.
14. Boh LE, Elliott ME. Osteoarthritis. In: DiPiro JT, et al, eds. *Pharmacotherapy: A Pathophysiologic Approach.* 5th ed. New York: McGraw-Hill; 2002.
15. Borchers AT, Keen CL, Cheema GS, Gershwin ME. The use of methotrexate in rheumatoid arthritis. *Semin Arthritis Rheum.* 2004;34:465–483.
16. Browning DJ. Hydroxychloroquine and chloroquine retinopathy: screening for drug toxicity. *Am J Ophthalmol.* 2002;133:649–656.
17. Buckbinder L, Robinson RP. The glucocorticoid receptor: molecular mechanism and new therapeutic opportunities. *Curr Drug Targets Inflamm Allergy.* 2002;1:127–136.
18. Buckwalter JA, Saltzman C, Brown T. The impact of osteoarthritis: implications for research. *Clin Orthop Relat Res.* 2004;(suppl 427):S6–S15.
19. Cannon GW, Kremer JM. Leflunomide. *Rheum Dis Clin North Am.* 2004;30:295–309.
20. Chabner B, Ryan DP, Paz-Ares L, et al. Antineoplastic agents. In: Hardman JG, et al, eds. *The Pharmacological Basis of Therapeutics.* 10th ed. New York: McGraw-Hill; 2001.
21. Choi HK. Dietary risk factors for rheumatic diseases. *Curr Opin Rheumatol.* 2005;17:141–146.
22. Christgau S, Henrotin Y, Tanko LB, et al. Osteoarthritic patients with high cartilage turnover show increased responsiveness to the cartilage protecting effects of glucosamine sulphate. *Clin Exp Rheumatol.* 2004;22: 36–42.
23. Cohen SB. The use of anakinra, an interleukin-1 receptor antagonist, in the treatment of rheumatoid arthritis. *Rheum Dis Clin North Am.* 2004;30:365–380.
24. Conn DL, Lim SS. New role for an old friend: prednisone is a disease-modifying agent in early rheumatoid arthritis. *Curr Opin Rheumatol.* 2003;15:193–196.
25. Constable S, Pirmohamed M. Drugs and the retina. *Expert Opin Drug Saf.* 2004;3:249–259.
26. Dahners LE, Mullis BH. Effects of nonsteroidal anti-inflammatory drugs on bone formation and soft-tissue healing. *J Am Acad Orthop Surg.* 2004;12: 139–143.
27. Eisler R. Chrysotherapy: a synoptic review. *Inflamm Res.* 2003;52:487–501.
28. Fajardo M, Di Cesare PE. Disease-modifying therapies for osteoarthritis: current status. *Drugs Aging.* 2005;22: 141–161.
29. Falgarone G, Jaen O, Boissier MC. Role for innate immunity in rheumatoid arthritis. *Joint Bone Spine.* 2005;72:17–25.

30. Felson DT. Risk factors for osteoarthritis: understanding joint vulnerability. *Clin Orthop Relat Res.* 2004;427:(suppl):S16–S21.

31. Finesilver AG. Newer approaches to the treatment of rheumatoid arthritis. *WMJ.* 2003;102:34–37.

32. Firestein GS, Corr M. Common mechanisms in immune-mediated inflammatory disease. *J Rheumatol Suppl.* 2005;73:8–13; discussion 29–30.

33. Fitzpatrick FA. Cyclooxygenase enzymes: regulation and function. *Curr Pharm Des.* 2004;10:577–588.

34. Fleischmann RM, Iqbal I, Stern RL. Considerations with the use of biological therapy in the treatment of rheumatoid arthritis. *Expert Opin Drug Saf.* 2004;3:391–403.

35. Fox, RI. Mechanism of action of hydroxychloroquine as an antirheumatic drug. *Semin Arthritis Rheum.* 1993;23(suppl 1):82–91.

36. Furst DE. Anakinra: review of recombinant human interleukin-I receptor antagonist in the treatment of rheumatoid arthritis. *Clin Ther.* 2004;26:1960–1975.

37. Furst, DE. The rationale use of methotrexate in rheumatoid arthritis and other rheumatic diseases. *Br J Rheumatol.* 1997;36:1196–1204.

38. Gabriel SE. The epidemiology of rheumatoid arthritis. *Rheum Dis Clin North Am.* 2001;27:269–281.

39. Garrood T, Scott DL. Combination therapy with disease modifying anti-rheumatic drugs in rheumatoid arthritis. *BioDrugs.* 2001;15:543–561.

40. Geletka R, St Clair EW. Treatment of early rheumatoid arthritis. *Best Pract Res Clin Rheumatol.* 2003;17:791–809.

41. Goldberg VM, Coutts RD. Pseudoseptic reactions to hylan viscosupplementation: diagnosis and treatment. *Clin Orthop Relat Res.* 2004;419:130–137.

42. Gossec L, Dougados M. Combination therapy in early rheumatoid arthritis.*Clin Exp Rheumatol.* 2003;21(suppl 31):S174–S178.

43. Gotzsche PC, Johansen HK. Short-term low-dose corticosteroids vs placebo and nonsteroidal antiinflammatory drugs in rheumatoid arthritis. *Cochrane Database Syst Rev.* 2004;CD000189.

44. Grainger R, Cicuttini FM. Medical management of osteoarthritis of the knee and hip joints. *Med J Aust.* 2004;180:232–236.

45. Haraoui B. The anti-tumor necrosis factor agents are a major advance in the treatment of rheumatoid arthritis. *J Rheumatol Suppl.* 2005;72:46–47.

46. Harder AT, An YH. The mechanisms of the inhibitory effects of nonsteroidal anti-inflammatory drugs on bone healing: a concise review. *J Clin Pharmacol.* 2003;43:807–815.

47. Hungerford DS, Jones LC. Glucosamine and chondroitin sulfate are effective in the management of osteoarthritis. *J Arthroplasty.* 2003;18(suppl 1):5–9.

48. Hyrich KL. Assessing the safety of biologic therapies in rheumatoid arthritis: the challenges of study design. *J Rheumatol Suppl.* 2005;72:48–50.

49. Issa SN, Ruderman EM. Damage control in rheumatoid arthritis. Hard-hitting, early treatment is crucial to curbing joint destruction. *Postgrad Med.* 2004;116:14–16, 21–24.

50. Jacobs JW, Geenen R, Evers AW, et al. Short term effects of corticosteroid pulse treatment on disease activity and the wellbeing of patients with active rheumatoid arthritis. *Ann Rheum Dis.* 2001;60:61–64.

51. Keystone EC. Safety of biologic therapies—an update. *J Rheumatol Suppl.* 2005;74:8–12.

52. Kirwan JR. Effects of long-term glucocorticoid therapy in rheumatoid arthritis. *Z Rheumatol.* 2000;59 (suppl 2):II, 85–89.

53. Klaassen CD. Heavy metals and heavy-metal antagonists. In: Hardman JG, et al, eds. *The Pharmacological Basis of Therapeutics.* 10th ed. New York: McGraw-Hill; 2001.

54. Krensky AM, Strom TB, Bluestone J.: Immunomodulators: immunosuppressive agents, tolerogens, and immunostimulants. In: Hardman JG, et al, eds. *The Pharmacological Basis of Therapeutics.* 10th ed. New York: McGraw-Hill; 2001.

55. Kvien TK. Epidemiology and burden of illness of rheumatoid arthritis. *Pharmacoeconomics.* 2004;22 (suppl 2):1–12.

56. Lee SJ, Kavanaugh A. Pharmacological treatment of established rheumatoid arthritis. *Best Pract Res Clin Rheumatol.* 2003;17:811–829.

57. Li EK, Tam LS, Tomlinson B. Leflunomide in the treatment of rheumatoid arthritis. *Clin Ther.* 2004;26:447–459.

58. Lorenz HM. T-cell-activation inhibitors in rheumatoid arthritis. *BioDrugs.* 2003;17:263–270.

59. Maddison P, Kiely P, Kirkham B, et al. Leflunomide in rheumatoid arthritis: recommendations through a process of consensus. *Rheumatology.* 2005;44:280–286.

60. Marmor MF. Hydroxychloroquine at the recommended dose (< or = 6.5 mg/kg/day) is safe for the retina in patients with rheumatoid arthritis and systemic lupus erythematosus. *Clin Exp Rheumatol.* 2004;22:143–144.

61. Martel-Pelletier J, Pelletier JP, Fahmi H. Cyclooxygenase-2 and prostaglandins in articular tissues. *Semin Arthritis Rheum.* 2003;33:155–167.

62. Matheson AJ, Perry CM. Glucosamine: a review of its use in the management of osteoarthritis. *Drugs Aging.* 2003;20:1041–1060.

63. Mavrikakis I, Sfikakis PP, Mavrikakis E, et al. The incidence of irreversible retinal toxicity in patients treated with hydroxychloroquine: a reappraisal. *Ophthalmology.* 2003;110:1321–1326.

64. McAlindon TE, LaValley MP, Gulin JP, Felson DT. Glucosamine and chondroitin for treatment of osteoarthritis: a systematic quality assessment and meta-analysis.*JAMA.* 2000;283:1469–1475.

65. Miceli-Richard C, Dougados M. Leflunomide for the treatment of rheumatoid arthritis. *Expert Opin Pharmacother.* 2003;4:987–997.

66. Morrow JD, Roberts LJ. Lipid-derived autacoids: eicosanoids and platelet-activating factor. In: Hardman JG, et al, eds. *The Pharmacological Basis of Therapeutics.* 10th ed. New York: McGraw-Hill; 2001.

67. Mullan RH, Bresnihan B. Disease-modifying antirheumatic drug therapy and structural damage in early

rheumatoid arthritis. *Clin Exp Rheumatol.* 2003;21 (suppl 31):S158–S164.

68. O'Dell JR. Therapeutic strategies for rheumatoid arthritis. *N Engl J Med.* 2004;350:2591–2602.

69. Olson JC. Juvenile idiopathic arthritis: an update. *WMJ.* 2003;102:45–50.

70. Olsen NJ, Stein CM. New drugs for rheumatoid arthritis. *N Engl J Med.* 2004;350:2167–2179.

71. Owens S, Wagner P, Vangsness CT, Jr. Recent advances in glucosamine and chondroitin supplementation. *J Knee Surg.* 2004;17:185–193.

72. Pattison DJ, Harrison RA, Symmons DP. The role of diet in susceptibility to rheumatoid arthritis: a systematic review. *J Rheumatol.* 2004;31:1310–1319.

73. Petersson IF, Jacobsson LT. Osteoarthritis of the peripheral joints. *Best Pract Res Clin Rheumatol.* 2002;16:741–760.

74. Peyron, JG. Intraarticular hyaluronan injections in the treatment of osteoarthritis: state-of-the-art review. *J Rheumatol.* 1993;39:10–15.

75. Pincus T. Clinical evidence for osteoarthritis as an inflammatory disease. *Curr Rheumatol Rep.* 2001;3:524–534.

76. Pincus T, Yazici Y, Sokka T, et al. Methotrexate as the "anchor drug" for the treatment of early rheumatoid arthritis. *Clin Exp Rheumatol.* 2003;21(suppl 31):S179–S185.

77. Porter DR, Sturrock RD. Fortnightly review: medical management of rheumatoid arthritis. *BMJ.* 1993;307:425–428.

78. Reginster JY, Deroisy R, Rovati LC, et al. Long-term effects of glucosamine sulphate on osteoarthritis progression: a randomised, placebo-controlled clinical trial. *Lancet.* 2001;357:251–256.

79. Reiff AO. Juvenile arthritis. In: Rakel RE, Bope ET, eds. *Conn's Current Therapy 2005.* New York: Elsevier Saunders; 2005.

80. Reiff AO. Developments in the treatment of juvenile arthritis. *Expert Opin Pharmacother.* 2004;5:1485–1496.

81. Rennie KL, Hughes J, Lang R, Jebb SA. Nutritional management of rheumatoid arthritis: a review of the evidence. *J Hum Nutr Diet.* 2003;16:97–109.

82. Richy F, Bruyere O, Ethgen O, et al. Structural and symptomatic efficacy of glucosamine and chondroitin in knee osteoarthritis: a comprehensive meta-analysis. *Arch Intern Med.* 2003;163:1514–1522.

83. Roberts L, McColl GJ. Tumour necrosis factor inhibitors: risks and benefits in patients with rheumatoid arthritis. *Intern Med J.* 2004;34:687–693.

84. Roberts LJ, Morrow JD. Analgesic-antipyretic and antiinflammatory agents and drugs employed in the treatment of gout. In: Hardman JG, et al, eds. *The Pharmacological Basis of Therapeutics.* 10th ed. New York: McGraw-Hill; 2001.

85. Ruxton C. Health benefits of omega-3 fatty acids. *Nurs Stand.* 2004;18:38–42.

86. Saag KG. Glucocorticoid use in rheumatoid arthritis. *Curr Rheumatol Rep.* 2002;4:218–225.

87. Saklatvala J, Dean J, Clark A. Control of the expression of inflammatory response genes. *Biochem Soc Symp.* 2003;70:95–106.

88. Scheinfeld N. A comprehensive review and evaluation of the side effects of the tumor necrosis factor alpha blockers etanercept, infliximab and adalimumab. *J Dermatolog Treat.* 2004;15:280–294.

89. Schimmer BP, Parker KL. Adrenocorticotropic hormone: adrenocortical steroids and their synthetic analogs; inhibitors of the synthesis and actions of adrenocortical hormones. In: Hardman JG, et al, eds. *The Pharmacological Basis of Therapeutics.* 10th ed. New York: McGraw-Hill; 2001.

90. Schuna AA. Rheumatoid arthritis. In: DiPiro JT, et al, eds. *Pharmacotherapy: A Pathophysiologic Approach.* 5th ed. New York: McGraw-Hill; 2002.

91. Scott DL. Etanercept in arthritis. *Int J Clin Pract.* 2005;59:114–118.

92. Seitz, M. Molecular and cellular effects of methotrexate. *Curr Opin Rheumatol.* 1999;11:226–232.

93. Singh G. Treatment options for osteoarthritis. *Surg Technol Int.* 2003;11:287–292.

94. Sivakumar B, Paleolog E. Immunotherapy of rheumatoid arthritis: past, present and future. *Curr Opin Drug Discov Devel.* 2005;8:169–176.

95. Snibbe JC, Gambardella RA. Use of injections for osteoarthritis in joints and sports activity. *Clin Sports Med.* 2005;24:83–91.

96. Strand V, Simon LS. Low dose glucocorticoids in early rheumatoid arthritis. *Clin Exp Rheumatol.* 2003;21(suppl 31):S186–S190.

97. Suarez-Almazor ME, Spooner C, Belseck E. Azathioprine for treating rheumatoid arthritis. *Cochrane Database Syst Rev.* 2000;CD001461.

98. Suarez-Almazor ME, Spooner C, Belseck E. Penicillamine for treating rheumatoid arthritis. *Cochrane Database Syst Rev.* 2000;CD001460.

99. Suresh E, Lambert CM. Combination treatment strategies in early rheumatoid arthritis. *Ann Rheum Dis.* 2005; 64:1252–1256.

100. Sweeney SE, Firestein GS. Rheumatoid arthritis: regulation of synovial inflammation.*Int J Biochem Cell Biol.* 2004;36:372–378.

101. Symmons DP. Epidemiology of rheumatoid arthritis: determinants of onset, persistence and outcome. *Best Pract Res Clin Rheumatol.* 2002;16:707–722.

102. Townsend HB, Saag KG. Glucocorticoid use in rheumatoid arthritis: benefits, mechanisms, and risks. *Clin Exp Rheumatol.* 2004;22(suppl 35):S77–S82.

103. Vane JR, Botting RM. The mechanism of action of aspirin. *Thromb Res.* 2003;110:255–258.

104. Van Ede AE, Laan RF, Blom HJ et al: Methotrexate in rheumatoid arthritis: an update with focus on mechanisms involved in toxicity. *Semin Arthritis Rheum.* 1998;27:277–292.

105. van Riel PL, Smolen JS, Emery P, et al. Leflunomide: a manageable safety profile. *J Rheumatol Suppl.* 2004; 71:21–24.

106. Waddell DD. The tolerability of viscosupplementation: low incidence and clinical management of local adverse events. *Curr Med Res Opin.* 2003;19: 575–580.

107. Wagner W, Khanna P, Furst DE. Nonsteroidal antiinflammatory drugs, disease-modifying antirheumatic drugs, nonopioid analgesics, and drugs used in gout.

In: Katzung BG, ed. *Basic and Clinical Pharmacology.* 9th ed. New York: Lange Medical Books/McGraw-Hill; 2004.

108. Wegman A, van der Windt D, van Tulder M, et al. Nonsteroidal antiinflammatory drugs or acetaminophen for osteoarthritis of the hip or knee? A systematic review of evidence and guidelines. *J Rheumatol.* 2004;31:344–354.

109. Weiss JE, Ilowite NT. Juvenile idiopathic arthritis. *Pediatr Clin North Am.* 2005;52:413–442.

110. Wienecke T, Gotzsche PC. Paracetamol versus nonsteroidal anti-inflammatory drugs for rheumatoid arthritis. *Cochrane Database Syst Rev.* 2004;CD003789.

111. Yamashita M, Ohuchi K, Takayanagi M. Effects of chrisotherapeutic gold compounds on prostaglandin E2 production. *Curr Drug Targets Inflamm Allergy.* 2003;2:216–223.

112. Zerkak D, Dougados M. The use of glucosamine therapy in osteoarthritis. *Curr Pain Headache Rep.* 2004;8:507–511.

Chapter 17

Patient-Controlled Analgesia

Patient-controlled analgesia (PCA) was first introduced into clinical practice in the early 1980s as an alternative way to administer analgesic medications. The basic principle behind PCA is that the patient can self-administer small doses of the drug (usually an opioid) at relatively frequent intervals to provide optimal pain relief.[32] These small doses are typically delivered intravenously or into the spinal canal by some type of machine (pump) that is controlled by the patient. Patient-controlled analgesia has several advantages over more traditional dosing regimens. In particular, PCA systems often provide equivalent or increased analgesic effects with a lower incidence of side effects while using less of the drug.[9,32] This fact has generated a great deal of interest and increased use of PCA in a variety of clinical situations. For instance, PCA systems have been used to help manage acute pain following surgery, and PCAs have also been used to treat pain in patients with cancer and other conditions associated with chronic pain.[10,19]

Hence, PCA continues to gain acceptance as an optimal method for treating pain. Because PCA is used extensively to treat acute and chronic pain, rehabilitation specialists should be aware of some of the fundamental principles governing PCA. This chapter begins by discussing the basic concepts and strategies of PCA, followed by some of its practical aspects, including the types of analgesics used, the possible routes of administration, and the types of machines used to administer the drugs. An indication of why PCA is often clinically superior to more traditional methods of analgesia is then presented. Finally, potential problems associated with PCA and the specific ways that PCA can affect patients receiving physical therapy and occupational therapy are discussed. It is hoped that this will provide the reader with a better understanding of why PCA

systems are often a preferred method of managing pain in contemporary practice.

Pharmacokinetic Basis for PCA

To provide optimal management of pain, analgesic drugs should be delivered into the bloodstream or other target tissues (epidural space, within joints, and so forth) in a predictable and fairly constant manner. The goal is to maintain drug levels within a fairly well-defined range, or therapeutic window.[32] Such a therapeutic window for systemic (intravenous) dosages is represented schematically by the shaded area in Figure 17–1. If drug levels are below this window, the analgesic is below the minimum analgesic concentration, and the patient is in pain. Drug levels above the window may produce adequate analgesia but may also produce side effects such as sedation. The traditional method of administering analgesics is to give relatively large doses with relatively large time intervals between each dosage. For instance, opioid analgesics are typically injected intramuscularly every 3 to 4 hours to manage severe pain, thus creating large fluctuations in the amount of drug present in the body. The dark solid lines in Figure 17–1 illustrate these large fluctuations. As illustrated in Figure 17–1, this traditional method of administration is associated with long periods of time when the drug concentration falls below the therapeutic window, allowing pain to occur, or above the therapeutic window, causing sedation.

Figure 17–1 also illustrates why PCA systems are better at maintaining drug levels within the therapeutic (analgesic) window. Systems using some form of PCA deliver small doses of the analgesic on a relative-

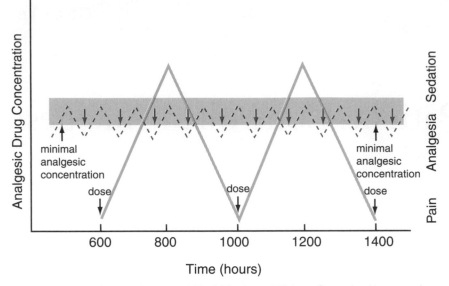

FIGURE 17–1 ▼ Pharmacokinetic model for PCA using opioid drugs. Conventional intramuscular injection is indicated by the long solid lines, PCA is indicated by the short dashed lines, and the therapeutic window for analgesia is indicated by the shaded area. (From Ferrante, et al. *Anesth Analg.* 1988;67: 457–461; with permission.)

ly frequent basis, as indicated by the dashed lines. Drug levels are maintained within the analgesic range; there are shorter periods of time when the drug concentration falls below the therapeutic window (i.e., below the shaded area), and there is virtually no time when side effects occur because the concentration rises above the therapeutic window. Hence, analgesia can be achieved more effectively with a reduced incidence of side effects.

PCA Dosing Strategies and Parameters

The fact that PCA enables the patient to self-deliver small doses of the analgesic at frequent intervals illustrates the need for specific dosing parameters that control the amount and frequency of analgesic administration. Several terms are used to describe these parameters and indicate each parameter's role in safeguarding against excessive drug delivery.[34,38] The basic terms that describe PCA dosing strategies are indicated below.

Loading Dose

A single large dose is given initially to establish analgesia. This loading dose is used to bring levels of the

analgesic to the therapeutic window, as illustrated by the shaded area in Figure 17–1.

Demand Dose

The amount of drug that is self-administered by the patient each time he or she activates the PCA delivery mechanism is known as the demand dose. The magnitude of these doses for some commonly used opioid analgesics is listed in Table 17–1.

Lockout Interval

The minimum amount of time allowed between each demand dose is called the lockout interval. After the patient self-administers a dose, the PCA delivery system will not deliver the next dose until the lockout interval has expired. Typical lockout intervals for commonly used opioids are listed in Table 17–1.

1- and 4-Hour Limits

Some PCA systems can be set to limit the total amount of drug given in a 1- or 4-hour period. The use of these parameters is somewhat questionable, however, because other parameters such as the demand dose and lockout interval automatically limit the total amount of drug that can be given in a specific period of time.

Table 17-1	PARAMETERS FOR INTRAVENOUS PCA USING OPIOID MEDICATIONS	
Drug (Concentration)	**Demand Dose**	**Lockout Interval (min)**
Alfentanil (0.1 mg/mL)	0.1–0.2 mg	5–8
Buprenorphine (0.03 mg/mL)	0.03–0.1 mg	8–20
Fentanyl (10 μg/mL)	10–20 μg	3–10
Hydromorphone (0.2 mg/mL)	0.05–0.25 mg	5–10
Meperidine (10 mg/mL)	5–25 mg	5–10
Methadone (1 mg/mL)	0.5–2.5 mg	8–20
Morphine (1 mg/mL)	0.5–2.5 mg	5–10
Nalbuphine (1 mg/mL)	1–5 mg	5–15
Oxymorphone (0.25 mg/mL)	0.2–0.4 mg	8–10
Pentazocine (10 mg/mL)	5–30 mg	5–15
Sufentanil (.2 μg/mL)	0.2–0.5 μg	3–10

Source: Ready,[38] p 2328, with permission.

Background Infusion Rate

In some patients, a small amount of the analgesic is infused continuously to maintain a low, background level of analgesia. Demand doses are superimposed on the background infusion whenever the patient feels an increase in pain (e.g., the so-called breakthrough pain that may occur when the patient coughs or changes position). The use of background infusion basically combines the technique of continuous infusion with PCA, which may provide optimal analgesia with minimal side effects.[38] Background infusion, for example, can maintain adequate analgesia even when patients are asleep or otherwise unable to activate the pump manually.

Nonetheless, routine use of background infusion has been questioned, especially when opioids are administered systemically (intravenously) by PCA. It appears that background infusions may not provide any additional analgesic benefits in most patients, but they can lead to an increased risk of side effects such as respiratory depression because patients ultimately receive a larger total amount of opioid (i.e., the background infusion plus the demand doses).[8,34] Hence, background infusion rates have been discouraged for most patients, but may still be used in specific cases such as patients who need larger amounts of opioids to control pain, especially during sleep.[34]

Successful Versus Total Demands

Successful demands occur when the patient activates the PCA delivery system and actually receives a demand dose of the drug. Demands made during the lockout interval are not considered successful, but are added to the number of successful demands to indicate the total demands. A large number of unsuccessful demands may indicate that the PCA parameters are not effective in providing adequate analgesia. Therefore, most PCA systems record the number of total demands so that the demand dose can be adjusted if a large number of unsuccessful demands are being made.

Types of Analgesics Used for PCA

Opioid analgesics (see Chapter 14) are the primary medications used during PCA.[9] Opioids such as morphine, meperidine, tramadol, fentanyl, and fentanyl derivatives (alfentanil, remifentanil) are powerful analgesics that act primarily on the spinal cord and brain to inhibit the transmission and perception of nociceptive impulses. Opioids must be used cautiously because these drugs can cause serious side effects and have the potential for patient overdose. As explained earlier, PCA often provides a safer and more effective way to administer these powerful drugs by preventing large fluctuations in plasma opioid levels.

Likewise, a number of nonopioid analgesics have been combined with opioids during systemic (intravenous) PCA to decrease the amount of opioid needed for adequate analgesia. This "opioid sparing" effect can be achieved by combining morphine or other opioids with ketorolac (an NSAID; see Chapter 15), ketamine (an anesthetic agent; see Chapter 11), or droperidol (an antipsychotic; see Chapter 8).[15,33,43] Alternatively, a very low dose of an opioid receptor antagonist (blocker) such as naloxone (see Chapter14) can also be administered along with the opioid during PCA. Preliminary evidence suggests that a low dosage of the opioid antagonist may block certain opioid side effects (nausea, pruritus) while still allowing an adequate level of analgesia.[11,36]

Local anesthetics such as bupivacaine and ropivacaine have also been used during PCA (see Chapter 12). These drugs, which block transmission along afferent sensory neurons, can be administered epidurally to block sensation at the spinal cord level. Local anesthetics are often administered when an epidural PCA is used during labor and childbirth.[23] These drugs have also been mixed with opioids to provide optimal epidural PCA during labor or following surgery.[2,4,25] Local anesthetics can also be applied to a specific site such as the subacromial space or around a specific peripheral nerve. This technique, known as patient controlled regional anesthesia (PCRA), is discussed later. Hence, local anesthetics serve as an alternative or adjunct to opioids during several types of PCA.

Administration Routes During PCA

Intravenous PCA

Patient controlled intravenous analgesia (PCIA) is perhaps the simplest and most common method of PCA administration. PCIA is typically administered by inserting a needle into a peripheral vein, and then connecting the needle to a catheter or intravenous

(IV) line. The catheter is then connected to a PCA pump (see later), and small intermittent doses of the analgesic are administered through the catheter and delivered directly into the systemic circulation. This technique is often effective in allowing the patient to regulate his or her level of analgesia for a short period of time (e.g., for the first few days after surgery).

When PCIA is needed for longer periods, a catheter can be implanted surgically in a large central vein, with the tip of the catheter advanced to the right atrium of the heart. The catheter is then tunneled through subcutaneous tissues and brought out through the patient's skin to allow administration of PCA. Alternatively, the catheter can be connected to a small container known as an *access port*, which is implanted subcutaneously within the patient's body (Fig. 17–2). This type of catheter-port system is used to provide a method of IV drug delivery that is located primarily within the patient's body. Injections can be made through the skin and into the port through a self-sealing silicone rubber septum located on the port. When these ports are used during PCA, the external PCA source is connected to the port via a special (Huber) needle that is inserted through the skin and into the port (see Fig. 17–2). The analgesic drug is then given from the PCA pump through a catheter into the port and ultimately into the systemic circulation. This provides an effective way of getting small, frequent doses of the drug into the bloodstream with less risk of infection or intravenous catheter displacement. This type of PCA-port delivery also enables the

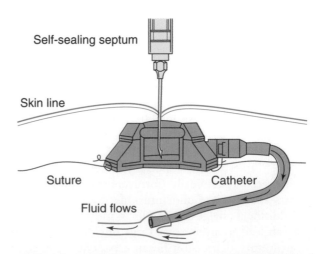

FIGURE 17–2 ▼ Schematic representation of an implantable vascular access port that can be used with PCA. The port can be connected to a PCA pump via a percutaneous needle, and a catheter leads from the port to a large central vein. (From Knox LS. *Crit Care Nurse.* 1987;7:71; with permission.)

patient to be disconnected from the PCA delivery system for short periods of time by removing the needle from the port. This allows the patient to bathe or get dressed without risking damage to the indwelling port-IV system.[17]

Epidural PCA

Patient controlled epidural analgesia (PCEI) is achieved by administering drugs directly into the area outside of the membranes (meninges) surrounding the spinal cord.[9] This is typically done by inserting a small catheter so that the tip of the catheter lies in the epidural space at a specific level of the spinal cord (Fig. 17–3). Alternatively, the tip of the catheter can be placed in the subarachnoid space—this type of delivery is known as spinal or **intrathecal administration**. That is, the drug is delivered into the space between the middle (arachnoid) layer of the meninges and the inner (pia mater) meningeal membrane (intrathecal

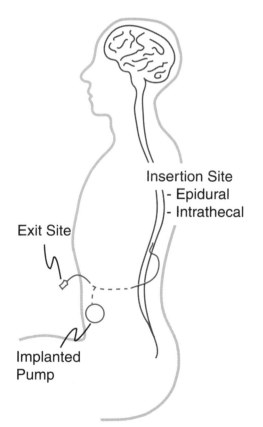

Insertion Site
- Epidural
- Intrathecal

Exit Site

Implanted
Pump

FIGURE 17–3 ▼ Schematic illustration of PCA spinal delivery. The catheter delivers the analgesic into either the epidural or intrathecal (subarachnoid) space. Catheters for long-term use are tunneled under the skin *(dashed line)* and can either be connected directly to an implanted PCA pump, or exit the anterior-lateral flank for connection to an external pump.

means "within a sheath"; see Chapter 2). Although intrathecal administration can be used in certain situations, the epidural route seems to be the preferred method during PCA because it is safer and there is less risk of damaging the meninges.

If PCEA is intended for short-term use, the catheter can be externalized through the skin on the midline of the patient's back and held in place by surgical tape. For long-term use, the catheter is often tunneled through the subcutaneous tissues in the patient's abdominal wall, after which the catheter can either be brought out through the skin on the patient's side (see Fig. 17–3) or connected to some type of implanted access port or drug reservoir. In either case, PCEA is achieved by using a pump to deliver the drug through the catheter and into the area directly surrounding the spinal cord.

Administration of drugs into the epidural space is obviously more difficult than simple intravenous delivery using a peripheral vein. Epidural delivery does, however, offer advantages in terms of providing more effective analgesia with a smaller amount of drug. For instance, it is estimated that epidural morphine is 5 to 10 times more potent than IV morphine, indicating that less drug needs to be administered by the epidural route to achieve adequate analgesia.[17] This fact makes sense, considering that PCEA administers the drug closer and more directly to the spinal cord compared with the amount of drug that must be added to the bloodstream via PCIA so that enough medication eventually reaches the spinal cord via the systemic circulation. Likewise, there have been numerous studies that directly compared PCEA with other parenteral administration routes, including PCIA. Although these studies varied in the type of analgesic drugs used and the clinical indication (i.e., pain control following various types of surgery), they routinely found that PCEA provided superior pain control without a significant increase in side effects.[6,26,40,49] By improving pain control after surgery, PCEA can also facilitate early recovery and rehabilitation in situations such as total knee arthroplasty.[24]

Transdermal PCA

Patient controlled transdermal analgesia (PCTA) is one of the newest variations on PCA. PCTA uses a delivery system consisting of a small patch that is approximately the size of a credit card.[29,45] This patch is adhered to the patient's skin, usually on the arm or upper chest. The patch is impregnated with an opioid such as fentanyl, and the patient can self-administer a small dose of the drug by pushing a button located on the patch. One such system is now commercially available, and will deliver 40 μg of fentanyl over a 10 minute period each time the patient activates the patch.[29,44]

Hence, PCTA is similar to other iontophoresis techniques that use a small amount of electric current to facilitate transdermal delivery. PCTA, however, offers the additional benefit of allowing the patient to activate drug delivery, thus helping to match the amount of medication delivered to each patient's specific needs. Because no needle is required, this technique also offers the obvious advantage of a noninvasive method for PCA. Patients can likewise remain more mobile because there is no IV line connecting the patient to a PCA pump.[13] Moreover, several studies have documented that PCTA using fentanyl can provide pain control that is superior to placebo and comparable to standard postoperative analgesic techniques such as morphine PCIA.[14,45] Thus, PCTA is one of the more exciting innovations in pain control, and future research will help clarify how this technique can be used effectively as an analgesic technique.

Regional PCA

Patient controlled regional analgesia (PCRA) occurs when the patient self-administers the medication directly into a specific anatomical site, such as a peripheral joint, near a peripheral nerve, or into a wound. This technique helps localize the drug to the site of administration, thereby providing adequate pain control with minimal effects on other tissues and organs. Although this technique has been used to administer analgesic medications such as morphine, PCRA typically uses some type of local anesthetic such as bupivacaine or ropivacaine. Hence, this technique is really analogous to patient-controlled regional *anesthesia* rather than a strictly analgesic intervention. Regardless, PCRA is an innovative way to provide safe and effective pain control.

PCRA is typically accomplished by inserting a small catheter into the affected site, and then attaching the catheter to some type of pump that enables the patient to self-administer small amounts of medication as needed. For example, a PCA system has been used to deliver local anesthetics such as bupivacaine and ropivacaine into the subacromial space following acromial decompression surgery.[3,27] Likewise, PCRA can be used to deliver a local anesthetic to the area around a peripheral nerve (sciatic, popliteal, and so forth), and

these perineural applications can help control pain following various types of surgery.[21,28] These regional administration techniques can, of course, also be accomplished by delivering a single (one-shot) dose of the medication, or via continuous infusion of the local anesthetic into the affected site.[9] Nonetheless, use of some type of patient-controlled pump offers the additional benefit of allowing the patient to regulate the amount of medication, and may improve patient satisfaction because the patient is more engaged in his or her own pain control. Hence, PCRA can be used alone or incorporated into more traditional analgesic regimens as an effective way to control local pain in a variety of situations.

PCA Pumps

The increase in popularity and use of PCA has largely been because of the development of infusion devices that can administer the analgesic in a safe and accurate manner. These devices, or *pumps*, vary in technologic sophistication and cost, but they all share common features (some are summarized in Table 17–2).[37] PCA pumps essentially allow the practitioner to set specific parameters of drug delivery (demand dose, lockout interval, etc.). The pump must then provide features to safeguard the patient against pump malfunction and to warn the patient or caregiver if drug delivery is interrupted.

Pumps used for PCA fall into two basic categories: external and internal (implantable).[39] The most basic type of external pump is a simple syringe driver (Fig. 17–4). A syringe containing the medication is placed in a viselike machine that advances the syringe a small amount when the patient activates the pump. A second type of pump uses some sort of peristaltic action that sequentially compresses a piece of tubing to milk the medication through the tubing toward the patient. A third pump, known as a cassette system, works by drawing the medication into a fluid container within the pump and expelling the selected amount of medication out of the chamber into tubing that leads to the patient. In most cases, these external pumps are activated when the patient pushes a button located on the end of a pendant that is connected to the pump (see Fig. 17–4).

Disposable models of external PCA pump are also available, offering a simple and less costly method for pain management.[32,42] Rather than using sophisticated electronic controls, these disposable pumps are typically activated when the patient squeezes a

Table 17–2	BASIC FEATURES OF SOME COMMON PCA PUMPS			
Feature	**Abbott AMP II**	**Abbott LifeCare 4100 PCA Plus II**	**Baxter 6060**	**Baxter PCA II**
Ambulatory Use	Yes	No	Yes	No
Size (inches)	6.75 × 4.0 × 2.3	8.25 × 13.4 × 6.0	4.7 × 3.9 × 2.3	13.0 × 6.3 × 2.8
Weight (lb)	1.3	15	1.0	4.2
Power source	Wall plug in AC; 2 × 9-volt alkaline battery; NiCd rechargeable battery pack	Wall plug in AC; one 8-volt sealed lead-acid battery	2 × 9-volt alkaline or lithium batteries; external lead-acid battery pack	Four D-cell alkaline batteries; AC power kit with two rechargeable NiCd batteries
Comments	Meets all basic requirements for performance, safety, and ease of use.	Performs adequately, but has a number of minor drawbacks in its ease of use and safety features.	Meets most requirements; has a mix of minor advantages and disadvantages; ease of use is only fair.	Meets most requirements and offers some advantages, but also has some drawbacks, most notably in its data logs and alarms.

Source: Adapted from Patient-controlled analgesic infusion pumps. *Health Devices.* 2001;30:168, 169, 182; with permission.

small bulb containing a small dose (i.e., the demand dose) of medication. As with other PCA pumps, safeguards are built in to limit how often these demand doses can be administered. Thus, disposable PCA pumps offer a cost-effective alternative that patients can use in the hospital or after discharge following surgery.[32,42]

Internal, or implantable, pumps are placed surgically beneath the patient's skin and connected to a catheter leading to the patient's bloodstream or perispinal spaces (epidural or intrathecal). This basically creates a closed system within the patient's body. These pumps typically contain a reservoir filled with medication. The reservoir can be refilled by inserting a Huber needle through the skin and into the pump via a resealable septum located on the outside of the pump (Fig. 17–5). Some implantable pumps use a rotatory peristaltic mechanism to milk the medication out of the pump. Other pumps use a bellows system to compress a chamber within the pump, thus expelling a given quantity of the drug. Implantable pumps are often programmed through the skin with some sort of electronic control device.

The type of pump that is selected depends primarily on which method (external or implantable) will best serve the patient's needs, as well as cost and availability of a given type of pump. Advances in pump technology will continue to improve the available devices, and future developments will undoubtedly provide devices that are even more efficient in providing PCA.

Comparison of PCA to Traditional Methods of Analgesic Administration

From the pharmacokinetic perspective discussed previously, it is apparent that giving small, frequent doses of analgesic through PCA is superior to administering large doses at infrequent intervals. Many clinical studies have attempted to verify this by comparing PCA using opioid drugs with traditional intramuscular (IM) opioid injection. Although some studies have not shown any clear advantages or disadvantages of PCIA,[34] most controlled trials indicate that PCA administered either intravenously or epidurally provides improved analgesia without a substantial increase in side effects.[5,6,7,12,22,46]

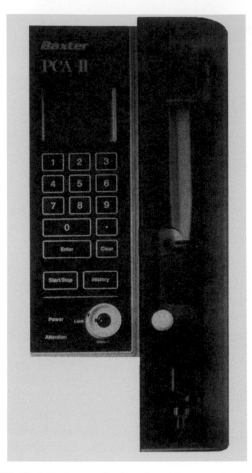

FIGURE 17-4 ▼ An example of a syringe driver pump that is commonly used with PCA.

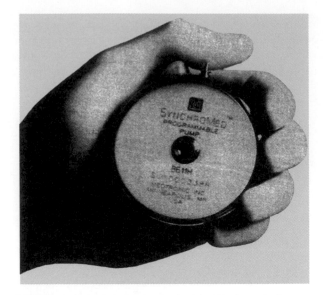

FIGURE 17-5 ▼ An example of an implantable, electronically controlled PCA pump. This pump is implanted surgically in the patient's abdomen and can be refilled periodically through a self-sealing septum.

Several studies also reported that patients were more satisfied with the pain control provided by PCA versus traditional dosing, which seems to be related to the increased feeling of control over pain.[19,30,46] Some studies also suggested that patients receiving opioid PCA are generally able to ambulate sooner and tend to have shorter hospital stays than patients receiving opioids by the traditional IM route.[20,24,48] Other studies, however, failed to find a significant difference in factors such as length of stay,[48] or in ability to ambulate sooner.[16] The discrepancies in the results from studies are understandable, considering that they often differed in research design and patient populations (various types of surgical procedures, and so forth). Nonetheless, the preponderance of evidence suggests that PCA systems afford some obvious advantages in certain patients over more traditional methods such as periodic IM injection.

One must then consider how PCA-like administration would compare with continuous infusion of an analgesic drug. As discussed in Chapter 14, it is sometimes feasible to administer opioid analgesics by slow, continuous infusion into the bloodstream or into some other area such as the epidural or intrathecal space. Continuous infusion would obviously provide the best way of maintaining drug concentration within a given therapeutic range. Several studies suggest that continuous epidural infusion of an opioid, local anesthetic, or some combination of these agents provides better pain control than techniques that allow the patient to self-administer the drug via the intravenous or epidural route.[35,41,47] Continuous infusion, however, tends to supply more total drug than patient-controlled techniques, and the additional drug quantities may pose unnecessary costs and expose patients to an increased risk of side effects.[1,31] Hence, continuous epidural infusion is an option for patients who do not achieve adequate pain control using PCEA or some other technique that enables the patient to self-administer the drug as needed.

Thus, PCA techniques have been shown to have certain advantages over more traditional methods such as intermittent IM injection or continuous epidural infusion. One must also consider that PCA decreases the need for other health professionals (physicians, nurses, pharmacists) to be directly involved in administering analgesics or adjusting the rate of analgesic delivery. Intramuscular injection, for instance, requires that the nurse be available at the proper time to inject the proper amount of the correct drug into the correct patient. This clearly takes the locus of control out of the patient's hands and makes the patient feel more dependent on an outside person to provide pain relief. When PCA systems are used appropriately, pain control is literally in the patient's hands. Likewise, continuous infusion often requires frequent adjustments by a qualified person who must attempt to match the dose of analgesic to the patient's pain level. This is especially difficult if pain levels are changing, such as in the patient recovering from surgery. With PCA, the patient is able to automatically adjust the amount of analgesia according to his or her pain. Again, this underscores a key advantage of PCA: it is superior to more traditional methods of analgesia because the person most qualified to judge his or her pain is empowered to self-administer the analgesic according to his or her own needs.

Problems and Side Effects of PCA

Pharmacologic Side Effects

Side effects typically seen when opioids are used for PCA include sedation, pruritus, and gastrointestinal problems (nausea, vomiting). The incidence of these side effects, however, is not significantly increased during PCA versus more traditional methods of opioid administration such as intermittent intramuscular dosing.[18] Respiratory depression is another common side effect of opioid use, but again, there is no increased incidence of this problem when appropriate amounts

of opioids are given via PCA.[9,32] In fact, the risk of respiratory depression is believed to be negligible when opioids are administered through spinal routes (epidural and intrathecal).[17] Hence, there does not seem to be an increase in the side effects commonly seen when PCA techniques are used to administer opioids, and the side effects commonly associated with these drugs may even be reduced during certain types of PCA application.

The incidence of side effects during PCA with local anesthetics is not well defined. Local anesthetics could conceivably cause sensory loss and motor weakness below the level of administration during PCEA. The possibility of these effects is directly dependent on the dose and type of local anesthetic, and efforts are usually made to use lower doses of agents such as bupivacaine and ropivacaine because these drugs tend to produce sensory effects with minimal motor loss. Also, local anesthetic side effects can be minimized during PCEA by combining the local anesthetic with an opioid, thus decreasing the total amount of each drug.[9] Some degree of sensory and motor loss will also occur when local anesthetics are administered into other peripheral sites, especially when these agents are administered near specific peripheral nerves (i.e., perineural PCRA). Hence, transient sensory and motor loss must always be considered as a potential side effect when local anesthetics are used during PCA.

Problems with PCA Delivery

Other problems that can occur with PCA systems include errors on the part of the operator (nurse, physician, etc.) or the patient, and mechanical problems with the pump-delivery system.[18] These problems are summarized in Table 17–3. Operator errors typically occur because the pump is not programmed correctly

Table **17–3**	**SUMMARY OF PROBLEMS THAT CAN OCCUR DURING PCA THERAPY**	
Operator Errors	**Patient Errors**	**Mechanical Problems**
Misprogramming PCA device	Failure to understand PCA therapy	Failure to deliver on demand
Failure to clamp or unclamp tubing	Misunderstanding PCA pump device	Cracked drug vials or syringes
Improperly loading syringe or cartridge	Intentional analgesic abuse	Defective one-way valve at Y connector
Inability to respond to safety alarms		Faulty alarm system
Misplacing PCA pump key		Malfunctions (e.g., lock)

Source: White,[48] p 81; with permission.

or some other error occurs in loading the analgesic.[18] Errors on the part of the patient can occur if the patient is not properly educated in PCA use or if the patient lacks adequate cognitive skills to use the PCA correctly. Problems can likewise occur if the patient intentionally tries to administer more drug than necessary to adequately control pain; that is, the patient attempts to use the PCA as a form of drug abuse. Although the safeguards provided by the device (small demand dose, appropriate lockout interval) should prevent addiction, these PCA systems are not usually as successful in controlling pain in people with a history of opioid addiction. Finally, mechanical problems, including pump malfunction and clogging or displacement of the delivery tubing, may preclude delivery of the analgesic. Members of the health-care team should be alert for signs that the drug is being overdelivered during PCA, as evidenced by an increase in analgesic side effects, or that the analgesic is being underdelivered, as indicated by inadequate pain control.

SUMMARY

PCA allows the patient to self-administer a small amount of analgesic medication on a relatively frequent basis. This technique has been used to administer drugs such as opioids and local anesthetics. PCA can often provide better pain control with smaller quantities of the drug and a lower incidence of side effects. The patient is allowed to self-administer a small dose of the drug by pressing a button that is connected to some type of pump. These PCA pumps vary in cost, level of sophistication, and location (external versus surgically implanted), but all pumps

Special Concerns for PCA in Rehabilitation Patients

■ ■ ■ When used appropriately, PCA offers several advantages to patients receiving physical therapy and occupational therapy. As discussed previously, PCA often provides analgesia with a lower chance of side effects such as sedation. Patients will be more alert and will have a clearer sensorium while still receiving optimal pain control. Likewise, PCA prevents large fluctuations in plasma analgesic concentration and helps maintain analgesic concentration within a more finite range (see Fig. 17–1). This decreases the need to schedule rehabilitation at a time when analgesic concentrations are at optimal levels because concentrations should always be within the appropriate range. Patients may also be more mobile using various PCA systems as compared with more traditional analgesic methods. The use of PCA may allow patients to begin ambulation sooner following surgery, and PCA systems can help decrease the need for the patient to be bed-bound for long periods because of severe pain or the side effects from high, intermittent doses of analgesics.[20,24] Rehabilitation specialists should therefore acknowledge the advantages of PCA and capitalize on these advantages whenever possible.

Rehabilitation specialists should also be aware of potential problems that can occur in patients receiving PCA. In particular, therapists should monitor the patient's signs and symptoms to help detect problems in PCA delivery. Therapists should use visual analog scales or some other valid measurement tool to routinely assess pain in patients receiving PCA. Patients exhibiting inadequate pain management or an unexplained increase in pain may be using a PCA system that is underdelivering the analgesic drug. The medical and nursing staff should be notified so that the delivery problem can be identified and rectified. Conversely, signs of respiratory depression or excessive sedation may indicate that the patient is being overdosed by the PCA system. This can obviously be a life-threatening situation that requires immediate attention. Hence, it is the responsibility of all health care workers, including rehabilitation specialists, to look for signs of PCA malfunction every time they interact with the patient.

CASE STUDY

Patient-Controlled Analgesia

Brief History. S.G., a 61-year-old man, was being treated for severe osteoarthritis in the right knee. Following an unsuccessful course of conservative therapy, S.G. was admitted to the hospital for a total knee replacement. The surgery was performed successfully, and PCA was instituted for postoperative pain management. PCA consisted of an external syringe pump connected to an IV catheter. The analgesic, meperidine (Demerol), was used at a concentration of 10 mg/mL. Parameters for PCA were set by the physician to allow a demand dose of 1 mL (10 mg) with a lockout interval of 10 minutes. An initial or loading dose of 10 mg was also provided at the conclusion of the surgery. Physical therapy was initiated at the patient's bedside on the afternoon following surgery. The therapist found the patient groggy, but the patient was coherent and able to understand simple commands. Pain, as assessed by a visual analog scale (VAS), was rated in the 4- to 5-cm range of a 10-cm scale (10 cm being equivalent to the "worst pain imaginable"). The patient was observed using his PCA during the therapy session,

and he seemed to understand how to use this device properly.

Problem/Influence of Drug Therapy. When seen at bedside on the day following surgery, the patient was in obvious discomfort. Pain was rated in the 8- to 9-cm range of the VAS. The patient stated that he had been using the PCA as instructed and that the device had been recording his successful attempts with an audible signal. Upon closer inspection, however, the therapist noticed that the syringe was not properly engaged in the pump mechanism. Hence, the syringe was not being propelled forward, and the demand dose was not being administered.

Decision/Solution. The PCA malfunction was brought to the attention of the nursing staff, and the problem was quickly rectified. The syringe containing the opioid had apparently been refilled earlier in the day and had not been installed properly in the pump's syringe driver. The patient was given an initial 10-mg infusion, and PCA was then resumed according to the original dosing parameters. The remainder of the patient's recovery was uneventful, and he was able to participate actively and enthusiastically in the rehabilitation sessions.

---

are capable of being programmed to prevent the patient from exceeding certain dosing parameters. PCA systems continue to increase in popularity and are now used in a variety of clinical situations to manage acute and chronic pain. Rehabilitation specialists should be aware that PCA can improve pain

control and enhance the patient's recovery. Human error or mechanical malfunction during PCA, however, may cause excessive or inadequate drug delivery, so therapists should also be alert for any signs that patients are receiving too much or too little analgesic during PCA.

References

1. Antok E, Bordet F, Duflo F, et al. Patient-controlled epidural analgesia versus continuous epidural infusion with ropivacaine for postoperative analgesia in children. *Anesth Analg.* 2003;97:1608–1611.
2. Aribogan A, Doruk N, Aridogan A, et al. Patient-controlled epidural analgesia after major urologic surgeries. A comparison of tramadol with or without bupivacaine. *Urol Int.* 2003;71:168–175.
3. Axelsson K, Nordenson U, Johanzon E, et al. Patient-controlled regional analgesia (PCRA) with ropivacaine after arthroscopic subacromial decompression. *Acta Anaesthesiol Scand.* 2003;47:993–1000.
4. Aygun S, Kocoglu H, Goksu S, et al. Postoperative patient-controlled analgesia with intravenous tramadol, intravenous fentanyl, epidural tramadol and epidural ropivacaine+fentanyl combination. *Eur J Gynaecol Oncol.* 2004;25:498–501.
5. Ballantyne JC, Carr DB, Chalmers TC, et al. Postoperative patient-controlled analgesia: meta-analyses of initial randomized control trials. *J Clin Anesth.* 1993; 5:182–193.
6. Block BM, Liu SS, Rowlingson AJ, et al. Efficacy of postoperative epidural analgesia: a meta-analysis. *JAMA.* 2003;290:2455–2463.
7. Boldt J, Thaler E, Lehmann A, et al. Pain management in cardiac surgery patients: comparison between standard therapy and patient-controlled analgesia regimen. *J Cardiothorac Vasc Anesth.* 1998; 12:654–658.
8. Boselli E, Debon R, Cimino Y, et al. Background infusion is not beneficial during labor patient-controlled analgesia with 0.1% ropivacaine plus 0.5 microg/ml sufentanil. *Anesthesiology.* 2004;100:968–972.
9. Brown AK, Christo PJ, Wu CL. Strategies for postoperative pain management. *Best Pract Res Clin Anaesthesiol.* 2004;18:703–717.

10. Carr DB, Reines HD, Schaffer J, et al. The impact of technology on the analgesic gap and quality of acute pain management. *Reg Anesth Pain Med.* 2005; 30:286–291.

11. Cepeda MS, Alvarez H, Morales O, Carr DB. Addition of ultralow dose naloxone to postoperative morphine PCA: unchanged analgesia and opioid requirement but decreased incidence of opioid side effects. *Pain.* 2004;107:41–46.

12. Chang AM, Ip WY, Cheung TH. Patient-controlled analgesia versus conventional intramuscular injection: a cost effectiveness analysis. *J Adv Nurs.* 2004;46: 531–541.

13. Chelly JE. An iontophoretic, fentanyl HCl patient-controlled transdermal system for acute postoperative pain management. *Expert Opin Pharmacother.* 2005; 6:1205–1214.

14. Chelly JE, Grass J, Houseman TW, et al. The safety and efficacy of a fentanyl patient-controlled transdermal system for acute postoperative analgesia: a multicenter, placebo-controlled trial. *Anesth Analg.* 2004; 98:427–433.

15. Chen JY, Wu GJ, Mok MS, et al. Effect of adding ketorolac to intravenous morphine patient-controlled analgesia on bowel function in colorectal surgery patients—a prospective, randomized, double-blind study. *Acta Anaesthesiol Scand.* 2005;49:546–551.

16. Choiniere M, Rittenhouse BE, Perreault S, et al. Efficacy and costs of patient-controlled analgesia versus regularly administered intramuscular opioid therapy. *Anesthesiology.* 1998;89:1377–1388.

17. Chrubasik J, Chrubasik S, Martin E. Patient-controlled spinal opiate analgesia in terminal cancer. Has its time really arrived? *Drugs.* 1992;43:799–804.

18. Cohen MR, Smetzer J. Patient-controlled analgesia safety issues. *J Pain Palliat Care Pharmacother.* 2005; 19:45–50.

19. Colwell CW, Jr. The use of the pain pump and patient-controlled analgesia in joint reconstruction. *Am J Orthop.* 2004;33(suppl):10–12.

20. Conner M, Deane D. Patterns of patient-controlled analgesia and intramuscular analgesia. *Appl Nurs Res.* 1995;8:67–72.

21. Duflo F, Qamouss Y, Remond C, et al. Patient-controlled regional analgesia is effective in children: a preliminary report. *Can J Anaesth.* 2004;51:928–930.

22. Etches RC. Patient-controlled analgesia. *Surg Clin North Am.* 1999;79:297–312.

23. Evron S, Glezerman M, Sadan O, et al. Patient-controlled epidural analgesia for labor pain: effect on labor, delivery and neonatal outcome of 0.125% bupivacaine vs 0.2% ropivacaine. *Int J Obstet Anesth.* 2004;13:5–10.

24. Farag E, Dilger J, Brooks P, Tetzlaff JE. Epidural analgesia improves early rehabilitation after total knee replacement. *J Clin Anesth.* 2005;17:281–285.

25. Gogarten W, Van de Velde M, Soetens E, et al. A multicentre trial comparing different concentrations of ropivacaine plus sufentanil with bupivacaine plus sufentanil for patient-controlled epidural analgesia in labour. *Eur J Anaesthesiol.* 2004;21:38–45.

26. Halpern SH, Muir H, Breen TW, et al. A multicenter randomized controlled trial comparing patient-controlled epidural with intravenous analgesia for pain relief in labor. *Anesth Analg.* 2004;99:1532–1538.

27. Harvey GP, Chelly JE, AlSamsam T, Coupe K. Patient-controlled ropivacaine analgesia after arthroscopic subacromial decompression. *Arthroscopy.* 2004; 20:451–455.

28. Ilfeld BM, Thannikary LJ, Morey TE, et al. Popliteal sciatic perineural local anesthetic infusion: a comparison of three dosing regimens for postoperative analgesia. *Anesthesiology.* 2004;101:970–977.

29. Koo PJ. Postoperative pain management with a patient-controlled transdermal delivery system for fentanyl. *Am J Health Syst Pharm.* 2005;62: 1171–1176.

30. Lebovits AH, Zenetos P, O'Neill DK, et al. Satisfaction with epidural and intravenous patient-controlled analgesia. *Pain Med.* 2001;2:280–286.

31. Ledin Eriksson S, Gentele C, Olofsson CH. PCEA compared to continuous epidural infusion in an ultra-low-dose regimen for labor pain relief: a randomized study. *Acta Anaesthesiol Scand.* 2003;47: 1085–1090.

32. Lehmann KA. Recent developments in patient-controlled analgesia. *J Pain Symptom Manage.* 2005; 29 (suppl):S72–S89.

33. Lo Y, Chia YY, Liu K, Ko NH. Morphine sparing with droperidol in patient-controlled analgesia. *J Clin Anesth.* 2005;17:271–275.

34. Macintyre PE. Intravenous patient-controlled analgesia: one size does not fit all. *Anesthesiol Clin North America.* 2005;23:109–123.

35. Maurer K, Bonvini JM, Ekatodramis G, et al. Continuous spinal anesthesia/analgesia vs. single-shot spinal anesthesia with patient-controlled analgesia for elective hip arthroplasty. *Acta Anaesthesiol Scand.* 2003;47: 878–883.

36. Maxwell LG, Kaufmann SC, Bitzer S, et al. The effects of a small-dose naloxone infusion on opioid-induced side effects and analgesia in children and adolescents treated with intravenous patient-controlled analgesia: a double-blind, prospective, randomized, controlled study. *Anesth Analg.* 2005;100:953–958.

37. Patient-controlled analgesic infusion pumps. *Health Devices.* 2001;30:157–185.

38. Ready LB. Acute perioperative pain. In: Miller RD, ed. *Anesthesia.* 5th ed. Philadelphia: Churchill Livingston; 2000.

39. Rosenthal K. Implantable pumps deliver innovative pain management. *Nurs Manage.* 2003;34:46–49.

40. Senagore AJ, Delaney CP, Mekhail N, et al. Randomized clinical trial comparing epidural anaesthesia and patient-controlled analgesia after laparoscopic segmental colectomy. *Br J Surg.* 2003;90:1195–1199.

41. Sucato DJ, Duey-Holtz A, Elerson E, Safavi F. Postoperative analgesia following surgical correction for adolescent idiopathic scoliosis: a comparison of continuous epidural analgesia and patient-controlled analgesia. *Spine.* 2005;30:211–217.

42. Sumikura H, van de Velde M, Tateda T. Comparison between a disposable and an electronic PCA device for labor epidural analgesia. *J Anesth.* 2004;18:262–266.

43. Sveticic G, Eichenberger U, Curatolo M. Safety of mixture of morphine with ketamine for postoperative patient-controlled analgesia: an audit with 1026 patients. *Acta Anaesthesiol Scand.* 2005;49:870–875.

44. Viscusi ER. Emerging techniques for postoperative analgesia in orthopedic surgery. *Am J Orthop.* 2004; 33(suppl):13–16.

45. Viscusi ER, Reynolds L, Chung F, et al. Patient-controlled transdermal fentanyl hydrochloride vs intravenous morphine pump for postoperative pain: a randomized controlled trial. *JAMA.* 2004;291: 1333–1341.

46. Walder B, Schafer M, Henzi I, Tramer MR. Efficacy and safety of patient-controlled opioid analgesia for acute postoperative pain. A quantitative systematic review. *Acta Anaesthesiol Scand.* 2001;45: 795–804.

47. Werawatganon T, Charuluxanun S. Patient controlled intravenous opioid analgesia versus continuous epidural analgesia for pain after intra-abdominal surgery. *Cochrane Database Syst Rev.* 2005;CD004088.

48. White PF. Mishaps with patient-controlled analgesia. *Anesthesiology.* 1987;66:81–83.

49. Yavuz L, Eroglu F, Ozsoy M. The efficacy of intravenous versus epidural tramadol with patient-controlled analgesia (PCA) in gynecologic cancer pain. *Eur J Gynaecol Oncol.* 2004;25:215–218.

Autonomic and Cardiovascular Pharmacology

Chapter 18

Introduction to Autonomic Pharmacology

The human nervous system can be divided into two major functional areas: the somatic nervous system and the autonomic nervous system (ANS). The somatic division is concerned primarily with voluntary function—that is, control of the skeletal musculature. The ANS is responsible for controlling bodily functions that are largely involuntary, or automatic, in nature. For instance, the control of blood pressure (BP) and other aspects of cardiovascular function is under the influence of the ANS. Other involuntary, or vegetative, functions such as digestion, elimination, and thermoregulation are also controlled by this system.

Considering the potential problems that can occur in various systems, such as the cardiovascular and digestive systems, the use of therapeutic drugs to alter autonomic function is one of the major areas of pharmacology. Drugs affecting autonomic function are prescribed routinely to patients, including those seen for physical therapy and occupational therapy. The purpose of this chapter is to review some of the primary anatomic and physiologic aspects of the ANS. This review is intended to provide rehabilitation specialists with a basis for understanding the pharmacologic effects and clinical applications of the autonomic drugs, which are discussed in subsequent chapters.

Anatomy of the Autonomic Nervous System: Sympathetic and Parasympathetic Divisions

The ANS can be roughly divided into two areas: the sympathetic and parasympathetic nervous systems.[6,9] The *sympathetic* or thoracolumbar, division arises pri-

marily from neurons located in the thoracic and upper lumbar regions of the spinal cord. The *parasympathetic*, or craniosacral, division is composed of neurons originating in the midbrain, brainstem, and sacral region of the spinal cord. There are many other anatomic and functional characteristics differentiating these two divisions these are briefly discussed later in this chapter. For a more detailed discussion of the anatomic and functional organization of the ANS, the reader is referred to several excellent sources listed at the end of this chapter.[7,9,11,17]

Preganglionic and Postganglionic Neurons

The somatic nervous system uses one neuron to reach from the central nervous system (CNS) to the periphery. In the somatic motor system, for instance, the alpha motor neuron begins in the spinal cord and extends all the way to the skeletal muscle; that is, it does not synapse until it reaches the muscle cell. In both the sympathetic and parasympathetic divisions, however, two neurons are used in sequence to reach from the CNS (i.e., brain or spinal cord) to the peripheral organ or tissue that is being supplied. The first neuron begins somewhere in the CNS and extends a certain distance toward the periphery before synapsing with a second neuron, which completes the journey to the final destination. The synapse of these two neurons is usually in one of the autonomic ganglia (see "Sympathetic Organization" and "Parasympathetic Organization"). Hence, the first neuron in sequence is termed the *preganglionic neuron* and the second is referred to as the *postganglionic neuron*.

In both the sympathetic and parasympathetic divisions, preganglionic fibers are myelinated type B fibers, and postganglionic fibers are the small, unmyelinated type C fibers. In the sympathetic division, preganglionic neurons tend to be short, while the sympathetic postganglionic neurons are long. The opposite is true for the parasympathetic division—preganglionic neurons are long and postganglionic neurons are short. The location of preganglionic and postganglionic fibers in each autonomic division is presented here.

Sympathetic Organization

The cell bodies for the sympathetic preganglionic fibers arise from the intermediolateral gray columns of the thoracic and upper lumbar spinal cord. The preganglionic fibers leave the spinal cord via the ventral root of the spinal nerve and end in a sympathetic ganglion. The sympathetic ganglia are located in three areas: (1) the paired paravertebral, or chain, ganglia, which lie bilaterally on either side of the vertebral column; (2) a group of unpaired prevertebral ganglia, which lie anterior to the aorta (e.g., the celiac plexus, the superior and inferior mesenteric ganglia); and (3) a small number of terminal ganglia, which lie directly in the tissue that is innervated (e.g., the bladder and rectum).

When the preganglionic fiber reaches one of the sympathetic ganglia, it synapses with a postganglionic fiber. Actually, one sympathetic preganglionic neuron may synapse with many postganglionic fibers. (The ratio of preganglionic to postganglionic fibers in the sympathetic chain ganglia is usually 1:15 to 20.)[17] The postganglionic fiber then leaves the ganglion to travel to the effector tissue that it supplies (i.e., the heart, peripheral arteriole, sweat gland, and so forth).

Parasympathetic Organization

Parasympathetic preganglionic neurons originate in the midbrain and brainstem (cranial portion) or the sacral region of the spinal cord. Neurons comprising the cranial portion of the parasympathetics exit the CNS via cranial nerves III, VII, IX, and X. Cranial nerve X (vagus nerve) is particularly significant because it contains approximately 75 percent of the efferent component of the entire parasympathetic division. Neurons composing the preganglionic fibers of the sacral portion exit the spinal cord via the pelvic splanchnic nerves.

As in the sympathetic division, parasympathetic preganglionic neurons synapse in the periphery with a postganglionic fiber. This synapse usually takes place in a terminal ganglion that is located directly in the organ or tissue supplied by the postganglionic neuron. Consequently, the parasympathetic ganglia are usually embedded directly in the innervated organ or tissue.

Functional Aspects of the Sympathetic and Parasympathetic Divisions

Except for skeletal muscle, virtually all tissues in the body are innervated in some way by the ANS.[9] Table 18–1 summarizes the innervation and effects of the sympathetic and parasympathetic divisions on some of the major organs and tissues in the body. As indicated in Table 18–1, some organs, such as the heart, are innervated by both sympathetic and parasympathetic neurons. Other tissues, however, may only be supplied by the sympathetic division. The peripheral arterioles, for instance, are innervated by the sympathetic division but receive no parasympathetic innervation.

If an organ *is* innervated by both the sympathetic and parasympathetic divisions, a physiologic antagonism typically exists between these divisions. That is, if both divisions innervate the tissue, one division usually increases function, whereas the other decreases activity. For instance, the sympathetics increase heart rate and stimulate cardiac output, whereas the parasympathetics cause bradycardia. However, it is incorrect to state that the sympathetics are always excitatory in nature and that the parasympathetics are always inhibitory. In tissues such as the gastrointestinal tract, the parasympathetics tend to increase intestinal motility and secretion, whereas the sympathetics slow down intestinal motility. The effect of each division on any tissue must be considered according to the particular organ or gland.

One generalization that can be made regarding sympathetic and parasympathetic function is that the sympathetic division tends to mobilize body energy, whereas the parasympathetic division tends to conserve and store it. Typically, sympathetic discharge is increased when the individual is faced with some stressful situation. This situation initiates the classic fight-or-flight scenario in which the person must either flee or defend himself or herself. Sympathetic discharge causes increased cardiac output, decreased visceral blood flow (thus leaving more blood available for skeletal muscle), increased cellular metabolism,

Table 18–1	RESPONSE OF EFFECTOR ORGANS TO AUTONOMIC STIMULATION	
Organ	**Sympathetic***	**Parasympathetic†**
Heart	Increased contractility (beta-1,-2)	Decreased heart rate (musc)
	Increased heart rate (beta-1,-2)	Slight decrease in contractility (musc)
Arterioles	Vasoconstriction of skin and viscera (alpha-1, -2)	No parasympathetic innervation
	Vasodilation of skeletal muscle and liver (beta-2)	
Lung	Bronchodilation (beta-2)	Bronchoconstriction (musc)
Eye		
Radial muscle	Contraction (alpha-1)	Relaxation (musc)
Ciliary muscle	Relaxation (beta-2)	Contraction (musc)
Gastrointestinal function	Decreased motility (alpha-1,-2; beta-1,-2)	Increased motility and secretion (musc)
Kidney	Increased renin secretion (alpha-1, beta-1)	No parasympathetic innervation
Urinary bladder		
Detrusor	Relaxation (beta-2)	Contraction (musc)
Trigone and sphincter	Contraction (alpha-1)	Relaxation (musc)
Sweat glands	Increased secretion (musc‡)	No parasympathetic innervation
Liver	Glycogenolysis and gluconeogenesis (alpha-1, beta-2)	No parasympathetic innervation
Fat cells	Lipolysis (alpha-2, beta-1,-2,-3)	No parasympathetic innervation

*The primary receptor subtypes mediating each response are listed in parentheses (e.g., alpha-1, beta-2).
†Note that all organ responses to parasympathetic stimulation are mediated via muscarinic (musc) receptors.
‡Represents response due to sympathetic postganglionic cholinergic fibers.

and several other physiologic changes that facilitate vigorous activity. In contrast, the parasympathetic division tends to have the opposite effect. Parasympathetic discharge slows down the heart and brings about changes that generally encourage inactivity. Parasympathetic discharge tends to increase intestinal digestion and absorption, an activity that stores energy for future needs.

Finally, activation of the sympathetic division tends to result in a more massive and diffuse reaction than does parasympathetic activation. Parasympathetic reactions tend to be fairly discrete and to affect only one organ or tissue. For instance, the parasympathetic fibers to the myocardium can be activated to slow down the heart without a concomitant emptying of the bowel through an excitatory effect on the lower gas-

trointestinal tract. When the sympathetic division is activated, effects are commonly observed on many tissues throughout the body. The more diffuse sympathetic reactions routinely produce a simultaneous effect on the heart, total peripheral vasculature, general cellular metabolism, and so on.

Function of the Adrenal Medulla

The adrenal medulla synthesizes and secretes norepinephrine and epinephrine directly into the bloodstream. Typically, the secretion from the adrenal medulla contains about 20 percent norepinephrine and 80 percent epinephrine.[7] These two hormones are fairly similar in action, except that epinephrine increases cardiac function and cellular metabolism to a greater extent because it has a higher affinity for certain receptors than norepinephrine (i.e., epinephrine binds more readily to the beta subtype of adrenergic receptors; see "Autonomic Receptors").[7]

The adrenal medulla is innervated by sympathetic neurons. During normal, resting conditions, the adrenal medulla secretes small amounts of epinephrine and norepinephrine. During periods of stress, however, a general increase in sympathetic discharge causes an increased release of epinephrine and norepinephrine from the adrenal medulla. Since these hormones are released directly into the bloodstream, they tend to circulate extensively throughout the body. Circulating epinephrine and norepinephrine can reach tissues that are not directly innervated by the sympathetic neurons, thus augmenting the general sympathetic effect. Also, the circulating epinephrine and norepinephrine are removed from the body more slowly than norepinephrine that is produced locally at the sympathetic postganglionic nerve terminals. As a result, adrenal release of epinephrine and norepinephrine tends to prolong the effect of the sympathetic reaction.

Consequently, the adrenal medulla serves to augment the sympathetic division of the ANS. In situations where a sudden increase in sympathetic function is required (i.e., the fight-or-flight scenario), the adrenal medulla works with the sympathetics to produce a more extensive and lasting response.

Autonomic Integration and Control

Most of the autonomic control over various physiologic functions is manifested through autonomic reflexes; that is, homeostatic control of BP, thermoregulation, and gastrointestinal function depend on the automatic reflex adjustment in these systems through the sympathetic and/or parasympathetic divisions.[9] Autonomic reflexes are based on the following strategy: a peripheral sensor monitors a change in the particular system. This information is relayed to a certain level of the CNS, where it is integrated. An adjustment is made in the autonomic discharge to the specific organ or tissue, which will alter its activity to return physiologic function back to the appropriate level.

A practical example of this type of autonomic reflex control is the so-called baroreceptor reflex, which is important in the control of BP. In this particular example, pressure sensors (i.e., baroreceptors) located in the large arteries of the thorax and neck monitor changes in BP and heart rate. A sudden drop in BP is sensed by the baroreceptors, and this information is relayed to the brainstem. In the brainstem, this information is integrated, and a compensatory increase occurs in sympathetic discharge to the heart and peripheral vasculature, and parasympathetic outflow to the heart is decreased. The result is an increase in cardiac output and an increase in peripheral vascular resistance, which effectively brings BP back to the appropriate level. The baroreceptor reflex also works in the opposite fashion—if BP were to suddenly increase, a decrease in sympathetic outflow and an increase in cardiac parasympathetic discharge would ultimately bring a return to normal pressure levels.

The baroreceptor response is just one example of the type of reflex activity employed by the ANS. The control of other involuntary functions usually follows a similar pattern of peripheral monitoring, central integration, and altered autonomic discharge. Body temperature, for instance, is monitored by thermoreceptors located in the skin, viscera, and hypothalamus. When a change in body temperature is monitored by these sensors, this information is relayed to the hypothalamus and appropriate adjustments are made in autonomic discharge in order to maintain thermal homeostasis (e.g., sweating is increased or decreased and blood flow is redistributed). Many other autonomic reflexes that control visceral and involuntary functions operate in a similar manner.

Integration of autonomic responses is often fairly complex and may occur at several levels of the CNS. Some reflexes, such as emptying of the bowel and bladder, are integrated primarily at the level of the sacral spinal cord. Other reflexes, such as the baroreceptor reflex, are integrated at higher levels in the so-called vasomotor center located in the brainstem. Also, the hypothalamus is important in regulating the ANS, and many functions including body temperature, water balance, and energy metabolism are controlled and integrated at the hypothalamus. To add to the complexity, higher levels of the brain such as the cortex and limbic system may also influence autonomic function through their interaction with the hypothalamus, brainstem, and spinal cord. This information is important pharmacologically because drugs that act on the CNS have the potential to alter autonomic function by influencing the central integration of autonomic responses. Drugs that affect the cortex, limbic system, and brainstem may indirectly alter the response of some of the autonomic reflexes by altering the relationship between afferent input and efferent sympathetic and parasympathetic outflow.

Autonomic Neurotransmitters

Acetylcholine and Norepinephrine

There are four sites of synaptic transmission in the efferent limb of the ANS: (1) the synapse between the preganglionic and postganglionic neurons in the sympathetic division, (2) the analogous preganglionic-postganglionic synapse in the parasympathetic division, (3) the synapse between the sympathetic postganglionic neuron and the effector cell, and (4) the parasympathetic postganglionic–effector cell synapse. Figure 18–1 summarizes the chemical neurotransmitter that is present at each synapse.

As indicated in Figure 18–1, the transmitter at the preganglionic-postganglionic synapse in both divisions is acetylcholine, as is the transmitter at the parasympathetic postganglionic–effector cell synapse. The transmitter at the sympathetic postganglionic–effector cell synapse is usually norepinephrine. A small number of sympathetic postganglionic fibers, however, also use acetylcholine as their neurotransmitter.

Consequently, all preganglionic neurons and parasympathetic postganglionic neurons are said to be cholinergic in nature because of the presence of acetylcholine at their respective synapses. Most sympathetic postganglionic neurons use norepinephrine and are referred to as **adrenergic**. (Norepinephrine is sometimes referred to as noradrenaline; hence the term "adrenergic.") An exception to this scheme is the presence of certain sympathetic postganglionic fibers that use acetylcholine as their neurotransmitter. These sympathetic cholinergic neurons innervate sweat glands and certain blood vessels in the face, neck, and lower extremities.

Other Autonomic Neurotransmitters

In recent years, it has become apparent that several nonadrenergic, noncholinergic neurotransmitters may also be present in the ANS. Purinergic substances such as adenosine and adenosine triphosphate have been implicated as possible transmitters in the gastrointestinal tract, cardiovascular system, and several other organs and systems influenced by autonomic nerves.[3,16] Several peptides such as substance P, vasoactive intestinal polypeptide, and angiotensin II have been identified as possibly participating in the autonomic control of various organs and systems.[10,11,13] Nitric oxide may also help regulate various peripheral autonomic responses, and this substance may also control CNS autonomic activity.[12,15,18]

It is still uncertain whether all of these nonadrenergic, noncholinergic substances are true neurotransmitters. They may act as cotransmitters that are

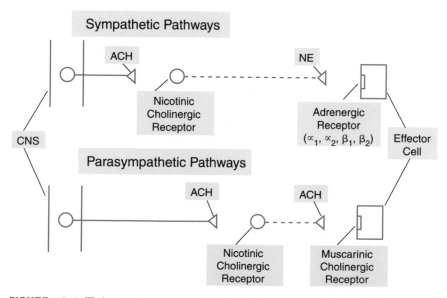

FIGURE 18–1 ▼ Autonomic neurotransmitters and receptors. Preganglionic neurons (solid lines) release acetylcholine (ACh). Postganglionic neurons (dashed lines) release ACh in the parasympathetic pathways and norepinephrine (NE) in the sympathetic pathways.

released from the synaptic terminal along with the classic autonomic transmitters (i.e., acetylcholine and norepinephrine). These other substances, however, may simply be produced locally and serve to modulate synaptic activity without actually being released from the presynaptic terminal. Additional information will be necessary to fully identify the role of these and other nonadrenergic, noncholinergic substances as autonomic neurotransmitters.

Autonomic Receptors

Since there are two primary neurotransmitters involved in autonomic discharge, there are two primary classifications of postsynaptic receptors. **Cholinergic** receptors are located at acetylcholine synapses, and **adrenergic** receptors are located at norepinephrine synapses. As indicated in Figure 18–2, each type of receptor has several subclassifications. The location and functional significance of these classifications and subclassifications are presented here.

Cholinergic Receptors

Cholinergic receptors are subdivided into two categories: **nicotinic** and **muscarinic**. Although acetylcholine will bind to all cholinergic receptors, certain receptors bind preferentially with the drug nicotine. Other receptors have a specific affinity for muscarine, a naturally occurring compound found in certain poisonous mushrooms. Thus the terms "nicotinic" and "muscarinic' were derived.

Nicotinic cholinergic receptors are located at the junction between preganglionic and postganglionic neurons in both the sympathetic and parasympathetic pathways (see Fig. 18–1). This fact is significant pharmacologically because any drug that affects these nicotinic receptors will affect activity in both divisions of the ANS. The cholinergic nicotinic receptor located in the ANS is sometimes referred to as a type I (or N_N) nicotinic receptor to differentiate it from the type II (or N_M) nicotinic receptors, which are located at the skeletal neuromuscular junction.

Muscarinic cholinergic receptors are located at all of the synapses between cholinergic postganglionic neurons and the terminal effector cell, including all the parasympathetic terminal synapses, as well as the sympathetic postganglionic cholinergic fibers, that supply sweat glands and some specialized blood vessels. Current research suggests that there may be five subtypes of muscarinic receptors, that is, muscarinic subtypes can be classified as M_1, M_2, M_3, and so forth, based on their structural and chemical characteristics.[9,19,22] Specific subtypes seem to predominate at certain organ systems. For example, the M_1, M_2, M_4, and M_5 receptors seem to be important in CNS responses,[20] whereas the M_3 subtype may be more prevalent in smooth muscle and heart tissue.[19,21] The exact role of these muscarinic receptor subtypes continues to be elucidated through ongoing research, and future studies will lend more insight to how each receptor subtype participates in normal function and specific diseases in humans.

Thus, cholinergic muscarinic receptors ultimately mediate the effect on the tissue itself. Table 18–2 summarizes the primary physiologic responses when muscarinic receptors are stimulated on various tissues in the body. Note that the specific response to stimulation of a muscarinic cholinergic receptor depends on

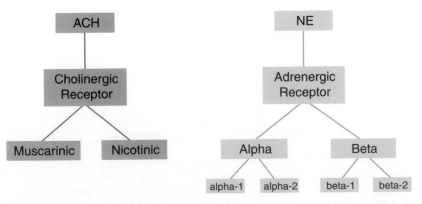

FIGURE 18–2 ▼ Receptor classifications and subclassifications for acetylcholine (ACh) and norepinephrine (NE), the two primary neurotransmitters used in the autonomic nervous system.

| Table 18-2 | AUTONOMIC RECEPTOR LOCATIONS AND RESPONSES |

Receptor	Primary Location(s)	Response*
	Cholinergic	
Nicotinic	Autonomic ganglia	Mediate transmission to postganglionic neuron
Muscarinic	All parasympathetic effector cells:	
	Visceral and bronchiole smooth muscle	Contraction (generally)
	Cardiac muscle	Decreased heart rate
	Exocrine glands (salivary, intestinal, lacrimal)	Increased secretion
	Sweat glands	Increased secretion
	Adrenergic	
Alpha-1	Vascular smooth muscle	Contraction
	Intestinal smooth muscle	Relaxation
	Radial muscle iris	Contraction (mydriasis)
	Ureters	Increased motility
	Urinary sphincter	Contraction
	Spleen capsule	Contraction
Alpha-2	CNS inhibitory synapses	Decreased sympathetic discharge from CNS
	Presynaptic terminal at peripheral adrenergic synapses	Decreased norepinephrine release
	Gastrointestinal tract	Decreased motility and secretion
	Pancreatic islet cells	Decreased insulin secretion
Beta-1	Cardiac muscle	Increased heart rate and contractility
	Kidney	Increased renin secretion
	Fat cells	Increased lipolysis
Beta-2	Bronchiole smooth muscle	Relaxation (bronchodilation)
	Some arterioles (skeletal muscle, liver)	Vasodilation
	Gastrointestinal smooth muscle	Decreased motility
	Skeletal muscle and liver cells	Increased cellular metabolism
	Uterus	Relaxation
	Gallbladder	Relaxation

the tissue in question. Stimulation of muscarinic receptors on the myocardium, for instance, causes a decrease in heart rate, whereas stimulation of muscarinic receptors in the intestinal wall leads to increases in smooth muscle contraction and glandular secretion.

Adrenergic Receptors

As shown in Figure 18–2, the adrenergic receptors are subdivided into two primary categories: alpha- and beta-adrenergic receptors. Alpha receptors are further subdivided into alpha-1 and alpha-2 receptors, and beta receptors are subdivided into beta-1, beta-2, and

beta-3 receptors.[9] These divisions are based on the different sensitivities of each receptor subcategory to different endogenous and exogenous agents. Alpha-1 receptors, for instance, bind more readily with certain agonists and antagonists, whereas alpha-2 receptors bind preferentially with other agents. Specific agents that bind to each adrenergic receptor subcategory are identified in Chapter 20.

In the ANS, the various types of adrenergic receptors are found on the effector cell in the innervated tissue. In other words, these receptors are located at the terminal synapse between sympathetic postganglionic adrenergic neurons and the tissue they supply.

The basic characteristics of each adrenergic receptor subtype are briefly outlined here.

Alpha-1 Receptors. A primary location of these receptors is the smooth muscle located in various tissues throughout the body. Alpha-1 receptors are located on the smooth muscle located in the peripheral vasculature, intestinal wall, radial muscle of the iris, ureters, urinary sphincter, and spleen capsule. The response of each tissue when the alpha-1 receptor is stimulated varies depending on the tissue (see Table 18-2). Research also suggests that there might be three subtypes of alpha-1 receptors, identified as alpha-1A, alpha-1B, and alpha-1D receptors.[4] Much of this research, however, has focused on the characteristics of alpha-1 receptor subtypes in various animal models. Studies are currently underway to determine the exact location and functional significance of these alpha-1 receptor subtypes in humans.

Alpha-2 Receptors. The alpha-2 receptors were originally identified by their presence on the presynaptic terminal of certain adrenergic synapses.[2] These presynaptic alpha-2 receptors appear to modulate the release of neurotransmitters from the presynaptic terminal; that is, they seem to decrease the release of norepinephrine and other chemicals, thus serving as a form of negative feedback limiting the amount of neurotransmitter released from the presynaptic terminal.[1,2] As discussed in Chapter 13, alpha-2 receptors have also been found on spinal interneurons, and stimulation of these alpha-2 receptors may cause decreased neurotransmitter release and diminished stimulation of the interneurons that influence the alpha motor neuron. Thus, alpha-2 stimulants (agonists) such as tizanidine have been used to decrease neuronal excitability in the spinal cord and thereby decrease muscle hyperexcitability in conditions such as spasticity. Also, alpha-2 receptors have been found postsynaptically on certain CNS adrenergic synapses involved in the control of sympathetic discharge.[9] Stimulation of these centrally located alpha-2 receptors is believed to inhibit sympathetic discharge from the brainstem. The importance of central alpha-2 receptors in controlling cardiovascular function and the possible use of alpha-2 agonists to control BP are discussed in Chapter 21. Alpha-2 receptors are also located in the gastrointestinal tract and pancreas, and stimulation of these receptors at these sites causes decreased intestinal motility and decreased insulin secretion, respectively.

As is the case with alpha-1 receptors, we now believe that at least three subtypes of alpha-2 receptors may exist, namely alpha-2A, alpha-2B, and alpha-2C.[4,14] The functional and pharmacological significance of these different alpha-2 receptor subtypes continues to be elucidated.

Beta-1 Receptors. These receptors predominate in the heart and kidneys (see Table 18–2).[9,24] The cardiac beta-1 receptors have received a tremendous amount of attention with regard to pharmacologic antagonism of their function through the use of the so-called beta blockers.

Beta-2 Receptors. Beta-2 receptors are found primarily on the smooth muscle of certain vasculatures, the bronchioles, the gallbladder, and the uterus.[9] Their presence in bronchiole smooth muscle is especially important in the pharmacologic management of respiratory conditions such as asthma (see Chapter 26). These receptors are also responsible for mediating changes in the metabolism of skeletal muscle and liver cells. Beta-2 receptors are also located on the heart, although the predominant effects on cardiac tissue seem to be mediated through the beta-1 subtype.

Beta-3 Receptors. Although it was originally thought that only two subtypes of beta receptors existed, we now know that a third subtype, the beta-3 receptor, plays a functional role in certain tissues. In particular, beta-3 receptors are located on adipose tissue, and stimulation of beta-3 receptors increases lipolysis (see Table 18-2).[9] In addition, beta-3 receptors are also found on the heart and some smooth muscles, and the functional significance of beta-3 receptors at these locations continues to be investigated.[5,23]

In summary, adrenergic receptors can be subclassified according to their location and affinity for specific pharmacologic agents. Table 18–2 summarizes the receptor subtypes that are located on the primary organs and tissues in the body, and the associated response when the receptor is stimulated. Exactly which receptor subtype is located on any given tissue depends on the tissue in question. Note that some tissues may have two or more different subtypes of adrenergic receptor (e.g., skeletal muscle arterioles appear to have alpha-1 and beta-2 receptors). Also, the response of a tissue when the receptor is stimulated is dependent on the specific receptor-cell interaction. Stimulation of the vascular alpha-1 receptor, for instance, results in smooth-muscle contraction and vasoconstriction, whereas stimulation of the intestinal alpha-1 receptor results in relaxation and decreased intestinal motility. This difference is caused by the way the receptor is coupled to the cell's internal biochemistry at each location. As discussed in Chapter 4, the surface receptor at one cell may be coupled to the cell's internal enzymatic machinery so that it stimulates cell function. The same receptor subtype at a different tissue will be linked to inhibitory enzymes that slow down cell function. Refer to Chapter 4 for a more detailed description of how surface receptors are coupled to cell function.

Pharmacologic Significance of Autonomic Receptors

Perhaps no area of research has contributed more to pharmacology than the identification, classification, and subclassification of autonomic receptors. The realization that various tissues have distinct subtypes of receptors has enabled the use of drugs affecting certain tissues and organs while causing minimal effects on other tissues. For instance, a beta-1 antagonist (i.e., a drug that specifically blocks the beta-1 adrenergic receptor) will slow down heart rate and decrease myocardial contractility without causing any major changes in the physiologic functions that are mediated by the other autonomic receptors.

However, several limitations of autonomic drugs must be realized. First, a drug that binds preferentially to one receptor subtype will bind to that receptor at all of its locations. For example, a muscarinic antagonist that decreases activity in the gastrointestinal tract may also decrease bronchial secretions in the lungs and cause urinary retention because of relaxation of the detrusor muscle of the bladder. Also, no drug is entirely specific for only one receptor subtype. For instance, the so-called beta-1–specific antagonists atenolol and metoprolol have a much greater affinity for beta-1 receptors than for beta-2 receptors.[8] At high enough concentrations, however, these drugs will affect beta-2 receptors as well. Finally, organs and tissues in the body do not contain only one subtype of receptor. For example, the predominant receptor in the bronchioles is the beta-2 subtype, but some beta-1 receptors are also present. Thus, a patient using a beta-1–specific drug such as metoprolol (Lopressor) may experience some respiratory effects as well.[8]

Consequently, the many side effects and beneficial effects of autonomic drugs can be attributed to the interaction of various agents with different receptors. The significance of autonomic receptor subtypes as well as the use of specific cholinergic and adrenergic drugs in treating various problems are covered in more detail in Chapters 19 and 20.

SUMMARY

The ANS is primarily responsible for controlling involuntary, or vegetative, functions in the body. The sympathetic and parasympathetic divisions of the ANS often function as physiologic antagonists to maintain homeostasis of various activities, including BP control, thermoregulation, digestion, and elimination. The primary neurotransmitters used in synaptic transmission within the ANS are acetylcholine and norepinephrine. These chemicals are found at specific locations in each autonomic division, as are their respective cholinergic and adrenergic receptors. The two primary types of autonomic receptors (cholinergic and adrenergic) are subdivided according to differences in drug affinity. Receptor subtypes are located in specific tissues throughout the body and are responsible for mediating the appropriate tissue response. Most autonomic drugs exert their effects by interacting in some way with autonomic synaptic transmission so that a fairly selective and isolated effect is achieved.

References

1. Brede M, Nagy G, Philipp M, et al. Differential control of adrenal and sympathetic catecholamine release by alpha 2-adrenoceptor subtypes. *Mol Endocrinol.* 2003; 17:1640–1646.
2. Brede M, Philipp M, Knaus A, et al. Alpha2-adrenergic receptor subtypes—novel functions uncovered in gene-targeted mouse models. *Biol Cell.* 2004;96: 343–348.
3. Burnstock G. Introduction: P2 receptors. *Curr Top Med Chem.* 2004;4:793–803.
4. Civantos Calzada B, Aleixandre de Artinano A. Alpha-adrenoceptor subtypes. *Pharmacol Res.* 2001; 44:195–208.
5. Gauthier C, Langin D, Balligand JL. Beta3-adrenoceptors in the cardiovascular system. *Trends Pharmacol Sci.* 2000;21:426–431.
6. Goldstein B. Anatomy of the peripheral nervous system. *Phys Med Rehabil Clin N Am.* 2001;12:207–236.
7. Guyton AC, Hall JE. *Textbook of Medical Physiology.* 11th ed. Philadelphia: WB Saunders; 2006.
8. Hoffman BB. Catecholamines, sympathomimetic drugs, and adrenergic receptor antagonists. In: Hardman, JG, et al, eds. *The Pharmacological Basis of Therapeutics.* 10th ed. New York: McGraw-Hill; 2001.
9. Hoffman BB, Taylor P. Neurotransmission: the autonomic and somatic motor nervous systems. In: Hardman, JG, et al, eds. *The Pharmacological Basis of Therapeutics.* 10th ed. New York: McGraw-Hill; 2001.

10. Johns EJ. Angiotensin II in the brain and the autonomic control of the kidney. *Exp Physiol.* 2005;90:163–168.

11. Katzung BG. Introduction to autonomic pharmacology. In: Katzung BG, ed. *Basic and Clinical Pharmacology.* 9th ed. New York: Lange Medical Books/McGraw Hill; 2004.

12. Mohan RM, Golding S, Heaton DA, et al. Targeting neuronal nitric oxide synthase with gene transfer to modulate cardiac autonomic function. *Prog Biophys Mol Biol.* 2004;84:321–344.

13. Pan HL. Brain angiotensin II and synaptic transmission. *Neuroscientist.* 2004;10:422–431.

14. Philipp M, Brede M, Hein L. Physiological significance of alpha(2)-adrenergic receptor subtype diversity: one receptor is not enough. *Am J Physiol Regul Integr Comp Physiol.* 2002;283:R287–R295.

15. Sartori C, Lepori M, Scherrer U. Interaction between nitric oxide and the cholinergic and sympathetic nervous system in cardiovascular control in humans. *Pharmacol Ther.* 2005;106:209–220.

16. Scislo TJ, O'Leary DS. Purinergic mechanisms of the nucleus of the solitary tract and neural cardiovascular control. *Neurol Res.* 2005;27:182–194.

17. Standring S, ed. *Gray's Anatomy.* 39th ed. New York: WB Saunders; 2005.

18. Stern JE. Nitric oxide and homeostatic control: an intercellular signalling molecule contributing to autonomic and neuroendocrine integration? *Prog Biophys Mol Biol.* 2004;84:197–215.

19. Uchiyama T, Chess-Williams R. Muscarinic receptor subtypes of the bladder and gastrointestinal tract. *J Smooth Muscle Res.* 2004;40:237–247.

20. Volpicelli LA, Levey AI. Muscarinic acetylcholine receptor subtypes in cerebral cortex and hippocampus. *Prog Brain Res.* 2004;145:59–66.

21. Wang Z, Shi H, Wang H. Functional M3 muscarinic acetylcholine receptors in mammalian hearts. *Br J Pharmacol.* 2004;142:395–408.

22. Yamada M, Basile AS, Fedorova I, et al. Novel insights into M5 muscarinic acetylcholine receptor function by the use of gene targeting technology. *Life Sci.* 2003;74:345–353.

23. Yamaguchi O. Beta3-adrenoceptors in human detrusor muscle. *Urology.* 2002;59(suppl 1):25–29.

24. Zheng M, Zhu W, Han Q, Xiao RP. Emerging concepts and therapeutic implications of beta-adrenergic receptor subtype signaling. *Pharmacol Ther.* 2005;108:257–268.

Chapter 19

Cholinergic Drugs

This chapter discusses drugs that affect the activity at cholinergic synapses—that is, synapses using acetylcholine as a neurotransmitter. Cholinergic synapses are important in a number of physiologic systems. As discussed in Chapter 18, acetylcholine is one of the primary neurotransmitters in the autonomic nervous system (ANS), especially in the parasympathetic autonomic division. Consequently, many drugs discussed in this chapter are administered to alter the response of various tissues to autonomic parasympathetic control. Acetylcholine is also the neurotransmitter at the skeletal neuromuscular junction. Certain cholinergic stimulants are used to treat a specific problem at the skeletal neuromuscular junction (i.e., myasthenia gravis). Cholinergic synapses are also found in specific areas of the brain, and some anticholinergic drugs are used to decrease the symptoms of diverse problems such as parkinsonism and motion sickness. Consequently, these drugs are used in a variety of clinical situations.

The purpose of this chapter is to present an overview of drugs sharing a common mode of action; that is, influencing cholinergic activity. Considering the diverse clinical applications of cholinergic and anticholinergic agents, physical therapists and occupational therapists will likely encounter patients taking these drugs. Knowledge of the pharmacodynamics of these medications will enable the rehabilitation specialist to understand the therapeutic rationale behind drug administration as well as the patient's response to the drug.

Autonomic cholinergic drugs can be divided into two general categories: cholinergic stimulants and anticholinergic drugs. Cholinergic stimulants effectively increase activity at acetylcholine synapses, whereas anticholinergic drugs decrease synaptic activity. Cholinergic stimulants and anticholinergic agents can be further characterized according to functional or pharmacodynamic criteria, and these criteria will be discussed in more detail in this chapter.

Cholinergic Receptors

Many autonomic cholinergic drugs affect synaptic activity by interacting with the acetylcholine receptor located on the postsynaptic membrane. At each cholinergic synapse, postsynaptic receptors are responsible for recognizing the acetylcholine molecule and transducing the chemical signal into a postsynaptic response. As discussed in Chapter 18, cholinergic receptors can be subdivided into muscarinic and nicotinic receptors according to their affinity for certain drugs.[12]

Muscarinic cholinergic receptors are generally found on the peripheral tissues supplied by parasympathetic postganglionic neurons—that is, on effector organs such as the gastrointestinal tract, urinary bladder, heart, eye, and so on. Acetylcholine synapses found in specific areas of the central nervous system (CNS) also use the muscarinic subtype of cholinergic receptor. Nicotinic cholinergic receptors are located in the autonomic ganglia (i.e., the N_N nicotinic subtype) and at the skeletal neuromuscular junction (the N_M nicotinic subtype). Refer to Chapter 18 for a more detailed discussion of cholinergic receptor subclassification.

The existence of different varieties of cholinergic receptors is important pharmacologically. Some drugs are relatively specific for a certain cholinergic receptor subtype, whereas others tend to bind rather indiscriminately to all cholinergic receptors. Obviously, specific drugs are preferable because they tend to produce a more precise response with fewer side effects. As this chapter will point out, however, specificity is only a relative term, and drugs that bind preferentially to one receptor subtype may produce a variety of responses.

Cholinergic Stimulants

Cholinergic stimulants increase activity at acetylcholine synapses. Chemically, many agents are capable of potently and effectively stimulating cholinergic activity. However, only a few drugs exhibit sufficient safety and relative specificity for use in clinical situations. These clinically relevant drugs can be subdivided into two categories depending on their mechanism of action. Direct-acting cholinergic stimulants exert their effects by binding directly with the cholinergic receptor (Fig. 19–1). Indirect-acting cholinergic stimulants increase synaptic activity by inhibiting the acetylcholinesterase enzyme located at the cholinergic synapse (Fig. 19–1). Table 19–1 lists specific direct-acting and indirect-acting cholinergic stimulants; the rationale for their use is presented below.

Direct-Acting Cholinergic Stimulants

Direct-acting stimulants bind directly to the cholinergic receptor to activate it, which in turn initiates a cellular response. These stimulants may be considered

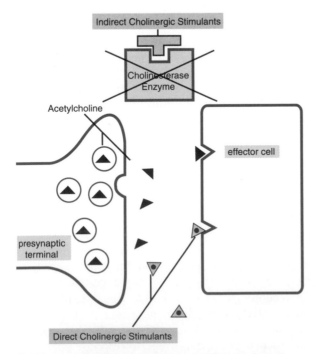

FIGURE 19–1 ▼ Mechanism of action of cholinergic stimulants. Direct-acting stimulants bind directly to the postsynaptic cholinergic receptor. Indirect-acting stimulants inhibit the cholinesterase enzyme, thus allowing acetylcholine to remain in the synaptic cleft.

true cholinergic agonists, and they function in a manner similar to the acetylcholine molecule. By definition, acetylcholine itself is a direct-acting cholinergic stimulant. Exogenously administered acetylcholine is not used therapeutically, however, because it is degraded rapidly and extensively by the acetylcholinesterase enzyme, which is found ubiquitously throughout the body.

As mentioned previously, there are many pharmacologic agents that can directly stimulate cholinergic receptors. A certain degree of drug specificity is desirable, however, when considering these agents for therapeutic purposes. For instance, drugs that have a greater specificity for the muscarinic cholinergic receptor are more beneficial. These muscarinic cholinergic stimulants will primarily affect the peripheral tissues while exerting a minimal effect on the cholinergic receptors located in the autonomic ganglia and the neuromuscular junction. (Recall that the cholinergic receptors found in the autonomic ganglia and at the skeletal neuromuscular junction are the N_N and N_M, respectively.)

Consequently, only a few agents are suitable for clinical use as direct-acting cholinergic stimulants. For systemic administration, bethanechol (Duvoid, others) is the primary direct-acting cholinergic stimulant (see Table 19–1). Bethanechol appears to preferentially stimulate muscarinic cholinergic receptors, especially those on gastrointestinal and bladder tissues.[5] Hence, this drug is sometimes used to increase gastrointestinal or bladder contractions, especially when motility in these tissues is reduced following abdominal surgery. Other direct-acting cholinergic stimulants such as carbachol and pilocarpine are limited to topical use in ophthalmologic conditions, especially glaucoma. These antiglaucoma drugs produce too many side effects if administered systemically, but are relatively specific when administered directly to the eye. Likewise, methacholine is a direct-acting cholinergic stimulant that can be administered locally to the lungs via inhalation to test for airway hyperresponsiveness when diagnosing patients for asthma. Clinical applications of direct-acting cholinergic stimulants are summarized in Table 19–1.

Indirect-Acting Cholinergic Stimulants

Indirect-acting stimulants increase activity at cholinergic synapses by inhibiting the acetylcholinesterase enzyme.[21] This enzyme is normally responsible for destroying acetylcholine after this neurotransmitter

Table 19-1	CHOLINERGIC STIMULANTS	
Generic Name	**Trade Name(s)**	**Primary Clinical Use(s)***
	Direct-Acting (Cholinergic Agonists)	
Bethanechol	Duvoid, Urabeth, Urecholine	Postoperative gastrointestinal and urinary atony
Carbachol	Isopto Carbachol, Carbastat, Miostat	Glaucoma
Pilocarpine	Pilocar, Adsorbocarpine, many others	Glaucoma
	Indirect-Acting (Cholinesterase Inhibitors)	
Ambenonium	Mytelase	Myasthenia gravis
Demecarium	Humorsol	Glaucoma
Donepezil	Aricept	Dementia of the Alzheimer's type
Echothiophate	Phospholine Iodide	Glaucoma
Edrophonium	Enlon, Reversol, Tensilon	Myasthenia gravis, reversal of neuromuscular blocking drugs
Galantamine	Reminyl	Dementia of the Alzheimer's type
Isoflurophate	Diflupyl	Glaucoma
Neostigmine	Prostigmin	Postoperative gastrointestinal and urinary atony, myasthenia gravis, reversal of neuro-muscular blocking drugs
Physostigmine	Antilirium, Eserine, Isopto Eserine	Glaucoma, reversal of CNS toxicity caused by anticholinergic drugs
Pyridostigmine	Mestinon	Myasthenia gravis, reversal of neuromuscular blocking drugs
Rivastigmine	Exelon	Dementia of the Alzheimer's type
Tacrine	Cognex	Dementia of the Alzheimer's type

*Agents used to treat glaucoma and other visual disturbances are administered topically, that is, directly to the eye. Agents used for other problems are given systemically by oral administration or injection.

is released from the presynaptic terminal. Indirectacting stimulants inhibit the acetylcholinesterase, thus allowing more acetylcholine to remain at the synapse. The result is an increase in cholinergic synaptic transmission.

Because of their effect on the acetylcholinesterase enzyme, indirect-acting stimulants are also referred to as *cholinesterase inhibitors* or *anticholinesterase agents*. The exact way in which these drugs inhibit the acetyl-

cholinesterase enzyme varies depending on the individual agent. The net effect is similar, however, in that the enzyme's ability to degrade acetylcholine is diminished by these drugs.

Unlike the systemic direct-acting cholinergic stimulants (e.g., bethanechol), cholinesterase inhibitors display a relative lack of specificity regarding which cholinergic synapses they stimulate. These drugs tend to inhibit the acetylcholinesterase found at all cholinergic synapses. Thus, they may exert a stimulatory effect on the peripheral muscarinic cholinergic synapses, as well as the cholinergic synapses found at the autonomic ganglia, at the skeletal neuromuscular junction, and within certain aspects of the CNS. In appropriate doses, however, certain agents exert some degree of specificity at peripheral versus CNS synapses. Indirect-acting stimulants such as neostigmine, for example, tend to predominantly affect the skeletal neuromuscular junction and peripheral tissues containing muscarinic receptors. In contrast, newer agents such as tacrine and donepezil show more specificity for cholinergic synapses in certain regions of the brain—hence, these newer drugs have been used to boost cholinergic function in conditions such as Alzheimer disease. Still, none of the indirect-acting cholinergic stimulants affect only one type of tissue, and some adverse side effects can be caused by their relatively nonspecific activity.

The primary indirect-acting cholinergic stimulants currently in use are neostigmine and pyridostigmine. Several other agents are also used therapeutically to treat systemic conditions such as myasthenia gravis, ophthalmologic disorders such as glaucoma, and diminished acetylcholine activity associated with degenerative brain syndromes such as Alzheimer disease. These indirect-acting agents are summarized in Table 19–1.

Clinical Applications of Cholinergic Stimulants

Direct- and indirect-acting cholinergic stimulants are used to treat the decrease in smooth-muscle tone that sometimes occurs in the gastrointestinal tract and urinary bladder following abdominal surgery or trauma. Indirect-acting stimulants are also used in the treatment of glaucoma and myasthenia gravis, in Alzheimer disease, and to reverse the effects from an overdose of other drugs such as neuromuscular blocking agents and anticholinergics. Each of these applications is briefly discussed here.

Alzheimer Disease. Alzheimer disease is a progressive neurodegenerative disorder that affects older adults. This disorder is characterized by neuronal atrophy and other pathological changes in neuron structure and function throughout the brain (neurofibrillary tangles, formation of plaques, and so forth). Included in this neuronal degeneration are cholinergic neurons that are critical in memory, cognition, and other higher cortical functions.[7] Although there is no cure for this disease, indirect cholinergic stimulants such as tacrine (Cognex), donepezil (Aricept), galantamine (Remingl), and rivastigmine (Exelon) (see Table 19–1) may help decrease some of the symptoms during the early stages of Alzheimer disease.[7,10] By inhibiting acetylcholine breakdown, these drugs prolong the effects of any acetylcholine released from neurons that are still functioning in the cerebral cortex.

Regrettably, these drugs do not alter the progression of Alzheimer disease, and they tend to lose effectiveness as the disease progresses into the advanced stages.[7] This loss of effectiveness makes sense when one considers that these drugs can only prolong the effects of endogenously released acetylcholine; they will have no effect when cortical neurons degenerate to the point where acetylcholine is no longer being synthesized and released within the brain. Nonetheless, drugs such as tacrine, donepezil, and other CNS cholinesterase inhibitors can help patients retain better cognitive function during the early stages of Alzheimer disease, which can help sustain a better quality-of-life for patients for as long as possible.[7]

Gastrointestinal and Urinary Bladder Atony. After surgical manipulation or other trauma to the viscera, there is often a period of atony (i.e., lack of tone) in the smooth muscle of these organs. As a result, intestinal peristalsis is diminished or absent, and the urinary bladder becomes distended, leading to urinary retention. Under normal circumstances, acetylcholine released from parasympathetic postganglionic neurons would stimulate smooth-muscle contraction in these tissues. Consequently, cholinergic agonists (i.e., drugs that mimic or enhance the effects of acetylcholine) are administered to treat this problem. Bethanechol and neostigmine, a direct-acting and an indirect-acting cholinergic stimulant, respectively, are the drugs most frequently used to treat this condition until normal gastrointestinal and urinary function is resumed.

Glaucoma. Glaucoma is an increase in intraocular pressure brought on by an accumulation of aqueous humor within the eye.[16] If untreated, this increased pressure leads to impaired vision and blindness. Cholinergic stimulation via the parasympathetic supply to the eye increases the outflow of aqueous humor, thus preventing excessive accumulation. If evidence of increased intraocular pressure exists, cholinergic stimulants are among the drugs that may be used to treat this problem.[15,16] Direct-acting and indirect-acting cholinergic drugs (see Table 19–1) are usually applied topically to the eye by placing the drug directly within the conjunctival sac to treat glaucoma. This application concentrates the action of the drug, thus limiting the side effects that might occur if these agents were given systemically. These agents are not typically the first drugs used to treat glaucoma, but they can be used if other agents are not effective.[6,15]

Myasthenia Gravis. Myasthenia gravis is a disease affecting the skeletal neuromuscular junction and is characterized by skeletal muscle weakness and profound fatigability.[14,23] As the disease progresses, fatigue increases in severity and in the number of muscles involved. In advanced stages, the patient requires respiratory support because of a virtual paralysis of the respiratory musculature. In myasthenia gravis, the number of functional cholinergic receptors located postsynaptically at the neuromuscular junction is diminished.[23] As a result, acetylcholine released from the presynaptic terminal cannot sufficiently excite the muscle cell to reach threshold. Thus, the decreased receptivity of the muscle cell accounts for the clinical symptoms of weakness and fatigue.

Myasthenia gravis appears to be caused by an autoimmune response whereby an antibody to the neuromuscular cholinergic receptor is produced.[23] Although no cure is available, cholinesterase inhibitors such as ambenonium, neostigmine, and pyridostigmine may help alleviate the muscular fatigue associated with this disease. These indirect-acting cholinergic agonists inhibit the acetylcholinesterase enzyme at the neuromuscular junction, allowing the endogenous acetylcholine released from the presynaptic terminal to remain at the myoneural junction for a longer period of time. The endogenously released acetylcholine is able to provide adequate excitation of the skeletal muscle cell and thus allow a more sustained muscular contraction.

Reversal of Neuromuscular Blockage. Drugs that block transmission at the skeletal neuromuscular junction are often used during general anesthesia to maintain skeletal muscle paralysis during surgical procedures (see Chapter 11). These skeletal muscle paralytic agents include curarelike drugs (e.g., tubocurarine, gallamine, pancuronium). Occasionally, the neuromuscular blockage caused by these drugs must be reversed. For instance, an accelerated recovery from the paralytic effects of these neuromuscular blockers may be desired at the end of the surgical procedure. Consequently, indirect-acting cholinergic stimulants are sometimes used to inhibit the acetyl-

cholinesterase enzyme at the neuromuscular junction, thus allowing endogenously released acetylcholine to remain active at the synaptic site and effectively overcome the neuromuscular blockade until the curarelike agents have been metabolized.

Reversal of Anticholinergic-Induced CNS Toxicity. Indirect-acting cholinergic stimulants (e.g., physostigmine) are sometimes used to reverse the toxic effects of anticholinergic drugs on the CNS. An overdose of anticholinergic drugs may produce toxic CNS effects such as delirium, hallucinations, and coma. By inhibiting acetylcholine breakdown, indirect-acting stimulants enable endogenously released acetylcholine to overcome the anticholinergic drug effects.

Adverse Effects of Cholinergic Stimulants

Cholinergic stimulants are frequently associated with a number of adverse side effects caused by the relative nonspecificity of these drugs. Even bethanechol, which is relatively specific for muscarinic receptors, may stimulate muscarinic receptors on many different tissues. For example, administering bethanechol to increase gastrointestinal motility may also result in bronchoconstriction if this drug reaches muscarinic receptors in the upper respiratory tract. Many indirect-acting stimulants (i.e., the cholinesterase inhibitors) show even less specificity and may increase synaptic activity at all synapses that they reach, including nicotinic cholinergic synapses.

The adverse effects associated with both the direct- and indirect-acting cholinergic stimulants mimic the effects that occur during exaggerated parasympathetic activity. This notion is logical considering that the parasympathetic autonomic division exerts its effects on peripheral tissues by releasing acetylcholine from postganglionic neurons. Consequently, the primary adverse effects of cholinergic stimulants include gastrointestinal distress (nausea, vomiting, diarrhea, abdominal cramping), increased salivation, bronchoconstriction, bradycardia, and difficulty in visual accommodation. Increased sweating and vasodilation of facial cutaneous blood vessels (flushing) may also occur because of an effect on the respective tissues supplied by special sympathetic postganglionic neurons that release acetylcholine. The incidence of these side effects varies from patient to patient, but the onset and severity increases as higher drug doses are administered.

Anticholinergic Drugs

In contrast to drugs that stimulate cholinergic activity, anticholinergic drugs attempt to diminish the response of tissues to cholinergic stimulation. In general, these drugs are competitive antagonists of the postsynaptic cholinergic receptors; that is, they bind reversibly to the cholinergic receptor but do not activate it. This binding blocks the receptor from the effects of endogenously released acetylcholine, thus diminishing the cellular response to cholinergic stimulation. (See Chapter 4 for a more detailed description of the mechanism by which drugs function as competitive antagonists.)

Anticholinergic drugs can be classified as antimuscarinic or antinicotinic agents, depending on their specificity for the two primary subtypes of cholinergic receptors. This chapter focuses on the antimuscarinic agents, with the antinicotinic drugs being discussed elsewhere in this text. Mecamylamine and trimethaphan, for example, are drugs that are relatively specific for the nicotinic receptor located in the autonomic ganglia (the N_N subtype). These N_N antagonists are sometimes used to treat extremely high blood pressure. The use of antinicotinic drugs in treating hypertensive emergencies is discussed in Chapter 21. Antinicotinic drugs that block the skeletal neuromuscular junction (i.e., the N_M antagonists) are sometimes used as an adjunct in general anesthesia and are used to produce skeletal muscle paralysis during surgery. These so-called neuromuscular blockers are discussed in Chapter 11.

Source and Mechanism of Action of Antimuscarinic Anticholinergic Drugs

The prototypical antimuscarinic anticholinergic drug is atropine (Fig. 19–2). Atropine is a naturally occurring substance that can be obtained from the extract of plants such as belladonna and jimsonweed. Other natural, semisynthetic, and synthetic antimuscarinic anticholinergic agents have been developed that are similar in structure or function to atropine.

As mentioned previously, antimuscarinic anticholinergic drugs all share the same basic mechanism of action: they block the postsynaptic cholinergic muscarinic receptor. However, certain antimuscarinic agents seem to preferentially affect some tissues more than others. For instance, certain antimuscarinics seem to preferentially antagonize gastrointestinal muscarinic receptors, whereas others have a predominant effect on CNS cholinergic synapses. This fact suggests

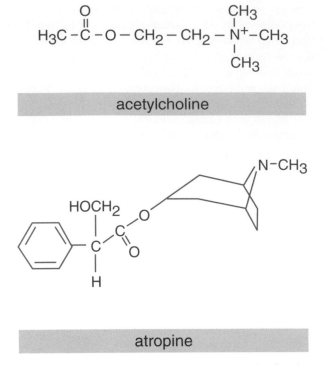

acetylcholine

atropine

FIGURE 19–2 ▼ Structures of acetylcholine and atropine. Atropine and similar agents antagonize the effects of acetylcholine by blocking muscarinic cholinergic receptors.

some degree of specificity of these drugs, which may be because of differences in the muscarinic receptor at gastrointestinal versus central synapses. Indeed, there is evidence that as many as five muscarinic receptor subtypes may exist at different locations in the body; these subtypes are designated M_1, M_2, M_3, M_4, and M_5 receptors.[24,25,26,28] Some drugs may be more selective for a certain receptor subtype than for others. This drug-receptor specificity is far from complete, however, and virtually every antimuscarinic drug will antagonize cholinergic receptors on a number of tissues, which leads to various side effects (see "Side Effects of Anticholinergic Drugs"). Perhaps as more is learned about muscarinic receptor subtypes, more selective anticholinergic drugs may be developed.

Clinical Applications of Antimuscarinic Drugs

The primary clinical applications of antimuscarinic anticholinergic drugs include the treatment of certain gastrointestinal disorders. These drugs may also be helpful in managing Parkinson disease. In addition, they have been used to treat a variety clinical disorders involving other physiologic systems.[5] The clinical ap-

Table 19–2	COMMON ANTICHOLINERGIC DRUGS*	

Generic Name	Trade Name(s)	Primary Clinical Use(s)*
Anisotropine	Generic	Peptic ulcer
Atropine	Generic	Peptic ulcer, irritable bowel syndrome, neurogenic bladder, bronchospasm, preoperative antisecretory agent, cardiac arrhythmias (e.g., sinus bradycardia, postmyocardial infarction, asystole), reversal of neuromuscular blockade, antidote to cholinesterase inhibitor poisoning
Belladonna	Generic	Peptic ulcer, irritable bowel syndrome, dysmenorrhea, nocturnal enuresis, antivertigo
Clidinium	Quarzan	Peptic ulcer, irritable bowel syndrome
Cyclopentolate	Pentolate, Cyclogyl, others	Induces mydriasis for ophthalmologic procedures
Dicyclomine	Bentyl, others	Irritable bowel syndrome
Glycopyrrolate	Robinul	Peptic ulcer, preoperative antisecretory agent, antidiarrheal, reversal of neuromuscular blockade
Homatropine	Homapin	Peptic ulcer, irritable bowel syndrome
Hyoscyamine	Cystospaz, Levsin, others	Peptic ulcer, irritable bowel syndrome, urinary bladder hypermotility, preoperative antisecretory agent
Ipratropium	Atrovent, others	Bronchodilator
Mepenzolate	Cantil	Peptic ulcer
Methantheline	Banthine	Peptic ulcer
Oxybutynin	Ditropan	Neurogenic or overactive bladder
Propantheline	Pro-Banthine	Peptic ulcer, irritable bowel syndrome, urinary incontinence
Scopolamine	Transderm-Scop, others	Motion sickness, preoperative antisecretory agent, postoperative nausea and vomiting, antivertigo
Tiotropium	Spinva	Bronchodilator
Tolterodine	Detrol	Overactive bladder

*Clinical uses listed for a specific agent reflect that agent's approved indication(s). Actual clinical use, however, may be limited because anticholinergics have often been replaced by agents that are more effective and better tolerated. Anticholinergic drugs used specifically to treat Parkinson disease are listed in Table 10–2, Chapter 10.

plications of antimuscarinic agents are discussed here, and specific drugs used in various clinical situations are outlined in Table 19–2.

Gastrointestinal System. Stimulation of the gastrointestinal tract via parasympathetic cholinergic neurons generally produces an increase in gastric secretions and an increase in gastrointestinal motility. Consequently, certain antimuscarinic anticholinergics tend to reverse this stimulation by blocking the effects of endogenously released acetylcholine. Clinically, these drugs are used as an adjunct in peptic ulcer. The rationale is that they will limit secretion of gastric acid, thus reducing irritation of the stomach mucosa. Also, antimuscarinic anticholinergic drugs have been approved for treatment of irritable bowel syndrome. This condition is characterized by hyperactivity of gastrointestinal smooth muscle and includes problems such as irritable colon and spastic colon. These antimuscarinic agents are sometimes referred to as *antispasmodics* because of their reported ability to decrease gastrointestinal smooth-muscle tone or spasms.

Drugs used to treat peptic ulcer and irritable bowel syndrome are listed in Table 19–2. Although these agents are approved for use in these conditions, considerable doubt exists as to how effective they are in actually resolving these gastrointestinal disorders. Their use in treating peptic ulcer has essentially been replaced by other agents such as the H_2 histamine receptor blockers and proton pump inhibitors (see Chapter 27), but antimuscarinic anticholinergics may still be used if other drugs are ineffective or poorly tolerated.[5] These drugs will not cure peptic ulcer or prevent its recurrence when the medication is discontinued. In essence, they only treat a symptom of the problem (e.g., increased gastric secretion), without really addressing the cause of the increased secretion (e.g., emotional stress).

Finally, antimuscarinic anticholinergic drugs used to treat gastrointestinal problems are often combined with other agents, such as antianxiety drugs. Librax, for instance, is the trade name for a combination of chlordiazepoxide and clidinium (an antianxiety agent and an anticholinergic agent, respectively). These combination products are supposedly better at relieving gastrointestinal problems where emotional factors are also present.

Parkinson Disease. The pharmacologic management of Parkinson disease is discussed in detail in Chapter 10. Consequently, the use of anticholinergic drugs in this disorder will only be mentioned briefly here. Parkinsonism is a movement disorder caused by a deficiency of the neurotransmitter dopamine in the basal ganglia. This deficiency leads to an overactivity of central cholinergic synapses. Hence, anticholinergic drugs should be beneficial in helping to resolve this increase in central cholinergic influence.[11]

Certain anticholinergic drugs such as benztropine, biperiden, and trihexyphenidyl are approved for use in treating Parkinson disease (see Chapter 10, Table 10–2 for a more complete list). These drugs seem to preferentially block the central muscarinic cholinergic synapses involved in parkinsonism. This does not mean that the drugs do not affect other peripheral muscarinic receptors. Indeed, antiparkinsonian drugs are associated with a number of side effects such as dry mouth, constipation, and urinary retention, which are caused by their antagonistic effect on muscarinic receptors located outside of the brain. Their primary effect, however, is to decrease the influence of central cholinergic synapses in parkinsonism.

Cardiovascular System. Atropine is sometimes used to block the effects of the vagus nerve (cranial nerve X) on the myocardium. Release of acetylcholine from vagal efferent fibers slows heart rate and the conduction of the cardiac action potential throughout the myocardium. Atropine reverses the effects of excessive vagal discharge and is used to treat the symptomatic bradycardia that may accompany myocardial infarction.[4] Atropine may also be useful in treating other cardiac arrhythmias such as atrioventricular nodal block and ventricular asystole.

Motion Sickness. Antimuscarinics (scopolamine in particular) are frequently used in the treatment of motion sickness.[22] Scopolamine appears to block cholinergic transmission from areas of the brain and brainstem that mediate motion-related nausea and vomiting (i.e., the vestibular system and reticular formation).[8] These drugs are often administered transdermally via small patches that adhere to the skin.[18]

Preoperative Medication. Atropine and related antimuscarinics are occasionally used preoperatively to decrease respiratory secretions during general anesthesia. Their use in this capacity has declined considerably, however, because the newer inhalation forms of general anesthesia do not stimulate bronchial secretions to the same extent as earlier general anesthetics (see Chapter 11).[5] Anticholinergic medications can sometimes be used preoperatively with other agents (sedatives, antianxiety agents, and so forth) to help control postoperative nausea and vomiting.[9,19] Antimuscarinics may also be administered to prevent bradycardia during surgery, especially in children.

Urinary Tract. Atropine and several synthetic antimuscarinics have been used to alleviate urinary frequency and incontinence caused by hypertonicity of the urinary bladder.[13,17] Increased bladder tone results if the normal reflex control of bladder function is disrupted (i.e., the so-called neurogenic bladder syndrome) or a urinary tract infection irritates the bladder. Some people might also exhibit increased urinary frequency and nocturia without any obvious pathological findings, a condition known as overactive bladder.[13,17] Regardless of the cause, antimuscarinics can help reduce bladder hypertonicity by inhibiting contraction of the bladder detrusor muscle, thus allowing the bladder to fill more normally, with a decrease in frequency of urination and a lesser chance of incontinence.

Respiratory Tract. Stimulation of the upper respiratory tract via the vagus causes bronchoconstriction. Anticholinergic drugs that block the effects of vagal-released acetylcholine will relax bronchial smooth muscle. Consequently, atropine and some synthetic derivatives (ipratropium, tiotropium) have been used to treat bronchospasms occurring in patients with asthma and chronic obstructive pulmonary disease (COPD).[3,5,20] Although anticholinergics are not usually the initial drugs used to treat bronchoconstriction, they may be used in combination with other drugs or as a second choice for patients who are unable to tolerate more conventional forms of bronchodilators such as the adrenergic agonists.[5] The use of anticholinergics in treating respiratory disorders is discussed in more detail in Chapter 26.

Eye. Atropine and similar antimuscarinics block the acetylcholine-mediated contraction of the pupillary sphincter muscle, thus causing dilation of the pupil (mydriasis).[1] During an ophthalmologic exam, these drugs may be applied topically in order to dilate the pupil, thus allowing a more detailed inspection of internal eye structures such as the retina.

Cholinergic Poisoning. Cholinergic poisoning can occur in several situations such as eating wild mushrooms, being exposed to certain pesticides, or being exposed to certain types of chemical warfare.[2,27] This type of poisoning often occurs because organophosphates and similar toxic compounds inhibit the acetylcholinesterase enzyme throughout the body, thereby causing severe overstimulation of nicotinic and muscarinic receptors in organs and physiologic systems. These potentially life-threatening occurrences typically require emergency treatment with atropine or an analogous anticholinergic agent. In cases of severe poisoning, fairly high doses of these drugs must often be administered for several days.

Side Effects of Anticholinergic Drugs

Considering the diverse uses of the previously named anticholinergics, these drugs can obviously affect a number of different tissues. A systemically adminis-

tered anticholinergic agent cannot be targeted for one specific organ without also achieving a response in other tissues as well. For instance, an antimuscarinic drug administered to decrease motility in the gastrointestinal tract may also affect other tissues containing muscarinic receptors (e.g., the bladder, bronchial smooth muscle, eye, heart). As higher doses are administered for any given problem, the chance of additional effects in tissues other than the target organ is also increased.

Consequently, antimuscarinic anticholinergic drugs are associated with a number of side effects. Exactly which symptoms (if any) will be encountered depends on a number of factors such as the specific anticholinergic agent, the dosage of the drug, and the individual response of each patient. The most common side effects include dryness of the mouth, blurred vision, urinary retention, constipation, and tachycardia. Each of these side effects is caused by the blockade of muscarinic receptors on the tissue or organ related to the effect. Some patients also report symptoms such as confusion, dizziness, nervousness, and drowsiness, presumably because of an interaction of antimuscarinic drugs with CNS cholinergic receptors. These CNS-related symptoms occur more frequently with anticholinergic drugs that readily cross the blood-brain barrier.

SUMMARY

Drugs affecting acetylcholine-mediated responses are classified as cholinergic stimulants and anticholinergic drugs. Cholinergic stimulants increase cholinergic activity by binding to the acetylcholine receptor and activating the receptor (direct-acting stimulants) or by inhibiting the acetylcholinesterase enzyme, thus allowing more acetylcholine to remain active at the cholinergic synapse (indirect-acting stimulants). Anticholinergic drugs inhibit cholinergic activity by acting as competitive antagonists; that is, they bind to the cholinergic receptor but do not activate it.

Cholinergic stimulants and anticholinergic drugs affect many tissues in the body and are used to treat a variety of clinical problems. Cholinergic stimulants are often administered to increase gastrointestinal and urinary bladder tone, to treat conditions such as glaucoma, myasthenia gravis, and Alzheimer disease, and to reverse the neuromuscular blockade produced by curarelike drugs. Anticholinergic drugs are used principally to decrease gastrointestinal motility and secretions, and to decrease the symptoms of Parkinson disease, but they may also be used to treat problems in several other physiologic systems. Because of the ability of cholinergic stimulants and anticholinergic drugs to affect different tissues, these drugs may be associated with a number of side effects. Considering the diverse clinical applications of cholinergic stimulants and anticholinergics, physical therapists and occupational therapists may frequently encounter patients taking these drugs. Rehabilitation specialists should be aware of the rationale for drug administration as well as possible side effects of cholinergic stimulants and anticholinergic agents.

References

1. Arnold RW, Gionet E, Hickel J, et al. Duration and effect of single-dose atropine: paralysis of accommodation in penalization treatment of functional amblyopia. *Binocul Vis Strabismus Q.* 2004;19:81–86.
2. Bajgar J. Organophosphates/nerve agent poisoning: mechanism of action, diagnosis, prophylaxis, and treatment. *Adv Clin Chem.* 2004;38:151–216.
3. Barr RG, Bourbeau J, Camargo CA, Ram FS. Inhaled tiotropium for stable chronic obstructive pulmonary disease. *Cochrane Database Syst Rev.* 2005;CD002876.
4. Brady WJ, Jr, Harrigan RA. Diagnosis and management of bradycardia and atrioventricular block associated with acute coronary ischemia. *Emerg Med Clin North Am.* 2001;19:371–384.
5. Brown JH, Taylor P. Muscarinic receptor agonists and antagonists. In: Hardman JG, et al, eds. *The Pharmacological Basis of Therapeutics.* 10th ed. New York: McGraw-Hill; 2001.
6. Duncan G, Collison DJ. Role of the non-neuronal cholinergic system in the eye: a review. *Life Sci.* 2003; 72:2013–2019.
7. Ellis JM. Cholinesterase inhibitors in the treatment of dementia. *J Am Osteopath Assoc.* 2005;105:145–158.
8. Flake ZA, Scalley RD, Bailey AG. Practical selection of antiemetics. *Am Fam Physician.* 2004;69: 1169–1174.
9. Golembiewski J, Chernin E, Chopra T. Prevention and treatment of postoperative nausea and vomiting. *Am J Health Syst Pharm.* 2005;62:1247–1260.
10. Kaduszkiewicz H, Zimmermann T, Beck-Bornholdt HP, van den Bussche H. Cholinesterase inhibitors for patients with Alzheimer's disease: systematic review of randomised clinical trials. *BMJ.* 2005; 331:321–327.
11. Katzenschlager R, Sampaio C, Costa J, Lees A. Anticholinergics for symptomatic management of Parkinson's disease. *Cochrane Database Syst Rev.* 2003; CD003735.
12. Katzung BG. Introduction to autonomic pharmacology. In: Katzung BG ed. *Basic and Clinical Pharmacology.* 9th ed. New York: Lange Medical Books/McGraw Hill; 2004.
13. Kavia R, Mumtaz F. Overactive bladder. *J R Soc Health.* 2005;125:176–179.
14. Kothari MJ. Myasthenia gravis. *J Am Osteopath Assoc.* 2004;104:377–384.
15. Lee DA, Higginbotham EJ. Glaucoma and its treatment: a review. *Am J Health Syst Pharm.* 2005;62: 691–699.
16. Marquis RE, Whitson JT. Management of glaucoma: focus on pharmacological therapy. *Drugs Aging.* 2005; 22:1–21.
17. Michel MC, de la Rosette JJ. Role of muscarinic receptor antagonists in urgency and nocturia. *BJU Int.* 2005;96(suppl 1):37–42.
18. Nachum Z, Shahal B, Shupak A, et al. Scopolamine bioavailability in combined oral and transdermal delivery. *J Pharmacol Exp Ther.* 2001;296:121–123.
19. Ozcan AA, Gunes Y, Haciyakupoglu G. Using diazepam and atropine before strabismus surgery to prevent postoperative nausea and vomiting: a randomized, controlled study. *J AAPOS.* 2003;7:210–212.
20. Saberi F, O'Donnell DE. The role of tiotropium bromide, a long-acting anticholinergic bronchodilator, in the management of COPD. *Treat Respir Med.* 2005;4: 275–281.
21. Silman I, Sussman JL. Acetylcholinesterase: 'classical' and 'non classical' functions and pharmacology. *Curr Opin Pharmacol.* 2005;5:293–302.
22. Spinks AB, Wasiak J, Villanueva EV, Bernath V. Scopolamine for preventing and treating motion sickness. *Cochrane Database Syst Rev.* 2004;CD002851.
23. Thanvi BR, Lo TC. Update on myasthenia gravis. *Postgrad Med J.* 2004;80:690–700.
24. Uchiyama T, Chess-Williams R. Muscarinic receptor subtypes of the bladder and gastrointestinal tract. *J Smooth Muscle Res.* 2004;40:237–247.
25. Volpicelli LA, Levey AI. Muscarinic acetylcholine receptor subtypes in cerebral cortex and hippocampus. *Prog Brain Res.* 2004;145:59–66.
26. Wang Z, Shi H, Wang H. Functional M3 muscarinic acetylcholine receptors in mammalian hearts. *Br J Pharmacol.* 2004;142:395–408.
27. Weinbroum AA. Pathophysiological and clinical aspects of combat anticholinesterase poisoning. *Br Med Bull.* 2005;72:119–133.
28. Yamada M, Basile AS, Fedorova I, et al. Novel insights into M5 muscarinic acetylcholine receptor function by the use of gene targeting technology. *Life Sci.* 2003;74: 345–353.

Chapter 20

Adrenergic Drugs

The purpose of this chapter is to describe drugs that either stimulate activity at norepinephrine synapses (adrenergic agonists) or inhibit norepinephrine influence (adrenergic antagonists). To be more specific, this chapter will focus on drugs primarily influencing activity in the sympathetic nervous system through their effect on adrenergic synapses. Norepinephrine is usually the neurotransmitter at the junction between sympathetic postganglionic neurons and peripheral tissues. Consequently, most of the adrenergic agonists discussed in this chapter will be used to augment sympathetic responses, while the adrenergic antagonists will be used to attenuate sympathetic-induced activity. In fact, adrenergic agonists are sometimes referred to as sympathomimetic, and antagonists are referred to as sympatholytic, because of their ability to increase and decrease sympathetic activity, respectively.

As in Chapter 19, drugs discussed here are categorized according to a common mode of action rather than according to common clinical applications. Most drugs introduced in this chapter will appear throughout this text when they are classified according to their use in treating specific problems. For instance, the beta-selective adrenergic antagonists (i.e., beta blockers; see "Beta Antagonists") are collectively introduced. Individual beta blockers, however, are also discussed in subsequent chapters with regard to their use in specific problems such as hypertension (see Chapter 21), angina pectoris (see Chapter 22), cardiac arrhythmias (see Chapter 23), and congestive heart failure (see Chapter 24).

The drugs described in this chapter are used to treat a variety of disorders, ranging from severe cardiovascular and respiratory problems to symptoms of the common cold. Because these drugs are widely used in cardiovascular disease and other disorders, many patients seen in physical therapy and occupational

therapy will be taking adrenergic agonists or antagonists. In this chapter, the basic pharmacodynamic mechanisms, clinical applications, and adverse effects of these drugs are introduced. The relevance of specific adrenergic drugs to physical rehabilitation is addressed in more detail in subsequent chapters categorizing their use according to specific disorders (hypertension, angina, asthma, etc.).

Many adrenergic agonists and antagonists exert their effects by binding directly to the appropriate postsynaptic receptor. Since a great deal of the specificity (or lack of specificity) of these drugs depends on the drug-receptor interaction, adrenergic receptor classes and subclasses are briefly reviewed here.

Adrenergic Receptor Subclassifications

As discussed in Chapter 18, adrenergic receptors can be divided into two primary categories: alpha and beta receptors. Each category can then be subdivided, so that five receptor subtypes are commonly identified: alpha-1, alpha-2, beta-1, beta-2, and beta-3.[16] Alpha-1 receptors have been further categorized as alpha 1a, 1b, and 1d receptors, and alpha-2 receptors have been subdivided into alpha 2a, 2b, and 2c receptors. The functional significance of these subclassifications remains unclear, so drugs affecting alpha receptors will be categorized according to the primary alpha receptor that they affect (i.e., alpha-1 or alpha-2). Adrenergic receptor subtypes are located on specific tissues throughout the body, and the response mediated by each receptor depends on the interaction between that receptor and the respective tissue. Refer to Chapter 18 for a more detailed description of adrenergic receptor locations and responses.

The primary uses of adrenergic agonists and antagonists according to their selectivity for individual receptor subtypes are summarized in Table 20–1. In general, a specific agonist is used to mimic or increase the receptor-mediated response, whereas the antagonist is used to decrease the receptor-mediated response.

Clinically useful adrenergic agonists and antagonists display variable amounts of specificity for each receptor subtype. Some drugs are fairly specific and bind to only one receptor subtype (e.g., a specific alpha-1 agonist like phenylephrine preferentially stimulates the alpha-1 subtype). Other drugs show a moderate amount of specificity, perhaps affecting one major receptor category. An example is the nonselective beta antagonist propranolol, which blocks beta-1 and beta-2 receptors but has little or no effect on alpha receptors. Finally, other drugs such as epinephrine are rather nonspecific and affect alpha and beta receptors equally. In some clinical situations, administering a selective drug may be desirable, whereas in others, a drug that interacts with more than one receptor sub-type is beneficial. Use of selective versus nonselective adrenergic drugs is considered in "Adrenergic Agonists" and "Adrenergic Antagonists" in this chapter.

"Receptor selectivity", however, is a relative term. Even though an adrenergic drug is reported to be selective for only one receptor subtype, a certain affinity for other receptor subtypes may also occur to a lesser degree. A beta-1–specific drug, for instance, binds preferentially to beta-1 receptors but may also show some slight affinity for beta-2 receptors. Selectivity is also dose-related, with the relative degree of receptor selectivity decreasing as higher doses are administered. Consequently, some side effects of the so-called selective drugs may be caused by stimulation of other receptor subtypes, especially at higher drug doses.

Adrenergic Agonists

Drugs that stimulate the adrenergic receptors are presented below according to their relative specificity for

Table 20–1	SUMMARY OF ADRENERGIC AGONIST/ANTAGONIST USE ACCORDING TO RECEPTOR SPECIFICITY		
Primary Receptor Location: Response When Stimulated	**Agonist Use(s)***		**Antagonist Use(s)***
Alpha-1 receptor			
Vascular smooth muscle: vasoconstriction	Hypotension Nasal congestion Paroxysmal supraventricular tachycardia		Hypertension
Alpha-2 receptor			
CNS synapses (inhibitory)	Hypertension Spasticity		No significant clinical use
Beta-1 receptor			
Heart: increased heart rate and force of contraction	Cardiac decompensation		Hypertension Arrhythmia Angina pectoris Heart failure Prevention of reinfarction
Beta-2 receptor			
Bronchioles: bronchodilation Uterus: relaxation	Prevent bronchospasm Prevent premature labor		No significant clinical use

*Primary clinical condition(s) that the agonists or antagonists are used to treat. See text for specific drugs in each category and a discussion of treatment rationale.

each receptor subtype. The drugs that primarily activate alpha receptors are discussed first, followed by beta-selective drugs, and drugs that have mixed alpha- and beta-agonist activity.

Alpha Agonists

Alpha-1–Selective Agonists

General Indications

Alpha-1 agonists bind directly to and activate the alpha-1 receptor located primarily on vascular smooth muscle, thus leading to smooth-muscle contraction and vasoconstriction. Because of their vasoconstrictive properties, these drugs are able to increase blood pressure by increasing peripheral vascular resistance. Consequently, certain alpha-1 agonists are administered systemically to treat acute hypotension occurring in emergencies such as shock or during general anesthesia. A second common clinical application of these drugs is the treatment of nasal congestion (i.e., runny nose and stuffy head feelings associated with the common cold). In appropriate doses, alpha-1 agonists preferentially constrict the vasculature in the nasal and upper respiratory mucosa, thus decreasing the congestion and mucosal discharge. A third application of alpha-1 agonists is to decrease heart rate during attacks of paroxysmal supraventricular tachycardia. By increasing peripheral vascular resistance, these drugs bring about a reflex decrease in heart rate through the cardiac baroreceptor reflex.

Specific Agents

Mephenteramine (Wyamine). This alpha-1 stimulant is used primarily to maintain or restore blood pressure during hypotensive episodes that may occur during spinal anesthesia. It is typically administered by intravenous or intramuscular injection.

Methoxamine (Vasoxyl). This drug is used primarily to increase and maintain blood pressure in severe, acute hypotension, especially during general anesthesia and spinal anesthesia. It is usually administered by injection (intramuscularly or intravenously) to allow a rapid onset.

Midodrine (ProAmatine). Midodrine can be administered orally to treat resistant cases of orthostatic hypotension. This drug can also prevent hypotension in patients undergoing dialysis, and it can offset the hypotensive effects of certain psychotropic drugs (e.g., antipsychotic medications).

Oxymetazoline (Afrin, Visine, many others). This drug is used in nose drops and nasal sprays to decrease nasal congestion through alpha-1–mediated vasoconstriction. Higher or systemic doses may also cause hypotension, presumably because central nervous system (CNS) alpha-2 receptors are stimulated in a manner similar to clonidine (see "Alpha-2–Selective Agonists"). Oxymetazoline can also be administered as eye drops to decrease redness and minor eye irritation.

Phenylephrine (Neo-Synephrine, others). Like methoxamine, phenylephrine can be administered systemically to treat hypotension, and phenylephrine can also be used to terminate certain episodes of supraventricular tachycardia. In addition, phenylephrine is administered topically to treat nasal congestion and is found in many over-the-counter spray decongestants.

Pseudoephedrine (Drixoral, Sudafed, many others). Pseudoephedrine is administered orally for its decongestant effects, is found in many over-the-counter preparations, and is commonly used to help relieve cold symptoms.

Xylometazoline (Otrivin, others). This drug is used primarily as a nasal spray to decrease congestion during colds and allergies.

Adverse Effects

The primary side effects associated with alpha-1–specific agonists are caused by excessive stimulation of alpha-adrenergic responses. Some of the more frequent side effects include increased blood pressure, headache, and an abnormally slow heart rate (because of reflex bradycardia). Some patients also report chest pain, difficulty breathing, and feelings of nervousness. These side effects are quite variable and are usually dose-related (i.e., they occur more frequently at higher doses).

Alpha-2–Selective Agonists

General Indications

Alpha-2–selective drugs are used primarily in the treatment of hypertension and spasticity. When treating hypertension, these drugs stimulate alpha-2 receptors located in the brain and brainstem. When stimulated, these central alpha-2 receptors exert an *inhibitory* effect on sympathetic discharge from the vasomotor center in the brainstem.[34] Diminished sympathetic discharge results in a decrease in blood pressure. The use of alpha-2 agonists in lowering blood pressure is discussed in more detail in Chapter 21.

Alpha-2 receptors have also been identified on interneurons in the spinal cord. Stimulation of these receptors causes interneuron inhibition, and a subsequent decrease in excitability of motor neurons supplied by the interneurons.[6,8] Alpha-2 agonists have therefore been used to normalize neuronal activity in conditions such as spasticity; the use of these drugs as antispasticity agents is discussed in more detail in Chapter 13.

Consequently, alpha-2 agonists appear to exert their antihypertensive effects and antispasticity effects by preferentially stimulating alpha-2 receptors in the brain and spinal cord, respectively. In both situations, it is unclear whether alpha-2 agonists exert their primary effects on presynaptic or postsynaptic receptors. Stimulation of presynaptic alpha-2 receptors located at adrenergic synapses results in a decrease in norepinephrine release from the presynaptic terminal.[8] Similarly, alpha-2 receptors have also been identified postsynaptically at specific central synapses, and these postsynaptic receptors are believed to directly inhibit neuronal excitation.[35] Thus, alpha-2 agonists may exert their effects by stimulating either central presynaptic or postsynaptic receptors, or by acting on inhibitory presynaptic and postsynaptic receptors simultaneously. Alpha-2 receptors may also exist on other tissues such as the eye, and the use of alpha-2 agonists continues to expand as more is learned about the location and function of these receptors.

Specific Agents

Brimonidine (Alphagan). This drug is administered locally to the eye to treat glaucoma. It stimulates ocular alpha-2 receptors, which decreases intraocular pressure by decreasing vitreous humor production and increasing drainage of vitreous humor from the eye.

Clonidine (Catapres, Duraclon). Clonidine is used as an antihypertensive as well as an analgesic. Clonidine's antihypertensive effects occur because the drug stimulates alpha-2 receptors in the vasomotor center of the brainstem and decreases sympathetic discharge to the heart and vasculature. Clonidine, however, is not usually successful when used alone in long-term treatment of essential hypertension. This drug is usually reserved for use in short-term management or in combination with other antihypertensive drugs, especially in patients who are unable to tolerate alpha-1 antagonists such as prazosin (Minipress) (see "Alpha Antagonists"). Clonidine also has sedative properties and has been used as an antianxiety drug, an adjunct in general

anesthesia, and an analgesic. In particular, this drug can be combined with other analgesics (opioids) for treating severe pain in people with cancer. Clonidine's analgesic effects are probably mediated by stimulation of alpha-2 receptors located in the spinal cord. Because of its effects on alpha-2 receptors in the spinal cord, clonidine has antispasticity effects. Use of this drug in spasticity, however, is often limited because it also causes hypotension.

Guanabenz (Wytensin). Guanabenz is used primarily to decrease blood pressure via its effect on alpha-2 receptors in the brainstem. This drug is similar to clonidine in efficacy and clinical use.

Guanfacine (Tenex). This drug is similar to guanabenz, and is typically used to treat advanced or resistant cases of high blood pressure.

Methyldopa (Aldomet). Methyldopa has been used as an antihypertensive drug for some time, but its mechanism of action is poorly understood. Currently, methyldopa is believed to exert its effects by being converted to alpha-methylnorepinephrine in the body.[26] Alpha-methylnorepinephrine is a potent alpha-2 agonist that lowers blood pressure by stimulating inhibitory central adrenergic receptors in a manner similar to clonidine and guanabenz.

Tizanidine (Zanaflex). Tizanidine is used primarily for treating spasticity.[14,24] This drug is similar to clonidine, but has less vasomotor effects and is therefore less likely to cause hypotension and other cardiovascular problems. As indicated earlier, tizanidine stimulates alpha-2 receptors in the spinal cord, which results in decreased excitatory input onto the alpha motor neuron. Decreased excitation of the alpha motor neuron results in decreased spasticity of the skeletal muscle supplied by that neuron.

Adverse Effects

Use of alpha-2–specific drugs may be associated with some relatively minor side effects such as dizziness, drowsiness, and dry mouth. More pronounced adverse effects such as difficult breathing, an unusually slow heart rate, and persistent fainting may indicate a toxic accumulation or overdose of these drugs.

Beta Agonists

Beta-1–Selective Agonists

General Indications

The beta-1 receptor is located primarily on the myocardium, and stimulation of the receptor results in increased heart rate and increased force of myocardial contraction (i.e., increased cardiac output). Consequently, beta-1 agonists are used primarily to increase cardiac output in emergency situations such as cardiovascular shock or if complications develop during cardiac surgery. Beta-1 agonists may also be used to increase cardiac function in the short-term treatment of certain types of heart disease, including heart failure.

Specific Agents

Dobutamine (Dobutrex). Dobutamine is used for short-term management of cardiac decompensation that sometimes occurs during exacerbations of heart disease or following cardiac surgery.[28] This drug is often administered via intravenous pump infusion to allow relatively stable plasma levels.

Dopamine (Intropin). In addition to its ability to stimulate dopamine receptors, this drug directly stimulates beta-1–adrenergic receptors. Depending on the dose, this drug also exerts complex effects on other dopaminergic and adrenergic receptors.[28] At low doses, for example, dopamine may cause peripheral vasodilation in the viscera and kidneys by stimulating dopamine receptors in the vasculature of these tissues. This effect may help sustain kidney function in people with heart failure because cardiac output is increased (beta-1 effect) as renal blood flow is also increased. At higher doses, however, dopamine may cause peripheral vasoconstriction by directly stimulating vascular alpha-1 receptors and increasing the release of norepinephrine from vascular sympathetic neurons. This effect can help sustain blood pressure in people with severe hypotension. Clinically, dopamine is used to treat cardiac decompensation in a manner similar to dobutamine. In particular, dopamine is used to increase cardiac output in acute or severe hypotension. That is, moderate to high doses of dopamine can stimulate the heart (beta-1 effect) while simultaneously increasing peripheral vascular resistance (alpha-1 effect). When used as a cardiac medication, dopamine is typically administered via intravenous (IV) drip to help maintain stable and consistent plasma levels.

Adverse Effects

Because of their cardiostimulatory effects, beta-1–selective drugs may induce side effects such as chest pain and cardiac arrhythmias in some patients. Shortness of breath and difficulty in breathing (i.e., feelings of chest constriction) have also been reported.

Beta-2–Selective Agonists

General Indications

One important location of beta-2 receptors is on bronchiole smooth muscle. When stimulated, the receptor mediates relaxation of the bronchioles. Consequently, most beta-2 agonists are administered to treat the bronchospasm associated with respiratory ailments such as asthma, bronchitis, and emphysema.[4,21] Since a nonselective beta agonist will also stimulate the myocardium (beta-1 effect), beta-2–selective agonists are often used preferentially in treating asthma, especially if the patient has a cardiac abnormality such as ischemia or arrhythmias.[21] Another clinically important location of beta-2 receptors is on uterine muscle. When stimulated, these receptors cause inhibition or relaxation of the uterus. As a result, drugs such as ritodrine and terbutaline are used to inhibit premature uterine contractions during pregnancy, thus preventing premature labor and delivery.[9,22]

Specific Agents

Beta-2-selective bronchodilators. This group of drugs includes albuterol (Proventil, Ventolin, others), fenoterol (Berotec), isoetharine (Bronkometer, Bronkosol, others), metaproterenol (Alupent, others), pirbuterol (Maxair), procaterol (Pro-Air), salmeterol (Serevent), and terbutaline (Brethaire, others). These agents are similar pharmacologically and are used to stimulate beta-2 receptors located on pulmonary smooth muscle, thus causing bronchodilation in patients with asthma and similar conditions. Isoproterenol (Isuprel) can also be included with this group, but this drug is somewhat less beta-2–selective and affects beta-1 receptors as well. Beta-2 bronchodilators are often administered by oral inhalation so that the drug is applied directly to bronchial membranes. Albuterol and similar agents, for example, are packaged in small aerosol inhalers so that the patient can self-administer the drug at the onset of a bronchospastic attack. The use of these drugs in treating respiratory conditions is addressed in more detail in Chapter 26.

Ritodrine (Yutopar). The primary clinical application of this drug is to inhibit premature labor.[22] Ritodrine activates uterine beta-2 receptors, which mediate relaxation of uterine muscle. This drug is usually administered initially via intravenous pump infusion, and maintenance therapy is accomplished through oral administration. There is little evidence, however, that ritodrine and other beta-selective agonists actually result in beneficial outcomes for the newborn child, and these drugs may actually be harmful to the mother (see "Adverse Effects" below).[9] Hence, it is not clear if beta-2 agonists will be used to prevent preterm labor in the future.

Adverse Effects

The primary side effects associated with beta-2–specific drugs include nervousness, restlessness, and trembling. These adverse symptoms may be caused by stimulation of central beta-adrenergic receptors. There is also some suggestion that excessive use of beta-2 agonists may cause increased airway hyperresponsiveness, which could lead to severe and possibly fatal asthmatic attacks.[21,33] This fact has generated debate about the safe and effective use of these drugs in treating asthma; contemporary use of beta-2 agonists along with other antiasthmatic drugs is described in Chapter 26. When used to prevent premature labor, drugs such as ritodrine have also been associated with increases in maternal heart rate and systolic blood pressure, as well as maternal pulmonary edema. These changes in maternal cardiopulmonary function can be quite severe and may be fatal to the mother.

Drugs with Mixed Alpha- and Beta-Agonist Activity

General Indications

Several drugs are available that display a rather mixed agonistic activity with regard to adrenergic receptor subtypes. Some drugs, like epinephrine, appear to be able to stimulate all four adrenergic receptor subtypes. Other drugs, such as norepinephrine, bind to both types of alpha receptors, bind to beta-1 receptors to a lesser extent, and show little or no affinity for beta-2 receptors. Another group of indirect adrenergic agonists (ephedrine, metaraminol) appear to act as nonselective agonists because of their ability to increase the release of norepinephrine from presynaptic storage sites. Because of the ability of many of these multiple-receptor drugs to affect a number of adrenoceptor subtypes, their clinical uses are quite varied. Specific agents with mixed agonistic activity and their respective applications are presented below.

Specific Agents

Amphetamines. Drugs such as amphetamine (generic), dextroamphetamine (Dexedrine, others),

and methamphetamine (Desoxyn) are known for their powerful sympathomimetic effects. These drugs appear to increase norepinephrine release, decrease norepinephrine reuptake and breakdown at adrenergic synapses, thus increasing activity at synapses with norepinephrine-sensitive receptors (i.e., alpha-1, alpha-2, and beta-1 receptors). These drugs may also exert similar effects on certain dopaminergic synapses. Amphetamines are used on a limited basis to treat attention-deficit disorder in children and to increase mental alertness in adults with narcolepsy. Use of these drugs to suppress appetite or to combat normal sleepiness is discouraged because of their high potential for abuse, and these drugs are classified in the United States as schedule II controlled substances (see Chapter 1 for a description of controlled substance classification).

Ephedrine (generic). Ephedrine appears to directly stimulate alpha-1, alpha-2, and beta-1 adrenoceptors, and may also stimulate these receptors indirectly by increasing the release of norepinephrine at synapses that use these receptor subtypes. This drug is used primarily for its alpha-1 effects and can be used to treat severe, acute hypotension. When treating hypotension in emergency situations (e.g., shock), ephedrine is administered systemically by injection (intravenously, intramuscularly, or subcutaneously). Because of its ability to stimulate alpha-1 receptors in the nasal mucosa, ephedrine is also used as a nasal decongestant. As a decongestant, ephedrine is typically combined with other agents (antitussives, antihistamines) to form cough/cold products. Ephedrine is also sometimes administered as a bronchodilator (beta-2 agonist effect), but the use of this drug in asthma and related conditions has generally been replaced by safer agents (see Chapter 26). Finally, ephedrine has been administered to produce a general excitatory effect on central adrenergic receptors and has been used to treat conditions associated with a decrease in CNS arousal (e.g., narcolepsy).

Epinephrine (Adrenalin, Bronkaid Mist, Primatene Mist, others). Epinephrine appears to directly stimulate all adrenergic receptor subtypes and is administered for a variety of reasons. Epinephrine is found in many antiasthmatic inhalation products because of its ability to stimulate beta-2 receptors on the bronchi. Because it stimulates vascular alpha-1 receptors, epinephrine may be applied topically to produce local vasoconstriction and control bleeding during minor surgical procedures (e.g., suturing superficial wounds). Likewise, epinephrine may be mixed with a local anesthetic when the anesthetic is injected during minor surgical and dental procedures. The vasoconstriction produced by epinephrine prevents the anesthetic from being washed away by the local blood flow, thus prolonging the anesthetic's effects. Because of a potent ability to stimulate the heart (beta-1 effect), epinephrine is frequently administered during cardiac arrest to reestablish normal cardiac rhythm. Finally, epinephrine is often the drug of choice in treating anaphylactic shock. Anaphylactic shock is a hypersensitive allergic reaction marked by cardiovascular collapse (decreased cardiac output, hypotension) and severe bronchoconstriction. Epinephrine is ideally suited to treat this problem because of its ability to stimulate the heart (beta-1 effect), vasoconstrict the periphery (alpha-1 effect), and dilate the bronchi (beta-2 effect).

Metaraminol (Aramine). Metaraminol appears to act like ephedrine; that is, metaraminol directly stimulates alpha-1, alpha-2, and beta-1 receptors, and indirectly stimulates them by increasing the release of presynaptic norepinephrine. This drug is usually administered by injection (intramuscularly, intravenously, or subcutaneously) to treat hypotension occurring in shock or general anesthesia.

Norepinephrine (Levophed). Norepinephrine stimulates both types of alpha receptors as well as beta-1 receptors but displays very little agonistic activity toward beta-2 receptors. It is usually administered intravenously to treat hypotension during shock or general anesthesia.

Phenylpropanolamine (Acutrim, Dexatrim, Propagest, others). The exact mechanism of this drug is unclear. Although it may directly stimulate alpha and beta receptors, this drug probably exerts its effects by increasing the release of presynaptic norepinephrine; thus, phenylpropanolamine is an indirect-acting, nonselective agonist. Because of its alpha-1 agonist properties, phenylpropanolamine can be used as a nasal decongestant. Phenylpropanolamine also appears to act as an appetite suppressant ("diet" drug) by increasing the release of norepinephrine within the hypothalamus. In this regard, it is similar to amphetaminelike compounds, which may also suppress feeding behavior by increasing adrenergic influence in the brain. Its use as a diet drug, however, has generated substantial concern because it may be abused by some individuals, and because excessive use may lead to hemorrhagic stroke.[17] Hence, efforts have been made to curtail the availability of this drug, especially in over-the-counter products. Finally, this drug can help treat urinary incontinence, presumably because of an effect on alpha receptors that inhibits contraction of the bladder. Phenylpropanolamine is taken orally for nasal decongestion, appetite suppression, or urinary incontinence.

Adverse Effects

Because of the general ability of many of the drugs previously described to produce CNS excitation, some of the primary side effects are nervousness, restlessness, and anxiety. Because these agents also tend to stimulate the cardiovascular system, prolonged or excessive use may also lead to complications such as hypertension, arrhythmias, and even cardiac arrest. When used to treat bronchospasm, prolonged administration via inhalation may also cause some degree of bronchial irritation with some agents.

Adrenergic Antagonists

Adrenergic antagonists or blockers bind to adrenergic receptors but do not activate them. These agents are often referred to as sympatholytic drugs because of their ability to block the receptors that typically mediate sympathetic responses (i.e., alpha and beta receptors). Clinically useful adrenergic antagonists usually show a fairly high degree of specificity for one of the major receptor classifications. They tend to bind preferentially to either alpha- or beta-adrenergic receptors. Specific drugs may show an additional degree of specificity within the receptor class. For instance, a beta blocker may bind rather selectively to only beta-1 receptors, or it may bind equally to both beta-1 and beta-2 receptors.

The general clinical applications of alpha and beta antagonists are presented below. Specific agents within each major group are also discussed.

Alpha Antagonists

General Indications

Alpha antagonists are administered primarily to reduce peripheral vascular tone by blocking the alpha-1 receptors located on vascular smooth muscle. When stimulated by endogenous catecholamines (norepinephrine, epinephrine), the alpha-1 receptor initiates vasoconstriction.

Consequently, alpha antagonists are used in conditions where peripheral vasodilation would be beneficial. A principal application of these agents, for instance, is in treating hypertension.[26,39] These drugs seem to attenuate the peripheral vasoconstriction mediated by excessive adrenergic influence, thus decreasing blood pressure through a decrease in peripheral vascular resistance. These agents may also be used in patients with a pheochromocytoma, a tumor that produces large quantities of epinephrine and norepinephrine. Alpha antagonists are often administered prior to and during the removal of such a tumor, thus preventing the hypertensive crisis that may occur from excessive alpha-1 stimulation from catecholamines released from the tumor. Similarly, alpha antagonists have been used to successfully prevent and treat the sudden increase in blood pressure occurring during an autonomic crisis. These drugs have been used to promote vasodilation in conditions of vascular insufficiency, including peripheral vascular disease and Raynaud phenomenon. However, the success of these drugs in treating vascular insufficiency has been somewhat limited.

Certain alpha-1 blockers such as doxazosin have been used extensively in treating benign prostatic hyperplasia (BPH).[23,32] Alpha-1 receptors located on smooth muscle in the prostate capsule, neck of the bladder, and urethra cause muscle constriction that restricts urine flow and the ability to empty the bladder. By blocking these receptors, alpha-1 antagonists relax these smooth muscles and allow men with BPH to void urine more easily and completely.[12,32]

A group of drugs known collectively as *ergot derivatives* display some alpha-blocking ability as well as other unique properties. Ergot alkaloids and ergoloid mesylates and are used clinically for diverse problems, including the treatment of vascular headache and improvement of mental function in presenile dementia.

Because the primary uses of alpha antagonists involve their ability to decrease vascular tone, the clinically useful alpha antagonists tend to be somewhat alpha-1 selective. Alpha-2 receptors should not be selectively antagonized because this event may ultimately lead to an *increase* in peripheral vascular tone through an increase in sympathetic discharge. Certain alpha-2 receptors are located in the brainstem, and stimulation of these receptors appears to decrease sympathetic outflow from the vasomotor center. Thus, blocking these centrally located alpha-2 receptors is counterproductive when a decrease in vascular tone is desired.

Specific Agents

Doxazosin (Cardura). This drug shows a high degree of alpha-1 selectively, and promotes relaxation of smooth muscle in the vasculature and other tissues. It was developed as an antihypertensive, and can be taken orally to reduce blood pressure because it decreases peripheral vascular resistance.[5,39] In addition, doxazosin may have beneficial effects on the plasma lipid profile (decreased total cholesterol, decreased triglycerides), and may decrease insulin resistance in people with type 2 diabetes mellitus (see Chapter 32).[7,19,36] Hence, this drug is useful in treating high blood pressure in people with metabolic problems including various hyperlipidemias and glucose intolerance. In addition, doxazosin has been successful in reducing urinary retention in men with BPH. As indicated above, this drug relaxes smooth muscle in the prostate and urethra, thereby allowing urine to flow more freely during micturition.

Ergot alkaloids. Ergotamine (Ergomar, others) and similar drugs such as dihydroergotamine (D. H. E. 45) and ergonovine (Ergotrate), exert several pharmacological effects. At higher doses, these drugs act as competitive alpha antagonists, hence their inclusion here. However, these drugs appear to produce vasoconstriction in blood vessels that have low vascular tone and vasodilation in blood vessels that have high vascular tone. Exactly how they accomplish these rather contradictory effects is unclear, but these drugs essentially function as partial agonists because they display agonistic (stimulatory) activity in vessels with low tone and antagonistic (inhibitory) activity in vessels with high tone. These drugs, however, can also block serotonin and dopamine receptors. Hence, they exert a number of complex effects throughout the body, and it is difficult to attribute their therapeutic effects to only one type of receptor. In the past, these drugs were used primarily for their ability to prevent or abort vascular headaches (migraine, cluster headaches) by vasoconstricting cerebral vessels.[37,38] Their antimigraine effects, however, may be due to their antagonistic effect on vascular serotonin receptors rather than an effect on cerebral alpha-1 receptors. Hence, use of these drugs in treating headaches has been replaced in many patients with serotonin-selective antagonists such as sumatriptan (Imitrex) and rizatriptin (Maxalt). Alpha-1 blockers are also used to prevent or treat postpartum hemorrhage because they stimulate the uterus to contract, thereby helping compress and occlude bleeding vessels in the uterine wall. Occasionally, these drugs can also be used to diagnosis angina pectoris because they cause transient constriction of the coronary arteries.

Ergoloid mesylate These compounds, which appear under trade names such as Gerimal and Hydergine, exhibit some ability to produce peripheral vasodilation by blocking peripheral alpha-1 receptors. The primary clinical application of ergoloid mesylates is to increase mental acuity and alertness in geriatric patients with dementia related to Alzheimer disease.[27] These drugs supposedly increase mental function by increasing cerebral blood flow or by increasing oxygen utilization in the brain. The mechanism of action of these drugs is probably a moot point, however, because there is little evidence that they produce any significant clinical benefits in treating Alzheimer dementia.[27] These drugs are usually administered orally or sublingually.

Phenoxybenzamine (Dibenzyline). Phenoxybenzamine is a noncompetitive alpha-1 blocker that binds irreversibly to the alpha-1 receptor. This drug tends to have a slow onset, but its effects last much longer than those of the competitive blockers (e.g., phentolamine and prazosin). Phenoxybenzamine is used primarily to control blood pressure prior to and during the removal of a pheochromocytoma. This drug is not typically used for the long-term management of hypertension, however, because it produces several side effects including reflex tachycardia. Other indications for phenoxybenzamine include treatment of urinary retention in benign prostatic hypertrophy and treatment of vasospastic disease (Raynaud phenomenon). Phenoxybenzamine is usually administered orally.

Phentolamine (Regitine). Phentolamine is a competitive alpha antagonist used primarily to control blood pressure during management of pheochromocytoma. The drug is usually administered via intravenous or intramuscular injection. Phentolamine is not usually used to treat essential hypertension because with prolonged use, effectiveness tends to decrease and patients begin to develop adverse side effects.

Prazosin (Minipress). Prazosin is a competitive alpha-1 antagonist that has emerged as one of the primary alpha-1 selective agents. It tends to produce vasodilation in both arteries and veins, and is used primarily in the long-term management of essential hypertension.[38] Prazosin has also been used to reduce alpha-1 receptor mediated activity in congestive heart failure, Raynaud phenomenon, pheochromocytoma, and BPH. Prazosin is administered orally.

Terazosin (Hytrin). This drug is similar to doxazosin.

Adverse Effects Of Alpha-1 Antagonists

One of the primary adverse effects associated with alpha antagonists is reflex tachycardia. By blocking alpha-1 receptors, these drugs tend to decrease blood pressure by decreasing peripheral vascular resistance. As blood pressure falls, a compensatory increase in cardiac output is initiated via the baroreceptor reflex. The increased cardiac output is mediated in part by an increase in heart rate, hence the reflex tachycardia. A second major problem with these drugs is orthostatic hypotension. Dizziness and syncope following changes in posture are quite common due to the decrease in peripheral vascular tone. With alpha antagonists, orthostatic hypotension may be a particular problem just after drug therapy is initiated, in geriatric patients, or following exercise.

Beta Antagonists

General Indications

Beta antagonists are generally administered for their effect on the beta-1 receptors that are located on the heart.[31] When stimulated, these receptors mediate an increase in cardiac contractility and rate of contraction. By blocking these receptors, beta antagonists reduce the rate and force of myocardial contractions. Consequently, beta antagonists are frequently used to decrease cardiac workload in conditions such as hypertension and certain types of angina pectoris. Beta blockers may also be used to normalize heart rate in certain forms of cardiac arrhythmias. Specific clinical applications of individual beta blockers are summarized in Table 20–2.

Another important function of beta blockers is their ability to limit the extent of myocardial damage following a heart attack and to reduce the risk of fatality following myocardial infarction.[11] Apparently, these drugs help reduce the workload of the damaged heart, thus allowing the heart to recover more completely following infarction. Likewise, there is substantial evidence that some beta blockers can help improve cardiac function in certain types of heart failure[3,13,15]; this idea is addressed in more detail in Chapter 24.

Clinically useful beta antagonists are classified as beta-1–selective if they predominantly affect the beta-1 subtype; they are classified as beta-nonselective if they have a fairly equal affinity for beta-1 and beta-2 receptors (see Table 20–2). Beta-1–selective drugs are also referred to as *cardioselective* because of their preferential effect on the myocardium. Even if a beta antagonist is nonselective (i.e., blocks both beta-1 and beta-2 receptors), the beta-1 blockade is clinically beneficial. When stimulated, beta-2 receptors, which

Table 20–2	SUMMARY OF COMMON BETA BLOCKERS		
Generic Name	**Trade Name(s)**	**Selectivity**	**Primary Indications***
Acebutolol	Sectral	Beta-1	Hypertension, arrhythmias
Atenolol	Tenormin	Beta-1	Angina pectoris, hypertension, prevent reinfarction
Betaxolol	Kerlone	Beta-1	Hypertension
Bisoprolol	Zebeta	Beta-1	Hypertension
Carteolol	Cartrol	Nonselective	Hypertension
Labetalol	Normodyne, Trandate	Nonselective	Hypertension
Metoprolol	Lopressor, Toprol-XL	Beta-1	Angina pectoris, hypertension, prevent reinfarction
Nadolol	Corgard	Nonselective	Hypertension, angina pectoris
Penbutolol	Levatol	Nonselective	Hypertension
Pindolol	Visken	Nonselective	Hypertension
Propranolol	Inderal	Nonselective	Angina pectoris, arrhythmias, hypertension, prevent reinfarction, prevent vascular headache
Sotalol	Betapace	Nonselective	Arrhythmias
Timolol	Blocadren	Nonselective	Hypertension, prevent reinfarction, prevent vascular headache

*Only indications listed in the United States product labeling are included in this table. All drugs are fairly similar pharmacologically, and some may be used for appropriate cardiovascular conditions not specifically listed in product labeling.

are found primarily on bronchial smooth muscle, cause bronchodilation. Blocking these beta-2 receptors may lead to smooth-muscle contraction and bronchoconstriction. Thus, drugs that selectively block beta-2 receptors have no real clinical significance because they promote bronchoconstriction.[2]

Currently, a number of beta blockers are used clinically; the selection of a specific agent depends on factors such as cardioselectivity, duration of action (half-life), and several other ancillary properties of each drug.[1,10] Certain beta blockers, for instance, produce added effects such as mild peripheral vasodilation or stabilization of cardiac membranes that can be beneficial in treating certain cardiovascular condi-

tions.[18,20,25] Primary indications and relative selectivity of these drugs are summarized in Table 20–2. Clinical applications of specific beta blockers are discussed in more detail in Chapters 21 through 24.

Specific Agents

Acebutolol (Sectral). Acebutolol is described as a relatively cardioselective beta blocker that tends to bind preferentially to beta-1 receptors at low doses, but binds to both types of beta receptors as the dosage increases. This drug also exerts mild to moderate intrinsic sympathomimetic activity, which means that acebutolol not only blocks the beta receptor from the effects of endogenous catecholamines, but also stimulates the receptor to some extent (i.e., it acts as a partial beta agonist). This advantage protects the beta receptor from excessive endogenous stimulation while still preserving a low level of background sympathetic activity. Primary clinical applications are for treatment of hypertension and prevention and treatment of cardiac arrhythmias. The drug is usually administered orally.

Atenolol (Tenormin). Like acebutolol, atenolol is regarded as beta-1 selective, but tends to be less beta-specific at higher doses. The drug is administered orally for the long-term treatment of hypertension and chronic, stable angina. Atenolol is also administered immediately following a myocardial infarction to prevent reinfarction and to promote recovery of the myocardium.

Betaxolol (Kerlone). This drug is a relatively beta-1 selective agent that is administered orally for treating hypertension.

Bisoprolol (Zebeta). This drug is similar to betaxolol.

Carteolol (Cartrol). Carteolol is a nonselective beta blocker that also has moderate intrinsic sympathomimetic activity. It is typically administered orally to treat hypertension.

Labetalol (Normodyne, Trandate). Labetalol is a nonselective beta blocker. This drug appears to have some alpha-1–selective blocking effects. Labetalol is used primarily in the management of hypertension and, while usually given orally, may be injected intravenously in emergency hypertensive situations.

Metoprolol (Lopressor, Toprol-XL). Metoprolol is considered a cardioselective beta blocker and has been approved for treating hypertension, preventing angina pectoris, and preventing myocardial reinfarction. As an antihypertensive and antianginal, metoprolol is usually administered orally. In the prevention of reinfarction, metoprolol is initiated by intravenous injection and then followed up by oral administration.

Nadolol (Corgard). Nadolol is a nonselective beta blocker that is administered orally as an antihypertensive and antianginal agent. This drug has an advantage over other nonselective beta blockers (propranolol) in that nadolol often needs to be taken only once each day.

Penbutolol (Levatol). This drug is similar to carteolol.

Pindolol (Visken). Pindolol is a nonselective beta blocker that exhibits the highest level of intrinsic sympathomimetic activity of all the beta blockers. Pin-

dolol is used primarily in the long-term management of hypertension, but this drug may also be used to prevent certain types of angina pectoris.

Propranolol (Inderal). Propranolol, the classic nonselective beta blocker, is approved for use in hypertension, angina pectoris, cardiac arrhythmias, and prevention of myocardial reinfarction. In addition, propranolol has been used in the prevention of vascular headache and as an adjunct to alpha blockers in treating pheochromocytoma. Propranolol is usually administered orally for the long-term management of the previously listed conditions, but it may be administered via intravenous injection for the immediate control of arrhythmias.

Sotalol (Betapace). This drug is a nonselective beta blocker that is administered primarily to treat arrhythmias, although it is sometimes used as an antihypertensive or antianginal agent. It is administered orally.

Timolol (Blocadren). This nonselective beta blocker is administered orally for the treatment of hypertension and prevention of myocardial reinfarction. It may also be used to treat angina or prevent vascular headaches.

Adverse Effects

When nonselective beta blockers are used, some antagonism of beta-2 receptors also occurs.[2,31] The antagonism of beta-2 receptors on bronchiole smooth muscle often leads to some degree of bronchoconstriction and an increase in airway resistance. Although this event is usually not a problem in individuals with normal pulmonary function, patients with respiratory problems such as asthma, bronchitis, and emphysema may be adversely affected by nonselective beta antagonists. In these patients, one of the beta-1–selective drugs should be administered.

Selective and nonselective beta blockers are also associated with several other adverse effects. The most serious of these effects results from excessive depression of cardiac function.[30] By slowing down the heart too much, these agents can lead to cardiac failure, especially if there is some preexisting cardiac disease. Because of their antihypertensive properties, beta blockers may produce orthostatic hypotension, and dizziness and syncope may occur following abrupt changes in posture. Patients taking beta blockers for prolonged periods have also been reported to have an increase in centrally related side effects such as depression, lethargy, and sleep disorders.[17,29] These behavioral side effects may be due to the interaction of beta blockers with CNS receptors.

Various other relatively minor side effects have also been reported, including gastrointestinal disturbances (nausea, vomiting) and allergic responses (fever, rash). However, these are fairly uncommon and tend to be resolved by adjusting the dosage or specific medication type.

Other Drugs That Inhibit Adrenergic Neurons

General Indications

Several agents are available that inhibit activity at adrenergic synapses by interfering with the release of norepinephrine. Rather than directly blocking the postsynaptic receptor, these drugs typically inhibit or deplete the presynaptic terminal of stored norepinephrine. These drugs are used primarily to decrease peripheral adrenergic influence and to treat problems such as hypertension and cardiac arrhythmias.

Specific Agents

Bretylium (Bretylol). Bretylium appears to directly inhibit the release of norepinephrine from adrenergic nerve terminals. With prolonged use, this drug may also replace presynaptic norepinephrine in a manner similar to guanadrel and guanethidine (see the next two agent listings in this section). Bretylium is used primarily in the treatment of cardiac arrhythmias (Chapter 23). In addition to its effect on norepinephrine release, bretlium also appears to have a direct stabilizing effect on cardiac muscle cells that contributes to this drug's antiarrhythmic properties. While usually given orally for the long-term management of ventricular arrhythmias, bretylium is also injected intravenously for the emergency treatment of ventricular tachycardia and ventricular fibrillation.

Guanadrel (Hylorel). Guanadrel is taken up by the presynaptic terminal and appears to directly inhibit the release of norepinephrine. With prolonged use, guanadrel slowly replaces norepinephrine in the presynaptic vesicles. This substitution of guanadrel for norepinephrine further inhibits activity at postsynaptic adrenergic synapses by creating a false neurotransmitter. Guanadrel also replaces stored norepinephrine in the adrenal medulla, thus decreasing adrenal influence on cardiovascular function. Guanadrel is administered orally for the management of hypertension.

Guanethidine (Ismelin). Similar in action and effects to guanadrel, this drug is actively transported into the presynaptic terminal by the norepinephrine pump, where it inhibits norepinephrine release and later replaces stored norepinephrine. Unlike guanadrel, guanethidine selectively affects postganglionic sympathetic adrenergic nerve terminals and does not affect release of norepinephrine from the adrenal medulla. Guanethidine is usually administered orally for the management of moderate-to-severe hypertension.

Metyrosine (Demser). Metyrosine inhibits the enzyme initiating catecholamine synthesis (epinephrine, norepinephrine); this drug is used to diminish catecholamine stores prior to removal of a catecholamine-producing tumor (pheochromocytoma).

Rauwolfia alkaloids. This chemical group includes reserpine (Serpalan), deserpidine (Harmonyl), and rauwolfia serpentina (Raudixin, Rauval, others). These drugs all inhibit the synthesis of catecholamines (norepinephrine, epinephrine) as well as 5-hydroxytryptamine (serotonin) in peripheral and CNS sympathetic nerve endings. This inhibition eventually causes a depletion of presynaptic neurotransmitter stores in several tissues including postganglionic nerve terminals, adrenal medulla, and brain. Unlike guanethidine and guanadrel, these agents do not appear to actually replace the presynaptic neurotransmitter, but simply prevent more transmitter from being resynthesized. Reserpine and the other rauwolfia alkaloids are administered orally to treat mild-to-moderate hypertension. The antihypertensive effects of these drugs are caused, in part, by the inhibition of peripheral adrenergic nerve terminals, although some of their antihypertensive effects may also be because of the inhibition of CNS catecholamine activity.

Adverse Effects

Orthostatic hypotension is occasionally a problem with the aforementioned drugs, and dizziness and syncope sometimes occur after a sudden change in posture. Some patients also experience gastrointestinal disturbances including nausea, vomiting, and diarrhea. Peripheral edema as evidenced by swelling in the feet and legs has also been reported.

SUMMARY

This chapter classifies and describes a variety of drugs according to their stimulatory (agonistic) or inhibitory (antagonistic) effects on adrenergic function. In general, adrenergic agonists are administered according to their ability to evoke specific tissue responses via specific adrenergic receptors. Alpha-1–adrenergic agonists are used as antihypotensive agents because of their ability to increase peripheral vascular resistance; they may also be used as nasal decongestants because of their ability to vasoconstrict the nasal mucosa. Agonists selective for alpha-2 receptors are administered to treat hypertension and spasticity because of their ability to inhibit neuronal activity in the brainstem and spinal cord, respectively. Cardioselective beta-1 agonists are used primarily for their ability to stimulate the heart, and beta-2 agonists are used in the treatment of asthma and premature labor because of their ability to relax bronchiole and uterine smooth muscle, respectively.

Alpha-adrenergic antagonists are used primarily as antihypertensive drugs because of their ability to block vascular alpha-1 receptors. Beta-adrenergic antagonists (beta blockers) are administered primarily for their inhibitory effects on myocardial function and are used in the prevention and treatment of hypertension, angina pectoris, arrhythmias, and myocardial reinfarction. Many of the drugs introduced in this chapter are discussed further in chapters that deal with the specific clinical conditions (e.g., hypertension, asthma, and other disorders).

References

1. Abraham WT, Iyengar S. Practical considerations for switching beta-blockers in heart failure patients. *Rev Cardiovasc Med.* 2004;5(suppl 1):S36–S44.
2. Andrus MR, Holloway KP, Clark DB. Use of beta-blockers in patients with COPD. *Ann Pharmacother.* 2004;38:142–145.
3. Bauman JL, Talbert RL. Pharmacodynamics of beta-blockers in heart failure: lessons from the carvedilol or metoprolol European trial. *J Cardiovasc Pharmacol Ther.* 2004;9:117–128.
4. Buhl R, Farmer SG. Current and future pharmacologic therapy of exacerbations in chronic obstructive pulmonary disease and asthma. *Proc Am Thorac Soc.* 2004;1:136–142.
5. Calvo C, Gil-Extremera B, Gomez-Fernandez P, et al. Doxazosin GITS versus standard doxazosin in mild to moderate hypertension. *Int J Cardiol.* 2005;101:97–104.
6. Coward DM. Tizanidine: neuropharmacology and mechanism of action. *Neurology.* 1994;44(suppl 9):S6–S10.
7. Dell'Omo G, Penno G, Pucci L, et al. The vascular effects of doxazosin in hypertension complicated by metabolic syndrome. *Coron Artery Dis.* 2005;16:67–73.
8. Delwaide PJ, Pennisi G. Tizanidine and electrophysiologic analysis of spinal control mechanisms in humans with spasticity. *Neurology.* 1994;44(suppl 9):S21–S28.
9. Doggrell SA. Recent pharmacological advances in the treatment of preterm membrane rupture, labour and delivery. *Expert Opin Pharmacother.* 2004;5:1917–1928.
10. Dulin B, Abraham WT. Pharmacology of carvedilol. *Am J Cardiol.* 2004;93:3B–6B.
11. Ellison KE, Gandhi G. Optimising the use of beta-adrenoceptor antagonists in coronary artery disease. *Drugs.* 2005;65:787–797.
12. Fitzpatrick JM, Desgrandchamps F. The clinical efficacy and tolerability of doxazosin standard and gastrointestinal therapeutic system for benign prostatic hyperplasia. *BJU Int.* 2005;95:575–579.
13. Fonarow GC. When to initiate beta-blockers in heart failure: is it ever too early? *Curr Heart Fail Rep.* 2005;2:94–99.
14. Gelber DA, Good DC, Dromerick A, et al. Open-label dose-titration safety and efficacy study of tizanidine hydrochloride in the treatment of spasticity associated with chronic stroke. *Stroke.* 2001;32:1841–1846.
15. Ghali JK. Beta-blockers in selected heart failure populations. *Curr Heart Fail Rep.* 2005;2:100–105.
16. Hoffman BB. Adrenoceptor-activating and other sympathomimetic drugs. In: Katzung BG, ed. *Basic and Clinical Pharmacology.* 9th ed. New York: Lange Medical Books/McGraw-Hill; 2004.
17. Hoffman BB. Catecholamines, sympathomimetic drugs, and adrenergic receptor antagonists. In: Hardman JG, et al, eds. *The Pharmacological Basis of Therapeutics.* 10th ed. New York: McGraw-Hill; 2001.
18. Ignarro LJ. Experimental evidences of nitric oxide-dependent vasodilatory activity of nebivolol, a third-generation beta-blocker. *Blood Press Suppl.* 2004;1:2–16.
19. Inukai T, Inukai Y, Matsutomo R, et al. Clinical usefulness of doxazosin in patients with type 2 diabetes complicated by hypertension: effects on glucose and lipid metabolism. *J Int Med Res.* 2004;32:206–213.
20. Jacob S, Henriksen EJ. Metabolic properties of vasodilating beta blockers: management considerations for hypertensive diabetic patients and patients with the metabolic syndrome. *J Clin Hypertens (Greenwich).* 2004;6:690–696.
21. Kelly HW. What is new with the beta2-agonists: issues in the management of asthma. *Ann Pharmacother.* 2005;39:931–938.
22. Kripke C. Use of beta agonists in preterm labor. *Am Fam Physician.* 2005;71:899–900.
23. Lowe FC. Role of the newer alpha-adrenergic-receptor antagonists in the treatment of benign prostatic hyperplasia-related lower urinary tract symptoms. *Clin Ther.* 2004;26:1701–1713.
24. Meythaler JM, Guin-Renfroe S, Johnson A, Brunner RM. Prospective assessment of tizanidine for spasticity

due to acquired brain injury. *Arch Phys Med Rehabil.* 2001;82:1155–1163.

25. Naccarelli GV, Lukas MA. Carvedilol's antiarrhythmic properties: therapeutic implications in patients with left ventricular dysfunction. *Clin Cardiol.* 2005;28:165–173.

26. Oates JA, Brown NJ. Antihypertensive agents and the drug therapy of hypertension. In: Hardman JG, et al, eds. *The Pharmacological Basis of Therapeutics.* 10th ed. New York: McGraw-Hill; 2001.

27. Olin J, Schneider L, Novit A, Luczak S. Hydergine for dementia. *Cochrane Database Syst Rev.* 2001;CD000359.

28. Ooi H, Colucci W. Pharmacological treatment of heart failure. In: Hardman JG, et al, eds. *The Pharmacological Basis of Therapeutics.* 10th ed. New York: McGraw-Hill; 2001.

29. Patten SB, Barbui C. Drug-induced depression: a systematic review to inform clinical practice. *Psychother Psychosom.* 2004;73:207–215.

30. Peel C, Mossberg KA. Effects of cardiovascular medications on exercise responses. *Phys Ther.* 1995;75:387–396.

31. Reiter MJ. Cardiovascular drug class specificity: beta-blockers. *Prog Cardiovasc Dis.* 2004;47:11–33.

32. Roehrborn CG, Schwinn DA. Alpha1-adrenergic receptors and their inhibitors in lower urinary tract symptoms and benign prostatic hyperplasia. *J Urol.* 2004;171:1029–1035.

33. Sitkauskiene B, Sakalauskas R. The role of beta(2)-adrenergic receptors in inflammation and allergy. *Curr Drug Targets Inflamm Allergy.* 2005;4:157–162.

34. Tank J, Diedrich A, Szczech E, et al. Alpha-2 adrenergic transmission and human baroreflex regulation. *Hypertension.* 2004;43:1035–1041.

35. Trendelenburg AU, Philipp M, Meyer A, et al. All three alpha-2-adrenoceptor types serve as autoreceptors in postganglionic sympathetic neurons. *Naunyn Schmiedebergs Arch Pharmacol.* 2003;368:504–512.

36. Ueshiba H, Miyachi Y. Effect of doxazosin on insulin resistance in hypertensive patients with obesity. *Horm Metab Res.* 2003;35:532–536.

37. Villalon CM, Centurion D, Valdivia LF, de Vries P, Saxena PR. Migraine: pathophysiology, pharmacology, treatment and future trends. *Curr Vasc Pharmacol.* 2003;1:71–84.

38. Zhang L, Hay JW. Cost-effectiveness analysis of rizatriptan and sumatriptan versus Cafergot in the acute treatment of migraine. *CNS Drugs.* 2005;19:635–642.

39. Zusman R. Patients with uncontrolled hypertension or concomitant hypertension and benign prostatic hyperplasia. *Clin Cardiol.* 2004;27:63–69.

Chapter 21

Antihypertensive Drugs

Hypertension is a sustained, reproducible increase in blood pressure. Hypertension is one of the most common diseases affecting adults living in industrialized nations. In the United States, for example, hypertension occurs in approximately 30% of the general population aged 20 and over.[44] The prevalence of this disease can be even higher in certain subpopulations (e.g., 41% in African Americans), and the incidence of hypertension increases with age.[44,45] If left untreated, the sustained increase in blood pressure associated with hypertension can lead to cardiovascular problems (stroke, heart failure), renal disease, and blindness.[15,22,108,111] These and other medical problems ultimately lead to an increased mortality rate in hypertensive individuals.

Although there is a general consensus regarding the adverse effects of hypertension, some debate exists as to exactly how much of an increase in blood pressure constitutes hypertension. Generally, diastolic values greater than 90 mm Hg and/or systolic values greater than 140 mm Hg warrant a diagnosis of hypertension. A more detailed classification scheme is shown in Table 21–1. Patients are classified as prehypertensive, stage 1, or stage 2 depending on the extent of their elevated blood pressure. As might be expected, the incidence of morbidity and mortality increases as the hypertension becomes more severe. Hence, pharmacologic and nonpharmacologic methods are implemented to decrease blood pressure to an optimal diastolic value of 80 mm Hg or less and an optimal systolic value less than 120 mm Hg (see Table 21–1).

Hypertension is often described as a silent killer because of the lack of symptoms throughout most of the disease course. Patients may feel fine into the advanced stages of hypertension. Rehabilitation specialists dealing with hypertensive patients are usually treating a problem other than the increased blood pressure (i.e., hypertension is not the reason the patient is referred to physical therapy and occupational therapy). Due to the prevalence of hypertension, however, many patients receiving therapy for other problems will also be taking antihypertensive drugs, so knowledge of the pharmacology of these agents is essential.

The pharmacologic management of hypertension has evolved to where blood pressure can be controlled for extended periods in most patients. There are currently several major categories of antihypertensive agents, and new drugs are continually being added to the antihypertensive arsenal. Each group of antihypertensive drugs is discussed under the appropriate section in this chapter, as well as how several different drugs can be used together when treating hyperten-

Table 21–1	CLASSIFICATION OF BP	
Category	**Systolic BP (mm Hg)**	**Diastolic BP (mm Hg)**
Optimal	<120	<80
Prehypertension	120–139	80–89
Hypertension		
Stage 1	140–159	90–99
Stage 2	≥160	≥100

BP = blood pressure.
Source: From The Seventh Report of the Joint National Committee on Prevention, Detection, Evaluation, and Treatment of High Blood Pressure (JNC-VII). *JAMA.* 2003;289:2560–2571, with permission.

sion. To better understand how these drugs work in decreasing blood pressure, the normal control of blood pressure and the possible mechanisms that generate a hypertensive state are briefly discussed.

Normal Control of Blood Pressure

Blood pressure is normally maintained by the complex interaction of several physiologic systems.[43] Rapid control of blood pressure is accomplished primarily by the baroreceptor reflex (see Chapter 18).[78] The baroreflex monitors and corrects changes in blood pressure within a matter of seconds by altering cardiac output and peripheral vascular resistance. The long-term management of blood pressure is accomplished primarily by the kidneys through their control of fluid balance. Changes in blood pressure through the renal handling of fluid and electrolytes usually take place over a period of several hours to several days. Humoral factors such as circulating catecholamines (from the adrenal gland), arginine-vasopressin (from the pituitary gland), and angiotensin II (from a reaction involving the kidneys) can also play a role in regulating blood pressure, especially if blood pressure decreases suddenly. Together these various systems interact to maintain blood pressure within a fairly narrow range.

Although the control of blood pressure is a fairly complex subject, the actual factors that determine blood pressure can be simplified. At any given time, blood pressure is the product of cardiac output and the total resistance in the peripheral vasculature. This relationship is illustrated by the following equation:

$$BP = (CO) \times (TPR)$$

where BP is blood pressure, CO is the cardiac output, and TPR is the total peripheral resistance in the systemic vasculature. As indicated by this equation, BP can be maintained at a relatively constant level by changes in either CO or TPR. A decrease in CO, for instance, can potentially be offset by an increase in TPR so that BP does not appreciably change. Conversely, a sudden fall in TPR will necessitate an increase in CO to maintain BP.

The relevance of this simple equation to antihypertensive therapy will become apparent as different drugs are discussed. Some antihypertensive drugs exert their effects by primarily acting on CO, others primarily affect TPR, and some agents decrease both factors.

Pathogenesis of Hypertension

Essential Versus Secondary Hypertension

Hypertension can be divided into two major categories: secondary hypertension and primary, or essential, hypertension. In secondary hypertension, the elevated blood pressure can be attributed to some specific abnormality such as renal artery stenosis, catecholamine-producing tumors, endocrine disorders, or cerebral damage. The treatment of secondary hypertension is rather straightforward, with efforts focusing on correcting the underlying pathology (e.g., the cause of the problem can be dealt with directly by surgery). Secondary hypertension, however, accounts for only about 5% of the patients diagnosed with hypertension.[13] The remaining 95% of hypertensive individuals are classified as having primary, or essential, hypertension. In essential hypertension, there is no clear, readily discernible cause of the elevated blood pressure.

Consequently, the exact cause of hypertension in the majority of patients is unknown. Many theories have been proposed to explain how blood pressure increases and eventually becomes sustained in essential hypertension. Some of the major factors that may account for the increased blood pressure in essential hypertension are presented here.

Possible Mechanisms in Essential Hypertension

The voluminous literature dealing with potential causes and mechanisms of essential hypertension cannot be fully reviewed here. As stated previously, the exact cause of hypertension in most patients is not known. There appears to be a rather complex interaction of genetic and environmental factors that ultimately leads to adaptive changes in the cardiovascular system of the patient with essential hypertension.[5,18,23,48,50] Diet, stress, and other external factors, for example, are associated with increased blood pressure. These factors seem to be more influential in certain patients, suggesting a possible genetic predisposition to hypertension. Other risk factors such as cigarette smoking and alcohol abuse clearly play a role in potentiating the onset and maintenance of hypertension. Obesity is also an important risk factor for hypertension and various other types of cardiovascular disease.[30,80] Essential hypertension is probably not caused by only one factor, but may be caused by a subtle, complex interaction of many factors. The exact way in which these factors interact probably varies from person to person, so that the cause of this disease really must be regarded individually rather than being based on one common etiology.

Despite the fact that the actual cause of hypertension is unknown, studies in humans and in animal models that mimic essential hypertension have suggested that the sympathetic nervous system may be a final common pathway in mediating and perpetuating the hypertensive state. That is, the factors described earlier may interact in such a way as to cause a general increase in sympathetic activity, which then becomes the common denominator underlying the elevated blood pressure in essential hypertension.[9,38,39] Increased sympathetic activity should produce a hypertensive effect because of the excitatory effect of sympathetic neurons on the heart and peripheral vasculature. Increased sympathetic drive may initially increase blood pressure by increasing cardiac output. In later stages, cardiac output often returns to normal levels, with the increased blood pressure being due to an increase in vascular resistance. The reasons for the shift from elevated cardiac output to elevated peripheral vascular resistance are somewhat unclear. A sustained increase in sympathetic activity, however, may be the initiating factor that begins a sequence of events ultimately resulting in essential hypertension.

Once blood pressure does become elevated, hypertension seems to become self-perpetuating to some extent. Mechanisms that control blood pressure (the baroreceptor reflex), for example, may decrease in sensitivity, thus blunting the normal response to elevated pressure.[60,96] Increased sympathetic discharge to the kidneys and altered renal hemodynamics may also cause changes in renal function contributing to the sustained increase in blood pressure.[40,41,57] Moreover, it is apparent that hypertension is often associated with metabolic abnormalities, including impaired glucose metabolism (due to insulin resistance), hyperinsulinemia, dyslipidemia, and abdominal obesity.[61,82,101] This cluster of problems, known commonly as metabolic syndrome, places the patient at risk for type 2 diabetes mellitus (see Chapter 32). Although the exact link between hypertension and metabolic syndrome is not clear, it is apparent that chronic elevations in blood pressure can lead to metabolic impairments that further jeopardize the health of patients with this disease.[32,101]

Increased blood pressure may also invoke adaptive changes in the peripheral vasculature so that peripheral vessels become less compliant and vascular resistance increases.[99,111] That is, increased pressure on the vascular wall actually causes thickening of the wall, which further increases the resistance to blood flow through the thickened vessels. The peripheral vasculature may also become more reactive to pressor substances such as norepinephrine and angiotensin II.[99] Hypertension is likewise associated with a defect in the production of vasoactive substances by the cells lining the peripheral vasculature (i.e., the vascular endothelium). The vascular endothelium normally produces several vasoactive substances including vasodilators (nitric oxide, bradykinin, prostaglandin I_2) and vasoconstrictors (angiotensin II, endothelin-I).[13,54,76] These endothelial-derived substances help maintain local control over vascular resistance.[54] In hypertension, however, there may be a defect in the production of these substances, especially a decreased production of nitric oxide.[13,54] A relative deficiency of this vasodilator would result in increased vascular resistance, which helps increase the hypertensive condition.

The possible factors involved in initiating and maintaining essential hypertension are summarized in Figure 21–1. Ultimately, certain environmental factors may turn on the sympathetic division of the autonomic nervous system in susceptible individuals. Increased sympathetic discharge then creates a vicious cycle whereby increased sympathetic effects—in conjunction with the increased blood pressure itself—help perpetuate hypertension. Exactly how various factors initiate the increased sympathetic discharge is not fully understood and may in fact vary from patient to patient. It is hoped that future studies will elaborate on the exact role of factors causing essential hypertension and that treatment can then be focused on preventing the changes that initially increase blood pressure.

Drug Therapy

Several major categories of drugs exist for the treatment of essential hypertension. These categories include diuretics, sympatholytic drugs, vasodilators, angiotensin-converting enzyme inhibitors, and calcium channel blockers. The primary sites of action and effects of each category are summarized in Table 21–2. The mechanism of action, rationale for use, specific agents, and adverse effects of drugs in each cate-

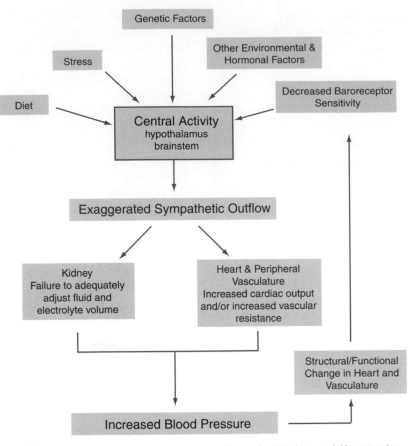

FIGURE 21–1 ▼ Schematic diagram of the possible mechanisms in essential hypertension. Various factors interact to turn on sympathetic outflow to the kidneys, heart, and peripheral vasculature, resulting in elevated blood pressure. Hypertension also causes structural and functional changes in the vasculature that help maintain the elevated pressure.

gory are discussed in the next few sections of this chapter.

Diuretics

Mechanism of Action and Rationale for Use

Diuretics increase the formation and excretion of urine. These drugs are used as antihypertensive agents because of their ability to increase the renal excretion of water and sodium, thus decreasing the volume of fluid within the vascular system. This situation is somewhat analogous to the decrease in pressure that would occur inside a balloon if some of the air inside were allowed to leak out. Consequently, diuretics appear to have a rather direct effect on blood pressure

through their ability to simply decrease the amount of fluid in the vascular system.

Diuretics are often the first type of drugs used to treat hypertension.[35,79] They are relatively inexpensive and seem to work well in a large percentage of patients with mild-to-moderate hypertension.[70] Likewise, a large clinical trial recently suggested that thiazide diuretics might be superior to calcium channel blockers and angiotensin converting enzyme inhibitors in preventing major cardiac events such as myocardial infarction, stroke, and heart failure in people with hypertension.[3] Hence, diuretics have been a mainstay in the treatment of hypertension for many years, and they remain one of the primary methods for treating this condition in a large number of people. The use of diuretics alone and in conjunction with other antihypertensives is discussed in more detail in "Stepped-Care Approach to Hypertension."

Table 21–2	ANTIHYPERTENSIVE DRUG CATEGORIES	
Category	**Primary Site(s) of Action**	**Primary Antihypertensive Effect(s)**
Diuretics	Kidneys	Decrease in plasma fluid volume
Sympatholytics	Various sites within the sympathetic division of the autonomic nervous system	Decrease sympathetic influence on the heart and/or peripheral vasculature
Vasodilators	Peripheral vasculature	Lower vascular resistance by directly vasodilating peripheral vessels
Inhibition of the renin-angiotensin system (ACE inhibitors and angiotensin II receptor blockers)	Peripheral vasculature and certain organs with a functional renin-angiotensin system (heart, kidneys)	ACE inhibitors: prevent the conversion of angiotensin I to angiotensin II. Angiotensin II receptor blockers: block the effects of angiotensin II on the vasculature and various other tissues
Calcium channel blockers	Limit calcium entry into vascular smooth muscle and cardiac muscle	Decrease vascular smooth-muscle contraction; decrease myocardial force and rate of contraction

ACE = angiotensin converting enzyme.

Although they differ chemically, all diuretics exert their beneficial effects by acting directly on the kidneys to increase water and sodium excretion.[13] Diuretic drugs can be subclassified according to their chemical structure or the manner in which they affect kidney function. The primary subclassifications of diuretics are listed here.

Classification of Diuretics

Thiazide Diuretics. Thiazide drugs share a common chemical nucleus as well as a common mode of action. These drugs act primarily on the early portion of the distal tubule of the nephron, where they inhibit sodium reabsorption. By inhibiting sodium reabsorption, more sodium is retained within the nephron, creating an osmotic force that also retains more water in the nephron. Since more sodium and water are passed through the nephron, where they will ultimately be excreted from the body, a diuretic effect is produced. Thiazides are the most frequently used type of diuretic for hypertension. Specific types of thiazide drugs are listed in Table 21–3.

Loop Diuretics. These drugs act primarily on the ascending limb of the loop of Henle (hence the term

Table 21–3	DIURETIC DRUGS USED TO TREAT HYPERTENSION

Thiazide diuretics

Bendroflumethiazide (Naturetin)
Chlorothiazide (Diuril)
Chlorthalidone (Hygroton, others)
Hydrochlorothiazide (Esidrix, others)
Hydroflumethiazide (Diucardin, Saluron)
Methyclothiazide (Enduron, others)
Metolazone (Diulo, Mykrox, Zaroxolyn)
Polythiazide (Renese)
Quinethazone (Hydromox)
Trichlormethiazide (Metahydrin, Naqua)

Loop diuretics

Bumetanide (Bumex)
Ethacrynic acid (Edecrin)
Furosemide (Lasix, others)

Potassium-sparing diuretics

Amiloride (Midamor)
Spironolactone (Aldactone)
Triamterene (Dyrenium)

"loop diuretic"). They exert their diuretic effect by inhibiting the reabsorption of sodium and chloride from the nephron, thereby preventing the reabsorption of the water that follows these electrolytes. Specific types of loop diuretics are listed in Table 21–3.

Potassium-Sparing Diuretics. Several different drugs with diuretic properties are classified as potassium-sparing because they are able to prevent the secretion of potassium into the distal tubule. Normally, a sodium-potassium exchange occurs in the distal tubule, where sodium is reabsorbed and potassium is secreted. Potassium-sparing agents interfere with this exchange in various ways (depending on the specific drug) so that potassium is spared from secretion and sodium remains in the tubule, where it is excreted. Although these agents do not produce a diuretic effect to the same extent as the loop and thiazide diuretics, potassium-sparing drugs have the advantage of reducing potassium loss and thus preventing hypokalemia. Specific potassium-sparing drugs are listed in Table 21–3.

Adverse Effects of Diuretics

The most serious side effects of diuretics are fluid depletion and electrolyte imbalance.[13,88] By the very nature of their action, diuretics decrease extracellular fluid volume as well as produce sodium depletion (hyponatremia) and potassium depletion (hypokalemia). Hypokalemia is a particular problem with the thiazide and loop diuretics, but occurs less frequently when the potassium-sparing agents are used. Hypokalemia and other disturbances in fluid and electrolyte balance can produce serious metabolic and cardiac problems and may even prove fatal in some individuals. Consequently, patients must be monitored closely, and the drug dosage should be maintained at the lowest effective dose. Also, potassium supplements are used in some patients to prevent hypokalemia.

Fluid depletion may also be a serious problem during diuretic therapy. A decrease in blood volume may cause a reflex increase in cardiac output and peripheral vascular resistance because of activation of the baroreflex (see Chapter 18). This occurrence may produce an excessive demand on the myocardium, especially in patients with cardiac disease. Decreased blood volume may also activate the renin-angiotensin system, thereby causing further peripheral vasoconstriction and increased cardiac workload. Again, the effects of fluid depletion may be especially serious in patients with certain types of heart failure.

Loop and thiazide diuretics may also impair glucose and lipid metabolism, and it has been suggested that high doses of these agents may predispose some patients to type 2 diabetes mellitus.[1,13] Although the exact risk of such metabolic disturbances is not known, the long-term use of these drugs has been questioned.[67] Nonetheless, concerns about metabolic side effects can be minimized if low doses are administered.[13]

Other less serious, but bothersome, side effects of diuretic therapy include gastrointestinal disturbances and weakness-fatigue. **Orthostatic hypotension** may occur because of the relative fluid depletion produced by these drugs. Changes in mood and confusion may also occur in some patients.

Sympatholytic Drugs

As discussed previously, the preponderance of evidence indicates that an increase in sympathetic activity may be an underlying factor in essential hypertension. Consequently, drugs that interfere with sympathetic discharge (i.e., sympatholytic agents) should be valuable as antihypertensive agents. These sympatholytic drugs can be classified according to where and how they interrupt sympathetic activity. Sympatholytic drugs used to treat hypertension include beta-adrenergic blockers, alpha-adrenergic blockers, presynaptic adrenergic neurotransmitter depletors, centrally acting drugs, and ganglionic blockers (Table 21–4). Each of these categories is discussed here.

Beta Blockers

Mechanism of Action and Rationale for Use

Beta-adrenergic blockers have been used extensively to decrease blood pressure and are a mainstay of antihypertensive therapy in many patients.[4,81] Beta blockers exert their primary effect on the heart, where they decrease heart rate and force myocardial contraction. In hypertensive patients, these drugs lower blood pressure by slowing down the heart and reducing cardiac output. This statement, however, is probably an oversimplification of how beta blockers produce an antihypertensive effect. In addition to their direct effect on the myocardium, beta blockers also produce a general decrease in sympathetic tone.[19,39] Although their exact effects on sympathetic activity remain to be determined, beta blockers may decrease sympathetic activi-

Table 21–4	SYMPATHOLYTIC DRUGS USED TO TREAT HYPERTENSION	

Beta blockers	*Presynaptic adrenergic inhibitors*
Acebutolol (Sectral)	Guanadrel (Hylorel)
Atenolol (Tenormin)	Guanethidine (Ismelin)
Betaxolol (Kerlone)	Reserpine (Serpalan,
Bisoprolol (Zebeta)	others)
Carteolol (Cartrol)	
Labetalol (Normodyne;	*Centrally Acting Agents*
Trandate)	Clonidine (Catapres)
Metoprolol (Lopressor,	Guanabenz (Wytensin)
others)	Guanfacine (Tenex)
Nadolol (Corgard)	Methyldopa (Aldomet)
Oxprenolol (Trasicor)	
Penbutolol (Levatol)	
Pindolol (Visken)	*Ganglionic Blockers*
Propranolol (Inderal)	Mecamylamine (Inversine)
Sotalol (Betapace)	Trimethaphan (Arfonad)
Timolol (Blocadren)	
Alpha blockers	
Doxazosin (Cardura)	
Phenoxybenzamine	
(Dibenzyline)	
Prazosin (Minipress)	
Terazosin (Hytrin)	

ty via the following: a central inhibitory effect on the brainstem, decreased renin release from the kidneys and within the central nervous system (CNS), impaired sympathetic activity in the ganglia or at the presynaptic adrenergic terminals, increased baroreceptor sensitivity, or via a combination of these and other factors.[19,74] Regardless of the exact mechanism of their action, beta blockers often compliment the effects of other antihypertensives (diuretics, angiotensin converting enzyme [ACE] inhibitors, and so forth) and are therefore included in the drug regimen of many patients with hypertension

Specific Agents

Beta-adrenergic blockers that are approved for use in hypertension are listed in Table 21–4. These drugs are all effective in decreasing blood pressure, but certain beta blockers have additional properties that make

them more suitable in specific patients.[68,81] As discussed in Chapter 20, some beta blockers are relatively selective for beta-1 receptors (cardioselective) and tend to affect the heart more than the lungs and other tissues (see Table 20–2). Certain beta blockers such as pindolol and acebutolol function as partial agonists and are said to have *intrinsic sympathomimetic activity* because they block the effects of excessive endogenous catecholamines while producing a normal background level of sympathetic stimulation to the heart.[13] Beta blockers such as labetalol and propranolol are able to normalize the excitability of the cardiac cell membrane; these drugs are said to have *membrane-stabilizing activity*—other beta blockers may also exhibit this membrane-stabilizing effect at higher doses.[13] Finally, some of the newer "third generation" beta blockers such as carvedilol and nebivolol produce peripheral vasodilation as well as a cardiac beta blockade, making these drugs especially useful in decreasing blood pressure.[17,55,97,112] Some newer agents may likewise have other beneficial effects, such as antioxidant properties and the ability to decrease lipid abnormalities and insulin resistance.[24,49,97] Hence, the selection of a specific beta blocker is based on these properties along with consideration for the individual needs of each patient.

Adverse Effects

Nonselective beta blockers (i.e., those with a fairly equal affinity for beta-1 and beta-2 receptors) may produce bronchoconstriction in patients with asthma and similar respiratory disorders. Cardiovascular side effects include excessive depression of heart rate and myocardial contractility as well as orthostatic hypotension. Some of the traditional beta blockers may impair glucose and lipid metabolism, but this effect can be reduced by using one of the newer vasodilating beta blockers such as carvedilol.[97] Other side effects include depression, fatigue, gastrointestinal disturbances, and allergic reactions. Beta blockers are generally well tolerated by most patients, however, and the incidence of side effects is relatively low.

Alpha Blockers

Mechanism of Action and Rationale for Use

Drugs that block the alpha-1–adrenergic receptor on vascular smooth muscle will promote a decrease in vascular resistance.[37,110] Since the total peripheral vascular resistance often increases in essential hypertension, blocking vascular adrenergic receptors should be an effective course of action. In a sense, alpha blockers act directly on the tissues that ultimately mediate the increased blood pressure—that is, the peripheral vasculature. In the past, the use of alpha blockers in mild-to-moderate essential hypertension was somewhat limited because these drugs are sometimes *too* effective and tend to cause problems with hypotension.[21]

It is now recognized that alpha-1 antagonists may offer specific advantages in treating hypertension, including an ability to improve blood lipid profiles (decreased triglycerides and total cholesterol, increased high-density lipoprotein–cholesterol ratio) and produce a favorable effect on glucose metabolism and insulin resistance.[12,20,102] Newer agents such as doxazosin (Cardura) also appear to have less adverse cardiovascular side effects—such as reflex tachycardia—presumably because these agents act longer and do not cause a sudden fall in blood pressure.[36] Likewise, a controlled-release formulation of this drug is now available. This formulation, known as doxazosin gastrointestinal therapeutic system (GITS), allows slower drug absorption into the bloodstream, thereby further reducing sudden adverse effects and improving tolerability.[13,91] Hence, alpha-1 blockers are gaining acceptance in certain patients with moderate hypertension, as well as being included in the antihypertensive regimen of patients having more severe cases of high blood pressure.

Alpha-1 blockers can also be used to treat the symptoms of benign prostatic hypertrophy because they decrease sympathetic-mediated contraction of smooth muscle located in the prostate gland.[34,91] Reduction of muscle tone in the prostate decreases constriction of the ureter, thereby improving urinary flow and the ability to empty the bladder.[58,83]

Specific Agents

The characteristics of individual alpha blockers are discussed in Chapter 20. Basically, these drugs can be differentiated according to their relative alpha-1 selectivity, their duration of action, and other pharmacokinetic properties. Prazosin (Minipress) has been the primary alpha blocker used in the past, but newer agents such as doxazosin and terazosin (Hytrin) are gaining acceptance in treating hypertension. Prazosin and other alpha blockers approved as antihypertensives are listed in Table 21–4.

Adverse Effects

One of the primary problems with alpha blockers is reflex tachycardia. When peripheral vascular resistance falls due to the effects of these drugs, the baroreceptor reflex often responds by generating a compensatory increase in heart rate. This tachycardia may be a significant problem, especially if there is a history of cardiac disease. To prevent reflex tachycardia, a beta blocker may be administered with the alpha blocker. The beta blocker will negate the increase in heart rate normally mediated through the sympathetic innervation to the heart. Alternatively, use of a longer-acting or controlled-release drug (doxazosin) may reduce the risk of reflex tachycardia because these agents produce a milder and more prolonged decrease in blood pressure following administration. Hence, reflex mechanisms controlling blood pressure (i.e., the baroreflex) are not suddenly activated as would be the case if blood pressure was reduced more rapidly with a shorter-acting drug.

Another major adverse effect with alpha blockers is orthostatic hypotension. Blockade of alpha-1 receptors in peripheral arteries and veins often promotes pooling of blood in the lower extremities when a patient stands up. Therapists should be alert for the symptoms of orthostatic hypotension (i.e., dizziness and syncope), especially for the first few days during alpha-blocker administration.

Finally, there is concern that alpha blockers may increase the risk of cardiac disease, including congestive heart failure.[2] By causing vasodilation, these drugs can increase plasma volume, thereby increasing the workload on the heart and predisposing certain patients to heart failure and other cardiac events (stroke, infarction). Hence, alpha blockers are not typically prescribed alone in treating hypertension, but are used in advanced cases along with diuretics (to control fluid balance) or other antihypertensives such as beta blockers and ACE inhibitors. Likewise, alpha blockers may be a good choice for men with advanced hypertension and benign prostatic hypertrophy because these drugs may help resolve both problems simultaneously.[91]

Presynaptic Adrenergic Inhibitors

Mechanism of Action and Rationale for Use

Drugs that inhibit the release of norepinephrine from the presynaptic terminals of peripheral adrenergic neurons may be used effectively in some individuals with hypertension. Some agents, such as reserpine, inhibit the presynaptic synthesis and storage of norepinephrine in peripheral and CNS adrenergic neurons.[21] Other agents (guanadrel, guanethidine) replace norepinephrine in peripheral sympathetic neurons, thus creating a false neurotransmitter.[21,74] In either case, depletion of norepinephrine from the presynaptic terminal decreases sympathetic-mediated excitation of the heart and peripheral vasculature, resulting in decreased blood pressure.

Specific Agents

Drugs that inhibit the presynaptic synthesis and storage of norepinephrine are discussed in Chapter 20. The drugs in this category used to treat hypertension are listed in Table 21–4. These drugs are often used in conjunction with other agents in the stepped-care approach to hypertension (see "Stepped-Care Approach to Hypertension").

Adverse Effects

Orthostatic hypotension is sometimes a problem with these agents. Other bothersome side effects include gastrointestinal disturbances such as nausea, vomiting, and diarrhea.

Centrally Acting Agents

Mechanism of Action and Rationale for Use

Several drugs currently available seem to inhibit sympathetic discharge from the brainstem. Sympathetic discharge from the vasomotor center appears to be influenced by two types of neuronal receptors located in the brainstem: alpha-2 adrenergic receptors and imidazoline type I1 receptors. Stimulation of these receptors results in a *decrease* in sympathetic discharge to the heart and vasculature. Centrally acting sympatholytics are therefore characterized as agonists for either one or possibly both types of these receptors. Clonidine, for example is considered to primarily be an alpha-2 agonist, although this drug also has some ability to stimulate imidazoline receptors.[21] Newer agents in this category (monoxidine, rilmenidine) seem to be more selective for imidazoline receptors.[51,62,94,104] In either case, stimulation of these centrally located receptors results in a decrease in sympathetic outflow and a subsequent decrease in car-

diovascular stimulation and blood pressure.[21,104] Consequently, centrally acting drugs offer a rather unique approach to hypertension because these drugs limit sympathetic activity at the source (brainstem vasomotor center) rather than at the periphery (cardiovascular neuroeffector junction).

Specific Agents

The primary drugs in this category are clonidine, guanabenz, guanfacine, and methyldopa (see Table 21–4). Clonidine, guanabenz, and guanfacine act directly on the alpha-2 receptor, whereas methyldopa acts as an alpha-2 agonist after being converted in vivo to alpha-methylnorepinephrine. As indicated, monoxidine and rilmenidine act primarily on imidazoline receptors.

Adverse Effects

At therapeutic doses, these drugs are associated with some troublesome but relatively minor side effects including dry mouth, dizziness, and sedation. The incidence of sedation seems to be related to these drug's alpha-2 stimulatory effects. Hence, agents that are more selective for imidazoline receptors may seem better tolerated because patients are more alert and have less psychomotor slowing.[104]

Ganglionic Blockers

Mechanism of Action and Rationale for Use

Drugs that block synaptic transmission at autonomic ganglia will dramatically and effectively reduce blood pressure by decreasing systemic sympathetic activity.[21,95] These agents are essentially nicotinic cholinergic antagonists (see Chapter 18), which block transmission at the junction between presynaptic and postsynaptic neurons in sympathetic and parasympathetic pathways. Because of the effect of these agents on both divisions of the autonomic nervous system, ganglionic blockers are used sparingly in treating hypertension. In the past, these drugs were used to reduce blood pressure in hypertensive emergencies.[100] Their routine use, however, has been largely replaced by vasodilators (nitroprusside; see "Vasodilators") and other agents that are safer and produce fewer side effects.[28,33] Still, ganglionic blockers may be used to decrease blood pressure rapidly in certain emergencies such as acute aortic dissection or autonomic crisis in people with spinal cord injury.[95,100]

Specific Agents

Ganglionic blockers currently used to decrease blood pressure in a hypertensive crisis are listed in Table 21–4.

Adverse Effects

As might be expected, ganglionic blockers produce a multitude of side effects because of the inhibition of both sympathetic and parasympathetic responses. Some adverse effects include gastrointestinal discomfort (nausea, constipation), urinary retention, visual disturbances, and orthostatic hypotension. At higher doses, they may even exhibit some neuromuscular blocking activity. These and other side effects may be quite severe in some patients. Fortunately, ganglionic blockers are usually not used for extended periods because the patient is placed on other antihypertensive drugs when the hypertensive crisis is resolved.

Vasodilators

Mechanism of Action and Rationale for Use

Drugs that directly vasodilate the peripheral vasculature will produce an antihypertensive effect by decreasing peripheral vascular resistance.[13] Although other drugs such as the alpha blockers may ultimately produce vasodilation by interrupting adrenergic supply to the vasculature, the vasodilators exert an inhibitory effect directly on vascular smooth-muscle cells. Vasodilators are believed to inhibit smooth-muscle contraction by increasing the intracellular production of second messengers such as cyclic guanosine monophosphate (cGMP; see Chapter 4). Increased amounts of cGMP inhibit the function of the contractile process in the vascular smooth-muscle cell, thus leading to vasodilation.

Specific Agents

The primary vasodilators used in hypertension are hydralazine (Apresoline) and minoxidil (Loniten) (Table 21–5). These drugs are not usually the first medications used in patients with hypertension, but tend to be added to the drug regimen if other agents (diuretics, beta blockers) fail.[89] Hydralazine is likewise used to lower blood pressure in emergency situations

Table 21–5	ANTIHYPERTENSIVE VASODILATORS, ACE INHIBITORS, ANGIOTENSIN II RECEPTOR BLOCKERS, AND CALCIUM CHANNEL BLOCKERS

Vasodilators

Diazoxide (Hyperstat)	Minoxidil (Loniten)
Hydralazine (Apresoline)	Nitroprusside (Nipride, Nitropress)

ACE inhibitors

Benazepril (Lotensin)	Moexipril (Univasc)
Captopril (Capoten)	Perindopril (Aceon)
Enalapril (Vasotec)	Quinapril (Accupril)
Fosinopril (Monopril)	Ramipril (Altace)
Lisinopril (Prinivil, Zestril)	Trandolapril (Mavik)

Angiotensin II receptor blockers

Candesartan (Atacand)	Telmisartan (Micardis)
Irbesartan (Avapro)	Valsartan (Diovan)
Losartan (Cozaar)	

Calcium channel blockers

Amlodipine (Norvasc)	Nicardipine (Cardene)
Bepridil (Vascor)	Nifedipine (Adalat, Procardia)
Diltiazem (Cardizem)	
Felodipine (Plendil)	Nimodipine (Nimotop)
Isradipine (DynaCirc)	Verapamil (Calan, Isoptin)

ACE = angiotensin converting enzyme.

such as severe preeclampsia or malignant hypertension.[56,100] Other vasodilators include diazoxide (Hyperstat) and nitroprusside (Nipride, Nitropress), but these drugs are usually given only in emergency situations to treat a patient in hypertensive crisis.[28]

Nitric oxide also produces vasodilation in vascular smooth muscle. As indicated earlier, hypertension may be perpetuated by a defect in the production of nitric oxide by the vascular endothelium. In follows that providing nitric oxide directly or administering precursors for nitric oxide production may help reduce vascular resistance and decrease arterial pressure in specific hypertensive syndromes.[6] To date, inhaled nitric oxide has been used to treat acute pulmonary hypertension associated with respiratory distress syndrome in newborns and adults.[10,52] Likewise, researchers are trying to determine if nitric oxide could be used to treat systemic (essential) hypertension, or if other drugs could be used to increase the production of endogenous nitric oxide in people with hypertension.[6] Future studies are needed to determine if manipulation of nitric oxide levels in the peripheral vasculature is a possible way to treat essential hypertension.

Adverse Effects

Although vasodilators are effective in lowering blood pressure, these drugs are associated with a number of adverse effects. Reflex tachycardia often occurs because baroreflex responses attempt to compensate for the fall in vascular resistance that these drugs produce. This side effect is analogous to the increased heart rate occurring when alpha blockers are used to decrease peripheral vascular resistance. Other common reactions include dizziness, postural hypotension, weakness, nausea, fluid retention, and headache. Minoxidil also increases hair growth on the face, ears, forehead,

and other hairy body surfaces. This increased hair growth is often a cause for the discontinuation of this drug in women. Some men, however, have applied minoxidil cutaneously to treat baldness, and a topical preparation of this drug (Rogaine) is marketed as a potential hair-growth stimulant.

Inhibition of the Renin-Angiotensin System

Mechanism of Action and Rationale for Use

The renin-angiotensin system involves several endogenous components that help regulate vascular tone in various organs and tissues.[25,84,109] In systemic circulation, the renin-angiotensin system acts by a sequence of events summarized in Figure 21–2. Renin is an enzyme produced primarily in the kidneys. When blood pressure falls, renin is released from the kidneys into the systemic circulation. Angiotensinogen is a peptide that is produced by the liver and circulates

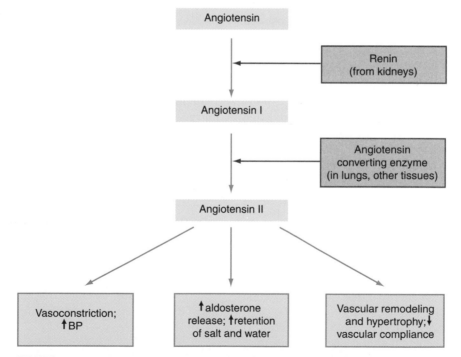

FIGURE 21–2 ▼ The renin-angiotensin system and the effects of angiotensin II. Angiotensin converting enzyme inhibitors interrupt this system by blocking the conversion of angiotensin I to angiotensin II, and angiotensin II receptor blockers prevent angiotensin II from stimulating cardiovascular tissues. *From:* Ciccone. Medications. In: DeTurk WE, Cahalin LP, eds. *Cardiovascular and Pulmonary Physical Therapy.* New York: McGraw-Hill; 2004: 193, with permission.

continually in the bloodstream. When renin contacts angiotensinogen, angiotensinogen is transformed into angiotensin I. The circulating angiotensin I is then transformed by angiotensin-converting enzyme into angiotensin II. The converting enzyme is located in the vasculature of many tissues, especially the lung. Angiotensin II is an extremely potent vasoconstrictor. Consequently, the fall in blood pressure that activated the renin-angiotensin system is rectified by the increase in vascular resistance caused by angiotensin II. Angiotensin II, or possibly its by-product angiotensin III, also increases aldosterone secretion from the adrenal cortex. Aldosterone directly increases sodium reabsorption from the kidneys, which creates osmotic forces in the kidneys that encourage water reabsorption, thus helping maintain plasma volume.

The sequence of events just described illustrate the role of the systemic renin-angiotensin system in normal blood pressure regulation. Exactly what goes wrong with this system in patients with essential hypertension is not fully understood. Some patients display increased levels of circulating renin, hence their classification as having high-renin hypertension. Why plasma renin production is elevated in these patients, however, is often unclear. In addition to problems in circulating levels of renin and angiotensin II, there may also be problems with the renin-angiotensin system in specific tissues or organs. For instance, a complete, functioning renin-angiotensin system has been identified within the brain[84,106] and in the heart and vascular walls.[86] This fact suggests that some of the hypertensive effects of this system may be mediated through CNS mechanisms or by changes directly in the vascular tissues.

Nonetheless, activation of the renin-angiotensin system is extremely detrimental in people with high blood pressure. Excess production of angiotensin II causes vascoconstriction that perpetuates the hypertensive condition. More importantly, angiotensin II is a powerful stimulant of vascular tissue growth, and sustained production of angiotensin II results in the thickening and hypertrophy of the vascular wall.[59] The thickened vascular wall causes a decrease in the lumen of the vessel, thereby causing additional resistance to blood flow and increased hypertension. Angiotensin II may have other detrimental effects on the vasculature, including inflammation of the vascular endothelium and increased lipid accumulation within the vascular wall.[14,53] Excessive production of angiotensin II is therefore associated with several detrimental changes in the vascular wall that can lead to hypertension and

related cardiovascular events (stroke, myocardial infarction, heart failure).[25]

Fortunately, two pharmacologic strategies have been developed to inhibit the effects of abnormal renin-angiotensin system activation. The first strategy involves drugs that inhibit the enzyme that converts angiotensin I to angiotensin II. These drugs are commonly referred to as angiotensin converting enzyme (ACE) inhibitors. ACE inhibitors decrease the hypertensive effects of angiotensin II by limiting the production of this compound. More recently, a second strategy has emerged in the form of drugs that block angiotensin II receptors on various tissues.[103,105] Angiotensin II stimulates vascular and other tissues by binding to a protein receptor (specifically, the AT1 angiotensin II receptor) on these tissues.[103] Newer drugs, known as angiotensin II blockers or antagonists, have been developed to block these receptors, thereby negating the harmful effects of angiotensin II on vascular and other tissues.

ACE inhibitors and angiotensin II blockers have been an important addition to the antihypertensive drug arsenal. These drugs can be used alone or in conjunction with other drugs for the long-term control of high blood pressure.[69,105] In fact, these drugs appear to have several advantages over other antihypertensives, such as a lower incidence of cardiovascular side effects (i.e., less reflex tachycardia and orthostatic hypotension).[64,105] The ability of these drugs to inhibit angiotensin II-induced vascular hypertrophy and remodeling is also recognized as an important benefit during the treatment of high blood pressure.[25,103] These drugs are likewise extremely beneficial in decreasing morbidity and mortality associated with congestive heart failure, and use of these drugs in heart failure will be addressed in Chapter 24.

Specific Agents

ACE inhibitors and angiotensin II blockers used to treat hypertension are listed in Table 21–5. These drugs have been shown to be effective in many cases of mild-to-moderate essential hypertension, and they may be used alone or in combination with beta blockers or diuretics.

Adverse Effects

ACE inhibitors are generally well-tolerated in most patients. Some individuals may experience an allergic reaction as evidenced by skin rash. This reaction usually disappears when the dosage is reduced or when administration is discontinued. Patients may also experience a persistent, dry cough that is annoying but relatively harmless. Although the incidence is rare, ACE inhibitors may cause hematological effects (neutropenia, agranulocytosis) and renal problems (glomerulonephritis, renal failure) in susceptible patients; these drugs should be use cautiously in certain patients with preexisting blood or kidney diseases. Other problems (gastrointestinal discomfort, dizziness, chest pain) may occur in some patients, but adverse effects are relatively rare.

Angiotensin II blockers are likewise well tolerated; these drugs do not cause the cough associated with ACE inhibitors.[64] Hence, angiotensin II blockers may be an effective alternative in patients who experience side effects such as coughing.[13]

Calcium Channel Blockers

Drugs that selectively block calcium entry into vascular smooth-muscle cells were originally developed to treat certain forms of angina pectoris and cardiac arrhythmias (Chapters 22 and 23, respectively). Calcium channel blockers are now recognized as being beneficial in the treatment of essential hypertension.[11,90] Calcium appears to play a role in activating the contractile element in smooth muscle much in the same way that calcium initiates actin-myosin interaction in skeletal muscle cells. Drugs that block calcium entry into vascular smooth muscle will inhibit the contractile process, leading to vasodilation and decreased vascular resistance.[74,90] Calcium channel blockers also tend to decrease heart rate and myocardial contraction force, and some of their antihypertensive properties may derive from their inhibitory effect on the heart.[65] These agents have a relatively small incidence of metabolic side effects, such as impaired glucose or lipid metabolism,[42,77] and they may help preserve renal function in people with hypertension-related kidney disease.[85,87,98] Consequently, calcium channel blockers have gained popularity over the last several decades as one of the primary treatments for high blood pressure.[7,11]

Some issues, however, have developed fairly recently regarding the safety of these drugs in treating hypertension. Several studies noted that use of certain calcium channel blockers (i.e., the short-acting form of nifedipine) was associated with an increased risk of myocardial infarction when these drugs were administered to certain hypertensive patients (older patients, patients with diabetes, patients with unstable angina).[66,107] The risk of infarction, however, seems minimal if long-acting or sustained-release formulations are used, presumably because these formulations do not cause a sudden change in blood pressure as do their shorter-acting counterparts.[27] Likewise, other studies suggested that calcium channel blockers may increase the risk of cancer, presumably because these drugs interfere with the normal role that calcium plays in regulating cell growth and turnover.[63] Subsequent studies, however, have failed to establish a clear link between calcium channel blockers and cancer.[63,92]

Consequently, calcium channel blockers still play an important role in the antihypertensive arsenal, but practitioners are more cautious about using these drugs to lower blood pressure in certain patients.[107] As mentioned above, the longer-acting or sustained-release forms of these drugs are somewhat safer and should be used whenever possible.[29,90]

Specific Agents

The primary calcium channel blockers used to treat hypertension are listed in Table 21–5. These agents differ somewhat from one another, and they can be subclassified in several categories according to their chemistry and how they block calcium channels.[42] Despite their chemical diversity, however, calcium channel blockers all act by limiting calcium entry into cardiovascular tissues.[13] These agents have all been shown to be effective in treating hypertension, and selection of a specific agent is typically based on the side-effect profile of each drug and the individual needs of each patient. As mentioned earlier, several agents are also available in longer-acting (sustained-release) forms, and use of these longer-acting agents may help reduce the risk of cardiovascular side effects (reflex tachycardia, orthostatic hypotension). Because calcium channel blockers are important in treating angina, the pharmacology of these drugs is discussed in more detail in Chapter 22.

Adverse Effects

These drugs may cause excessive vasodilation as evidenced by swelling in the feet and ankles, and some patients may also experience orthostatic hypotension. Abnormalities in heart rate (too fast, too slow, irregular) may also occur, and reflex tachycardia—caused by excessive peripheral vasodilation—has been noted with certain drugs such as the short-acting form of nifedipine. Other bothersome side effects include dizziness, headache, and nausea.

Stepped–Care Approach to Hypertension

In many hypertensive patients, more than one type of drug must be given to successfully control blood pressure.[31,113] In general, the more severe the hypertension, the greater the need for a combination of several agents. To provide some type of rationale for effective drug use, a stepped-care approach is often implemented. The object of a stepped-care approach is to begin drug therapy with certain types of drugs and then, if additional drugs are needed, to follow a logical progression in each patient. One type of stepped-care system is outlined in Table 21–6. Typically, drug therapy is initiated with either a thiazide diuretic, a beta blocker, an ACE inhibitor, or a calcium channel blocker (step 1). If blood pressure is not adequately controlled, other types of antihypertensive drugs are instituted as outlined in steps 2 through 4 (see Table 21–6).

Table 21–6	STEPPED-CARE APPROACH TO HYPERTENSION

STEP 1: In patients with mild hypertension, drug therapy is usually initiated with a single agent (monotherapy) from one of the following classes: a diuretic, a beta blocker, an angiotensin converting enzyme (ACE) inhibitor, or a calcium channel blocker.

STEP 2: If a single drug is unsuccessful in reducing blood pressure, a second agent is added. The second drug can be from one of the initial classes not used in step 1, or it can be from a second group that includes the centrally acting agents (clonidine, guanabenz), presynaptic adrenergic inhibitors (reserpine, guanethidine), alpha-1 blockers (prazosin, doxazosin), and vasodilators (hydralazine, minoxidil).

STEP 3: A third agent is added, usually from one of the classes listed in step 2 that has not already been used. Three different agents from three different classes are often administered concurrently in this step.

STEP4: A fourth drug is added from still another class.

A stepped-care approach is generally regarded as an effective way to use different types of antihypertensive drugs.[31] However, the stepped-care approach is not a set protocol—it only acts as a guideline for drug administration. It has also been suggested that initial treatment should be more aggressive in many patients, and that two agents should be used concurrently during initial treatment.[16,72] That is, treatment may be more successful if two antihypertensive drugs from different categories are used in the first step rather than a single drug.[46,113] Clearly, specific programs can (and should) be tailored to individual patients by providing various drugs at each step.[16,46]

Nonpharmacologic Treatment of Hypertension

Although several effective and relatively safe drugs exist for treating hypertension, the use of nondrug methods in decreasing blood pressure should not be overlooked, especially in cases of mild or borderline hypertension.[73,93] Certain dietary modifications, such as sodium restriction, low-fat diets, and diets high in certain fish oils, have been helpful in some patients.[47,71] Decreasing the use of alcohol and tobacco may also help lower blood pressure. Generally, a decrease in body weight will produce an antihypertensive effect[26,71]; regular exercise may help decrease blood pressure by decreasing body weight or by mechanisms unrelated to weight loss.[8,75] Many forms of behavior modification and stress management techniques have also been suggested as nonpharmacologic methods of blood pressure control.

Considerable debate exists as to whether or not mild hypertension should be treated initially with drugs, or if a trial with one or more nonpharmacologic technique should be employed first.[73] This decision must be made on an individual basis with consideration given to the patient's lifestyle and chance of compliance with a nondrug approach. There is ample evidence, however, that optimal results are obtained when lifestyle changes are combined with antihypertensive drug therapy.[73,74] Hence, changes in lifestyle and behavior should be encouraged in all hypertensive patients, regardless of whether drug therapy is initiated. Patients should be encouraged to quit smoking, lose weight, manage stress, and modify their diet, even if blood pressure is reduced pharmacologically.

Special Concerns in Rehabilitation Patients

■ ■ ■ Considering the prevalence of hypertension, therapists will undoubtedly work with many patients taking blood pressure medications. These drugs produce a diverse array of side effects that can influence the rehabilitation session. Primary among these are hypotension and orthostatic hypotension. Since the major action of these drugs is to lower blood pressure, physical therapists and occupational therapists should be cautious when their patients change posture suddenly or engage in other activities that may lower blood pressure.

Activities producing widespread vasodilation must be avoided or used very cautiously, especially if vasodilating drugs are being taken. Systemically applied heat (whirlpool, Hubbard tank), for instance, may cause blood pressure to fall precipitously if alpha blockers, calcium channel blockers, or direct-acting vasodilators are being administered. Similarly, exercise may cause vasodilation in skeletal musculature, which may potentiate the peripheral vasodilation induced by antihypertensive drugs. Additionally, if beta blockers are given, cardiac responses to exercise (i.e., increased heart rate and cardiac output) may be somewhat blunted because the myocardial response to sympathetic stimulation will be diminished.

Aside from being aware of the side effects of antihypertensive drugs, therapists may also play an important role in encouraging patient compliance in dealing with high blood pressure. Although drug therapy can control blood pressure, patients are often forgetful or hesitant about taking their medications, largely because hypertension is usually asymptomatic until the late stages of this disease. The patient will probably feel fine even when the drug is not taken, or the patient may actually avoid taking the drug because of some bothersome side effect (i.e., the patient may actually feel better without the drug). The idea that hypertension is a silent killer must be reinforced continually. Through their close contact with the patient, rehabilitation specialists are often in a good position to remind the patient of the consequences of noncompliance. In addition, therapists can help suggest and supervise nonpharmacologic methods of lowering blood pressure (e.g., exercise programs, stress management, relaxation techniques). Physical therapists and occupational therapists can play a valuable role in helping patients realize the importance of long-term pharmacologic and nonpharmacologic management of hypertension.

CASE STUDY

Hypertension

Brief History. H.C. is a 55-year-old man who works as an attorney for a large corporation. He is consistently faced with a rather demanding work schedule, often working 12- to 14-hour days, 6 days each week. In addition, he is 25 to 30 pounds overweight and is a habitual cigarette smoker. He has a long history of high blood pressure, which has been managed fairly successfully over the past 15 years through the use of different drugs. Currently, H.C. is in step 3 of the stepped-care approach to hypertensive therapy, and three drugs are being administered to control his blood pressure. He is receiving a diuretic (furosemide, [Lasix] 100 mg/d), a cardioselec-

tive beta blocker (metoprolol, [Lopressor] 200 mg/d), and a vasodilator (minoxidil, [Loniten] 20 mg/d).

While rushing to a business luncheon, H.C. was hit by an automobile as he was crossing the street. He was admitted to the hospital, where radiologic examination revealed a fracture of the right pelvis. Further examination did not reveal any other significant internal injuries. The pelvic fracture appeared stable at the time of admission, and internal fixation was not required. H.C. remained in the hospital and was placed on bed rest. Two days after admission, a physical therapist was called in to consult on the case. The physical therapist suggested a progressive ambulation program using the facility's therapeutic pool. The buoyancy provided by the pool would allow a gradual increase in weight bearing while protecting the fracture site.

Problem/Influence of Medication. To guard against patient hypothermia, the water temperature in the therapeutic pool was routinely maintained at 95°F. The therapist was concerned that immersing the patient in the pool would cause excessive peripheral vasodilation. Because the patient was taking a vasodilating drug (minoxidil), the additive effect of the warm pool and vasodilating agent might cause profound hypotension because of a dramatic decrease in total peripheral resistance. Also, because this patient was taking a cardioselective beta blocker (metoprolol), his heart would not be able to sufficiently increase cardiac output to offset the decreased peripheral resistance.

Decision/Solution. When the patient was in the pool, the therapist monitored heart rate and blood pressure at frequent, regular intervals. Blood pressure did decrease when the patient was ambulating in the pool, but not to a point of con-

cern because the patient's active leg muscle contractions facilitated venous return, and the buoyancy of the water decreased the effects of gravity on venous pooling in the lower extremities. In fact, only at the end of the rehabilitation session, when the patient came out of the pool, did hypotension became a potential problem. The patient was still experiencing peripheral vasodilation because of the residual effects of the warm water, but he no longer had the advantage of active muscle contractions and water buoyancy to help maintain his blood pressure. To prevent a hypotensive episode at the end of the session, the therapist placed the patient supine on a stretcher as soon as he came out of the water. Also, the patient's legs were quickly toweled dry, and vascular support stockings were placed on the patient's legs. These precautions allowed the patient to progress rapidly through his rehabilitation without any adverse incidents. When he was eventually discharged from the hospital, he was ambulating with crutches, with partial weight bearing on the side of the pelvic fracture.

SUMMARY

Hypertension is a common disease marked by a sustained increase in blood pressure. If untreated, hypertension leads to serious problems such as stroke, renal failure, and problems in several other physiologic systems. Although the cause of hypertension is discernible in a small percentage of patients, the majority of hypertensive individuals are classified as having essential hypertension, which means that the cause of their elevated blood pressure is unknown. Fortunately, several types of drugs are currently available to adequately control blood pressure in essential hypertension. Drugs such as diuretics, sympatholytics (alpha blockers, beta blockers, etc.), vasodilators, angiotensin-converting enzyme inhibitors, and calcium channel blockers have all been used in treating hypertension. These agents are usually prescribed according to a stepped-care protocol, where therapy is initiated with one drug, and subsequent agents are added as required. Rehabilitation specialists should be aware of the potential side effects of these drugs. Physical therapists and occupational therapists assume an important role in making patients aware of the sequelae of hypertension, and therapists should actively encourage patients to comply with pharmacologic and nonpharmacologic methods of lowering blood pressure.

References

1. Aksnes TA, Reims HM, Kjeldsen SE, Mancia G. Antihypertensive treatment and new-onset diabetes mellitus. *Curr Hypertens Rep.* 2005;7:298–303.
2. ALLHAT Collaborative Research Group. Major cardiovascular events in hypertensive patients randomized to doxazosin vs. chlorthalidone: the antihypertensive and lipid-lowering treatment to prevent heart attack trial (ALLHAT). *JAMA.* 2000;283:1967–1975.
3. ALLHAT Officers and Coordinators for the ALLHAT Collaborative Research Group. Major outcomes in high-risk hypertensive patients randomized to angiotensin-converting enzyme inhibitor or calcium channel blocker vs. diuretic: the antihypertensive and lipid-lowering treatment to prevent heart attack trial (ALLHAT). *JAMA.* 2002;288:2981–2997.
4. Ambrosioni E, Bacchelli S, Esposti DD, Borghi C. Beta-blockade in hypertension and congestive heart failure. *J Cardiovasc Pharmacol.* 2001;38(suppl 3):S25–S31.
5. Aneja A, El-Atat F, McFarlane SI, Sowers JR. Hypertension and obesity. *Recent Prog Horm Res.* 2004;59:169–205.
6. Augustyniak RA, Thomas GD, Victor RG, Zhang W. Nitric oxide pathway as new drug targets for refractory hypertension. *Curr Pharm Des.* 2005;11:3307–3315.
7. Basile J. The role of existing and newer calcium channel blockers in the treatment of hypertension. *J Clin Hypertens.* 2004;6:621–629.
8. Baster T, Baster-Brooks C. Exercise and hypertension. *Aust Fam Physician.* 2005;34:419–424.
9. Biaggioni I. Sympathetic control of the circulation in hypertension: lessons from autonomic disorders. *Curr Opin Nephrol Hypertens.* 2003;12:175–180.

10. Bizzarro M, Gross I, Bizzarro M. Inhaled nitric oxide for the postoperative management of pulmonary hypertension in infants and children with congenital heart disease. *Cochrane Database Syst Rev.* 2005;CD005055.

11. Black HR. Calcium channel blockers in the treatment of hypertension and prevention of cardiovascular disease: results from major clinical trials. *Clin Cornerstone.* 2004;6:53–66.

12. Calvo C, Gil-Extremera B, Gomez-Fernandez P, et al. Doxazosin GITS versus standard doxazosin in mild to moderate hypertension. *Int J Cardiol.* 2005;101: 97–104.

13. Carter BL, Saseen JJ. Hypertension. In: DiPiro JT, et al, eds. *Pharmacotherapy: A Pathophysiological Approach.* 5th ed. New York: McGraw-Hill; 2002.

14. Cheng ZJ, Vapaatalo H, Mervaala E. Angiotensin II and vascular inflammation. *Med Sci Monit.* 2005;11: RA194–RA205.

15. Chobanian AV, Bakris GL, Black HR, et al. The Seventh Report of the Joint National Committee on Prevention, Detection, Evaluation, and Treatment of High Blood Pressure: the JNC 7 report. *JAMA.* 2003;289: 2560–2572.

16. Choi KL, Bakris GL. Hypertension treatment guidelines: practical implications. *Semin Nephrol.* 2005;25: 198–209.

17. Cockcroft J. Nebivolol: a review. *Expert Opin Pharmacother.* 2004;5:893–899.

18. Coy V. Genetics of essential hypertension. *J Am Acad Nurse Pract.* 2005;17:219–224.

19. de Champlain J. Do most antihypertensive agents have a sympatholytic action? *Curr Hypertens Rep.* 2001;3: 305–313.

20. Dell'Omo G, Penno G, Pucci L, et al. The vascular effects of doxazosin in hypertension complicated by metabolic syndrome. *Coron Artery Dis.* 2005;16:67–73.

21. DeQuattro V, Li D. Sympatholytic therapy in primary hypertension: a user friendly role for the future. *J Hum Hypertens.* 2002;16(suppl 1):S118–S123.

22. Diamond JA, Phillips RA. Hypertensive heart disease. *Hypertens Res.* 2005;28:191–202.

23. Doris PA, Fornage M. The transcribed genome and the heritable basis of essential hypertension. *Cardiovasc Toxicol.* 2005;5:95–108.

24. Dulin B, Abraham WT. Pharmacology of carvedilol. *Am J Cardiol.* 2004;93:3B–6B.

25. Dzau V. The cardiovascular continuum and renin-angiotensin–aldosterone system blockade. *J Hypertens Suppl.* 2005;23:S9–S17.

26. Ebrahim S, Smith GD. Lowering blood pressure: a systematic review of sustained effects of non-pharmacological interventions. *J Public Health Med.* 1998;20:441–448.

27. Eisenberg MJ, Brox A, Bestawros AN. Calcium channel blockers: an update. *Am J Med.* 2004;116:35–43.

28. Elliot WJ. Clinical features and management of selected hypertensive emergencies. *J Clin Hypertens.* 2004;6: 587–592.

29. Epstein M, Campese VM. Evolving role of calcium antagonists in the management of hypertension. *Med Clin North Am.* 2004;88:149–165.

30. Eslami P, Tuck M. The role of the sympathetic nervous system in linking obesity with hypertension in white versus black Americans. *Curr Hypertens Rep.* 2003;5:269–272.

31. Fahey T, Schroeder K, Ebrahim S. Interventions used to improve control of blood pressure in patients with hypertension. *Cochrane Database Syst Rev.* 2005; CD005182.

32. Farmer JA. Hypertension and the metabolic syndrome. *Curr Cardiol Rep.* 2004;6:427–433.

33. Fenves AZ, Ram CV. Drug treatment of hypertensive urgencies and emergencies. *Semin Nephrol.* 2005;25: 272–280.

34. Fitzpatrick JM, Desgrandchamps F. The clinical efficacy and tolerability of doxazosin standard and gastrointestinal therapeutic system for benign prostatic hyperplasia. *BJU Int.* 2005;95:575–579.

35. Fuchs FD. Diuretics: drugs of choice for the initial management of patients with hypertension. *Expert Rev Cardiovasc Ther.* 2003;1:35–41.

36. Fulton B, Wagstaff AJ, Sorkin EM. Doxazosin. An update of its clinical pharmacology and therapeutic applications in hypertension and benign prostatic hyperplasia. *Drugs.* 1995;49:295–320.

37. Garcia-Sainz JA, Villalobos-Molina R. The elusive alpha(1D)-adrenoceptor: molecular and cellular characteristics and integrative roles. *Eur J Pharmacol.* 2004;500:113–120.

38. Grassi G. Sympathetic and baroreflex function in hypertension: implications for current and new drugs. *Curr Pharm Des.* 2004;10:3579–3589.

39. Grassi G. Counteracting the sympathetic nervous system in essential hypertension. *Curr Opin Nephrol Hypertens.* 2004;13:513–519.

40. Grisk O. Sympatho-renal interactions in the determination of arterial pressure: role in hypertension. *Exp Physiol.* 2005;90:183–187.

41. Grisk O, Rettig R. Interactions between the sympathetic nervous system and the kidneys in arterial hypertension. *Cardiovasc Res.* 2004;61:238–246.

42. Grossman E, Messerli FH. Calcium antagonists. *Prog Cardiovasc Dis.* 2004;47:34–57.

43. Guyton AC, Hall JF. *Textbook of Medical Physiology.* 11th ed. Philadelphia: WB Saunders Co; 2006.

44. Hajjar I, Kotchen TA. Trends in prevalence, awareness, treatment, and control of hypertension in the United States, 1988–2000. *JAMA.* 2003;290:199–206.

45. Hertz RP, Unger AN, Cornell JA, Saunders E. Racial disparities in hypertension prevalence, awareness, and management. *Arch Intern Med.* 2005;165:2098–2104.

46. Holzgreve H. Combination versus monotherapy as initial treatment in hypertension. *Herz.* 2003;28: 725–732.

47. Hooper L, Bartlett C, Davey SG, Ebrahim S. Advice to reduce dietary salt for prevention of cardiovascular disease. *Cochrane Database Syst Rev.* 2004;CD003656.

48. Imumorin IG, Dong Y, Zhu H, et al. A gene-environment interaction model of stress-induced hypertension. *Cardiovasc Toxicol.* 2005;5:109–132.

49. Jacob S, Henriksen EJ. Metabolic properties of vasodilating beta blockers: management considerations for

hypertensive diabetic patients and patients with the metabolic syndrome. *J Clin Hypertens.* 2004;6:690–696.

50. Johnson JA, Turner ST. Hypertension pharmacogenomics: current status and future directions. *Curr Opin Mol Ther.* 2005;7:218–225.

51. Kaaja R, Manhem K, Tuomilehto J. Treatment of postmenopausal hypertension with moxonidine, a selective imidazoline receptor agonist. *Int J Clin Pract Suppl.* 2004;139:26–32.

52. Kinsella JP, Abman SH. Inhaled nitric oxide therapy in children. *Paediatr Respir Rev.* 2005;6:190–198.

53. Kon V, Jabs K. Angiotensin in atherosclerosis. *Curr Opin Nephrol Hypertens.* 2004;13:291–297.

54. Kunes J, Hojna S, Kadlecova M, et al. Altered balance of vasoactive systems in experimental hypertension: the role of relative NO deficiency. *Physiol Res.* 2004;53 (suppl 1):S23–S34.

55. Kuroedov A, Cosentino F, Luscher TF. Pharmacological mechanisms of clinically favorable properties of a selective beta1-adrenoceptor antagonist, nebivolol. *Cardiovasc Drug Rev.* 2004;22:155–168.

56. Lew M, Klonis E. Emergency management of eclampsia and severe pre-eclampsia. *Emerg Med.* 2003;15:361–368.

57. Lohmeier TE, Hildebrandt DA, Warren S, et al. Recent insights into the interactions between the baroreflex and the kidneys in hypertension. *Am J Physiol Regul Integr Comp Physiol.* 2005;288:R828–R836.

58. Lowe FC. Role of the newer alpha(1)-adrenergic-receptor antagonists in the treatment of benign prostatic hyperplasia-related lower urinary tract symptoms. *Clin Ther.* 2004;26:1701–1713.

59. Mahmud A, Feely J. Arterial stiffness and the renin-angiotensin–aldosterone system. *J Renin Angiotensin Aldosterone Syst.* 2004;5:102–108.

60. Malpas SC. What sets the long-term level of sympathetic nerve activity: is there a role for arterial baroreceptors? *Am J Physiol Regul Integr Comp Physiol.* 2004;286:R1–R12.

61. Manrique C, Lastra G, Whaley-Connell A, Sowers JR. Hypertension and the cardiometabolic syndrome. *J Clin Hypertens.* 2005;7:471–476.

62. Martin U, Hill C, O' Mahony D. Use of moxonidine in elderly patients with resistant hypertension. *J Clin Pharm Ther.* 2005;30:433–437.

63. Mason RP. Effects of calcium channel blockers on cellular apoptosis: implications for carcinogenic potential. *Cancer.* 1999;85:2093–2102.

64. Meier P, Maillard M, Burnier M. The future of angiotensin II inhibition in cardiovascular medicine. *Curr Drug Targets Cardiovasc Haematol Disord.* 2005;5:15–30.

65. Messerli FH. Calcium antagonists and beta-blockers: impact on cardiovascular and cerebrovascular events. *Clin Cornerstone.* 2004;6:18–27.

66. Messerli FH, Grossman E. The calcium antagonist controversy: a posthumous commentary. *Am J Cardiol.* 1998; 82(suppl 9B):35R–39R.

67. Messerli FH, Grossman E. Therapeutic controversies in hypertension. *Semin Nephrol.* 2005;25:227–235.

68. Messerli FH, Grossman E. Beta-blockers in hypertension: is carvedilol different? *Am J Cardiol.* 2004; 93:7B–12B.

69. Mogensen CE. New concepts in blood pressure-lowering management in diabetic patients: the case for early ACE inhibitor combination therapy with diuretics. *J Hum Hypertens.* 2005;19(suppl 1): S15–S20.

70. Moser M, Setaro J. Continued importance of diuretics and beta-adrenergic blockers in the management of hypertension. *Med Clin North Am.* 2004;88: 167–187.

71. Mulrow CD, Chiquette E, Angel L, et al. Dieting to reduce body weight for controlling hypertension in adults. *Cochrane Database Syst Rev.* 2000; CD000484.

72. Neutel JM. The use of combination drug therapy in the treatment of hypertension. *Prog Cardiovasc Nurs.* 2002;17:81–88.

73. Nicolson DJ, Dickinson HO, Campbell F, Mason JM. Lifestyle interventions or drugs for patients with essential hypertension: a systematic review. *J Hypertens.* 2004;22:2043–2048.

74. Oates JA, Brown NJ. Antihypertensive agents and the drug treatment of hypertension. In: Hardman JG, et al, eds. *The Pharmacological Basis of Therapeutics.* 10th ed. New York: McGraw-Hill; 2001.

75. Pescatello LS, Franklin BA, Fagard R, et al. American College of Sports Medicine position stand. Exercise and hypertension. *Med Sci Sports Exerc.* 2004;36: 533–553.

76. Pollock DM, Pollock JS. Endothelin and oxidative stress in the vascular system. *Curr Vasc Pharmacol.* 2005;3:365–367.

77. Pontremoli R, Leoncini G, Parodi A. Use of nifedipine in the treatment of hypertension. *Expert Rev Cardiovasc Ther.* 2005;3:43–50.

78. Prakash ES, Madanmohan, Pal GK. What is the ultimate goal in neural regulation of cardiovascular function? *Adv Physiol Educ.* 2004;28:100–101.

79. Psaty BM, Lumley T, Furberg CD, et al. Health outcomes associated with various antihypertensive therapies used as first-line agents: a network meta-analysis. *JAMA.* 2003;289:2534–2544.

80. Rahmouni K, Correia ML, Haynes WG, Mark AL. Obesity-associated hypertension: new insights into mechanisms. *Hypertension.* 2005;45:9–14.

81. Reiter MJ. Cardiovascular drug class specificity: beta-blockers. *Prog Cardiovasc Dis.* 2004;47:11–33.

82. Roche HM, Phillips C, Gibney MJ. The metabolic syndrome: the crossroads of diet and genetics. *Proc Nutr Soc.* 2005;64:371–377.

83. Roehrborn CG, Schwinn DA. Alpha1-adrenergic receptors and their inhibitors in lower urinary tract symptoms and benign prostatic hyperplasia. *J Urol.* 2004;171:1029–1035.

84. Sakai K, Sigmund CD. Molecular evidence of tissue renin-angiotensin systems: a focus on the brain. *Curr Hypertens Rep.* 2005;7:135–140.

85. Segura J, Garcia-Donaire JA, Ruilope LM. Calcium channel blockers and renal protection: insights from the latest clinical trials. *J Am Soc Nephrol.* 2005;16 (suppl 1):S64–S66.

86. Shirani J, Loredo ML, Eckelman WC, et al. Imaging the renin-angiotensin–aldosterone system in the heart. *Curr Heart Fail Rep.* 2005;2:78–86.

87. Sica DA. Calcium channel blockers and the kidney. *Clin Cornerstone.* 2004;6:39–52.

88. Sica DA. Diuretic-related side effects: development and treatment. *J Clin Hypertens.* 2004;6:532–540.

89. Sica DA. Minoxidil: an underused vasodilator for resistant or severe hypertension. *J Clin Hypertens.* 2004;6:283–287.

90. Sica DA. Calcium channel blocker class heterogeneity: select aspects of pharmacokinetics and pharmacodynamics. *J Clin Hypertens.* 2005;7(suppl 1):21–26.

91. Steers WD, Kirby RS. Clinical ease of using doxazosin in BPH patients with and without hypertension. *Prostate Cancer Prostatic Dis.* 2005;8:152–157.

92. Steffen HM. Use of calcium channel antagonists for the treatment of hypertension in the elderly. *Drugs Aging.* 2004;21:565–581.

93. Svetkey LP, Erlinger TP, Vollmer WM, et al. Effect of lifestyle modifications on blood pressure by race, sex, hypertension status, and age. *J Hum Hypertens.* 2005; 19:21–31.

94. Szabo B. Imidazoline antihypertensive drugs: a critical review on their mechanism of action. *Pharmacol Ther.* 2002;93:1–35.

95. Taylor P. Agents acting at the neuromuscular junction and autonomic ganglia. In: Hardman JG, et al, eds. *The Pharmacological Basis of Therapeutics.* 10th ed. New York: McGraw-Hill; 2001.

96. Thrasher TN. Baroreceptors, baroreceptor unloading, and the long-term control of blood pressure. *Am J Physiol Regul Integr Comp Physiol.* 2005;288:R819–R827.

97. Toda N. Vasodilating beta-adrenoceptor blockers as cardiovascular therapeutics. *Pharmacol Ther.* 2003;100: 215–234.

98. Toto RD. Management of hypertensive chronic kidney disease: role of calcium channel blockers. *J Clin Hypertens.* 2005;7(suppl 1):15–20.

99. Touyz RM. Intracellular mechanisms involved in vascular remodelling of resistance arteries in hypertension: role of angiotensin II. *Exp Physiol.* 2005;90: 449–455.

100. Tuncel M, Ram VC. Hypertensive emergencies: etiology and management. *Am J Cardiovasc Drugs.* 2003;3:21–31.

101. Tuomilehto J. Cardiovascular risk: prevention and treatment of the metabolic syndrome. *Diabetes Res Clin Pract.* 2005;68(suppl 2):S28–S35.

102. Ueshiba H, Miyachi Y. Effect of doxazosin on insulin resistance in hypertensive patients with obesity. *Horm Metab Res.* 2003;35:532–536.

103. Unger T. Blood pressure lowering and renin-angiotensin system blockade. *J Hypertens Suppl.* 2003;21:S3–S7.

104. van Zwieten PA. Centrally acting imidazoline I1-receptor agonists: do they have a place in the management of hypertension? *Am J Cardiovasc Drugs.* 2001;1:321–326.

105. Volpe M, Ruilope LM, McInnes GT, Waeber B, Weber MA. Angiotensin-II receptor blockers: benefits beyond blood pressure reduction? *J Hum Hypertens.* 2005;19:331–339.

106. von Bohlen, Halbach O. The renin-angiotensin system in the mammalian central nervous system. *Curr Protein Pept Sci.* 2005;6:355–371.

107. Weber MA. Calcium channel antagonists in the treatment of hypertension. *Am J Cardiovasc Drugs.* 2002;2: 415–431.

108. White WB. Update on the drug treatment of hypertension in patients with cardiovascular disease. *Am J Med.* 2005;118:695–705.

109. Wong J, Patel RA, Kowey PR. The clinical use of angiotensin-converting enzyme inhibitors. *Prog Cardiovasc Dis.* 2004;47:116–130.

110. Yasuda G, Hasegawa K, Kuji T, et al. Effects of doxazosin on ambulatory blood pressure and sympathetic nervous activity in hypertensive type 2 diabetic patients with overt nephropathy. *Diabet Med.* 2005;22:1394–1400.

111. Yudkin JS. Mechanisms of vascular disease in hypertension with special reference to diabetes. *Semin Vasc Med.* 2002;2:139–148.

112. Zanchetti A. Clinical pharmacodynamics of nebivolol: new evidence of nitric oxide-mediated vasodilating activity and peculiar haemodynamic properties in hypertensive patients. *Blood Press Suppl.* 2004;1:17–32.

113. Zannad F. Managing hypertension: a question of STRATHE. *J Hum Hypertens.* 2005;19(suppl 1): S3–S7.

Chapter 22

Treatment of Angina Pectoris

Angina pectoris is pain that occurs in the chest region during ischemic heart disease. Attacks of angina pectoris begin suddenly and are often described as a sensation of intense compression and tightness in the retrosternal region, with pain sometimes radiating to the jaw or left arm. In many patients, episodes of angina pectoris are precipitated by physical exertion. Some forms of angina, however, may occur spontaneously even when the patient is at rest or asleep.

The basic problem in angina pectoris is that the supply of oxygen to the heart is insufficient to meet myocardial demands at a given point in time, which results in an imbalance between myocardial oxygen supply and demand (Fig. 22–1).[6,34] This imbalance leads to myocardial ischemia, which results in several metabolic, electrophysiologic, and contractile changes in the heart. The painful symptoms inherent to angina pectoris seem to result from the accumulation of metabolic by-products such as lactic acid. Presumably, these metabolic by-products act as nociceptive substances and trigger the painful compressive sensations characteristic of angina pectoris.

Although angina pectoris is believed to be caused by the buildup of lactic acid and other metabolites, the exact mechanisms responsible for mediating anginal pain remain unknown. Also, the emotional state of the patient and other factors that influence central pain perception play an obvious role in angina pectoris.[20,34] In fact, the majority of anginal attacks may be silent in many patients, and myocardial ischemia may fre-

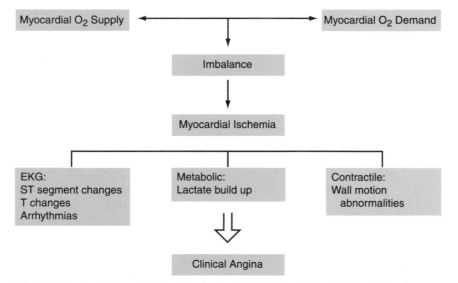

FIGURE 22–1 ▼ Myocardial ischemia equation. (*Adapted from:* Miller AB. Mixed ischemic subsets. Comparison of the mechanism of silent ischemia and mixed angina. *Am J Med.* 1985;79 [suppl 3a]:25, with permission.)

quently occur without producing any symptoms.[7,31] Certain patients may also exhibit symptoms of angina even though their coronary arteries appear to be normal and there is no obvious obstruction to coronary blood flow.[5,57] Clearly, there is much information regarding the nature of angina pectoris still remaining to be clarified.

Considering the prevalence of ischemic heart disease in the United States, many patients receiving physical therapy and occupational therapy may suffer from angina pectoris. These patients may be undergoing rehabilitation for a variety of clinical disorders, including (but not limited to) coronary artery disease. This chapter describes the primary drug groups used to treat angina pectoris, as well as the pharmacologic management of specific forms of angina. Physical therapists and occupational therapists should be aware of the manner in which these drugs work and the ways in which antianginal drugs can influence patient performance in rehabilitation sessions.

Drugs Used to Treat Angina Pectoris

Three drug groups are typically used to treat the symptoms of angina pectoris: organic nitrates, beta blockers, and calcium channel blockers. These drugs exert various effects that help restore or maintain the balance between myocardial oxygen supply and myocardial oxygen demand. The effects of these drug categories and specific agents within each category are presented here.

Organic Nitrates

Mechanism of Action and Rationale for Use

Organic nitrates consist of drugs such as nitroglycerin, isosorbide dinitrate, and isosorbide mononitrate (Table 22–1). The ability of these agents to dilate vascular smooth muscle is well established. Nitrates are actually drug precursors (prodrugs) that become activated when they are converted to nitric oxide within vascular smooth muscle.[16,26] Nitric oxide causes vasodilation by increasing the production of cyclic guanosine monophosphate (cGMP) within the muscle cell. Cyclic GMP acts as a second messenger that inhibits smooth-

Table 22–1	ORGANIC NITRATES	
Dosage Form	Onset of Action	Duration of Action
Nitroglycerin		
Oral	20–45 min	4–6 hr
Buccal (extended release)	2–3 min	3–5 hr
Sublingual/lingual	1–3 min	30–60 min
Ointment	30 min	4–8 hr
Transdermal patches	Within 30 min	8–24 hr
Isosorbide dinitrate		
Oral	15–40 min	4–6 hr
Oral (extended release)	30 min	12 hr
Chewable	2–5 min	1–2 hr
Sublingual	2–5 min	1–2 hr
Isosorbide mononitrate		
Oral	30–60 min	6–8 hr
Amyl nitrite		
Inhaled	30 sec	3–5 min

muscle contraction, probably by initiating the phosphorylation of specific contractile proteins.[41]

For years nitrates were believed to relieve angina attacks by dilating the coronary arteries; that is, they supposedly increased blood flow to the myocardium, thereby increasing myocardial oxygen supply. We now know, however, that these drugs exert their primary antianginal effects by producing a general vasodilation in the vasculature throughout the body, not just in the coronary vessels.[31] By producing dilation in the systemic venous system, nitrates decrease the amount of blood returning to the heart (cardiac preload). By dilating systemic peripheral arterioles, these drugs decrease the pressure against which the heart must pump (cardiac afterload). A decrease in cardiac preload and afterload decreases the amount of work the heart must perform; hence, myocardial oxygen demand decreases.

Consequently, nitroglycerin and other organic nitrates seem to primarily decrease myocardial oxygen demand rather than directly increase oxygen supply. Nitrates can also dilate the coronary arteries to some extent; these drugs are documented to have an increase in coronary artery flow.[31] The *primary* way that these drugs relieve angina pectoris, however, is through their ability to decrease cardiac work, thus decreasing myocardial oxygen demand.

Specific Agents

Nitroglycerin (Nitro-Bid, Nitrostat, Nitro-Dur, many others). In addition to being used as a powerful explosive, nitroglycerin is perhaps the most well known antianginal drug. The explosive nature of this agent is rendered inactive by diluting it with lactose, alcohol, or propylene glycol. Nitroglycerin is administered for both the prevention and treatment of anginal attacks and is available in oral, buccal, sublingual, and transdermal forms (see Table 22–1).

Sublingual administration of nitroglycerin is the best method to treat an acute attack of angina. Placed under the tongue, the drug is rapidly absorbed through the oral mucosa into the systemic circulation. Therapeutic effects usually begin within 2 minutes when nitroglycerin is administered sublingually. Sublingual administration also spares the nitroglycerin from the first-pass effect because the drug is able to reach the systemic circulation before first passing through the liver, where it is inactivated (see Chapter 2).

Extended-release versions of this drug, which can be taken buccally (between the cheek and gum), have been developed for the prevention of angina. Likewise, nitroglycerin can be delivered via an aerosol form that is sprayed on or under the tongue (lingual spray). Oral preparations have also been developed, but this method of administration is limited because—as previously mentioned—nitroglycerin undergoes extensive first-pass degradation in the liver when absorbed directly from the intestines.

For prophylaxis of angina, nitroglycerin can also be administered transdermally via ointment or medicated patches placed on the skin (see Table 22–1). Nitroglycerin-impregnated patches or disks are applied cutaneously like a small bandage, with the drug slowly and continuously absorbed through the skin and into the systemic circulation.[31] Transdermal administration of nitroglycerin using these patches has been regarded favorably because of its ease and convenience. By providing fairly continuous and sustained administration, nitroglycerin can also help prevent the onset of an anginal episode in many patients.

One problem associated with the nitroglycerin patch is that continuous nitroglycerin administration will cause drug tolerance, thus reducing the antianginal effectiveness of this medication.[8,33] The exact reasons for this tolerance are not fully understood and may involve a decrease in the ability to convert nitroglycerin to nitric oxide, a decrease in the responsiveness of the vasculature to nitric oxide, an increased sensitivity to endogenous vasoconstrictors, or a combination of these and other factors.[33,41,53] Tolerance to nitrate drugs is rather short-lived, however, and normal responses to nitrate drugs can be restored within only a few hours after withdrawing these agents.[47]

Consequently, patients may benefit from having at least an 8-hour interval each day when they do not wear their patches. Daily administration, for example, might be optimized by wearing the patch for 12 to 14 hours followed by a 10- to 12-hour nitrate-free interval.[47] This method of intermittent nitroglycerin administration may provide beneficial effects with less chance of developing drug tolerance.[1] The drawback, of course, is that the patient will be more susceptible to angina attacks during the nitrate-free interval. Hence, intermittent nitrate use must be monitored carefully in each patient to make sure that the patch provides adequate protection during the part of day or night when angina is likely to occur, without leaving the patient especially vulnerable during the nondrug interval.

Nitroglycerin ointment is another way to provide continuous transdermal administration.[47] The ointment is applied directly to the skin on the patient's chest or back, in much the same way as any topical ointment or skin cream. Although somewhat messy and inconvenient, nitroglycerin ointment may be helpful in preventing angina in certain situations, such as when the patient is sleeping.[31] This method is not as popular as transdermal patches, however, because patches are more convenient and easier to apply. Likewise, tolerance may occur if nitroglycerin is applied continually through topical ointments.

Isosorbide Dinitrate Like nitroglycerin, isosorbide dinitrate is used for the treatment of acute episodes of angina as well as for the prevention of anginal attacks. The antianginal and hemodynamic effects last longer with isosorbide dinitrate, however, so this drug is often classified as a long-acting nitrate.[31] For acute attacks, isosorbide dinitrate is administered sublingually, buccally, or by chewable tablets (see Table 22–1). For prevention of angina, oral tablets are usually given.

Isosorbide Mononitrate This drug is another long-acting nitrate that is similar in structure and function to isosorbide dinitrate. It is typically given orally for prevention of anginal attacks.

Amyl Nitrite This drug is supplied in small ampules that can be broken open to inhale during acute anginal attacks. Absorption of the drug through the nasal membranes causes peripheral vasodilation and decreased cardiac preload and afterload. Clinical use of inhaled amyl nitrite is very limited, however, and this type of antianginal treatment has generally been replaced by safer and more convenient methods of nitrate administration (e.g., nitroglycerin patches).

Adverse Side Effects of Nitrates

The primary adverse effects associated with organic nitrates are headache, dizziness, and orthostatic hypotension.[47] These effects are related to the drugs' ability to dilate peripheral blood vessels and decrease peripheral resistance. Nausea may also be a problem in some patients. As indicated earlier, tolerance to the beneficial effects of nitrates can occur during continuous administration, but providing daily nitrate-free intervals should prevent this problem.

Beta-Adrenergic Blockers

Mechanism of Action and Rationale for Use

By antagonizing beta-1 receptors on the myocardium, beta blockers tend to decrease the heart rate and force of myocardial contraction,[12] thus producing an obvious decrease in the work that the heart must perform and a decrease in myocardial oxygen demand. Beta block-

ers help maintain an appropriate balance between myocardial oxygen supply and demand by preventing an increase in myocardial oxygen demand.

Consequently, beta blockers are given to certain patients with angina to limit the oxygen demands of the heart.[12,31] This prophylactic administration prevents the onset of an anginal attack. The use of beta blockers in specific forms of angina is reviewed later in this chapter.

Specific Agents

Individual beta blockers were discussed in Chapter 20; beta blockers effective in treating angina pectoris are listed in Table 22–2. Various beta blockers seem to display a fairly equal ability to decrease episodes of stable angina pectoris.[31] However, certain beta-blockers may be more favorable in some patients because the side effects are more tolerable, or because the dosing schedule is more convenient (i.e., the drug needs to be given only once each day rather than in several doses). Likewise, some of the newer beta blockers may have other properties that might provide additional benefits. Newer agents such as carvedilol (Coreg), for example, produce peripheral vasodilation that can be advantageous in patients with angina who also have hypertension.[49] Certain beta blockers are also helpful in preventing sudden death after myocardial infarction, so these agents may be especially useful in treating angina in a patient recovering from a heart attack.[12,31] The choice of a specific beta blocker therefore depends on the pharmacologic profile of each drug in conjunction the particular needs of each patient.[47]

Table 22–2	BETA BLOCKERS USED TO TREAT ANGINA PECTORIS	
Generic Name	**Trade Name**	**Usual Oral Dose**
Acebutolol	Sectral	200–600 mg 2 times a day
Atenolol	Tenormin	50–100 mg once a day
Carteolol	Cartrol	2.5–10.0 mg once a day
Labetalol	Normodyne, Trandate	200–400 mg 2 times a day
Metoprolol	Lopressor, others	50–200 mg 2 times a day
Nadolol	Corgard	40–240 mg once a day
Penbutolol	Levatol	20 mg once a day
Pindolol	Visken	5–20 mg 2 times a day
Propranolol	Inderal	40–80 mg 2–4 times a day
Sotalol	Betapace	80–160 mg 2 times a day
Timolol	Blocadren	10–30 mg 2 times a day

Adverse Side Effects

Beta blockers that bind to both beta-1 and beta-2 receptors (nonselective agents, see Table 20–2) may induce bronchoconstriction in patients with asthma or similar respiratory problems. These patients should be given one of the more cardioselective beta antagonists, such as atenolol (Tenormin) or metoprolol (Lopressor, others). Beta blockers may also produce excessive cardiac depression in individuals with certain types of cardiac disease. Beta blockers are generally well tolerated in most patients, however, and major problems are infrequent.

Calcium Channel Blockers

Mechanism of Action and Rationale for Use

These drugs block the entry of calcium into vascular smooth muscle.[9,39] In vascular smooth muscle, calcium ions facilitate contraction by initiating actin-myosin interaction. Calcium channel blockers decrease the entry of calcium into vascular smooth-muscle cells, thus causing relaxation and vasodilation. By blocking calcium entry into coronary artery smooth muscle, these drugs mediate coronary vasodilation, with a subsequent increase in the supply of oxygen to the myocardium. Consequently, a primary role of calcium channel blockers in angina pectoris is to directly increase coronary blood flow, thus increasing myocardial oxygen supply.[24,31]

Calcium channel blockers also cause some degree of systemic vasodilation, and some of their antianginal effects may be related to a decrease in myocardial oxygen demand caused by a decrease in cardiac preload and afterload; that is, they may exert some of their beneficial effects in a manner similar to that of organic nitrates.[47] Also, calcium channel blockers limit the entry of calcium into cardiac striated cells, thus decreasing myocardial contractility and oxygen demand. The *primary* beneficial effects of these drugs in angina pectoris, however, are related to their ability to dilate the coronary arteries and peripheral vasculature. Certain calcium channel blockers can also affect myocardial excitability by altering the conduction of electrical activity throughout the myocardium.[9] This effect seems to be more important when these drugs are used to treat cardiac arrhythmias (see Chapter 23).

The calcium channel blockers currently used to treat angina pectoris are listed in Table 22–3. Although the chemistry and exact mechanism of action of each drug are somewhat distinct, all of these agents exert their effects by limiting calcium entry into specific cardiovascular tissues. Certain calcium channel blockers are said to be "selective" if they affect vascular smooth muscle, but have little or no affect on the heart. Nonselective calcium channel blockers affect the vasculature and inhibit calcium entry into cardiac muscle cells. Individual agents are discussed below.

Specific Agents

Bepridil (Vascor). Bepridil is a nonselective calcium channel blocker that inhibits calcium influx into vascular smooth muscle and cardiac striated muscle. It can vasodilate coronary and peripheral vessels, hence its use in angina pectoris. Bepridil also decreases heart rate (negative chronotropic effect) and cardiac contractility (negative inotropic effect) through an inhibitory effect on the myocardium. These negative chronotropic and negative inotropic effects can be problematic, especially if this drug is combined with beta blockers or other drugs that inhibit heart rate and contractility.[45]

Table 22–3	CALCIUM CHANNEL BLOCKERS	
Generic Name	**Trade Name**	**Usual Oral Antianginal Dose**
Amlodipine	Norvasc	5–10 mg once a day
Bepridil	Vascor	200–300 mg once a day
Diltiazem	Cardizem, Dilacor	30–90 mg 3 or 4 times a day
Felodipine	Plendil	10 mg once a day
Isradipine	DynaCirc	2.5–10 mg 2 times a day
Nicardipine	Cardene	20 mg 3 times a day
Nifedipine	Adalat, Procardia	10–30 mg 3 or 4 times a day
Verapamil	Calan, Isoptin, Verelan	80–160 mg 3 times a day

Diltiazem (Cardizem, Dilacor). Like the other calcium channel blockers, diltiazem is able to vasodilate the coronary arteries and the peripheral vasculature. Diltiazem also produces some depression of electrical conduction in the sinoatrial and atrioventricular nodes, an effect that may cause slight bradycardia. This bradycardia can be worsened by beta blockers or in patients with myocardial conduction problems, and diltiazem should probably be avoided in these individuals.[32,45]

Nifedipine (Adalat, Procardia) and Other Dihydropyridines. Nifedipine and similar drugs are members of the dihydropyridine class of calcium channel blockers. This class is distinguished by drugs with an *-ipine* suffix, including felodipine (Plendil), isradipine (DynaCirc), and nicardipine (Cardene). These drugs are relatively selective for vascular smooth muscle as compared to cardiac striated muscle, and they vasodilate the coronary arteries and peripheral vasculature without exerting any direct effects on cardiac excitability or contractility.[31] These drugs are therefore advantageous when treating patients with angina who also have certain types of cardiac arrhythmias or problems with cardiac excitation and conduction.[9] Nifedipine and similar drugs may, however, produce reflex tachycardia, which is a compensatory increase in heart rate occurring when peripheral vascular resistance decreases because of the drug-induced vasodilation. Other nondihydropyridine drugs (diltiazem, verapamil) also lower vascular resistance, but reflex tachycardia is prevented because these drugs also have an inhibitory effect on heart rate (negative chronotropic effect). If reflex tachycardia does occur with nifedipine, this problem can be controlled by using sustained-release or long-acting forms of these drugs (see "Adverse Side Effects").

Verapamil (Calan, Isoptin). Verapamil has been used to treat angina because of its ability to vasodilate the coronary vessels. Verapamil, however, seems to be moderately effective compared to the other antianginal drugs, and verapamil also depresses myocardial excitability and decreases heart rate.[9,32] Because of its negative effects on cardiac excitation, verapamil is probably more useful in controlling certain cardiac arrhythmias (see Chapter 23).

Adverse Side Effects

The primary problems associated with the calcium channel blockers are related to the peripheral vasodilation produced by these agents. Headache, flushing or feelings of warmth, and dizziness may occur in some patients. Peripheral edema, as evidenced by swelling in the feet and legs, may also occur, and nausea is fairly common. Nonselective calcium channel blockers that affect the myocardium (e.g., bepridil, diltiazem, verapamil) can cause disturbances in cardiac rhythm. As indicated, reflex tachycardia can also be a problem, especially with nifedipine and other dihydropyridine calcium channel blockers ("-ipine" drugs) that selectively decrease vascular resistance without simultaneously inhibiting heart rate.

There has been some concern about the safety of the calcium channel blockers. In particular, reports indicated that certain calcium channel blockers, such as the short-acting form of nifedipine, may be associated with an increased risk of myocardial infarction in certain patients (older patients with hypertension, patients with unstable angina).[21,29]

The short-acting or immediate-release form of nifedipine and other "-ipine" calcium channel blockers can be problematic because these drugs may cause a fairly rapid decrease in peripheral vascular resistance and blood pressure.[46] A rapid fall in vascular resistance and blood pressure can precipitate reflex hemodynamic changes (increased heart rate, decreased myocardial perfusion), which leads to ischemia and infarction in susceptible patients. Sustained-release or longer-acting forms of nifedipine and similar agents may be somewhat safer because they do not cause as rapid a change in vascular resistance as the short-acting drugs.[11,24]

Preliminary studies also suggested that calcium channel blockers my increase the risk of cancer.[10,28] Intracellular calcium levels are important in regulating cell division. By modifying calcium influx, calcium channel blockers could conceivably accelerate cell proliferation and lead to cancerous growths. Fortunately, the carcinogenic potential of these drugs has not been proven conclusively by subsequent studies.[21] Hence, calcium channel blockers continue to be used cautiously but effectively in large numbers of patients.

Use of Anticoagulants in Angina Pectoris

Angina pectoris is typically associated with some degree of coronary artery occlusion. To help prevent further blockage of the coronary arteries, certain anticoagulant drugs can be administered so that a partially occluded artery does not become completely blocked and cause myocardial infarction.[15,52] The most common agents used in this situation are heparin and platelet inhibitors such as aspirin.[23,52] The pharmacology and anticoagulant effects of these drugs are discussed in detail in Chapter 25, and their use in angina is addressed briefly here.

Heparin is often used during the initial or acute phase of unstable angina to prevent clot formation at atherosclerotic plaques that may have ruptured in the coronary arteries.[14,15] Heparin is a fast-acting anticoagulant that leads to the inhibition of thrombin, a key component of the clotting mechanism. With regard to their use in angina, low molecular weight heparins (LMWH) such as enoxaparin (Lovenox) seem to be especially advantageous because they produce a more predictable anticoagulant response and are tolerated better than more traditional (unfractionated) heparin.[14,23,56] Heparin must, however, be administered parenterally, and LMWHs are usually given via subcutaneous injection.

Aspirin and other drugs that reduce platelet activity are essential in preventing platelet-induced clotting in the coronary arteries and other vascular tissues.[50] As discussed in Chapter 15, aspirin inhibits the biosynthesis of prostaglandins, and certain prostaglandins are responsible for activating platelets during the clotting process. In angina pectoris, aspirin administration can prevent platelets from becoming activated in partially occluded coronary vessels, and therefore helps maintain blood flow through these vessels.[36]

Aspirin is administered orally, and is often used for the long-term management of platelet-induced clotting in people with angina. Aspirin, however, only produces a moderate amount of platelet inhibition, and stronger antiplatelet drugs are also available. Drugs such as clopidogrel (Plavix), for example, block the effects of adenosine diphosphate (ADP) on the platelet, thereby reducing the ability of ADP to activate the platelet.[19,27] These stronger antiplatelet drugs can be used alone or added to aspirin therapy in patients who are at high risk for infarction.[3,50]

Heparin and antiplatelet drugs are therefore used in various forms of angina to help prevent infarction. When administered with the traditional anti-anginal medications, these anticoagulants can help decrease morbidity and mortality in people with ischemic heart disease. For more details on the effects of anticoagulant medications, please refer to Chapter 25.

Treatment of Specific Types of Angina Pectoris

All forms of angina pectoris are not the same. Traditionally, angina has been subclassified according to factors that precipitate the angina and the pathophysiologic mechanisms responsible for producing myocardial ischemia.[6] The major forms of angina and the primary drugs used to treat each type are discussed here and summarized in Table 22–4.

Table 22–4	TYPES OF ANGINA PECTORIS	
Classification	**Cause**	**Drug Therapy**
Stable angina	Myocardial oxygen demand exceeds oxygen supply; usually brought on by physical exertion	Sublingual/lingual nitroglycerin is typically used at the onset of an acute episode; a beta blocker or a long-acting nitrate is often used to prevent attacks
Variant angina	Myocardial oxygen supply decreases due to coronary vasospasm; may occur while patient is at rest	Treated primarily with a calcium channel blocker
Unstable angina	Myocardial oxygen supply decreases at the same time oxygen demand increases; can occur at any time secondary to atherosclerotic plaque rupture within the coronary artery	May require a combination of drugs—that is, a calcium channel blocker plus a beta blocker. Anticoagulant drugs are also helpful in preventing thrombogenesis and coronary occlusion

Stable Angina

Stable angina is the most common form of ischemic heart disease.[47] The primary problem in stable angina is that myocardial oxygen demand greatly exceeds oxygen supply. Stable angina is also frequently referred to as effort, or exertional, angina, since attacks are usually precipitated by a certain level of physical exertion. If the patient exercises beyond a certain level of his or her capacity, the coronary arteries are unable to deliver the oxygen needed to sustain that level of myocardial function, and an anginal episode occurs. The inability of the coronary arteries to adequately deliver oxygen in stable angina is usually caused by some degree of permanent coronary artery occlusion (e.g., coronary artery atherosclerosis or stenosis).

Because stable angina is caused primarily by an increase in myocardial oxygen demand, treatment of this form of angina has mainly consisted of beta blockers and organic nitrates.[13,47] Beta blockers are often the first drugs used in the long-term management of stable angina because they decrease the workload of the heart, thus limiting myocardial oxygen requirements.[12] Hence, beta-blockers are often taken orally on a daily basis to prevent the onset of an angina episode.

The primary drug strategy for managing an acute attack consists of an organic nitrate in the form of nitroglycerin.[13] Nitroglycerin is often applied via sublingual tablets or lingual sprays at the onset of an attack or just before exercise or other activities that routinely precipitate an attack. As previously mentioned, the sublingual route allows rapid drug effects while avoiding the first pass effect. Nitrates can also be given as a preventive measure to blunt myocardial oxygen needs, and nitroglycerin can be administered transdermally through patches or ointments, or a long-acting nitrate (isosorbide dinitrate, isosorbide mononitrate) can be administered orally. As discussed earlier, however, long-term use of nitrates can cause tolerance, and an intermittent dosing procedure (i.e., daily nitrate-free intervals) should be instituted when these drugs are taken regularly to prevent angina.[13]

Calcium channel blockers can also be given to treat stable angina, especially if beta blockers are not tolerated or are contraindicated in specific patients.[13] These drugs decrease cardiac workload directly by limiting calcium entry into myocardial cells and indirectly by producing peripheral vasodilation, thus decreasing cardiac preload and afterload.[47] Hence, calcium channel blockers are administered in stable angina primarily for their effect on the myocardium and peripheral vasculature rather than for their ability to dilate the coronary arteries. Nonetheless, these drugs also produce some degree of coronary vasodilation, and this action may produce additional beneficial effects in certain patients with stable angina.[47]

The drugs discussed above can be used separately, but a combination of these antianginal drugs is also used in many patients with stable angina.[22] For example, a beta blocker and long-acting nitrate may be administered together, especially when either drug by itself is not completely successful in managing anginal episodes. Likewise, a beta blocker and calcium channel blocker may be used in combination,[22] but care must be taken to avoid excessive negative chronotropic and negative ionotropic effects on the heart (that is, nondihydropyridine calcium channel blockers can decrease heart rate and contraction force, which can add to the inhibitory effects of beta blockers on the heart).[45] Hence, beta blockers are typically combined with nifedipine or another dihydropyridine agent ("-ipine" drugs) when these two types of antianginal agents are used together.[36,45]

Finally, other drugs can be included to improve the general health and outcome in patient with stable angina. In particular, low-dose aspirin therapy or other antiplatelet strategies are important in decreasing the risk of thrombus formation and coronary infarction.[25,48] Drugs that decrease plasma lipids (e.g., statin drugs, see Chapter 25), and certain antihypertensives (e.g., angiotensin converting enzyme inhibitors, see Chapter 21), also play a prominent role in decreasing mortality in people with stable angina.[17,25] Clearly, a comprehensive medication regimen is needed for optimal management, and this regimen should be tailored to meet the individual needs of each patient.

Variant Angina (Prinzmetal Ischemia)

In variant angina, the primary problem is that oxygen supply to the myocardium *decreases* because of coronary artery vasospasm.[6,51] Vasospasm causes oxygen supply to decrease even though oxygen demand has not changed, and this phenomenon can occur even when the patient is at rest. In some patients with variant angina, the coronary arteries appear to be supersensitive to endogenous vasoconstrictive agents, and a variety of emotional or environmental stimuli may trigger coronary vasospasm.[18,30] In many patients, however, the reason for this spontaneous coronary vasoconstriction is unknown.

Calcium channel blockers are usually the drugs of choice in treating the variant form of angina.[18,51] These drugs limit the entry of calcium into the coronary vessels, thus attenuating or preventing the vasospasm underlying variant angina.[9] If calcium channel blockers are not tolerated, long-acting nitrates may be used instead. Calcium channel blockers are especially effective in treating variant angina, however, and most patients with this form of angina respond well to these agents. If patients do not respond to a single calcium channel blocker, long-acting nitrates may be added for management of severe variant angina.[18,51]

Unstable Angina

The more severe form of angina is often classified as "unstable" angina. This type of angina is often initiated by sudden rupture of atherosclerotic plaques within the coronary arteries, which precipitates coronary vasoconstriction and thrombus formation.[4,6] Plaque rupture can be brought on by exertion, or it may occur spontaneously when the patient is at rest. The primary defect in unstable angina, therefore, is a decrease in myocardial oxygen supply, although myocardial oxygen demand may be increasing simultaneously if the patient is exercising. Because unstable angina is also associated with thrombosis and increased platelet aggregation in the affected coronary arteries, this type of angina is often a precursor to acute myocardial infarction.[6] Together, unstable angina and myocardial infarction comprise the category of acute coronary syndromes.[2,38] Unstable angina is therefore regarded as the most serious and potentially dangerous form of angina.[43]

Various traditional antianginal drugs have been used alone or in combination to treat the ischemic symptoms of unstable angina.[35,47] Beta blockers, for example, are among the primary drugs because they decrease cardiac workload and thereby prevent subsequent damage to the ischemic myocardium.[12,31] Beta blockers can likewise be combined with the two other types of traditional antianginal medications (nitrates and calcium channel blockers), depending on the specific needs and responses of each patient.[47] Most

important, however, is the recognition that unstable angina is often associated with coronary artery thrombosis, and that anticoagulant and antiplatelet therapy is critical in preventing this type of angina from progressing to myocardial infarction.[44,47] Hence, anticoagulant drugs are often administered in the early stages of unstable angina, with antiplatelet drugs (aspirin, clopidogrel) being continued indefinitely to help prevent coronary occlusion.[54,55] Likewise, lipid lowering drugs such as the statins (see Chapter 25) are instrumental in providing long term benefits and preventing coronary occlusion in patients with unstable angina.[40,42]

Nonpharmacologic Management of Angina Pectoris

The primary drugs used to treat angina (nitrates, beta blockers, calcium channel blockers) are effective and relatively safe for long-term use. These agents, however, really only treat a symptom of heart disease, namely, the pain associated with myocardial ischemia. Traditional antianginal drugs do not cure any cardiac conditions, nor do they exert any beneficial long-term effects on cardiac function. Consequently, efforts are made in many patients with angina to resolve the underlying disorder responsible for causing an imbalance in myocardial oxygen supply and demand.

Nonpharmacologic treatment usually begins by identifying any potentiating factors that might initiate or exacerbate anginal attacks. For instance, hypertension, congestive heart failure, anemia, and thyrotoxicosis may all contribute to the onset of angina. In some cases, treatment of one of these potentiating factors may effectively resolve the angina, thus making subsequent drug therapy unnecessary. Lifestyle changes, including exercise, weight control, giving up smoking, and stress management, may also be helpful in decreasing or even eliminating the need for antianginal drugs. Finally, a number of surgical techniques that try to increase coronary blood flow may be attempted. Revascularization procedures such as coronary artery bypass and coronary artery angioplasty may be successful in increasing myocardial oxygen supply, thus attenuating anginal attacks in some patients. Regardless of what strategy is pursued, a permanent solution to the factors that precipitate myocardial ischemia should be explored in all patients with angina pectoris.

Special Concerns in Rehabilitation Patients

■ ■ ■ Physical therapists and occupational therapists must be aware of patients who are taking medications for angina pectoris and whether the medications are taken prophylactically or during an attack. For the patient with stable angina taking nitroglycerin at the onset of an anginal episode, therapists must make sure the drug is always nearby during therapy sessions. Since many activities in rehabilitation (exercise, functional training, etc.) increase myocardial oxygen demand, anginal attacks may occur during the therapy session. If the nitroglycerin tablets are in the patient's hospital room (inpatients) or were left at home (outpatients), the anginal attack will be prolonged and possibly quite severe. A little precaution in making sure patients bring their nitroglycerin to therapy can prevent some tense movements while waiting to see if an anginal attack will subside.

For patients taking antianginal drugs prophylactically (i.e., at regular intervals), having the drug actually present during the rehabilitation session is not as crucial, providing that the patient has been taking the medication as prescribed. Therapists must still be aware, however, that many rehabilitation activities may disturb the balance between myocardial oxygen supply and demand, particularly by increasing oxygen demand beyond the ability of the coronary arteries to increase oxygen supply to the heart. Consequently, therapists must be aware of the cardiac limitations in their patients with angina and use caution in not overtaxing the heart to the extent that the antianginal drugs are ineffective.

Another important consideration in rehabilitation is the effect of antianginal drugs on the response to an exercise bout. Some patients taking these drugs may experience an *increase* in exercise tolerance because the patient is not as limited by symptoms of angina.[37] Certain drugs, however, may blunt the ability of the heart to respond to an acute exercise bout. Beta blockers and certain calcium channel blockers, for instance, slow down heart rate and decrease myocardial contractility during exercise.[37] At any absolute exercise workload, the myocardial response (e.g., heart rate) of the patient taking these drugs will be lower than if the drug was not taken. Consequently, the heart may not be able to handle some workloads. This blunted exercise response must be taken into account when patients engage in cardiac conditioning activities, and exercise workloads should be adjusted accordingly.

Finally, therapists should be aware of how the side effects of the antianginal drugs may impact the therapy session. The nitrates and calcium channel blockers both produce peripheral vasodilation and can lead to hypotension. This decrease in blood pressure may be exaggerated when the patient suddenly sits or stands up (orthostatic hypotension). Also, conditions that produce peripheral vasodilation, such as heat or exercise, may produce an additive effect on the drug-induced hypotension, thus leading to dizziness and syncope. Therapists should be aware that patients taking nitrates and calcium channel blockers may experience hypotension when systemic heat is applied or when patients perform exercises that use large muscle groups.

CASE STUDY

Antianginal Drugs

Brief History. T.M. is a 73-year-old man who is retired from his job as an accountant. He has a long history of type 2 diabetes mellitus, which has progressively worsened over the past decade despite oral antidiabetic medication and insulin treatment. He also has a history of stable (classic) angina that has been managed by nitroglycerin. The patient self-administers a nitroglycerin tablet sublingually (0.4 mg per tablet) at the onset of an anginal attack. Recently, the patient was admitted to the hospital for treatment of a gangrenous lesion on his left foot. When this lesion failed to respond to conservative treatment, a left below-knee amputation was performed. Following the amputation, the patient was referred to physical therapy for strengthening and a preprosthetic evaluation.

Problem/Influence of Medication. A program of general conditioning and strengthening was initiated at the patient's bedside the day following surgery. On the third day, the therapist decided to bring the patient to the physical therapy department for a more intensive program, including standing activities with the parallel bars. The patient arrived in the department via wheelchair and began complaining immediately of chest pains. The patient had not brought his nitroglycerin tablets with him to the therapy session. The therapist immediately phoned the nursing floor, and the patient's medication was rushed to the physical therapy department. While waiting for the nitroglycerin to arrive, the patient's vital signs

were monitored and he was placed in a supine position on a mat table. The drug was administered sublingually while the patient remained supine, and his chest pain subsided.

Decision/Solution. Evidently, the exertion and apprehension of merely being transported to the physical therapy department was sufficient to trigger an attack of angina in this patient. The fact that his medication was not readily available created a rather anxious situation, which was fortunately resolved without any serious incident. To prevent a repeat of this predicament, the therapist contacted the nursing staff and requested that the patient always bring his medication with him to physical therapy. On subsequent occasions when the patient did experience the onset of angina, he was immediately placed in a supine position and the drug was administered sublingually. The patient was placed supine to prevent any orthostatic hypotension that may occur with nitroglycerin. He was eventually fitted with a temporary prosthesis and transferred to an extended-care facility to continue rehabilitation.

SUMMARY

Pain in the chest region, or angina pectoris, is a common symptom of ischemic heart disease. Anginal pain usually occurs because of an imbalance between myocardial oxygen supply and myocardial oxygen demand. Organic nitrates, beta blockers, and calcium channel blockers are the primary drugs used to treat angina pectoris. Organic nitrates and beta blockers primarily exert their effects by decreasing myocardial oxygen demand, whereas calcium channel blockers primarily increase myocardial oxygen supply. Several forms of angina pectoris can be identified, and specific types of antianginal drugs are used alone or in combination with each other to treat or prevent various forms of angina.

Rehabilitation specialists must be aware of any patients who have angina pectoris and the possibility of patients having an anginal attack during a therapy session. Therapists should also be cognizant of what drugs are being taken to control the patient's angina, as well as any side effects that may influence certain rehabilitation procedures.

References

1. Abrams J. How to use nitrates. *Cardiovasc Drugs Ther.* 2002;16:511–514.
2. Achar SA, Kundu S, Norcross WA. Diagnosis of acute coronary syndrome. *Am Fam Physician.* 2005;72: 119–126.
3. Atwater BD, Roe MT, Mahaffey KW. Platelet glycoprotein IIb/IIIa receptor antagonists in non-ST segment elevation acute coronary syndromes: a review and guide to patient selection. *Drugs.* 2005;65:313–324.
4. Boyle JJ. Macrophage activation in atherosclerosis: pathogenesis and pharmacology of plaque rupture. *Curr Vasc Pharmacol.* 2005;3:63–68.
5. Bugiardini R, Bairey Merz CN. Angina with "normal" coronary arteries: a changing philosophy. *JAMA.* 2005;293:477–484.
6. Cassady SL. Cardiovascular pathophysiology. In: DeTurk WE, Cahalin LP, eds. *Cardiovascular and Pulmonary Physical Therapy.* New York: McGraw-Hill; 2004.
7. Cohn PF. Silent myocardial ischemia: recent developments. *Curr Atheroscler Rep.* 2005;7:155–163.
8. Csont T, Ferdinandy P. Cardioprotective effects of glyceryl trinitrate: beyond vascular nitrate tolerance. *Pharmacol Ther.* 2005;105:57–68.
9. DeWitt CR, Waksman JC. Pharmacology, pathophysiology and management of calcium channel blocker and beta-blocker toxicity. *Toxicol Rev.* 2004;23:223–238.
10. Dong EW, Connelly JE, Borden SP, et al. A systematic review and meta-analysis of the incidence of cancer in randomized, controlled trials of verapamil. *Pharmacotherapy.* 1997;17:1210–1219.
11. Eisenberg MJ, Brox A, Bestawros AN. Calcium channel blockers: an update. *Am J Med.* 2004;116:35–43.
12. Ellison KE, Gandhi G. Optimising the use of beta-adrenoceptor antagonists in coronary artery disease. *Drugs.* 2005;65:787–797.

13. Fihn SD, Williams SV, Daley J, et al. Guidelines for the management of patients with chronic stable angina: treatment. *Ann Intern Med.* 2001;135:616–632.

14. Gouin-Thibault I, Pautas E, Siguret V. Safety profile of different low-molecular weight heparins used at therapeutic dose. *Drug Saf.* 2005;28:333–349.

15. Granger CB, Weaver WD. Reducing cardiac events after acute coronary syndromes. *Rev Cardiovasc Med.* 2004;5(suppl 5):S39–S46.

16. Hashimoto S, Kobayashi A. Clinical pharmacokinetics and pharmacodynamics of glyceryl trinitrate and its metabolites. *Clin Pharmacokinet.* 2003;42:205–221.

17. Jain A, Wadehra V, Timmis AD. Management of stable angina. *Postgrad Med J.* 2003;79:332–336.

18. Keller KB, Lemberg L. Prinzmetal's angina. *Am J Crit Care.* 2004;13:350–354.

19. Kerr JL, Oppelt TF, Rowen RC. Role of clopidogrel in unstable angina and non-ST-segment elevation myocardial infarction: from literature and guidelines to practice. *Pharmacotherapy.* 2004;24:1037–1049.

20. Ketterer MW, Mahr G, Cao JJ, et al. What's "unstable" in unstable angina? *Psychosomatics.* 2004;45: 185–196.

21. Kizer JR, Kimmel SE. Epidemiologic review of the calcium channel blocker drugs. An up-to-date perspective on the proposed hazards. *Arch Intern Med.* 2001; 161:1145–1158.

22. Klein WW, Jackson G, Tavazzi L. Efficacy of monotherapy compared with combined antianginal drugs in the treatment of chronic stable angina pectoris: a meta-analysis. *Coron Artery Dis.* 2002;13:427–436.

23. Korkmaz ME. Low-molecular-weight heparins in acute coronary syndromes. *Curr Vasc Pharmacol.* 2003;1:259–271.

24. Kumar S, Hall RJ. Drug treatment of stable angina pectoris in the elderly: defining the place of calcium channel antagonists. *Drugs Aging.* 2003;20:805–815.

25. Lettino M, Falcone C, Tavazzi L. Therapeutic approach in patients with stable angina. *Ital Heart J.* 2005;6:1–8.

26. Li H, Cui H, Liu X, Zweier JL. Xanthine oxidase catalyzes anaerobic transformation of organic nitrates to nitric oxide and nitrosothiols: characterization of this mechanism and the link between organic nitrate and guanylyl cyclase activation. *J Biol Chem.* 2005;280: 16594–16600.

27. Manoharan G, Adgey AA. Current management of unstable angina: lessons from the TACTICS-TIMI 18 trial. *Am J Cardiovasc Drugs.* 2002;2:237–243.

28. Mason RP. Effects of calcium channel blockers on cellular apoptosis: implications for carcinogenic potential. *Cancer.* 1999;85:2093–2102.

29. Massie BM. The safety of calcium-channel blockers. *Clin Cardiol.* 1998;21(suppl 2):II12–II17.

30. Mayer S, Hillis LD. Prinzmetal's variant angina. *Clin Cardiol.* 1998;21:243–246.

31. Michel T. Treatment of myocardial ischemia. In: Brunton L, et al, eds. *The Pharmacologic Basis of Therapeutics.* 10th ed. New York: McGraw-Hill; 2006.

32. Mills TA, Kawji MM, Cataldo VD, et al. Profound sinus bradycardia due to diltiazem, verapamil, and/or beta-adrenergic blocking drugs. *J La State Med Soc.* 2004;156:327–331.

33. Munzel T, Daiber A, Mulsch A. Explaining the phenomenon of nitrate tolerance. *Circ Res.* 2005;97: 618–628.

34. Noronha B, Duncan E, Byrne JA. Optimal medical management of angina. *Curr Cardiol Rep.* 2003;5: 259–265.

35. O'Connor R, Persse D, Zachariah B, et al. Acute coronary syndrome: pharmacotherapy. *Prehosp Emerg Care.* 2001;5:58–64.

36. Parmley WW. Optimum treatment of stable angina pectoris. *Cardiovasc Drugs Ther.* 1998;12(suppl 1): 105–110.

37. Peel C, Mossberg, KA. Effects of cardiovascular medications on exercise responses. *Phys Ther.* 1995;75: 387–396.

38. Pollack CV, Jr, Gibler WB. 2000 ACC/AHA guidelines for the management of patients with unstable angina and non-ST-segment elevation myocardial infarction: a practical summary for emergency physicians. *Ann Emerg Med.* 2001;38:229–240.

39. Romero M, Sanchez I, Pujol MD. New advances in the field of calcium channel antagonists: cardiovascular effects and structure-activity relationships. *Curr Med Chem Cardiovasc Hematol Agents.* 2003;1: 113–141.

40. Rondina MT, Muhlestein JB. Early initiation of statin therapy in acute coronary syndromes: a review of the evidence. *J Interv Cardiol.* 2005;18:55–63.

41. Schulz E, Tsilimingas N, Rinze R, et al. Functional and biochemical analysis of endothelial (dys)function and NO/cGMP signaling in human blood vessels with and without nitroglycerin pretreatment. *Circulation.* 2002;105:1170–1175.

42. Schwartz GG, Olsson AG. The case for intensive statin therapy after acute coronary syndromes. *Am J Cardiol.* 2005;96:45F–53F.

43. Shah PK. Pathophysiology of plaque rupture and the concept of plaque stabilization. *Cardiol Clin.* 2003;21: 303–314.

44. Shin J, Edelberg JE, Hong MK. Vulnerable atherosclerotic plaque: clinical implications. *Curr Vasc Pharmacol.* 2003;1:183–204.

45. Spaulding C, Cabanes L, Weber S. Pharmacological and therapeutic basis for combined administration of beta blockers and calcium channel blockers in the treatment of stable chronic angina. *Br J Clin Pract Suppl.* 1997;88:17–22.

46. Stason WB, Schmid CH, Niedzwiecki D, et al. Safety of nifedipine in angina pectoris: a meta-analysis. *Hypertension.* 1999;33(1):24–31.

47. Talbert RL. Ischemic heart disease. In: DiPiro JT, et al, eds. *Pharmacotherapy: A Pathophysiologic Approach.* 5th ed. New York: McGraw-Hill; 2002.

48. Thadani U. Current medical management of chronic stable angina. *J Cardiovasc Pharmacol Ther.* 2004;9 (suppl 1):S11–S29.

49. Toda N. Vasodilating beta-adrenoceptor blockers as cardiovascular therapeutics. *Pharmacol Ther.* 2003;100: 215–234.

50. Tran H, Anand SS. Oral antiplatelet therapy in cerebrovascular disease, coronary artery disease, and peripheral arterial disease. *JAMA*. 2004;292: 1867–1874.

51. Van Spall HG, Overgaard CB, Abramson BL. Coronary vasospasm: a case report and review of the literature. *Can J Cardiol*. 2005;21:953–957.

52. Wallentin L. Prevention of cardiovascular events after acute coronary syndrome. *Semin Vasc Med*. 2005;5: 293–300.

53. Warnholtz A, Tsilimingas N, Wendt M, Munzel T. Mechanisms underlying nitrate-induced endothelial dysfunction: insight from experimental and clinical studies. *Heart Fail Rev*. 2002;7:335–345.

54. Wiviott SD, Braunwald E. Unstable angina and non-ST-segment elevation myocardial infarction: part I. Initial evaluation and management, and hospital care. *Am Fam Physician*. 2004;70:525–532.

55. Wiviott SD, Braunwald E. Unstable angina and non-ST-segment elevation myocardial infarction: part II. Coronary revascularization, hospital discharge, and post-hospital care. *Am Fam Physician*. 2004;70: 535–538.

56. Yan AT, Goodman SG. Low-molecular-weight heparins in ischemic heart disease. *Curr Opin Cardiol*. 2004;19:309–316.

57. Yang EH, Lerman A. Angina pectoris with a normal coronary angiogram. *Herz*. 2005;30:17–25.

Chapter 23

Treatment of Cardiac Arrhythmias

An *arrhythmia* can be broadly defined as any significant deviation from normal cardiac rhythm.[6] Various problems in the origination and conduction of electrical activity in the heart can lead to distinct types of arrhythmias. If untreated, disturbances in normal cardiac rhythm result in impaired cardiac pumping ability, and certain arrhythmias are associated with cerebrovascular accidents, cardiac failure, and other sequelae that can be fatal.[1,2,16] Fortunately, a variety of drugs are available to help establish and maintain normal cardiac rhythm.

This chapter presents the primary antiarrhythmic drugs and therapeutic rationale for their use. Many patients seen in rehabilitation are given these drugs to help control and prevent the onset of arrhythmias. Physical therapists and occupational therapists often work directly with cardiac patients in cardiac rehabilitation and fitness programs. Likewise, cardiac patients taking antiarrhythmic drugs may be seen in rehabilitation for any number of other neuromuscular or musculoskeletal disorders. Consequently, therapists should have some knowledge of the clinical use of these drugs.

To understand how antiarrhythmic drugs exert their effects, we first review the origin and spread of electrical activity throughout the heart. This chapter begins with a brief discussion of cardiac electrophysiology, followed by a presentation of the basic mechanisms responsible for producing disturbances in cardiac rhythm and the common types of arrhythmias seen clinically. Finally, antiarrhythmic drugs are presented according to their mechanism of action and clinical use.

Cardiac Electrophysiology

Cardiac Action Potentials

The action potential recorded from a cardiac Purkinje fiber is shown in Figure 23–1. At rest, the interior of the cell is negative relative to the cell's exterior. As in other excitable tissues (neurons, skeletal muscle), an action potential occurs when the cell interior suddenly becomes positive (*depolarizes*), primarily because of sodium ion influx. The cell interior then returns to a negative potential (*repolarizes*), primarily because of

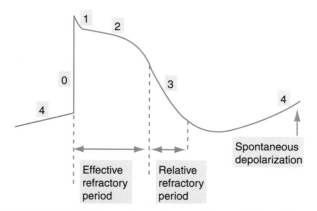

FIGURE 23–1 ▼ The cardiac action potential recorded from a Purkinje cell. The effective refractory period is the time during which the cell cannot be depolarized, and the relative refractory period is the time in which a supranormal stimulus is required to depolarize the cell. Action potential phases (0–4) and the ionic basis for each phase are discussed in the text. (*From:* Keefe DLD, Kates RE, Harrison DC. New antiarrhythmic drugs: their place in therapy. *Drugs.* 1981; 22:363; with permission.)

the efflux of potassium ions. The cardiac action potential, however, has several features that distinguish it from action potentials recorded in other nerves and muscles.[5,37] The cardiac action potential is typically divided into several phases (see Fig. 23–1). The ionic movement that occurs in each phase is outlined here.

Phase 0. Rapid depolarization occurs because of the sudden influx of sodium ions into the cell. At some threshold level, the cell membrane suddenly becomes permeable to sodium ions because of the opening of sodium channels or gates, similar to the spike seen in skeletal muscle depolarization.

Phase 1. An early, brief period of repolarization occurs because specific potassium channels in the cell membrane open to allow potassium to leave the cell.

Phase 2. The action potential undergoes a plateau phase, primarily because the calcium channels open, and there is a slow, prolonged influx of calcium ions into the cell. There is no net change in the charge within the cell because the efflux of positively charged potassium ions that occurred in phase 1 is balanced by the influx of positively charged calcium ions. Thus, the cell's potential remains relatively constant for a brief period, which creates the distinctive plateau that can be seen in Figure 23–1. The phase 2 plateau is important in cardiac cells because it prolongs the cell's effective refractory period (i.e., the time interval between successive action potentials). The plateau basically enables the heart to enter a period of rest (*diastole*) so that the cardiac chambers can fill with blood before the next contraction (*systole*).

Phase 3. At the end of the plateau, repolarization is complete. This is primarily because of the closing (*inactivation*) of the calcium channels, which terminates the entry of calcium into the cell. Repolarization is completed by the unopposed exit of potassium ions.

Phase 4. Phase 4 consists of a slow, spontaneous depolarization in certain cardiac cells (such as the one shown in Fig. 23–1). This spontaneous depolarization probably occurs because of the continuous leak of sodium ions into the cell, combined with a gradual decrease in potassium exit from the cell. This combination of sodium entry and decreased potassium exit causes a progressive accumulation of positive charge within the cell, which causes the cell to become more and more positive until it reaches threshold and phase 0 is initiated again.[37]

Action potentials recorded from various cardiac cells may vary somewhat from the action potential described previously. Some cells, for instance, totally lack phase 1 and have a slower phase 0. Such cells are said to have a slow response as opposed to the fast response just described. Also, action potentials from the nodal cells (see the next section, "Normal Cardiac Rhythm") differ somewhat from the fast response cells. Nonetheless, the fundamental ionic fluxes occurring during cardiac action potentials are similar in all cardiac cells. This ionic activity is pharmacologically significant because various antiarrhythmic drugs will affect the movement of sodium and other ions in an attempt to establish and maintain normal cardiac rhythm.

Normal Cardiac Rhythm

Certain cardiac cells are able to initiate and maintain a spontaneous automatic rhythm. Even in the absence of any neural or hormonal input, these cells will automatically generate an action potential. They are usually referred to as *pacemaker cells* in the myocardium. Pacemaker cells have the ability to depolarize spontaneously because of a rising phase 4 in the cardiac action potential (see Fig. 23–1). As described previously, the resting cell automatically begins to depolarize during phase 4 until the cell reaches threshold and an action potential is initiated.

Pacemaker cells are found primarily in the sinoatrial (SA) node and the atrioventricular (AV) node (Fig. 23–2). Although many other cardiac cells also have the ability to generate an automatic rhythm, the pacemaker cells in the SA node usually dominate and control cardiac rhythm in the normal heart.

Normal Conduction of the Cardiac Action Potential

The cardiac action potential is normally conducted throughout the heart in a coordinated and predictable pattern (Fig. 23–2).[5] The action potential originates in the SA node and is conducted throughout both atria via the atrial muscle cells. While spreading through the atria, the action potential reaches the AV node. From the AV node, the action potential

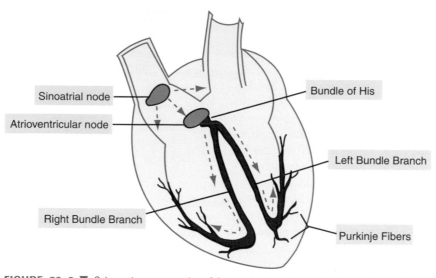

FIGURE 23–2 ▼ Schematic representation of the conduction system of the heart. Conduction normally follows the pathways indicated by the dashed lines. Impulses originate in the sinoatrial node and are transmitted to the atrioventricular node. Impulses are then conducted from the atrioventricular node to the ventricles by the bundle of His and bundle branches.

is passed on to the ventricles via a specialized conducting system known as the *bundle of His*. The bundle of His is composed primarily of specialized conducting cells known as *Purkinje fibers*. As the bundle leaves the AV node, it divides into left and right branches, which supply the respective ventricles. The action potential is distributed to all parts of the ventricles via the bundle branches and Purkinje fibers (see Fig. 23–2).

Mechanisms of Cardiac Arrhythmias

The origin of the cardiac action potential and system of action potential propagation represents normal cardiac excitation and conduction. Any number of factors can disrupt the normal cardiac excitation process, thus resulting in arrhythmic contractions. Such factors include disease, metabolic and electrolyte imbalances, abnormal autonomic influence on the heart, toxicity to other drugs (e.g., digitalis), and myocardial ischemia and infarction.[10,20,24,32,33] In addition, it is now recognized that genetic factors can predispose individuals to certain arrhythmias.[13,35,36] Specifically, mutations is certain genes can cause altered expression and function of channel proteins that control movements of sodium, potassium, or calcium ions across

the cardiac cell membrane.[19,36,42] Thus, inherited alterations in ion channel function can affect cardiac action potential initiation or conduction, especially when the heart is damaged (e.g., ischemic) or exposed to other factors that stress the heart.[32,34,35]

Regardless of what the initiating factor is in producing arrhythmias, the mechanism underlying a disturbance in cardiac rhythm can be attributed to one of the three basic abnormalities listed below.[5]

1. *Abnormal impulse generation.* The normal automatic rhythm of the cardiac pacemaker cells has been disrupted. Injury and disease may directly render the SA and AV cells incapable of maintaining normal rhythm. Also, cells that do not normally control cardiac rhythm may begin to compete with pacemaker cells, thus creating multiple areas of automaticity.
2. *Abnormal impulse conduction.* The conduction of impulses throughout the myocardium has been interrupted. Various diseases and local damage may result in the delay or failure of an action potential to reach certain areas. These conduction impairments or heart blocks can prevent a smooth and synchronous contraction, thus creating an abnormal rhythm.
3. *Simultaneous abnormalities of impulse generation and conduction.* A combination of both previously listed factors may cause cardiac arrhythmias.

Types of Arrhythmias

Cardiac arrhythmias are described by many different terms according to their site of origin, nature of disturbed heartbeat, or impairment in cardiac conduction.[5] This text cannot fully describe all of the various forms of the clinically occurring arrhythmias. To understand when various antiarrhythmic drugs are used, however, some basic terms describing cardiac arrhythmias must be defined. Some of the more commonly occurring arrhythmias are listed in Table 23–1. For a more detailed description of the electrophysiologic nature and diagnosis of these arrhythmias, the reader is referred to several other sources on this topic.[6,17,18]

Classification of Antiarrhythmic Drugs

Drugs used to treat cardiac arrhythmias are traditionally placed in one of four distinct classes according to their mechanism of action.[5,9] These classifications are summarized in Table 23–2. The classification system has been criticized somewhat because it has several limitations, including the fact that certain drugs may have characteristics from more than one class, and that certain drugs with antiarrhythmic properties (e.g., digitalis) do not fit into this system. Nonetheless, this method of categorizing antiarrhythmic drugs is still commonly used.[5,18] The mechanism of action and specific agents within each class are described here.

Class I: Sodium Channel Blockers

Mechanism of Action and Rationale for Use

Class I antiarrhythmic drugs are essentially sodium channel blockers.[5,27,29] These drugs bind to membrane sodium channels in various excitable tissues, including myocardial cells. In cardiac tissues, class I drugs normalize the rate of sodium entry into cardiac tissues and thereby help control cardiac excitation and conduction.[8,27] Certain class I agents (e.g., lidocaine) are also used as local anesthetics; the way that these drugs bind to sodium channels is discussed in more detail in Chapter 12.

Because sodium influx plays an important role during action potential generation during phase 0 of

Table 23–1	COMMON FORMS OF ARRHYTHMIAS
Classification	**Characteristic Rhythm**
Sinus arrhythmias	
Sinus tachycardia	> 100 beats/min
Sinus bradycardia	< 60 beats/min
Sick sinus syndrome	Severe bradycardia (<50 beats/min); periods of sinus arrest
Supraventricular arrhythmias	
Atrial fibrillation and flutter	Atrial rate > 300 beats/min
Atrial tachycardia	Atrial rate > 140–200 beats/min
Premature atrial contractions	Variable
Atrioventricular junctional arrhythmias	
Junctional rhythm	40–55 beats/min
Junctional tachycardia	100–200 beats/min
Conduction disturbances	
Atrioventricular block	Variable
Bundle branch block	Variable
Fascicular block	Variable
Ventricular arrhythmias	
Premature ventricular contractions	Variable
Ventricular tachycardia	140–200 beats/min
Ventricular fibrillation	Irregular; totally uncoordinated rhythm

the cardiac action potential, inhibition of sodium channels tends to decrease membrane excitability. Thus, class I drugs help stabilize the cardiac cell membrane and normalize the rate of cardiac cell firing. Although all class I drugs exert their antiarrhythmic effects by inhibiting sodium channel function, various agents affect myocardial excitation and conduction in slightly different ways. Class I drugs are typically subclassified according to how they influence cardiac electrophysi-

Table 23–2	CLASSIFICATION OF ANTIARRHYTHMIC DRUGS

Generic Names	Trade Names
Class I: Sodium channel blockers	
Subclass A	
Disopyramide	Norpace
Procainamide	Promine, Pronestyl, Procan
Quinidine	Cardioquin, Quinidex, others
Subclass B	
Lidocaine	Xylocaine
Mexiletine	Mexitil
Moricizine*	Ethmozine
Subclass C	
Flecainide	Tambocor
Propafenone	Rythmol
Class II: Beta blockers	
Acebutolol	Sectral
Atenolol	Tenormin
Esmolol	Brevibloc
Metoprolol	Lopressor
Nadolol	Corgard
Propranolol	Inderal
Sotalol	Betapace
Timolol	Blocadren
Class III: Drugs that prolong repolarization	
Amiodarone†	Cordarone
Bretylium	Bretylol
Dofetilide	Tikosyn
Ibutilide	Corvert
Class IV: Calcium channel blockers	
Diltiazem	Cardizem, Dilacor
Verapamil	Calan, Isoptin, Verelan

*Also has some class IC properties.

†Also has some properties from the other three drug classes.

ology (see Table 23–2).[5,25] These subclassifications and specific agents in each group are presented below.

Specific Agents

Class IA. Drugs in this group are similar in that they produce a moderate slowing of phase 0 depolarization and a moderate slowing of action potential propagation throughout the myocardium. These drugs also prolong repolarization of the cardiac cell, thus lengthening the interval before a second action potential can occur (i.e., they increase the effective refractory period). Class IA agents include quinidine, procainamide, and disopyramide (see Table 23–2); these drugs are used to treat a variety of arrhythmias originating in the ventricles or atria.

Class IB. These drugs display a minimal ability to slow phase 0 depolarization, and produce a minimal slowing of cardiac conduction. In contrast to IA drugs, class IB drugs usually shorten cardiac repolarization; that is, the effective refractory period is decreased. Class IB drugs include lidocaine, mexiletine, and moricizine (see Table 23–2); These drugs are primarily used to treat ventricular arrhythmias such as ventricular tachycardia and premature ventricular contractions (PVCs). However, Class IB drugs are typically reserved for people with more severe types of ventricular arrhythmias, and their use in relatively minor or asymptomatic arrhythmias has been replaced by safer drugs or nonpharmacological management (see "Nonpharmacologic Treatment of Arrhythmias" later in this chapter).

Class IC. These drugs produce both a marked decrease in the rate of phase 0 depolarization and a marked slowing of cardiac conduction. They have little effect on repolarization. Class IC drugs include flecainide and propafenone (see Table 23–2), and appear to be best suited to treat ventricular arrhythmias such as ventricular tachycardia and PVCs.

Adverse Side Effects

Despite their use in treating arrhythmias, the most common side effect of all antiarrhythmic drugs is their tendency to *increase* rhythm disturbances (proarrhythmic effects). While attempting to control one type of arrhythmia, these agents can aggravate or initiate other cardiac rhythm abnormalities.[3,9] This fact seems especially true with all class I agents.[8,31] Because these drugs affect sodium channel function and cardiac excitability, they may produce some serious proarrhythmic effects in certain patients. For example, patients with heart failure, myocardial ischemia, and structural heart disease (including previous infarction) seem to be especially prone to class I–induced arrhythmias, and these drugs should be avoided in these patients.[9,41] Likewise, people with inherited mutations in myocardial sodium channel function may be susceptible to proarrhythmic effects of class I agents.[4] Class I drugs are also associated with a variety of side effects such as dizziness, visual disturbances, and nausea.[5] These symptoms are often important, however, because they may indicate the presence of arrhythmias even when the pulse or electrocardiogram (ECG) is not being directly monitored. Hence, class I drugs are still important in treating certain arrhythmias, but they are used less and with more caution than in the past.[8,9]

Class II: Beta Blockers

Mechanisms of Action and Rationale for Use

Drugs that block beta-1 receptors on the myocardium are one of the mainstays in arrhythmia treatment. Beta blockers are effective because they decrease the excitatory effects of the sympathetic nervous system and related catecholamines (norepinephrine and epinephrine) on the heart.[5,28] This effect typically decreases cardiac automaticity and prolongs the effective refractory period, thus slowing heart rate.[5] Beta blockers also slow down conduction through the myocardium, and are especially useful in controlling function of the atrioventricular node.[21] Hence, these drugs are most effective in treating atrial tachycardias such as atrial fibrillation.[23] Some ventricular arrhythmias may also respond to treatment with beta blockers.

Specific Agents

Individual beta blockers are presented in Chapter 20. Beta blockers shown to be effective in treating arrhythmias include acebutolol, atenolol, esmolol, metoprolol, nadolol, propranolol, sotalol, and timolol (see Table 23–2). Choice of a specific beta blocker depends to a large extent on the exact type of arrhythmia present and the individual patient's response to the drug.

Adverse Side Effects

Nonselective beta blockers affect beta-2 receptors on the lungs as well as beta-1 receptors on the heart, and these nonselective agents can increase bronchoconstriction in patients with asthma and chronic obstructive pulmonary disease. Hence, a drug that is more specific for beta-1 receptors is preferred in these patients. Beta blockers can also produce excessive slowing of cardiac conduction in some patients, resulting in an increase in arrhythmias. Severe adverse reactions are rare, however, and beta blockers are well-tolerated by most patients when used appropriately to treat arrhythmias.

Class III: Drugs That Prolong Repolarization

Mechanism of Action and Rationale for Use

Class III agents delay repolarization of cardiac cells, which prolongs the effective refractory period of the cardiac action potential.[5,28] This delay lengthens the time interval before a subsequent action potential can be initiated, thus slowing and stabilizing the heart rate. The effects of class III drugs are complex, but their ability to lengthen the cardiac action potential is most likely mediated by inhibition of potassium efflux during repolarization.[5] That is, these drugs limit the ability of potassium to leave the cell during phase 2 and 3 of the action potential, which prolongs repolarization and prevents the cell from firing another action potential too rapidly. Class III drugs are used to treat ventricular arrhythmias such as ventricular tachycardia and ventricular fibrillation, and supraventricular arrhythmias such as postoperative atrial fibrillation.[22,30] Interest in using these drugs and developing new class III agents has increased recently because they affect both atrial and ventricular problems and are relatively safe compared to other agents such as the class I drugs.[11,38,40]

Specific Agents

Class III drugs currently in use include amiodarone, bretylium, dofetilide, and ibutilide (see Table 23–2). These drugs all exert their primary effects by prolonging repolarization in cardiac cells. Amiodarone, however, also appears to have some properties similar to drugs in other classes, and may help control arrhythmias by inhibiting sodium channel function (class I effect), by beta blockade (class II effect), or even by blocking calcium channels (class IV effect).[5]

Adverse Side Effects

An initial increase in cardiac arrhythmias (proarrhythmic effect) may occur when class III drugs are instituted. The most important proarrhythmia is known as torsades de pointes, which is a form of ventricular tachycardia that can be fatal.[11,40] Specific class III agents are associated with various other side effects. Amiodarone, for example, is associated with pulmonary toxicity and liver damage. Other class III drugs may have a more favorable side-effect profile but may not be as effective as amiodarone in controlling arrhythmias. Side effects of class III drugs therefore vary from agent to agent, and any untoward effects should be monitored carefully.

Class IV: Calcium Channel Blockers

Mechanism of Action and Rationale for Use

Class IV drugs have a selective ability to block calcium entry into myocardial and vascular smooth-muscle cells. These drugs inhibit calcium influx by binding to specific channels in the cell membrane.[12,15] As discussed previously, calcium entry plays an important role in the generation of the cardiac action potential, especially during phase 2. By inhibiting calcium influx into myocardial cells, calcium channel blockers can alter the excitability and conduction of cardiac tissues.

Calcium channel blockers decrease the rate of discharge of the SA node and inhibit conduction velocity through the AV node.[5] These drugs are most successful in treating arrhythmias caused by atrial dysfunction, such as supraventricular tachycardia and atrial fibrillation.[15,39]

Specific Agents

The pharmacology of specific calcium channel blockers is presented in Chapter 22. Of the calcium channel blockers currently in use, verapamil and diltiazem are currently approved for treating arrhythmias (Table 23–2). Although these drugs differ chemically, both normalize heart rate by reducing calcium effects on SA and AV nodal tissues. Preliminary studies suggested that verapamil might be more effective that diltiazem, but their antiarrhythmic effects seem to be fairly similar when administered orally at therapeutic doses.[18] Other calcium channel blockers, however, such as nifedipine and similar dihydropyridines (see Chapter 22), do not have any substantial effects on cardiac rhythm. These other calcium channel blockers are more effective in dilating vascular smooth muscle and are used more frequently to treat hypertension and angina pectoris (see Chapters 21 and 22).

Adverse Side Effects

Because drugs like verapamil slow down the heart rate by inhibiting calcium entry into cardiac muscle cells, excessive bradycardia (less than 50 beats per minute) may occur in some patients receiving these drugs. Calcium channel blockers also limit calcium entry into vascular smooth muscle, which may cause peripheral vasodilation and lead to dizziness and headaches in some patients.

Other Drugs Used to Treat Arrhythmias

Several other drug strategies can be used to treat certain arrhythmias even though these drugs are not classified according to the traditional categories described above.[18] Digitalis glycosides, for example, are typically used to treat congestive heart failure (see Chapter 24), but these drugs can also be used to prevent or treat certain arrhythmias, including severe atrial fibrillation and paroxysmal AV nodal reentrant tachycardia. The pharmacology of digitalis is addressed in detail in Chapter 24. Large doses of magnesium (1–2 gms) can be infused intravenously to treat severe ventricular arrhythmias such as torsades de pointes. Magnesium is thought to control these arrhythmias by normalizing cardiac ion channel function, but the exact mechanism of magnesium's effects is not fully understood. Adenosine, a substance found naturally in the body, can also be administered intravenously to terminate severe arrhythmias such as reentrant supraventricular tachycardia. This substance binds to specific adenosine receptors on the heart, and affects heart rate by decreasing calcium entry into myocardial tissues.

Nonpharmacologic Treatment of Arrhythmias

Antiarrhythmic drugs often help normalize cardiac rhythm and decrease the symptoms associated with cardiac arrhythmias. These drugs, however, do not usually cure these conditions because they do not typically resolve the source of the arrhythmia. As indicated earlier, many antiarrhythmic drugs are also associated with potentially serious side effects, including the risk of increased arrhythmias.[9] Hence, other interventions have been used to try to treat the cause of the rhythm disturbance. In particular, the use of implantable electronic devices (cardioverter defibrillators) and other surgeries (electrode catheter ablation) have been used increasingly to supplement or replace drug therapy in helping control certain arrhythmias.[7,14,26,43] Drug therapy remains a common treatment for people with arrhythmias, but many patients may also use a nonpharmacological approach to help provide a more long-term solution for certain rhythm disturbances.

Special Concerns in Rehabilitation Patients

■ ■ ■ The primary problems associated with antiarrhythmic drugs in rehabilitation patients are related to the side effects of these agents. Therapists should be aware of the potential for increased arrhythmias or changes in the nature of arrhythmias with these drugs. This concern may be especially important in patients involved in exercise and cardiac rehabilitation programs. Therapists who supervise such patients can often detect the presence of arrhythmias by monitoring ECG recordings. If an ECG recording is not available, palpation of pulses for rate and regularity may detect rhythm disturbances. Also, the presence of other side effects such as faintness or dizziness may signal the presence of cardiotoxic drug effects and increased arrhythmias. Consequently, therapists treating patients for both cardiac and noncardiac disorders may help detect the cardiotoxic effects of antiarrhythmic drugs by staying alert for any side effects. By playing a role in the early detection of increased arrhythmias, therapists can alert the physician to a problem and avert any potentially serious or even fatal consequences.

Other concerns related to side effects are fairly minor. Hypotension may occur with some agents, especially with bretylium (class III) and calcium channel blockers (class IV). Therapists should be aware that patients may become dizzy, especially after sudden changes in posture.

CASE STUDY

Antiarrhythmic Drugs

Brief History. M.R. is a 48-year-old man with a history of coronary artery disease and cardiac rhythm disturbances. Specifically, he has experienced episodes of paroxysmal supraventricular tachycardia, with his heart rate often exceeding 180 beats per minute. He has been treated for several years with the nonspecific beta blocker propranolol (Inderal). Oral propranolol (60 mg/d) has successfully diminished his episodes of tachycardia. In an effort to improve his myocardial function and overall cardiovascular fitness, M.R. recently enrolled as an outpatient in a cardiac rehabilitation program. Under the supervision of a physical therapist, he attended cardiac training sessions three times each week. A typical session consisted of warm-up calisthenics, bicycle ergometry, and cool-down stretching activities. Each session lasted approximately 45 minutes.

Problem/Influence of Medication. Propranolol and the other beta blockers are successful in reducing various supraventricular arrhythmias. These drugs, however, also attenuate the cardiac response to exercise. Heart rate and cardiac output are lower at any absolute workload, and maximal heart rate and cardiac output are attenuated by beta blockade. Consequently, the exercise response of a patient taking a beta blocker will be less than if the patient is not tak-

ing the drug. This consideration is important because the exercise prescription for any given patient must take into account the patient's maximal exercise capacity. Typically, patients exercise at some submaximal percentage of their maximal ability. If maximal exercise capacity is influenced by the beta blocker, the exercise prescription must be adjusted accordingly.

Decision/Solution. Prior to beginning the rehabilitation program, the patient underwent a graded exercise test (GXT). All patients with cardiac disorders should undergo a GXT before beginning a cardiac rehabilitation program. Patients taking beta blockers and other drugs that affect cardiac function must also be tested under the conditions in which they will eventually be exercising. The GXT accurately determined the patient's exercise workload while he was taking his normal dosage of propranolol. Consequently, the prescribed exercise workload was adjusted by the therapist for the effect of the beta blocker.

During the cardiac rehabilitation sessions, the therapist periodically monitored heart rate, blood pressure, and ECG. No significant episodes of arrhythmias were noted, and the patient progressed rapidly through the program. He was eventually discharged from the formal program with instructions of how to continue his rehabilitation exercises at home and at a local health club.

SUMMARY

Cardiac arrhythmias may arise due to disturbances in the origination and conduction of electrical activity in the heart. These changes in cardiac rhythm can be controlled to a large extent by several groups of drugs including sodium channel blockers, beta blockers, calcium channel blockers, and drugs that prolong the cardiac action potential. These agents work by differ-ent cellular mechanisms to stabilize heart rate and improve the conduction of electrical impulses throughout the myocardium. Although these drugs are often successful in preventing or resolving arrhythmias, rehabilitation specialists should be cognizant of patients who are taking these agents. Therapists should also be alert for any changes in cardiac function or other side effects that may signal toxicity of these drugs.

References

1. Adamson PB, Barr RC, Callans DJ, et al. The perplexing complexity of cardiac arrhythmias: beyond electrical remodeling. *Heart Rhythm.* 2005;2:650–659.
2. Agarwal A, York M, Kantharia BK, Ezekowitz M. Atrial fibrillation: modern concepts and management. *Annu Rev Med.* 2005;56:475–494.
3. Albrecht CA. Proarrhythmia with non-antiarrhythmics. A review. *Cardiology.* 2004;102:122–139.
4. Balser JR. Inherited sodium channelopathies: novel therapeutic and proarrhythmic molecular mechanisms. *Trends Cardiovasc Med.* 2001;11:229–237.
5. Bauman JL, Schoen MD. Arrhythmias. In: DiPiro JT, et al, eds. *Pharmacotherapy: A Pathophysiologic Approach.* 5th ed New York: McGraw-Hill; 2002.
6. Berne RM, Levy MN. *Cardiovascular Physiology.* 8th ed. St Louis: Mosby; 2001.
7. Brennan TD, Haas GJ. The role of prophylactic implantable cardioverter defibrillators in heart failure: recent trials usher in a new era of device therapy. *Curr Heart Fail Rep.* 2005;2:40–45.
8. Campbell TJ, Williams KM. Therapeutic drug monitoring: antiarrhythmic drugs. *Br J Clin Pharmacol.* 1998;46:307–319.
9. Chaudhry GM, Haffajee CI. Antiarrhythmic agents and proarrhythmia. *Crit Care Med.* 2000;28(suppl): N158–N164.
10. Chiang CE. Congenital and acquired long QT syndrome. Current concepts and management. *Cardiol Rev.* 2004;12:222–234.
11. Elming H, Brendorp B, Pehrson S, et al. A benefit-risk assessment of class III antiarrhythmic agents. *Expert Opin Drug Saf.* 2004;3:559–577.
12. Elmslie KS. Calcium channel blockers in the treatment of disease. *J Neurosci Res.* 2004;75:733–741.
13. Francis J, Antzelevitch C. Brugada syndrome. *Int J Cardiol.* 2005;101:173–178.
14. Gillinov AM, Wolf RK. Surgical ablation of atrial fibrillation. *Prog Cardiovasc Dis.* 2005;48:169–177.
15. Grossman E, Messerli FH. Calcium antagonists. *Prog Cardiovasc Dis.* 2004;47:34–57.
16. Gutierrez A, Lopez JE. Update in atrial fibrillation. *P R Health Sci J.* 2004;23:279–284.
17. Guyton AC, Hall JE. Cardiac arrhythmias and their electrocardiographic interpretation. In: *Textbook of Medical Physiology.* 11th ed. Philadelphia: WB Saunders; 2006.
18. Hume JR, Grant AO. Agents used in cardiac arrhythmias. In: Katzung BG, ed. *Basic and Clinical Pharmacology.* 9th ed. New York: Lange Medical Books/McGraw-Hill; 2004.
19. Ji S, Cesario D, Valderrabano M, Shivkumar K. The molecular basis of cardiac arrhythmias in patients with cardiomyopathy. *Curr Heart Fail Rep.* 2004;1:98–103.
20. Khan IA. Long QT syndrome: diagnosis and management. *Am Heart J.* 2002;143:7–14.
21. Khan IA, Nair CK, Singh N, et al. Acute ventricular rate control in atrial fibrillation and atrial flutter. *Int J Cardiol.* 2004;97:7–13.
22. Khan MH. Oral class III antiarrhythmics: what is new? *Curr Opin Cardiol.* 2004;19:47–51.
23. Kuhlkamp V, Bosch R, Mewis C, Seipel L. Use of beta-blockers in atrial fibrillation. *Am J Cardiovasc Drugs.* 2002;2:37–42.
24. Leonardi M, Bissett J. Prevention of atrial fibrillation. *Curr Opin Cardiol.* 2005;20:417–423.
25. Marcus GM, Sung RJ. Antiarrhythmic agents in facilitating electrical cardioversion of atrial fibrillation and promoting maintenance of sinus rhythm. *Cardiology.* 2001;95:1–8.
26. Marine JE, Dong J, Calkins H. Catheter ablation therapy for atrial fibrillation. *Prog Cardiovasc Dis.* 2005;48: 178–192.
27. Nattel S, Kneller J, Zou R, Leon LJ. Mechanisms of termination of atrial fibrillation by Class I antiarrhythmic drugs: evidence from clinical, experimental, and mathematical modeling studies. *J Cardiovasc Electrophysiol* 2003;14(suppl):S133–S139.
28. Nattel S, Singh BN. Evolution, mechanisms, and classification of antiarrhythmic drugs: focus on class III actions. *Am J Cardiol.* 1999;84(suppl 9A):11R–19R.
29. Ohmura K, Kobayashi Y, Miyauchi Y, et al. Electrocardiographic and electrophysiological characteristics of atrial fibrillation organized into atrial flutter by oral administration of class I antiarrhythmic agents. *Pacing Clin Electrophysiol.* 2003;26:692–702.
30. Purerfellner H. Recent developments in cardiovascular drug therapy: treatment of atrial arrhythmias with new class III drugs and beyond. *Curr Med Chem Cardiovasc Hematol Agents.* 2004;2:79–91.
31. Roden DM. Mechanisms and management of proarrhythmia. *Am J Cardiol.* 1998;82(4A):49I–57I.
32. Roden DM, Viswanathan PC. Genetics of acquired long QT syndrome. *J Clin Invest.* 2005;115: 2025–2032.

33. Roffi M, Cattaneo F, Brandle M. Thyrotoxicosis and the cardiovascular system. *Minerva Endocrinol.* 2005; 30:47–58.

34. Rubart M, Zipes DP. Mechanisms of sudden cardiac death. *J Clin Invest.* 2005;115:2305–2315.

35. Sarkozy A, Brugada P. Sudden cardiac death and inherited arrhythmia syndromes. *J Cardiovasc Electrophysiol.* 2005;16(suppl 1):S8–S20.

36. Schwartz PJ. Management of long QT syndrome. *Nat Clin Pract Cardiovasc Med.* 2005;2:346–351.

37. Seifter J, Ratner A, Sloane D. The electrical activity of the heart. In: *Concepts in Medical Physiology.* Philadelphia: Lippincott, Williams and Wilkins; 2005

38. Singh BN, Wadhani N. Antiarrhythmic and proarrhythmic properties of QT-prolonging antianginal drugs. *J Cardiovasc Pharmacol Ther.* 2004;9(suppl 1):S85–S97.

39. Tamargo J, Caballero R, Delpon E. Pharmacological approaches in the treatment of atrial fibrillation. *Curr Med Chem.* 2004;11:13–28.

40. Tsikouris JP, Cox CD. A review of class III antiarrhythmic agents for atrial fibrillation: maintenance of normal sinus rhythm. *Pharmacotherapy.* 2001;21: 1514–1529.

41. Van Gelder IC, Brugemann J, Crijns HJ. Current treatment recommendations in antiarrhythmic therapy. *Drugs.* 1998;55:331–346.

42. Viswanathan PC, Balser JR. Inherited sodium channelopathies: a continuum of channel dysfunction. *Trends Cardiovasc Med.* 2004;14:28–35.

43. Willems R, Heidbuchel H. Nonpharmacologic treatment of atrial fibrillation in elderly persons. *Am J Geriatr Cardiol.* 2005;14:68–72.

Chapter 24

Treatment of Congestive Heart Failure

Congestive heart failure is a chronic condition in which the heart is unable to pump a sufficient quantity of blood to meet the needs of peripheral tissues.[13,16] Essentially, the heart's pumping ability has been compromised by some form of myocardial disease or dysfunction. The congestive aspect of heart failure arises from the tendency for fluid to accumulate in the lungs and peripheral tissues because the heart is unable to maintain proper circulation. The pathophysiology of congestive heart failure is fairly complex; the possible causes and mechanisms are addressed in more detail below in "Pathophysiology of Congestive Heart Failure."

The primary symptoms associated with congestive heart failure are peripheral edema and a decreased tolerance for physical activity.[39,60] Dyspnea and shortness of breath are also common, especially if the left heart is failing and pulmonary congestion is present (see the next section). In severe cases, cyanosis develops because the heart cannot deliver oxygen to peripheral tissues.

Congestive heart failure represents one of the major illnesses present in industrialized nations.[32,34,53] In the United States, approximately 5 million people have been diagnosed with this disease,[34] and the incidence of heart failure (number of new cases each year) is approximately 400,000 to 700,000.[39] The prevalence of heart failure also increases in the elderly, and the number of people with heart failure will undoubtedly increase as a larger percentage of our population reaches advanced age.[53] This disease is likewise associated with serious consequences, and the prognosis for congestive heart failure is often poor.[32,53] Despite recent advances in medical treatment, approximately 50 percent of patients die within 5 years after they are diagnosed with heart failure.[34]

Consequently, effective treatment of congestive heart failure is a critical and challenging task. Pharmacotherapy represents one of the primary methods of treating congestive heart failure, and the drugs discussed in this chapter play a vital role in the optimal management of this disease. As with other cardiac problems, the prevalence of congestive heart failure necessitates that members of the health care community be aware of the pharmacologic management of this disease. Rehabilitation specialists will often treat patients with heart failure, and therapists should be cognizant of the drugs used to treat this problem.

Pathophysiology of Congestive Heart Failure

Vicious Cycle of Heart Failure

The mechanisms underlying chronic heart failure are complex and may include biochemical disturbances in the cardiac cell, altered genetic expression of myocardial proteins, and systemic changes in hemodynamic and neurohormonal factors.[10,16,60] Heart failure also tends to be self-perpetuating because an aberration in cardiac function often initiates a vicious cycle leading to further decrements in cardiac function.[53] Figure 24–1 illustrates the way in which a vicious cycle might be generated by the interaction of cardiac and neurohumoral factors. The sequence of events depicted in Figure 24–1 is discussed briefly here.

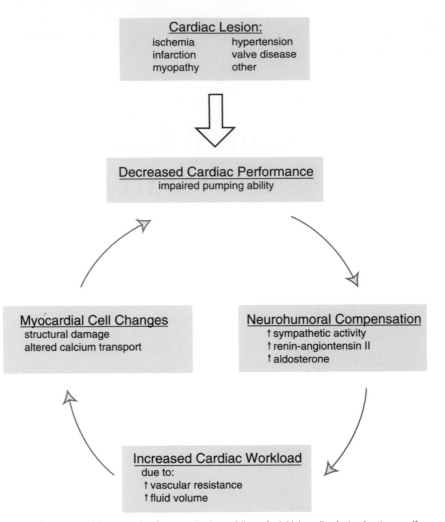

FIGURE 24–1 ▼ Vicious cycle of congestive heart failure. An initial cardiac lesion begins a self-perpetuating decrease in myocardial performance.

1. *Decreased cardiac performance.* Any number of factors that affect cardiac pumping ability may be responsible for initiating a change in myocardial performance. Factors such as ischemic heart disease, myocardial infarction, valve dysfunction, and hypertension may all compromise the heart's pumping ability.[29,53,71] Also, cardiomyopathy may result from other diseases and infections.[13]

2. *Neurohumoral compensations.* The body responds to the decreased cardiac pumping ability in a number of ways. In the early stages of failure, cardiac output decreases, and the delivery of oxygen and nutrients to tissues and organs is diminished. To compensate for this initial decrease, several neural and humoral changes occur, increasing cardiac contractility and helping maintain blood pressure. In particular, the sympathetic nervous system and renin-angiotensin system are activated, and secretion of aldosterone and antidiuretic hormone increases.[2,15,42,61] Although these compensations are initially helpful in maintaining cardiac function, they actually place more stress on the failing heart.[18] This increased stress initiates a vicious cycle because it causes more damage to the myocardium, which further compromises cardiac pumping ability, causing more neurohumoral activation, more stress to the heart, and so on (see Fig. 24–1).

3. *Increased cardiac workload.* The neurohumoral changes previously described contribute to peripheral vasoconstriction, as well as a general increase in sodium and water retention.[15] These effects place additional strain on the heart by increasing cardiac preload (the volume of blood returning to the heart) and cardiac afterload (the pressure that the heart must pump against).[13]

4. *Changes in myocardial cell function.* The increased workload on the heart can lead to, or cause exaggerated alterations, in cell function. Increased cardiac workload may lead to further structural damage to the already compromised myocardial cell.[25,28] Also, studies on the molecular basis of heart failure have suggested that alterations in calcium transport, contractile protein function, energy production and utilization, free-radical production, and beta-receptor density may occur.[2,28,60] Continued stress on the heart may exacerbate these changes, leading to more cellular dysfunction and inappropriate adaptive changes in myocardial cell structure and function, which ultimately leads to abnormal changes in the size, shape, and function of the heart (cardiac remodeling).[25,50,67] Increased dysfunction on the cellular level therefore leads to pathological remodeling, resulting in a further decrease in cardiac performance, thus completing the cycle shown in Figure 24–1.

The changes in cardiac function previously described represent a simplification of the interaction of central and peripheral factors in congestive heart failure. This description does, however, illustrate the primary problems that occur in this disease, as well as the manner in which heart failure tends to self-perpetuate.

Likewise, heart failure is not always associated with systolic dysfunction and an obvious decline in cardiac pumping ability. In approximately half the cases of symptomatic heart failure, systolic function and cardiac output may appear normal when the patient is at rest.[53,63] In this type of heart failure, cardiac function is impaired because the left ventricle is stiff and unable to relax during the filling phase, resulting in increased pressures at the end of diastole.[31] This condition is often described as "diastolic" heart failure, but it is also identified by other names such as heart failure with preserved left ventricular function and heart failure with normal ejection fraction.[63] In diastolic heart failure, systolic function may appear normal at rest, but increased stress on the myocardium leads to progressive changes in cellular function and cardiac remodeling that are detrimental to cardiac function.

Diastolic heart failure is more common in older adults, especially older women.[51] The pathophysiology of this type of heart failure might also differ from heart failure associated with left ventricular or systolic dysfunction, with hypertension being relatively more important in the cause of diastolic heart failure.[35] Drug therapy for diastolic heart failure therefore focuses on lowering blood pressure and using other agents to reduce stress on the heart (see "Agents that Decrease Cardiac Workload").[31] The causes of systolic and diastolic heart failure continue to be investigated, and future research will help clarify the factors responsible for specific forms of cardiac dysfunction.

Congestion in Left and Right Heart Failure

The primary problem in advanced heart failure is that the heart is unable to push blood forward through the circulatory system, thus causing pressure to build up in the veins returning blood to the heart. In effect, blood begins to back up in the venous system, increasing the pressure gradient for fluid to move out of the capillary beds. The net movement of fluid out of the capillaries causes the edema or congestion typically found in advanced stages of heart failure.

Although heart disease commonly affects the entire myocardium, congestive heart failure is sometimes divided into left and right heart failure (Fig. 24–2). In *left heart failure*, the left atrium and ventricle are unable to adequately handle the blood returning from the lungs. This causes pressure to build up in the pulmonary veins, and fluid accumulates in the lungs. Consequently, left heart failure is associated with pulmonary edema (see Fig. 24–2 *A*).

In *right heart failure*, the right atrium and ventricle are unable to handle blood returning from the systemic circulation. This causes fluid to accumulate in the peripheral tissues, and ankle edema and organ congestion (liver, spleen) are typical manifestations (see Fig. 24–2 *B*). If both left and right heart failure occur simultaneously, congestion is found in the lungs as well as the periphery.

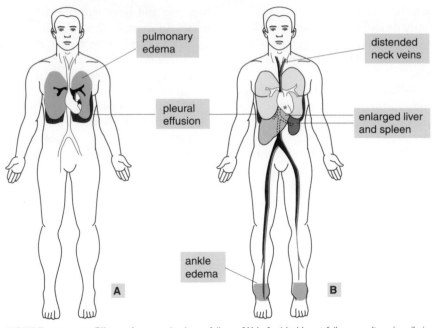

FIGURE 24–2 ▼ Effects of congestive heart failure. *(A)* Left-sided heart failure results primarily in pulmonary edema. *(B)* Right-sided heart failure results in peripheral edema (swollen ankles, enlarged organs). *(Adapted from:* Kent TH, Hart MN. *Introduction to Human Disease.* 2nd ed. Norwalk, CT: Appleton-Century-Crofts; 1987: 141, with permission.)

Pharmacotherapy

One of the basic goals in congestive heart failure is to improve the heart's pumping ability. Drug administration should selectively increase cardiac contractile performance and produce what is referred to as a *positive inotropic effect.* "Inotropic" refers to the force of muscular contraction; the primary drugs used to exert a positive inotropic effect are the cardiac glycosides such as digitalis. In addition to increasing cardiac contractility, drugs that decrease cardiac workload through an effect on the heart or peripheral vasculature, or by controlling fluid volume, are recognized as beneficial in congestive heart failure. Angiotensin-converting enzyme inhibitors, beta blockers, diuretics, and vasodilators are included in this group.

The primary drug groups used to treat congestive heart failure are listed in Table 24–1. These drugs are described according to their primary goal in treating heart failure—that is, drugs that improve myocardial contraction force (positive inotropic agents) and agents that decrease cardiac workload. The mechanism of action and specific agents within each group are presented below.

Drugs That Increase Myocardial Contraction Force (Positive Inotropic Agents)

Digitalis

The cardiac glycosides are digoxin, digitoxin, and similar agents (Table 24–1). For simplicity, the term "digitalis" is used to represent these drugs. Although the widespread use of digitalis has been questioned, it continues to be one of the primary drugs used to treat congestive heart failure.[14,19,37] There is little doubt that digitalis improves cardiac pumping ability and therefore improves the primary symptoms of congestive heart failure.[66] Digitalis typically increases cardiac output at rest and during exercise, and exercise tolerance often increases because the heart is able to pump blood more effectively.[14,19] There is little evidence, however, that digitalis prolongs life expectancy in people with heart failure.[36,53] Also, the use of digitalis is limited to some extent by the toxic effects of this drug (see "Adverse Side Effects," later).

Nonetheless, the consensus is that digitalis is a useful drug because it can decrease the symptoms of

Table 24–1	PRIMARY DRUGS USED IN CONGESTIVE HEART FAILURE
Drug Group	**Primary Effect**
Agents that increase myocardial contraction force (positive inotropic agents)	

Digitalis glycosides
  Digoxin (Lanoxin)
  Digitioxin (Digitaline)
	Increase myocardial contractility by elevating intracellular calcium levels and facilitating actin-myosin interaction in cardiac cells; may also help normalize autonomic effects on the heart

Other positive inotropes
  Inamrinone (generic)
  Milrinone (Primacor)
	Enhance myocardial contractility by prolonging effects of cyclic adenosine monophosphate (cAMP), which increases intracellular calcium levels and promotes stronger actin-myosin interaction in cardiac cells

Dopamine (Intropin) Dobutamine (Dobutrex)	Stimulate cardiac beta-1 adrenergic receptors, which selectively increases myocardial contraction force
Agents that decrease cardiac workload	

Angiotensin-converting enzyme inhibitors*
  Benazepril (Lotensin)
  Captopril (Capoten)
  Enalapril (Vasotec)
  Fosinopril (Monopril)
  Lisinopril (Prinivil, Zestril)
  Quinapril (Accupril)
  Ramipril (Altace)
  Trandolapril (Mavik)
	Reduce peripheral vascular resistance by preventing angiotensin II–induced vasoconstriction and vascular hypertrophy/remodeling; also help prevent sodium and water retention by limiting aldosterone secretion, and promote vasodilation by prolonging the effects of bradykinin

Angiotensin II receptor blockers**
  Eprosartan (Teveten)
  Losartan (Cozaar)
  Valsartan (Diovan)
	Reduce angiotensin II–induced peripheral vascular resistance and cardiovascular hypertrophy/remodeling by blocking angiotensin II receptors on the heart and vasculature

Beta adrenergic blockers
  Acebutolol (Sectral)
  Atenolol (Tenormin)
  Carteolol (Cartrol)
  Carvedilol (Coreg)
  Labetolol (Normodyne, Trandate)
  Metoprolol (Lopressor)
  (others, see Table 20–2)
	Prevent sympathetic-induced overload on the heart by blocking the effects of epinephrine and norepinephrine on the myocardium; some agents (e.g., carvedilol) may also produce peripheral vasodilation

Diuretics***	Decrease the volume of fluid the heart must pump by promoting the excretion of excess sodium and water; also reduce fluid accumulation (congestion) in the lungs and other tissues

(Continued on following page)

Table 24–1	PRIMARY DRUGS USED IN CONGESTIVE HEART FAILURE *(Continued)*
Drug Group	**Primary Effect**
Vasodilators Hydralazine (Apresoline) Nesiritide (Natrecor) Nitrates (isosorbide dinitrate, others) Prazosin (Minipress)	Promote dilation in the peripheral vasculature, which decreases the amount of blood returning to the heart (cardiac preload) and decreases the pressure the heart must pump against (cardiac afterload)

*Only the Angiotensin-converting enzyme (ACE) inhibitors currently approved for treating heart failure are listed here. See Chapter 21, Table 21–5 for a more complete list of ACE inhibitors.
**Angiotensin II–receptor blockers are not currently approved for treating heart failure; they are used primarily as an alternative if patients cannot tolerate ACE inhibitors.
***Various thiazide, loop, or potassium-sparing diuretics can be used depending on the needs of each patient; see Chapter 21, Table 21–3 for specific diuretic agents.

heart failure as well as the number of hospitalizations and other aspects of morbidity associated with this disease.[19,36,53] Digitalis must, however, be used cautiously and specifically in certain cases of congestive heart failure, rather than as a panacea for all forms of this disease.[19,60] Specifically, digitalis is often added to the pharmacological regimen in patients with heart failure who remain symptomatic despite treatment with other agents such as diuretics, angiotensin-converting enzyme (ACE) inhibitors, and beta blockers (see the respective headings later in this chapter).[19,37] In such patients, combining digitalis with these drugs will clearly provide better clinical effects than can be achieved by using digitalis alone.[14,37]

Effects and Mechanism of Action

Mechanical Effects

Digitalis and the other cardiac glycosides increase the heart's mechanical pumping ability by bringing about an increase in intracellular calcium concentration. Increased intracellular calcium enhances contractility by facilitating the interaction between thick (myosin) and thin (actin) filaments in the myocardial cell.[60,66] Digitalis probably increases intracellular calcium concentration by a complex mechanism, which is illustrated in Figure 24–3. Details of this mechanism are also briefly outlined below.

1. Digitalis exerts its primary effect by inhibiting the sodium-potassium pump on the myocardial cell membrane.[66] The sodium-potassium pump is an active transport system that normally transports sodium out of the cell and potassium into it. Sodium enters the cardiac cell during the depolarization phase of each action potential, and the sodium-potassium pump is responsible for removing this sodium from the cell (see Chapter 23 for a description of ion movements during cardiac excitation). Inhibition of the sodium-potassium pump therefore causes sodium to accumulate within the cell.

2. An increase in intracellular sodium concentration leads to an increase in intracellular calcium.[51] During cardiac excitation, calcium ions normally enter the myocardial cell through specific calcium channels during each action potential (see Chapter 23). An enzyme known as the sodium-calcium exchange protein removes some of the calcium that enters. This enzyme uses the ionic gradient for sodium entry to help remove calcium from the cell, thus exchanging sodium entry for calcium exit from the cell. Because intracellular sodium concentration has increased, there is a smaller driving force (electrochemical gradient) for sodium to enter the cell. If less sodium enters, there is a reduction in the ability of the sodium-calcium exchange protein to remove calcium. Hence, intracellular calcium concentration increases.

3. The increased availability of calcium within the cardiac cell enables it to store more calcium in the sarcoplasmic reticulum.[60] As in any type of muscle cell, calcium is normally stored within the sarcoplasmic reticulum and released during each action potential to facilitate actin-myosin

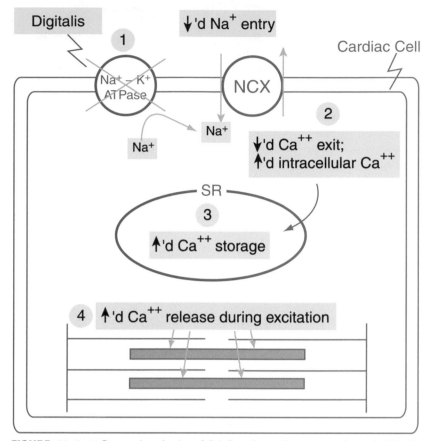

FIGURE 24–3 ▼ Proposed mechanism of digitalis action on the sarcomere located within the myocardial cell. Digitalis inhibits the Na+, K+-ATPase *(1)* resulting in increased intracellular sodium (Na+). Increased intracellular sodium alters the Na+, Ca++ exchange (NCX) mechanism so that intracellular Ca++ also increases *(2)*. As intracellular calcium increases, more calcium is available for storage in the sarcoplasmic reticulum (SR) *(3)*. During cardiac excitation, more calcium is released from storage sites in the sarcoplasmic reticulum, which facilitates contractile protein binding, resulting in increased myocardial contractility *(4)*. See text for additional details.

interaction and initiate muscle contraction. Because more calcium is stored in the cardiac cell, the sarcoplasmic reticulum releases more calcium during each action potential, thereby initiating greater actin-myosin interaction and a stronger cardiac contraction.

Autonomic and Electrophysiologic Effects

In addition to its effects on cardiac contractility, digitalis has a direct inhibitory effect on sympathetic nervous system activity.[37,60] This effect is beneficial because it decreases stress on the failing heart by decreasing excessive sympathetic stimulation of the heart and peripheral vasculature[2]. Therapeutic levels of digitalis likewise stabilize heart rate and slow impulse conduc-

tion through the myocardium. In fact, digitalis is used to prevent and treat certain arrhythmias such as atrial tachycardia and atrial fibrillation (see Chapter 23).[8] Some of these electrical properties may be caused by the direct effect of digitalis on the sodium-potassium pump and can be attributed to alterations in sodium, potassium, and calcium fluxes. As indicated, digitalis also decreases excessive sympathetic stimulation of the heart, and this effect helps normalize cardiac excitation and conduction. Digitalis likewise causes reflex stimulation of the vagus nerve, thus further slowing heart rate and conduction.[60] The autonomic and electrical properties of digitalis therefore improve cardiac excitation and function, and these effects generally complement the mechanical effects of this drug in treating congestive heart failure.

Adverse Side Effects

Digitalis toxicity is a fairly common and potentially fatal adverse reaction to high blood levels of this drug.[20,57] Common signs of toxicity include gastrointestinal distress (nausea, vomiting, diarrhea) and central nervous system (CNS) disturbances (drowsiness, fatigue, confusion, visual disturbances; Table 24–2). Because digitalis alters the electrophysiologic properties of the heart, abnormalities in cardiac function are also common during digitalis toxicity. Common adverse cardiac effects include arrhythmias such as premature atrial and ventricular contractions, paroxysmal atrial tachycardia, ventricular tachycardia, and high degrees of atrioventricular block. As toxicity increases, severe arrhythmias such as ventricular fibrillation can occur and may result in death.

To prevent digitalis toxicity, a low drug dosage should be maintained if possible. Plasma levels of digitalis should be monitored in suspected cases of toxicity to determine an appropriate decrease in dosage.[19] Health care personnel should also be encouraged to look for early signs of toxicity so that digitalis can be discontinued before the effects become life-threatening.

Other Positive Inotropic Agents

Phosphodiesterase Inhibitors

Phosphodiesterase inhibitors include drugs such as inamrinone (known formally as amrinone) and milrinone. Inamrinone and milrinone exert their effects by inhibiting the phosphodiesterase enzyme that breaks down cyclic adenosine monophosphate (cAMP) in cardiac cells. Cyclic-AMP is a common second messenger in many cells (see Chapter 4), and drugs that inhibit the phosphodiesterase enzyme allow cAMP concentrations to increase in the cell.[4,45] In cardiac cells, cAMP acts on membrane calcium channels to allow more calcium to enter the cell.[41] Thus, inamrinone and milrinone cause a cAMP-mediated increase in intracellular calcium, which subsequently increases the force of contraction within the myocardial cell. These drugs also have some vasodilating properties, and some of their beneficial effects in congestive heart failure may be due to their ability to decrease cardiac preload and afterload.[45,60]

Hence, phosphodiesterase inhibitors such as inamrinone and milrinone are classified as positive inotropic agents because they increase myocardial con-

Table 24–2	SIGNS AND SYMPTOMS OF DIGITALIS TOXICITY[a]

Gastrointestinal symptoms
  anorexia
  nausea
  vomiting
  abdominal pain
Visual disturbances
  halos
  photophobia
  problems with color perception
  scotomata
CNS effects
  headache
  confusion
  delirium
  confusion
  psychosis
  fatigue
  weakness
Cardiac effects[b]
  ventricular arrhythmias
  premature ventricular depolarizations, bigeminy, trigeminy, ventricular tachycardia, ventricular fibrillation
  atrioventricular (A-V) block
  first degree, second degree (Mobitz type I), third degree block
  A-V junctional escape rhythms, junctional tachycardia
  atrial rhythms with slowed A-V conduction or A-V block
  particularly paroxysmal atrial tachycardia with A-V block
  sinus bradycardia

[a] Some adverse effects may be difficult to distinguish from the signs/symptoms of heart failure.

[b] Digitalis toxicity has been associated with almost every rhythm abnormality; only the more common manifestations are listed.

Adapted from: Johnson JA, Parker RB, Patterson JH. Heart failure. In: DiPiro JT, et al, eds. *Pharmacotherapy: A Pathophysiologic Approach.* 5th ed. New York: McGraw-Hill; 2002, with permission.

tractility in a relatively selective manner.[41] These drugs, however, must be administered parenterally by intravenous infusion; hence, they are usually limited to short-term treatment of patients with severe congestive heart failure.[9,45] There is also little evidence that these drugs are more effective than digitalis in producing positive inotropic effects, and there is concern that these agents may actually result in more serious side effects, including an increase in patient mortality compared with other drug treatments.[1,4,9] Therefore, inamrinone and milrinone have limited use in treating heart failure and are usually administered in severe or acute cases of heart failure, or in patients with severe heart failure who are awaiting a heart transplant.[4,6,9,26] It is hoped that newer forms of phosphodiesterase inhibitors will be developed in the future that are safer and more effective than the existing drugs.[43,54]

Dopamine and Dobutamine

Dopamine and dobutamine are sometimes used to stimulate the heart in cases of acute or severe heart failure (see Chapter 20). Dopamine and dobutamine exert a fairly specific positive inotropic effect, presumably through their ability to stimulate beta-1 receptors on the myocardium.[60] Other beta-1 agonists (epinephrine, prenalterol, etc.) will also increase myocardial contractility, but most of these other beta-1 agonists will also increase heart rate or have other side effects that prevent their use in congestive heart failure. Dopamine and dobutamine are usually reserved for patients with advanced cases of congestive heart failure who do not respond to other positive inotropic drugs (e.g., digitalis).[6,72]

Agents That Decrease Cardiac Workload

Drugs Affecting the Renin-Angiotensin System

As discussed previously in this chapter, the renin-angiotensin system is often activated in congestive heart failure. Activation of this system results in increased production of a powerful vasoconstrictor known as angiotensin II (see Chapter 21 for details of the renin-angiotensin system). Excess production of angiotensin II is extremely detrimental to the cardiovascular system because it causes increased workload on the heart and abnormal structural changes (remodeling) of the heart and vasculature. Fortunately, two drug strategies have been developed to deal with abnormal activation of the renin-angiotensin system. These strategies are the ACE inhibitors and angiotensin II receptor blockers—each strategy is addressed below.

ACE inhibitors

Angiotensin-converting enzyme (ACE) inhibitors have been used successfully to treat hypertension (see Chapter 21) and are now recognized as critical in treating congestive heart failure.[14,17,33] ACE inhibitors interrupt the renin-angiotensin system and help decrease morbidity and mortality in patients with congestive heart failure by improving the patient's neurohormonal and hemodynamic function.[60,70] The ACE inhibitors commonly used in congestive heart failure include captopril (Capoten), enalapril (Vasotec), and several similar drugs listed in Table 24–1. In severe congestive heart failure, these drugs are often given in combination with diuretics and digitalis.

ACE inhibitors are now considered one of the mainstays of treatment in congestive heart failure. These drugs are the first agents shown to prolong the life span of people with this disease [60]; that is, digitalis, diuretics, and other drugs commonly used to treat heart failure may all produce symptomatic improvements, but the use of ACE inhibitors alone or in combination with these drugs actually results in decreased mortality.[32,60]

The use of ACE inhibitors in treating heart failure has therefore increased dramatically over the last several years.[53] There is evidence that these drugs should be used even more extensively and in higher doses, especially in the early stages of this disease.[32,48] By reducing the detrimental effects of angiotensin II on the vascular system, early use of ACE inhibitors may prevent or delay the progression of this disease (see the next section, "Effects and Mechanism of Action of ACE Inhibitors").

Effects and Mechanism of Action of ACE Inhibitors

As discussed in Chapter 21, ACE inhibitors suppress the enzyme that converts angiotensin I to angiotensin II in the bloodstream. Angiotensin II is a potent vasoconstrictor. By inhibiting the formation of angiotensin II, ACE inhibitors limit peripheral vasoconstriction. This effect results in a decrease in cardiac workload primarily by decreasing the pressure against which the heart must pump (cardiac afterload).[13,41] Decreased cardiac afterload eases the strain on the failing heart, resulting in improved cardiac performance and increased exercise tolerance.[39]

Angiotensin II also promotes abnormal growth and remodeling of the heart, and this substance is thought to be responsible for many of the pathological changes in left ventricular function in heart failure.[5,14] Angiotensin II likewise stimulates growth and hypertrophy of vascular tissues, which results in the thickening of peripheral blood vessels' walls.[21,49] This thickening reduces the size of the vessel lumen, which further increases cardiac afterload because the heart must force blood into these narrowed vessels. ACE inhibitors therefore prevent angiotensin II–induced cardiovascular remodeling, which helps reduce the workload on the heart and prevents the progression of heart failure.[11,60]

By directly inhibiting angiotensin II formation, ACE inhibitors also inhibit aldosterone secretion.[42] Angiotensin II promotes aldosterone secretion from the adrenal cortex (it is probably a by-product of angiotensin II—that is, angiotensin III, which directly stimulates aldosterone secretion). Aldosterone increases renal sodium reabsorption, with a subsequent increase in water reabsorption (i.e., the exact opposite effect produced by a diuretic). Inhibition of aldosterone secretion is beneficial in congestive heart failure because vascular fluid volume does not increase and overtax the failing heart. Consequently, ACE inhibitors may help decrease cardiac workload in congestive heart failure by both hemodynamic mechanisms (prevention of vasoconstriction by angiotensin II) and fluid-electrolyte mechanisms (inhibition of aldosterone secretion).

Finally, ACE inhibitors exert some of their beneficial effects by increasing bradykinin levels in the bloodstream.[17,70] Bradykinin is a vasodilator, and increased levels of this compound decrease cardiac workload in people with heart failure. Normally, ACE is responsible for the enzymatic destruction of bradykinin in the bloodstream. ACE inhibitors reduce the breakdown of bradykinin, thereby prolonging the vasodilating effects of this substance.[17,70]

Hence, ACE inhibitors reduce the detrimental effects of excess angiotensin II and aldosterone, and prolong the beneficial effects of bradykinin. These effects work in combination to sustain cardiovascular health in people with heart failure.

Angiotensin II Receptor Blockers

Angiotensin II receptor blockers (ARBs) represent a second strategy for treating disorders associated with the renin-angiotensin system.[24] These drugs include agents such as candesartan, losartan and valsartan. As indicated in Chapter 21, these drugs prevent angiotensin II from binding to receptors on vascular tissues,

thus inhibiting angiotensin II–induced damage of the cardiovascular system. It appears that ARBs are as effective as ACE inhibitors in treating heart failure and preventing mortality.[24,46,47] It has also been suggested that combining an ARB with an ACE inhibitor might provide more benefits than using either drug alone.[5,24,52] This idea remains controversial, however, because some studies failed to observe a supplemental effect when an ARB was added to ACE inhibitor in the treatment of patients with heart failure.[17,59]

Consequently, ARBs are used primarily as an alternative for people who are unable to tolerate traditional ACE inhibitors.[17,46,47] Future studies comparing ACE inhibitors with these newer angiotensin II receptor blockers should help clarify which type of drug—or perhaps a combination of the two—provides optimal treatment in heart failure.[17]

Adverse Side Effects of Drugs Affecting the Renin-Angiotensin System

Adverse effects with ACE inhibitors are relatively rare. In fact, one of the primary advantages of these drugs over more toxic compounds such as digitalis is the low incidence of serious effects. ACE inhibitors are occasionally associated with bothersome side effects such as skin rashes, gastrointestinal discomfort, and dizziness; these effects are often transient or can be resolved with an adjustment in dosage. Some patients taking ACE inhibitors develop a persistent dry cough, and this side effect is often the reason for discontinuing the drug or seeking an alternative treatment. As indicated above, the newer angiotensin II receptor blockers can be used as an alternative to ACE inhibitors if patients are not able to tolerate a dry cough or other ACE inhibitor–induced side effects.

Beta Blockers

In the past, beta blockers were considered detrimental in patients with heart failure.[60] As indicated in Chapter 20, these drugs decrease heart rate and myocardial contraction force by blocking the effects of epinephrine and norepinephrine on the heart. Common sense dictated that a decrease in myocardial contractility would be counterproductive in heart failure, and beta blockers were therefore contraindicated in heart failure.[60,69] It is now recognized that beta blockers are actually beneficial in people with heart failure because these drugs attenuate the excessive sympathetic activity associated with this disease.[56,64] As indicated earlier, increased sympathetic activity and other neurohumoral changes often contribute to the vicious cycle associated with heart failure, and excessive sympathetic stimulation can accelerate the pathologic changes in the failing heart.[7,62,65] Beta blockers reduce the harmful effects of excessive sympathetic stimulation, and use of these drugs has been shown to reduce the morbidity and mortality associated with heart failure.[3,38,65] Hence, beta blockers are now considered one of the principal treatments of this disease, and use of these drugs along with ACE inhibitors and traditional agents (digitalis, diuretics, and so forth) is advocated as state-of-the-art therapy for providing optimal treatment in heart failure.[27,53]

Effects and Mechanism of Action

Beta blockers bind to beta-1 receptors on the myocardium and block the effects of norepinephrine and epinephrine (see Chapter 20). These drugs therefore normalize sympathetic stimulation of the heart and help reduce heart rate (negative chronotropic effect) and myocardial contraction force (negative inotropic effect). Beta blockers may also prevent angina by stabilizing cardiac workload, and they may prevent certain arrhythmias by stabilizing heart rate.[40] These additional properties can be useful to patients with heart failure who also have other cardiac symptoms.

Finally, it has been suggested that some of the newer "third-generation" beta blockers such as carvedilol (Coreg) may be especially useful in heart failure because these drugs block beta-1 receptors on the heart while also blocking alpha-1 receptors on the vasculature, thus causing peripheral vasodilation.[30,55] Vasodilation of peripheral vessels could further reduce myocardial stress by decreasing the pressure that the heart must work against in the peripheral vessels (cardiac afterload).

Adverse Side Effects

The side effects and problems associated with beta blockers were addressed in Chapter 20. The primary problem associated with these drugs is that they may cause excessive inhibition of the heart, resulting in an abnormally slow heart rate and reduced contraction force. This effect is especially problematic in heart failure because the heart is already losing its ability to pump blood. Nonetheless, the risk of this and other side effects is acceptable in most people with heart failure, and this risk is minimized by adjusting the dosage

so that sympathetic activity is normalized rather than reduced to unacceptably low levels.

Diuretics

Diuretics increase the excretion of sodium and water (see Chapter 21). These agents are useful in congestive heart failure primarily because of their ability to reduce congestion in the lungs and peripheral tissues by excreting excess fluid retained in these tissues.[32,60] Diuretics also decrease the amount of fluid the heart must pump (cardiac preload), thereby reducing the workload on the failing heart.[60] Diuretics help improve the symptoms of heart failure, and they are often used with other agents (ACE inhibitors, beta blockers, digitalis) to provide optimal treatment of this disease.[14,32] Diuretic drugs, which are also used to treat hypertension, are discussed in more detail in Chapter 21. Diuretics that can be used in the treatment of congestive heart failure and hypertension are listed in Chapter 21, Table 21–3.

Effects and Mechanism of Action

Diuretics work by inhibiting the reabsorption of sodium from the nephron, which, in turn, decreases the amount of water that is normally reabsorbed with sodium, thus increasing water excretion. This effect reduces congestion caused by fluids retained in the body and decreases cardiac preload by excreting excess fluid in the vascular system. Chapter 21 provides a more detailed discussion on the mechanism of action of diuretic drugs.

It has also been suggested that certain diuretics such as spironolactone (Aldactone) might be especially helpful in heart failure.[14,42] Spironolactone blocks aldosterone receptors in the kidneys and other tissues, thereby producing a diuretic effect as well as preventing adverse cardiovascular changes associated with excess aldosterone production. Future studies will help clarify whether spironolactone should be used preferentially in heart failure because of its ability to reduce fluid volume and protect against aldosterone-induced damage.[53]

Adverse Side Effects

By the very nature of their action, diuretics are often associated with disturbances in fluid and electrolyte balance. Volume depletion, hyponatremia, hypokalemia, and altered pH balance are among the most frequent problems.[68] These electrolyte and pH changes can produce serious consequences by affecting cardiac excitability and precipitating arrhythmias. Patients on diuretics should be monitored closely for symptoms such as fatigue, confusion, and nausea, which may indicate the presence of drug-induced disturbances in fluid-electrolyte balance. Some patients may also become resistant to diuretic drugs; the effectiveness of the diuretic is diminished primarily because the kidneys adapt to the drug-induced sodium excretion.[23,44] Resistance can often be prevented, however, by altering the dose and type of diuretic or by adding a second diuretic.[23,39]

Vasodilators

Various drugs that vasodilate peripheral vessels have been successful in treating patients with cases of severe congestive heart failure.[22,60] By reducing peripheral vascular resistance, these agents decrease the amount of blood returning to the heart (cardiac preload) and reduce the pressure that the heart must pump against (cardiac afterload). Reduced cardiac preload and afterload helps alleviate some of the stress on the failing heart, thus slowing the disease progression. Vasodilators commonly used in heart failure include prazosin, hydralazine, and organic nitrates (e.g., nitroglycerin, isosorbide dinitrate, sodium nitroprusside; see Table 24–1). In particular, a combination of hydralazine and isosorbide dinitrate has been found to be helpful in reducing symptoms and improving survival in patients with advance heart failure.[22,53]

In addition to these traditional vasodilators, nesiritide (Natrecor) was developed as a newer method for producing arterial and venous dilation in people with heart failure.[58] This substance was derived from human B-type natriuretic peptide (BNP) using recombinant DNA techniques. BNP is a naturally occurring substance that is released from the ventricles when the heart is subjected to increased blood volume and pressure.[12] This substance dilates peripheral arteries and veins, thus reducing cardiac afterload and preload, respectively. Hence, nesiritide can be administered intravenously to reduce cardiac workload in certain patients with severe or acute heart failure.[12,58]

Effects and Mechanism of Action

Prazosin produces vasodilation by blocking alpha-1 receptors on vascular smooth muscle (see Chapter 20);

hydralazine, organic nitrates, and BNP produce vasodilation by a direct inhibitory effect on the vascular smooth-muscle cells (see Chapters 21 and 22). Although these vasodilators work by different mechanisms, they all can decrease cardiac workload by decreasing peripheral vascular resistance. These drugs may be combined with other agents (digoxin, ACE inhibitors, beta blockers) to provide optimal benefits in patients with varying degrees of congestive heart failure.[53,60]

Adverse Side Effects

The primary side effects associated with vasodilators include headache, dizziness, hypotension, and orthostatic hypotension. These effects are all related to the tendency of these drugs to increase peripheral blood flow and decrease peripheral vascular resistance. Vasodilators may also cause reflex tachycardia in certain patients if the baroreceptor reflex increases heart rate in an attempt to maintain adequate blood pressure.

Summary of Drug Therapy

The treatment of heart failure has undergone substantial changes over the past few years. Digitalis, once the cornerstone of treatment, is associated with a number of serious side effects, and there is considerable doubt as to whether digitalis actually increases the rate of survival of patients with congestive heart failure.[36,53] Standard treatment is now centered on using drugs that decrease cardiac workload, such as ACE inhibitors and beta blockers.[53] These drugs not only help resolve the symptoms of heart failure, but can also slow the progression of this disease and help prolong life expectancy. Other drugs such as digitalis, diuretics, and vasodilators can be added to the ACE inhibitor/beta blocker regimen as needed to help resolve symptoms, or as heart failure becomes more pronounced. Regardless of which drugs are used, there is consensus that early intervention in the treatment of congestive heart failure is crucial in providing the best outcome.[60]

SUMMARY

Congestive heart failure is a serious cardiac condition in which the ability of the heart to pump blood becomes progressively worse. Decreased myocardial performance leads to a number of deleterious changes, including peripheral edema (i.e., congestion) and in-

Special Concerns in Rehabilitation Patients

■ ■ ■ Therapists should be aware of the potential for drugs used to treat congestive heart failure to affect the patient's welfare and response to rehabilitation. Acute congestive heart failure may occur in patients with myocardial disease because of a lack of therapeutic drug effects or because of the toxic effects of some cardiac drugs. Therapists should remain alert for signs of acute congestive heart failure such as increased cough, difficulty in breathing (dyspnea), abnormal respiratory sounds (rales), and frothy sputum. Therapists should also remain alert for signs of digitalis toxicity such as dizziness, confusion, nausea, and arrhythmias. Early recognition by the therapist may prevent serious or even fatal consequences. Likewise, patients taking diuretics sometimes exhibit excessive fatigue and weakness — these may be the early signs of fluid and electrolyte depletion. Therapists may help detect serious metabolic and electrolyte imbalances that result from problems with diuretic drugs. Finally, use of vasodilators often causes hypotension and postural hypotension. Therapists must use caution when patients suddenly sit up or stand up. Also, therapeutic techniques that produce systemic vasodilation (whirlpool, exercise) may produce profound hypotension in patients taking vasodilators, and these modalities should therefore be used cautiously.

CASE STUDY

Congestive Heart Failure

Brief History. D.S. is a 67-year-old woman with a long history of congestive heart failure caused by myocarditis. She has been treated successfully with digitalis glycosides (digoxin [Zanoxin], 0.5 mg/d) for several years. Despite some swelling in her ankles and feet and a tendency to become winded, she has maintained a fairly active lifestyle and enjoys gardening and other hobbies. Recently, she developed some weakness and incoordination that primarily affected her right side. Subsequent testing revealed that she had suffered a cerebral vascular accident (stroke). She was not admitted to the hospital but remained living at home with her husband. Physical therapy, however, was provided in the home to facilitate optimal recovery from her stroke. The therapist began seeing her three times each week for a program of therapeutic exercise and functional training.

Problem/Influence of Medication. The therapist initially found D.S. to be alert, coherent, and eager to begin therapy. Although there was some residual weakness and decreased motor skills, the prognosis for a full recovery appeared good. The therapist was impressed by the patient's enthusiasm and pleasant nature during the first two sessions.

By the end of the first week, however, the therapist noted a distinct change in the patient's demeanor. She was confused and quite lethargic. The therapist initially suspected that she might have had another stroke. However, physical examination did not reveal any dramatic decrease in strength or coordination. Realizing that the patient was still taking digitalis for the treatment of heart failure, the therapist began to suspect the possibility of digitalis toxicity.

Decision/Solution. The therapist immediately notified the physician about the change in the patient's status. The patient was admitted to the hospital, where a blood test confirmed the presence of digitalis toxicity (i.e., blood levels of digitalis were well above the therapeutic range). Apparently, the stroke had sufficiently altered the metabolism and excretion of the digitalis so that the therapeutic dosage was now accumulating in the patient's body. The altered pharmacokinetic profile was probably caused in part by the decrease in the patient's mobility and level of activity that occurred after the stroke. The digitalis dosage was reduced, and a diuretic was added to provide management of the congestive heart failure. The patient was soon discharged from the hospital and resumed physical therapy at home. Her rehabilitation progressed without further incident.

creased fatigue during physical activity. Treatment of congestive heart failure consists primarily of drug therapy. Certain drugs such as digitalis and other positive inotropic agents attempt to directly increase cardiac pumping ability. Other drugs such as diuretics and vasodilators decrease cardiac workload by decreasing vascular fluid volume or dilating peripheral blood vessels, respectively.

ACE inhibitors and beta blockers have gained widespread acceptance in treating heart failure because these drugs decrease the abnormal neurohumoral changes associated with this disease. Specifically, ACE inhibitors decrease activity in the renin-angiotensin system, and beta blockers prevent excessive cardiovascular stimulation from the sympathetic nervous system. These effects help prevent abnormal stimulation of the heart and vasculature, and early treatment with ACE inhibitors and beta blockers is now recognized as critical in delaying the progression of this disease and decreasing mortality in people with heart failure. Even with optimal treatment, however, the prognosis for patients with congestive heart failure is often poor. Therapists should be aware of the drugs used to treat this disorder and that certain side effects may adversely affect rehabilitation or signal a problem with drug treatment.

References

1. Abraham WT, Adams KF, Fonarow GC, et al. In-hospital mortality in patients with acute decompensated heart failure requiring intravenous vasoactive medications: an analysis from the Acute Decompensated Heart Failure National Registry (ADHERE). *J Am Coll Cardiol.* 2005;46:57–64.
2. Adams KF, Jr. Pathophysiologic role of the renin-angiotensin-aldosterone and sympathetic nervous systems in heart failure. *Am J Health Syst Pharm.* 2004;61(suppl 2):S4–S13.
3. Ahmed A, Dell'Italia LJ. Use of beta-blockers in older adults with chronic heart failure. *Am J Med Sci.* 2004; 328:100–111.
4. Amsallem E, Kasparian C, Haddour G, et al. Phosphodiesterase III inhibitors for heart failure. *Cochrane Database Syst Rev.* 2005;CD002230.
5. Anavekar NS, Solomon SD. Angiotensin II receptor blockade and ventricular remodelling. *J Renin Angiotensin Aldosterone Syst.* 2005;6:43–48.
6. Aranda JM, Jr, Schofield RS, Pauly DF, et al. Comparison of dobutamine versus milrinone therapy in hospitalized patients awaiting cardiac transplantation: a prospective, randomized trial. *Am Heart J.* 2003; 145:324–329.
7. Bader FM, MacGregor JF, Gilbert EM. Initiation and use of beta-blockers in class IV heart failure. *Curr Heart Fail Rep.* 2004;1:72–76.
8. Bauman JL, Schoen MD. Arrhythmias. In: DiPiro JT, et al, eds. *Pharmacotherapy: A Pathophysiologic Approach.* 5th ed. New York: McGraw-Hill; 2002.
9. Bayram M, De Luca L, Massie MB, Gheorghiade M. Reassessment of dobutamine, dopamine, and milrinone in the management of acute heart failure syndromes. *Am J Cardiol.* 2005;96:47G–58G.
10. Bleumink GS, Schut AF, Sturkenboom MC, et al. Genetic polymorphisms and heart failure. *Genet Med.* 2004;6:465–474.
11. Brown NJ, Vaughan, DE. Angiotensin-converting enzyme inhibitors. *Circulation.* 1998;97:1411–1420.
12. Burger AJ. A review of the renal and neurohormonal effects of B-type natriuretic peptide. *Congest Heart Fail.* 2005;11:30–38.
13. Cassady SL. Cardiovascular pathophysiology. In: DeTurk WE, Cahalin LP, eds. *Cardiovascular and Pulmonary Physical Therapy.* New York: McGraw-Hill; 2004.
14. Chatterjee K. Congestive heart failure: what should be the initial therapy and why? *Am J Cardiovasc Drugs.* 2002;2:1–6.
15. Chatterjee K. Neurohormonal activation in congestive heart failure and the role of vasopressin. *Am J Cardiol.* 2005;95:8B–13B.
16. Colucci WS, Braunwald E. Pathophysiology of heart failure. In: Braunwald E, Zipes DP, Libby P, eds. *Heart Disease.* Vol. 1. 6th ed. Philadelphia: WB Saunders; 2001.
17. Cruden NL, Newby DE. Angiotensin antagonism in patients with heart failure: ACE inhibitors, angiotensin receptor antagonists or both? *Am J Cardiovasc Drugs.* 2004;4:345–353.
18. Davila DF, Nunez TJ, Odreman R, de Davila CA. Mechanisms of neurohormonal activation in chronic congestive heart failure: pathophysiology and therapeutic implications. *Int J Cardiol.* 2005;101:343–346.
19. Dec GW. Digoxin remains useful in the management of chronic heart failure. *Med Clin North Am.* 2003;87: 317–337.
20. Demiryurek AT, Demiryurek S. Cardiotoxicity of digitalis glycosides: roles of autonomic pathways, autacoids and ion channels. *Auton Autacoid Pharmacol.* 2005;25:35–52.
21. Dzau V. The cardiovascular continuum and renin-angiotensin-aldosterone system blockade. *J Hypertens Suppl.* 2005;23:S9–S17.
22. Elkayam U, Bitar F. Effects of nitrates and hydralazine in heart failure: clinical evidence before the African American heart failure trial. *Am J Cardiol.* 2005;96: 37i–43i.
23. Ellison DH. Diuretic resistance: physiology and therapeutics. *Semin Nephrol.* 1999;19:581–597.

24. Erhardt LR. A review of the current evidence for the use of angiotensin-receptor blockers in chronic heart failure. *Int J Clin Pract.* 2005;59:571–578.

25. Fedak PW, Verma S, Weisel RD, Li RK. Cardiac remodeling and failure: from molecules to man (part I). *Cardiovasc Pathol.* 2005;14:1–11.

26. Felker GM, O'Connor CM. Inotropic therapy for heart failure: an evidence-based approach. *Am Heart J.* 2001;142:393–401.

27. Fonarow GC. When to initiate beta-blockers in heart failure: is it ever too early? *Curr Heart Fail Rep.* 2005; 2:94–99.

28. Francis GS. Pathophysiology of chronic heart failure. *Am J Med.* 2001;110(suppl 7A):37S–46S.

29. Gheorghiade M, De Luca L, Fonarow GC, et al. Pathophysiologic targets in the early phase of acute heart failure syndromes. *Am J Cardiol.* 2005;96: 11G–17G.

30. Greenberg B. Nonselective versus selective beta-blockers in the management of chronic heart failure: clinical implications of the carvedilol or Metoprolol European Trial. *Rev Cardiovasc Med.* 2004;5(suppl 1):S10–S17.

31. Gutierrez C, Blanchard DG. Diastolic heart failure: challenges of diagnosis and treatment. *Am Fam Physician.* 2004;69:2609–2616.

32. Guyatt GH, Devereaux PJ. A review of heart failure treatment. *Mt Sinai J Med.* 2004;71:47–54.

33. Hebert PR, Foody JM, Hennekens CH. The renin-angiotensin system: the role of inhibitors, blockers, and genetic polymorphisms in the treatment and prevention of heart failure. *Curr Vasc Pharmacol.* 2003; 1:33–39.

34. Hobbs RE. Guidelines for the diagnosis and management of heart failure. *Am J Ther.* 2004;11:467–472.

35. Hogg K, Swedberg K, McMurray J. Heart failure with preserved left ventricular systolic function; epidemiology, clinical characteristics, and prognosis. *J Am Coll Cardiol.* 2004;43:317–327.

36. Hood WB, Jr, Dans AL, Guyatt GH, et al. Digitalis for treatment of congestive heart failure in patients in sinus rhythm. *Cochrane Database Syst Rev.* 2004; CD002901.

37. Hoppe UC, Erdmann E. Digitalis in heart failure! Still applicable? *Z Kardiol.* 2005;94:307–311.

38. Jafri SM. The effects of beta blockers on morbidity and mortality in heart failure. *Heart Fail Rev.* 2004; 9:115–121.

39. Johnson JA, Parker RB, Patterson JH. Heart failure. In: DiPiro JT, et al, eds. *Pharmacotherapy: A Pathophysiologic Approach.* 5th ed. New York: McGraw-Hill; 2002.

40. Joseph J, Gilbert EM. The sympathetic nervous system in chronic heart failure. *Prog Cardiovasc Dis.* 1998;41 (suppl 1):9–16.

41. Katzung BG, Parmley WW. Drugs used in heart failure. In: Katzung BG, ed. *Basic and Clinical Pharmacology.* 9th ed. New York: Lange Medical Books/ McGraw-Hill; 2004.

42. Khan NU, Movahed A. The role of aldosterone and aldosterone-receptor antagonists in heart failure. *Rev Cardiovasc Med.* 2004;5:71–81.

43. Kivikko M, Lehtonen L. Levosimendan: a new inodilatory drug for the treatment of decompensated heart failure. *Curr Pharm Des.* 2005;11:435–455.

44. Kramer BK, Schweda F, Riegger GA. Diuretic treatment and diuretic resistance in heart failure. *Am J Med.* 1999;106:90–96.

45. Lehtonen LA, Antila S, Pentikainen PJ. Pharmacokinetics and pharmacodynamics of intravenous inotropic agents. *Clin Pharmacokinet.* 2004;43:187–203.

46. Levine TB, Levine AB. Rationale for the use of angiotensin II receptor blockers in patients with left ventricular dysfunction (part I of II). *Clin Cardiol.* 2005;28:215–218.

47. Levine TB, Levine AB. Clinical update: the role of angiotensin II receptor blockers in patients with left ventricular dysfunction (part II of II). *Clin Cardiol.* 2005;28:277–280.

48. Luzier AB, DiTusa L. Underutilization of ACE inhibitors in heart failure. *Pharmacotherapy.* 1999; 19:1296–1307.

49. Mahmud A, Feely J. Arterial stiffness and the renin-angiotensin-aldosterone system. *J Renin Angiotensin Aldosterone Syst.* 2004;5:102–108.

50. Mann DL. Basic mechanisms of left ventricular remodeling: the contribution of wall stress. *J Card Fail.* 2004;10(suppl 6):S202–S206.

51. McDonough AA, Velotta JB, Schwinger RH, et al. The cardiac sodium pump: structure and function. *Basic Res Cardiol.* 2002;97(suppl 1):I19–I24.

52. McMurray JJ. Angiotensin inhibition in heart failure. *J Renin Angiotensin Aldosterone Syst.* 2004;5(suppl 1): S17–S22.

53. McMurray JJ, Pfeffer MA. Heart failure. *Lancet.* 2005; 365:1877–1889.

54. Mebazaa A, Barraud D, Welschbillig S. Randomized clinical trials with levosimendan. *Am J Cardiol.* 2005; 96:74G–79G.

55. Metra M, Cas LD, di Lenarda A, Poole-Wilson P. Beta-blockers in heart failure: are pharmacological differences clinically important? *Heart Fail Rev.* 2004; 9:123–130.

56. Ohlstein EH, Romanic AM. New developments in the use of beta-blockers for the management of heart failure. *Expert Opin Investig Drugs.* 2004;13:999–1005.

57. Pickett JR, Dickinson ET. Dealing with DIG. A comprehensive review of digoxin and its therapeutic and toxic effects. *JEMS.* 2005;30:70–78, 82, 84.

58. Richards AM, Lainchbury JG, Troughton RW, et al. Clinical applications of B-type natriuretic peptides. *Trends Endocrinol Metab.* 2004;15:170–174.

59. Ripley TL. Valsartan in chronic heart failure. *Ann Pharmacother.* 2005;39:460–469.

60. Rocco TP, Fang JC. Pharmacotherapy of congestive heart failure. In: Brunton LL, ed. *The Pharmacological Basis of Therapeutics.* 11th ed. New York: McGraw-Hill; 2006.

61. Russell SD, DeWald T. Vasopressin receptor antagonists. Therapeutic potential in the management of acute and chronic heart failure. *Am J Cardiovasc Drugs.* 2003;3:13–20.

62. Sabbah HN. Biologic rationale for the use of beta-blockers in the treatment of heart failure. *Heart Fail Rev.* 2004;9:91–97.

63. Sanderson JE. Diastolic heart failure or heart failure with a normal ejection fraction. *Minerva Cardioangiol* 2006; 54: 715–724.

64. Satwani S, Dec GW, Narula J. Beta-adrenergic blockers in heart failure: review of mechanisms of action and clinical outcomes. *J Cardiovasc Pharmacol Ther.* 2004;9: 243–255.

65. Sauls JL, Rone T. Emerging trends in the management of heart failure: beta blocker therapy. *Nurs Clin North Am.* 2005;40:135–148.

66. Schwinger RH, Bundgaard H, Muller-Ehmsen J, Kjeldsen K. The Na, K-ATPase in the failing human heart. *Cardiovasc Res.* 2003;57:913–920.

67. Sharpe N. Pharmacologic effects on cardiac remodeling. *Curr Heart Fail Rep.* 2004;1:9–13.

68. Sica DA. Diuretic-related side effects: development and treatment. *J Clin Hypertens.* 2004;6: 532–540.

69. Sorrentino MJ. Beta-blockers for congestive heart failure. *Compr Ther.* 2003;29:210–214.

70. Unger T, Li J. The role of the renin-angiotensin-aldosterone system in heart failure. *J Renin Angiotensin Aldosterone Syst.* 2004;5(suppl 1): S7–S10.

71. Volpe M, Pagannone E, Tocci G, Rubattu S. Hypertension and heart failure: role of neurohormonal mechanisms. *Clin Exp Hypertens.* 2004;26:603–610.

72. Yamani MH, Haji SA, Starling RC, et al. Comparison of dobutamine-based and milrinone-based therapy for advanced decompensated congestive heart failure: Hemodynamic efficacy, clinical outcome, and economic impact. *Am Heart J.* 2001; 142:998–1002.

Chapter 25

Treatment of Coagulation Disorders and Hyperlipidemia

Blood coagulation, or *hemostasis*, is necessary to prevent excessive hemorrhage from damaged blood vessels. Under normal conditions, clotting factors in the bloodstream spontaneously interact with damaged vessels to create a blood clot that plugs the leaking vessel. Obviously, inadequate blood clotting is harmful in that even minor vessel damage can lead to excessive blood loss. Overactive clotting is also detrimental because it will lead to *thrombogenesis* (i.e., the abnormal formation of blood clots, or thrombi).[92,108] Thrombus formation may lead directly to vessel occlusion and tissue infarction. Also, a piece of a thrombus may dislodge, creating an embolism that causes infarction elsewhere in the body, for example, in the lungs or brain.

Consequently, normal hemostasis can be regarded as a balance between too much and too little blood coagulation.[133,140] This balance is often disrupted by a number of factors. Insufficient levels of blood clotting factors typically cause inadequate clotting, as in patients with hemophilia. Excessive clotting often occurs during prolonged bed rest or when blood flow through vessels is partially obstructed, as in coronary atherosclerosis.

Restoration of normal hemostasis is accomplished through pharmacologic methods. Excessive clotting and thrombus formation are rectified by drugs that prevent clot formation (anticoagulants, antithrombotics) or facilitate the removal of previously formed clots (*thrombolytics*). Inadequate clotting is resolved by replacing the missing clotting factors or by drugs that facilitate the synthesis of specific clotting factors.

Hemostasis can also be influenced by *hyperlipidemia*, which is a chronic and excessive increase in plasma lipids. With hyperlipidemia, cholesterol and other lipids are progressively deposited onto arterial walls, forming plaquelike lesions indicative of atherosclerosis. These atherosclerotic lesions progressively occlude the arterial lumen, and atherosclerotic plaques can suddenly rupture, thus leading to thrombosis and infarction. Atherosclerotic heart disease is one of the leading causes of morbidity and mortality in the United States, and pharmacologic methods to lower plasma lipids are often used in conjunction with dietary and lifestyle modifications to treat hyperlipidemia and prevent atherosclerosis.

Drugs used to normalize blood clotting or reduce hyperlipidemia are among the most common medications used clinically, and rehabilitation specialists will deal with many patients taking these agents. Many patients, in fact, will be treated in therapy for problems relating directly to thrombus formation (e.g., ischemic stroke, myocardial infarction, pulmonary embolism). Individuals with inadequate clotting, such as patients with hemophilia, are also seen routinely in rehabilitation because of the intrajoint hemorrhaging and other problems associated with this disease. Consequently, the purpose of this chapter is to acquaint therapists with several common and important groups of drugs used to treat coagulation disorders and hyperlipidemia.

Normal Mechanism of Blood Coagulation

To understand how various drugs affect hemostasis, it is necessary to review the normal way in which blood clots are formed. The physiologic mechanisms involved in hemostasis are outlined in Figure 25–1, with

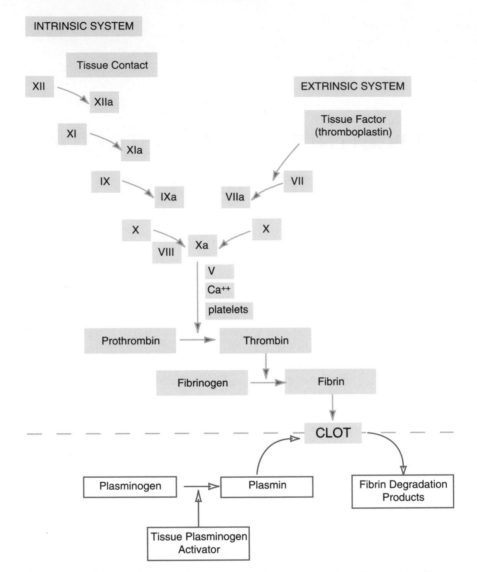

FIGURE 25–1 ▼ Mechanism of blood coagulation. Factors involved in clot formation are shown above the dashed line; factors involved in clot breakdown are shown below the dashed line. See text for further discussion.

clot formation and breakdown illustrated in the upper and lower parts of the figure, respectively.

Clot Formation

Clot formation involves the activation of various clotting factors circulating in the bloodstream.[108,135] The clotting factors are proteolytic enzymes synthesized in the liver that remain inactive until there is some injury to a blood vessel. Blood vessel damage begins a cascade effect, whereby one of the clotting factors is activated, which leads to the next factor's activation, and so forth.[128,135] As shown in Figure 25–1, clot formation occurs through two systems: an intrinsic and an extrinsic system. In the intrinsic system, the direct contact of the first clotting factor (factor XII) with the damaged vessel wall activates the clotting factor and initiates the cascade. In the extrinsic system, a substance known as *tissue factor* (known also as *thromboplastin*) is released from the damaged vascular cell. Tissue factor directly activates clotting factor VII, which then activates subsequent factors in the clotting mechanism. For optimal coagulation to occur in vivo, both the intrinsic and extrinsic systems must be present.

Both the intrinsic and extrinsic systems ultimately lead to the conversion of prothrombin to thrombin.[92] *Thrombin* is an enzyme that quickly converts the inactive fibrinogen molecule to *fibrin*. Individual strands of fibrin bind together to form a meshlike structure, which ultimately forms the framework for the blood clot. Other cellular components, especially platelets, help reinforce the clot by sticking to the fibrin mesh.

Clot Breakdown

The breakdown of blood clots is illustrated in the lower part of Figure 25–1. *Tissue plasminogen activator (t-PA)* converts plasminogen to plasmin. *Plasmin*, also known as fibrinolysin, is an enzyme that directly breaks down the fibrin mesh, thus destroying the clot.

The balance between clot formation and breakdown is crucial in maintaining normal hemostasis. Obviously, clots should not be broken down as quickly as they are formed because then no coagulation will occur. Likewise, a lack of breakdown would enable clots to proliferate at an excessive rate, leading to thrombus formation.

The complex interaction of the factors described above, and a number of endogenous anticoagulant proteins such as protein C, protein S, and antithrombin III normally control the balance between clot formation and clot breakdown.[36,61] Disease or inactivity, however, can alter this balance, leading to exaggerated clotting and venous or arterial thrombosis. Drugs used to treat overactive clotting are addressed in the next section.

Drugs Used to Treat Overactive Clotting

Drugs used to treat excessive clot formation can be grouped into three primary categories: anticoagulant, antithrombotic, and thrombolytic agents (Table 25–1). Anticoagulants exert their effect by controlling the function and synthesis of clotting factors; these drugs are used primarily to prevent clot formation in the venous system—that is, venous thrombosis. Antithrombotic drugs act primarily by inhibiting platelet function, and primarily prevent thrombus formation in arteries. Thrombolytic drugs facilitate the destruction of blood clots, and are used to reestablish blood flow through vessels that have been occluded by thrombi. Specific agents discussed below are listed in Table 25–1.

Anticoagulants

The primary anticoagulants are heparin and a group of orally acting agents including warfarin (Coumadin) and other coumarin derivatives. These drugs are used primarily in the treatment of abnormal clot formation in the venous system. Venous clots typically form in the deep veins of the legs because of the relatively sluggish blood flow through those vessels. Hence, deep vein thrombosis is a primary indication for anticoagulant therapy.[103] When a piece of the clot breaks off and travels through the circulation to lodge elsewhere in the vascular system, deep vein thrombosis results in thromboembolism. Emboli originating in the venous system typically follow the venous flow back to the right side of the heart, where they are then pumped to the lungs. They finally lodge in the smaller vessels within the lungs, thus creating a pulmonary embolism.[122] Consequently, the pathologic condition that initiates anticoagulant therapy is often pulmonary embolism secondary to venous thrombosis.

Anticoagulant drugs are administered for the acute treatment of venous thrombosis and thromboembolism; they may also be given prophylactically to individuals who are at high risk to develop venous thrombosis. For instance, these drugs are often administered after surgical procedures (joint replacement, mechanical heart valve replacement, and so forth), following certain cardiovascular incidents (myocardial infarction, ischemic stroke), and during medical conditions when patients will be relatively inactive for extended periods of time.[72,79,86,120]

Heparin

Heparin is the primary drug used in the initial treatment of venous thrombosis.[100,103] The anticoagulant effects of heparin are seen almost instantly after administration. Heparin works by potentiating the activity of a circulating protein known as antithrombin III.[24,76] Antithrombin III binds to several of the active clotting factors (including thrombin) and renders the clotting factors inactive. Heparin accelerates the antithrombin III–induced inactivation of these clotting factors, thus reducing the tendency for clotting and thrombogenesis.

Heparin is a large, sugarlike molecule that is poorly absorbed from the gastrointestinal tract. Consequently, heparin must be administered parenterally. The agent was traditionally administered through intravenous (IV) infusion or repeated IV injection

Table 25–1	DRUGS USED TO TREAT OVERACTIVE CLOTTING

Drug Category	Primary Effect and Indication

Anticoagulants
Heparins
  Unfractionated heparin (Calciparin,
    Liquaemin, others)
Low molecular weight heparins:
  Ardeparin (Normiflo)
  Dalteparin (Fragmin)
  Enoxaparin (Lovenox)
  Tinzaparin (Innohep)
Oral anticoagulants
  Anisindione (Miradon)
  Dicumarol (generic)
  Warfarin (Coumadin)
	Inhibit synthesis and function of clotting factors; used primarily to prevent and treat venous thromboembolism

Antithrombotics
Aspirin
ADP receptor inhibitors
  Clopidogrel (Plavix)
  Ticlopidine (Ticlid)
Glycoprotein IIb-IIIa receptor inhibitors:
  Abciximab (ReoPro)
  Eptifibatide (Integrilin)
  Tirofiban (Aggrastat)
Others
  Dipyridamole (Persantine, others)
  Sulfinpyrazone (Anturane)
	Inhibit platelet aggregation and platelet-induced clotting; used primarily to prevent arterial thrombus formation

Thrombolytics
  Alteplase, recombinant (Activase)
  Anistreplase (Eminase)
  Streptokinase (Streptase)
  Urokinase (Abbokinase)
	Facilitate clot dissolution; used to reopen occluded vessels in arterial and venous thrombosis

through a rubber-capped indwelling needle called a *heparin lock*. In the past, heparin preparations were also somewhat heterogeneous and contained various forms of compounds with heparinlike activity. In recent years, efforts have been made to chemically extract certain types of heparin from the more general (unfractionated) forms of this compound.[76,103] These efforts have led to the extraction and clinical use of specific forms of heparin known as *low-molecular-weight heparins (LMWHs)*. These agents are enoxaparin, (Lovenox), dalteparin (Fragmin), tinzaparin (Innohep), and other drugs identified by the "-parin" suffix.

The LMWHs appear to be as effective as unfractionated (mixed) heparins, but they offer certain advantages. For example, LMWHs can be administered by subcutaneous injection into fat tissues, thereby decreasing the need for repeated intravenous administration. Subcutaneous administration offers an easier and more convenient route, especially for people who are being treated at home or as outpatients.[98,118] Dosing schedules of LMWHs are typically easier (once per day), compared to 2 or more daily injections of unfractioned heparin.[132] The anticoagulant effects of LMWHs are also more predictable, and these agents tend to normalize clotting with less risk of adverse effects such as hemorrhage and death.[142] The more predictable response to LMWHs also decreases or eliminates the need for repeated laboratory monitoring of partial thromboplastin time, international normalized ratio (INR), or other indicators of clotting time.[98,103]

The use of traditional (unfractionated) heparin has therefore been replaced by LMWHs to a large extent.[18,100] LMWHs are clearly safer and more convenient to their unfractionated counterparts, and these drugs have become the primary method of treating acute venous thrombosis.[47,100] LMWHs are now used routinely to prevent or treat deep vein thrombosis (DVT) following various types of surgery or medical conditions (ischemic stroke, cancer).[70,127] It has also been suggested that LMWHs will produce optimal effects if they are administered for more than a few days, and some patients who are at high risk for thrombosis may receive LMWHs via subcutaneous injection for several weeks or months.[80] Future research will help determine the best way to use LMWHs to prevent or treat venous thrombosis in specific clinical situations.

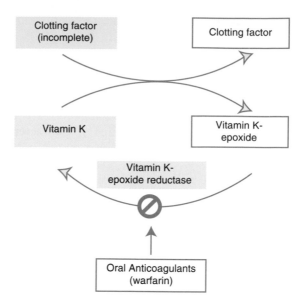

FIGURE 25–2 ▼ Role of vitamin K in the synthesis of vitamin K–dependent clotting factors (II, VII, IX, and X). Vitamin K catalyzes the reaction necessary for completion of clotting factor synthesis, but it is oxidized in the process to vitamin K epoxide. Regeneration of vitamin K occurs via vitamin K epoxide reductase. Oral anticoagulants such as warfarin (Coumadin) block the regeneration of the vitamin K, thus halting the further synthesis of the vitamin K–dependent factors.

Oral Anticoagulants

Drugs that are structurally and functionally similar to dicumarol constitute a group of orally active anticoagulant agents (see Table 25–1). The primary drug in this group is warfarin (Coumadin). These drugs exert their anticoagulant effects by impairing the hepatic synthesis of several clotting factors.[19,134] The specific mechanism of coumarin drugs is illustrated in Figure 25–2. In the liver, vitamin K acts as a catalyst in the final step of the synthesis of clotting factors II, VII, IX, and X. In the process, vitamin K is oxidized to an altered form known as vitamin K epoxide. For the process to continue, vitamin K epoxide must be reduced to its original form.[134] As shown in Figure 25–2, coumarin drugs block the conversion of vitamin K epoxide to vitamin K, thus impairing the synthesis of several clotting factors. With time, a decrease in the level of circulating clotting factors results in a decrease in blood coagulation and in thrombogenesis.

Unlike heparin, the primary advantage of coumarin drugs is that they are administered orally.[72] However, because of the nature of their action, there is often a lag time of several days before the decreased production of clotting factors is sufficient to interrupt the clotting cascade and an anticoagulant effect is appreciated.[21] Consequently, anticoagulant therapy often begins with parenteral administration of heparin, followed by oral administration of coumarin drugs.[75,122] Heparin is administered for the first few days to achieve an immediate effect. Coumarin drugs are then initiated, and heparin is discontinued after the coumarin drugs have had time to exert their anticoagulant effect. Oral administration of coumarin drugs may then be continued for several weeks to several months following an incident of thrombosis or pulmonary embolism.[75,122]

Other Anticoagulants

In addition to heparin and the oral anticoagulants, drugs have been developed that inhibit specific components in the clotting mechanism. Lepirudin (Refludan), for example, is a drug that directly inhibits thrombin; it can be administered intravenously to prevent excessive clotting in conditions such as heparin-induced thrombocytopenia (see next section, "Adverse Effects of Anticoagulant Drugs).[101]

Fondaparinux (Arixtra) is a newer agent that can be administered by subcutaneous injection to prevent DVT following orthopedic procedures (hip, knee replacement) and other surgeries.[5,15] Unlike other anticoagulants that inhibit thrombin activity, fonda-parinux inhibits clotting factor Xa (see Fig. 25–1). Moreover, preliminary studies suggest that fonda-parinux may be more effective in preventing DVT than heparin (including LMWHs).[5,70] In addition, fondaparinux may be safer because it does not appear to cause heparin-induced thrombocytopenia.[76] Hence, fondaparinux will probably continue to gain accept-ance as a primary way to prevent DVT in many clini-cal situations.

Finally, ximelagatran is new drug that is current-ly being developed to prevent or treat DVT.[109] Xime-lagatran directly inhibits thrombin, but has the advantage of oral administration. If approved, this drug could offer a convenient alternative to other oral coagulants such as warfarin in the long-term manage-ment of DVT and pulmonary embolism (PE).[2,5] Future research should determine the optimal use of this agent—either alone or in combination with exist-ing anticoagulants.

Adverse Effects of Anticoagulant Drugs

Predictably, hemorrhage is the primary and most seri-ous problem with drugs used to decrease blood clot-ting.[58,75,90] Increased bleeding may occur with heparin, warfarin, and other anticoagulants; this bleeding may be quite severe in some patients. Any unusual bleed-ing, such as blood in the urine or stools, unexplained nosebleeds, or an unusually heavy menstrual flow, may indicate a problem. Also, back pain or joint pain may be an indication of abdominal or intrajoint hemor-rhage, respectively. To prevent excessive bleeding, lab-oratory tests that measure hemostasis are sometimes used to monitor patients taking anticoagulants. Tests such as partial thromboplastin time and prothrombin time can indicate the effectiveness of drugs that alter blood coagulation, and adjustments in drug dosage are based on whether coagulation time falls within an acceptable range.[47,75]

Heparin may also produce a decrease in platelets (thrombocytopenia) in some patients.[13,84] This condi-tion, known commonly as heparin-induced thrombo-cytopenia (HIT), is less common with LMWHs versus unfractionated heparin, but HIT can occur with any type of heparin treatment.[101,145]

Heparin-induced thrombocytopenia (HIT) can likewise be asymptomatic and resolve spontaneously (type I HIT), or it can be severe (type II HIT). Type II HIT is mediated by an immune reaction, which can lead to serious complications including *increased* thrombosis in vascular tissues throughout the body.[101,119] Development of type II HIT is therefore an emergency situation typically resolved by discon-tinuing heparin and substituting an alternative type of anticoagulant (e.g., lepirudin).[101]

Finally, oral anticoagulants may produce some gastrointestinal distress (nausea, stomach cramps, diar-rhea); these side effects are more common with dicumarol than with the other oral anticoagulants.

Antithrombotic Drugs

Whereas anticoagulants affect the synthesis and func-tion of clotting factors, antithrombotics primarily inhibit the function of platelets.[117,152] In the blood stream, platelets respond to vascular injury by chang-ing their shape and adhering to one another (aggrega-tion) at the site of clot formation. Platelets may sometimes aggregate inappropriately, however, thus forming a thrombus and occluding certain blood ves-sels. In particular, arterial thrombi are often formed by abnormal platelet aggregation, especially in arteries with atherosclerotic plaques that rupture suddenly and initiate platelet clotting at the site of the rupture.[97] Hence, antithrombotic drugs are primarily used to prevent the formation of arterial clots, such as those that cause coronary artery occlusion or cerebral infarction.

Aspirin

Aspirin suppresses platelet aggregation by inhibiting the synthesis of prostaglandins and thromboxanes.[94,151] As discussed in Chapter 15, aspirin exerts virtually all of its effects by inhibiting the cyclooxygenase enzyme that initiates the synthesis of lipidlike hormones known as prostaglandins and thromboxanes. Certain prosta-glandins and thromboxanes, especially thromboxane A_2, have a potent ability to induce platelet aggregation. By inhibiting the synthesis of these proaggregation substances, aspirin prevents platelet-induced thrombus formation.

Although the exact dose may vary in specific clinical situations, patients typically experience a meaningful antithrombotic effect at very low aspirin doses. For example, many antithrombotic regimens suggest a daily dosage between 75 and 325 mg/d.[81,123] Considering that an adult aspirin tablet typically con-tains 325 mg of drug, these antithrombotic dosages represent taking the equivalent of one tablet or less each day. A pediatric (baby) aspirin tablet typical-ly contains 160 mg of drug, and many patients achieve adequate antithrombotic effects with one baby aspirin tablet each day. Antithrombotic effects can be achieved at these remarkably low doses because aspirin inhibits platelet function irreversibly.[94] That is, when aspirin reaches a given platelet, that platelet is inhibited for the remainder of its lifespan (about 7–8 days).

Because of its antithrombotic effects, aspirin has received a great deal of attention regarding its use in treating and preventing myocardial infarction. During the acute phase of an infarction, aspirin is critical in helping to limit the progression of platelet-induced occlusion, thereby reducing the extent of damage to the myocardium.[55] Following the acute phase, aspirin is often administered for prolonged periods to maintain coronary artery patency and prevent reinfarction.[65,94] Also, low doses of aspirin may decrease the incidence of an initial infarction in susceptible individuals—that is, people who have not yet sustained an infarction but have one or more risk factors for coronary artery disease.[94]

These rather remarkable findings have prompted a great deal of debate about the chronic use of aspirin and possible side effects such as increased hemorrhage. In particular, the incidence of intracranial hemorrhage (hemorrhagic stroke) may be increased when aspirin is administered to decrease thrombosis.[62] Nonetheless, aspirin is considered standard therapy during the acute phase of myocardial infarction, and prolonged use of aspirin is one of the primary pharmacologic methods used to prevent reinfarction.

Although increasing the risk of hemorrhagic stroke, aspirin may help prevent the type of stroke caused by cerebral ischemia and infarction.[3,59,107] The rationale is that aspirin will prevent infarction in cerebral vessels in the same manner that it prevents coronary infarction in heart attacks. Clearly, the use of aspirin must be limited to the types of stroke that result from insufficient blood flow, as opposed to hemorrhagic stroke. In particular, aspirin seems especially helpful in reducing the risk of ischemic stroke in people with atrial fibrillation.[3,107] Even so, the antithrombotic benefits of aspirin in some cerebral vessels must be weighed against the possible side effects such as increased bleeding in other vessels. Long-term aspirin therapy is probably beneficial to a certain percentage of stroke patients, but should be used selectively.[59,107]

Consequently, the role of chronic aspirin administration in helping to prevent myocardial and cerebral infarction remains an area of intense investigation. There seems to be little doubt that aspirin can be a very cost-effective method for decreasing the morbidity and mortality associated with these types of infarction. Nonetheless, the long-term effects of aspirin on other organs such as the liver, kidneys, and gastrointestinal tract must be considered. In addition, the therapeutic effects of low-dose aspirin therapy vary substantially from person to person, and some people may appear resistant to aspirin's antithrombotic effects.[48,138] Although the reasons are not clear, the antithrombotic effects of low-dose aspirin therapy may also differ between men and women—men experience greater protection against heart attack and women experience greater protection against ischemic stroke.[17] Hence, continued analysis of this topic promises to be an exciting and productive area of pharmacologic research.

Finally, aspirin has also been used to prevent thrombus formation in peripheral veins (deep vein thrombosis [DVT]), and aspirin is sometimes used as an adjunct or alternative to anticoagulants (heparin, warfarin) that are routinely used to treat DVTs.[8] Aspirin can likewise be administered to prevent thromboembolism following surgical procedures such as coronary artery bypass, arterial grafts, endarterectomy, and valve replacement.[45,78] By preventing platelet-induced thrombogenesis, aspirin helps maintain patency and prevent reocclusion of vessels following these procedures.

Other Antithrombotic Drugs

Although aspirin remains the primary antithrombotic agent, this drug is a relatively weak inhibitor of platelet activity.[48] As indicated, aspirin may also increase the risk of intracranial hemorrhage, and may be poorly tolerated in some patients due to gastric irritation, an allergic response, and so forth.[48,123] Efforts have therefore been made to develop stronger and safer antiplatelet drugs.

One antiplatelet strategy that has shown considerable promise is the use of drugs that inhibit the ability of fibrinogen and other chemical mediators to activate platelets.[63,40] These drugs are known as glycoprotein (GP) IIb-IIIa inhibitors because they block (antagonize) the GP receptor on the platelet membrane that is stimulated by fibrinogen and other chemical mediators.[7,35] Fibrinogen is unable to bind to the platelet, thereby decreasing platelet activation and reducing platelet-induced clotting.[64] Agents that are currently available include abciximab (ReoPro), eptifibatide (Integrilin), and tirofiban (Aggrastat) (see Table 25–1).[21] GP IIb-IIIa inhibitors are the post powerful inhibitors of platelet activity,[129] and these drugs are used primarily during balloon angioplasty and other percutaneous coronary interventions that help reestablish coronary artery blood flow.[23,35] Administering these drugs intravenously during such procedures can help maintain coronary flow and decrease mortality, especially in people at high risk for reinfarction.[7,22] GP IIb-IIIa inhibitors, however, are not typically administered orally for the long-term prevention of myocardial infarction and similar thrombotic events.[123]

Another antiplatelet strategy involves drugs that inhibit the adenosine diphosphate (ADP) receptor on the platelet membrane.[63,104] ADP is another compound that increases platelet activity, and platelet-induced clotting is reduced by drugs that inhibit the receptor for this compound.[93,104] Such drugs include clopidogrel (Plavix) and ticlopidine (Ticlid); these drugs are used primarily to prevent myocardial infarction and ischemic stroke (see Table 25–1). They produce moderate inhibition of platelet activity, making them somewhat more effective than aspirin but not as strong as the GP IIb-IIIa inhibitors.[129] Likewise, these ADP receptor inhibitors seem to be well-tolerated, and they therefore provide an option for decreasing platelet-induced clotting in patients who cannot tolerate other antiplatelet drugs such as aspirin.[48] ADP inhibitors such as clopidogrel (Plavix) can also be added to low-dose aspirin therapy in cases where aspirin alone does not provide adequate antithrombotic effects.[31,93,124]

Dipyridamole (Persantine, other names) has been used alone or in combination with aspirin to decrease platelet-induced clotting. This drug may affect platelet function by impairing adenosine metabolism and/or by increasing the concentration of cyclic adenosine monophosphate within the platelet.[1] The exact mechanism of dipyridamole, however, is poorly understood. Although it is not used as commonly as other antiplatelet drugs, dipyridamole has shown benefits in preventing ischemic stroke and myocardial infarction.[85,87] It has also been suggested that dipyridamole can be combined with aspirin to provide greater benefits compared to using either drug alone.[85] Hence, dipyridamole is a potential alternative or adjunct to other antiplatelet agents (aspirin, ADP receptor inhibitors) in treating arterial thrombosis.

Finally, sulfinpyrazone (Anturane) is usually administered to treat gouty arthritis, but has also shown some antithrombotic properties because of an ability to decrease platelet function. Sulfinpyrazone decreases platelet aggregation by inhibiting prostaglandin synthesis in a manner similar to aspirin. Sulfinpyrazone can be used as an alternative to aspirin in preventing reinfarction after a heart attack, especially in patients who are not able to tolerate aspirin or other antithrombotic drugs.

Adverse Effects of Antithrombotic Drugs

The primary concern with aspirin and other antithrombotic drugs is an increased risk of bleeding. Patients taking these agents should be especially alert for any unexplained or heavy bleeding or any other symptoms that might indicate hemorrhage (sudden increases in joint or back pain, severe headaches, and so forth). Aspirin can likewise cause gastric irritation, and high doses of aspirin may be toxic to the liver and kidneys (see Chapter 15). However, the likelihood of severe gastric disturbances and liver or renal toxicity is relatively low at the doses needed to create an antithrombotic effect. Other potential side effects of non-aspirin antithrombotics include hypotension for the GP IIb-IIIa inhibitors (abciximab, eptifibatide), gastrointestinal distress for clopidogrel and dipyridamole, blood dyscrasias (neutropenia, agranulocytosis, thrombocytopenia) for ticlopidine, and formation of kidney stones for sulfinpyrazone.

Thrombolytic Drugs

Thrombolytics facilitate the breakdown and dissolution of clots that have already formed. These drugs work by converting plasminogen (profibrinolysin) to plasmin (fibrinolysin).[34] As shown in Figure 25–1, plasmin is the active form of an endogenous enzyme that breaks down fibrin clots. Thrombolytic drugs activate this enzyme by various mechanisms and can be used to dissolve clots that have already formed, thus reopening occluded blood vessels.

Thrombolytic drugs are extremely valuable in treating acute myocardial infarction.[14,102] When administered at infarction onset, these drugs can reestablish blood flow through occluded coronary vessels, often preventing or reversing myocardial damage, which decreases the morbidity and mortality normally associated with a heart attack.[39] These drugs can help reopen occluded coronary vessels when administered within 12 hours after symptom onset.[102] Thrombolytics seem to produce the best results, however, when they are administered soon after the symptom onset. Administration within 1 hour after symptom onset, for example, can result in a 50 percent reduction in mortality in patients with acute myocardial infarction.[105]

Consequently, thrombolytic agents are administered whenever possible during the first few hours after an acute myocardial infarction. It was originally believed that these drugs had to be administered directly into the coronary arteries to reopen occluded coronary vessels.[6] However, it is now realized that these drugs will produce beneficial effects when injected intravenously into the systemic circulation; that is, the drug can be injected into any accessible vein and eventually reach the coronary clot through the general circulation.[137] The intravenous route is a much more practical method of administration because it is easier, faster, and safer than the intracoronary route.

Thrombolytic drugs offer an attractive method of preventing—or even reversing—myocardial damage during acute myocardial infarction. Intracranial hemorrhage and other bleeding problems are the primary drawbacks to thrombolytic treatment because these drugs can also stimulate clot breakdown in other vessels, including the cerebral vasculature.[16,116] Thrombolytics are therefore contraindicated in certain situations, including in patients with a history of hemorrhagic stroke, intracranial neoplasm, active internal bleeding, possible aortic dissection, and several other factors representing the increased risk of hemorrhage.[102,137] Also, thrombolytic therapy may not be curative, and reocclusion occurs in certain patients.

Thrombolytic agents may also be used to treat specific cases of ischemic stroke.[4,74] It was originally thought that these drugs should not be used to treat ischemic stroke because of the risk of intracranial hemorrhage.[111] It appears, however, that thrombolytic treatment can be used carefully in selected patients to dissolve clots within cerebral vessels and allow reperfusion of the brain, thus limiting the amount of damage from the infarction.[146] The window of opportunity for administration, however, is smaller when treating ischemic stroke compared to myocardial infarction, and thrombolytic agents must typically be administered within 3 hours after cerebral infarction.[4] Also, certain thrombolytics, such as recombinant tissue plasminogen activator (see below), may be better than other thrombolytics when treating ischemic stroke.[4,146] Nonetheless, thrombolytic treatment is regarded as an important option for patients who are experiencing an ischemic stroke, and who have minimal risk factors for intracranial or systemic hemorrhage.

Finally, thrombolytic drugs are gaining acceptance in treating other types of arterial and venous occlusion. For example, thrombolytic therapy can help dissolve clots in peripheral arteries (femoral, popliteal, and so forth)[56]; these drugs can help resolve thrombus formation in the large veins (DVT).[68] This treatment is especially helpful during severe, limb-threatening occlusion, or when surgical removal of the thrombus is not possible.[68,113]

To minimize the risk of side effects, thrombolytic drugs can be administered directly to the site of the clot through an intravascular catheter.[68,112] Thrombolytics may also play a role in treating acute, massive pulmonary embolism (PE).[60,82] Use of these drugs in PE is typically reserved for life-threatening situations, especially when the PE is so severe that function of the right ventricle is compromised.[82] Bypass grafts and shunts that have become occluded because of clot formation may also be cleaned out with thrombotic drug use.[21]

The most common thrombolytic agents are listed below. Although these drugs differ chemically, they all ultimately activate fibrinolysis in some way. There has likewise been considerable debate about which agent provides optimal long-term benefits following myocardial infarction. With regard to myocardial infarction, these agents are fairly similar in terms of efficacy and safety profile.[116] Selecting a specific agent seems less important than simply making sure that the agent is used in a timely fashion; that is, the time elapsed before beginning treatment is probably more important than the actual type of thrombolytic agent administered to treat myocardial infarction.[137] Some of the newer agents, however, can be administered by rapid (bolus) infusion, and may therefore help decrease the time between when a patient arrives at the hospital and when meaningful amounts of the drug are able to reach the clot.[14,50] The relative benefits and unique aspects of each agent are presented here.

Streptokinase and Urokinase

Streptokinase and urokinase both bring about the activation of plasmin. Streptokinase indirectly activates plasmin (fibrinolysin) by binding to the precursor molecule plasminogen (profibrinolysin) and facilitating activation by endogenous mechanisms. Urokinase directly converts plasminogen to plasmin by enzymatically cleaving a peptide bond within the plasminogen molecule. Both agents have been used successfully to resolve acute clot formation in coronary arteries and peripheral vessels. Streptokinase, however, tends to be the most commonly used type of thrombolytic because it is relatively inexpensive and because the incidence of intracranial hemorrhage may be somewhat lower with streptokinase than with other thrombolytics.[116]

Tissue Plasminogen Activator

In the endogenous control of hemostasis, plasminogen is activated by an intrinsic substance known as tissue plasminogen activator (t-PA) (see Fig. 25–1). Intravenous administration of t-PA rapidly and effectively initiates clot breakdown by directly activating plasmin (fibrinolysin). Although extraction of t-PA from human blood is costly and impractical, the commercial synthesis of t-PA has been made possible through the use of recombinant DNA techniques. Consequently, t-PA (also known by the generic name alteplase) is now available in commercial forms (Activase), and this agent joins streptokinase as one of the primary thrombolytic agents.

Tissue plasminogen activator has been used successfully to treat acute myocardial infarction, and the benefits of this treatment are well documented.[102,116] This drug, however, does not seem to be superior to other thrombolytics when treating coronary artery thrombosis, and streptokinase may be a more cost-effective method of treating myocardial infarction. Alternatively, t-PA may be more effective than other thrombolytics in its ability to initially reopen cerebral vessels; this drug is often used preferentially during ischemic stroke.[4,44] Hence, the added cost of t-PA may be justified in this situation.

Anistreplase

Anistreplase (Eminase)—also known as anisoylated plasminogen-streptokinase activator complex (APSAC)—is formed by combining plasminogen with streptokinase, and then chemically altering (anisoylating) the catalytic site on this complex so that plasminogen remains inactive until it is administered. When administered systemically, anistreplase binds to fibrin, where it is chemically activated so that streptokinase can modify plasminogen and initiate clot breakdown. The supposed advantage of using anistreplase is that this compound will be more selective for clots that have already formed and have less effect on systemic fibrinolysis. Anistreplase causes considerable systemic fibrinolysis, however, and the advantages of this compound over streptokinase alone remain to be determined.

Reteplase and Tenecteplase

Reteplase (Retavase) and tenecteplase (TNKase) are newer thrombolytics. These agents are derived of human tissue plasminogen activator, and therefore have actions similar to t-PA (alteplase).[38,149] Reteplase and tenecteplase offer the advantage of more rapid (bolus) infusion, and may be somewhat easier to administer than other thrombolytics that need to be infused slowly over several hours.[14] These newer agents, however, are not shown to be superior to more traditional agents (streptokinase, urokinase).[16,39] Reteplase and tenecteplase therefore offer another therapeutic option, and future studies should help determine if these drugs provide advantages in specific patient subgroups or types of occlusive disease.

Adverse Effects of Thrombolytic Drugs

Hemorrhage is the major adverse effect associated with thrombolytic agents. As indicated, intracranial hemorrhage may occur following thrombolytic therapy, especially in patients who have predisposing risk factors such as advanced age, severe or untreated hypertension, or a history of hemorrhagic stroke.[137] Excessive bleeding may also occur during dressing changes, wound care, and other invasive procedures following thrombolytic treatment. Thrombolytic drugs may cause fever and an allergic reaction (itching, nausea, headache, other symptoms). The risk and severity of fever and allergic response seems greatest for streptokinase, but all the thrombolytics can potentially cause these reactions.

Treatment of Clotting Deficiencies

Hemophilia

Hemophilia is a hereditary disease in which an individual is unable to synthesize adequate amounts of a specific clotting factor. The two most common forms of hemophilia are hemophilia A, which is caused by deficiency of clotting factor VIII, and hemophilia B, which is a deficit in clotting factor IX.[25] In either form of this disease, patients are missing adequate amounts of a key clotting factor and have problems maintaining normal hemostasis. Even trivial injuries can produce serious or fatal hemorrhage. Also, patients with hemophilia often develop joint problems because of intraarticular hemorrhage (hemarthrosis).

Treatment of hemophilia consists of replacing the missing clotting factor. Depending on the severity of the disease, clotting factors can be administered on a regular basis (prophylaxis) or during an acute hemorrhagic episode.[26,53,67] Although this treatment seems relatively straightforward, obtaining sufficient amounts of the missing factor is a very costly procedure. At present, the primary source of clotting factors VIII and IX is human blood extract. Obtaining an adequate supply can cost more than $30,000 per patient per year.

A more serious problem is the potential for clotting factor extract to contain viruses such as hepatitis B, or HIV, which causes AIDS. The lack of proper blood screening has resulted in tragic consequences; for example, clotting factors extracted from patients infected with HIV have served as a vehicle for viral transmission to patients with hemophilia. More stringent screening procedures and other techniques such as heat treatment of clotting factor extracts have decreased the risk of transmission, but patients with hemophilia receiving exogenous factors remain at risk for viral infection. New methods of drug production, such as genetic engineering and recombinant DNA techniques, are currently being used to manufacture specific clotting factors such as factor VIII.[21] It is hoped that these techniques will provide a safer, cheaper source of missing clotting factors for patients with hemophilia.

Deficiencies of Vitamin K–Dependent Clotting Factors

As indicated earlier in this chapter, the liver needs adequate amounts of vitamin K to synthesize clotting factors II, VII, IX, and X. As shown in Figure 25–2, vitamin K catalyzes the final steps in the synthesis of these factors. Normally, vitamin K is supplied through the diet or synthesized by intestinal bacteria and subsequently absorbed from the gastrointestinal tract into the body. However, any defect in vitamin K ingestion, synthesis, or absorption may result in vitamin K deficiency. Insufficient vitamin K in the body results in an inadequate hepatic synthesis of the clotting factors listed previously, thus resulting in poor hemostasis and excessive bleeding.

Deficiencies in vitamin K and the related synthesis of the vitamin K–dependent clotting factors are treated by administering exogenous vitamin K.[20] Various commercial forms of this vitamin are available for oral or parenteral (intramuscular or subcutaneous) administration. Specifically, individuals with a poor diet, intestinal disease, or impaired intestinal absorption may require vitamin K to maintain proper hemostasis.

Vitamin K is routinely administered to newborn infants to prevent hemorrhage.[10,121] For the first 5 to 8 days following birth, newborns lack the intestinal bacteria necessary to help synthesize vitamin K. Vitamin K is administered to facilitate clotting factor synthesis until the newborn is able to produce sufficient endogenous vitamin K. Finally, vitamin K can be administered to accelerate clotting factor production when clotting time is excessively long (e.g., INR between 4.5 and 10.0).[69,148] Specifically, patients with delayed blood clotting due to excess warfarin levels can be administered vitamin K either orally or by parenteral routes to help reestablish normal clotting time.[69]

Antifibrinolytics

The excessive bleeding that sometimes occurs following surgery, trauma, or advanced cancer may be caused by an overactive fibrinolytic system—that is, *hyperfibrinolysis*.[27,115,130] Hyperfibrinolysis results in excessive clot destruction and ineffective hemostasis. Likewise, patients with hemophilia who undergo surgery, including dental procedures (tooth extractions, restorations, etc.), will benefit if clot breakdown is inhibited because hemorrhage and the need for additional clotting factors are reduced. Antifibrinolytic agents such as aminocaproic acid (Amicar) and tranexamic acid (Cyklokapron) are often used in these situations.[27,106,130,115] These drugs appear to inhibit activation of plasminogen (profibrinolysin) to plasmin (fibrinolysin). Plasmin is the enzyme responsible for breaking down fibrin clots (see Fig. 25–1). Antifibrinolytics prevent the activation of this enzyme, thus preserving clot formation.

Aminocaproic acid and tranexamic acid are administered either orally or intravenously for the acute treatment of hyperfibrinolysis or to prevent clot breakdown in patients with hemophilia who are undergoing surgery. Some adverse effects such as nausea, diarrhea, dizziness, and headache may occur when these drugs are administered, but these problems are relatively minor and usually disappear when the drug is discontinued.

Agents Used to Treat Hyperlipidemia

Hyperlipidemia, an abnormally high concentration of lipids in the bloodstream, is one of the primary causes of cardiovascular disease in industrialized nations. This condition typically causes deposition of fatty plaquelike lesions on the walls of large and medium-sized arteries (*atherosclerosis*), which can lead to thrombosis and infarction. Hence, elevated plasma lipids are related to some of the events discussed previously in this chapter because atherosclerosis can precipitate increased clotting and thromboembolic disease.

Hyperlipidemia is often caused by poor diet and lifestyle, as well as by several genetic conditions that cause disorders in lipid metabolism.[83,89] It is not possible to review the endogenous control of lipid metabolism or the various pathologic processes involved in hyperlipidemia here—these topics are addressed in other sources.[89,139] It should be realized, however, that lipids such as cholesterol are transported in the bloodstream as part of a lipid-protein complex known as a *lipoprotein*. Certain lipoproteins are considered beneficial because they may decrease the formation of atherosclerotic plaques by removing cholesterol from the arterial wall. These beneficial complexes are known as high-density lipoproteins (HDLs) because of the relatively large amount of protein in the complex. Other lipoproteins are considered harmful because they transport and deposit cholesterol on the arterial wall. These atherogenic lipoproteins include intermediate-density lipoproteins (IDLs), low-density lipoproteins (LDLs), and very-low-density lipoproteins (VLDLs). Pharmacologic and nonpharmacologic strategies to reduce hyperlipidemia typically focus on reducing these atherogenic lipoproteins and increasing the beneficial HDLs.

Drugs that can be used to treat hyperlipidemia are summarized in Table 25–2 and are discussed briefly below. These agents are typically used when plasma lipid levels are unsuccessfully controlled by nonpharmacologic methods such as low-fat diets, weight reduction, regular exercise, and smoking cessation.[41,136,143] However, these drugs can be used in conjunction with nonpharmacologic methods, and optimal results are often realized through a combination of drug therapy and various dietary and lifestyle modifications.[136]

HMG-CoA Reductase Inhibitors (Statins)

This category includes atorvastatin (Lipitor), fluvastatin (Lescol), lovastatin (Mevacor), pravastatin (Pravachol), and simvastatin (Zocor) (Table 25–2). These drugs, known commonly as statins, are characterized by their ability to inhibit an enzyme known as 3-hydroxy-3-methylglutaryl coenzyme A (HMG-CoA) reductase.[96] This enzyme catalyzes one of the early steps of cholesterol synthesis, and drugs that inhibit HMG-CoA reductase decrease cholesterol produc-

tion, especially in liver cells. Decreased hepatic cholesterol biosynthesis also causes more surface receptors for LDL cholesterol to be synthesized; this increase in surface receptors triggers an increase in the breakdown of LDL cholesterol and a decrease in the synthesis of VLDL, which serves as a precursor for LDL synthesis.[57] HMG-CoA reductase inhibitors can also decrease triglyceride levels,[57] and produce a modest increase in HDL levels.[89] However, the exact reasons for the beneficial effects on triglycerides and HDL levels are not entirely clear.

The HMG-CoA reductase inhibitors therefore improve several aspects of the plasma lipid profile. These agents may produce several favorable effects that are independent of their ability to affect plasma lipid levels.[9,96] It appears that certain by-products of cholesterol metabolism act directly or influence the production of other chemical signals that adversely affect cellular function in various tissues.[9] Increased production of these by-products could therefore influence a variety of pathological conditions. By controlling the production of these by-products, statins may produce a wide range of beneficial effects in addition to their ability to improve plasma lipids.

Statins, for example, might produce direct beneficial effects on the vascular endothelium by increasing the production and vasodilating effects of nitric oxide, and they may help stabilize atherosclerotic plaques on the arterial wall.[37,51,150] These drugs may likewise have anti-inflammatory and antioxidant effects that contribute to their ability to improve the vascular wall's function.[37,96] Statins may even have anticancer effects, and investigators continue to explore their potential in preventing and treating certain malignancies.[40,54] Statins therefore seem to exert several complex effects, and their ability to reduce the risk of cardiovascular disease is probably the result of a combination of their favorable effects on plasma lipids combined with their ability to improve the function of the vascular endothelium.

Statins are helpful in decreasing morbidity and mortality in people with high cholesterol, as well as individuals who have normal cholesterol but other risk factors for cardiovascular disease.[66] It is estimated that these drugs decrease the risk of a major cardiac event by approximately 30 to 35 percent, although the benefits depend on the extent that cholesterol is reduced and the influence of other risk factors.[91,95,126] Nonetheless, statins are now regarded as a mainstay in treating cardiovascular disease, and efforts are underway to expand the use of these medications and to explore the

Table 25–2	DRUGS USED TO TREAT HYPERLIPIDEMIA		
Generic Name	**Trade Name(s)**	**Dosage***	**Primary Effect**
Atorvastatin	Lipitor	10–80 mg once each day	Decreases total cholesterol and plasma LDL-C; may also decrease triglycerides and increase HDL-C somewhat
Cholestyramine	Questran	4 g 2–6 times each day before meals and at bedtime	Decreases total cholesterol and LDL-C
Clofibrate	Abitrate, Atromid-S	1.5–2.0 g each day in 2–4 divided doses	Lowers triglycerides and VLDL-C; may also increase HDL-C levels
Ezetimibe	Zetia	10 mg once each day	Lowers total cholesterol, LDL-C, and triglycerides; increases HDL-C levels
Fenofibrate	Tricor	54–160 mg once each day	Similar to clofibrate
Fluvastatin	Lescol	20–40 mg once each day in the evening	Similar to atorvastatin
Gemfibrozil	Lopid	1.2 g each day in 2 divided doses 30 min before morning and evening meal	Similar to clofibrate
Lovastatin	Mevacor	20–80 mg each day as a single dose or in divided doses with meals	Similar to atorvastatin
Niacin	Niaspan, others	1–2 g 3 times each day	Lowers total cholesterol, triglycerides, LDL-C, and VLDL-C; increases HDL-C
Pravastatin	Pravachol	10–40 mg once each day at bedtime	Similar to atorvastatin
Simvastatin	Zocor	5–80 mg once each day in the evening	Similar to atorvastatin

*Doses represent typical adult oral maintenance dose.
HDL-C = high-density lipoprotein cholesterol; LDL-C = low-density lipoprotein cholesterol, VLDL-C = very low-density lipoprotein cholesterol.

optimal use of these drugs with other pharmacologic and nonpharmacologic interventions in cardiovascular disease.[66,91]

Fibric Acids

Fibric acids or "fibrates" include clofibrate (Abitrate, Atromid) and gemfibrozil (Lopid). These drugs pri-marily decrease triglyceride levels, and are therefore most helpful in hyperlipidemias that are characterized by increased triglycerides.[49,147] Fibrates also produce beneficial increases in HDL production, and can help lower LDL levels.[42,147] Fibrates are therefore helpful in treating a combination of lipid abnormalities (i.e., mixed hyperlipidemias) that include increased triglyc-erides and LDL levels along with low HDL lev-els.[43,49,52]

The exact mechanism of these drugs is unclear, but they probably work by binding to a specific nuclear receptor known as the peroxisome proliferator activated receptor.[52,141] This receptor, found primarily in the liver and adipose tissues, affects the transcription of genes that affect lipid metabolism.[89] Fibrates activate this receptor, thereby mediating several changes at the nuclear level that ultimately cause a decrease in triglycerides and other beneficial changes in plasma lipid metabolism.[30,52] In a manner similar to the statins, fibrates may also exert anti-inflammatory, antioxidant, and other beneficial effects in addition to their positive effects on plasma lipids.[42,49]

Although it is not exactly clear how much these agents can reduce the risk of a major cardiac event (e.g., infarction, stroke), these drugs will probably remain the first choice for people with certain hyperlipidemias (e.g., increased triglycerides). These drugs are likewise advocated for mixed hyperlipidemias that are common in metabolic disorders such as type 2 diabetes mellitus (see Chapter 32).[32,141] Certain fibrates can be used with other drugs, such as statins, to provide more comprehensive pharmacologic control of certain lipid disorders.[30,147]

Other Lipid-Lowering Agents

Several other agents have beneficial effects on plasma lipid profiles occurring through various cellular mechanisms.[89] Cholestyramine (Questran), for example, attaches to bile acids within the gastrointestinal lumen and increases the fecal excretion of these acids. This action leads to decreased plasma cholesterol concentrations because cholesterol breakdown is accelerated to replace the bile acids that are lost in the feces.

Niacin (nicotinic acid, vitamin B_3, Niaspan, other names) has received considerable attention as a "broad spectrum" antilipidemic because this drug produces beneficial effects on virtually all aspects of the lipid profile.[28,99] That is, high doses of niacin (several grams each day) help decrease LDL and triglyceride levels while raising HDL levels.[71,99] This drug apparently binds to a specific nicotinic acid receptor in fat cells and initiates a number of metabolic effects, which leads to decreased lipid synthesis and increased lipolysis.[29] Likewise, niacin may be used in combination with statins to produce optimal benefits in certain patients without increasing the risk of stain-induced myopathy (see next section, "Adverse Effects of Antihyperlipidemia Agents").[71] Hence, niacin continues to gain acceptance as an important drug in treating hyperlipidemia.

Finally, ezetimibe (Zetia) is a relatively new agent that inhibits cholesterol absorption from the gastrointestinal (GI) tract.[33,110] This action produces many beneficial effects including reduced LDL and triglyceride levels, and increased HDL levels.[12] Ezetimibe seems especially useful in complimenting the effects of the statin drugs, and it can be combined safely with a statin to produce optimal benefits in many patients.[114,131] Additional drugs limiting cholesterol absorption may ultimately be developed as part of the treatment against hyperlipidemia.

Adverse Effects of Antihyperlipidemia Agents

Most of the drugs used to treat hyperlipidemia are well tolerated. Some gastrointestinal distress (nausea, diarrhea) is common with most of the drugs, but these problems are usually minor and do not require the discontinuation of drug therapy.

Other bothersome side effects are related to specific agents. Niacin, for instance, is often associated with cutaneous vasodilation and a sensation of warmth when doses are administered, but administering an extended-release form of this drug can reduce these sensations.[71,99] Some fairly serious problems, including liver dysfunction, gallstones, and pancreatitis, can occur with many antihyperlipidemia drugs, but the incidence of these side effects is rare. Cardiovascular problems such as arrhythmias, blood dyscrasias, and angioneurotic syndrome may also occur with fibric acids.

Neuromuscular problems have been noted with certain agents. In particular, myopathy (muscular pain, inflammation, weakness) is a rare, but potentially serious side effect of statin drugs. The reasons for these effects are unclear, but statin-induced myopathy is associated with several risk factors such as high statin doses, advanced age, multiple diseases, frail stature, and immunosuppressant drugs.[125,144] Combining a statin with certain fibric acids (gemfibrozil) may also increase the risk of myopathy. Although statin-induced myopathy is usually reversible, this syndrome should be recognized early before it can progress to more severe forms of muscle disease and muscle damage (rhabdomyolysis).[11,77] Treatment typically consists of discontinuing the statin, and allowing an adequate period of rest and recovery—4 to 6 weeks in most cases. Preliminary studies suggest that statins may also affect nervous tissue, and that sensory and motor neuropathies may occur in certain patients.[11] Future studies are needed to clarify the effects of these drugs on

Special Concerns in Rehabilitation Patients

■ ■ ■ Therapists will frequently encounter patients taking drugs to alter hemostasis. Many patients on prolonged bed rest have a tendency for increased thrombus formation and are particularly susceptible to deep vein thrombosis. These patients will often be given anticoagulant drugs. Heparin followed by warfarin may be administered prophylactically or in response to the symptoms of thrombophlebitis in patients who have undergone hip surgery, heart valve replacement, and other surgical procedures. Therapists should be aware that the primary problem associated with anticoagulant drugs is an increased tendency for bleeding. Any rehabilitation procedures that deal with open wounds (dressing changes, debridement, etc.) should be carefully administered. Rigorous manual techniques, such as deep tissue massage or chest percussion, must also be used with caution since these procedures may directly traumatize tissues and induce bleeding in patients taking anticoagulants. Certain manual techniques such as upper cervical manipulation should be avoided or used very cautiously because of increased risk of damage to the vertebral artery in patients taking anticlotting drugs.

Anticoagulants and antithrombotic drugs (e.g., aspirin) may also be given to rehabilitation patients to prevent the recurrence of myocardial infarction. As discussed previously, aspirin appears to be especially attractive in preventing an initial incident or the recurrence of infarction. Aspirin is relatively free from any serious side effects that may influence the rehabilitation session. Long-term anticoagulant and antithrombotic therapy is also frequently employed in specific cases of cerebrovascular accidents (strokes) that are due to recurrent cerebral embolism and occlusion. Obviously, giving anticoagulant and antithrombotic drugs to patients with a tendency toward the hemorrhagic type of stroke is counterproductive, because these drugs would only exacerbate this condition. However, stroke cases in which hemorrhage has been ruled out may benefit from prolonged anticoagulant or antithrombotic therapy. Again, therapists should be cognizant of the tendency for increased bleeding with these agents. However, the long-term use of these agents, especially aspirin, usually does not create any significant problems in the course of rehabilitation.

Thrombolytic drugs (streptokinase, t-PA, others) usually do not have a direct impact on physical therapy or occupational therapy. Thrombolytics are typically given in acute situations, immediately following myocardial infarction. Therapists may, however, benefit indirectly from the effects of these drugs because patients may recover faster and more completely from heart attacks. Thrombolytics may also help reopen occluded peripheral vessels, thus improving tissue perfusion and wound healing in rehabilitation patients.

Therapists will often work with individuals who have chronic clotting deficiencies, such as patients with hemophilia. Intrajoint hemorrhage (*hemarthrosis*) with subsequent arthropathy is one of the primary problems associated with hemophilia.[46,88] The joints most often affected are the knees, ankles, elbows, hips, and shoulders.[88] Hemarthrosis is usually treated by replacing the missing clotting factor and by rehabilitating the affected joints. Therapists often employ a judicious program of exercise, joint support, and pain management to help improve joint function following hemarthrosis.[73] Consequently, the therapist often works in conjunction with pharmacologic management to help improve function in hemophilia-related joint disorders.

Finally, therapists may encourage patients to comply with pharmacologic and nonpharmacologic methods used to lower plasma lipids. Drugs used to treat hyperlipidemia are typically used in conjunction with diet, exercise, and other lifestyle changes that reduce fat intake and improve plasma lipid profiles. Therapists can help design and implement exercise programs that enable patients to lose weight and increase plasma levels of antiatherogenic components such as HDL, thus maximizing the effects of drug therapy.

CASE STUDY

Clotting Disorders

Brief History. C.W. is an obese, 47-year-old woman who sustained a compression fracture of the L-1 and L-2 vertebrae during a fall from a second-story window. (There was some suggestion that she may have been pushed during an argument with her husband, but the details remain unclear.) She was admitted to the hospital, where her medical condition was stabilized, and surgical procedures were performed to treat her vertebral fracture. Her injuries ultimately resulted in a partial transection of the spinal cord, with diminished motor and sensory function in both lower extremities. She began an extensive rehabilitation program, including physical therapy and occupational therapy. She was progressing well when she developed shortness of breath and an acute pain in her right thorax. A diagnosis of massive pulmonary embolism was made. Evidently she had developed deep vein thrombosis in both lower extremities, and a large embolism from the venous clots had lodged in her lungs, producing a pulmonary infarction.

Drug Treatment. Because of the extensive nature of the pulmonary infarction, a thrombolytic agent was used to attempt to resolve the clot. An initial dosage of 250,000 units of streptokinase (Streptase) was administered intravenously within 2 hours after the onset of symptoms. Streptokinase was continued via intravenous infusion at a rate of 100,000 units/hr for 24 hours after the initial dose.

To prevent further thromboembolism, streptokinase infusion was followed by heparin. A low-molecular weight heparin (enoxaparin [Lovenox], 1.5 mg/kg body weight) was administered subcutaneously once each day. Clotting time was monitored by periodic blood tests during the heparin treatment. After 7 days of heparin therapy, C.W. was switched to warfarin. Warfarin (Coumadin) was administered orally, and the dosage was adjusted until she was receiving 5 mg/d. Oral warfarin was continued throughout the remainder of the patient's hospital stay, as well as after discharge.

Impact on Rehabilitation. The drugs used to resolve the thromboembolic episode greatly facilitated the patient's recovery. The use of a thrombolytic agent (streptokinase) enabled the patient to resume her normal course of rehabilitation within 2 days of the pulmonary embolism. Thus, the use of these drugs directly facilitated physical therapy and occupational therapy by allowing the patient to resume therapy much sooner than if the embolism had been treated more conservatively (i.e., rest and anticoagulants) or more radically (i.e., surgery). Because the patient remained on anticoagulant drugs for an extended period of time, the therapists dealing with the patient routinely looked for signs of excessive bleeding such as skin bruising and hematuria. The patient remained free from any further thromboembolic episodes, however, and was eventually discharged to an extended-care rehabilitation facility to continue her progress.

---

nervous tissue, and to lend more insight to the prevention and treatment of statin-induced neuromuscular toxicity.

SUMMARY

Normal hemostasis is a balance between excessive and inadequate blood clotting. Overactive blood clotting is harmful because of the tendency for thrombus formation and occlusion of arteries and veins. Vessels may become directly blocked by the thrombus, or a portion of the thrombus may break off and create an embolism that lodges elsewhere in the vascular system. The tendency for excessive thrombus formation in the venous system is usually treated with anticoagulant drugs such as heparin and warfarin. Platelet inhibitors such as aspirin help prevent arterial thrombogenesis. Thrombolytic drugs (streptokinase, t-PA) that facilitate the dissolution of harmful clots may successfully reopen

vessels that have suddenly become occluded because of acute thrombus formation.

The inadequate blood clotting and excessive bleeding that occur in patients with hemophilia are treated by replacing the missing clotting factor. Other conditions associated with inadequate coagulation may be treated by administering either vitamin K, which helps improve the synthesis of certain clotting factors, or antifibrinolytic agents (aminocaproic acid, tranexamic acid), which inhibit clot breakdown.

Hyperlipidemia can lead to atherosclerosis and subsequent cardiovascular incidents such as thrombosis and infarction. This condition is often treated by a combination of drug therapy and diet and life-style modifications. Pharmacologic interventions are typically targeted toward decreasing the synthesis of harmful (atherogenic) plasma components, including certain lipoproteins (IDL, LDL, VLDL) that are associated with atherosclerotic plaque formation.

References

1. Abrams CS. Intracellular signaling in platelets. *Curr Opin Hematol.* 2005;12:401–405.
2. Agnelli G, Sonaglia F, Becattini C. Direct thrombin inhibitors for the prevention of venous thromboembolism after major orthopaedic surgery. *Curr Pharm Des.* 2005;11:3885–3891.
3. Aguilar M, Hart R, Hart RM. Antiplatelet therapy for preventing stroke in patients with non-valvular atrial fibrillation and no previous history of stroke or transient ischemic attacks. *Cochrane Database Syst Rev.* 2005;CD001925.
4. Albers GW, Amarenco P, Easton JD, et al. Antithrombotic and thrombolytic therapy for ischemic stroke: the Seventh ACCP Conference on Antithrombotic and Thrombolytic Therapy. *Chest.* 2004;126(suppl):483S–512S.
5. Andersen JC. Advances in anticoagulation therapy: the role of selective inhibitors of factor Xa and thrombin in thromboprophylaxis after major orthopedic surgery. *Semin Thromb Hemost.* 2004;30:609–618.
6. Anderson JL, Marshall HW, Bray BE, et al. A randomized trial of intracoronary streptokinase in the treatment of acute myocardial infarction. *N Engl J Med.* 1983;308:1312–1318.
7. Anne G, Gruberg L. Platelet glycoprotein IIb/IIIa inhibitors during percutaneous coronary interventions: a pharmacological and clinical review. *Expert Opin Pharmacother.* 2004;5:335–348.
8. Antiplatelet Trialists' Collaboration. Collaborative overview of randomised trials of antiplatelet therapy—III: reduction in venous thrombosis and pulmonary embolism by antiplatelet prophylaxis among surgical and medical patients. *BMJ.* 1994;308:235–246.
9. Arnaud C, Veillard NR, Mach F. Cholesterol-independent effects of statins in inflammation, immunomodulation and atherosclerosis. *Curr Drug Targets Cardiovasc Haematol Disord.* 2005;5:127–134.
10. Autret-Leca E, Jonville-Bera AP. Vitamin K in neonates: how to administer, when and to whom. *Paediatr Drugs.* 2001;3:1–8.
11. Baker SK, Tarnopolsky MA. Statin-associated neuromyotoxicity. *Drugs Today.* 2005;41:267–293.
12. Ballantyne CM. Role of selective cholesterol absorption inhibition in the management of dyslipidemia. *Curr Atheroscler Rep.* 2004;6:52–59.
13. Bartholomew JR. The incidence and clinical features of heparin-induced thrombocytopenia. *Semin Hematol.* 2005;42(suppl 3):S3–S8.
14. Baruah DB, Dash RN, Chaudhari MR, Kadam SS. Plasminogen activators: a comparison. *Vascul Pharmacol.* 2006;44:1–9.
15. Bauersachs RM. Fondaparinux: an update on new study results. *Eur J Clin Invest.* 2005;35(suppl 1):27–32.
16. Bell WR. Present-day thrombolytic therapy: therapeutic agents—pharmacokinetics and pharmacodynamics. *Rev Cardiovasc Med.* 2002;3(suppl 2):S34–S44.
17. Berger JS, Roncaglioni MC, Avanzini F, et al. Aspirin for the primary prevention of cardiovascular events in women and men: a sex-specific meta-analysis of randomized controlled trials. *JAMA.* 2006;295:306–313.
18. Bergqvist D. Low-molecular-weight heparin for the prevention of postoperative venous thromboembolism after abdominal surgery: a review. *Curr Opin Pulm Med.* 2005;11:392–397.
19. Berkner KL. The vitamin K-dependent carboxylase. *Annu Rev Nutr.* 2005;25:127–149.
20. Bern M. Observations on possible effects of daily vitamin K replacement, especially upon warfarin therapy. *JPEN J Parenter Enteral Nutr.* 2004;28:388–398.
21. Bickert B, Kwiatkowski JL. Coagulation disorders. In: DiPiro JT, et al, eds. *Pharmacotherapy: A Pathophysiologic Approach.* 5th ed. New York: McGraw-Hill; 2002.
22. Boersma E, Westerhout CM. Intravenous glycoprotein IIb/IIIa inhibitors in acute coronary syndromes: lessons from recently conducted randomized clinical trials. *Curr Opin Investig Drugs.* 2004;5:313–319.
23. Brophy JM, Joseph L. Medical decision making with incomplete evidence—choosing a platelet glycoprotein IIbIIIa receptor inhibitor for percutaneous coronary interventions. *Med Decis Making.* 2005;25:222–228.
24. Bussey H, Francis JL, Heparin Consensus Group. Heparin overview and issues. *Pharmacotherapy.* 2004;24(Pt 2):103S–107S.
25. Butenas S, Mann KG. Blood coagulation. *Biochemistry.* 2002;67:3–12.
26. Carcao MD, Aledort L. Prophylactic factor replacement in hemophilia. *Blood Rev.* 2004;18:101–113.
27. Carley S, Sen A. Best evidence topic report. Antifibrinolytics for the initial management of sub arachnoid haemorrhage. *Emerg Med J.* 2005;22:274–275.
28. Carlson LA. Niaspan, the prolonged release preparation of nicotinic acid (niacin), the broad-spectrum lipid drug. *Int J Clin Pract.* 2004;58:706–713.
29. Carlson LA. Nicotinic acid: the broad-spectrum lipid drug. A 50th anniversary review. *J Intern Med.* 2005;258:94–114.
30. Chapman MJ. Fibrates in 2003: therapeutic action in atherogenic dyslipidaemia and future perspectives. *Atherosclerosis.* 2003;171:1–13.
31. Chopra V, Marmur JD, Cavusoglu E. The role of clopidogrel in the management of patients with ischemic heart disease. *Cardiovasc Drugs Ther.* 2003;17:467–477.
32. Choy PC, Siow YL, Mymin D, O K. Lipids and atherosclerosis. *Biochem Cell Biol.* 2004;82:212–224.
33. Clader JW. Ezetimibe and other azetidinone cholesterol absorption inhibitors. *Curr Top Med Chem.* 2005;5:243–256.
34. Collen D, Lijnen HR. Thrombolytic agents. *Thromb Haemost.* 2005;93:627–630.
35. Curtin R. Intravenous glycoprotein IIb/IIIa antagonists: their benefits, problems and future developments. *Curr Pharm Des.* 2004;10:1577–1585.
36. Dahlback B. Progress in the understanding of the protein C anticoagulant pathway. *Int J Hematol.* 2004;79:109–116.
37. Davignon J. Beneficial cardiovascular pleiotropic effects of statins. *Circulation.* 2004;109(suppl 1):III39–III43.
38. Davydov L, Cheng JW. Tenecteplase: a review. *Clin Ther.* 2001;23:982–997.

39. Deitcher SR, Jaff MR. Pharmacologic and clinical characteristics of thrombolytic agents. *Rev Cardiovasc Med.* 2002;3(suppl 2):S25–S33.

40. Demierre MF, Higgins PD, Gruber SB, et al. Statins and cancer prevention. *Nat Rev Cancer.* 2005;5:930–942.

41. Denke MA. Diet, lifestyle, and nonstatin trials: review of time to benefit. *Am J Cardiol.* 2005;96:3F–10F.

42. Despres JP, Lemieux I, Robins SJ. Role of fibric acid derivatives in the management of risk factors for coronary heart disease. *Drugs.* 2004;64:2177–2198.

43. Devroey D, Velkeniers B, Duquet W, Betz W. The benefit of fibrates in the treatment of 'bad HDL-C responders to statins'. *Int J Cardiol.* 2005;101:231–235.

44. Doggrell SA. Alteplase: descendancy in myocardial infarction, ascendancy in stroke. *Expert Opin Investig Drugs.* 2001;10:2013–2029.

45. Dorffler-Melly J, Koopman MM, Prins MH, Buller HR. Antiplatelet and anticoagulant drugs for prevention of restenosis/reocclusion following peripheral endovascular treatment. *Cochrane Database Syst Rev.* 2005;CD002071.

46. Dunn AL. Management and prevention of recurrent hemarthrosis in patients with hemophilia. *Curr Opin Hematol.* 2005;12:390–394.

47. Eichinger S. Treatment of venous thromboembolism. *Wien Med Wochenschr.* 2005;15:7–10.

48. Eikelboom JW, Hankey GJ. Failure of aspirin to prevent atherothrombosis: potential mechanisms and implications for clinical practice. *Am J Cardiovasc Drugs.* 2004;4:57–67.

49. Elisaf M. Effects of fibrates on serum metabolic parameters. *Curr Med Res Opin.* 2002;18:269–276.

50. Ellis K, Brener S. New fibrinolytic agents for MI: as effective as current agents, but easier to administer. *Cleve Clin J Med.* 2004;71:20, 23–25, 29–30.

51. Elrod JW, Lefer DJ. The effects of statins on endothelium, inflammation and cardioprotection. *Drug News Perspect.* 2005;18:229–236.

52. Fazio S, Linton MF. The role of fibrates in managing hyperlipidemia: mechanisms of action and clinical efficacy. *Curr Atheroscler Rep.* 2004;6:148–157.

53. Fischer K, Van Den Berg M. Prophylaxis for severe haemophilia: clinical and economical issues. *Haemophilia.* 2003;9:376–381.

54. Fritz G. HMG-CoA reductase inhibitors (statins) as anticancer drugs (review). *Int J Oncol.* 2005;27:1401–1409.

55. Gensini GF, Comeglio M, Falai M. Advances in antithrombotic therapy of acute myocardial infarction. *Am Heart J.* 1999;138(Pt 2):S171–S176.

56. Giannini D, Balbarini A. Thrombolytic therapy in peripheral arterial disease. *Curr Drug Targets Cardiovasc Haematol Disord.* 2004;4:249–258.

57. Ginsberg HN. Effects of statins on triglyceride metabolism. *Am J Cardiol.* 1998;81(4A):32B–35B.

58. Glasheen JJ. Preventing warfarin-related bleeding. *South Med J.* 2005;98:96–103.

59. Go AS, Fang MC, Singer DE. Antithrombotic therapy for stroke prevention in atrial fibrillation. *Prog Cardiovasc Dis.* 2005;48:108–124.

60. Goldhaber SZ, Bounameaux H. Thrombolytic therapy in pulmonary embolism. *Semin Vasc Med.* 2001;1:213–220.

61. Gomez K, McVey JH, Tuddenham E. Inhibition of coagulation by macromolecular complexes. *Haematologica.* 2005;90:1570–1576.

62. Gorelick PB, Weisman SM. Risk of hemorrhagic stroke with aspirin use: an update. *Stroke.* 2005;36:1801–1807.

63. Goto S. Understanding the mechanism and prevention of arterial occlusive thrombus formation by antiplatelet agents. *Curr Med Chem Cardiovasc Hematol Agents.* 2004;2:149–156.

64. Goto S. Understanding the mechanism of platelet thrombus formation under blood flow conditions and the effect of new antiplatelet agents. *Curr Vasc Pharmacol.* 2004;2:23–32.

65. Granger CB, Weaver WD. Reducing cardiac events after acute coronary syndromes. *Rev Cardiovasc Med.* 2004;5(suppl 5):S39–S46.

66. Green ML. Management of dyslipidemias in the age of statins. *Prim Care.* 2003;30:641–669.

67. Gringeri A. Long-term aspects of hemophilia B treatment: part II. *Blood Coagul Fibrinolysis.* 2004;15(suppl 2):S15–S6.

68. Grunwald MR, Hofmann LV. Comparison of urokinase, alteplase, and reteplase for catheter-directed thrombolysis of deep venous thrombosis. *J Vasc Interv Radiol.* 2004;15:347–352.

69. Gunther KE, Conway G, Leibach L, Crowther MA. Low-dose oral vitamin K is safe and effective for outpatient management of patients with an INR:10. *Thromb Res.* 2004;113:205–209.

70. Gutt CN, Oniu T, Wolkener F, et al. Prophylaxis and treatment of deep vein thrombosis in general surgery. *Am J Surg.* 2005;189:14–22.

71. Guyton JR. Extended-release niacin for modifying the lipoprotein profile. *Expert Opin Pharmacother.* 2004;5:1385–1398.

72. Hardwick ME, Colwell CW, Jr. Advances in DVT prophylaxis and management in major orthopaedic surgery. *Surg Technol Int.* 2004;12:265–268.

73. Heijnen L, Buzzard BB. The role of physical therapy and rehabilitation in the management of hemophilia in developing countries. *Semin Thromb Hemost.* 2005;31:513–517.

74. Higashida RT, Furlan AJ, Roberts H, et al. Trial design and reporting standards for intra arterial cerebral thrombolysis for acute ischemic stroke. *Stroke.* 2003;34:e109–e137.

75. Ho WK, Hankey GJ, Lee CH, Eikelboom JW. Venous thromboembolism: diagnosis and management of deep venous thrombosis. *Med J Aust.* 2005;182:476–481.

76. Hyers TM. Heparin and other rapidly acting anticoagulants. *Semin Vasc Surg.* 2005;18:130–133.

77. Jamal SM, Eisenberg MJ, Christopoulos S. Rhabdomyolysis associated with hydroxymethylglutaryl-coenzyme A reductase inhibitors. *Am Heart J.* 2004;147:956–965.

78. Kadakia RA, Ferguson JJ. Optimal antithrombotic treatment for percutaneous coronary intervention. *Minerva Cardioangiol.* 2005;53:15–42.

79. Kamphuisen PW, Agnelli G, Sebastianelli M. Prevention of venous thromboembolism after acute ischemic stroke. *J Thromb Haemost.* 2005;3:1187–1194.

80. Kher A, Samama MM. Primary and secondary prophylaxis of venous thromboembolism with low-molecular-weight heparins: prolonged thromboprophylaxis, an alternative to vitamin K antagonists. *J Thromb Haemost.* 2005;3:473–481.

81. Kong DF. Aspirin in cardiovascular disorders. What is the optimum dose? *Am J Cardiovasc Drugs.* 2004;4: 151–158.

82. Konstantinides S. Should thrombolytic therapy be used in patients with pulmonary embolism? *Am J Cardiovasc Drugs.* 2004;4:69–74.

83. Krauss RM. Dietary and genetic probes of atherogenic dyslipidemia. *Arterioscler Thromb Vasc Biol.* 2005;25: 2265–2272.

84. Larned ZL, O'Shea SI, Ortel TL. Heparin-induced thrombocytopenia: clinical presentations and therapeutic management. *Clin Adv Hematol Oncol.* 2003;1: 356–364.

85. Leonardi-Bee J, Bath PM, Bousser MG, et al. Dipyridamole for preventing recurrent ischemic stroke and other vascular events: a meta-analysis of individual patient data from randomized controlled trials. *Stroke.* 2005;36:162–168.

86. Lieberman JR, Hsu WK. Prevention of venous thromboembolic disease after total hip and knee arthroplasty. *J Bone Joint Surg Am.* 2005;87:2097–2112.

87. Ling GS, Ling SM. Preventing ischemic stroke in the older adult. *Cleve Clin J Med.* 2005;72(suppl 3): S14–S25.

88. Luck JV, Jr, Silva M, Rodriguez-Merchan EC, et al. Hemophilic arthropathy. *J Am Acad Orthop Surg.* 2004;12:234–245.

89. Mahley RW, Bersot TP. Drug therapy for hypercholesterolemia and dyslipidemia. In: Brunton LL, et al, eds. *The Pharmacological Basis of Therapeutics.* 11th ed. New York: McGraw-Hill; 2006.

90. Makris M. Management of excessive anticoagulation or bleeding. *Semin Vasc Med.* 2003;3:279–284.

91. Malik S, Kashyap ML. Dyslipidemia treatment: current considerations and unmet needs. *Expert Rev Cardiovasc Ther.* 2003;1:121–134.

92. Mann KG, Butenas S, Brummel K. The dynamics of thrombin formation. *Arterioscler Thromb Vasc Biol.* 2003;23:17–25.

93. Manolis AS, Tzeis S, Andrikopoulos G, et al. Aspirin and clopidogrel: a sweeping combination in cardiology. *Curr Med Chem Cardiovasc Hematol Agents.* 2005;3: 203–219.

94. Maree AO, Fitzgerald DJ. Aspirin and coronary artery disease. *Thromb Haemost.* 2004;92:1175–1181.

95. Maron DJ, Fazio S, Linton MF. Current perspectives on statins. *Circulation.* 2000;101:207–213.

96. Mason RP, Walter MF, Day CA, Jacob RF. Intermolecular differences of 3-hydroxy-3-methylglutaryl coenzyme a reductase inhibitors contribute to distinct pharmacologic and pleiotropic actions. *Am J Cardiol.* 2005;96:11F–23F.

97. Massberg S, Schulz C, Gawaz M. Role of platelets in the pathophysiology of acute coronary syndrome. *Semin Vasc Med.* 2003;3:147–162.

98. Matsagas MI. Outpatient treatment of venous thromboembolism using low molecular weight heparins. An overview. *Int Angiol.* 2004;23:305–316.

99. McKenney J. New perspectives on the use of niacin in the treatment of lipid disorders. *Arch Intern Med.* 2004;164:697–705.

100. McRae SJ, Ginsberg JS. Initial treatment of venous thromboembolism. *Circulation.* 2004;110(suppl 1): I3–I9.

101. Menajovsky LB. Heparin-induced thrombocytopenia: clinical manifestations and management strategies. *Am J Med.* 2005;118(suppl 8A):21S–30S.

102. Menon V, Harrington RA, Hochman JS, et al. Thrombolysis and adjunctive therapy in acute myocardial infarction: the Seventh ACCP Conference on Antithrombotic and Thrombolytic Therapy. *Chest.* 2004;126(suppl):549S–575S.

103. Merli G. Anticoagulants in the treatment of deep vein thrombosis. *Am J Med.* 2005;118(suppl 8A):13S–20S.

104. Murugappan S, Shankar H, Kunapuli SP. Platelet receptors for adenine nucleotides and thromboxane A2. *Semin Thromb Hemost.* 2004;30: 411–418.

105. Nee PA. Thrombolysis after acute myocardial infarction. *J Accid Emerg Med.* 1997;14:2–9.

106. Neilipovitz DT. Tranexamic acid for major spinal surgery. *Eur Spine J.* 2004;13(suppl 1):S62–S65.

107. Norris JW. Antiplatelet agents in secondary prevention of stroke: a perspective. *Stroke.* 2005;36: 2034–2036.

108. Norris LA. Blood coagulation. *Best Pract Res Clin Obstet Gynaecol.* 2003;17:369–383.

109. Nutescu EA. Emerging options in the treatment of venous thromboembolism. *Am J Health Syst Pharm.* 2004;61(suppl 7):S12–S17.

110. Nutescu EA, Shapiro NL. Ezetimibe: a selective cholesterol absorption inhibitor. *Pharmacotherapy.* 2003;23:1463–1474.

111. O'Connor CM, Califf RM, Massey EW, et al. Stroke and acute myocardial infarction in the thrombolytic era: clinical correlates and long-term prognosis. *J Am Coll Cardiol.* 1990;16:533–540.

112. Ouriel K, Gray B, Clair DG, Olin J. Complications associated with the use of urokinase and recombinant tissue plasminogen activator for catheter-directed peripheral arterial and venous thrombolysis. *J Vasc Interv Radiol.* 2000;11:295–298.

113. Ouriel K, Kaul AF, Leonard MC. Clinical and economic outcomes in thrombolytic treatment of peripheral arterial occlusive disease and deep venous thrombosis. *J Vasc Surg.* 2004;40:971–977.

114. Patel SB. Ezetimibe: a novel cholesterol-lowering agent that highlights novel physiologic pathways. *Curr Cardiol Rep.* 2004;6:439–442.

115. Pereira J, Phan T. Management of bleeding in patients with advanced cancer. *Oncologist.* 2004;9:561–570.

116. Perler B. Thrombolytic therapies: the current state of affairs. *J Endovasc Ther.* 2005;12:224–232.

117. Phillips DR, Conley PB, Sinha U, Andre P. Therapeutic approaches in arterial thrombosis. *J Thromb Haemost.* 2005;3:1577–1589.

118. Pineo GF, Hull RD. Low-molecular-weight heparin for the treatment of venous thromboembolism in the elderly. *Clin Appl Thromb Hemost.* 2005;11: 15–23.

119. Poncz M. Mechanistic basis of heparin-induced thrombocytopenia. *Semin Thorac Cardiovasc Surg.* 2005;17:73–79.

120. Prandoni P, Sabbion P, Tanduo C, et al. Prevention of venous thromboembolism in high-risk surgical and medical patients. *Semin Vasc Med.* 2001;1:61–70.

121. Puckett RM, Offringa M. Prophylactic vitamin K for vitamin K deficiency bleeding in neonates. *Cochrane Database Syst Rev.* 2000;CD002776.

122. Rees M, Williams TJ. Pulmonary embolism—assessment and management. *Aust Fam Physician.* 2005;34: 555–561.

123. Rezkalla SH, Benz M. Antiplatelet therapy from clinical trials to clinical practice. *Clin Med Res.* 2003; 1:101–104.

124. Ringleb PA, Schellinger PD, Schwark C. Clopidogrel in the management of cerebrovascular events. *Int J Clin Pract.* 2004;58:402–410.

125. Rosenson RS. Current overview of statin-induced myopathy. *Am J Med.* 2004;116:408–416.

126. Ross SD, Allen IE, Connelly JE, et al. Clinical outcomes in statin treatment trials: a meta-analysis. *Arch Intern Med.* 1999;159:1793–1802.

127. Sandercock P, Counsell C, Stobbs SL. Low-molecular-weight heparins or heparinoids versus standard unfractionated heparin for acute ischaemic stroke. *Cochrane Database Syst Rev.* 2005;CD000119.

128. Schenone M, Furie BC, Furie B. The blood coagulation cascade. *Curr Opin Hematol.* 2004;11:272–277.

129. Schror K. Antithrombotic drugs in vascular medicine: a historical perspective. *Semin Vasc Med.* 2003;3: 97–105.

130. Serna DL, Thourani VH, Puskas JD. Antifibrinolytic agents in cardiac surgery: current controversies. *Semin Thorac Cardiovasc Surg.* 2005;17:52–58.

131. Shepherd J. Lipids in health and disease. *Biochem Soc Trans.* 2004;32(Pt 6):1051–1056.

132. Siddiqui MA, Wagstaff AJ. Enoxaparin: a review of its use as thromboprophylaxis in acutely ill, nonsurgical patients. *Drugs.* 2005;65:1025–1036.

133. Sidelmann JJ, Gram J, Jespersen J, Kluft C. Fibrin clot formation and lysis: basic mechanisms. *Semin Thromb Hemost.* 2000;26:605–618.

134. Stafford DW. The vitamin K cycle. *J Thromb Haemost.* 2005;3:1873–1878.

135. Stassen JM, Arnout J, Deckmyn H. The hemostatic system. *Curr Med Chem.* 2004;11:2245–2260.

136. Stone NJ, Bilek S, Rosenbaum S. Recent National Cholesterol Education Program Adult Treatment Panel III update: adjustments and options. *Am J Cardiol.* 2005;96(4A):53E–59E.

137. Stringer KA, Lopez LM. Uncomplicated myocardial infarction. In: DiPiro JT, et al, eds. *Pharmacotherapy: A Pathophysiologic Approach.* 5th ed. New York: McGraw-Hill; 2002.

138. Szczeklik A, Musial J, Undas A, Sanak M. Aspirin resistance. *J Thromb Haemost.* 2005;3:1655–1662.

139. Talbert RL. Hyperlipidemia. In: DiPiro JT, et al, eds. *Pharmacotherapy: A Pathophysiologic Approach.* 5th ed. New York: McGraw-Hill; 2002.

140. Thiagarajan P. New targets for antithrombotic drugs. *Am J Cardiovasc Drugs.* 2002;2:227–235.

141. Tsimihodimos V, Miltiadous G, Daskalopoulou SS, et al. Fenofibrate: metabolic and pleiotropic effects. *Curr Vasc Pharmacol.* 2005;3:87–98.

142. van Dongen CJ, van den Belt AG, Prins MH, Lensing AW. Fixed dose subcutaneous low molecular weight heparins versus adjusted dose unfractionated heparin for venous thromboembolism. *Cochrane Database Syst Rev.* 2004;CD001100.

143. Varady KA, Jones PJ. Combination diet and exercise interventions for the treatment of dyslipidemia: an effective preliminary strategy to lower cholesterol levels? *J Nutr.* 2005;135:1829–1835.

144. Vasudevan AR, Hamirani YS, Jones PH. Safety of statins: effects on muscle and the liver. *Cleve Clin J Med.* 2005;72:990–993, 996–1001.

145. Walenga JM, Prechel M, Jeske WP, Bakhos M. Unfractionated heparin compared with low-molecular-weight heparin as related to heparin-induced thrombocytopenia. *Curr Opin Pulm Med.* 2005;11:385–391.

146. Wardlaw JM, Zoppo G, Yamaguchi T, Berge E. Thrombolysis for acute ischaemic stroke. *Cochrane Database Syst Rev.* 2003;CD000213.

147. Wierzbicki AS, Mikhailidis DP, Wray R. Drug treatment of combined hyperlipidemia. *Am J Cardiovasc Drugs.* 2001;1:327–336.

148. Wilson SE, Watson HG, Crowther MA. Low-dose oral vitamin K therapy for the management of asymptomatic patients with elevated international normalized ratios: a brief review. *CMAJ.* 2004;170:821–824.

149. Wooster MB, Luzier AB. Reteplase: a new thrombolytic for the treatment of acute myocardial infarction. *Ann Pharmacother.* 1999;33:318–324.

150. Wright DG, Lefer DJ. Statin mediated protection of the ischemic myocardium. *Vascul Pharmacol.* 2005;42:265–270.

151. Wu KK. Aspirin and other cyclooxygenase inhibitors: new therapeutic insights. *Semin Vasc Med.* 2003;3: 107–112.

152. Wu KK, Matijevic-Aleksic N. Molecular aspects of thrombosis and antithrombotic drugs. *Crit Rev Clin Lab Sci.* 2005;42:249–277.

Respiratory and Gastrointestinal Pharmacology

Chapter 26

Respiratory Drugs

The respiratory system is responsible for mediating gas exchange between the external environment and the bloodstream. The upper respiratory tract conducts air to the lower respiratory passages and ultimately to the lungs. It also humidifies and conditions inspired air and serves to protect the lungs from harmful substances. In the lungs, gas exchange takes place between the alveoli and the pulmonary circulation.

The drugs discussed in this chapter are directed primarily at maintaining proper airflow through the respiratory passages. Agents that treat specific problems in the lungs themselves are not discussed here but are covered in other areas of this text. For instance, drugs used to treat infectious diseases of the lower respiratory tract and lungs are presented in Section 8 (Chapters 33 to 35).

The respiratory agents presented here are divided into two primary categories. The first group includes drugs that treat acute and relatively minor problems, such as nasal congestion, coughing, and seasonal **allergies.** The second category includes drugs that treat more chronic and serious airway obstructions, such as bronchial asthma, chronic bronchitis, and emphysema. Physical therapists and occupational therapists will frequently treat patients with both acute and chronic respiratory conditions. Consequently, the overview of the drugs presented in this chapter is of interest.

Drugs Used to Treat Respiratory Tract Irritation and Control Respiratory Secretions

The drugs presented below are used to treat symptomatic coughing and irritation resulting from problems such as the common cold, seasonal allergies, and upper respiratory tract infections. Many of these drugs are found in over-the-counter preparations. Often, several different agents are combined in the same commercial preparation; for example, a decongestant, an antitussive, and an expectorant may be combined and identified by a specific trade name. Also, agents within a specific category may have properties that overlap into other drug categories. Certain antihistamines, for instance, may also have antitussive properties.

Antitussives

Antitussive drugs are used to suppress coughing associated with the common cold and other minor throat irritations. When used to treat cold and flu symptoms, these drugs are often combined with aspirin or acetaminophen, as well as with other respiratory tract agents.[93] Antitussives are usually recommended for short-term use in relieving symptomatic coughing.[13] Nonetheless, the extensive use of antitussives has been questioned in our society. Coughing is a type of defense mechanism that can help expel mucus and foreign material from the upper respiratory tract.[83] By inhibiting this mechanism, antitussives may reduce the ability of coughing to raise secretions. Hence, antitussives may be helpful in treating an annoying dry cough, but use of these drugs to treat an active and productive cough may not be justified.[47]

There is also concern that many antitussives are not really effective in treating cough. In particular, over-the-counter products may not contain an adequate amount of the active medication, and it appears that these products may be no more effective than placebo in treating cough.[92,93] Doses that are effective in treating cough may also produce serious side effects.[20,83] Hence, mechanisms underlying the cough reflex continue to be studied so that safer and more effective antitiussives can be developed.[26,59]

Some of the commonly used antitussives are listed in Table 26–1. As shown in the table, codeine and similar opiate derivatives suppress the cough reflex by a central inhibitory effect.[21,124] Other nonopioid antitussives work by inhibiting the irritant effects of histamine on the respiratory mucosa or by a local anesthetic action on the respiratory epithelium. The primary adverse effect associated with most antitussives is sedation. Dizziness and gastrointestinal upset may also occur.

Decongestants

Congestion within and mucous discharge from the upper respiratory tract are familiar symptoms of many conditions. Allergies, the common cold, and various respiratory infections often produce a runny nose and a stuffy head sensation. Decongestants used to treat these symptoms are usually alpha-1–adrenergic agonists (see Chapter 20).[36] These agents bind to alpha-1 receptors located on the blood vessels of the nasal mucosa and stimulate vasoconstriction, thus effectively drying up the mucosal vasculature and decreasing local congestion in the nasal passages.[35]

Alpha-1 agonists used as decongestants are listed in Table 26–2. Depending on the preparation, these agents may be taken systemically or applied locally to the nasal mucosa via aerosol sprays. It appears that occasional use of these drugs can help the symptoms related to nasal congestion.[35,108] These drugs, however, can mimic the effects of increased sympathetic nervous system activity, and can cause serious cardiovascular and central nervous system (CNS) excitation. Excessive use or abuse should therefore be avoided.

The primary adverse effects associated with decongestants are headache, dizziness, nervousness, nausea, and cardiovascular irregularities (increased blood pressure, palpitations). As indicated, these effects become more apparent at higher doses and during prolonged or excessive drug use.[90]

Antihistamines

Antihistamines are used for reasons ranging from sedation to the treatment of parkinsonism. One of the most common applications of antihistamines, however, is the treatment of the respiratory allergic response to seasonal allergies (hay fever, and so forth) and other allergens (hence their inclusion in this chapter).[44,46,64]

Histamine is an endogenous chemical that is involved in the normal regulation of certain physiologic functions (gastric secretion, CNS neural modulation), as well as various hypersensitivity (allergic)

Table 26–1	COMMON ANTITUSSIVE AGENTS	
Generic Name	**Trade Name(s)***	**Method of Action**
Benzonatate	Tessalon	Local anesthetic effect on respiratory mucosa
Codeine	Many trade names	Inhibits cough reflex by direct effect on brainstem cough center
Dextromethorphan	Many trade names	Inhibits cough reflex (similar to codeine), but is non-narcotic
Diphenhydramine	Benadryl (others)	Antihistamine
Hydrocodone	Donatussin DC, Hydropane, Tussigon, many others	Similar to codeine
Hydromorphone	Dilaudid Cough	Similar to codeine

*Trade names often reflect combination of the antitussive with other agents (i.e., expectorants, decongestants).

Table 26–2	COMMON NASAL DECONGESTANTS	
Generic Name	**Trade Name(s)***	**Dosage Forms**
Ephedrine	Rynatuss, others	Oral
Oxymetazoline	Afrin, Dristan 12-Hr Nasal Spray, others	Nasal spray
Phenylephrine	Neo-Synephrine Nasal Spray, others	Nasal spray
Pseudoephedrine	Dimetapp Decongestant, Sudafed, many others	Oral
Xylometazoline	Otrivin	Nasal Spray

*Trade names often reflect combination of the decongestant with other ingredients.

reactions.[50,96] Histamine exerts its effects on various cells through four primary receptor subtypes: the H_1, H_2, H_3, and H_4 receptors.[97] By definition, antihistamines are drugs that specifically block the H_1 subtype of histamine receptors; that is, the effects of histamine during allergic reactions, respiratory infections, and so forth are mediated primarily through the H_1 receptor located on vascular, respiratory, and other tissues.[39]

H_2 receptors are involved primarily in the regulation of gastric acid secretion. Drugs that selectively block the H_2 receptor (referred to simply as H_2 antagonists) may help control gastric secretion in conditions such as peptic ulcer; these drugs are discussed in Chapter 27.

A third receptor subtype, the H_3 receptor, has been identified, and this subtype may be involved in the local regulation of histamine release from CNS nerve terminals.[109] Likewise, a new H_4 receptor has been identified on blood cells or cells derived from blood cells.[97] The clinical and pharmacologic significance of H_3 and H_4 receptors remains to be determined.[97]

Antihistamines used in the symptomatic treatment of hay fever and similar allergies are listed in Table 26–3. By blocking the effects of histamine on the upper respiratory tissues, these drugs help decrease nasal congestion, mucosal irritation and discharge (rhinitis, sinusitis), and conjunctivitis that are caused by inhaled allergens.[96,97] Similarly, antihistamines may decrease the coughing and sneezing associated with the common cold. Although these drugs do not reverse bronchospasm associated with asthma, antihistamines may be used as an adjunct in patients with asthma to help control rhinitis and sinusitis (see "Treatment of Bronchial Asthma").[61,130]

The primary adverse effects associated with antihistamines are sedation, fatigue, dizziness, blurred vision, and incoordination. Gastrointestinal distress (nausea, vomiting) is also quite common. Certain side effects, however, are related directly to each drug's ability to cross the blood-brain barrier (see Chapter 5 for a description of the blood-brain barrier). The original or "first-generation" antihistamines readily cross the blood-brain barrier and enter the brain, thus causing CNS-related side effects such as sedation and psychomotor slowing.[39,110] Newer "second-generation" antihistamines, however, do not easily cross the blood-brain barrier, and the risk of sedation and other CNS side effects is reduced substantially.[110,119] These newer agents, also known as nonsedating antihistamines, include cetirizine (Zyrtec), loratadine (Claritin), desloratidine (Clarinex), and fexofenadine (Allegra) (see Table 26–3). Newer antihistamines also seem to be more selective for the H_1 receptor subtype, and produce fewer side effects related to other histamine receptors and receptors for other neurotransmitters (e.g., acetylcholine, serotonin, and norepinephrine).[38,119]

The newer drugs therefore represent a substantial improvement over original antihistamines. They are not, however, devoid of side effects. For example, certain nonsedating antihistamines such as astemizole and terfenadine may be cardiotoxic, and problems such as severe ventricular arrhythmias (torsades de pointes) have occurred when these drugs are taken in high doses or taken by individuals with preexisting cardiac and liver problems.[70,71] These cardiac effects, however,

Table 26-3	ANTIHISTAMINES		
Generic Name	**Trade Name(s)**[#]	**Dosage**[*]	**Sedation Potential**[†]
Azatadine	Optimine	1–2 mg every 8–12 hr	Low
Brompheniramine	Bromphen, Dimetapp, others	4 mg every 4–6 hr	Low
Carbinoxamine	Rondec, others	4–8 mg every 6–8 hr	Low to moderate
Cetirizine	Zyrtec	5–10 mg/d	Very low
Chlorpheniramine	Chlor-Trimeton, Telachlor, others	4 mg every 4–6 hr	Low
Clemastine	Tavist	1.34 mg twice daily or 2.68 mg 1–3 times daily	Low
Cyproheptadine	Periactin	4 mg every 6–8 hr	Moderate
Desloratidine	Clarinex, Aerius	5 mg once a day	Very low
Dexchlorpheniramine	Polaramine, Dexchlor	2 mg every 4–6 hr	Low
Dimenhydrinate	Dramamine, others	50–100 mg every 4–6 hr	High
Diphenhydramine	Benadryl, others	25–50 mg every 4–6 hr	High
Doxylamine	Unisom Nighttime Sleep-Aid	12.5–25 mg every 4–6 hr	High
Fexofenadine	Allegra	60 mg twice daily or 180 mg/d	Very low
Hydroxyzine	Atarax, Vistaril	25–100 mg 3–4 times a day	Moderate
Loratadine	Claritin	10 mg once a day	Very low
Phenindamine	Nolahist	25 mg every 4–6 hr	Low
Pyrilamine	Codimal, others	25–50 mg every 8 hr	Moderate
Tripelennamine	PBZ	25–50 mg every 4–6 hr	Moderate
Triprolidine	Actifed, others	2.5 mg every 6–8 hr	Low

[#]Some trade names reflect the combination of the antihistamine with other agents (decongestants, antitussives, and so forth).
[*]Normal adult dosage when taken orally for antihistamine effects.
[†]Sedation potential is based on comparison to other antihistamines and may vary considerably from person to person.

do not seem to occur with other nonsedating antihist-amines, and drugs other than astemizole and terfena-dine can be used in patients at risk for cardioxicity.[71,127] Likewise, the nonsedating effects of the newer agents vary according to the drug and the patient, and efforts should be made to find the drug and dose that pro-duces antihistamine effects with the fewest side effects for each patient.[12,38] Nonetheless, several newer nonsedating agents are currently available, and these drugs have become the agents of choice for many peo-ple because they decrease histamine-related symptoms without producing excessive sedation and other neu-ropsychiatric effects.

Mucolytics and Expectorants

Mucolytic drugs attempt to decrease the viscosity of respiratory secretions. Expectorant drugs facilitate the production and ejection of mucus. These drugs are used to prevent the accumulation of thick, viscous secretions that can clog respiratory passages and lead to pulmonary problems. Expectorants and mucolytics are used in acute disorders ranging from the common cold to pneumonia, as well as in chronic disorders such as emphysema and chronic bronchitis.[74,85] These drugs are often used in combination with other agents (e.g., antitussives, decongestants, bronchodilators). Although mucolytics and expectorants are widely used, there is some question about whether these drugs actually produce beneficial effects in various types of respiratory disease.[85,93] Some studies have documented that these drugs can improve the ability to expel mucus and increase pulmonary function, but the extent of these benefits may vary widely according to the specif-ic patient and type of respiratory illness.[53,74]

The primary mucolytic drug currently in use is acetylcysteine (Mucomyst, Mucosil).[128] This drug is thought to work by splitting the disulfide bonds of res-piratory mucoproteins, thus forming a less viscous secretion. There is, however, some evidence that this drug also has antioxidant effects, and some of acetyl-cysteine's benefits may be due to its ability to decrease free-radical damage in the respiratory tissues.[129] Acetylcysteine is usually administered directly to the respiratory mucosa by inhalation or intratracheal instillation (through a tracheostomy). The primary adverse effects associated with this drug include nau-sea, vomiting, inflammation of the oral mucosa (stom-atitis), and rhinorrhea. However, serious adverse effects are relatively rare.

Several expectorant agents have been used in the past, but guaifenesin is the only drug currently acknowledged by the FDA to have evidence of thera-peutic effects.[27,128] This drug is administered to increase the production of respiratory secretions, thus encouraging ejection of phlegm and sputum. Exactly how guaifenesin exerts this effect, however, is not fully understood. Guaifenesin, which is usually adminis-tered orally in some form of syrup or elixir, is often combined with other agents in over-the-counter pre-parations, which are known by many different trade names. The primary adverse effect associated with guaifenesin is gastrointestinal upset, which is exacer-bated if excessive doses are taken or if this drug is taken on an empty stomach.

Drugs Used to Maintain Airway Patency in Obstructive Pulmonary Disease

Airway obstruction is a major problem in respiratory disorders such as bronchial asthma, chronic bronchitis, and emphysema. The latter two disorders are usually grouped under the heading of *chronic obstructive pul-monary disease (COPD)*.[55] Asthma and COPD are char-acterized by bronchospasm, airway inflammation, and mucous plugging of the airways.[55,121] One of the pri-mary goals of drug treatment is to prevent or reverse the bronchial constriction and subsequent obstruction of the airways in these disorders by using bronchodila-tors (beta-adrenergic agonists, xanthine derivatives, anticholinergics) and anti-inflammatory agents (gluco-corticoids, others). These agents are discussed in the next section.

Beta-Adrenergic Agonists

Rationale for Use and Mechanism of Action

Respiratory smooth-muscle cells contain the beta-2 subtype of adrenergic receptors.[76] (See Chapter 18 for a discussion of adrenergic receptor classifications.) Stimulation of these beta-2 receptors results in *relax-ation* of bronchiole smooth muscle. Hence, drugs that stimulate these beta-2 adrenergic receptors (i.e., beta-adrenergic agonists) produce bronchodilation and can be used to prevent or inhibit airway obstruction in bronchospastic diseases.[22,99]

Beta-adrenergic agonists are believed to induce smooth-muscle relaxation by the mechanism illustrat-

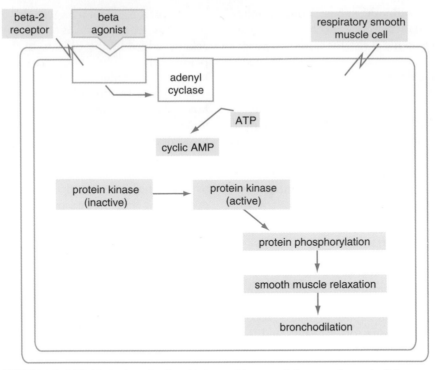

FIGURE 26–1 ▼ Mechanism of action of beta agonists on respiratory smooth muscle. Beta agonists facilitate bronchodilation by stimulating adenyl cyclase activity, which in turn increases intracellular cyclic AMP production. Cyclic AMP activates protein kinase, which appears to add an inhibitory
phosphate group to contractile proteins, thus causing muscle relaxation and bronchodilation.

ed in Figure 26–1. As shown in the figure, stimulation
of the beta-2 receptor increases activity of the adenyl
cyclase enzyme. This enzyme increases the production
of intracellular cyclic adenosine monophosphate
(cAMP). The cAMP acts as an intracellular second
messenger, which then increases the activity of other
enzymes such as protein kinase. The increased protein
kinase activity ultimately inhibits smooth-muscle contraction, probably by adding a phosphate group to
specific contractile proteins.

Specific Agents and Method of Administration

Beta-adrenergic agonists used to induce bronchodilation are listed in Table 26–4. As shown in the table,
some drugs are nonselective and stimulate alpha and
beta receptors fairly equally. Other agonists are more
selective and preferentially stimulate the beta-adrenergic receptors. Finally, the beta-2–specific agents are
the most selective and tend to bind preferentially to
beta-2 receptors. Beta-2–selective agonists offer an advantage when administered systemically because there

is less chance of side effects caused by stimulation of
other adrenergic receptors located on other tissues
(e.g., beta-1 receptors on the myocardium).[94] When
administered via inhalation, however, the issue of
adrenergic receptor selectivity becomes less important
because the drug is applied directly to the respiratory
tissues that primarily contain the beta-2 subtype.[76]
These agents also have different durations of action;
some of the newer drugs (formoterol, salmeterol) are
considered to be long-acting beta-adrenergic agonists.[94,99] These long-acting agents may provide more
stable and sustained bronchodilation in conditions
such as asthma.[22,99]

Beta-adrenergic drugs can be administered
orally, subcutaneously, or by inhalation. Inhalation of
these drugs is often the preferred method of administration in treating respiratory disorders. Inhalation
allows the drug to be delivered directly to the respiratory tissues with a minimum of systemic side effects
because of its absorption into the systemic circulation.[4] The onset of action is also more rapid with
inhalation.

Table 26–4	**BETA-ADRENERGIC BRONCHODILATORS**					
Drug	**Primary Receptor**	**Route of Administration**	**Onset of Action (min)**	**Time to Peak Effect**	**Duration of Action (hr)**
Albuterol	Beta-2	Inhalation Oral	5–15 15–30	1–1.5 2–3	3–6 8 or more
Epinephrine	Alpha, beta-1,2	Inhalation Intramuscular Subcutaneous	3–5 Variable 6–15	— — 0.3	1–3 <1–4 <1–4
Formoterol	Beta-2	Inhalation	1–3	—	12
Isoetharine	Beta-2	Inhalation	1–6	0.25–1	1–4
Isoproterenol	Beta-1,2	Inhalation Intravenous Sublingual	2–5 Immediate 15–30	— — —	0.5–2 <1 1–2
Metaproterenol	Beta-2	Inhalation (aerosol) Oral	Within 1 Within 15–30	1 Within 1	1–5 Up to 4
Pirbuterol	Beta-2	Inhalation	Within 5	0.5–1	5
Salmeterol	Beta-2	Inhalation	10–20	3–4	12
Terbutaline	Beta-2	Inhalation Oral Parenteral	15–30 Within 60–120 Within 15	1–2 Within 2–3 Within 0.5–1	3–6 4–8 1.5–4

Oral or subcutaneous administration is usually associated with more side effects. However, when administered orally or subcutaneously, beta agonists may reach the more distal branches of the airway to a greater extent. The bronchioles are usually constricted during an asthmatic attack, and the drug may not reach the distal respiratory passages when administered by inhalation.

Several beta agonists are available in metered-dose inhalers (MDIs) for inhalation administration. MDIs contain the drug in a small aerosol canister, and a specific amount is dispensed each time the patient depresses the canister.[33,81] Although MDIs are convenient because of their small size and portability, there is a certain amount of coordination required on the part of the patient to ensure adequate delivery of the drug. Some patients (e.g., young children) may have trouble timing the inhaled dose with a proper inspiratory effort.[37] In these patients, drug delivery can be facili-tated by using a spacer or reservoirlike attachment that sequesters the drug between the MDI and the patient's mouth.[17] The patient can first dispense the drug into the reservoir and then take a deep breath, thus improving delivery to the respiratory tissues.

Another method of inhaling beta agonists is through a *nebulizer*.[33,81] These devices mix the drug with air to form a fine mist that is inhaled through a mask, thus reaching the lungs over a more prolonged period (10 minutes). Nebulizers originally needed to be used in the home because they were large and needed an electrical outlet. Newer devices, however, are portable and use batteries. It was thought that nebulizers would provide a more effective treatment than MDIs because the nebulizer provides a fine mist and longer time for administration, which would enable better delivery of the drug to the more distal bronchioles. This fact, however, has not been proven conclusively, and the therapeutic benefits from nebulizers and MDIs seem to be equivalent if the patient uses either device appropriately.[17,78] Still, nebulizers may be a useful alternative for people who cannot master the technique needed for MDI delivery.

Finally, beta-2 drugs can be delivered via a dry powder inhaler (DPI).[33,81] This method offers the portability and convenience similar to an MDI. Again, the therapeutic effects of delivering a beta-2 drug via a DPI are not superior to other methods of inhalation (MDI, nebulizer), but DPIs may be easier for certain patients who lack the coordination and timing needed to use an MDI.[33,78]

Adverse Side Effects

With prolonged or excessive use, inhaled adrenergic agonists may actually increase bronchial responses to allergens and other irritants.[2,22] Although the exact reasons are not clear, excessive use of beta-2 drugs may promote airway irritation, thus increasing the incidence and severity of bronchospastic attacks.[57,126] Prolonged use of beta-2 drugs may also cause tolerance; the dose must be increased to achieve therapeutic effects when this occurs.[22,99] Hence, the regular and repeated use of adrenergic agonists has been questioned somewhat in recent years (see "Treatment of Bronchial Asthma").

Other side effects depend on the relative selectivity and route of administration of specific agents.[1] Adrenergic agonists that also stimulate beta-1 receptors may cause cardiac irregularities if they reach the myocardium through the systemic circulation. Similarly, stimulation of CNS adrenergic receptors may produce symptoms of nervousness, restlessness, and tremor. Adverse effects are relatively infrequent, however, when beta-adrenergic agonists are used as directed and administered locally via inhalation.

Xanthine Derivatives

Rationale for Use and Mechanism of Action

Xanthine derivatives are a group of chemically similar compounds that exert a variety of pharmacologic effects. Common xanthine derivatives include theophylline, caffeine, and theobromine (Fig. 26–2); these compounds are frequently found in various foods and beverages (tea, coffee, soft drinks). Theophylline and several theophylline derivatives are also administered therapeutically to produce bronchodilation in asthma and other forms of reversible airway obstruction (bronchitis, emphysema).[65,79] Theophylline and caffeine are also potent CNS stimulants, and some of the more common side effects of these drugs are related to this CNS excitation (see "Adverse Side Effects," later in this chapter).

Although the ability of xanthine derivatives to produce bronchodilation has been recognized for some time, the exact mechanism of action of theophylline and similar agents has been the subject of much debate. These drugs may enhance bronchodilation by inhibiting the phosphodiesterase (PDE) enzyme located in bronchial smooth-muscle cells.[113] PDE breaks down cAMP; inhibiting this enzyme results in higher intracellular cAMP concentrations. As discussed previously in this section (see "Beta-Adrenergic Agonists"), cAMP is the second messenger that brings about respiratory smooth-muscle relaxation and subsequent bronchodilation. By inhibiting PDE, theophylline can prolong the effects of this second messenger and increase bronchodilation. More important, PDE inhibition may decrease the function of inflammatory cells and inhibit the production of inflammatory mediators, thus accounting for theophylline's anti-inflammatory properties.[6,54] There is, in fact, considerable evidence that much of theophylline's beneficial effects are relat-

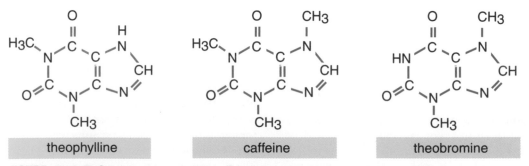

FIGURE 26–2 ▼ Common xanthine derivatives. Theophylline is often administered therapeutically to reduce bronchoconstriction.

ed to this drug's anti-inflammatory properties rather than to a direct bronchodilating effect.[24,43] The importance of controlling airway inflammation is addressed in more detail later in this chapter.

Theophylline may also act as an adenosine antagonist.[86,113] Adenosine is thought to bind to specific receptors on the smooth-muscle cells and to stimulate contraction. By blocking this effect, theophylline would facilitate smooth-muscle relaxation. Theophylline may likewise help produce bronchodilation by other mechanisms, such as inhibition of intracellular calcium release and stimulation of catecholamine release.[115] In reality, theophylline and similar drugs may induce bronchodilation and help protect the airways through a combination of several mechanisms, but the relative importance of each cellular effect remains to be determined.

Specific Agents and Method of Administration

Xanthine derivatives used in the treatment of bronchospastic disease are listed in Table 26–5. In general, these drugs are administered orally, although certain drugs may be given rectally or by injection if the oral route is not tolerated. When the oral route is used, sustained-release preparations of theophylline are available (see Table 26–5). These preparations enable the patient to take the drug just once or twice each day, thus improving patient compliance.

Table 26–5	XANTHINE DERIVATIVE BRONCHODILATORS	
Generic Name	**Trade Name(s)**	**Dosage Forms**
Aminophylline	Phyllocontin	Oral; extended-release oral; rectal; injection
Dyphylline	Dilor, Lufyllin	Oral; injection
Oxtriphylline	Choledyl	Oral; extended-release oral
Theophylline	Aerolate, Lanophyllin, Theo-Dur, many others	Oral; extended-release oral; injection

Adverse Side Effects

The most serious limitation in the use of xanthine bronchodilators is the possibility of toxicity.[95,113] Toxicity may appear when plasma levels are between 15 and 20 µg/mL. Because the recommended levels are between 10 and 20 µg/mL, signs of toxicity may occur in some patients even when blood levels are in the therapeutic range. Early signs of toxicity include nausea, confusion, irritability, and restlessness. When blood levels exceed 20 µg/mL, serious toxic effects such as cardiac arrhythmias and seizures may occur. In some patients, the serious toxic effects may be the first indication that there is a problem, because these effects are not always preceded by the more innocuous signs of toxicity. Theophylline-induced seizures are a life-threatening phenomenon, especially in patients who have been ingesting high levels of theophylline for prolonged periods.[95,113]

Consequently, during long-term use, care should be taken to avoid a toxic accumulation of theophylline. Patients in whom the metabolism of this drug is altered are especially prone to toxicity. In particular, factors such as liver disease, heart failure, alcohol consumption, cigarette smoking, concomitant use of other drugs (e.g., cimetidine), and patient age (older than 55) have all been identified as possible predisposing factors in theophylline toxicity.[113] To prevent toxicity, the dosage should be individualized for each patient, using the lowest possible dose (see "Treatment of Bronchial Asthma").

Anticholinergic Drugs

Rationale for Use and Mechanism of Action

The lungs receive extensive parasympathetic innervation via the vagus nerve.[76] The efferent fibers of the vagus nerve release acetylcholine onto respiratory smooth-muscle cells, which contain muscarinic cholinergic receptors. When stimulated, these receptors mediate bronchoconstriction. Consequently, drugs that block muscarinic cholinergic receptors prevent acetylcholine-induced bronchoconstriction, thus improving airflow in certain types of bronchospastic disease. In particular, anticholinergics are often the drugs of choice in treating COPD.[7,29] The primary factors that mediate bronchoconstriction in emphysema and chronic bronchitis appear to be increased vagal tone and acetylcholine release.[7,32] Drugs that reduce this vagal influence are therefore the cornerstone of controlling bronchoconstriction in COPD. Anticholinergics are not typically the first-line treatment of asthma because the primary pathophysiological feature of asthma is airway inflammation rather than increased vagal tone.[32] Nonetheless, these drugs can also be used to supplement anti-inflammatory and other medications in treating acute episodes of moderate to severe asthma.[84]

Specific Agents and Route of Administration

The anticholinergic bronchodilators include ipratropium and tiotropium, which are muscarinic receptor blockers that are similar in structure and function to atropine. Although atropine is the prototypical muscarinic antagonist, its use in respiratory conditions is usually limited because it is readily absorbed into the systemic circulation and tends to produce many side effects even when administered by inhalation. Alternatively, ipratropium (Atrovent) is an anticholinergic agent that is poorly absorbed into the systemic circulation and can be administered by an aerosol inhaler.[110] Thus, inhaled ipratropium is associated with substantially fewer systemic side effects.

Tiotropium (Spiriva) was also developed as an anticholinergic bronchodilator that is similar to ipratropium, but with longer lasting effects.[88] Tiotropium only needs to be inhaled once each day, whereas ipratropium is often inhaled 3 or 4 times each day.[8,98] It appears that tiotropium may also be superior to ipratropium in improving pulmonary function and reducing the frequency and severity of exacerbations in people with COPD.[41,51] Future studies will continue to clarify how tiotropium and other anticholinergics can be used to provide optimal treatment of COPD.[7]

Adverse Side Effects

Systemic side effects associated with atropine include dry mouth, constipation, urinary retention, tachycardia, blurred vision, and confusion. As stated previously, these effects appear to occur much less often with inhaled anticholinergics like ipratropium and tiotropium, which are not absorbed as readily into the systemic circulation.

Glucocorticoids

Rationale for Use and Mechanism of Action

Inflammation appears to be a key underlying factor in the exaggerated responsiveness of the respiratory passages in asthma and other obstructive pulmonary disorders.[111,116] Because of their powerful anti-inflammatory effects, glucocorticoids are used to control inflammation-mediated bronchospasm and are undoubtedly the most effective agents for controlling asthma.[49,68]

Glucocorticoids (also known as corticosteroids) inhibit the inflammatory response in several important ways.[10,118] These drugs directly affect the genes and transcription factors that produce inflammatory components.[77,91] As a result, the drugs inhibit the production of proinflammatory products (cytokines, prostaglandins, leukotrienes, and so forth) while increasing the production of anti-inflammatory proteins. Glucocorticoids also reverse the increase in vascular permeability and inhibit the migration of neutrophils and monocytes typically occurring during the inflammatory response.[18,118] The mechanism of action of glucocorticoids and cellular responses mediated by the glucocorticoids is discussed in more detail in Chapter 29.

Specific Agents and Routes of Administration

Glucocorticoids used to treat asthma are listed in Table 26–6. During severe, acute episodes of bronchoconstriction (e.g., status asthmaticus), glucocorticoids are usually administered intravenously. For more prolonged use, glucocorticoids are given orally or by inhalation. As with the beta agonists, the inhaled route is preferable because of the decreased chance of systemic side effects.[69,112] Glucocorticoids that are currently available via inhalation include beclomethasone, budesonide, flunisolide, and triamcinolone (see Table 26–6). Inhalation of a glucocorticoid allows the drug to be applied directly to the respiratory mucosa, and any glucocorticoid that is absorbed into the systemic circulation is rapidly metabolized. When these drugs are administered appropriately by the inhalation route, the chance of adverse effects is greatly reduced, compared with the possible effects associated with systemic administration (see "Adverse Side Effects").[69,112] Patients should be advised to rinse their mouth cavities with water after using oral glucocorticoid inhalers to prevent local irritation of the oral mucosa.

Adverse Side Effects

The major limitation of the glucocorticoids in any disease is the risk of serious adverse effects. Because of the general catabolic effect of these drugs on supporting tissues, problems with osteoporosis, skin breakdown, and muscle wasting can occur during prolonged

Table 26–6	CORTICOSTEROIDS USED IN OBSTRUCTIVE PULMONARY DISEASE	
Generic Name	**Trade Name(s)**	**Dosage Forms**[*]
Beclomethasone	Beclovent, Vanceril	Inhalation
Betamethasone	Celestone	Oral; intravenous or intramuscular injection
Budesonide	Pulmicort	Inhalation
Cortisone	Cortone	Oral; intramuscular injection
Dexamethasone	Decadron, others	Oral; intravenous or intramuscular injection
Flunisolide	AeroBid	Inhalation
Hydrocortisone	Cortef	Oral; intravenous or intramuscular injection
Methylprednisolone	Medrol	Oral; intravenous injection
Prednisolone	Prelone, others	Oral
Prednisone	Deltasone, others	Oral
Triamcinolone	Azmacort, others	Inhalation; oral, intramuscular injection

*Dosage forms that use the inhalation route are often preferred in asthma and other obstructive pulmonary diseases. Systemic administration by the oral route or by injection is typically reserved for acute or severe bronchoconstrictive disease (see text for details).

systemic administration.[14,125] Other possible systemic effects include retardation of growth in children, cataracts, glaucoma, hyperglycemia, aggravation of diabetes mellitus, and hypertension.[69,125] Patients may also become resistant to anti-inflammatory effects during repeated exposure to these drugs, especially when they are used to treat COPD.[5] Prolonged or excessive use can have a negative feedback effect on the adrenal gland, resulting in loss of adrenal function (adrenal suppression) while these drugs are being administered.[30]

Fortunately, the risk of these adverse effects is minimal when these drugs are administered by inhalation. Inhalation provides a more direct and topical application of the glucocorticoid to the respiratory tissues, with fairly limited absorption of the drug into the systemic circulation. The risk of adverse effects is also minimized when the total dose of the glucocorticoid is kept below certain levels.[69,113] Consequently, prolonged systemic drug administration should be avoided, and glucocorticoids should be administered by inhalation using the lowest effective dose. It is also prudent to periodically examine patients for bone min-

eral loss and other side effects when these drugs are used for prolonged periods.[14] Nonetheless, these drugs are extremely effective in treating various types of bronchoconstriction, and they should be used judiciously whenever possible.[49,68]

Cromones

Rationale for Use and Mechanism of Action

Cromones such as cromolyn sodium (Intal, Nasalcrom) and nedocromil sodium (Tilade) can help prevent bronchospasm in people with asthma. These drugs are not bronchodilators and will not reverse bronchoconstriction during an asthmatic attack. Hence, these agents must be taken prior to the onset of bronchoconstriction, and they must typically be administered prophylactically to prevent asthma attacks that are initiated by specific, well-defined activities (e.g., exercise, exposure to a friend's pet, pollen).[107] Likewise, the regular use of these drugs several times each day for several months may decrease airway hyperresponsiveness so that the incidence of asthmatic attacks decreases.[102,113]

Cromolyn and nedocromil are believed to prevent bronchoconstriction by inhibiting the release of inflammatory mediators such as histamine and leukotrienes from pulmonary mast cells.[56,102] Both agents can be administered by MDI; cromolyn can also be administered through a nebulizer. In addition, cromolyn is available in a nonprescription nasal spray (Nasalcrom) that can be helpful in preventing allergic rhinitis associated with seasonal allergies such as hay fever.[80]

Adverse Side Effects

Some irritation of the nasal and upper respiratory passages may occur following inhalation, but these drugs are remarkably free of serious adverse reactions. Hence, cromolyn and nedocromil are often used preferentially to treat mild persistent asthma, especially in children or in individuals who are unable to tolerate the side effects of other antiasthma drugs.[102,113]

Leukotriene Inhibitors

Rationale for Use and Mechanism of Action

Leukotrienes are inflammatory compounds that are especially important in mediating the airway inflammation that underlies bronchoconstrictive disease.[3,45] As indicated in Chapter 15, leukotrienes are 20-carbon fatty acids (eicosanoids) that are similar in structure and function to prostaglandins. Leukotrienes are actually derived from the same precursor as prostaglandins (arachidonic acid), but leukotrienes are synthesized by the lipoxygenase enzyme rather than by the cyclooxygenase enzyme (see Chapter 15, Fig. 15–2). Recently, strategies have been developed to selectively decrease the effects or synthesis of leukotrienes. For example, zileuton (Zyflo) inhibits the lipoxygenase enzyme, thereby reducing the production of leukotrienes.[63] Other drugs such as montelukast (Singulair) and zafirlukast (Accolate) block the receptor for leukotrienes on respiratory tissues.[11,67] These drugs offer a fairly selective method for controlling a specific aspect of inflammation in bronchoconstrictive disease.[42,100]

Evidence also suggests that leukotriene inhibitors can be combined with other drugs (glucocorticoids, beta agonists) to provide optimal management in specific patients with asthma and COPD.[11,60] In particular, it appears that these drugs may enhance the anti-inflammatory effects of glucocorticoids, and may therefore provide therapeutic effects at a relatively lower dose of glucocorticoid (glucocorticoid sparing effect).[52,123] Hence, the combination of a glucocorticoid and antileukotriene drug has become a popular option for many patients with bronchoconstrictive disease.[52]

Adverse Side Effects

Leukotriene inhibitors are safer than other anti-inflammatory agents such as the glucocorticoids. Some hepatic impairment has been reported with these drugs, but cases of severe toxicity are relatively rare.

Treatment of Bronchial Asthma

Pathophysiology of Bronchial Asthma

Asthma is a disease of the respiratory system characterized by bronchial smooth-muscle spasm, airway inflammation, and mucous plugging of the airways.[111,116] Patients with asthma have an exaggerated bronchoconstrictor response of the airways to various stimuli.[23,111] In some patients, the stimuli that trigger an asthmatic attack are well-defined (e.g., allergens like dust, pollen, chemicals, or certain drugs). Other factors such as exercise, cold, psychologic stress, and viral infections may trigger an asthmatic attack in some individuals. In other patients, the initiating factor may be unknown.

Although the exact cause of asthma remains to be determined, the basis for the increased airway reactivity has been elucidated somewhat. Airway inflammation is the critical factor in initiating the exaggerated bronchial reactions associated with this disease.[116,117] In asthmatic airways, there seems to be a complex interaction between several different cells including macrophages, neutrophils, eosinophils, platelets, and the airway epithelial cells themselves.[10,32] These cells release proinflammatory chemical mediators such as prostaglandins, leukotrienes, bradykinin, histamine, and platelet activating factor.[10] The chemicals irritate the respiratory epithelium and stimulate the contraction of bronchiole smooth muscle. Thus, the localized inflammation appears to sensitize airway structures to asthmatic triggers, and the bronchoconstriction and other features of asthma seem to be related directly to the inflammatory response underlying this disease.

Long-Term Management of Asthma

The primary focus of treating asthma has undergone a shift within the past few years. In the past, treatment consisted primarily of bronchodilators such as the beta-adrenergic agonists and the xanthine derivatives, with systemic anti-inflammatory steroids (glucocorticoids) added only in more advanced and severe cases. The use of glucocorticoids has increased, however, and these drugs are now used as first-line agents in most patients, including cases of newly detected, mild asthma.[68,87] The increased use of glucocorticoids is largely due to the fact that certain types of glucocorticoids can now be administered by inhalation. As indicated previously, inhaled glucocorticoids are not absorbed readily into the systemic circulation, and the risk of systemic side effects is therefore substantially reduced. Another reason for the shift toward increased glucocorticoid use is the recognition that these drugs directly reduce the inflammation that underlies asthmatic disease, whereas bronchodilators merely treat the secondary manifestations of this disease.[68] Put more simply, glucocorticoids directly affect the underlying disease process by decreasing the inflammation causing airway hyperresponsiveness.

Glucocorticoids have assumed the leading role in treating asthma. In addition, the role of leukotriene inhibitors has recently expanded to help control inflammation in asthma.[11,52] As indicated earlier, leukotrienes play a key role in mediating airway inflammation, and drugs that block leukotriene receptors (montelukast, zafirlukast), or inhibit the formation of leukotrienes (zileuton) can be extremely helpful in the long term control of asthma. These leukotriene inhibitors are nonsteroidal, and they can be especially helpful when combined with an anti-inflammatory steroid (glucocorticoid). The combination can provide optimal anti-inflammatory effects using lower doses of the glucocorticoid, thus preventing the systemic adverse effects associated with higher doses of steroids.[52,123] Hence, guidelines now advocate dual therapy using a glucocorticoid and leukotriene inhibitor for the long-term management of many patients with asthma.[52,114]

Beta-2 agonists are still used frequently as the primary method of *symptomatically* treating asthma attacks. Many patients, for example, inhale beta-2 agonists through MDIs as "rescue" therapy at the onset of a bronchospastic attack; this technique is a mainstay in managing acute episodes of asthma.[22,49] Nonetheless, the use of beta-2 agonists as long-term maintenance therapy for asthma has been questioned. Prolonged and excessive use of beta-2 agonists may actually *increase* airway hyperresponsiveness, thus increasing the risk of bronchoconstrictive attacks.[2,22]

The current philosophy is that beta-2 agonists still serve an important role in the treatment of periodic or acute bronchospasm[22]; that is, the intermittent use of a short-acting beta-2 agonist can help decrease the severity of an acute asthma attack. The role of beta-2 agonists in the long-term treatment of asthma is less obvious. These drugs are clearly not the primary form of treatment, but long-acting beta-2 agonists such as salmeterol and formoterol can be combined with glucocorticoids to provide optimal results in certain patients.[25,82] Long-acting beta-2 agonists are therefore considered supplemental to glucocorticoid therapy, and the addition of these beta agonists should be considered if glucocorticoid treatment alone is not successful in the long-term management of asthma.[25,82] Combining a long-acting beta-2 drug with a glucocorticoid can also reduce the dosage of the glucocorticoid, thus reducing the risk of side effects associated with high doses of glucocorticoids.[25]

The role of theophylline in treating asthma has been reexamined. Once considered the foundation for drug therapy, theophylline is now used sparingly compared to glucocorticoids and other antiasthmatic drugs (beta-2 agonists, antileukotriene drugs). Theophylline is a powerful bronchodilator, but problems with toxicity often limit its use in the long-term management of asthma.[43,103] Currently, low doses of theophylline are sometimes added to the drug regimen of patients who are resistant to treatment using glucocorticoids and beta agonists.[43] The combination of theophylline with a glucocorticoid may likewise provide optimal effects at lower doses.[43] As indicated earlier, it is also recognized that theophylline may have anti-inflammatory effects, and some of the renewed interest in using low-dose theophylline therapy is based on this drug's ability to control airway inflammation rather than actually produce bronchodilation.[24] Hence, theophylline remains an important adjunct in treating certain patients with asthma, and this drug may be used more extensively as more is learned about the synergistic effects of theophylline and glucocorticoids.

Inhaled glucocorticoids are therefore the cornerstone of drug therapy for patients with asthma. Leukotriene inhibitors, beta agonists, and theophylline can be used to supplement glucocorticoids as needed, with the specific drug regimen determined on a patient-by-patient basis. In addition, other drugs such as the cromones (cromolyn sodium, nedocromil) and antihistamines can be used to prevent the release or block the irritant effects of histamine in people with asthma.[102,130] Efforts should be made to find the optimal combination of agents for each patient, and the drug regimen must be reviewed constantly and adjusted in response to the patient's needs and the clinical course of the asthmatic disease.

Along with drug therapy, several nonpharmacologic interventions should be employed. Efforts should be made to determine the initiating factors of an asthmatic attack, and patients should be taught how to avoid these factors whenever possible. Also, considerable evidence exists that aerobic conditioning can improve the overall health and well-being of people with asthma.[62,122] Of course, exercise itself may be an asthmatic trigger in some individuals.[73] However, certain forms of aerobic exercise such as swimming may be an excellent way to improve the cardiorespiratory status of patients with asthma without causing excessive risk of bronchospastic attacks.[62]

Treatment of Reversible Bronchospasm in COPD

As indicated previously, bronchospasm is often present in COPD—that is, in chronic bronchitis and emphysema.[121] *Chronic bronchitis* is a clinical diagnosis applied to a long-standing inflammation of the bronchial tree. *Emphysema* is a pathologic condition marked by the destruction of alveolar walls and enlargement of the terminal air spaces.

Drug therapy for COPD is directed primarily toward maintaining airway patency and preventing airflow restriction.[7,55] Thus, anticholinergics (ipratropium, tiotropium) are typically the first drugs used, followed by other bronchodilators such as long-acting beta-2 agonists.[29,106] Theophylline can also be used as a bronchodilator in COPD, but it is usually reserved for acute exacerbations or for patients who have not responded adequately to other bronchodilators.[9,79] It has been suggested that at relatively low doses, theophylline may also produce beneficial effects in COPD because of its anti-inflammatory effects rather than its bronchodilating properties.[6,54] Hence, there has been renewed interest in using theophylline as a part of COPD treatment.[54]

Glucocorticoids have also been used to treat airway inflammation in COPD, but their use in this situation remains controversial. In contrast to their beneficial effects in asthma, glucocorticoids have not always produced clear therapeutic benefits in the long-term treatment of COPD.[10,14] Hence, these drugs are not typically prescribed on a routine basis but are usually reserved for the more severe cases or acute exacerbations of COPD-related bronchospasm.[32,58]

Treatment of Respiratory Problems in Cystic Fibrosis

Cystic fibrosis is one of the most common hereditary diseases in Caucasian populations—the autosomal-recessive trait is found in approximately 1 of every 2000 Caucasian births.[15] Cystic fibrosis essentially affects all the major exocrine glands, resulting in very thick, viscous secretions. These thickened secretions often form mucous plugs, which obstruct major ducts in various glands and organs.[15,66] For instance, the pancreatic and bile ducts are often obstructed, resulting in problems with nutrient digestion and absorption. Mucous plugging of the bronchioles occurs quite frequently, leading to pulmonary problems such as pneumonia, bronchiectasis, pulmonary fibrosis, and various pulmonary infections (especially *Staphylococcus*). These respiratory problems are usually the primary health threat to individuals with cystic fibrosis.[15]

Pharmacologic management of respiratory problems in cystic fibrosis is focused on maintaining airway patency as much as possible. Bronchodilators and mucolytic and/or expectorant drugs may help limit the formation of mucous plugs. Systemic glucocorticoids (e.g., prednisone) may also be beneficial in some patients in limiting airway inflammation and improving pulmonary function.[28] The side effects and risks of systemic glucocorticoids, however, may outweigh any benefits, especially in children.[19,28] Inhaled glucocorticoids could reduce the likelihood of severe adverse effects, but their beneficial effects are limited because inhaled forms of these drugs cannot penetrate through the thick mucus secretions in the airways of people with cystic fibrosis.[28] Other nonsteroidal anti-inflammatory interventions, including high doses of NSAIDs (e.g., ibuprofen), might also be helpful, but additional studies will be needed to clarify the role of these interventions in people with cystic fibrosis.[19,75]

Anti-infective agents also play a key role in the treatment of cystic fibrosis, and respiratory infections are treated with appropriate antibiotic agents.[16,89] In particular, azithromycin has shown considerable promise because it is an antibacterial drug with anti-inflammatory properties.[75,89] In addition to drug therapy, daily maintenance of respiratory hygiene (postural drainage, breathing exercises, etc.) is a key component in the management of cystic fibrosis. Evidence for the beneficial effects of chest physical therapy has been questioned somewhat, but there seems little doubt that a regular exercise program can help improve cardiovascular health and musculoskeletal function in people with cystic fibrosis.[31] With recent advances in medical treatment, many people with cystic fibrosis are living into their third or fourth decade, and an exercise program seems especially important in helping maintain quality-of-life for these individuals.[31]

Although there is still no cure for cystic fibrosis, several pharmacologic techniques have been recently developed that may help decrease the viscosity of respiratory secretions in patients with this disease. One technique uses aerosol preparations that contain enzymes known as *deoxyribonucleases*. These enzymes can be inhaled to break down the large quantities of DNA that are present in respiratory secretions of patients with cystic fibrosis.[48,104] Respiratory secretions in these patients often contain large amounts of DNA because the genetic material contained in airway in-

flammatory cells is deposited into the airway lumen when these cells are destroyed. DNA increases the viscosity and thickness of the respiratory secretions, and preparations that contain recombinant human deoxyribonuclease (rhDNAse, dornase alfa, Pulmozyme) can lyse this DNA, thus decreasing the viscosity of these secretions, thereby improving pulmonary function and reducing the chance of lung collapse (atelectasis) and infection.[48,104] This treatment is typically administered by inhalation via a nebulizer, with the dose and frequency adjusted according to the needs of each patient. Researchers continue to investigate the optimal and most cost effective way to incorporate deoxyribonuclease therapy into a drug for people with cystic fibrosis.[104,105]

Many other drug and nutritional interventions have also been attempted as part of the treatment for cystic fibrosis, but most of these interventions lack conclusive evidence of beneficial effects.[75] On the other hand, considerable progress has been made to develop strategies to correct the defective gene causing cystic fibrosis.[72,107] This gene therapy may someday provide an effective long-term treatment by replacing the defective gene with a functionally correct gene.[40,107] These strategies and other new tech-

Special Concerns in Rehabilitation Patients

■ ■ ■ Proper respiratory hygiene is crucial in preventing the serious adverse effects of respiratory infection and obstructive pulmonary disease. The accumulation of bronchial secretions can lead to decreased gas exchange, atelectasis, and additional infection. Rehabilitation specialists often play a critical role in preventing pulmonary mucus accumulation.[31,34] Therapists can facilitate the pharmacotherapeutic effects of mucolytic and expectorant drugs by performing postural drainage and breathing exercises. Even if patients are not being treated directly with chest physical therapy and respiratory hygiene, rehabilitation specialists should always encourage patients to cough and raise secretions for expectoration. Physical therapists and occupational therapists should also coordinate their treatments with respiratory therapy. Often, mucolytic and expectorant drugs are administered by the respiratory therapist through a nebulizer or positive-pressure ventilator. A program of chest physical therapy may be most effective when administered 30 minutes to 1 hour after these agents are administered (i.e., after the drugs have had some time to exert an effect on respiratory secretions).

Therapists should be aware of which patients are prone to bronchospastic attacks. If patients use some sort of portable aerosol bronchodilator, they should be encouraged to bring their medication to therapy. Rehabilitation procedures involving exercise may trigger a bronchospastic attack in some individuals, so the medication should be close at hand.

Continued on following page

Therapists should also be aware of the potential side effects of bronchodilator drugs. In particular, the cardiac side effects of the beta-adrenergic agonists and xanthine derivatives (theophylline, others) should be considered. Therapists may notice cardiac arrhythmias while monitoring the electrocardiogram (ECG) or while taking the patient's pulse; these cardiac abnormalities may indicate a problem with bronchodilator medications. Noncardiac symptoms such as nervousness, confusion, and tremors may also indicate bronchodilator toxicity and should be brought to the physician's attention. Early recognition of toxicity may be lifesaving, especially when xanthine derivatives such as theophylline are used. Finally, patients receiving systemic glucocorticoid treatment may be prone to the well-known catabolic effects of these drugs. Therapists should be especially alert for skin breakdown, and care should be taken not to overstress the bones and musculotendinous structures that may be weakened by the prolonged use of glucocorticoids.

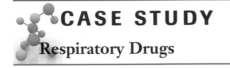

CASE STUDY

Respiratory Drugs

Brief History. V.C., a 63-year-old man, has a long history of COPD and hypertension. Twelve years ago, he was diagnosed with emphysema. During the past 5 years, his symptoms of shortness of breath, wheezing, and bronchospasm have become progressively worse. He is also a chronic cigarette smoker and has had a cough for many years, which produces large amounts of sputum daily. Although his physician advised him repeatedly to quit smoking, the patient was unable to kick the habit. To control his bronchospasm, the patient self-administers an inhaled anticholinergic agent (tiotropium) once each day. To help resolve acute bronchospasm, he also uses an inhaled beta-2 agonist (albuterol) via an MDI at the onset of an attack. He is also taking a diuretic and beta-1 blocker to control his hypertension. Two days ago, he was admitted to the hospital with weakness and incoordination in his left arm and leg. Subsequent medical tests indicated that he had suffered a cerebral vascular accident. Physical therapy was ordered to begin at the patient's bedside to facilitate optimal recovery from the stroke. The physical therapist began treating the patient with passive and active exercises to encourage motor return. The patient was also being seen by a respiratory therapist. The respiratory therapy treatments included administration of the mucolytic drug acetylcysteine via a nebulizer three times daily. The patient continued to self-administer the beta-2 agonist at the onset of bronchospasms.

Problem/Influence of Medication. Despite the program of respiratory therapy, bronchial secretions began to accumulate in the patient's airways. The patient had also been instructed in deep-breathing and coughing exercises, and he was told by the respiratory therapist to perform these exercises periodically throughout the day. However, no postural drainage was being performed to encourage ejection of sputum.

Decision/Solution. In addition to the neuromuscular facilitation activities, the physical therapist initiated a program of chest physical therapy including postural drainage and deep-breathing exercises. The physical therapist coordinated these activities with the respiratory therapist so that the patient first received a treatment of the mucolytic agent. Also, the physical therapist had the patient self-administer a dose of the inhaled beta-2 bronchodilator approximately 1 hour prior to the chest therapy session, thus allowing the bronchodilator to produce maximal airway dilation and permit optimal clearance of bronchial secretions.

niques are still experimental at present, but there is hope that these interventions may someday provide a means to alleviate the primary respiratory complications that often lead to illness and death in patients with cystic fibrosis.

SUMMARY

The drugs discussed in this chapter are used to control irritation and maintain airflow through the respiratory passages. Drugs such as the antitussives, decongestants, antihistamines, mucolytics, and expectorants are used primarily for the temporary relief of cold, flu, and seasonal allergy symptoms. These agents are frequently found in over-the-counter preparations, and several different agents are often combined in the same commercial product. Airway obstruction in chronic disorders such as bronchial asthma, chronic bronchitis, and emphysema is treated primarily with bronchodilator agents (beta-adrenergic agonists, xanthine derivatives, anticholinergics) and anti-inflammatory drugs (glucocorticoids, cromones, leukotriene inhibitors). Rehabilitation specialists should also be cognizant of which patients suffer from bronchospastic disorders (e.g., asthma) and of what medications are being used to control airway obstruction. Therapists can help facilitate the pharmacotherapeutic goals in patients with obstructive pulmonary disease by encouraging proper respiratory hygiene and breathing exercises and by helping improve overall cardiorespiratory endurance whenever possible.

References

1. Abramson MJ, Walters J, Walters EH. Adverse effects of beta-agonists: are they clinically relevant? *Am J Respir Med.* 2003;2:287–297.
2. Anderson SD, Brannan JD. Long-acting beta 2-adrenoceptor agonists and exercise-induced asthma: lessons to guide us in the future. *Paediatr Drugs.* 2004; 6:161–175.
3. Arm JP. Leukotriene generation and clinical implications. *Allergy Asthma Proc.* 2004;25:37–42.
4. Barnes PJ. Distribution of receptor targets in the lung. *Proc Am Thorac Soc.* 2004;1:345–351.
5. Barnes PJ. Corticosteroid resistance in airway disease. *Proc Am Thorac Soc.* 2004;1:264–268.
6. Barnes PJ. Theophylline in chronic obstructive pulmonary disease: new horizons. *Proc Am Thorac Soc.* 2005;2:334–341.
7. Barnes PJ. The role of anticholinergics in chronic obstructive pulmonary disease. *Am J Med.* 2004; 117(suppl 12A):24S–32S.
8. Barr RG, Bourbeau J, Camargo CA, Ram FS. Inhaled tiotropium for stable chronic obstructive pulmonary disease. *Cochrane Database Syst Rev.* 2005; CD002876.
9. Barr RG, Rowe BH, Camargo CA. Methylxanthines for exacerbations of chronic obstructive pulmonary disease. *Cochrane Database Syst Rev.* 2003;CD002168.
10. Belvisi MG. Regulation of inflammatory cell function by corticosteroids. *Proc Am Thorac Soc.* 2004;1: 207–214.
11. Bisgaard H. Pathophysiology of the cysteinyl leukotrienes and effects of leukotriene receptor antagonists in asthma. *Allergy.* 2001;56 (suppl 66):7–11.
12. Blaiss MS. Antihistamines: treatment selection criteria for pediatric seasonal allergic rhinitis. *Allergy Asthma Proc.* 2005;26:95–102.
13. Bolser DC. Cough suppressant and pharmacologic protussive therapy: ACCP evidence-based clinical practice guidelines. *Chest.* 2006;129(suppl): 238S–2349S.
14. Bonay M, Bancal C, Crestani B. The risk/benefit of inhaled corticosteroids in chronic obstructive pulmonary disease. *Expert Opin Drug Saf.* 2005;4:251–271.
15. Bosso JA, Milavetz G. Cystic fibrosis. In: DiPiro JT, et al, eds. *Pharmacotherapy: A Pathophysiologic Approach.* 5th ed. New York: McGraw-Hill; 2002.
16. Canton R, Cobos N, de Gracia J, et al. Antimicrobial therapy for pulmonary pathogenic colonisation and infection by Pseudomonas aeruginosa in cystic fibrosis patients. *Clin Microbiol Infect.* 2005;11:690–703.
17. Cates CC, Bara A, Crilly JA, Rowe BH. Holding chambers versus nebulisers for beta-agonist treatment of acute asthma. *Cochrane Database Syst Rev.* 2003; CD000052.
18. Chanez P, Bourdin A, Vachier I, et al. Effects of inhaled corticosteroids on pathology in asthma and chronic obstructive pulmonary disease. *Proc Am Thorac Soc.* 2004;1:184–190.
19. Chmiel JF, Konstan MW. Anti-inflammatory medications for cystic fibrosis lung disease: selecting the most appropriate agent. *Treat Respir Med.* 2005; 4:255–273.
20. Chung KF. Current and future prospects for drugs to suppress cough. *IDrugs.* 2003;6:781–786.
21. Chung KF, Chang AB. Therapy for cough: active agents. *Pulm Pharmacol Ther.* 2002;15:335–338.
22. Cockcroft DW. As-needed inhaled beta2-adrenoceptor agonists in moderate-to-severe asthma: current recommendations. *Treat Respir Med.* 2005;4:169–174.
23. Courtney AU, McCarter DF, Pollart SM. Childhood asthma: treatment update. *Am Fam Physician.* 2005; 71:1959–1968.
24. Culpitt SV, de Matos C, Russell RE, et al. Effect of theophylline on induced sputum inflammatory indices and neutrophil chemotaxis in chronic obstructive pulmonary disease. *Am J Respir Crit Care Med.* 2002; 165:1371–1376.
25. Currie GP, Lee DK, Wilson AM. Effects of dual therapy with corticosteroids plus long acting beta2-agonists in asthma. *Respir Med.* 2005;99:683–694.
26. Dicpinigaitis PV. Potential new cough therapies. *Pulm Pharmacol Ther.* 2004;17:459–462.
27. Dicpinigaitis PV, Gayle YE. Effect of guaifenesin on cough reflex sensitivity. *Chest.* 2003;124:2178–2181.
28. Dinwiddie R. Anti-inflammatory therapy in cystic fibrosis. *J Cyst Fibros.* 2005;4(suppl 2):45–48.
29. Disse B. Antimuscarinic treatment for lung diseases from research to clinical practice. *Life Sci.* 2001; 68:2557–2564.
30. Dluhy RG. Clinical relevance of inhaled corticosteroids and HPA axis suppression. *J Allergy Clin Immunol.* 1998;101(part 2):S447–S450.

31. Dodd ME, Prasad SA. Physiotherapy management of cystic fibrosis. *Chron Respir Dis.* 2005;2:139–149.

32. Doherty DE. The pathophysiology of airway dysfunction. *Am J Med.* 2004;117(suppl 12A):11S–23S.

33. Dolovich MB, Ahrens RC, Hess DR, et al. Device selection and outcomes of aerosol therapy: evidence-based guidelines: American College of Chest Physicians/American College of Asthma, Allergy, and Immunology. *Chest.* 2005;127:335–371.

34. Downs AM, Lindsay KLB. Physical therapy associated with airway clearance dysfunction. In: DeTurk WE, Cahalin LP, eds. *Cardiovascular and Pulmonary Physical Therapy.* New York: McGraw-Hill; 2004.

35. Eccles R, Jawad MS, Jawad SS, et al. Efficacy and safety of single and multiple doses of pseudoephedrine in the treatment of nasal congestion associated with common cold. *Am J Rhinol.* 2005;19:25–31.

36. Erickson CH, McLeod RL, Mingo GG, et al. Comparative oral and topical decongestant effects of phenylpropanolamine and d-pseudoephedrine. *Am J Rhinol.* 2001;15:83–90.

37. Geller DE. Comparing clinical features of the nebulizer, metered-dose inhaler, and dry powder inhaler. *Respir Care.* 2005;50:1313–1322.

38. Golightly LK, Greos LS. Second-generation antihistamines: actions and efficacy in the management of allergic disorders. *Drugs.* 2005;65:341–384.

39. Grant JA. Molecular pharmacology of second-generation antihistamines. *Allergy Asthma Proc.* 2000;21:135–140.

40. Griesenbach U, Geddes DM, Alton EW. Gene therapy for cystic fibrosis: an example for lung gene therapy. *Gene Ther.* 2004;11(suppl 1):S43–S50.

41. Gross NJ. Tiotropium bromide. *Chest.* 2004;126: 1946–1953.

42. Hallstrand TS, Henderson WR, Jr. Leukotriene modifiers. *Med Clin North Am.* 2002;86:1009–1033.

43. Hansel TT, Tennant RC, Tan AJ, et al. Theophylline: mechanism of action and use in asthma and chronic obstructive pulmonary disease. *Drugs Today.* 2004; 40:55–69.

44. Hansen J, Klimek L, Hormann K. Pharmacological management of allergic rhinitis in the elderly: safety issues with oral antihistamines. *Drugs Aging.* 2005; 22:289–296.

45. Holgate ST, Peters-Golden M, Panettieri RA, Henderson WR, Jr. Roles of cysteinyl leukotrienes in airway inflammation, smooth muscle function, and remodeling. *J Allergy Clin Immunol.* 2003;111(suppl): S18–S36.

46. Hore I, Georgalas C, Scadding G. Oral antihistamines for the symptom of nasal obstruction in persistent allergic rhinitis—a systematic review of randomized controlled trials. *Clin Exp Allergy.* 2005;35:207–212.

47. Irwin RS, Boulet LP, Cloutier MM, et al. Managing cough as a defense mechanism and as a symptom. A consensus panel report of the American College of Chest Physicians. *Chest.* 1998;114(suppl):133S–181S.

48. Jones AP, Wallis CE. Recombinant human deoxyribonuclease for cystic fibrosis. *Cochrane Database Syst Rev.* 2003;CD001127.

49. Joos GF, Brusselle GG, Van Hoecke H, et al. Positioning of glucocorticosteroids in asthma and allergic rhinitis guidelines (versus other therapies). *Immunol Allergy Clin North Am.* 2005;25:597–612.

50. Jutel M, Blaser K, Akdis CA. Histamine in chronic allergic responses. *J Investig Allergol Clin Immunol.* 2005;15:1–8.

51. Keam SJ, Keating GM. Tiotropium bromide. A review of its use as maintenance therapy in patients with COPD. *Treat Respir Med.* 2004;3:247–268.

52. Kemp JP. Recent advances in the management of asthma using leukotriene modifiers. *Am J Respir Med.* 2003;2:139–156.

53. King M, Rubin BK. Pharmacological approaches to discovery and development of new mucolytic agents. *Adv Drug Deliv Rev.* 2002;54:1475–1490.

54. Kobayashi M, Nasuhara Y, Betsuyaku T, et al. Effect of low-dose theophylline on airway inflammation in COPD. *Respirology.* 2004;9:249–254.

55. Konzem SL, Stratton MA. Chronic obstructive lung disease. In: DiPiro JT, et al, eds. *Pharmacotherapy: A Pathophysiologic Approach.* 5th ed. New York: McGraw-Hill; 2002.

56. Krishnaswamy G, Kelley J, Johnson D, et al. The human mast cell: functions in physiology and disease. *Front Biosci.* 2001;6:D1109–D1127.

57. Larj MJ, Bleecker ER. Effects of beta2-agonists on airway tone and bronchial responsiveness. *J Allergy Clin Immunol.* 2002;110(Suppl):S304–S312.

58. Larj MJ, Bleecker ER. Therapeutic responses in asthma and COPD. Corticosteroids. *Chest.* 2004;126 (suppl 2):138S–149S.

59. Lee LY, Undem BJ. Mechanisms of chronic cough. *Pulm Pharmacol Ther.* 2004;17:463–464.

60. Leff AR. Regulation of leukotrienes in the management of asthma: biology and clinical therapy. *Annu Rev Med.* 2001;52:1–14.

61. Lordan JL, Holgate ST. H1-antihistamines in asthma. *Clin Allergy Immunol.* 2002;17:221–248.

62. Lucas SR, Platts-Mills TA. Physical activity and exercise in asthma: relevance to etiology and treatment. *J Allergy Clin Immunol.* 2005;115:928–934.

63. McMillan RM. Leukotrienes in respiratory disease. *Paediatr Respir Rev.* 2001;2:238–244.

64. Meltzer EO. Evaluation of the optimal oral antihistamine for patients with allergic rhinitis. *Mayo Clin Proc.* 2005;80:1170–1176.

65. Mitra A, Bassler D, Goodman K, et al. Intravenous aminophylline for acute severe asthma in children over two years receiving inhaled bronchodilators. *Cochrane Database Syst Rev.* 2005;CD001276.

66. Moskowitz SM, Gibson RL, Effmann EL. Cystic fibrosis lung disease: genetic influences, microbial interactions, and radiological assessment. *Pediatr Radiol.* 2005;35:739–757.

67. Nayak A. A review of montelukast in the treatment of asthma and allergic rhinitis. *Expert Opin Pharmacother.* 2004;5:679–686.

68. O'Byrne PM. Initiation, dose reduction, and duration of inhaled corticosteroid therapy. *Immunol Allergy Clin North Am.* 2005;25:511–521.

69. O'Connell EJ. Optimizing inhaled corticosteroid therapy in children with chronic asthma. *Pediatr Pulmonol.* 2005;39:74–83.

70. Oppenheimer JJ, Casale TB. Next generation antihistamines: therapeutic rationale, accomplishments and advances. *Expert Opin Investig Drugs.* 2002;11:807–817.

71. Paakkari I. Cardiotoxicity of new antihistamines and cisapride. *Toxicol Lett.* 2002;127:279–284.

72. Parsons DW. Airway gene therapy and cystic fibrosis. *J Paediatr Child Health.* 2005;41:94–96.

73. Parsons JP, Mastronarde JG. Exercise-induced bronchoconstriction in athletes. *Chest.* 2005;128:3966–3974.

74. Poole PJ, Black PN. Mucolytic agents for chronic bronchitis or chronic obstructive pulmonary disease. *Cochrane Database Syst Rev.* 2003;CD001287.

75. Prescott WA, Jr, Johnson CE. Antiinflammatory therapies for cystic fibrosis: past, present, and future. *Pharmacotherapy.* 2005;25:555–573.

76. Proskocil BJ, Fryer AD. Beta2-agonist and anticholinergic drugs in the treatment of lung disease. *Proc Am Thorac Soc.* 2005;2:305–312.

77. Pujols L, Mullol J, Torrego A, Picado C. Glucocorticoid receptors in human airways. *Allergy.* 2004;59:1042–1052.

78. Ram FS, Brocklebank DM, Muers M, et al. Pressurised metered-dose inhalers versus all other hand-held inhalers devices to deliver bronchodilators for chronic obstructive pulmonary disease. *Cochrane Database Syst Rev.* 2002;CD002170.

79. Ram FS, Jardin JR, Atallah A, et al. Efficacy of theophylline in people with stable chronic obstructive pulmonary disease: a systematic review and meta-analysis. *Respir Med.* 2005;99:135–144.

80. Ratner PH, Ehrlich PM, Fineman SM, et al. Use of intranasal cromolyn sodium for allergic rhinitis. *Mayo Clin Proc.* 2002;77:350–354.

81. Rau JL. The inhalation of drugs: advantages and problems. *Respir Care.* 2005;50:367–382.

82. Remington TL, Digiovine B. Long-acting beta-agonists: anti-inflammatory properties and synergy with corticosteroids in asthma. *Curr Opin Pulm Med.* 2005;11:74–78.

83. Reynolds SM, Mackenzie AJ, Spina D, Page CP. The pharmacology of cough. *Trends Pharmacol Sci.* 2004;25:569–576.

84. Rodrigo GJ, Castro-Rodriguez JA. Anticholinergics in the treatment of children and adults with acute asthma: a systematic review with meta-analysis. *Thorax.* 2005;60:740–746.

85. Rogers DF. Mucoactive drugs for asthma and COPD: any place in therapy? *Expert Opin Investig Drugs.* 2002;11:15–35.

86. Rorke S, Holgate ST. Targeting adenosine receptors: novel therapeutic targets in asthma and chronic obstructive pulmonary disease. *Am J Respir Med.* 2002;1:99–105.

87. Rowe BH, Edmonds ML, Spooner CH, et al. Corticosteroid therapy for acute asthma. *Respir Med.* 2004;98:275–284.

88. Saberi F, O'Donnell DE. The role of tiotropium bromide, a long-acting anticholinergic bronchodilator, in the management of COPD. *Treat Respir Med.* 2005;4:275–281.

89. Saiman L. The use of macrolide antibiotics in patients with cystic fibrosis. *Curr Opin Pulm Med.* 2004;10:515–523.

90. Salerno SM, Jackson JL, Berbano EP. The impact of oral phenylpropanolamine on blood pressure: a meta-analysis and review of the literature. *J Hum Hypertens.* 2005;19:643–652.

91. Schleimer RP. Glucocorticoids suppress inflammation but spare innate immune responses in airway epithelium. *Proc Am Thorac Soc.* 2004; 1:222–230.

92. Schroeder K, Fahey T. Should we advise parents to administer over the counter cough medicines for acute cough? Systematic review of randomised controlled trials. *Arch Dis Child.* 2002;86:170–175.

93. Schroeder K, Fahey T. Over-the-counter medications for acute cough in children and adults in ambulatory settings. *Cochrane Database Syst Rev.* 2004;CD001831.

94. Sears MR, Lotvall J. Past, present and future—beta2-adrenoceptor agonists in asthma management. *Respir Med.* 2005;99:152–170.

95. Shannon M. Life-threatening events after theophylline overdose: a 10-year prospective analysis. *Arch Intern Med.* 1999;159:989–994.

96. Simons FE. H1-Antihistamines: more relevant than ever in the treatment of allergic disorders. *J Allergy Clin Immunol.* 2003;112(suppl):S42–S52.

97. Skidgel RA, Erdos EG. Histamine, bradykinin, and their antagonists. In: Brunton LL, et al, eds. *The Pharmacological Basis of Therapeutics* 11th ed. New York: McGraw-Hill; 2006.

98. Somand H, Remington TL. Tiotropium: a bronchodilator for chronic obstructive pulmonary disease. *Ann Pharmacother.* 2005;39:1467–1475.

99. Sovani MP, Whale CI, Tattersfield AE. A benefit-risk assessment of inhaled long-acting beta2-agonists in the management of obstructive pulmonary disease. *Drug Saf.* 2004;27:689–715.

100. Spahr JE, Krawiec ME. Leukotriene receptor antagonists—risks and benefits for use in paediatric asthma. *Expert Opin Drug Saf.* 2004;3:173–185.

101. Spooner CH, Saunders LD, Rowe BH. Nedocromil sodium for preventing exercise-induced bronchoconstriction. *Cochrane Database Syst Rev.* 2002;CD001183.

102. Storms W, Kaliner MA. Cromolyn sodium: fitting an old friend into current asthma treatment. *J Asthma.* 2005;42:79–89.

103. Suessmuth S, Freihorst J, Gappa M. Low-dose theophylline in childhood asthma: a placebo-controlled, double-blind study. *Pediatr Allergy Immunol.* 2003;14:394–400.

104. Suri R. The use of human deoxyribonuclease (rhDNase) in the management of cystic fibrosis. *BioDrugs.* 2005;19:135–144.

105. Suri R, Grieve R, Normand C, et al. Effects of hypertonic saline, alternate day and daily rhDNase on healthcare use, costs and outcomes in children with cystic fibrosis. *Thorax.* 2002;57:841–846.

106. Tashkin DP. Is a long-acting inhaled bronchodilator the first agent to use in stable chronic obstructive pulmonary disease? *Curr Opin Pulm Med.* 2005; 11:121–128.

107. Tate S, Elborn S. Progress towards gene therapy for cystic fibrosis. *Expert Opin Drug Deliv.* 2005;2: 269–280.

108. Taverner D, Latte J, Draper M. Nasal decongestants for the common cold. *Cochrane Database SystRev.* 2004; CD001953.

109. Taylor-Clark T, Foreman J. Histamine-mediated mechanisms in the human nasal airway. *Curr Opin Pharmacol.* 2005;5:214–220.

110. Ten Eick AP, Blumer JL, Reed MD. Safety of antihistamines in children. *Drug Saf.* 2001;24:119–147.

111. Tillie-Leblond I, Gosset P, Tonnel AB. Inflammatory events in severe acute asthma. *Allergy.* 2005;60:23–29.

112. Uings IJ, Farrow SN. A pharmacological approach to enhancing the therapeutic index of corticosteroids in airway inflammatory disease. *Curr Opin Pharmacol.* 2005;5:221–226.

113. Undem BJ. Pharmacotherapy of asthma. In: Brunton LL, et al, eds. *The Pharmacological Basis of Therapeutics.* 11th ed. New York: McGraw-Hill; 2006.

114. van den Toorn LM. Clinical implications of airway inflammation in mild intermittent asthma. *Ann Allergy Asthma Immunol.* 2004;92:589–594.

115. Vassallo R, Lipsky JJ. Theophylline: recent advances in the understanding of its mode of action and uses in clinical practice. *Mayo Clin Proc.* 1998;73:346–354.

116. Vignola AM. Effects of inhaled corticosteroids, leukotriene receptor antagonists, or both, plus long-acting beta2-agonists on asthma pathophysiology: a review of the evidence. *Drugs.* 2003;63(suppl 2): 35–51.

117. Walsh GM. Novel therapies for asthma—advances and problems. *Curr Pharm Des.* 2005;11:3027–3038.

118. Wanner A, Horvath G, Brieva JL, et al. Nongenomic actions of glucocorticosteroids on the airway vasculature in asthma. *Proc Am Thorac Soc.* 2004; 1:235–238.

119. Welch MJ, Meltzer EO, Simons FE. H1-antihistamines and the central nervous system. *Clin Allergy Immunol.* 2002;17:337–388.

120. Wellington K. Ipratropium bromide HFA. *Treat Respir Med.* 2005;4:215–222.

121. Wells CL. Pulmonary pathology. In: DeTurk WE, Cahalin LP, eds. *Cardiovascular and Pulmonary Physical Therapy.* New York: McGraw-Hill; 2004.

122. Welsh L, Kemp JG, Roberts RG. Effects of physical conditioning on children and adolescents with asthma. *Sports Med.,* 2005;35:127–141.

123. Wenzel SE. The role of leukotrienes in asthma. *Prostaglandins Leukot Essent Fatty Acids.* 2003; 69:145–155.

124. Widdicombe J, Kamath S. Acute cough in the elderly: aetiology, diagnosis and therapy. *Drugs Aging.* 2004; 21:243–258.

125. Woodcock A. Effects of inhaled corticosteroids on bone density and metabolism. *J Allergy Clin Immunol.* 1998;101(part 2):S456–S459.

126. Wraight JM, Smith AD, Cowan JO, et al. Adverse effects of short-acting beta-agonists: potential impact when anti-inflammatory therapy is inadequate. *Respirology.* 2004;9:215–221.

127. Yap YG, Camm AJ. Potential cardiac toxicity of H1-antihistamines. *Clin Allergy Immunol.* 2002;17: 389–419.

128. Yuta A, Baraniuk JN. Therapeutic approaches to mucus hypersecretion. *Curr Allergy Asthma Rep.* 2005; 5:243–251.

129. Zafarullah M, Li WQ, Sylvester J, Ahmad M. Molecular mechanisms of N-acetylcysteine actions. *Cell Mol Life Sci.* 2003;60:6–20.

130. Zitt MJ. The role of nonsedating antihistamines in asthma therapy. *Allergy Asthma Proc.* 2003;24: 239–252.

Chapter 27

Gastrointestinal Drugs

This chapter discusses drugs that are used to treat specific problems in the gastrointestinal (GI) system. The GI tract is responsible for food digestion and the absorption of nutrients and water. Dietary constituents normally undergo a series of digestive processes as they progress through the GI system. Under normal conditions, the transit time of food and water is adequate to allow the processes of digestion and absorption to take place. Indigestible and nonabsorbable products are eliminated by defecation.

The primary disorders that occur in the GI tract are related to damage from gastric acid secretion and abnormal food movement through the GI tract. Problems may develop if digestive secretions in the stomach begin to damage the upper GI mucosa and cause a peptic ulcer. Certain drugs attempt to prevent or heal peptic ulcers by controlling gastric acid secretion and protecting the mucosal lining. Problems with gastrointestinal motility may also respond to pharmacologic management. Excessive motility (*diarrhea*) and inadequate bowel evacuation (*constipation*) are treated with various agents that normalize peristalsis and facilitate normal bowel movements. Drugs are also available to treat other problems with digestion and vomiting (*emesis*). The GI system is susceptible to various infectious and parasitic invasions. The drugs used to treat these disorders are presented in Chapters 33 through 35, which deal with the chemotherapy of infectious diseases.

Rehabilitation specialists will often treat patients taking some form of GI agent. These medications are commonly used by the general public, as well as by hospitalized individuals and outpatients receiving physical therapy and occupational therapy. Although the direct impact of most GI drugs on physical rehabilitation is relatively small, an understanding of how these drugs are used will help therapists recognize their role in the patient's pharmacotherapeutic regimen.

Drugs Used to Control Gastric Acidity and Secretion

The acidic nature of the gastric juices is essential for activating digestive protease activity and controlling intestinal bacteria. The gastric acids, however, can cause severe ulceration and hemorrhage of the stomach lining if excessive amounts of acid are produced or if the normal protection of the stomach mucosa is disturbed by irritants, drugs, or bacterial infection.[54,56] Consequently, several different types of drugs are available that attempt to control or prevent the detrimental effects of gastric acid. These agents are used to treat *peptic ulcers*—that is, ulcerations of the mucosal lining of the esophagus, stomach, and duodenum.[37,51] These drugs may also be helpful in treating general problems related to indigestion and epigastric pain (dyspepsia) and to heartburn sensations caused by the leakage of gastric acid into the distal esophagus, called *gastroesophageal reflux*.[1] Agents used to control gastric acidity and secretion are presented below.

Antacids

Rationale for Use and Mechanism of Action

Antacids attempt to chemically neutralize stomach acids. These drugs typically contain a base such as carbonate or hydroxide combined with aluminum, magnesium, or calcium.[34] The base combines with excess hydrogen ions (H^+) in the stomach to increase intragastric pH. The basic strategy of this chemical neutralization is illustrated in Figure 27–1.

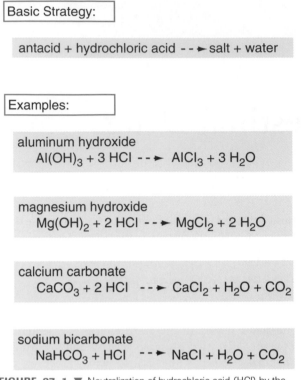

Basic Strategy:

antacid + hydrochloric acid - - ► salt + water

Examples:

aluminum hydroxide
$$Al(OH)_3 + 3\ HCl\ \text{- - ►}\ AlCl_3 + 3\ H_2O$$

magnesium hydroxide
$$Mg(OH)_2 + 2\ HCl\ \text{- - ►}\ MgCl_2 + 2\ H_2O$$

calcium carbonate
$$CaCO_3 + 2\ HCl\ \text{- - ►}\ CaCl_2 + H_2O + CO_2$$

sodium bicarbonate
$$NaHCO_3 + HCl\ \text{- - ►}\ NaCl + H_2O + CO_2$$

FIGURE 27–1 ▼ Neutralization of hydrochloric acid (HCl) by the primary forms of antacids. In each reaction, the antacid combines with HCl to form a salt and water. Carbon dioxide (CO_2) is also produced by calcium carbonate and sodium bicarbonate antacids.

Antacids are frequently used to treat episodic minor gastric discomfort (indigestion, heartburn) often accompanying overeating or indulging in certain incompatible foods. One concern regarding antacids is that they may be abused because the public has come to regard antacids as a panacea for poor eating habits. Antacids can also be used in the more serious and chronic conditions of peptic ulcer and chronic gastroesophageal reflux, but large amounts of antacids must be used for prolonged periods.[9] Hence, the use of antacids in these more serious conditions has been replaced to a large extent by other drugs such as H_2 receptor blockers and proton pump inhibitors (see later).[34,38] Consequently, antacids are used primarily to treat fairly minor and transient dyspepsia occurring from overeating, eating spicy foods, and so forth.[48]

Specific Agents

Antacids are identified by many trade names and frequently appear in over-the-counter products. There is such a plethora of antacids on the market that even a partial listing of commercial preparations is difficult.

The primary antacids can be classified as: aluminum-containing, magnesium-containing, calcium carbonate–containing, sodium bicarbonate–containing, or a combination of any of these classifications. These drugs are typically taken orally, either as tablets or as a liquid oral suspension.

Adverse Side Effects

Constipation is the most common side effect associated with the aluminum-containing antacids, whereas diarrhea often occurs with magnesium-containing preparations. Acid-rebound phenomenon is a potential problem with antacids, especially with those containing calcium.[20] That is, acid production may increase because antacids increase the pH of the gastric fluids, which serves as the normal stimulus for increased acid secretion. This situation does not present a problem while the antacid is in the stomach, because most of the excess acid will be neutralized. Gastric secretion may remain elevated, however, even after the antacid effects diminish and stomach pH returns to normal levels. The unopposed rebound of acid secretion may then cause increased gastric distress, necessitating increased use of the antacid.

Because antacids alter gastric pH, these drugs can affect the metabolism of other medications that rely on gastric acidity to help dissolve the medication or activate the drug.[34] Likewise, excessive use of antacids can alter the absorption of electrolytes (especially phosphate) and other drugs from the GI tract, and antacids can cause changes in urinary pH affecting drug elimination. Therefore, electrolyte imbalances and altered pharmacokinetics can occur if antacids are used in high doses for prolonged periods.[34]

H_2 Receptor Blockers

Rationale for Use and Mechanism of Action

The regulation of gastric acid secretion involves the complex interaction of many endogenous chemicals, including histamine.[21] Histamine stimulates specific receptors on stomach parietal cells to increase gastric acid secretion. These histamine receptors are classified as H_2 receptors in order to differentiate them from the H_1 receptors located on vascular, respiratory, and gastrointestinal smooth muscle.[32] Drugs have been developed that selectively bind to H_2 receptors without activating it. These H_2 antagonists, or blockers, prevent the histamine-activated release of gastric acid under basal conditions and during stimulation by food and other factors.[31,53]

The H$_2$ blockers are therefore used for both acute and long-term management of peptic ulcer and other problems such as dyspepsia and gastroesophageal reflux disease (GERD).[59] These drugs have a good safety profile, and many of the H$_2$ blockers originally introduced as prescription agents are now available as over-the-counter preparations. Nonetheless, the use of H$_2$ blockers have diminished somewhat because of the superior effects achieved with proton pump inhibitors (see below).[23] H$_2$ blockers remain an option for treating mild or occasional gastric irritation, but the routine use of these drugs in serious gastric disease has been largely replaced by more effective drugs such as proton pump inhibitors.

Specific Agents

The primary H$_2$ blockers used to control gastric secretions are listed in Table 27–1. Cimetidine was the first H$_2$ blocker to be widely used as an antiulcer agent. Newer drugs such as famotidine, nizatidine, and ranitidine appear to be at least as effective as cimetidine; they differ from one another primarily in their phar-

Table 27-1	H$_2$ RECEPTOR BLOCKERS	
Generic Name	**Trade Name**	**Adult Oral Dosage***
Cimetidine	Tagamet	300 mg 4 times each day with meals and at bedtime, 400 or 600 mg in the morning and at bedtime, or 800 mg at bedtime
Famotidine	Pepcid	40 mg once daily at bedtime or 20 mg BID
Nizatidine	Axid	300 mg once daily at bedtime or 150 mg BID
Ranitidine	Zantac	150 mg twice daily or 300 mg at bedtime

*Represents typical dose for treatment of gastric or duodenal ulcers. Doses for preventing ulcer recurrence or treating gastroesophageal reflux disease (heartburn) may be somewhat lower.

macokinetics (absorption, metabolism, and so forth) and their potential for interacting with other drugs.[21] Hence, all H$_2$ blockers seem to be essentially similar when used at moderate doses to control excess gastric acid secretion.

Adverse Side Effects

These drugs are generally well-tolerated in most patients, and adverse effects are rare during short-term or periodic use. Problems that may occur include headache and dizziness. Mild, transient GI problems (nausea, diarrhea, constipation) may also occur with the H$_2$ blockers, and arthralgia and myalgia have been reported with cimetidine use. Tolerance may occur during long-term use, and acid rebound can occur after discontinuation from prolonged use.[23]

Proton Pump Inhibitors

Rationale for Use and Mechanism of Action

These drugs inhibit the H$^+$, K$^+$-ATPase enzyme that is ultimately responsible for secreting acid from gastric parietal cells into the lumen of the stomach.[21] This enzyme is also known as the "proton pump"; hence these drugs are often referred to as proton pump inhibitors (PPIs). PPIs are extremely effective at inhibiting the proton pump, and therapeutic doses can virtually eliminate gastric acid secretion.[6,14] There is some evidence that PPIs also have antibacterial effects against *Helicobacter pylori* infection and that these drugs may have some anti-inflammatory properties that help decrease gastric irritation.[10] Evidence indicates that PPIs are more effective than H$_2$ blockers and antacids in controlling acid secretion and promoting the healing of ulcers.[8,47,55] PPIs have therefore gained prominence in treating gastric problems, and are now the drug of choice in the long-term treatment of patients with gastric and duodenal ulcers and GERD.[12,47]

Specific Agents

Omeprazole (Prilosec) was the original PPI; this drug is now joined by esomeprazole (Nexium), lansoprazole (Prevacid), pantoprazole (Protonix), and rabeprazole (AcipHex) (see Table 27–2). All of these drugs are similar, with selection often depending on cost, availability, and the drug interaction potential of each agent.[15] Likewise, nonprescription forms of certain PPIs are now available, and these forms offer a convenient,

Table 27–2	PROTON PUMP INHIBITORS					
		Typical Daily Dose*				
		Gastroesophageal Reflux Disease		*Gastric or Duodenal Ulcer*		
Generic Name	**Trade Name**	**Treatment: Healing**	**Maintenance: Prevent Recurrence**	**Treatment: Healing**	**Maintenance: Prevent Recurrence**	
Esomeprazole	Nexium	20–40 mg	20 mg	40 mg	20–40 mg	
Lansoprazole	Prevacid	15–30 mg	15 mg	15–30 mg	15 mg	
Omeprazole	Prilosec	20–40 mg	20 mg	20–40 mg	20–40 mg	
Pantoprazole	Protonix	40 mg	20–40 mg	40 mg	40 mg	
Rabeprazole	AcipHex	20 mg	20 mg	20 mg	20 mg	

*Doses are usually administered once each day. Time of administration (morning, bedtime, and so forth) is determined according to each patient's symptoms and disease characteristics.

effective, and remarkably safe option for patients who need to suppress gastric irritation and treat GERD.[24]

Adverse Side Effects

PPIs are usually well-tolerated. As with antacids and H_2 blockers, increased secretion of gastric acid (acid rebound) can occur when PPIs are discontinued after prolonged use.[21] It has also been suggested that long-term use is associated with gastric polyps and gastrointestinal tumors.[46] This suggestion, however, arises from studies on animals, and no causative link between PPIs and gastrointestinal hyperplasia has been established in humans.[21] On the other hand, there is substantial evidence that PPIs can decrease the morbidity associated with increased gastric acid secretion, and PPIs can decrease the risk of esophageal damage and carcinoma associated with GERD.[30] Hence, the benefits of these drugs seem to outweigh the risks, and PPIs do not usually produce any adverse effects during the long-term treatment of peptic ulcer and gastrointestinal reflux disease.[3]

Treatment of *H. Pylori* Infection in Gastric Ulcer Disease

Helicobacter pylori (*H. pylori*) is a gram-negative bacterium that is often present in the upper GI tract in people with gastric ulcer disease.[42] It has been sug-

gested that this bacterium may cause or potentiate gastroduodenal ulcers, and that the treatment of an *H. pylori* infection is essential in order to treat these types of ulcers.[7,54] Use of antibiotics results in an increased healing rate and a decreased recurrence of gastric ulcers in many people who test positive for *H. pylori* infection.[16,42] The fact that *H. pylori* is present in certain patients should not eliminate the possibility that other factors (stress, diet, and so forth) may also be contributing to gastric ulcer disease.[41] There are patients who are infected with *H. pylori* who do *not* develop gastric ulcers.[2] Hence, the exact role of this bacterium as a causative factor in gastric ulcers remains uncertain. Nonetheless, *H. pylori* may contribute to the development of gastric ulcers in susceptible individuals, and antibacterial drugs should be considered in patients with ulcers who are infected with this bacterium.

Treatment of *H. pylori* infection typically consists of a combination therapy, using several drugs simultaneously.[42] For example, one common form of "triple therapy" consists of two antibacterials (amoxicillin and clarithromycin) and one of the PPIs described earlier in this chapter.[17,36] Alternatively, various "quadruple therapies" have been used combining bismuth compound (described later in the section on "Treatment of Diarrhea") with a PPI and two antibacterials (e.g., tetracycline and metronidazole).[5,36] These drug regimens are typically administered for 1 to 2 weeks; and antibacterial drugs are discontinued after this period. Some patients, however, may need to remain on maintenance doses of the PPI or other antiulcer drugs to facilitate ulcer healing and prevent recurrence.[18]

Consequently, treatment of *H. pylori* infection may improve the prognosis of people with gastric ulcers and other forms of upper GI distress (dyspepsia, gastroesophageal reflux disease). Patients with clinical signs of ulcers who also test positive for this infection should receive a treatment regimen attempting to eradicate the infection. Successful treatment of an *H. pylori* infection may reduce or eliminate the need for subsequent antiulcer medications in patients with gastric ulcer disease.[42]

Other Agents Used to Control and Treat Gastric Ulcers

Several other agents besides the antacids, H_2 blockers, and PPIs have proved successful in preventing or treating problems associated with gastric acidity and mucosal breakdown. Some of the more frequently used agents are discussed below.

Anticholinergics. The role of muscarinic cholinergic antagonists in treating peptic ulcers was discussed in Chapter 19. Cholinergic stimulation of the gut via vagal efferent fibers produces a general increase in GI motility and secretion. Drugs that block the effects of acetylcholine on stomach parietal cells will decrease the release of gastric acid. Nonetheless, atropine and similar anticholinergics are rarely used to control gastric acid secretion because most cholinergic muscarinic inhibitors cause many side effects, such as dry mouth, constipation, urinary retention, and confusion.[21] One possible exception is the antimuscarinic drug pirenzepine (Gastrozepin), which is fairly selective for muscarinic receptors located on the stomach mucosa, and effectively decreases gastric secretion at a dose that does not cause excessive side effects.[21] Although this drug is not as effective as newer agents (PPIs, H_2 blockers), it can be used when treatment with other agents is not possible.

Metoclopramide (Reglan). This drug is officially classified as a dopamine receptor antagonist but also appears to enhance the peripheral effects of acetylcholine. Primarily because of this latter effect, metoclopramide stimulates motility in the upper GI tract (prokinetic effect), which may be useful in moving the stomach contents toward the small intestine, thus decreasing the risk of gastric acid moving backward

into the esophagus. This drug may therefore be helpful in treating gastroesophageal reflux disease.[44] The primary side effects associated with metoclopramide are related to its antagonistic effects on central nervous system (CNS) dopamine receptors. Restlessness, drowsiness, and fatigue are fairly common. Some extrapyramidal symptoms (i.e., parkinsonismlike tremor and rigidity) may also occur because of the central antidopamine effects.

Prostaglandins. There is little doubt that certain prostaglandins such as PGE_2 and PGI_2 inhibit gastric secretion and help protect the stomach mucosa by stimulating gastric mucus secretion.[4,29] The problem has been determining exactly how the prostaglandins are involved and whether exogenous prostaglandin analogs can be used to help treat peptic ulcer. Two prostaglandin analogs, enprostil and misoprostol, have been studied as possible treatments for peptic ulcer.[11,39] The general consensus from clinical trials has been that these drugs are successful in treating ulcers, but they do not seem to offer any advantages over more traditional antiulcer drugs such as PPIs.[21] Also, prostaglandin analogs may be effective only at doses that also cause other GI effects, such as diarrhea.[21]

Consequently, prostaglandin analogs have not gained overwhelming acceptance as antiulcer drugs. Currently, only misoprostol (Cytotec) is available for clinical use, and this drug is typically reserved for the treatment of gastric damage caused by aspirin and similar nonsteroidal anti-inflammatory drugs (NSAIDs).[21] The use of misoprostol to reduce or prevent NSAID-induced gastropathy is discussed in more detail in Chapter 15.

Sucralfate (Carafate, Sulcrate). Sucralfate is a disaccharide that exerts a cytoprotective effect on the stomach mucosa.[26,37] Although the exact mechanism is unclear, sucralfate may form a protective gel within the stomach that adheres to ulcers and shields them from the contents of the stomach. The protective barrier formed by the drug prevents further erosion and permits healing of duodenal and gastric ulcers. Sucralfate is well tolerated, although constipation may occur in some patients.

Antidiarrheal Agents

Normal propulsion of food through the GI tract is crucial for proper absorption of nutrients and water. If transit time is too fast, diarrhea occurs, resulting in poor food absorption and dehydration. Diarrhea is often a temporary symptom of many relatively minor GI disorders, but it may also occur with more serious conditions such as dysentery, ulcerative colitis, and cholera. If diarrhea is sustained for even a few days, the resulting dehydration can be a serious problem, especially in infants or debilitated patients. Consequently, efforts should be made to control diarrhea as soon as possible. Antidiarrheal agents are listed in Table 27–3, and their pharmacology is discussed in the following sections.

Opioid Derivatives

Rationale for Use and Mechanism of Action

The constipating effects of morphine and certain other opioid derivatives have been recognized for some time. These drugs produce a general decrease in GI motility, and they may also reduce fluid loss by increasing the absorption of salt and water or by decreasing fluid and electrolyte excretion from the GI tract.[44] The exact manner in which opioids exert these effects, however, is not known. As indicated in Chapter 14, opioids bind to CNS receptors and mediate analgesic effects, which may help decrease symptoms of cramping and abdominal discomfort. The primary effects of opioids on GI motility (antiperistalsis), however, seem to occur because opioids bind to neuronal receptors on the enteric nerve plexus within the gut wall or by a direct effect of opioids on GI epithelial and smooth muscle cells.[13,19] In particular, the mu subtype of the opioid receptor seems to be important in mediating the GI effects of opioid drugs; stimulation of these receptors is the primary method for reducing GI motility and treating diarrhea.[13]

Specific Agents

Opioid derivatives used to treat diarrhea are listed in Table 27–3. Opium tincture (laudanum) and camphorated opium tincture (paregoric) are naturally occurring opiates that are very potent inhibitors of peristalsis. These natural agents are still available for treating diarrhea, but they have essentially been replaced by newer opioids such as diphenoxylate and loperamide. These newer opioids are somewhat less potent but may produce fewer side effects.

Table 27–3 ANTIDIARRHEAL AGENTS

Generic Name	Trade Names	Dosage
Adsorbents		
Attapulgite	Donnagel, others	1.2–1.5 gm after each loose bowel movement
Kaolin, Pectin	Kao-Spen, Kapectolin*	60–120 mL regular-strength suspension after each loose, bowel movement
Bismuth salicylate	Pepto-Bismol, others	525 mg every half hour to 1 hour or 1050 mg every hour if needed
Opioid derivatives		
Difenoxine	Motofen†	2 mg initially, 1 mg after each loose stool or every 3–4 hrs
Diphenoxylate	Lomotil, others†	5 mg 3 or 4 times daily
Loperamide	Imodium, others	4 mg initially, 2 mg after each loose stool
Opium tincture	—	0.3–1.0 mL 4 times daily
Paregoric	—	5–10 mL 1–4 times daily

*Commercial products typically contain both kaolin and pectin.
†Commercial products often combine difenoxine or diphenoxylate (an opioid) with atropine (an anticholinergic).

Adverse Side Effects

The primary side effects with these drugs are nausea, abdominal discomfort, constipation, and other GI disturbances. Drowsiness, fatigue, and dizziness have also been reported. Although addiction is a potential problem when opioids are administered, the risk of tolerance and physical dependence is fairly small when these drugs are used in recommended dosages for the short-term treatment of diarrhea.

Adsorbents

Rationale for Treatment and Mechanism of Action

Adsorbents such as kaolin, pectin, or attapulgite are administered to take up and hold harmful substances such as bacteria and toxins in the intestinal lumen.[44] Theoretically, these adsorbents sequester the harmful products that cause the diarrhea. These products are used frequently in minor diarrhea, although there is some doubt as to whether they really help decrease stool production and water loss.

Specific Agents

Adsorbents used to treat diarrhea are listed in Table 27–3. These agents frequently appear as the active ingredients in over-the-counter products and may be combined with each other or with other drugs such as antacids.

Adverse Side Effects

Adsorbents are essentially free from side effects, although constipation may follow prolonged or excessive use.

Bismuth Salicylate

Rationale for Treatment and Mechanism of Action

Bismuth salicylate has a number of properties contributing to its antidiarrheal effects. This drug may stimulate water and electrolyte absorption from the lower GI tract, thus decreasing fecal fluid loss. In addition, the bismuth component of this compound may have antibacterial effects, and the salicylate component may inhibit the production of prostaglandins that irritate the intestinal lining. The combination of these properties makes this drug fairly effective in treating mild-to-moderate diarrhea.[44] Bismuth salicylate also decreases gastric acid secretion and exerts antacid effects, hence its use in stomach upset and minor gastric irritation. As indicated earlier, bismuth compounds are also part of the antibacterial regimen in *H. pylori* infection.

Specific Agents

Bismuth salicylate is the active ingredient in Pepto-Bismol, a fairly inexpensive and readily available over-the-counter commercial product.

Adverse Side Effects

This drug is relatively free from serious side effects. Problems with salicylate intoxication may occur during overdose or in people who are sensitive to aspirin and other salicylates.

Miscellaneous Agents Used to Treat Diarrhea

Various other drug strategies have been used in specific cases of diarrhea or in situations where conventional drug therapy is unsuccessful. Clonidine (Catapres) for example, is a CNS alpha-2 receptor agonist that is normally used to treat hypertension (see Chapters 20 and 21). This drug, however, can also stimulate alpha-2 receptors in the GI tract, thereby decreasing secretion, increasing absorption, and normalizing GI movement.[25] Octreotide (Sandostatin) is a complex drug that mimics the effects of endogenously produced somatostatin. Octreotide inhibits the secretion of serotonin and other peptides that stimulate GI function, and this drug is especially useful in treating diarrhea caused by tumors that secrete these substances into the GI tract.[25,50] Finally, cholestyramine (Questran) and colestipol (Colestid) are drugs that sequester and bind bile acids within the GI tract; these agents can be useful in treating diarrhea caused by excess bile acid secretion.[50]

Laxatives and Cathartics

Rationale for Use

Laxatives are used to promote evacuation of the bowel and defecation. Cathartics, or purgatives, are also used to promote lower GI evacuation, but in a somewhat more rapid fashion than with typical laxatives. For this discussion, the term "laxative" will be used to include both relatively slow-acting and fast-acting agents.

Laxatives are typically used whenever normal bowel movements have been impaired but no obstruction exists in the GI system. For instance, laxatives may benefit patients on prolonged bed rest, patients with infrequent or painful bowel movements, patients with spinal cord injuries, or patients who should avoid straining during defecation (e.g., postpartum patients and those recovering from surgical procedures). Laxatives are also indicated for bowel evacuation prior to surgical or diagnostic procedures.

The problem with laxatives is that they are frequently abused. The long-term, chronic use of laxatives is usually unnecessary and often unhealthy. These agents are self-administered by individuals who are obsessed with maintaining daily bowel movements. The individuals may have the misconception that daily bowel evacuation is needed to maintain normal GI function. Also, laxatives are often relied on instead of other factors that promote normal bowel evacuation, such as a high-fiber diet, adequate hydration, and physical activity.[22] Consequently, laxatives serve an important but finite role in GI function, and their role in helping maintain daily evacuation should be deemphasized.

Specific Agents and Mechanism of Action

The many available types of laxatives are usually classified by their apparent mode of action.[22,27,35] Often, two different laxatives, either from the same class or from two different classes, are combined in the same commercial preparation. Some of the more common laxatives, listed by their apparent mechanisms of action, are in Table 27–4. The major laxative classes and rationales for their use are outlined in the next few sections.

Bulk-Forming Laxatives. These agents absorb water and swell within the lower GI tract. The increased size of the water-laden laxative stretches the bowel, thus stimulating intestinal movement (peristalsis). Bulk laxatives commonly contain natural and semisynthetic dietary fiber such as bran, psyllium, and methylcellulose.

Stimulant Laxatives. The precise mechanism of stimulant laxatives is not known. They may activate peristalsis by a direct irritant effect on the intestinal mucosa or by stimulating the nerve plexus within the

Table 27–4	LAXATIVES*
Bulk-forming	
Methylcellulose	Citrucel
Psyllium	Fiberall, Metamucil
Stimulants	
Bisacodyl	Correctol, Dulcolax, Feen-A-Mint
Casanthranol	Doxidan Liquid Gels; Peri-Colace
Casanthrol	Agoral
Castor oil	Purge
Senna	Senokot; Ex-Lax
Hyperosmotic	
Glycerin	Sani-Supp; Fleet Glycerin Laxative
Lactulose	Cholac; Constilac; Constulose
Magnesium hydroxide	Phillips' Milk of Magnesia, Haley's MO
Magnesium sulfate	Epsom salts
Polyethylene glycol	MiraLax
Sodium phosphate	Fleet Phospho-Soda
Lubricants and stool softeners	
Docusate	Colace
Mineral oil	Fleet Mineral Oil, Nujol

*Some of the more common agents are listed as examples in each laxative category. Common trade names are listed in the right-hand column. Many other preparations are available that combine two or more laxatives in the same commercial product.

gut wall. Some evidence suggests that they may work by increasing fluid accumulation within the small intestine. Common stimulant laxatives are castor oil, bisacodyl, and plant extracts such as senna and cascara.

Hyperosmotic Laxatives. Administration of osmotically active substances produces a gradient that draws water into the bowel and small intestine. This gradient increases stool fluid content and stimulates peristalsis. A variety of hyperosmotic substances—including magnesium salts, sodium salts, potassium salts, lactulose, polyethylene glycol, and glycerin—can be used to achieve this effect.

Lubricants and Stool Softeners. Agents like mineral oil and docusate facilitate the entry of water into the fecal mass, thus softening the stool and permitting easier defecation. These agents may also exert a laxative effect because of the increased pressure in the bowel secondary to the increased stool size.

Adverse Effects

Disturbances in the GI system, such as nausea and cramps, may occur with laxative use. With prolonged use, serious lower GI irritation, including spastic colitis, may occur. Fluid and electrolyte abnormalities are also a potential problem. Excessive loss of water and the concomitant loss of electrolytes may transpire, resulting in dehydration and possible acid-base imbalances.[44] These abnormalities are especially significant in older or debilitated patients. Finally, chronic administration may result in a laxative dependence when bowel evacuation has become so subservient to laxative use that the normal mechanisms governing evacuation and defecation are impaired.

Miscellaneous Gastrointestinal Drugs

Several other types of drugs are administered for specific purposes in controlling GI function. These other drugs are introduced here only to alert the reader to their existence. For a more detailed description of the use of any of these agents, one of the drug indexes such as the *Physician's Desk Reference (PDR)* should be consulted.

Digestants

These agents are administered to aid in the digestion of food. The primary digestant preparations contain pancreatic enzymes or bile salts. Pancreatic enzymes such as amylase, trypsin, and lipase are responsible for digestion of carbohydrates, proteins, and lipids, respectively. These enzymes are normally synthesized in the pancreas and secreted into the duodenum via the pancreatic duct. Bile salts are synthesized in the liver, stored in the gallbladder, and released into the duodenum via the common bile duct. Bile salts serve to emulsify lipids in the intestinal tract and are important in lipid digestion and absorption.

Digestant preparations are used to replace digestive constituents in the stomach and upper small intestine whenever the endogenous production of these constituents is impaired. In particular, digestants are often administered to individuals with cystic fibrosis.[49] As discussed in Chapter 26, cystic fibrosis is a hereditary disease that affects all the major exocrine glands, resulting in thick, viscous secretions. These thickened secretions may form mucous plugs that obstruct certain ducts such as the pancreatic and bile ducts. This condition leads to a chronic deficiency of pancreatic enzymes and bile salts; as a result, patients cannot digest and absorb nutrients from the GI tract. Preparations containing these digestants may be administered orally to replace the missing compounds, thus improving digestion and nutrient absorption.

Emetics

Emetics are used to induce vomiting and are frequently administered to help empty the stomach of poisons or ingested toxins. The two primary emetics are apomorphine and ipecac. Both agents seem to work by stimulating the medullary emetic center, and ipecac also exerts a direct emetic effect on the stomach.

Antiemetics

Antiemetics are used to decrease the nausea and vomiting that are associated with motion sickness and recovery from surgery or that develop in response to other medical treatments, such as cancer chemotherapy and radiation treatment.[33,40,43] Antiemetic agents include antihistamines (dimenhydrinate, meclizine, others), anticholinergics (scopolamine), drugs that block specific CNS dopamine (D_2) and serotonin (5-HT_3) receptors, cannabinoids, and several other drugs that act at various sites in the CNS to suppress nausea and vomiting.[44] Other antiemetic drugs such as antacids and adsorbents act locally to soothe the gastric mucosa and decrease the irritation that may cause vomiting.

Cholelitholytic Agents

Drugs like chenodeoxycholic acid (chenodiol) and ursodeoxycholic acid (ursodiol) can dissolve certain types of gallstones.[28,45] These drugs decrease the cholesterol content of bile and may help dissolve gallstones that are supersaturated with cholesterol; these drugs do not appear effective in the treatment of calcified gallstones.[28]

Special Concerns in Rehabilitation Patients

■ ■ ■ Drugs affecting the GI system are important in rehabilitation patients by virtue of their frequent use. Critically ill patients will suffer some degree of stress-related damage to the stomach mucosa, especially if they are managed in the intensive care unit.[52,57] This stress ulceration syndrome appears to be especially prevalent in patients with burns, multiple traumas, renal failure, and CNS trauma. Drugs such as the PPIs (omeprazole, others) and H_2 receptor blockers (cimetidine, ranitidine, others) are often helpful in controlling gastric acid secretions, thus preventing damage to the mucosal lining.[57,58]

Patients seen in rehabilitation are often relatively inactive and suffer from many adverse effects of prolonged bed rest, including constipation. Constipation and fecal impaction may also be a recurrent and serious problem in patients with spinal cord injuries. Laxatives are used routinely in these patients to facilitate adequate bowel evacuation. Patients receiving cancer chemotherapy often have problems with nausea and vomiting, and antiemetic drugs may be helpful to these individuals. Various other GI disorders, including diarrhea and chronic indigestion, occur frequently in many rehabilitation patients and are often treated effectively with the appropriate agents.

Despite their frequent use, most GI drugs do not produce any significant side effects that will impair rehabilitation. Some dizziness and fatigue may occur with agents such as the opiates used to treat diarrhea or the antiulcer H_2 blockers, but these effects are fairly mild. Other problems with GI drugs are generally related to transient GI disturbances. In general, GI drugs are well tolerated and safe in most patients. In effect, these drugs indirectly facilitate physical rehabilitation by resolving annoying and uncomfortable GI symptoms, thus allowing the patient to participate more readily in the program.

CASE STUDY

Gastrointestinal Drugs

Brief History. M.B. is a 48-year-old insurance sales representative with a long history of back pain. He has had recurrent episodes of sciatica because of a herniated disk at the L5-S1 interspace. Currently, he is being seen as an outpatient in a private physical therapy practice. Despite several treatments, his back pain did not improve. In fact, his pain was recently exacerbated when he was straining to pass a stool during a period of constipation. Evidently, this occurrence had been repeated often, and the patient's back problems were increased by the bowel-related problems causing straining during defecation.

Decision/Solution. The physical therapist consulted with the 'patient's physician and recommended that a brief trial with a bulk-forming laxative might be helpful during the acute episode of back pain in this patient. The therapist also explained to the patient that straining during defecation exacerbated his back problems. To prevent the recurrence of this problem, the patient was encouraged to ingest a high-fiber diet and adequate amounts of water to prevent constipation. M.B. was also informed that the short-term use of a laxative might be necessary to avoid constipation and straining. The therapist warned the patient, however, about the laxative dependence that can occur during chronic use.

SUMMARY

A variety of pharmacologic agents are used to maintain proper function in the GI system. Drugs such as antacids, H_2 receptor antagonists and PPIs help control gastric acid secretion and protect the stomach mucosa. These agents are widely used to prevent and treat peptic ulcer. Specific drugs are used to control GI motility. Drugs that inhibit excessive peristalsis (i.e., diarrhea) include the opiate derivatives, adsorbents, and bismuth salicylate. Decreased motility (constipation) is usually treated with various laxatives. Other GI agents attempt to treat specific problems such as poor digestion, emesis, or gallstones. GI drugs are used frequently in rehabilitation patients and, it is hoped, will produce beneficial effects that will allow the patient to participate more actively in the rehabilitation program.

References

1. Armstrong D. Gastroesophageal reflux disease. *Curr Opin Pharmacol.* 2005;5:589–595.
2. Berardi RR. Peptic ulcer disease. In: DiPiro JT, et al, eds. *Pharmacotherapy: A Pathophysiologic Approach.* 5th ed. New York: McGraw-Hill; 2002.
3. Bixquert M. Maintenance therapy in gastro-esophageal reflux disease. *Drugs.* 2005;65(suppl 1):59–66.
4. Brzozowski T, Konturek PC, Konturek SJ, et al. Role of prostaglandins in gastroprotection and gastric adaptation. *J Physiol Pharmacol.* 2005;56(suppl 5):33–55.
5. Bytzer P, O'Morain C. Treatment of Helicobacter pylori. *Helicobacter.* 2005;10(suppl 1):40–46.
6. Calvet X, Gomollon F. What is potent acid inhibition, and how can it be achieved? *Drugs.* 2005;65 (suppl 1): 13–23.
7. Candelli M, Nista EC, Carloni E, et al. Treatment of *H. pylori* infection: a review. *Curr Med Chem.* 2005;12: 375–384.
8. Carballo F. Efficiency of potent gastric acid inhibition. *Drugs.* 2005;65(suppl 1):105–111.
9. Ching CK, Lam SK. Antacids. Indications and limitations. *Drugs.* 1994;47:305–317.
10. Dattilo M, Figura N. Helicobacter pylori infection, chronic gastritis, and proton pump inhibitors. *J Clin Gastroenterol.* 1998;27(suppl 1):S163–S169.
11. Davies NM, Longstreth J, Jamali F. Misoprostol therapeutics revisited. *Pharmacotherapy.* 2001;21:60–73.
12. Dekel R, Morse C, Fass R. The role of proton pump inhibitors in gastro-esophageal reflux disease. *Drugs.* 2004;64:277–295.
13. De Schepper HU, Cremonini F, Park MI, Camilleri M. Opioids and the gut: pharmacology and current clinical experience. *Neurogastroenterol Motil.* 2004; 16:383–394.
14. Dominguez-Munoz JE, Sobrino M. Clinical response (remission of symptoms) in erosive and non-erosive gastro-esophageal reflux disease. *Drugs.* 2005;65 (suppl 1):43–50.
15. Esplugues JV. A pharmacological approach to gastric acid inhibition. *Drugs.* 2005;65(suppl 1):7–12.
16. Fennerty MB. *Helicobacter pylori*: why it still matters in 2005. *Cleve Clin J Med.* 2005;72(suppl 2):S1–S7.
17. Gisbert JP. Potent gastric acid inhibition in Helicobacter pylori eradication. *Drugs.* 2005;65(suppl 1): 83–96.
18. Gisbert JP. The recurrence of *Helicobacter pylori* infection: incidence and variables influencing it. A critical review. *Am J Gastroenterol.* 2005;100:2083–2099.
19. Greenwood-Van Meerveld B, Gardner CJ, Little PJ, et al. Preclinical studies of opioids and opioid antagonists on gastrointestinal function. *Neurogastroenterol Motil.* 2004;16(suppl 2):46–53.
20. Hade JE, Spiro HM. Calcium and acid rebound: a reappraisal. *J Clin Gastroenterol.* 1992;15:37–44.
21. Hoogerwerf WA, Pasricha PJ. Pharmacotherapy of gastric acidity, peptic ulcers, and gastroesophageal reflux disease. In: Brunton LL, et al, eds. *The Pharmacological Basis of Therapeutics.* 11th ed. New York: McGraw-Hill; 2006.
22. Hsieh C. Treatment of constipation in older adults. *Am Fam Physician.* 2005;72:2277–2284.
23. Huang JQ, Hunt RH. Pharmacological and pharmacodynamic essentials of H(2)-receptor antagonists and proton pump inhibitors for the practising physician. *Best Pract Res Clin Gastroenterol.* 2001;15:355–370.
24. Inadomi JM, Fendrick AM. PPI use in the OTC era: who to treat, with what, and for how long? *Clin Gastroenterol Hepatol.* 2005;3:208–215.
25. Ippoliti C. Antidiarrheal agents for the management of treatment-related diarrhea in cancer patients. *Am J Health Syst Pharm.* 1998;55:1573–1580.
26. Itoh T, Kusaka K, Kawaura K, et al. Selective binding of sucralfate to endoscopic mucosal resection-induced gastric ulcer: evaluation of aluminum adherence. *J Int Med Res.* 2004;32:520–529.
27. Klaschik E, Nauck F, Ostgathe C. Constipation— modern laxative therapy. *Support Care Cancer.* 2003; 11:679–685.
28. Konikoff FM. Gallstones—approach to medical management. *Med Gen Med.* 2003;5:8.
29. Konturek SJ, Konturek PC, Brzozowski T. Prostaglandins and ulcer healing. *J Physiol Pharmacol.* 2005; 56(suppl 5):5–31.
30. Lanas A. Potent gastric acid inhibition in the management of Barrett's esophagus. *Drugs.* 2005;65(suppl 1): 75–82.
31. Lazzaroni M, Bianchi Porro G. Non-steroidal anti-inflammatory drug gastropathy: clinical results with H$_2$ antagonists and proton pump inhibitors. *Ital J Gastroenterol Hepatol.* 1999;31 (suppl 1):S73–S78.
32. Lehmann F, Hildebrand P, Beglinger C. New molecular targets for treatment of peptic ulcer disease. *Drugs.* 2003;63:1785–1797.
33. Maranzano E, Feyer PCh, Molassiotis A, et al. Evidence-based recommendations for the use of antiemetics in radiotherapy. *Radiother Oncol.* 2005; 76:227–233.
34. Maton PN, Burton ME. Antacids revisited: a review of their clinical pharmacology and recommended therapeutic use. *Drugs.* 1999;57:855–870.
35. McClung HJ, Potter C. Rational use of laxatives in children. *Adv Pediatr.* 2004;51:231–262.
36. McLoughlin RM, O'Morain CA, O'Connor HJ. Eradication of Helicobacter pylori: recent advances in treatment. *Fundam Clin Pharmacol.* 2005;19: 421–427.

37. Metz DC. Preventing the gastrointestinal consequences of stress-related mucosal disease. *Curr
Med Res Opin.* 2005;21:11–18.

38. Mossner J, Caca K. Developments in the inhibition
of gastric acid secretion. *Eur J Clin Invest.* 2005;35:
469–475.

39. Murata H, Kawano S, Tsuji S, et al. Combination
of enprostil and cimetidine is more effective than
cimetidine alone in treating gastric ulcer: prospective
multicenter randomized controlled trial. *Hepatogastroenterology.* 2005;52:1925–1929.

40. Olver IN. Update on anti-emetics for chemotherapy-
induced emesis. *Intern Med J.* 2005;35:478–481.

41. O'Mahony R, Vaira D, Holton J, Basset C. Helicobacter pylori: current status and future prospects. *Sci Prog.*
2004;87:269–296.

42. Ong SP, Duggan A. Eradication of *Helicobacter pylori*
in clinical situations. *Clin Exp Med.* 2004;4:30–38.

43. Oo TH, Hesketh PJ. Drug insight: new antiemetics in
the management of chemotherapy-induced nausea and
vomiting. *Nat Clin Pract Oncol.* 2005;2:196–201.

44. Pasricha PJ. Treatment of disorders of bowel motility
and water flux; antiemetics; agents used in biliary and
pancreatic disease. In: Brunton LL, et al, eds. *The
Pharmacological Basis of Therapeutics.* 11th ed. New
York: McGraw-Hill; 2006.

45. Petroni ML, Jazrawi RP, Pazzi P, et al. Ursodeoxycholic acid alone or with chenodeoxycholic acid for
dissolution of cholesterol gallstones: a randomized
multicentre trial. The British-Italian Gallstone Study
group. *Aliment Pharmacol Ther.* 2001;15:123–128.

46. Raghunath AS, O'Morain C, McLoughlin RC. Review
article: the long-term use of proton-pump inhibitors.
Aliment Pharmacol Ther. 2005;22(suppl 1):55–63.

47. Robinson M. Proton pump inhibitors: update on their
role in acid-related gastrointestinal diseases. *Int J Clin
Pract.* 2005;59:709–715.

48. Robinson M, Rodriguez-Stanley S, Miner PB, et
al. Effects of antacid formulation on postprandial
oesophageal acidity in patients with a history of
episodic heartburn. *Aliment Pharmacol Ther.* 2002;
16:435–443.

49. Schibli S, Durie PR, Tullis ED. Proper usage of pancreatic enzymes. *Curr Opin Pulm Med.* 2002;8:542–546.

50. Schiller LR. Chronic Diarrhea. *Curr Treat Options
Gastroenterol.* 2005;8:259–266.

51. Smoot DT, Go MF, Cryer B. Peptic ulcer disease.
Prim Care. 2001;28:487–503.

52. Stollman N, Metz DC. Pathophysiology and prophylaxis of stress ulcer in intensive care unit patients. *J
Crit Care.* 2005;20:35–45.

53. Tutuian R, Katz PO, Ahmed F, et al. Over-the-counter
H(2)-receptor antagonists do not compromise intragastric pH control with proton pump inhibitors. *Aliment Pharmacol Ther.* 2002;16:473–477.

54. Vaira D, Gatta L, Ricci C, et al. Peptic ulcer and *Helicobacter pylori:* update on testing and treatment. *Postgrad Med.* 2005;117:17–22, 46.

55. van Pinxteren B, Numans ME, Bonis PA, Lau J. Short-
term treatment with proton pump inhibitors, H$_2$-
receptor antagonists and prokinetics for
gastro-esophageal reflux disease-like symptoms and
endoscopy negative reflux disease. *Cochrane Database
Syst Rev.* 2004;CD002095.

56. Wallace JL. Recent advances in gastric ulcer therapeutics. *Curr Opin Pharmacol.* 2005;5:573–577.

57. Welage LS. Overview of pharmacologic agents for acid
suppression in critically ill patients. *Am J Health Syst
Pharm.* 2005;62(suppl 2):S4–S10.

58. Yang YX, Lewis JD. Prevention and treatment of stress
ulcers in critically ill patients. *Semin Gastrointest Dis.*
2003;14:11–19.

59. Zacny J, Zamakhshary M, Sketris I, et al. Systematic
review: the efficacy of intermittent and on-demand
therapy with histamine H$_2$-receptor antagonists or
proton pump inhibitors for gastro-esophageal reflux
disease patients. *Aliment Pharmacol Ther.* 2005;21:
1299–1312.

Endocrine
Pharmacology

Chapter 28

Introduction to Endocrine Pharmacology

The endocrine system helps to maintain internal homeostasis through the use of endogenous chemicals known as hormones. A *hormone* is typically regarded as a chemical messenger that is released into the bloodstream to exert an effect on target cells located some distance from the hormonal release site.[2] Various endocrine glands manufacture and release specific hormones that help regulate physiologic processes such as reproduction, growth and development, energy metabolism, fluid and electrolyte balance, and response to stress and injury.[2,20]

The use of drugs to help regulate and control endocrine function is an important area of pharmacology. In one sense, hormones can be considered drugs that are manufactured by the patient's body. This situation presents an obvious opportunity to use exogenous chemicals to either mimic or attenuate the effects of specific hormones during endocrine dysfunction.

Drugs can be used as replacement therapy during hormonal deficiency—for example, insulin administration in diabetes mellitus. Likewise, exogenous hormone analogs can be administered to accentuate the effects of their endogenous counterparts, such as using glucocorticoids to help treat inflammation. Conversely, drugs can be administered to treat endocrine hyperactivity—for example, the use of antithyroid drugs in treating hyperthyroidism. Finally, drugs can be used to regulate normal endocrine function to achieve a desired effect, as is done through the inhibition of ovulation by oral contraceptives.

The purpose of this chapter is to review the basic aspects of endocrine function, including the primary hormones and their effects. The factors regulating hormonal release and the cellular mechanisms of hormone action are also briefly discussed. Finally, the basic ways in which drugs can be used to alter endocrine function are presented. This overview is intended to provide rehabilitation specialists with a general review of endocrine and hormone activity; subsequent chapters deal with specific endocrine drugs and the problems they are used to treat.

Primary Endocrine Glands and Their Hormones

The primary endocrine glands and the hormones they produce are briefly discussed here. These glands and the physiologic effects of their hormones are also summarized in Tables 28–1 and 28–2. For the purpose of this chapter, only the primary endocrine glands and their respective hormones are discussed. Substances such as prostaglandins and kinins, which are produced locally by a variety of different cells, are not discussed here, but are referred to elsewhere in this text (e.g., see Chapter 15). Also, chemicals such as norepinephrine, which serve a dual purpose as hormones and neurotransmitters, are discussed in this chapter only with regard to their endocrine function.

Hypothalamus and Pituitary Gland

The pituitary gland is a small, pea-shaped structure located within the sella turcica at the base of the brain. The pituitary lies inferior to the hypothalamus and is attached to the hypothalamus by a thin stalk of tissue known as the *infundibulum*. The structural and functional relationships between the hypothalamus and pituitary gland are briefly discussed later in this section. A more detailed presentation of the anatomic and physiologic functions of the hypothalamus and pituitary gland can be found in several sources.[8,14,32]

The pituitary can be subdivided into an anterior, an intermediate, and a posterior lobe. These subdivi-

Table 28-1	HYPOTHALAMIC AND PITUITARY HORMONES

Hypothalamic Hormones and Releasing Factors	Effect
Growth hormone–releasing hormone (GHRH)	↑ GH release
Growth hormone–inhibitory hormone (GHIH)	↓ GH release
Gonadotropin-releasing hormone (GnRH)	↑ LH and FSH release
Thyrotropin-releasing hormone (TRH)	↑ TSH release
Corticotropin-releasing hormone (CRH)	↑ ACTH release
Prolactin-inhibitory factor (PIF)	↓ Pr release

Pituitary Hormones	Principal Effects
Anterior lobe	
Growth hormone (GH)	↑ tissue growth and development
Luteinizing hormone (LH)	Female: ↑ ovulation; ↑ estrogen and progesterone synthesis from corpus luteum
	Male: ↑ testosterone synthesis
Follicle-stimulating hormone (FSH)	Female: ↑ follicular development and estrogen synthesis
	Male: enhance spermatogenesis
Thyroid-stimulating hormone (TSH)	↑ synthesis of thyroid hormones (T_3, T_4)
Adrenocorticotropic hormone (ACTH)	↑ adrenal steroid synthesis (e.g., cortisol)
Prolactin (Pr)	Initiates lactation
Posterior lobe	
Antidiuretic hormone (ADH)	↑ renal reabsorption of water
Oxytocin	↑ uterine contraction; ↑ milk ejection during lactation

Table 28-2	OTHER PRIMARY ENDOCRINE GLANDS

Gland	Hormone(s)	Principal Effects
Thyroid	Thyroxine (T_4), Triiodothyronine (T_3)	Increase cellular metabolism; facilitate normal growth and development
Parathyroids	Parathormone (PTH)	Increase blood calcium
Pancreas	Glucagon	Increase blood glucose
	Insulin	Decrease blood glucose; increase carbohydrate, protein, and fat storage
Adrenal cortex	Glucocorticoids	Regulate glucose metabolism; enhance response to stress
	Mineralocorticoids	Regulate fluid and electrolyte levels
Adrenal medulla	Epinephrine, Norepinephrine	Vascular and metabolic effects that facilitate increased physical activity
Testes	Testosterone	Spermatogenesis; male sexual characteristics
Ovaries	Estrogens, Progesterone	Female reproductive cycle and sexual characteristics

sions and their respective hormones are listed in Table 28–1 and briefly discussed below.

Anterior Lobe. The anterior pituitary, or adenohypophysis, secretes six important peptide hormones. The anterior pituitary releases: growth hormone (GH), luteinizing hormone (LH), follicle-stimulating hormone (FSH), thyroid-stimulating hormone (TSH), adrenocorticotropic hormone (ACTH), and prolactin (Pr). The physiologic effects of these hormones are listed in Table 28–1.

Hormonal release from the anterior pituitary is controlled by specific hormones or releasing factors from the hypothalamus.[2,15] Basically, a releasing factor is sent from the hypothalamus to the anterior pituitary via local vascular structures known as the hypothalamic-hypophysial portal vessels. For example, to increase the secretion of growth hormone, the hypothalamus first secretes growth hormone–releasing hormone (GHRH) into the portal vessels. The GHRH travels a short distance to the anterior pituitary via the hypothalamic-hypophysial portal system. Upon arriving at the pituitary, the GHRH causes the anterior pituitary to release growth hormone into the systemic circulation, where it can then travel to various target tissues in the periphery. Other hypothalamic-releasing factors that have been identified are listed in Table 28–1. Specific releasing factors are still being investigated, and the identification of additional factors (including those that inhibit anterior pituitary hormone release) will undoubtedly be forthcoming.

Intermediate Lobe. In mammals, there is a small intermediate lobe of the pituitary (pars intermedia) that may secrete melanocyte-stimulating hormone (MSH). Although it can influence skin pigmentation in lower vertebrates, the intermediate lobe does not produce MSH in meaningful amounts in humans. Humans can, however, produce MSH from a precursor protein (proopiomelacortin) that is synthesized in central tissues (anterior pituitary, hypothalamus) and the periphery (skin, lymphoid tissues).[32] MSH may play a role in controlling several diverse functions such as appetite, energy homeostasis, and inflammation.[5,21,38] MSH and similar hormones such as ACTH are key components of a neuroendocrine arrangement known as the melanocortin system; investigators continue to determine if this system can be manipulated pharmacologically to help control various physiological systems.

Posterior Lobe. The posterior pituitary, or neurohypophysis, secretes two hormones: antidiuretic hormone (ADH) and oxytocin.[2,12] ADH exerts its effect primarily on the kidneys, where it increases the reabsorption of water from the distal renal tubules. Oxytocin is important in parturition and stimulates the uterus to contract. It also promotes lactation by stimulating the ejection of milk from the mammary glands.

The hypothalamic control of the posterior pituitary is quite different than that of the anterior and intermediate lobes. Specific neurons have their cell bodies in certain hypothalamic nuclei. Cell bodies in the paraventricular nuclei manufacture oxytocin, whereas the supraoptic nuclei contain cell bodies that synthesize ADH. The axons from these cells extend downward through the infundibulum to terminate in the posterior pituitary. Hormones synthesized in the hypothalamic cell bodies are transported down the axon to be stored in neurosecretory granules in their respective nerve terminals (located in the posterior pituitary). When an appropriate stimulus is present, these neurons fire an action potential, which causes the hormones to release from their pituitary nerve terminals. The hormones are ultimately picked up by the systemic circulation and transported to their target tissues.

Thyroid Gland

The thyroid gland is located in the anterior neck region, approximately at the level of the fifth cervical to first thoracic vertebrae.[22] This gland consists of bilateral lobes that lie on either side of the trachea and are connected by a thin piece of the gland known as the isthmus. The thyroid synthesizes and secretes two hormones: thyroxine (T_4) and triiodothyronine (T_3). The synthesis of these hormones is controlled by the hypothalamic-pituitary system via thyroid-releasing hormone from the hypothalamus, which causes thyroid-stimulating hormone release from the anterior pituitary. Thyroid-stimulating hormone increases T_3 and T_4 synthesis and release from the thyroid gland.

The primary effect of the thyroid hormones is to increase cellular metabolism in most body tissues.[24,39] These hormones stimulate virtually all aspects of cellular function, including protein, fat, and carbohydrate metabolism. By exerting a stimulatory effect on the cellular level, thyroid hormones play a crucial role in helping maintain and regulate body heat (*thermogenesis*) in the whole organism. T_3 and T_4 also play an important role in growth and development, especially in the growth and maturation of normal bone. Finally, thyroid hormones play a permissive role in allowing other hormones, such as steroids, to exert their effects. The physiology and pharmacology of thyroid hormones are further discussed in Chapter 31.

Parathyroid Gland

Parathyroid glands are small, egg-shaped structures embedded in the posterior surface of the thyroid gland. There are usually four parathyroid glands, with two glands located on each half of the thyroid gland. The parathyroids synthesize and release parathyroid hormone (PTH). PTH is essential in maintaining normal calcium homeostasis in the body; the primary effect of PTH is to increase the concentration of calcium in the bloodstream.[33,34] PTH increases circulating calcium levels primarily by mobilizing calcium from storage sites in bone.

The primary factor regulating PTH release is the level of calcium in the bloodstream.[42] Parathyroid gland cells appear to act as calcium sensors that monitor circulating calcium levels. As circulating calcium levels fall below a certain point, PTH secretion is increased. Conversely, elevated plasma calcium titers inhibit PTH secretion. The ability of PTH to control plasma calcium levels and regulate bone mineral metabolism is discussed in more detail in Chapter 31

Pancreas

The pancreas is located behind the stomach in the lower left area of the abdomen. This gland is unique in that it serves both endocrine and exocrine functions.[4,19] The exocrine aspect of this gland involves digestive enzymes that are excreted into the duodenum. As an endocrine gland, the pancreas primarily secretes two peptide hormones: insulin and glucagon. These hormones are synthesized and secreted by cells located in specialized clusters known as the *islets of Langerhans*. In the islets of Langerhans, glucagon and insulin are synthesized by alpha and beta cells, respectively.

Pancreatic hormones are involved in the regulation of blood glucose, and the glucose concentration in the blood serves as the primary stimulus for hormone release. For example, following a fast, glucagon is released from pancreatic alpha cells as blood glucose levels fall. Glucagon mobilizes the release of glucose from storage sites in the liver, thus bringing blood glucose levels back to normal. An increase in blood glucose after eating a meal stimulates insulin release from the beta cells. Insulin facilitates the storage of glucose in the liver and muscle, thus removing glucose from

the bloodstream and returning blood glucose to normal levels. Insulin also exerts a number of other effects on protein and lipid metabolism. The effects of insulin and its pharmacologic replacement in diabetes mellitus are discussed in more detail in Chapter 32

Adrenal Gland

Adrenal glands are located at the superior poles of each kidney. Each adrenal gland is composed of an outer cortex and an inner medulla. The hormones associated with the adrenal cortex and adrenal medulla are described in the following sections.

Hormones of the Adrenal Cortex. The adrenal cortex synthesizes and secretes two primary groups of steroidal hormones: the glucocorticoids and the mineralocorticoids.[41] Small amounts of sex steroids (estrogens, androgens, progesterone) are also produced, but these amounts are essentially insignificant during normal adrenal function.

Glucocorticoids such as cortisol have a number of physiologic effects.[1] Glucocorticoids are involved in the regulation of glucose metabolism and are important in enhancing the body's ability to handle stress. They also have significant anti-inflammatory and immunosuppressive properties and are often used therapeutically to control inflammation or suppress the immune response in various clinical situations. Glucocorticoid synthesis is controlled by the hypothalamic-pituitary system. Corticotropin-releasing hormone (CRH) from the hypothalamus stimulates ACTH release from the anterior pituitary, which in turn stimulates the synthesis of glucocorticoids.

Mineralocorticoids are involved in controlling electrolyte and fluid levels.[9,44] The primary mineralocorticoid produced by the adrenal cortex is *aldosterone*. Aldosterone increases the reabsorption of sodium from the renal tubules. By increasing sodium reabsorption, aldosterone facilitates the reabsorption of water. Aldosterone also inhibits the renal reabsorption of potassium, thus increasing potassium excretion. Mineralocorticoid release is regulated by fluid and electrolyte levels in the body and by other hormones, such as the renin-angiotensin system.

The pharmacologic aspects of the glucocorticoids and mineralocorticoids are discussed in more detail in Chapter 29

Hormones of the Adrenal Medulla. The adrenal medulla synthesizes and secretes epinephrine and norepinephrine.[11,37] These hormones have a number of physiologic effects, which are discussed in Chapters 18 and 20. Small amounts of epinephrine and norepinephrine are released under resting, basal conditions. The primary significance of these hormones, however, seems to be in helping to prepare the body for sudden physical activity. The classic function of the adrenal medulla can be illustrated by the fight-or-flight reaction, in which a stressful challenge is presented to the individual and interpreted as requiring either a defense or a need to flee.

The release of epinephrine and norepinephrine from the adrenal medulla is controlled by the sympathetic division of the autonomic nervous system. As discussed in Chapter 18, sympathetic cholinergic preganglionic neurons directly innervate this gland. An increase in sympathetic activity causes increased firing in these neurons, which in turn stimulates the release of epinephrine and norepinephrine from the adrenal medulla.

Gonads

Reproductive organs are the primary source of the steroid hormones that influence sexual and reproductive functions. In men, the testes produce *testosterone* and similar androgens that are responsible for spermatogenesis and the secondary sexual characteristics of adult males.[7,26] In women, sexual maturation and reproductive function are governed by the production of estrogens and progestins from the ovaries.[27] The release of male and female sex steroids is controlled by hormones from the hypothalamus and anterior pituitary.[32] The control of male and female hormone activity and the pharmacologic implications of these hormones are discussed in Chapter 30.

Endocrine Physiology and Pharmacology

Hormone Chemistry

Hormones can be divided into several primary categories according to their basic chemical structure. *Steroid hormones* share a common chemical framework that is derived from lipids such as cholesterol.[28] Examples of steroids include the sex hormones (androgens, estrogens, progesterone), the glucocorticoids, and the mineralocorticoids. *Peptide hormones* consist of amino acids linked together in a specific sequence. These peptide chains can range in length from 3 to 180 amino acids. Primary examples of peptide hormones

are the hypothalamic releasing factors and the pituitary hormones. Finally, several hormones are modified from a single amino acid. For instance, the thyroid hormones (T_3 and T_4) are manufactured from the amino acid tyrosine. In addition, hormones from the adrenal medulla (epinephrine, norepinephrine) are synthesized from either phenylalanine or tyrosine.

The basic chemical structure of various hormones is significant in determining how the hormone will exert its effects on target tissues (see "Hormone Effects on the Target Cell," later). Different hormones that are fairly similar in structure can often have similar physiologic and pharmacologic effects. This is especially true for the steroids, in which one category of steroidal agents may have some of the same properties of a different category.[36] For instance, the endogenous glucocorticoids (e.g., cortisol) also exert some mineralocorticoid effects, presumably because of their similar chemical structure. The overlapping effects and their consequences are discussed in more detail in Chapters 29 through 32, which deal with specific endocrine systems.

Synthesis and Release of Hormones

Hormones are typically synthesized within the cells of their respective endocrine glands. Most hormones are synthesized and packaged in storage granules within the gland. When the gland is stimulated, the storage granule fuses with the cell membrane, and the hormone is released by exocytosis. Notable exceptions to this are the steroid hormones, which are not stored to any great extent but are synthesized on demand when an appropriate stimulus is present.[2]

Hormone synthesis and release can be initiated by both extrinsic and intrinsic factors.[2] Extrinsic factors include various environmental stimuli such as pain, temperature, light, and smell. Intrinsic stimuli include various humoral and neural factors. For instance, release of a hormone can be initiated by other hormones. These occurrences are particularly typical of the anterior pituitary hormones, which are controlled by releasing hormones from the hypothalamus. Hormonal release can be influenced by neural input; a primary example is the sympathetic neural control of epinephrine and norepinephrine release from the adrenal medulla. Other intrinsic factors that affect hormone release are the levels of ions and metabolites within the body. For instance, parathyroid hormone release is governed directly by the calcium concentration in the bloodstream, and the release of glucagon from pancreatic alpha cells is dependent on blood glucose levels.

Feedback Control Mechanisms in Endocrine Function

As mentioned previously, the endocrine system is concerned with maintaining homeostasis in the body. When a disturbance in physiologic function occurs, hormones are released to rectify the disturbance. As function returns to normal, hormone release is attenuated and homeostasis is resumed. For example, an increase in the blood glucose level initiates the release of insulin from pancreatic beta cells. Insulin increases the incorporation into and storage of glucose in liver, skeletal muscle, and other tissues. Blood glucose levels then return to normal, and insulin release is terminated.

Hormonal release is also frequently regulated by some form of negative feedback system.[2,23] In these feedback systems, an increase in the release of a specific hormone ultimately serves to inhibit its own release, thus preventing the amount of the released hormone from becoming excessive. An example of a negative feedback system involving the hypothalamic-pituitary axis is illustrated in Figure 28–1. The endocrine hormone ultimately inhibits its own release by inhibiting the secretion of specific hypothalamic releasing factors and pituitary hormones. Numerous examples of such negative feedback loops are present in various endocrine pathways.

There are also a few examples of positive feedback mechanisms in the endocrine system.[25,43] In a positive feedback loop, rising concentrations of one hormone cause an increase in other hormones, which, in turn, facilitates increased production of the first hormone. The primary example of this type of feedback occurs in the female reproductive system, where low levels of estrogen production increase the release of pituitary hormones (LH, FSH).[10,43] Increased LH and FSH then facilitate further estrogen production, which further increases pituitary hormone secretion, and so on (see Chapter 30). Positive feedback mechanisms are relatively rare, however, compared with negative feedback controls in the endocrine system.

The presence of feedback systems in endocrine function is important from a pharmacologic perspective. Drugs can be administered that act through the intrinsic feedback loops to control endogenous hormone production. A primary example is the use of oral contraceptives, when exogenous estrogen and proges-

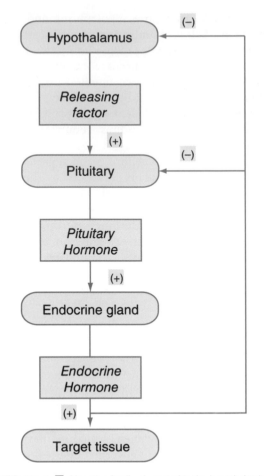

FIGURE 28–1 ▼ Negative feedback control in the hypothalamic–pituitary–endocrine pathways. Excitatory and inhibitory effects are indicated by (+) and (–), respectively. Negative feedback loops occur owing to inhibition of the endocrine hormone on the pituitary and hypothalamus.

terone are administered in controlled amounts to inhibit ovulation (see Chapter 30). Therapeutic administration of hormonal agents may create problems, however, because of these negative feedback effects. For instance, glucocorticoid administration may act as negative feedback to suppress the normal endogenous production of adrenal steroids.[16] If the body is unable to produce its own supply of adrenal steroids, abrupt withdrawal of the exogenous compounds can result in severe or even fatal consequences. Adrenocortical suppression is discussed in more detail in Chapter 29.

Hormone Transport

Hormones are usually carried from their site of origin to the target cell via the systemic circulation.[2] During transport in the bloodstream, certain hormones such as steroids are bound to specific plasma proteins. These protein carriers appear to help prolong the half-life of the hormone and prevent premature degradation. Other protein carriers may be important in the local effects of hormone function. For instance, the testes produce androgen-binding protein, which helps transport and concentrate testosterone within the seminiferous tubules of the testes (see Chapter 30).

Hormone Effects on the Target Cell

Most hormones affect their target cell by interacting with a specific receptor. Hormone receptors are located at three locations, shown in Figure 28–2. These primary locations are on the surface membrane of the cell, within the cytosol of the cell, or within the cell's nucleus.[2] Receptors at each location tend to be specific for different types of hormones and also tend to affect cell function in a specific manner. Each type of receptor is briefly discussed below.

Surface Membrane Receptors. These receptors are located on the outer surface of the plasma membrane (see Fig. 28–2).[6] Surface receptors tend to recognize the peptide hormones and some amino acid derivatives (e.g., pituitary hormones, catecholamines). They are typically linked to specific intracellular enzymes. When stimulated by a peptidelike hormone, the receptor initiates some change in the enzymatic machinery located within the cell. This event usually results in a change in the production of some intracellular chemical second messenger such as cyclic adenosine monophosphate (cAMP).[6]

An example of a hormone that exerts its effects through a surface receptor–second messenger system is ACTH.[36] ACTH is a polypeptide that binds to a surface receptor on adrenal cortex cells. The surface receptor then stimulates the adenylate cyclase enzyme to increase production of cAMP, which acts as a second messenger (the hormone was the first messenger), and increases the activity of other enzymes within the cell to synthesize adrenal steroids such as cortisol. For a more detailed description of surface receptor–second messenger systems, see Chapter 4.

Cytosolic Hormone Receptors. Steroid hormones typically bind to protein receptors, which are located directly within the cytosol (see Fig. 28–2).[17] Of course, this means that the hormone must first enter the cell, which is easily accomplished by the steroid hormones because they are highly lipid soluble. After entering the cell, the hormone initiates a series of events that are depicted in Figure 28–3. Basically, the hormone and receptor form a large activated steroid-receptor complex.[17] This complex travels to the cell's nucleus, where it binds to specific genes located within the DNA sequence.[31,40] This process initiates gene expres-

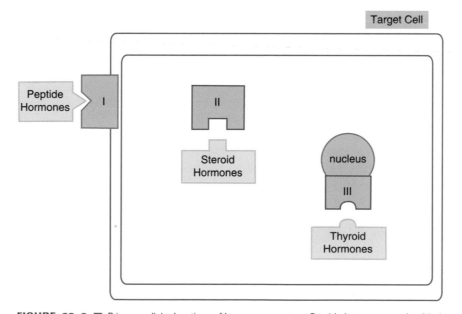

FIGURE 28–2 ▼ Primary cellular locations of hormone receptors. Peptide hormones tend to bind to surface membrane receptors (site I); steroid hormones bind to cytosolic receptors (site II); and thyroid hormones bind to receptors in the cell nucleus (site III).

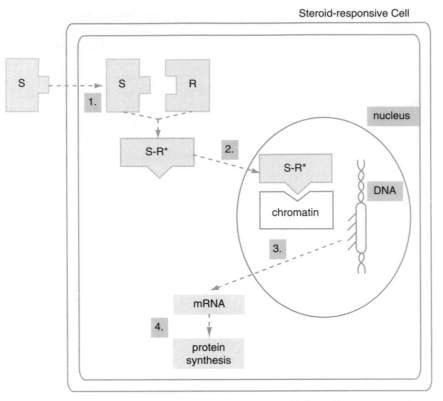

FIGURE 28–3 ▼ Sequence of events of steroid hormone action. (1) Steroid hormone enters the cell, binds to a cytosolic receptor, and creates an activated steroid-receptor complex (S-R). (2) S-R complex travels to the cell's nucleus, where it binds to specific gene segments on nuclear chromatin. (3) DNA undergoes transcription into messenger RNA (mRNA) units. (4) mRNA undergoes translation in the cytosol into specific proteins that alter cell function.

sion and transcription of messenger RNA units, which go back to the cytosol and are translated into specific proteins by the endoplasmic reticulum.[40] These newly manufactured proteins are usually enzymes or structural proteins that change cell function in a specific manner. For instance, anabolic steroids increase muscle size by facilitating the production of more contractile proteins. Thus, steroids tend to exert their effects on target cells by directly affecting the cell's nucleus and subsequently altering the production of certain cellular proteins.

Hence, steroids exert their primary effects by acting on receptors located within the cell. As discussed in Chapter 4, it is apparent that these substances exert some of their effects by binding to a second set of receptors located on the cell surface.[13,18] Studies continue to define the exact role of steroidal surface receptors and their contribution to the effects of each type of steroid

Nuclear Hormone Receptors. Certain hormones interact directly with hormonal receptors that are located on the chromatin within the cell nucleus (see Fig. 28–2).[3] Thyroid hormones (T_3 and T_4) are a primary example of hormones that bind directly to nuclear receptors.[29] After binding, thyroid hormones invoke a series of changes similar to those caused by the steroid–cytosolic receptor complex; that is, the nucleus begins to transcribe messenger RNA, which is ultimately translated into specific proteins. In the case of the thyroid hormones, these new proteins usually alter the cell's metabolism. Thyroid hormones are discussed in more detail in Chapter 31.

Hormone receptors have some obvious and important pharmacologic distinctions. Drugs that can bind to and activate specific hormonal receptors (agonists) will mimic the effects of the endogenous compounds. Drugs that block the receptors (antagonists) will attenuate any unwanted hormonal effects. In fact, drugs may be produced that are even more specific for hormonal receptors than their endogenous counterparts. For instance, synthetic glucocorticoids, such as dexamethasone, exert anti-inflammatory effects in a manner similar to that of endogenous glucocorticoids, but with diminished mineralocorticoid-like side effects such as water and sodium retention. This increased specificity is presumably brought about by a more precise action of the synthetic compound on the glucocorticoid receptors rather than the mineralocorticoid receptors.

Clinical Use of Endocrine Drugs

The general ways in which pharmacologic agents can be used to alter endocrine activity are as follows.

Replacement Therapy. If the endogenous production of a hormone is deficient or absent, therapeutic administration of the hormone can be used to restore normal endocrine function.[30,35] The exogenous hormone can be obtained from natural sources, such as extracts from animal tissues, or from chemical synthesis. In addition, new recombinant DNA techniques are being used to produce hormones from cell cultures, and these techniques have shown great promise in being able to generate hormones like human insulin.

Hormone substitution is sometimes referred to as simple replacement therapy. However, the use of exogenous hormones to replace normal endocrine function can be a complicated task. Problems such as regulation of optimal dosage, the interaction of the exogenous drug with other endogenous hormone systems, and drug-induced side effects are frequently encountered.

Diagnosis of Endocrine Disorders. Hormones or their antagonists can be administered to determine the presence of excess endocrine function or endocrine hypofunction. For example, hormones or their synthetic analogs can be administered that either increase or decrease pituitary secretion to determine if pituitary function is normal. Likewise, antagonists to specific hormones can be administered to see if symptoms are caused by excessive hormone production. Specific examples of how hormones are used to diagnose endocrine abnormalities are presented in subsequent chapters.

Treatment of Excessive Endocrine Function. Hyperactive or inappropriate endocrine function is often treated pharmacologically. Inhibition of hormone function can occur at several levels. For instance, drugs that directly inhibit the synthesis of the hormone or inhibit its release through various negative feedback mechanisms (see previous section, "Feedback Control Mechanisms in Endocrine Function") may be administered. Also, hormone antagonists (drugs that block hormone receptors) may be used for prolonged periods to attenuate the effects of excessive hormone production.

Exploitation of Beneficial Hormone Effects. Hormones and their synthetic analogs are often administered to exaggerate the beneficial effects of their endogenous counterparts. The classic example is the use of glucocorticoids to treat inflammation. Doses of glucocorticoids that are much higher than the physiologic levels produced by the body can be very effective in decreasing inflammation in a variety of clinical conditions (e.g., rheumatoid arthritis, allergic reactions). Of course, the use of high doses of hormones to accentuate beneficial effects may also cause some side effects and impair various aspects of endocrine function. However, short-term use of hormones in this capacity is often a useful therapeutic intervention.

Use of Hormones to Alter Normal Endocrine Function. Because of the intrinsic control mechanisms in the endocrine system, administration of exogenous hormones can often affect the normal release of hormones. This fact can be exploited in certain situations to cause a desired change in normal endocrine function. For instance, oral contraceptives containing estrogen and progesterone inhibit ovulation by inhibiting the release of LH and FSH from the anterior pituitary.

Use of Hormones in Nonendocrine Disease. There are many examples of how various hormones and hormone-related drugs can be used to treat conditions that are not directly related to the endocrine system. For instance, certain forms of cancer respond to treatment with glucocorticoids (see Chapter 36). Drugs that block the cardiac beta-1 receptors may help control angina and hypertension by preventing excessive stimulation from adrenal medulla hormones (epinephrine, norepinephrine; see Chapters 21 and 22).

SUMMARY

The endocrine glands regulate a variety of physiologic processes through the release of specific hormones. Hormones are the equivalent of endogenously produced drugs that usually travel through the bloodstream to exert an effect on specific target tissues. Hormones typically alter cell function by binding to receptors located at specific sites on or within the target cell. Pharmacologic agents can be administered to mimic or exaggerate hormonal effects, inhibit exces-

sive hormonal activity, and produce other desirable changes in endocrine activity. The use of hormones and hormone-related substances in the pharmacologic management of specific disorders is discussed in Chapters 29 through 32.

References

1. Barnes PJ. Molecular mechanisms and cellular effects of glucocorticosteroids. *Immunol Allergy Clin North Am.* 2005;25:451–468.
2. Barrett EJ. Organization of the endocrine system. In: Boron WF, Boulpaep EL, eds. *Medical Physiology: A Cellular and Molecular Approach.* New York: Saunders; 2003.
3. Berkenstam A, Gustafsson JA. Nuclear receptors and their relevance to diseases related to lipid metabolism. *Curr Opin Pharmacol.* 2005;5:171–176.
4. Bertelli E, Bendayan M. Association between endocrine pancreas and ductal system. More than an epiphenomenon of endocrine differentiation and development? *J Histochem Cytochem.* 2005;53: 1071–1086.
5. Bohm M, Luger TA. Melanocortins in fibroblast biology—current update and future perspective for dermatology. *Exp Dermatol.* 2004;13(suppl 4):16–21.
6. Bourne HR, von Zasrtow M. Drug receptors and pharmacodynammics. In: Katzung BG, ed. *Basic and Clinical Pharmacology.* 9th ed. New York: Lange Medical Books/McGraw-Hill; 2004.
7. Collins LL, Lee HJ, Chen YT, et al. The androgen receptor in spermatogenesis. *Cytogenet Genome Res.* 2003;103:299–301.
8. Cone RD, Low MJ, Elmquist JK, Cameron JL. Neuroendocrinology. In: Larsen PR, et al, eds. *Williams Textbook of Endocrinology.* 10th ed. Philadelphia: WB Saunders; 2003.
9. Connell JM, Davies E. The new biology of aldosterone. *J Endocrinol.* 2005;186:1–20.
10. Dafopoulos K, Mademtzis I, Vanakara P, et al. Evidence that termination of the estradiol-induced luteinizing hormone surge in women is regulated by ovarian factors. *J Clin Endocrinol Metab.* 2006;91: 641–645.
11. Eisenhofer G, Kopin IJ, Goldstein DS. Catecholamine metabolism: a contemporary view with implications for physiology and medicine. *Pharmacol Rev.* 2004;56: 331–349.
12. Engelmann M, Ludwig M. The activity of the hypothalamo-neurohypophysial system in response to acute stressor exposure: neuroendocrine and electrophysiological observations. *Stress.* 2004;7:91–96.
13. Farach-Carson MC, Davis PJ. Steroid hormone interactions with target cells: cross talk between membrane and nuclear pathways. *J Pharmacol Exp Ther.* 2003;307: 839–845.
14. Fitzgerald PA. Hypothalamic and pituitary hormones. In: Katzung BG, ed. *Basic and Clinical Pharmacology.* 9th ed. New York: Lange Medical Books/McGraw-Hill; 2004
15. Guillemin R. Hypothalamic hormones a.k.a. hypothalamic releasing factors. *J Endocrinol.* 2005;184:11–28.
16. Gulliver T, Eid N. Effects of glucocorticoids on the hypothalamic–pituitary–adrenal axis in children and adults. *Immunol Allergy Clin North Am.* 2005;25:541–555.
17. Hayashi R, Wada H, Ito K, Adcock IM. Effects of glucocorticoids on gene transcription. *Eur J Pharmacol.* 2004;500:51–62.
18. Jacob J, Sebastian KS, Devassy S, et al. Membrane estrogen receptors: genomic actions and post transcriptional regulation. *Mol Cell Endocrinol.* 2006; [Epub ahead of print].
19. Kang SY, Go VL. Pancreatic exocrine-endocrine interrelationship. Clinical implications. *Gastroenterol Clin North Am.* 1999;28:551–569.
20. Kronenberg HM, Melmed S, Larsen PR, Polonsky KS. Principles of endocrinology. In: Larsen PR, et al, eds. *Williams Textbook of Endocrinology.* 10th ed. Philadelphia: WB Saunders; 2003.
21. Lam CW, Getting SJ. Melanocortin receptor type 3 as a potential target for anti-inflammatory therapy. *Curr Drug Targets Inflamm Allergy.* 2004;3:311–315.
22. Larsen PR, Davies TF, Schlumberger MJ, Hay ID. Thyroid physiology and diagnostic evaluation of patients with thyroid disorders. In: Larsen PR, et al, eds. *Williams Textbook of Endocrinology.* 10th ed. Philadelphia: WB Saunders; 2003.
23. Laugero KD. Reinterpretation of basal glucocorticoid feedback: implications to behavioral and metabolic disease. *Vitam Horm.* 2004;69:1–29.
24. Laurberg P, Andersen S, Karmisholt J. Cold adaptation and thyroid hormone metabolism. *Horm Metab Res.* 2005;37:545–549.
25. Lin KC, Sagawa N, Yura S, Itoh H, Fujii S. Simultaneous increases of leptin and gonadotropin-releasing hormone following exogenous estrogen administration in women with normally menstrual cycle. *Endocr J.* 2005;52:449–454.
26. Lombardo F, Sgro P, Salacone P, et al. Androgens and fertility. *J Endocrinol Invest.* 2005;28(suppl): 51–55.
27. Loose DS, Stancel GM. Estrogens and progestins. In: Brunton LL, et al, eds. *The Pharmacological Basis of Therapeutics.* 11th ed. New York: McGraw-Hill; 2006.

28. Miller WL. Disorders of androgen synthesis—from cholesterol to dehydroepiandrosterone. *Med Princ Pract.* 2005;14(suppl 1):58–68.

29. Moore JM, Guy RK. Coregulator interactions with the thyroid hormone receptor. *Mol Cell Proteomics.* 2005; 4:475–482.

30. Morley JE, Haren MT, Kim MJ, et al. Testosterone, aging and quality of life. *J Endocrinol Invest.* 2005; 28(suppl):76–80.

31. Ozawa H. Steroid hormones, their receptors and neuroendocrine system. *J Nippon Med Sch.* 2005;72: 316–325.

32. Parker KL, Schimmer BO. Pituitary hormones and their hypothalamic releasing factors. In: Brunton LL, et al, eds. *The Pharmacological Basis of Therapeutics.* 11th ed. New York: McGraw-Hill; 2006.

33. Poole KE, Reeve J. Parathyroid hormone—a bone anabolic and catabolic agent. *Curr Opin Pharmacol.* 2005;5:612–617.

34. Potts JT. Parathyroid hormone: past and present. *J Endocrinol.* 2005;187:311–325.

35. Prelevic GM, Kocjan T, Markou A. Hormone replacement therapy in postmenopausal women. *Minerva Endocrinol.* 2005;30:27–36.

36. Schimmer BP, Parker KL. Adrenocorticotropic hormone; adrenocortical steroids and their synthetic analogs; inhibitors of the synthesis and actions of adrenocortical hormones. In: Brunton LL, et al, eds.

The Pharmacological Basis of Therapeutics. 11th ed. New York: McGraw-Hill 2006.

37. Schinner S, Bornstein SR. Cortical-chromaffin cell interactions in the adrenal gland. *Endocr Pathol.* 2005;16:91–98.

38. Seeley RJ, Drazen DL, Clegg DJ. The critical role of the melanocortin system in the control of energy balance. *Annu Rev Nutr.* 2004;24:133–149.

39. Silvestri E, Schiavo L, Lombardi A, Goglia F. Thyroid hormones as molecular determinants of thermogenesis. *Acta Physiol Scand.* 2005;184:265–283.

40. Smoak KA, Cidlowski JA. Mechanisms of glucocorticoid receptor signaling during inflammation. *Mech Ageing Dev.* 2004;125:697–706.

41. Stewart PM. The adrenal cortex. In: Larsen PR, et al, eds. *Williams Textbook of Endocrinology.* 10th ed. Philadelphia: WB Saunders; 2003.

42. Tfelt-Hansen J, Brown EM. The calcium-sensing receptor in normal physiology and pathophysiology: a review. *Crit Rev Clin Lab Sci.* 2005;42:35–70.

43. Unsworth WP, Taylor JA, Robinson JE. Prenatal programming of reproductive neuroendocrine function: the effect of prenatal androgens on the development of estrogen positive feedback and ovarian cycles in the ewe. *Biol Reprod.* 2005;72:619–627.

44. Wehling M. Effects of aldosterone and mineralocorticoid receptor blockade on intracellular electrolytes. *Heart Fail Rev.* 2005;10:39–46.

Chapter 29

Adrenocorticosteroids

This chapter discusses the pharmacology of the steroid hormones that are produced by the adrenal cortex. The two primary types of adrenal steroids are the glucocorticoids and mineralocorticoids. Small amounts of other steroids such as the sex hormones (androgens, estrogens, and progestins) are also produced by the adrenal cortex. These steroids are discussed in Chapter 30.

The **adrenocorticosteroids** have several important physiologic and pharmacologic functions. The **glucocorticoids** (cortisol, corticosterone) are primarily involved in the control of glucose metabolism and the body's ability to deal with stress. Glucocorticoids have other attributes, such as their ability to decrease inflammation and suppress the immune system. **Mineralocorticoids,** such as aldosterone, are involved in maintaining fluid and electrolyte balance in the body.

Adrenal steroids and their synthetic analogs can be administered pharmacologically to mimic the effects of their endogenous counterparts. This approach is frequently used as replacement therapy in various hormonal deficiencies. The quantity administered during hormonal replacement is roughly equivalent to the normal endogenous production and is often referred to as a **physiologic dose.** In higher doses, adrenal steroids can be used to capitalize on a particular beneficial effect, such as using glucocorticoids as anti-inflammatory agents. These larger doses are typically referred to as **pharmacologic doses** in order to differentiate them from the amount used to maintain normal endocrine function.

Physical and occupational therapists will encounter many patients who are receiving adrenal steroids for hormone replacement or for various other therapeutic reasons. This chapter discusses the biosynthesis of the adrenal steroids in an effort to show some of the structural and functional similarities between various steroid groups. The basic physiologic and pharmacologic properties of the glucocorticoids are then addressed, followed by a description of mineralocorticoid function. This chapter should provide therapists with a better understanding of the pharmacotherapeutic and toxic characteristics of these compounds.

Steroid Synthesis

The primary pathways involved in steroid biosynthesis are shown in Figure 29–1. These hormones are manufactured by enzymes located in the cytosol of adrenocortical cells. As shown in Figure 29–1, there are three primary pathways, each leading to one of the major types of steroid hormone.[16,62] The mineralocorticoid pathway synthesizes aldosterone, the glucocorticoid pathway synthesizes cortisol, and the androgen/estrogen pathway leads to the synthesis of sex hormones. Although all three pathways are present in the adrenal cortex, the mineralocorticoid and glucocorticoid pathways predominate. The appropriate enzymes for sex hormone are biosynthesis are also present in the gonads, where hormones are synthesized in the testes (men) or ovaries (women).

Steroid hormones bear a remarkable structural similarity to one another (see Fig. 29–1). The precursor for steroid biosynthesis is cholesterol. Consequently, all of the steroid hormones share the same basic chemical configuration as their parent compound. This fact has several important physiologic and pharmacologic implications. First, even relatively minor changes in the side chains of the parent compound create steroids with dramatically different physiologic effects. For instance, the addition of only one hydrogen atom in the sex steroid pathway changes testosterone (the primary male hormone) to estradiol

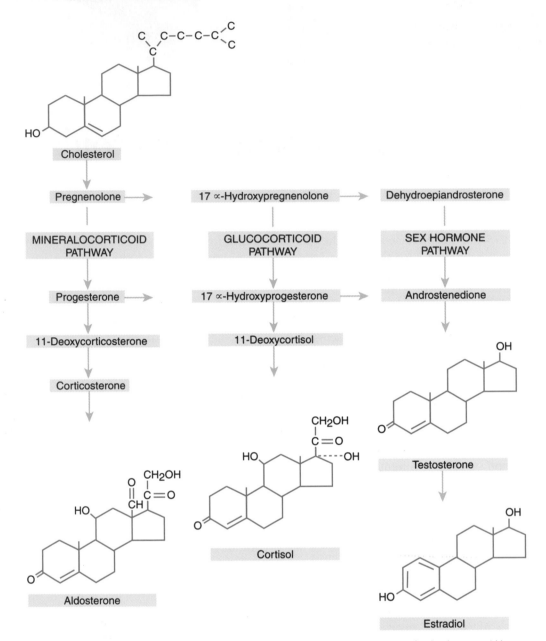

FIGURE 29–1 ▼ Pathways of adrenal steroid biosynthesis. Cholesterol is the precursor for the three steroid hormone pathways. Note the similarity between the structures of the primary mineralocorticoid (aldosterone), the primary glucocorticoid (cortisol), and the sex hormones (testosterone, estradiol). See text for further discussion.

(one of the primary female hormones). Second, the structural similarity between different types of steroids helps explain why there is often some crossover in the physiologic effects of each major category. One can readily understand how aldosterone has some glucocorticoidlike activity and cortisol has some mineralocorticoidlike effects when one considers the similarity in their organic configuration. Cor-

ticosterone (a glucocorticoid) is even the precursor to aldosterone (a mineralocorticoid).

Steroid structure and biosynthesis have been used from a pharmacologic standpoint. Pharmacologists have tried to develop more effective and less toxic synthetic steroids by manipulating the chemical side groups of these compounds. An example is the synthetic glucocorticoid dexamethasone, which is 25 times more potent than cortisol in reducing inflammation, but has a smaller tendency to cause sodium retention than the naturally occurring glucocorticoid.[62] Also, excessive steroid synthesis can be rectified in certain situations by using drugs that inhibit specific enzymes shown in the biosynthetic pathways.

Glucocorticoids

Role of Glucocorticoids in Normal Function

The primary glucocorticoid released in humans is *cortisol* (also known as hydrocortisone). Cortisol synthesis and secretion are under the control of specific hypothalamic and pituitary hormones.[7,24,31] Corticotropin-releasing hormone (CRH) from the hypothalamus stimulates the release of adrenocorticotropic hormone (ACTH) from the anterior pituitary. ACTH travels in the systemic circulation to reach the adrenal cortex, where it stimulates cortisol synthesis. Cortisol then travels in the bloodstream to various target tissues to exert a number of physiologic effects (see "Physiologic Effects of Glucocorticoids," later).

Cortisol also plays a role in controlling the release of CRH and ACTH from the hypothalamus and pituitary, respectively. As illustrated in Figure 29–2, the relationship between plasma cortisol and CRH and ACTH release is a classic example of a negative feedback control system. Increased plasma cortisol levels serve to inhibit subsequent release of CRH and ACTH, thus helping to maintain homeostasis by moderating glucocorticoid activity.

Under normal conditions, cortisol release occurs on a cyclic basis, as shown in Figure 29–3. In an unstressed human, plasma cortisol levels rise slowly throughout the early morning hours and peak at approximately 8 AM.[16] This type of physiologic event is often referred to as a *circadian rhythm*, indicating that the cycle is repeated over a 24-hour period. The fact that plasma cortisol levels progressively increase as the individual is preparing to arise suggests that cortisol helps prepare the organism for increased activity. Indeed, this belief is supported by the observation that in a rat, plasma glucocorticoid levels peak at around midnight, which corresponds to the time when nocturnal animals become active.

In addition to their normal circadian release, glucocorticoids are also released in response to virtually any stressful stimulus. For instance, trauma, infection,

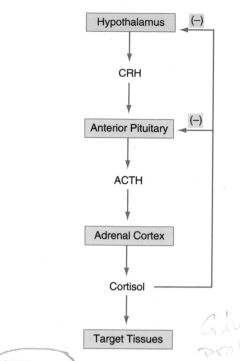

FIGURE 29–2 ▼ Negative feedback control of glucocorticoid synthesis. Cortisol limits its own synthesis by inhibiting the release of corticotropin-releasing hormone (CRH) from the hypothalamus and adrenocorticotropic hormone (ACTH) from the anterior pituitary.

hemorrhage, temperature extremes, food and water deprivation, and any perceived psychologic stress can increase cortisol release.[8,55,71,80] Various stressful events generate afferent input to the hypothalamus, thus evoking CRH and ACTH release from the hypothalamus and anterior pituitary, respectively.

Mechanism of Action of Glucocorticoids

Glucocorticoids affect various cells in a manner that is characteristic of steroid hormones (see Chapter 28, Fig. 28–3). In general, steroids alter protein synthesis in responsive cells through a direct effect on the cell's nucleus. These hormones alter the transcription of specific DNA genes, which results in subsequent changes in RNA synthesis and the translation of RNA into cellular proteins.[6,73]

Specifically, glucocorticoids exert their classic cellular effects first by entering the target cell and binding to a receptor located in the cytosol.[19,33] Binding the glucocorticoid to the receptor creates an activated hormone-receptor complex. This activated complex then travels (translocates) to the nucleus of

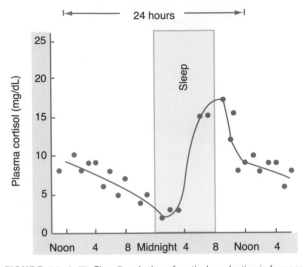

FIGURE 29–3 ▼ Circadian rhythm of cortisol production in humans. Peak plasma cortisol levels normally occur approximately at the time an individual awakens (6 to 8 AM). (*Adapted from:* Katzung BG. *Basic and Clinical Pharmacology.* 2nd ed. Lange Medical Publications; New York 1984:454; after Liddle, 1966. Reproduced with permission of the McGraw-Hill Companies.)

the cell, where it binds directly to specific DNA gene segments that control inflammation.[33,73] The activated hormone-receptor complex basically acts as a "transcription factor" because it modulates the transcription of DNA into messenger RNA (mRNA) units.[22,73] The activated hormone-receptor complex can also inhibit other transcription factors (nuclear factor-kappa B, activator protein-1) that normally activate inflammatory genes.[1,73] By inhibiting these transcription factors, glucocorticoids turn off pro-inflammatory genes and ultimately suppress the production of various inflammatory products.

Hence, glucocorticoids affect the activity of specific genes associated with the inflammatory response, thereby altering mRNA transcription for products related to inflammation.[33,73] Changes in mRNA transcription ultimately lead to a change in protein synthesis in the cell.[19] For example, glucocorticoids exert their anti-inflammatory effects by increasing the transcription of proteins that decrease inflammation while decreasing the transcription of inflammatory cytokines, enzymes, and other inflammatory proteins (see "Anti-Inflammatory Effects").[19,23,72] Other physiologic and therapeutic effects of glucocorticoids are likewise mediated by altering the expression of proteins acting as cellular enzymes, membrane carriers, receptors, structural proteins, and so on.

Consequently, glucocorticoids induce their primary effects by binding to specific genes that ultimately alter protein synthesis and lead to a change in the physiologic status of the cell. This genomic effect often takes several hours or days to occur because of the time required to alter protein synthesis and to create new proteins that reach meaningful concentrations in the cell. However, glucocorticoids may also have a more immediate effect on cell function that is independent of the hormonal action at the cell's nucleus.[19,76] This more rapid nongenomic effect is probably mediated through a different set of glucocorticoid receptors that are located on the cell membrane.[25,76] By binding to these surface receptors, glucocorticoids could induce rapid changes in cell function by altering membrane permeability, enzyme activity, and other factors.[76] Hence, glucocorticoids may actually affect cell function through two mechanisms: a rapid effect that is mediated by surface receptors and a delayed but more prolonged effect that is mediated by intracellular receptors affecting transcription at the genomic level.[19] Future research should lend insight to the importance of the rapid effects and will increase our understanding of how these two effects may interact in producing glucocorticoid-related responses.

Physiologic Effects of Glucocorticoids

Glucocorticoids exert a number of diverse physiologic effects, which are briefly discussed below.

Effects on Glucose, Protein, and Lipid Metabolism

Cortisol and other glucocorticoids increase blood glucose and liver glycogen.[62] This fact is something of a metabolic paradox because circulating levels of glucose are increased at the same time that glucose storage is enhanced. This situation is analogous to being able to draw money out of a savings account while increasing the amount of money in the savings account. The withdrawn money is available to spend (i.e., the increased blood glucose is readily available as an energy source) while the savings account accrues additional funds (i.e., liver glycogen is increased).

Glucocorticoids accomplish this paradox by affecting the metabolism of glucose, fat, and protein (see Figure 29–4). Cortisol facilitates the breakdown of muscle into amino acids and lipids into free fatty acids, which can be transported to the liver to form

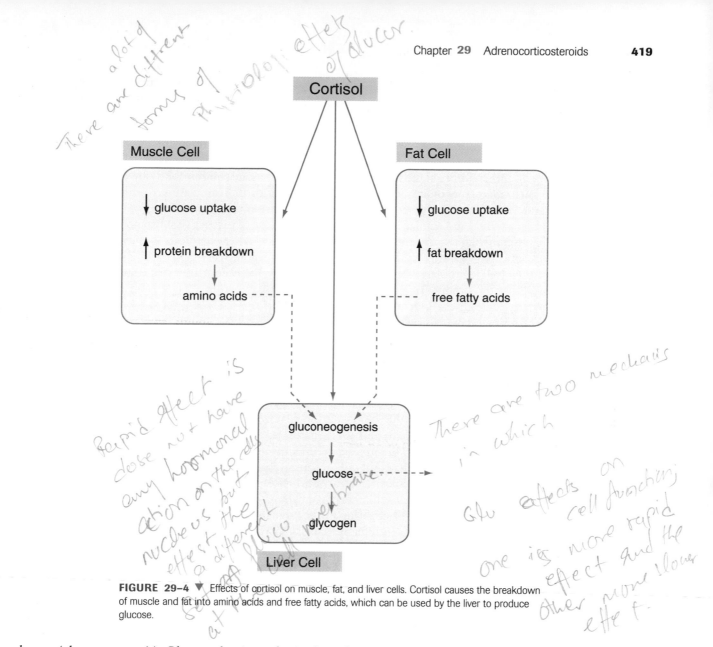

FIGURE 29–4 ▼ Effects of cortisol on muscle, fat, and liver cells. Cortisol causes the breakdown of muscle and fat into amino acids and free fatty acids, which can be used by the liver to produce glucose.

glucose (gluconeogenesis). Glucose that is synthesized in the liver can either be stored as glycogen or released back into the bloodstream to increase blood glucose levels. Cortisol also inhibits the uptake of glucose into muscle and fat cells, thus allowing more glucose to remain available in the bloodstream.

Consequently, one of the primary effects of glucocorticoids is to maintain blood glucose and liver glycogen levels to enable a supply of this energy substrate to be readily available for increased activity. This effect occurs during the daily basal release of cortisol and to an even greater extent when high levels of cortisol are released in response to stress. However, the beneficial effects on glucose titers occur largely at

the expense of muscle breakdown. This muscle catabolism is one of the primary problems that occurs when glucocorticoids are administered for long periods as a therapeutic agent (see "Adverse Effects of Glucocorticoids," later).

Anti-Inflammatory Effects

Glucocorticoids are effective and potent anti-inflammatory agents. Regardless of the cause of the inflammation, glucocorticoids attenuate the heat, erythema, swelling, and tenderness of the affected area. The exact way that these agents intervene in the inflammatory process is complex and not completely understood. Some of the primary anti-inflammatory mechanisms are addressed here.

As indicated earlier, glucocorticoids often inhibit transcription factors that normally stimulate genes within specific cells to express inflammatory components.[1,33] Glucocorticoids—for example—act on macrophages, lymphocytes, and endothelial cells to inhibit the expression of inflammatory proteins (cytokines) such as interleukin-1, interleukin-6, tissue necrosis factor alpha, interferon gamma, and similar inflammatory cytokines.[62] These cytokines are the primary chemical signal for activating various inflammatory cells such as T lymphocytes, fibroblasts, and natural killer cells.[62] By inhibiting the production and release of these inflammatory cytokines, glucocorticoids inhibit the function of key cells comprising the inflammatory response.

Glucocorticoids also inhibit the transcription and expression of adhesion molecules such as endothelial leukocyte adhesion molecule-1 and intracellular adhesion molecule-1.[64,72] These adhesion molecules are responsible for attracting leukocytes in the bloodstream to endothelial cells at the site of inflammation.[13,62] Glucocorticoids inhibit the production of adhesion molecules, thereby diminishing the ability of leukocytes to find and enter inflamed tissues. Likewise, glucocorticoids inhibit the production of other chemoattractive chemicals, such as platelet-activating factor and interleukin-1.[13] By limiting the production of factors attracting leukocytes to the site of inflammation, glucocorticoids inhibit a critical step in the initiation of the inflammatory process.[62]

Glucocorticoids inhibit the production of other pro-inflammatory substances such as prostaglandins and leukotrienes.[15,74] The role of these substances in mediating the inflammatory response was discussed in Chapter 15. Glucocorticoids activate specific genes that promote the synthesis of a family of proteins known as *annexins*.[51,74] Annexins (known previously as lipocortins) inhibit the phospholipase A_2 enzyme, which is responsible for liberating phospholipids from cell membranes so that they can be transformed into prostaglandins and leukotrienes (see Chapter 15, Fig. 15–1). By inhibiting this enzyme, glucocorticoids eliminate the precursor for prostaglandin and leukotriene biosynthesis, thus preventing the production of these pro-inflammatory substances.

Finally, high doses of glucocorticoids appear to stabilize lysosomal membranes, thereby making them less fragile and susceptible to rupture.[35] Lysosomes are subcellular organelles that contain a variety of degra-

dative enzymes. When lysosomes are ruptured, these enzymes begin to digest cellular components, thus contributing to the local damage present at a site of inflammation. Glucocorticoids may help prevent lysosomal rupture and subsequent damage contributing to the inflammatory response. Glucocorticoids also decrease vascular permeability by either increasing the reactivity of the vasculature to other vasoconstrictors (epinephrine, norepinephrine) or by suppressing the local release of vasoactive substances such as histamine, kinins, and other chemicals that cause increased capillary permeability.[16,85] This reduction in vascular permeability helps control swelling and erythema at the site of inflammation.

Immunosuppression

Glucocorticoids have long been recognized for their ability to inhibit hypersensitivity reactions, especially delayed or cell-mediated allergic reactions. The exact way in which this immunosuppression occurs is unclear, but many immunosuppressive effects are mediated by the same actions that explain the anti-inflammatory effects of these drugs. As indicated previously, glucocorticoids inhibit the transcription of various factors that signal and direct other cells in the inflammatory and immune responses. Loss of these key signals results in decreased migration of leukocytes and macrophages to the location of a foreign tissue or antigen.[62] These drugs also suppress the ability of immune cells to synthesize or respond to chemical mediators such as interleukins and interferons.[26,62] Chemicals such as interleukin-1, gamma interferon, and related substances normally mediate the communication between immune system cells such as T cells, B cells, and other lymphocytes.[56,62] By suppressing the synthesis and effects of these mediators, glucocorticoids interrupt cellular interaction and inhibit activation of key cellular components that cause the immune response. The effects of glucocorticoids on the immune response and the clinical applications of glucocorticoid-induced immunosuppression are discussed further in Chapter 37.

Other Effects of Glucocorticoids

Cortisol and similar glucocorticoids affect a variety of other tissues.[62] These hormones affect renal function by enhancing sodium and water reabsorption and by impairing the ability of the kidneys to excrete a water load. They alter central nervous system (CNS) function, with abnormal glucocorticoid levels (either too high or too low) producing changes in behavior and mood. Glucocorticoids alter the formed elements in the blood by facilitating an increase in erythrocytes, neutrophils, and platelets while decreasing the number of lymphocytes, eosinophils, monocytes, and basophils. Adequate amounts of glucocorticoids are needed for normal cardiac and skeletal muscle function. Vascular reactivity diminishes and capillary permeability increases if glucocorticoids are not present. Clearly, these hormones are involved in regulating a number of diverse and important physiologic functions.

Therapeutic Glucocorticoid Agents

The primary glucocorticoids used pharmacologically are listed in Table 29–1. These drugs are either chemically identical to the naturally occurring hormones, or they are synthetic analogs of cortisol. The clinical choice of a particular agent depends on the problem being treated and the desired effect in each patient.

As indicated in Table 29–1, glucocorticoids are available in various preparations corresponding to the specific route of administration. For instance, systemic preparations can be administered either orally or parenterally to treat systemic disorders such as collagen diseases and adrenocortical insufficiency. In more localized problems, these agents may be applied directly to a specific area using other preparations (e.g., topical, ophthalmic). Glucocorticoids are sometimes injected into a specific tissue or anatomic space to treat a localized problem. For instance, certain types of back and neck pain may be treated by injection into the epidural space,[21,47] and local glucocorticoid injections have been used to treat problems such as carpal tunnel syndrome.[2] Likewise, glucocorticoids may be injected directly into a joint (knee, shoulder, and so forth) to treat severe acute inflammation that is isolated to a particular joint.[5,9,65] The repeated intra-articular administration of glucocorticoids is not advisable, however, because of the catabolic effect of these hormones on supporting tissues (see "Adverse Effects of Glucocorticoids"). In addition, the repeated injection of glucocorticoids in and around tendons is not recommended because glucocorticoids can cause breakdown and rupture of these structures.[52] Hence, a general rule of thumb is to limit the number of glucocorticoid injections into a specific joint to four or fewer per year.[17]

Clinical Uses of Glucocorticoids

Glucocorticoids are used in two primary situations: to evaluate and treat endocrine disorders and to help resolve the symptoms of a variety of nonendocrine problems. These two major applications are discussed below.

Glucocorticoid Use in Endocrine Conditions

Replacement Therapy

Glucocorticoids are administered to help restore normal function in conditions of adrenal cortical hypofunction. Glucocorticoid replacement is instituted in both primary and secondary adrenal insufficiency. In primary insufficiency (Addison disease), glucocorticoid production is deficient because of the destruction of the adrenal cortex. In secondary insufficiency, adrenal cortex function is diminished because of other factors, such as a lack of adequate ACTH release from the anterior pituitary. Replacement therapy can also be initiated after the removal of the adrenals or pituitary gland because of disease and tumors. For instance, adrenalectomy or destruction of the pituitary to resolve adrenal cortical hypersecretion (Cushing syndrome) is typically followed by long-term glucocorticoid administration. Replacement therapy is needed to maintain optimum health whenever normal physiologic function of the adrenal cortex is disrupted.

Evaluation of Endocrine Dysfunction

Glucocorticoids may be given for diagnostic purposes to evaluate hormonal disorders. Exogenous glucocorticoids (especially the synthetic hormones such as dexamethasone) are potent inhibitors of ACTH secretion from the anterior pituitary. By suppressing the secretion of ACTH, glucocorticoids can help determine whether an endocrine imbalance is influenced by ACTH secretion. Favorable changes in the endocrine profile during ACTH suppression indicate that ACTH and ACTH-related hormones have a role in mediating the abnormality.

Use in Nonendocrine Conditions

Glucocorticoids are used primarily for their anti-inflammatory and immunosuppressive effects to treat

Table 29–1	THERAPEUTIC GLUCOCORTICOIDS						
		Type of Preparation Available					
Generic Name	**Common Trade Name(s)**	**Systemic**	**Topical**	**Inhalation**	**Ophthalmic**	**Otic**	**Nasal**
Alclometasone	Aclovate		X				
Amcinonide	Cyclocort		X				
Beclomethasone	Beclovent, Vanceril, others		X	X			X
Betamethasone	Celestone, Diprosone, others	X	X		X	X	
Budesonide	Pulmicort Turbohaler, Rhinocort			X			X
Clobetasol	Dermovate, Temovate		X				
Clocortolone	Cloderm		X				
Cortisone	Cortone	X					
Desonide	DesOwen, Tridesilon		X				
Desoximetasone	Topicort		X				
Dexamethasone	Decadron, Dexasone, others	X	X		X	X	X
Diflorasone	Florone, Maxiflor		X				
Flunisolide	AeroBid, Nasalide			X			X
Fluocinolone	Flurosyn, Synalar, others		X				
Fluocinonide	Lidex, others		X				
Fluorometholone	FML S.O.P., Fluor-Op, others				X		
Flurandrenolide	Cordran		X				
Fluticasone	Cultivate, Flonase		X				X
Halcinonide	Halog		X				
Halobetasol	Ultravate		X				
Hydrocortisone	Cortef, Dermacort, Hydrocortone, many others	X	X		X		
Medrysone	HMS Liquifilm				X		

Generic Name	Common Trade Name(s)	Type of Preparation Available					
		Systemic	Topical	Inhalation	Ophthalmic	Otic	Nasal
Methylprednisolone	Medrol, others	X					
Mometasone	Elocon, Nasonex		X				X
Prednicarbate	Dermatop		X				
Prednisolone	Pediapred, Prelone, others	X			X		
Prednisone	Deltasone, Meticorten, others	X					
Triamcinolone	Azmacort, Aristocort, Nasacort, others	X	X	X			X

a long and diverse list of nonendocrine conditions. Some of the approved indications for glucocorticoid administration are listed in Table 29–2. Of particular interest to rehabilitation specialists is the use of these agents in treating collagen diseases and rheumatic disorders, including rheumatoid arthritis.

As indicated in Table 29–2, these drugs are generally used to control inflammation or suppress the immune system for relatively short periods of time, regardless of the underlying pathology. The very fact that these drugs are successful in such a wide range of disorders illustrates that glucocorticoids do not cure the underlying problem. In a sense, they only treat a symptom of the original disease—that is, inflammation. This fact is important because the patient may appear to be improving, with decreased symptoms of inflammation, while the disease continues to worsen. Also, glucocorticoids are often administered in fairly high dosages to capitalize on their anti-inflammatory and immunosuppressive effects. These high dosages may create serious adverse effects when given for prolonged periods (see the next section, "Adverse Effects of Glucocorticoids"). Despite these limitations, glucocorticoids can be extremely helpful and even lifesaving in the short-term control of severe inflammation and various allergic responses.

Adverse Effects of Glucocorticoids

The effectiveness and extensive clinical use of natural and synthetic glucocorticoids must be tempered by the serious side effects these agents produce. Some of the more common problems associated with glucocorticoid use are described below.

Adrenocortical Suppression

Adrenocortical suppression occurs because of the negative feedback effect of the administered glucocorticoids on the hypothalamic–anterior pituitary system and the adrenal glands.[20,32] Basically, the patient's normal production of glucocorticoids is shut down by the exogenous hormones. The magnitude and duration of this suppression are related to the dosage, route of administration, and duration of glucocorticoid therapy.[4,62] Some degree of adrenocortical suppression can even occur after a single large dose.[45] This suppression will become more pronounced as systemic administration is continued for longer periods. Also, topical glucocorticoid administration over an extensive area of the body (especially in infants) may provide enough systemic absorption to suppress adrenocortical function.[69] Adrenocortical suppression can be a serious problem when glucocorticoid therapy is terminated. Patients who have experienced complete suppression will not be able to immediately resume production of glucocorticoids. Because abrupt withdrawal can be life-threatening, glucocorticoids must be withdrawn slowly by tapering the dose.[36,62]

Drug-Induced Cushing Syndrome

In drug-induced Cushing syndrome, patients begin to exhibit many of the symptoms associated with the

Table 29–2	NONENDOCRINE DISORDERS TREATED WITH GLUCOCORTICOIDS	

General Indication	Principal Desired of Glucocorticoids	Examples of Specific Disorders
Allergic disorders	Decreased inflammation	Anaphylactic reactions, drug-induced allergic reactions, severe hay fever, serum sickness
Collagen disorders	Immunosuppression	Acute rheumatic carditis, dermatomyositis, systemic lupus erythematosus
Dermatologic disorders	Decreased inflammation	Alopecia areata, dermatitis (various forms), keloids, lichens, mycosis fungoides, pemphigus, psoriasis
Gastrointestinal disorders	Decreased inflammation	Crohn disease, ulcerative colitis
Hematologic disorders	Immunosuppression	Autoimmune hemolytic anemia, congenital hypoplastic anemia, erythroblastopenia, thrombocytopenia
Nonrheumatic inflammation	Decreased inflammation	Bursitis, tenosynovitis
Neoplastic disease	Antilymphocytic effects	Leukemias, lymphomas, nasal polyps, cystic tumors
Neurologic disease	Decreased inflammation and immunosuppression	Tuberculous meningitis, multiple sclerosis, myasthenia gravis
Neurotrauma	Decreased edema;* inhibit free radical-induced neuronal damage	Brain surgery, closed head injury, certain brain tumors, spinal cord injury
Ophthalmic disorders	Decreased inflammation	Chorioretinitis, conjunctivitis, herpes zoster ophthalmicus, iridocyclitis, keratitis, optic neuritis
Organ transplant	Immunosuppression	Transplantation of liver, kidney, heart, and so forth
Renal diseases	Decreased inflammation	Nephrotic syndrome, membranous glomerulonephritis
Respiratory disorders	Decreased inflammation	Bronchial asthma, berylliosis, aspiration pneumonitis, symptomatic sarcoidosis, pulmonary tuberculosis
Rheumatic disorders	Decreased inflammation and immunosuppression	Ankylosing spondylitis, psoriatic arthritis, rheumatoid arthritis, gouty arthritis, osteoarthritis

*Efficacy of glucocorticoid use in decreasing cerebral edema has not been conclusively proved.

adrenocortical hypersecretion typical of naturally occurring Cushing syndrome.[36] These patients commonly exhibit symptoms of roundness and puffiness in the face, fat deposition and obesity in the trunk region, muscle wasting in the extremities, hypertension, osteoporosis, increased body hair (*hirsutism*), and glucose intolerance. These changes are all caused by the metabolic effects of the glucocorticoids. The adverse effects can be alleviated somewhat by reducing the glucocorticoid dosage. Some of the Cushing syndrome effects must often be tolerated, however, to allow the glucocorticoids to maintain a therapeutic effect (decreased inflammation or immunosuppression).

Breakdown of Supporting Tissues

Glucocorticoids exert a general catabolic effect not only on muscle (as described previously) but also on other tissues. Bone, ligaments, tendons, and skin are also subject to a wasting effect from prolonged glucocorticoid use. Although the exact mechanisms are complex and not well understood, glucocorticoids appear to weaken these supporting tissues by inhibiting the genes responsible for production of collagen and other tissue components, and by increasing the expression of substances that promote breakdown of bone, muscle, and so forth.[22,44] Glucocorticoids, for example, probably interfere with muscle protein synthesis by altering the muscle's ability to retain and use amino acids.[14,57] Thus, these drugs cause atrophy of skeletal muscle by increasing the rate of protein breakdown and decreasing the rate of protein synthesis.[60,68] In severe cases, glucocorticoids can induce a steroid myopathy that is characterized by proximal muscle weakness, which can affect ambulation and functional ability.[53,62] This type of myopathy is typically resolved by discontinuing the glucocorticoid, but symptoms may persist long after the drug has been withdrawn.[62]

Glucocorticoids also have negative effects on bone; loss of bone strength is considered one of the most common side effects of prolonged, systemic glucocorticoid administration.[3,46] Again, the exact reasons for these effects are unclear, but glucocorticoids probably suppress the production of substances that stimulate bone formation (e.g., insulin-like growth factor-I), and increase the expression of substances that promote bone loss (e.g., colony-stimulating factor-1, nuclear factor k-B ligand).[12] The result is a loss of bone mineral content that can lead to osteoporosis and fractures, particularly in the ribs and vertebral bodies.[62]

The magnitude of the wasting effect caused by systemic glucocorticoids is dependent on many factors, including the patient's overall health and the duration and dosage of drug therapy. Nonetheless, it is apparent that significant bone and muscle loss can occur even when these drugs are given in low doses.[67] Likewise, moderate to high doses will almost certainly cause some degree of muscle and bone loss when glucocorticoids are administered continuously for more than a few weeks.[77,79]

The potential for tissue breakdown must always be considered during the rehabilitation of patients taking these drugs, and therapists must be especially careful to avoid overstressing tissues that are weakened by the prolonged use of systemic glucocorticoids. Likewise, bone loss and risk of osteoporosis should be evaluated periodically in patients receiving long-term systemic glucocorticoids.[38,67] Patients with evidence of excessive bone loss can be treated with drugs such as the bisphosphonates (etidronate, pamidronate).[61,77] Estrogen replacement may also be helpful in minimizing bone loss in women receiving glucocorticoids, although the beneficial effects on bone mineral content must be balanced against the risks of estrogen replacement (cancer, cardiovascular disease; see Chapter 30).[86] Other interventions such as calcium supplements, vitamin D supplements, and calcitonin may help prevent bone loss in people receiving long-term glucocorticoid therapy.[61,86] The ability of various drugs to stabilize bone and prevent osteoporosis is addressed in Chapter 31.

Other Adverse Effects

Several other problems can occur during prolonged glucocorticoid use. Peptic ulcer may develop because of the breakdown of supporting proteins in the stomach wall or direct mucosal irritation by the drugs. An increased susceptibility to infection often occurs because of the immunosuppressive effect of glucocorticoids. These drugs may retard growth in children because of their inhibitory effect on bone and muscle growth and because they inhibit growth hormone.[11,29] Glucocorticoids may cause glaucoma by impairing the normal drainage of aqueous fluid from the eye, and cataract formation is also associated with prolonged use.[39,41] Mood changes and even psychoses have been reported, but the reasons for these occurrences are not clear.[59,84] Glucocorticoids with some mineralocorticoidlike activity may cause hypertension because of sodium and water retention. Some of the newer synthetic drugs have fewer mineralocorticoid effects, however, and hypertension occurs less frequently with these. Finally, glucocorticoids alter glucose metabolism, and people with diabetes mellitus will have an increased risk of hyperglycemia, insulin resistance, and decreased control of blood glucose levels.[37,48]

Drugs That Inhibit Adrenocortical Hormone Biosynthesis

Occasionally, the production of adrenal steroids must be inhibited because of adrenocortical hyperactivity. Several agents are available that block specific enzymes in the glucocorticoid biosynthetic pathway. Aminoglutethimide (Cytadren) inhibits the first step in adrenal corticoid synthesis by blocking the conversion of cholesterol to subsequent hormone precursors (see Fig. 29–1). Metyrapone (Metopirone) inhibits the hydroxylation reaction of several intermediate compounds in the adrenal corticoid pathway. Ketoconazole (Nizoral) is an antifungal drug that is used primarily to treat candidiasis and other local and systemic fungal infections (see Chapter 35). This agent also inhibits several enzymes responsible for steroid biosynthesis, and high doses may be used to suppress adrenocortical hormone production in Cushing's disease. Finally, mitotane (Lysodren) is an antineoplastic drug used in treating adrenal tumors (see Chapter 36), but can also be used to reduce hyperactivity of the adrenal gland in endocrine disorders. Mitotane directly suppresses the adrenal gland, although the exact mechanism of this suppression is unclear.

These drugs therefore reduce adrenal corticoid hypersecretion in conditions such as adrenal tumors. Adrenal hypersecretion caused by increased pituitary ACTH release (Cushing syndrome of pituitary origin) may also be resolved temporarily by these drugs. However, a longer term solution to pituitary ACTH hypersecretion, such as pituitary irradiation, is usually desirable.[50] Metyrapone is also used to test hypothalamic–anterior pituitary function. Specifically, this drug is used to evaluate the ability of the anterior pituitary to release ACTH. When this drug attenuates the production of adrenal glucocorticoids, the anterior pituitary should respond by secreting ACTH into the bloodstream. If ACTH response is too low, pituitary hypofunction is indicated. If ACTH response is exaggerated, pituitary hyperfunction or Cushing syndrome of pituitary origin is indicated.

Mineralocorticoids

Mineralocorticoids are also steroid hormones that are produced by the adrenal cortex. The principal mineralocorticoid in humans is *aldosterone*. Aldosterone is primarily involved in maintaining fluid and electrolyte balance in the body. This hormone works on the kidneys to increase sodium and water reabsorption and potassium excretion.

Regulation of Mineralocorticoid Secretion

Aldosterone release is regulated by several factors that are related to the fluid and electrolyte status in the body.[27] A primary stimulus for aldosterone release is increased levels of *angiotensin II*.[75,83] Angiotensin II is part of the renin-angiotensin system, which is concerned with maintaining blood pressure (see Chapter 21). Basically, a sudden fall in blood pressure initiates a chain of events that generates increased circulating levels of angiotensin II. Angiotensin II helps maintain blood pressure by vasoconstricting peripheral vessels. Angiotensin II (and probably also its metabolic byproduct angiotensin III) helps exert a more prolonged antihypotensive effect by stimulating aldosterone secretion from the adrenal cortex. Aldosterone can then facilitate sodium and water retention, thus maintaining adequate plasma volume.

In addition to the angiotensin II effects, aldosterone secretion is regulated by increased plasma potassium levels.[75,83] Presumably, elevated plasma potassium serves as a stimulus to increase aldosterone release, thus causing increased potassium excretion and a return to normal plasma levels. Finally, there is evidence that ACTH may also play a role in aldosterone release. Although ACTH is primarily involved in controlling glucocorticoid secretion, this hormone may also stimulate mineralocorticoid release to some extent.[75]

Mechanism of Action and Physiologic Effects of Mineralocorticoids

Aldosterone exerts its effects on the kidneys by binding to specific receptors in epithelial cells that line the distal tubule of the nephron.[18] These receptors have a high affinity for mineralocorticoid hormones. They also have a moderate affinity for many of the natural glucocorticoid hormones (e.g., cortisol) and a low affinity for the newer synthetic glucocorticoids, such as dexamethasone. This accounts for the finding that certain glucocorticoids exert some mineralocorticoidlike effects, whereas others have relatively minor effects on electrolyte and fluid balance.[10,54]

Mineralocorticoids are believed to increase sodium reabsorption by affecting sodium channels and sodium pumps on the epithelial cells lining the renal tubules.[18,58] Mineralocorticoids' ability to increase the expression of sodium channels is illustrated in Figure 29–5. These hormones enter the tubular epithelial cell, bind to receptors in the cell, and create an activated hormone-receptor complex.[18] This complex then travels to the nucleus to initiate transcription of messenger RNA units, which are translated into specific membrane-related proteins.[27,58] These proteins in some way either create or help open sodium pores on the cell membrane, thus allowing sodium to leave the tubule and enter the epithelial cell by passive diffusion.[27,83] Sodium is then actively transported out of the cell and reabsorbed into the bloodstream. Water reabsorption is increased as water follows the sodium movement back into the bloodstream. As sodium is reabsorbed, potassium is secreted by a sodium-potassium exchange, thus increasing potassium excretion (see Fig. 29–5).

In addition to their effects on the synthesis of membrane sodium channels, mineralocorticoids also have a more rapid and immediate effect on sodium reabsorption.[28,43] This effect was originally thought to occur because the hormone binds to a different set of receptors on the epithelial cell membrane that increases the activity of existing sodium channels and pumps such as the Na^+-K^+ ATPase.[63] At this point, however, efforts to identify a specific mineralocorticoid receptor on the cell membrane have been unsuccessful, and there is still debate about how mineralocorticoids exert their rapid, nonnuclear effects.[28,49] Nonetheless, the effects of mineralocorticoids (like the glucocorticoids discussed earlier) seem to occur in two phases: a rapid phase that is mediated by nonnuclear mechanisms and a delayed, but prolonged phase that is mediated by intracellular receptors binding to the cell's nucleus and increasing the transcription of specific proteins.[18,49] The two phases of mineralocorticoid action both play a role in the physiologic action of these hormones, and future research should help to define how these actions can be affected by various drugs and diseases.

In addition to its normal role in controlling fluid and electrolyte balance, aldosterone can have detrimental effects on the heart and vasculature. Excess or prolonged aldosterone production can cause hypertrophy and fibrosis of cardiac and vascular tissues and lead to detrimental changes in these tissues.[30,78] Moreover, it is now apparent that aldosterone can be produced locally within certain tissues including the heart and vascular endothelium.[78,83] That is, these tissues may produce their own supply of aldosterone as well as receive circulating levels of aldosterone from the

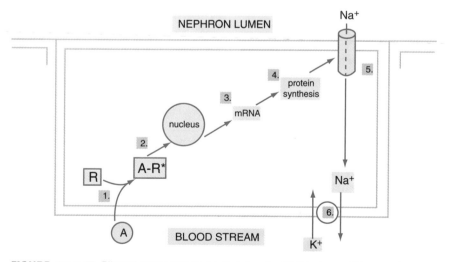

FIGURE 29–5 ▼ Effect of aldosterone on renal tubule cells. (*1*) Aldosterone (A) enters the cell and binds to a cytosolic receptor (R), creating an activated hormone-receptor complex (A–R). (*2*) A–R complex travels to the cell's nucleus, where it induces mRNA synthesis. (*3*) mRNA units undergo translation in the cytosol. (*4*) Specific proteins are synthesized that increase membrane permeability to sodium (Na^+). (*5*) Na^+ leaves the nephron lumen and enters the cell down an electrochemical gradient. (*6*) Na^+ is actively reabsorbed into the body, and potassium (K^+) is actively secreted from the bloodstream by the cellular Na^+-K^+ pump.

adrenal cortex. It therefore appears that high levels of aldosterone may adversely affect cardiovascular tissues and contribute to cardiovascular disease. Hence, certain drugs such as the aldosterone antagonists (see below) may help control the detrimental effects of aldosterone on cardiovascular tissues, and these drugs are gaining acceptance in the treatment of certain cardiovascular diseases such as hypertension and heart failure.[27,40]

Therapeutic Use of Mineralocorticoid Drugs

Drugs with mineralocorticoidlike activity (aldosterone agonists) are frequently administered as replacement therapy whenever the natural production of mineralocorticoids is impaired. Mineralocorticoid replacement is usually required in patients with chronic adrenocortical insufficiency (Addison disease), following adrenalectomy, and in other forms of adrenal cortex hypofunction. These conditions usually require both mineralocorticoid and glucocorticoid replacement.

Fludrocortisone (Florinef) is the primary aldosteronelike agent that is used in replacement therapy. This compound is chemically classified as a glucocorticoid, but it has high levels of mineralocorticoid activity and is used exclusively as a mineralocorticoid. Fludrocortisone is administered orally.

Adverse Effects of Mineralocorticoid Agonists

The primary problem associated with mineralocorticoid agonists is hypertension. Because these drugs increase sodium and water retention, blood pressure may increase if the dosage is too high. Other adverse effects may include peripheral edema, weight gain, and hypokalemia. These problems are also caused by the effects of these drugs on electrolyte and fluid balance, and are usually resolved by adjusting the dosage.

Mineralocorticoid Antagonists

The mineralocorticoid antagonists used clinically include spironolactone (Aldactone) and eplerenone (Inspra). These drugs are competitive antagonists of the aldosterone receptor; that is, they bind to the receptor but do not activate it. When bound to the receptor, these drugs block the effects of endogenous mineralocorticoids (aldosterone) by preventing the aldosterone from binding to renal cells and other tissues. Consequently, spironolactone and eplerenone antagonize the normal physiologic effects of aldosterone, resulting in increased sodium and water excretion and decreased potassium excretion.

Spironolactone and eplerenone are used primarily as diuretics in treating hypertension and heart failure. These drugs are classified as potassium-sparing diuretics because they help increase sodium and water excretion without increasing the excretion of potassium (see Chapter 21). Spironolactone is also used to help diagnose hyperaldosteronism. The drug is given for several days to antagonize the effects of excessive aldosterone production. When the drug is discontinued, serum potassium levels will decrease sharply if hyperaldosteronism is present; that is, plasma potassium levels will fall when aldosterone is again permitted to increase potassium excretion.

As indicated above, mineralocorticoid antagonists, such as spironolactone and eplerenone, can help decrease the detrimental effects of aldosterone on the heart and vasculature. By blocking aldosterone receptors in cardiac and vascular cells, these drugs prevent adverse cellular changes (fibrosis, hypertrophy) that can contribute to hypertension, heart failure, and other cardiovascular diseases.[27,40] Preliminary evidence suggests that mineralocorticoid receptor antagonists may help reduce the progression of these diseases, and future studies will help clarify how these drugs can be best used as part of the pharmacological regimen for patients with cardiovascular dysfunction.[82]

Mineralocorticoid antagonists may cause an increase in plasma potassium levels (hyperkalemia), which could be life-threatening if prolonged or severe.[70] Spironolactone can also interfere with the function of the endogenous sex hormones, thereby producing side effects such as increased body hair, deepening of the voice, decreased libido, menstrual irregularities, and breast enlargement in men. It appears, however, that eplerenone has a lower incidence of these sexual side effects, and this drug may preferentially suppress mineralocorticoid function without also affecting the sex hormones.[81] Finally, mineralocorticoid antagonists can cause gastrointestinal disturbances (diarrhea, stomach pain, gastric ulcers), and spironolactone can also cause CNS effects (drowsiness, lethargy, confusion, headache).

Special Concerns of Adrenal Steroid Use in Rehabilitation Patients

■ ■ ■ Adrenal steroids play an important role in the pharmacologic management of many patients seen in rehabilitation. As indicated in Table 29–2, systemic conditions such as rheumatoid arthritis, ankylosing spondylitis, and lupus erythematosus are often treated with glucocorticoid drugs. More localized musculoskeletal conditions, such as acute bursitis and tenosynovitis, may also be treated for short periods with glucocorticoids. Because these problems are often being treated simultaneously in a rehabilitation setting, therapists must be especially cognizant of the effects and implications of glucocorticoids.

The primary aspect of glucocorticoid administration that concerns therapists is the catabolic effect of these hormones on supporting tissues. As discussed previously, glucocorticoids cause a general breakdown in muscle, bone, skin, and other collagenous structures. The glucocorticoid-induced catabolism of these tissues can be even greater than expected in the presence of other contributing factors such as inactivity, poor nutrition, and the effects of aging. For instance, a certain amount of osteoporosis would be expected in an elderly, sedentary woman with rheumatoid arthritis. The use of glucocorticoids, however, may greatly accelerate the bone dissolution in such a patient, even when the drugs are used for relatively limited periods.[67]

Therapists can help attenuate some of the catabolic effects of these drugs. Strengthening activities help maintain muscle mass and prevent severe wasting of the musculotendinous unit.[34,42,66] Various strengthening and weight-bearing activities may also reduce bone loss to some extent. In general, any activity that promotes mobility and ambulation will be beneficial during and after glucocorticoid therapy. Therapists must use caution, however, to avoid injuring structures that are weakened by glucocorticoid use. The load placed on the musculoskeletal system must be sufficient to evoke a therapeutic response but not so excessive that musculoskeletal structures are damaged. The difference between therapeutic stress and harmful stress may be rather small in some patients taking glucocorticoids; therapists must use sound clinical judgment when developing and implementing exercise routines for these patients. Because glucocorticoids also cause thinning and wasting of skin, therapists should ensure that extra efforts are made to prevent skin breakdown in patients on prolonged glucocorticoid therapy.

Other aspects of prolonged adrenocorticoid administration also concern physical therapists and occupational therapists. Therapists should be aware of the sodium- and water-retaining properties of both glucocorticoids and mineralocorticoids. When used in acute situations or in long-term replacement therapy, both groups of adrenal steroids may cause hypertension. Therapists should routinely monitor blood pressure in patients taking either type of agent. Because of their immunosuppressive effects, glucocorticoids increase patients' susceptibility to infection. Therapists must be especially cautious about exposing these patients to any possible sources of infection. Finally, therapists should be alert for any other signs of toxicity to adrenal steroids, such as mood changes or psychoses. Therapists may recognize the early stages of such toxic reactions and prevent serious consequences by alerting medical staff.

CASE STUDY

Adrenocorticosteroids

Brief History. E.M. is a 58-year-old woman with a history of rheumatoid arthritis. She has involvement of many joints in her body, but her knees are especially affected by this disease. Her symptoms of pain, swelling, and inflammation are fairly well controlled by nonsteroidal anti-inflammatory drugs. She does experience periods of exacerbation and remission, however. During periods of exacerbation, she receives physical therapy as an outpatient at a private practice. The therapy typically consists of heat, ultrasound, range of motion, and strengthening activities to both knees. During a recent exacerbation, her symptoms were more severe than usual, and the patient began to develop flexion contractures in both knees. The therapist suggested that she consult her physician. Upon noting the severe inflammation, the physician elected to inject both knees with a glucocorticoid agent. Methylprednisolone (Depo-Medrol) was injected into the knee joints. The patient was advised to continue physical therapy on a daily basis.

Problem/Influence of Medication. Glucocorticoid administration produced a dramatic decrease in the swelling and inflammation in both knees. The therapist was tempted to begin aggressive stretching activities to resolve the knee flexion contractures and restore normal range of motion. The therapist was aware, however, that glucocorticoids may weaken ligaments, tendons, and other supporting structures because of an inhibitory effect on collagen formation. The therapist also realized that this effect may be present for some time after glucocorticoid administration. Even though only a single intra-articular injection was used, the drug may be retained locally within fat and other tissues because of the high degree of lipid solubility of steroid agents. Consequently, the injected glucocorticoid may continue to exert a catabolic effect on knee joint structures for some time.

Decision/Solution. The therapist was especially careful to use low-intensity, prolonged-duration stretching forces when trying to resolve the knee flexion contractures. Gentle stretching, massage, and other manual techniques were continued until full active and passive knee extension was achieved.

SUMMARY

The two principal groups of adrenal steroids are the glucocorticoids and mineralocorticoids. These hormones are synthesized from cholesterol within cells of the adrenal cortex. The primary glucocorticoid produced in humans is cortisol (hydrocortisone), and the primary mineralocorticoid is aldosterone. Glucocorticoids exert a number of effects such as regulation of glucose metabolism, attenuation of the inflammatory response, and suppression of the immune system. Mineralocorticoids are involved primarily in the control of fluid and electrolyte balance.

Pharmacologically, natural and synthetic adrenal steroids are often used as replacement therapy to resolve a deficiency in adrenal cortex function. The glucocorticoids are also administered primarily for their anti-inflammatory and immunosuppressive effects in a diverse group of clinical problems. These agents can be extremely beneficial in controlling the symptoms of various rheumatic and allergic disorders. Prolonged glucocorticoid use, however, is limited by a number of serious effects, such as adrenocortical suppression and breakdown of muscle, bone, and other tissues. Physical therapists and occupational therapists should be especially aware of the potential side effects of glucocorticoids, which are used in many disorders that are seen in a rehabilitation setting.

References

1. Adcock IM, Ito K, Barnes PJ. Glucocorticoids: effects on gene transcription. *Proc Am Thorac Soc.* 2004;1: 247–254.
2. Agarwal V, Singh R, Sachdev A, et al. A prospective study of the long-term efficacy of local methyl prednisolone acetate injection in the management of mild carpal tunnel syndrome. *Rheumatology.* 2005; 44:647–650.
3. Alesci S, De Martino MU, Ilias I, et al. Glucocorticoid-induced osteoporosis: from basic mechanisms to clinical aspects. *Neuroimmunomodulation.* 2005;12:1–19.

4. Allen DB. Inhaled steroids for children: effects on growth, bone, and adrenal function. *Endocrinol Metab Clin North Am.* 2005;34:555–564.

5. Arroll B, Goodyear-Smith F. Corticosteroid injections for painful shoulder: a meta-analysis. *Br J Gen Pract.* 2005;55:224–228.

6. Barnes PJ. Corticosteroids: the drugs to beat. *Eur J Pharmacol.* 2006; 533:2–14.

7. Barrett EJ. Organization of the endocrine system. In: Boron WF, Boulpaep EL, eds. *Medical Physiology: A Cellular and Molecular Approach.* New York: Saunders; 2003.

8. Beishuizen A, Thijs LG. The immunoneuroendocrine axis in critical illness: beneficial adaptation or neuroendocrine exhaustion? *Curr Opin Crit Care.* 2004;10: 461–467.

9. Bell AD, Conaway D. Corticosteroid injections for painful shoulders. *Int J Clin Pract.* 2005;59:1178–1186.

10. Bhargava A, Pearce D. Mechanisms of mineralocorticoid action: determinants of receptor specificity and actions of regulated gene products. *Trends Endocrinol Metab.* 2004;15:147–153.

11. Brown JJ, Zacharin MR. Proposals for prevention and management of steroid-induced osteoporosis in children and adolescents. *J Paediatr Child Health.* 2005; 41:553–557.

12. Canalis E. Mechanisms of glucocorticoid action in bone. *Curr Osteoporos Rep.* 2005;3:98–102.

13. Caramori G, Adcock I. Anti-inflammatory mechanisms of glucocorticoids targeting granulocytes. *Curr Drug Targets Inflamm Allergy.* 2005;4:455–463.

14. Carballo-Jane E, Pandit S, Santoro JC, et al. Skeletal muscle: a dual system to measure glucocorticoid-dependent transactivation and transrepression of gene regulation. *J Steroid Biochem Mol Biol.* 2004;88: 191–201.

15. Chivers JE, Cambridge LM, Catley MC, et al. Differential effects of RU486 reveal distinct mechanisms for glucocorticoid repression of prostaglandin E release. *Eur J Biochem.* 2004;271:4042–4052.

16. Chrousos GP. Adrenocorticosteroids and adrenocortical antagonists. In: Katzung BG, ed *Basic and Clinical Pharmacology.* 9th ed. New York: Lange Medical Books/McGraw-Hill; 2004.

17. Cole BJ, Schumacher HR, Jr. Injectable corticosteroids in modern practice. *J Am Acad Orthop Surg.* 2005;13: 37–46.

18. Connell JM, Davies E. The new biology of aldosterone. *J Endocrinol.* 2005;186:1–20.

19. Czock D, Keller F, Rasche FM, Haussler U. Pharmacokinetics and pharmacodynamics of systemically administered glucocorticoids. *Clin Pharmacokinet.* 2005;44:61–98.

20. Dahl R. Systemic side effects of inhaled corticosteroids in patients with asthma. *Respir Med.* 2006; 100: 1307–1317.

21. DePalma MJ, Bhargava A, Slipman CW. A critical appraisal of the evidence for selective nerve root injection in the treatment of lumbosacral radiculopathy. *Arch Phys Med Rehabil.* 2005;86: 1477–1483.

22. Dostert A, Heinzel T. Negative glucocorticoid receptor response elements and their role in glucocorticoid action. *Curr Pharm Des.* 2004;10: 2807–2816.

23. Elenkov IJ. Glucocorticoids and the Th1/Th2 balance. *Ann N Y Acad Sci.* 2004;1024:138–146.

24. Enyeart JJ. Biochemical and ionic signaling mechanisms for ACTH-stimulated cortisol production. *Vitam Horm.* 2005;70:265–279.

25. Farach-Carson MC, Davis PJ. Steroid hormone interactions with target cells: cross talk between membrane and nuclear pathways. *J Pharmacol Exp Ther.* 2003;307: 839–845.

26. Franchimont D. Overview of the actions of glucocorticoids on the immune response: a good model to characterize new pathways of immunosuppression for new treatment strategies. *Ann N Y Acad Sci.* 2004;1024: 124–137.

27. Fuller PJ, Young MJ. Mechanisms of mineralocorticoid action. *Hypertension.* 2005;46:1227–1235.

28. Funder JW. The nongenomic actions of aldosterone. *Endocr Rev.* 2005;26:313–321.

29. Gallagher MP, Levine LS, Oberfield SE. A review of the effects of therapy on growth and bone mineralization in children with congenital adrenal hyperplasia. *Growth Horm IGF Res.* 2005;15(suppl A): S26–S30.

30. Goodfriend TL. Aldosterone—a hormone of cardiovascular adaptation and maladaptation. *J Clin Hypertens.* 2006;8:133–139.

31. Guillemin R. Hypothalamic hormones a.k.a. hypothalamic releasing factors. *J Endocrinol.* 2005;184: 11–28.

32. Gulliver T, Eid N. Effects of glucocorticoids on the hypothalamic–pituitary–adrenal axis in children and adults. *Immunol Allergy Clin North Am.* 2005;25: 541–555.

33. Hayashi R, Wada H, Ito K, Adcock IM. Effects of glucocorticoids on gene transcription. *Eur J Pharmacol.* 2004;500:51–62.

34. Hickson RC, Marone JR. Exercise and inhibition of glucocorticoid-induced muscle atrophy. *Exerc Sport Sci Rev.* 1993;21:135–167.

35. Hinz B, Hirschelmann R. Dexamethasone megadoses stabilize rat liver lysosomal membranes by non-genomic and genomic effects. *Pharm Res.* 2000;17:1489–1493.

36. Hopkins RL, Leinung MC. Exogenous Cushing's syndrome and glucocorticoid withdrawal. *Endocrinol Metab Clin North Am.* 2005;34:371–384.

37. Iwamoto T, Kagawa Y, Naito Y, et al. Steroid-induced diabetes mellitus and related risk factors in patients with neurologic diseases. *Pharmacotherapy.* 2004;24: 508–514.

38. Kanis JA, Borgstrom F, De Laet C, et al. Assessment of fracture risk. *Osteoporos Int.* 2005;16:581–589.

39. Kersey JP, Broadway DC. Corticosteroid-induced glaucoma: a review of the literature. *Eye.* 2006;20: 407–416.

40. Khan NU, Movahed A. The role of aldosterone and aldosterone-receptor antagonists in heart failure. *Rev Cardiovasc Med.* 2004;5:71–81.

41. Kuo HK, Lai IC, Fang PC, Teng MC. Ocular complications after a sub-tenon injection of triamcinolone acetonide for uveitis. *Chang Gung Med J.* 2005;28: 85–89.

42. LaPier TK. Glucocorticoid-induced muscle atrophy. The role of exercise in treatment and prevention. *J Cardiopulm Rehabil.* 1997;17:76–84.

43. Losel R, Schultz A, Boldyreff B, Wehling M. Rapid effects of aldosterone on vascular cells: clinical implications. *Steroids.* 2004;69:575–578.

44. Ma K, Mallidis C, Bhasin S, et al. Glucocorticoid-induced skeletal muscle atrophy is associated with upregulation of myostatin gene expression. *Am J Physiol Endocrinol Metab.* 2003;285:E363–E371.

45. Mader R, Lavi I, Luboshitzky R. Evaluation of the pituitary-adrenal axis function following single intraarticular injection of methylprednisolone. *Arthritis Rheum.* 2005;52:924–928.

46. Maricic M. Glucocorticoid-induced osteoporosis: treatment options and guidelines. *Curr Osteoporos Rep.* 2005;3:25–29.

47. McLain RF, Kapural L, Mekhail NA. Epidural steroid therapy for back and leg pain: mechanisms of action and efficacy. *Spine J.* 2005;5:191–201.

48. Midtvedt K, Hjelmesaeth J, Hartmann A, et al. Insulin resistance after renal transplantation: the effect of steroid dose reduction and withdrawal. *J Am Soc Nephrol.* 2004;15:3233–3239.

49. Mihailidou AS, Funder JW. Nongenomic effects of mineralocorticoid receptor activation in the cardiovascular system. *Steroids.* 2005;70:347–351.

50. Mondok A, Szeifert GT, Mayer A, et al. Treatment of pituitary tumors: radiation. *Endocrine.* 2005;28: 77–85.

51. Mulla A, Leroux C, Solito E, Buckingham JC. Correlation between the antiinflammatory protein annexin 1 (lipocortin 1) and serum cortisol in subjects with normal and dysregulated adrenal function. *J Clin Endocrinol Metab.* 2005;90:557–562.

52. Nichols AW. Complications associated with the use of corticosteroids in the treatment of athletic injuries. *Clin J Sport Med.* 2005;15:370–375.

53. Owczarek J, Jasinska M, Orszulak-Michalak D. Drug-induced myopathies. An overview of the possible mechanisms. *Pharmacol Rep.* 2005;57:23–34.

54. Pascual-Le Tallec L, Lombes M. The mineralocorticoid receptor: a journey exploring its diversity and specificity of action. *Mol Endocrinol.* 2005;19:2211–2221.

55. Rasmusson AM, Vythilingam M, Morgan CA, 3rd. The neuroendocrinology of posttraumatic stress disorder: new directions. *CNS Spectr.* 2003;8:651–656, 665–667.

56. Reichardt HM. Immunomodulatory activities of glucocorticoids: insights from transgenesis and gene targeting. *Curr Pharm Des.* 2004;10:2797–2805.

57. Rieu I, Sornet C, Grizard J, Dardevet D. Glucocorticoid excess induces a prolonged leucine resistance on muscle protein synthesis in old rats. *Exp Gerontol.* 2004;39:1315–1321.

58. Rogerson FM, Brennan FE, Fuller PJ. Mineralocorticoid receptor binding, structure and function. *Mol Cell Endocrinol.* 2004;217:203–212.

59. Sacks O, Shulman M. Steroid dementia: an overlooked diagnosis? *Neurology.* 2005;64:707–709.

60. Salehian B, Kejriwal K. Glucocorticoid-induced muscle atrophy: mechanisms and therapeutic strategies. *Endocr Pract.* 1999;5:277–281.

61. Sambrook PN. How to prevent steroid induced osteoporosis. *Ann Rheum Dis.* 2005;64:176–178.

62. Schimmer BP, Parker KL. Adrenocorticotropic hormone; adrenocortical steroids and their synthetic analogs; inhibitors of the synthesis and actions of adrenocortical hormones. In: Brunton LL, et al, eds. *The Pharmacological Basis of Therapeutics* 11th ed. New York: McGraw-Hill; 2006.

63. Schmidt BM, Christ M, Falkenstein E, Wehling M. Nongenomic steroid actions: completing the puzzle. Aldosterone as an example. *Exp Clin Endocrinol Diabetes.* 1998;106:441–445.

64. Schramm R, Thorlacius H. Neutrophil recruitment in mast cell-dependent inflammation: inhibitory mechanisms of glucocorticoids. *Inflamm Res.* 2004; 53:644–652.

65. Schumacher HR, Chen LX. Injectable corticosteroids in treatment of arthritis of the knee. *Am J Med.* 2005; 118:1208–1214.

66. Seene T. Turnover of skeletal muscle contractile proteins in glucocorticoid myopathy. *J Steroid Biochem Mol Biol.* 1994;50:1–4.

67. Shaker JL, Lukert BP. Osteoporosis associated with excess glucocorticoids. *Endocrinol Metab Clin North Am.* 2005;34:341–356.

68. Sheffield-Moore M, Urban RJ. An overview of the endocrinology of skeletal muscle. *Trends Endocrinol Metab.* 2004;15:110–115.

69. Shohat M, Mimouni M, Shuper A, Varsano I. Adrenocortical suppression by topical application of glucocorticoids in infants with seborrheic dermatitis. *Clin Pediatr (Phila).* 1986;25:209–212.

70. Sica DA. The risks and benefits of aldosterone antagonists. *Curr Heart Fail Rep.* 2005;2:65–71.

71. Silverman MN, Pearce BD, Biron CA, Miller AH. Immune modulation of the hypothalamic–pituitary–adrenal (HPA) axis during viral infection. *Viral Immunol.* 2005;18:41–78.

72. Sloka JS, Stefanelli M. The mechanism of action of methylprednisolone in the treatment of multiple sclerosis. *Mult Scler.* 2005;11:425–432.

73. Smoak KA, Cidlowski JA. Mechanisms of glucocorticoid receptor signaling during inflammation. *Mech Ageing Dev.* 2004;125:697–706.

74. Smyth EM, Burke A, FitzGerald GA. Lipid-derived autocoids: eicosanoids and platelet-activating factor. In: Brunton LL, et al, eds. *The Pharmacological Basis of Therapeutics.* 11th ed. New York: McGraw-Hill; 2006.

75. Spat A, Hunyady L. Control of aldosterone secretion: a model for convergence in cellular signaling pathways. *Physiol Rev.* 2004;84:489–539.

76. Stellato C. Post-transcriptional and nongenomic effects of glucocorticoids. *Proc Am Thorac Soc.* 2004; 1:255–263.
77. Summey BT, Yosipovitch G. Glucocorticoid-induced bone loss in dermatologic patients: an update. *Arch Dermatol.* 2006;142:82–90.
78. Takeda Y. Role of cardiovascular aldosterone in hypertension. *Curr Med Chem Cardiovasc Hematol Agents.* 2005;3:261–266.
79. Tamura Y, Okinaga H, Takami H. Glucocorticoid-induced osteoporosis. *Biomed Pharmacother.* 2004;58: 500–504.
80. Webster JI, Sternberg EM. Role of the hypothalamic–pituitary–adrenal axis, glucocorticoids and glucocorticoid receptors in toxic sequelae of exposure to bacterial and viral products. *J Endocrinol.* 2004;181: 207–221.
81. Weinberger MH. Eplerenone: a new selective aldosterone receptor antagonist. *Drugs Today.* 2004;40: 481–485.
82. Williams GH. Cardiovascular benefits of aldosterone receptor antagonists. *Climacteric.* 2003;6(suppl 3): 29–35.
83. Williams GH. Aldosterone biosynthesis, regulation, and classical mechanism of action. *Heart Fail Rev.* 2005;10:7–13.
84. Wolkowitz OM, Lupien SJ, Bigler E, et al. The "steroid dementia syndrome": an unrecognized complication of glucocorticoid treatment. *Ann N Y Acad Sci.* 2004;1032:191–194.
85. Yang S, Zhang L. Glucocorticoids and vascular reactivity. *Curr Vasc Pharmacol.* 2004;2:1–12.
86. Zizic TM. Pharmacologic prevention of osteoporotic fractures. *Am Fam Physician.* 2004;70: 1293–1300.

Male and Female Hormones

In this chapter, the pharmacology of male and female hormones is discussed. Male hormones, such as testosterone, are usually referred to collectively as androgens. The female hormones consist of two principal groups: the estrogens (e.g., estradiol) and the progestins (e.g., progesterone). Androgens, estrogens, and progestins are classified as steroid hormones; their chemical structure is similar to those of the other primary steroid groups, the glucocorticoids and mineralocorticoids (see Chapter 29). The principal functions, however, of male and female hormones are to control reproductive function and secondary sexual characteristics in their respective gender groups.

Male and female hormones are produced primarily in the gonads. Androgens are synthesized in the testes in the male. In the female, the ovaries are the principal sites of estrogen and progestin production. As discussed in Chapter 29, small amounts of sex-related hormones are also produced in the adrenal cortex in both sexes, which accounts for the fact that small amounts of hormones of the opposite sex are seen in females and males; that is, low testosterone levels are seen in females, and males produce small quantities of estrogen. However, under normal conditions, the amounts of sex-related hormones produced by the adrenal cortex are usually too small to produce significant physiologic effects.

This chapter first discusses the physiologic role of the male hormones and the pharmacologic use of natural and synthetic androgens. The physiologic and pharmacologic characteristics of the female hormones are then addressed. As these discussions indicate, there are several aspects of male and female hormones that should concern physical therapists and occupational therapists. Rehabilitation patients may use these agents for approved purposes, for example, female hormones as contraceptives. These agents may also be used for illicit reasons, such as the use of male hormones to enhance athletic performance. Hence, rehabilitation specialists should be aware of the therapeutic and potential toxic effects of these drugs.

Androgens

Source and Regulation of Androgen Synthesis

In adult males, *testosterone* is the principal androgen produced by the testes.[39,40,144] Testosterone is synthesized by Leydig cells located in the interstitial space between the seminiferous tubules (Fig. 30–1). The *seminiferous tubules* are the convoluted ducts within the testes in which sperm production (*spermatogenesis*) takes place. Testosterone produced by the Leydig cells exerts a direct effect on the seminiferous tubules, as well as systemic effects on other physiologic systems (see "Physiologic Effects of Androgens").

Production of testosterone by the Leydig cells is regulated by the pituitary **gonadotropins** *luteinizing hormone* (LH) and *follicle-stimulating hormone* (FSH).[71,159] LH and FSH appear to control spermatogenesis, as shown in Figure 30–1. LH is the primary hormone that stimulates testosterone production. LH released from the anterior pituitary binds to receptors on the surface of Leydig cells and directly stimulates testosterone synthesis.[61,144] FSH is also released from the anterior pituitary; this hormone primarily affects the Sertoli cells that line the seminiferous tubules and are responsible for the development and maturation of normal sperm (see Fig. 30–1).[1,159] FSH stimulates the growth and function of Sertoli cells, and this hormone induces Sertoli cells to produce several products that influence spermatogenesis and androgen function.

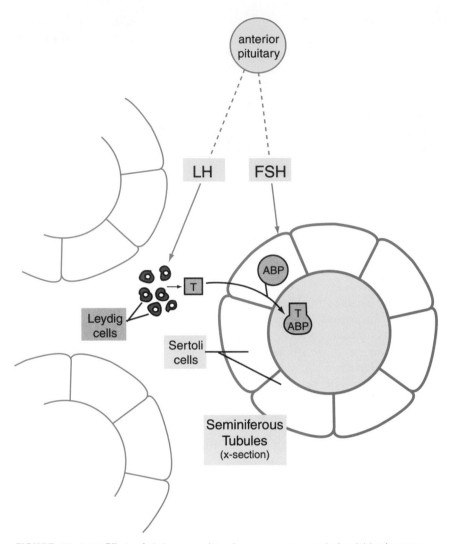

FIGURE 30–1 ▼ Effects of pituitary gonadotropins on spermatogenesis. Luteinizing hormone (LH) stimulates testosterone (T) production from Leydig cells. Follicle-stimulating hormone (FSH) acts primarily on Sertoli cells to increase synthesis of androgen-binding protein (ABP). ABP appears to bind with T and facilitate transport into the seminiferous tubule, where spermatogenesis takes place.

FSH, for example, increases the expression of a polypeptide known as androgen-binding protein (ABP). ABP helps concentrate testosterone within the seminiferous tubules and helps transport testosterone to the epididymis.[39] FSH may also affect Leydig cell function indirectly by increasing the production of other chemical messengers from the Sertoli cells that enhance differentiation and function of Leydig cells.[146,147]

Therefore, both pituitary gonadotropins are required for optimal androgen function. LH acts on the Leydig cells to stimulate testosterone synthesis, whereas FSH acts on the Sertoli cells to stimulate their function and help testosterone reach target tissues within the seminiferous tissues. Other hormones may also play a synergistic role in steroidogenesis in the male. For instance, growth hormone, thyroid hormones, insulin-like growth factor 1, and prolactin may also affect the functions of Leydig and Sertoli cells, thereby influencing the production and effects of testosterone.[21,98]

Release of the pituitary gonadotropins (LH, FSH) is regulated by gonadotropin-releasing hormone (GnRH) from the hypothalamus.[21,144] A classic negative feedback system exists between the GnRH/pituitary gonadotropins and testosterone synthesis. Increased plasma levels of testosterone inhibit the release of GnRH, LH, and FSH, thus maintaining testosterone levels within a relatively finite range. In addition, testosterone production is fairly tonic in normal men. Fluctuations may occur in the amount of testosterone produced over a given period, and androgen production tends to diminish slowly as part of normal aging.[108] Androgen production, however, does not correspond to a regular monthly cycle similar to hormonal production in women; that is, testosterone is produced more or less constantly, whereas female hormones are typically produced according to the stages of the menstrual cycle (see "Estrogen and Progesterone," later).

Physiologic Effects of Androgens

Testosterone and other androgens are involved in the development of the sexual characteristics in males and in the stimulation of spermatogenesis. These two primary effects are described below.

Development of Male Characteristics

The influence of testosterone on sexual differentiation begins in utero. In the fetus, the testes produce small amounts of testosterone that affect the development of the male reproductive organs. Androgen production then remains relatively unimportant until puberty. At the onset of puberty, a complex series of hormonal events stimulates the testes to begin to synthesize significant amounts of testosterone. The production of testosterone brings about the development of most of the physical characteristics associated with men. Most notable are increased body hair, increased skeletal muscle mass, voice change, and maturation of the external genitalia.

These changes are all caused by the effect of androgenic steroids on their respective target tissues. Like other steroids, androgens enter the target cell and bind to a cytoplasmic receptor.[123,128,158] The activated steroid-receptor complex then travels to the cell's nucleus, where it binds to specific chromatin units. Protein synthesis increases through the transcription/translation of RNA by binding the activated complex to DNA gene segments. The proteins produced then cause a change in cellular function, which is reflected as one of the maturational effects of the androgens. For instance, testosterone increases pro-

tein synthesis in skeletal muscle, thus increasing muscle mass in certain situations, such as at the onset of puberty. This particular androgenic effect (increased muscle mass) as it relates to androgen abuse in athletes is discussed in more detail under "Androgen Abuse" later in this chapter.

Role in Spermatogenesis

As discussed previously, androgens are essential for the production and development of normal sperm.[39,69] Testosterone is produced by the Leydig cells located in the interstitial space between the seminiferous tubules. LH serves as the primary stimulus to increase androgen production from Leydig cells. Testosterone enters the tubules to directly stimulate the production of sperm through an effect on protein synthesis within the tubule cells. FSH must also be present in the testes to facilitate testosterone transport into the Sertoli cells and to work synergistically with testosterone to allow full growth and maturation of developing sperm.[100,159]

Pharmacologic Use of Androgens

Clinical Use of Androgens

Androgens and their synthetic derivatives are approved for administration in several clinical situations, which are presented below.

Replacement Therapy. Testosterone and other androgens are administered as replacement therapy when the endogenous production of testosterone is impaired. Such conditions include removal of the testes (orchiectomy), various intrinsic forms of testicular failure (cryptorchidism, orchitis), and problems in the endocrine regulation of testosterone production, such as lack of LH production and other forms of hypogonadism.[32,144]

Because androgen production also diminishes slowly with aging, relatively small or "physiologic" doses of androgens have been used to replace the age-related decline in endogenous production in some older men.[105,108] This type of replacement has been reported to produce beneficial effects on body composition, strength, bone mineralization, mood, libido, and other characteristics associated with normal androgen production.[68,85,107] The primary concern, however, is that androgens can increase prostate growth and perhaps increase the risk of prostate cancer in susceptible older men.[106,152] Hence, androgen replacement continues to be evaluated as a therapeutic option in certain men who are experiencing an excessive decline in androgen production during aging.[85,108] Future studies should help clarify how these hormones might be used to promote optimal health in older men.[105]

Catabolic States. Androgens can be administered for their anabolic properties in conditions where there is substantial muscle catabolism and protein loss.[101] Such conditions include chronic infections, severe traumas, severe burns, and recovery from extensive surgeries.[35,115] However, the use of androgens in these situations is somewhat controversial. These agents are not typically used as a primary treatment, but as adjuncts to more conventional treatments such as dietary supplementation and exercise.

Androgens can also be used to increase lean body mass in men who are infected with human immunodeficiency virus (HIV). Men with HIV infection may have muscle wasting because of low testosterone production combined with the catabolic effects of this infection and subsequent anti-HIV therapies (see Chapter 34).[38,150] Physiologic dosages of androgens have therefore been used to maintain or increase muscle mass and bone density in these individuals. The effects of this treatment, however, have not been overwhelmingly successful; only modest increases in lean body mass were seen in some studies.[83] Larger (supraphysiologic) dosages of androgens, such as oxandrolone, have been reported to produce beneficial effects on muscle mass and strength in men with HIV infection, especially if drug therapy is combined with resistance training.[149] Hence, androgens may be a possible option to help reduce muscle wasting and maintain muscle strength and function in men who experience severe muscle loss during HIV infection and AIDS.[83,150]

Delayed Puberty. In males, androgens may be administered on a limited basis to accelerate the normal onset of puberty.[124,125] These drugs are typically used when puberty is anticipated to occur spontaneously but at a relatively late date—that is, when puberty is not delayed because of some pathologic condition.

Breast Cancer. Androgens have been used to treat a limited number of hormone-sensitive tumors, such as certain cases of breast cancer in women. Other drugs such as the antiestrogens, however, have largely replaced the use of androgens in such cancers. The

role of various hormones in the treatment of cancer is discussed in more detail in Chapter 36.

Anemia. Testosterone and similar compounds are potent stimulators of erythropoietin synthesis from the kidneys and other tissues.[109] Erythropoietin, in turn, stimulates production of red blood cell synthesis in bone marrow. Human erythropoietin, however, can now be synthesized using recombinant DNA techniques. Hence, various types of anemia that occur secondary to renal disease, cancer chemotherapy, and so forth are usually treated directly with recombinant erythropoietin.[109] Nonetheless, androgens may be used as an adjunct to erythropoietin and other drugs to stimulate red blood cell production in certain patients with severe or recalcitrant anemia.[10]

Hereditary Angioedema. This hereditary disorder is characterized by a defect in the control of clotting factors that ultimately leads to increased vascular permeability.[114] Loss of vascular fluid from specific capillary beds causes localized edema in various tissues such as the skin, upper respiratory tract, and gastrointestinal tract. Certain androgens act on the liver to restore production of several clotting factors and to increase production of a glycoprotein inhibiting the initial stages of the clotting sequence that leads to increased vascular permeability.[114] Hence, androgens are typically given prophylactically to decrease the frequency and severity of angioedema attacks.

Specific Agents

Androgens that are used clinically are listed in Table 30–1. Specific agents are usually administered orally or intramuscularly, as indicated, to replace endogenous androgen production, or to treat various medical problems. Androgens can also be classified according to their relative androgenic and anabolic properties; that is, certain androgens are given primarily to mimic male sexual characteristics (androgenic effects), whereas other androgens are given primarily to enhance tissue metabolism (anabolic effects; see Table 30–1). This distinction is not absolute, however, because all compounds given to produce anabolism will also produce some androgenic effects. Many other androgenic and anabolic steroids exist and can be acquired relatively easily on the black market by individuals engaging in androgen abuse (see "Androgen Abuse"). Nonetheless, the agents listed in Table 30–1 are the principal androgens approved for clinical use; these drugs are used to treat catabolic states, anemias, and similar conditions.

Table 30–1	CLINICAL USE OF ANDROGENS		

Generic Name	Trade Name(s)	Primary Indication(s)	Routes of Administration
Fluoxymesterone	Android-F, Halotestin	Androgen deficiency; breast cancer in women; delayed puberty in boys; anemia	Oral
Methyltestosterone	Android, Oreton, Testred, Virilon	Androgen deficiency; breast cancer in women; delayed puberty in boys	Oral
Nandrolone	Durabolin, Deca-Durabolin, others	Anemia; breast cancer in women	Intramuscular
Oxandrolone	Oxandrin	Catabolic states	Oral
Oxymetholone	Anadrol	Anemia; Angioedema	Oral
Stanozolol	Winstrol	Angioedema	Oral
Testosterone injectable suspension	Testamone, Testaqua	Androgen deficiency; breast cancer; delayed puberty in boys	Intramuscular
Testosterone cypionate injection	Andronate, Depo-Testosterone, others	Androgen deficiency; breast cancer in women; delayed puberty in boys	Intramuscular
Testosterone enanthate injection	Delatest, Delatestryl, others	Androgen deficiency; breast cancer in women; delayed puberty in boys; anemia	Intramuscular
Testosterone propionate injection	Testex	Androgen deficiency; breast cancer in women; delayed puberty in boys	Intramuscular
Testosterone implants	Testopel pellets	Androgen deficiency; delayed puberty in boys	Subcutaneous
Testosterone gel	Testoderm, Andro-derm	Androgen deficiency	Transdermal
Testosterone transdermal systems	AndroGel	Androgen deficiency	Transdermal

Adverse Effects of Clinical Androgen Use

The primary problems associated with androgens are related to the masculinizing effects of these drugs.[136,139] In women, androgen administration can produce hirsutism, hoarseness or deepening of the voice, and changes in the external genitalia (enlarged clitoris). Irregular menstrual periods and acne may also occur in women undergoing androgen therapy. In men, these drugs may produce bladder irritation, breast swelling and soreness, and frequent or prolonged erections. When used in children, androgens may cause accelerated sexual maturation and impairment of normal bone development due to premature closure of epiphyseal plates. Consequently, these drugs are used very cautiously in children.

The described adverse effects are related to the dose and duration of androgen use; problems are seen more frequently during prolonged androgen administration at relatively high doses. In adults, most of these adverse effects are reversible, and symptoms will diminish once the agent is discontinued. A few effects, however—such as vocal changes in females—may persist even after the drugs are withdrawn. Skeletal changes are irreversible, and permanent growth impairment may occur if these drugs are used in children.

As indicated earlier, androgens may increase the risk of prostate cancer, especially in older men who are susceptible to this disease.[106] Other side effects of long-term, high-dose androgen use include liver damage and hepatic carcinoma. Hypertension may occur because of the salt-retaining and water-retaining effects of these drugs, and androgens can adversely affect plasma lipids (increased total cholesterol, decreased levels of high density lipoproteins). Although these hepatic and cardiovascular problems may occur during therapeutic androgen use, their incidence is even more prevalent when extremely large doses of androgens are used to enhance athletic performance. The use and abuse of androgens in athletes are discussed later in "Androgen Abuse."

Antiandrogens

Antiandrogens are drugs that inhibit the synthesis or effects of endogenous androgen production.[144] These agents can be helpful in conditions such as prostate cancer and other conditions aggravated by excessive androgen production.[31,112] Specific antiandrogens affect endogenous male hormones in several different ways. Finasteride (Proscar) and dutasteride (Avodart) inhibit the conversion of testosterone to dihydrotestosterone. Dihydrotestosterone accelerates the growth and development of the prostate gland; these antiandrogens may be helpful in attenuating this effect in conditions such as benign prostate hypertrophy. Flutamide (Eulexin), bicalutamide (Casodex), and nilutamide (Nilandron) act as antagonists (blockers) of the cellular androgen receptor; these drugs are used to decrease hirsutism in women or to help treat prostate cancer.

Advanced prostate cancer is also treated with a number of drugs that mimic or block the effects of

GnRH. GnRH analogs include buserelin (Suprefact), goserelin (Zoladex), leuprolide (Lupron), and nafarelin (Synarel). When first administered, these agents cause an increase in pituitary LH release, which—in turn—stimulates testicular androgen production. However, continued administration of GnRH analogs desensitizes pituitary GnRH receptors, thus decreasing LH and testosterone production from the pituitary and testes, respectively.[89] A newer agent, abarelix (Plenaxis), directly antagonizes (blocks) the GnRH receptor on the pituitary.[144] This drug is especially helpful in certain patients because it will cause a more direct and immediate decrease in LH production compared to the GnRH analogs.

Androgen Abuse

Nature of Androgen Abuse

The use of androgens or anabolic steroids to increase athletic performance is an issue of controversy and concern. The fact that certain athletes self-administer large doses of androgens in an effort to increase muscle size and strength has been known for some time. Typically, androgen use is associated with athletes involved in strength and power activities such as weight lifting, bodybuilding, shot put, and the like. Androgen abuse, however, has infiltrated many aspects of athletic competition at both the amateur and professional levels. There also appears to be a contingent of men, women, and adolescents who are not athletes, but take anabolic steroids to increase lean body mass for cosmetic purposes; that is, these individuals take these drugs to simply appear more muscular.[37,47]

Individuals who admit to using anabolic steroids or who test positive for androgen abuse represent some of the top performers in their respective sports.[103] Also, the use of anabolic steroids among the general athletic population may be reaching alarming proportions, including younger athletes.[19] A comprehensive survey of male high school students indicated that over 6 percent had taken anabolic steroids at least once in their lifetime.[126] Clearly, androgen abuse is one of the major problems affecting the health and welfare of athletes of various ages and athletic pursuits.

Athletes engaging in androgen abuse usually obtain these drugs from various illicit but readily available sources.[155] Some examples of anabolic steroids that are used by athletes are listed in Table 30–2. These agents include testosterone, synthetic analogs of testosterone, and precursors that are converted to ana-

Table 30–2	EXAMPLES OF ANABOLIC ANDROGENS THAT ARE ABUSED BY ATHLETES

Generic Name	Trade Name
Orally active androgens	
Chlorodehydromethyltestosterone	Turinabol
Fluoxymesterone	Halotestin
Methandrostenolone	Dianabol
Methyl Testosterone	Android
Oxandrolone	Anavar
Oxymetholone	Anadrol
Stanozolol	Winstrol
Androgens administered by intramuscular injection	
Boldenone	Equipoise
Drostanolone	Masteron
Methenolone	Primobolan
Nandrolone decanoate	Deca-Durabolin
Stanozolol	Winstrol-V
Testosterone cypionate	
Testosterone enanthate	
Testosterone propionate	
Testosterone suspension	

Adapted from: Parkinson AB, Evans NA. Anabolic androgenic steroids: a survey of 500 users. *Med Sci Sports Exerc.* 2006; 38:644–651.

bolic substances within the body. In addition, several different androgens are often taken simultaneously for a combined dose that is 10 to 100 times greater than the therapeutic dose.[62,156] This "stacking" of different anabolic steroids often consists of combining oral and injectable forms of these drugs (see Table 30–2). Athletes often self-administer these drugs in cycles that last between 7 and 14 weeks, and the dosage of each drug is progressively increased during the cycle. An example of a dosing cycle using stacked anabolic steroids is shown in Table 30–3.

To help control anabolic steroid abuse, drug testing at the time of a specific competition has been instituted in many sports. To prevent detection, an athlete will employ a complex pattern of high-dosage androgen administration followed with washout periods. Washouts are scheduled a sufficient amount of time prior to the competition, thus allowing the drug to be eliminated from the body before testing. The practice of planned schedules can be negated to some extent, however, through randomized drug testing that subjects the athlete to testing at any point in the training period, as well as at the time of the competition.[103]

Two primary questions usually arise concerning anabolic steroids: do these agents really enhance athletic performance, and what are the adverse effects of androgen abuse? Definitive answers to these questions are difficult because of the illicit nature of androgen abuse and because of the ethical and legal problems of administering large doses of androgens to healthy ath-

Table 30–3	EXAMPLE OF A STEROID DOSING CYCLE USED DURING ANDROGEN ABUSE*

	Dosage (mg) Week							
Drug Name	*1*	*2*	*3*	*4*	*5*	*6*	*7*	*8*
Testosterone cypionate	200	400	600	1200	2400	4200	4200	4200
Nandrolone (Deca-Durabolin)	100	100	100	200	400	600	600	600
Oxymetholone (Anadrol)	100	150	200	250	300	500	750	1000
Methandrostenolone (Dianabol)	25	30	35	50	60	75	100	125
Methandrostenolone (Dianabol injectable)	25	25	50	50	100	100	100	100
Oxandrolone (Anavar)	25	30	35	50	50	50	50	50

*This regimen was used by a bodybuilder who went through three cycles each year for 8 years. The subject also reported taking 600 mg of testosterone per week between cycles. This subject ultimately developed avascular necrosis in both femoral heads.
Source: From Pettine, p 96, with permission.[118]

letes as part of controlled research studies. The effects of androgens on athletic performance and the potential adverse effects of these drugs are discussed briefly here.

Effects of Androgens on Athletic Performance

There is little doubt that androgens can promote skeletal muscle growth and increase strength in people who do not synthesize meaningful amounts of endogenous androgens (women, prepubescent males). The question has often been whether large amounts of exogenous androgens can increase muscle size, strength, and athletic performance in healthy men. In general, it appears that athletic men taking androgens during strength training may experience greater increments in lean body mass and muscle strength than athletes training without androgens.[47,50,64] The extent of the increase, however, will vary considerably depending on the dosage and type of androgens used.[6,64]

It also remains unclear what magnitude of any strength gains can be directly attributed to anabolic steroids. For instance, the anabolic effects of steroids cannot be isolated easily from the other factors that produce increments in strength and muscle size (e.g., weight training). In particular, androgens appear to increase aggressiveness, and individuals taking these drugs may train longer and more intensely than athletes who are not taking them.[63] Consequently, strength increments in the athlete taking androgens may be brought about by the enhanced quality and quantity of training rather than as a direct effect of anabolic steroids on muscle protein synthesis.

Thus, the effects of androgens on athletic performance in men remain unclear. It seems probable that high dosages of androgens would increase muscle size and strength, which might ultimately translate to improved athletic performance.[64] Nonetheless, we may never know the exact ergogenic effects of these drugs in men because of the illicit nature of androgen abuse and the ethical problems involved in performing clinical studies of these drugs in humans.[64,87]

Adverse Effects of Androgen Abuse

Virtually any drugs that are taken at extremely high dosages can be expected to produce serious side effects. Exactly how harmful androgen abuse is in an athletic population remains somewhat uncertain, however.[64] The illicit nature of androgen abuse and the various dosage regimens have made it difficult to determine the precise incidence and type of adverse effects.[64] Also, the long-term effects of androgen abuse may not be known for some time; that is, pathologies may not be fully realized until several years after the drugs are discontinued.[50,117] Nonetheless, there is considerable evidence, often in the form of individual reports and case studies, that androgen abuse can have severe and possibly fatal consequences. Some of the more common adverse effects associated with androgen administration are presented below. Further discussion of the potential adverse effects in athletes can be found in several reviews listed at the end of this chapter.[50,64,99,117]

High doses of androgens can produce liver damage, including the formation of hepatic tumors and peliosis hepatis (blood-filled cysts within the liver).[17,99,145] In some individuals, these liver abnormalities have proved fatal. Androgens can also produce detrimental changes in cardiac structure and function that result in cardiomyopathy, ischemic heart disease, arrhythmias, and heart failure.[48,157] Furthermore, these hormones pose additional cardiovascular risks by producing unfavorable changes in blood lipid profiles, such as decreased high-density lipoprotein cholesterol levels.[6,99] These effects on plasma lipids predispose the athlete to atherosclerotic lesions and subsequent vessel occlusion, and specific cases of stroke and myocardial infarction in athletes using androgens have been attributed to the atherogenic effects of these drugs.[48,64] Androgens also cause hypertension because of direct effects on the myocardium and because of the salt- and water-retaining properties of these drugs.[99] Problems with glucose metabolism brought about by insulin resistance have also been reported.[24]

Androgens can affect bone metabolism, and avascular necrosis of the femoral heads has been documented in a weight lifter using these drugs.[118] Androgens also accelerate closure of epiphyseal plates and can lead to impaired skeletal growth in young children. This effect on skeletal development is important because athletes may begin to self-administer anabolic steroids at a relatively young age (i.e., prior to age 16).[19] As previously mentioned, androgens may produce behavioral changes, including increased aggression, leading to radical mood swings and violent episodes in some individuals.[99,103,116]

Androgens can produce changes in reproductive function and secondary sexual characteristics. In males, high levels of androgens act as negative feedback and lead to testicular atrophy and impaired sperm production. Infertility in males may result because of an inability to form sperm (*azoospermia*).[75,93] In females, androgens produce certain masculinizing effects, such as an increase in body hair, a deepening of the voice, and changes in the external genitalia. Androgens may also impair the normal female reproductive (menstrual) cycle. Some changes in male and female sexual and reproductive function appear to be reversible, but changes such as male infertility and azoospermia may take 4 months or longer to return to normal.[75] Other effects, such as vocal changes in females, may be permanent.

In summary, anabolic steroids may produce some ergogenic benefits in a limited subset of athletes, but rather serious consequences may occur. Nonetheless, athletes may be so driven to succeed that the adverse effects are disregarded. Also, athletes may suspect that their competitors are using steroids and feel that they must also take these drugs to remain competitive. Clearly, there is a need for governing agencies to try to eliminate the illicit use of these substances from athletic competition. Health care professionals can also discourage androgen abuse by informing athletes that the risks of androgen abuse exceed any potential benefits.[154]

Estrogen and Progesterone

In women, the ovaries produce two major categories of steroid hormones: estrogens and progestins. The primary estrogen produced in humans is *estradiol*, and the primary progestin is *progesterone*. For simplicity, the terms *estrogen* and *progesterone* will be used to indicate these two primary forms of female hormones. Small amounts of male hormones (androgens) are also produced by the ovaries, and these androgens may play a role in the development of some secondary sexual characteristics in the female during puberty, for example, increased body hair and growth spurts. Nonetheless, the hormones exerting the major influence on sexual development and reproduction in the female are estrogen and progesterone. The physiologic effects of these hormones are presented here.

Effects of Estrogen and Progesterone on Sexual Maturation

Estrogen and progesterone play a primary role in promoting sexual differentiation in the developing female fetus. These hormones also become important in completing female sexual maturation during puberty. At the onset of puberty, a complex series of hormonal events stimulates the ovaries to begin producing estrogen and progesterone. Ovarian production of these hormones initiates the maturation of reproductive function and development of secondary sexual characteristics in the female.

Estrogen is the primary hormone that initiates the growth and development of the female reproductive system during puberty. Changes in the external genitalia and maturation of the internal reproductive organs (e.g., uterus, oviducts, vagina) are primarily brought about by the influence of estrogen. Estrogen also produces several other characteristic changes in females, such as breast development, deposition of subcutaneous fat stores, and changes in the skeletal system (for example, closure of epiphyseal plates, widening of the pelvic girdle). Progesterone is less important in sexual maturation and is involved to a greater extent in facilitating and maintaining pregnancy.

Regulation and Effects of Hormonal Synthesis During the Menstrual Cycle

In the nonpregnant, postpubescent female, production of estrogen and progesterone is not tonic in nature but follows a pattern or cycle of events commonly referred to as the *menstrual cycle*. The menstrual cycle usually occurs over a 28-day period. The primary function of this cycle is to stimulate the ovaries to produce an ovum that is available for fertilization, while simultaneously preparing the endometrium of the uterus for implantation of the ovum, should fertilization occur. These events are illustrated in Figure 30–2. The cycle is characterized by several specific phases and events that are briefly outlined below. A more detailed description of the regulation of female reproduction can be found in several sources listed at the end of this chapter.[33,88,94,113]

Follicular Phase. The first half of the menstrual cycle is influenced by hormonal release from a developing ovarian follicle, hence the term "follicular phase." In the follicular phase, the anterior pituitary releases FSH. As its name implies, FSH stimulates the maturation of several follicles within the ovary. Usually, one such follicle undergoes full maturation and ultimately yields an ovum. Because of the effect of FSH, the developing follicle also begins to secrete increasing amounts of estrogen. Estrogen produced by the ovarian follicle causes proliferation and thickening of the endometrial lining of the uterus. The follicular phase is also referred to as the proliferative phase.

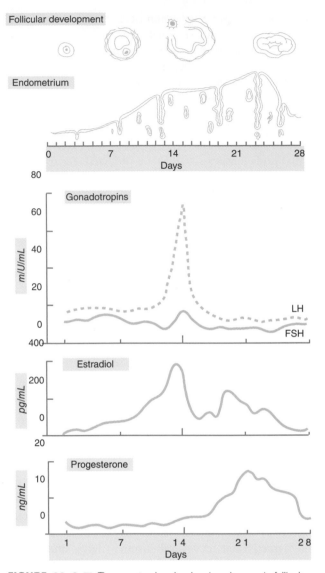

FIGURE 30–2 ▼ The menstrual cycle, showing changes in follicular development, uterine endometrium, pituitary gonadotropins (LH, FSH), and ovarian hormones. (*From:* Katzung BG. *Basic and Clinical Pharmacology.* 9th ed. New York: Lange Medical Books/McGraw-Hill; 2004: 662. Reproduced with permission of the McGraw-Hill Companies.)

Endometrial vascularization is also increased, and glandular structures begin to develop in the uterine wall. The uterine glands, however, do not begin to function (secrete mucus) to any great extent during the follicular phase.

Ovulation. Just prior to the cycle's midpoint, the anterior pituitary secretes a sudden, large burst of LH. A smaller burst of FSH secretion also occurs around the midpoint of the cycle, as shown in Figure 30–2.

The LH surge is the primary impetus for ovulation. During ovulation, the mature follicle ruptures, releasing the ovum from the ovary. At this point, the ovum should begin to travel toward the uterus via the fallopian tubes. The ruptured follicle remains in the ovary and continues to play a vital role in the reproductive cycle. After releasing the ovum, the follicle becomes infiltrated with lipids and is referred to as the *corpus luteum* (yellow body). The role of the corpus luteum is described next.

Luteal Phase. The *luteal phase* refers to the fact that the corpus luteum governs the events in the second half of the menstrual cycle. In response to the residual effects of the LH-FSH surge, the corpus luteum continues to grow and develop for approximately 1 week after ovulation. During this time, the corpus luteum secretes both estrogen and progesterone. The combined effects of estrogen and progesterone cause further thickening in the uterine lining, as well as an increase in the vascularization and glandular secretion of the endometrium. During the luteal phase, progesterone is the primary stimulus that causes the uterine glands to fully develop and secrete a mucous substance that provides a favorable environment for implantation of the fertilized egg. Hence, the luteal phase is also referred to as the *secretory phase* because of the enhanced function of the uterine glands.

Corpus Luteum Regression and Termination of the Cycle. If the egg is not fertilized or implantation does not occur, the corpus luteum begins to regress, primarily because of a lack of continued support for the corpus luteum from the pituitary gonadotropins (LH, FSH). Because the corpus luteum regresses, it can no longer produce adequate amounts of estrogen and progesterone to maintain the endometrium of the uterus. Consequently, the endometrium begins to slough off, creating the menstrual bleeding that typifies the female reproductive cycle. The onset of menstrual bleeding marks the end of one reproductive cycle and the beginning of the next.

In summary, the menstrual cycle is primarily regulated by the interaction between pituitary and ovarian hormones. Also, releasing hormones from the hypothalamus plays a role in controlling female reproduction through their effects on LH and FSH release from the anterior pituitary.[7] A complex series of positive and negative feedback mechanisms control the cyclic release of various female hormones.[22,81,97] For instance, increased estrogen secretion in the follicular phase stimulates the LH surge that evokes ovulation. This event is considered an example of positive feedback because low estrogen levels increase LH release, which further increases estrogen secretion, thus further increasing LH release, and so on. Conversely, secretion of the pituitary gonadotropins (LH, FSH) is inhibited toward the latter part of the luteal phase, presumably because of the negative feedback influence of high levels of estrogen and progesterone.

Pharmacologic intervention can take advantage of these complex feedback systems in certain situations. Most notable is the use of estrogen and progesterone as hormonal contraceptives. By altering the normal control between pituitary and ovarian hormones and uterine function, preparations containing these two steroids are an effective means of birth control. The pharmacologic use of female hormones is discussed in more detail in "Pharmacologic Use of Estrogen and Progesterone."

Female Hormones in Pregnancy and Parturition

Estrogen and progesterone also play a significant role in pregnancy and childbirth. For successful implantation and gestation of the fertilized egg to occur, synthesis of these two steroids must be maintained to prevent the onset of menstruation. As just mentioned, menstruation begins when the corpus luteum is no longer able to produce sufficient estrogen and progesterone to sustain the endometrium. When fertilization does occur, however, some hormonal response must transpire to maintain steroid production from the corpus luteum and to ensure that the endometrium remains ready for implantation. This response is caused by the release of human chorionic gonadotropin (HCG) from the fertilized ovum. HCG takes over the role of LH and rescues the corpus luteum from destruction.[82,133] The corpus luteum then continues to produce steroids (especially progesterone), which maintain the uterine lining in a suitable state for implantation and gestation of the fertilized egg.

Eventually, the corpus luteum does begin to degenerate between the 9th and 14th week of gestation. By that point, the placenta has assumed estrogen and progesterone production. Generally speaking, maternal progesterone helps to maintain the uterus and placenta throughout the rest of the pregnancy. Progesterone also increases the growth and develop-ment of the maternal mammary glands in preparation for lactation. Although the role of estrogen is less clear, increased estrogen production may play a pivotal part in setting the stage for parturition. Clearly, both steroids are needed for normal birth and delivery.

Pharmacologic Use of Estrogen and Progesterone

The most frequent and prevalent use of the female hormones is in contraceptive preparations (see "Hormonal Contraceptives"). The other primary indications for estrogen and progesterone are replacement of endogenous hormone production and subsequent resolution of symptoms related to hormonal deficiencies. This replacement can be especially important following menopause—that is, when the female reproductive cycle ceases and the associated cyclic production of the ovarian hormones ends. Specific clinical conditions that may be resolved by estrogen and progesterone are listed below.

Conditions Treated with Estrogen and Progesterone

Replacement Therapy. Estrogen and progesterone are often used to replace the endogenous production of hormones following menopause or in women who have had an ovariectomy. Hormone replacement therapy—that is, the replacement of both estrogen and progesterone, or the replacement of only estrogen—has been used in certain women to control perimenopausal and postmenopausal symptoms such as atrophic vaginitis, atrophic dystrophy of the vulva, and vasomotor effects such as hot flashes.[46,90,151] Likewise, there is little doubt that estrogens are essential in preventing and treating postmenopausal osteoporosis.[28,92,148] Women receiving hormone replacements with estrogen are able to maintain or increase bone mineral density, and estrogen replacement is often associated with a decreased incidence of vertebral fractures and other osteoporosis-related problems.[25,53,92] Estrogen can also be combined with other interventions such as calcium supplements, physical activity, and other medications (see Chapter 31) to provide optimal protection against osteoporosis following menopause.[28,78]

Nonetheless, the benefits of estrogen or hormone replacement therapy must be balanced against the potential risks of these interventions (see "Adverse Effects of Estrogen and Progesterone," later). Certain benefits that previously were reported from observational studies have been challenged recently by randomized controlled trials carefully investigating the effects of hormonal replacement.[11,127] For example, low doses of estrogen cause favorable changes in plasma lipid profiles (decreased levels of low-density lipoproteins and increased levels of high-density lipoproteins), and it was thought that the beneficial effects on plasma lipoproteins might decrease the risk of atherosclerotic lesions and reduce the incidence of coronary heart disease in postmenopausal women.[121,134,160] The idea that estrogen replacement offers protection against coronary heart disease was challenged somewhat by a study known as the Heart and Estrogen/Progesterone Replacement Study (HERS).[74] According to the HERS findings, estrogen combined with progesterone did not decrease the incidence of infarction and death in postmenopausal women with a history of coronary heart disease.[74] In addition, the Women's Health Initiative (WHI)—a large, randomized controlled trial—failed to find a beneficial effect on the incidence of coronary heart disease in postmenopausal women receiving estrogen replacement.[3,134]

Hence, it appears that hormone replacement can play a role in modifying certain risk factors associated with coronary heart disease in postmenopausal women, but the actual outcomes (heart attack, death) do not seem to be affected significantly by these hormonal interventions. Clearly, continued research in this area is needed to clarify if hormone replacement therapy can help decrease cardiac morbidity and mortality in certain postmenopausal women.[60,121]

Finally, it has been suggested that estrogen replacement may offer some protection against cognitive decline in conditions such as Alzheimer disease and other forms of dementia.[65,96] Estrogen may, for example, have several neuroprotective effects, including the ability to decrease free radical–induced damage, sustain cholinergic function in the brain, and inhibit the neuronal degeneration associated with Alzheimer disease.[73] Conclusive evidence of the beneficial effects, however, is lacking.[11,65] On the contrary, there is some evidence that estrogen replacement may increase the incidence of dementia in older postmenopausal women.[65,138] Estrogen replacement is therefore not currently accepted as standard treatment for Alzheimer disease, and additional studies are needed to determine the exact relationship between hormone replacement therapy and dementia in older women.

Hypogonadism. Estrogens, or a combination of estrogen and progesterone, may be used to treat abnormally low ovarian function. Appropriate use of these hormones induces the uterine changes and cyclic bleeding associated with the normal female reproductive cycle.

Failure of Ovarian Development. Occasionally, the ovaries fail to undergo normal development because of hypopituitarism or other disorders. Estrogens may be given at the time of puberty to encourage development of secondary sexual characteristics (e.g., breast development).

Menstrual Irregularities. Various problems with normal menstruation are treated by estrogen and progesterone. These hormones are used either separately or are combined to resolve amenorrhea, dysmenorrhea, and other types of functional uterine bleeding that are caused by a hormonal imbalance.

Endometriosis. Endometriosis is a condition characterized by growths of uterinelike tissue that occur at various locations within the pelvic cavity. Progesterone and estrogen-progesterone combinations help suppress bleeding from these tissues and may help shrink the size of these growths.

Carcinoma. Estrogen has been used to treat metastatic breast cancer in men and postmenopausal women. Advanced prostate cancer in men may also respond to estrogen treatment. Progesterone is helpful in treating uterine cancer and several other types of metastases, such as breast, renal, and endometrial carcinoma.

Specific Agents

Therapeutically used types of estrogens and progestins are listed in Tables 30–4 and 30–5. Both types of hormones can be administered in their natural form (estradiol and progesterone), and several synthetic derivatives of each type are also available. Most of the drugs listed in Tables 30–4 and 30–5 are available as oral preparations, and many conditions can be conveniently treated by oral administration. These hormones may also be administered transdermally via patches, creams, or gels; the transdermal route may offer certain advantages, such as decreased side effects and liver problems.[86,130] Certain preparations can be

Table 30–4	CLINICAL USE OF ESTROGENS	
Generic Name	**Trade Name(s)**	**Primary Indication(s)**
Dienestrol	Ortho Dienestrol	Estrogen replacement (vaginal)
Estradiol	Depo-Estradiol, Estrace, Estraderm, Vivelle, many others	Estrogen replacement, antineoplastic, prevention of osteoporosis
Conjugated estrogens	Premarin	Estrogen replacement, antineoplastic, prevention of osteoporosis, prevention of abnormal uterine bleeding
Esterified estrogens	Menest	Estrogen replacement, antineoplastic, prevention of osteoporosis
Estrone	Estro-A, Estragyn, others	Estrogen replacement, antineoplastic, prevention of abnormal uterine bleeding
Estropipate	Ogen, Ortho-Est	Estrogen replacement, prevention of osteoporosis
Ethinyl estradiol	Estinyl	Estrogen replacement, antineoplastic

Table 30–5	CLINICAL USE OF PROGESTINS	
Generic Name	**Trade Name(s)**	**Primary Indication(s)**
Hydroxyprogesterone	Hylutin, Prodrox, others	Amenorrhea, dysfunctional uterine bleeding
Levonorgestrel	Norplant	Contraception
Medroxyprogesterone	Cycrin, Provera, others	Secondary amenorrhea, dysfunctional uterine bleeding, breast or endometrial carcinoma
Megestrol	Megace	Breast or endometrial carcinoma, advanced prostate cancer, anorexia/cachexia
Norethindrone	Aygestin, Micronor, others	Secondary amenorrhea, dysfunctional uterine bleeding, endometriosis
Norgestrel	Ovrette	Contraception
Progesterone	Gesterol, Prometrium, others	Secondary amenorrhea, dysfunctional uterine bleeding

administered by vaginal suppositories, and vaginal administration can be helpful in treating dysfunction of the endometrium of the uterus.[23,86] Finally, several preparations are also available for injection, and parenteral routes may be used in some situations, such as severe uterine bleeding.

Adverse Effects of Estrogen and Progesterone

Cardiovascular disease is a primary risk factor during estrogen and progesterone therapy. Higher doses or prolonged exposure to estrogen has been associated with serious cardiovascular problems, including myocardial infarction, stroke, and thromboembolism.[140,160] These problems are significant when relatively large doses are administered to men for the treatment of breast and prostate cancer. Cardiovascular disease, however, can also occur in women receiving estrogen or estrogen combined with progesterone as hormone replacement therapy. In particular, an increased risk of stroke was documented in postmenopausal women who were treated with estrogen compared to a placebo during the WHI trial.[3,16] Other cardiovascular problems (myocardial infarction, venous thrombosis) are also risk factors, especially in women with atherosclerosis or other factors that accelerate blood clotting.[41,102]

The primary problems associated with progesterone also involve abnormal blood clotting, which may lead to thrombophlebitis, pulmonary embolism, and cerebral infarction.[5] Progesterone may alter the normal menstrual cycle, leading to unpredictable changes in the bleeding pattern. The adverse effects of progesterone, however, may vary depending on the exact type of progesterone administered.[141,142]

Hormonal therapies are also associated with an increased risk of certain cancers, but the carcinogenic potential of estrogen and progesterone replacement is not completely clear. Estrogen replacement, for example, may increase the risk of ovarian and endometrial cancers in certain postmenopausal women, but this risk seems to depend on many other factors including the patient's age, additional cancer risks, prolonged use of estrogen, and concomitant use of progesterone.[4] Regarding breast cancer, there is little doubt that certain breast cancers are estrogen sensitive, and that estrogen replacement is contraindicated in women with these cancers. However, the risk of developing new breast cancer during hormone therapy is difficult to determine. Some evidence suggests that hormone replacement therapy (estrogen combined with progesterone) may slightly increase the risk of breast cancer.[26,36] Other reports, including the WHI, suggest that estrogen replacement in postmenopausal women does not increase the risk of breast cancer, and may even confer a slight reduction in the risk of such cancers.[3] Clearly, more research is needed to clarify the effects of hormonal therapies on various types of cancer.

Finally, therapeutic use of estrogen and progesterone may cause nausea, which is usually transient. Swelling of the feet and ankles may also occur because of sodium and water retention.

Selective Estrogen Receptor Modulators

Selective estrogen receptor modulators (SERMs) bind to and activate estrogen receptors on certain tissues, while blocking the effects of estrogen on other tissues.[29,129] Specifically, these agents activate estrogen receptors on bone and vascular tissues (including plasma lipids) while acting as estrogen antagonists (blockers) on uterine and breast tissues. SERMs therefore have the obvious advantage of producing favorable effects on bone mineralization and cardiovascular function while reducing the potential carcinogenic effects of estrogen on breast and uterine tissues.

Tamoxifen (Nolvadex) was the first SERM developed for clinical use; this drug is approved for the prevention and treatment of breast cancer because it has strong antiestrogen effects on breast tissues. The anticancer effect is achieved while simultaneously stimulating other estrogen receptors that help maintain bone mineral density and improve cardiovascular function and plasma lipid profiles.[29,104] Tamoxifen, however, does not completely block estrogen receptors on uterine tissues, and this drug may actually stimulate endometrial proliferation and increase the incidence of uterine cancers.[29,95,111] Likewise, this agent may lower the risk factors associated with cardiovascular disease (plasma lipid profile, vascular reactivity); however, the risk of venous thromboembolism may be increased somewhat.[15] Tamoxifen can also produce symptoms that mimic estrogen withdrawal (hot flashes, vaginitis), especially when this drug is first administered to women. These symptoms often diminish, however, with continued use.

More recently, another SERM, known as raloxifene (Evista), was developed. Raloxifene is similar to tamoxifen except that it blocks estrogen receptors on breast *and* uterine tissues and may therefore produce beneficial effects (inhibiting breast cancer, improving bone and cardiovascular function) without increasing the risk of endometrial cancers.[30,51,57] Raloxifene is currently approved for treating osteoporosis, and the use of this drug is associated with increased vertebral bone density and a reduced risk of vertebral fractures.[30,77]

As indicated, raloxifene may also reduce the incidence of breast and uterine cancers.[20,57] This drug may cause several bothersome side effects, including hot flashes, joint or muscle pain, depression, insomnia, and gastrointestinal disturbances. More serious problems with raloxifene may be indicated by symptoms such as chest pain, flulike syndrome, leg cramping, venous thromboembolism, skin rash, and cystitis or urinary tract infections.

Efforts continue to develop other SERMs that will capitalize on the beneficial effects of estrogen while minimizing or even reducing the carcinogenic effects of estrogen on other tissues. As newer agents are developed, SERMs may have an expanded role in the treatment of various diseases and perhaps provide a safer and more effective method of estrogen replacement.[54,59]

Antiestrogens

In addition to the SERMs, a limited number of drugs directly antagonize all the effects of estrogen and are considered to be true antiestrogens. These antiestrogens appear to bind to estrogen receptors in the cytosol but do not cause any subsequent changes in cellular function. Hence, these drugs block the effects of estrogen by occupying the estrogen receptor and preventing estrogen from exerting a response. Clomiphene (Clomid, Serophene) is an antiestrogen that is sometimes administered to women to treat infertility.[8,72] The mechanism of clomiphene as a fertility drug is somewhat complex. Relatively high levels of estrogen normally produce an inhibitory or negative feedback effect on the release of pituitary gonadotropins (LH and FSH). As an antiestrogen, clomiphene blocks this inhibitory effect, thus facilitating gonadotropin release.[72] Increased gonadotropins (especially LH) promote ovulation, thus improving the chance of fertilization. The primary adverse effects associated with clomiphene are vascular hot flashes. Enlarged ovaries may also occur because of the stimulatory effect of increased gonadotropin release.

More recently, fulvestrant (Faslodex) was introduced as an antiestrogen. This drug binds to and blocks estrogen receptors, and may also result in the receptors' degradation.[42,58] Hence, fulvestrant is used to treat estrogen-sensitive breast cancers.[27,58] This drug is administered monthly by intramuscular injection, and some redness and irritation can occur at the injection site. Other common side effects include gastrointestinal symptoms (nausea, vomiting, loss of appetite) and vasomotor symptoms (hot flashes).

Antiprogestins

Agents that specifically block progesterone receptors were first developed in the early 1980s.[94] The primary clinical application of these drugs is the termination of pregnancy; that is, these drugs can be used to induce abortion during the early stages of gestation. Because progesterone is largely responsible for sustaining the placenta and fetus, the blockade of progesterone receptors in the uterus negates the effects of this hormone, with subsequent detachment of the placenta and loss of placental hormones such as human chorionic gonadotropin. Detachment of the placenta from the uterine lining results in loss of the fetus and termination of the pregnancy.

The primary antiprogestin is mifepristone, known also as RU486. This drug can be administered orally during the first 7 weeks of pregnancy, with abortion typically occurring within the next 2 to 3 days. To stimulate uterine contraction and ensure complete expulsion of the detached embryo, a prostaglandin analog such as misoprostol or prostaglandin E_1 is typically administered orally or intravaginally 48 hours after mifepristone administration.[135] This regimen of mifepristone followed by a prostaglandin agent is successful in terminating pregnancy in approximately 95 percent of cases.[135]

Mifepristone has been used as an abortive agent in China and parts of Europe for some time, and this drug recently received FDA approval for use in the United States. This drug is marketed in the United States under the trade name Mifeprex. When used to induce abortion, the primary physical side effects of mifepristone are excessive uterine bleeding and cramping, although these side effects may be related more to the use of prostaglandins following mifepristone treatment.[94] The chance of incomplete abortion must also be considered, and a follow-up physician visit approximately 2 weeks after administration is needed to ensure that the pregnancy was terminated.

Consequently, the major focus on this drug at present is its potential for use in terminating pregnancy. In the future, mifepristone may also be used for other reasons. This drug could, for example, have contraceptive potential because it prevents ovulation and blocks the effects of progesterone on endometrial proliferation and vascularization, thus rendering the endometrium less favorable for implantation of the fertilized egg. Mifepristone may likewise be useful as a "morning after" pill to prevent conception after unprotected sex (see "Types of Contraceptive Preparations," later).[55,132] In addition to its effects on progesterone receptors, mifepristone can also block cellular glucocorticoid receptors; the clinical significance of this effect remains to be explored.[18] Finally, mifepristone may be useful in treating certain growths and tumors that are exacerbated by progesterone, including endometriosis, leiomyoma, meningioma, and breast cancer.[94] It will be interesting to see how this drug is ultimately used to prevent or terminate pregnancy and perhaps manage progesterone-related diseases as well.

Hormonal Contraceptives

During the 1960s, oral contraceptives containing estrogens and progestins were approved for use in preventing pregnancy. The introduction of these birth control pills provided a relatively easy and effective method of contraception. Today, oral contraceptives are taken routinely by many women of child-bearing age, and these drugs are among the most commonly prescribed medications in the United States and throughout the world.[94] Hormonal alternatives to oral contraceptives are also gaining popularity, and administration of various compounds by injection, transdermal patch, subcutaneous implants, vaginal inserts, and intrauterine devices are now available. These agents are addressed below.

Types of Contraceptive Preparations

The most common form of hormonal preparation is the oral contraceptive or "birth control pill," which typically contains a fixed amount of estrogen and progesterone in the same pill. Examples of some common estrogen-progestin contraceptives are listed in Table 30–6. When taken appropriately, these preparations appear to be 99 to 100 percent effective in preventing pregnancy.[94] Typically, the contraceptive pill is taken each day for 3 weeks, beginning at the onset of menstruation. This intake is followed by 1 week in which either no pill or a "blank" pill that lacks the hormones is taken. For convenience and improved adherence, these preparations are usually packaged in some form of dispenser that encourages the user to remember to take one pill each day.

More recently, a variation on the length of the oral contraceptive cycle was introduced in which women take the active form of the pill for 84 days, and then take a 7-day placebo.[66,70] This provides a 3-month cycle before menstruation, thus reducing the number of menstrual periods to only 4 per year. These long cycle regimens seem to be as effective as the more traditional (monthly) cycle regimens, although the longer cycles may cause more unscheduled bleeding or "spotting," especially during the first few cycles.[2,66,110] Still, long cycle regimens may be preferred by some women because they offer the convenience of fewer periods and menstrual symptoms (cramps, etc.).[43,161]

Contraceptive hormones can also be administered via nonoral routes. A contraceptive patch containing ethinyl estradiol (an estrogen) and norelgestromin (a progestin) can be applied to the skin once a week, to allow the slow, transdermal administration of these hormones.[49,79] A vaginal ring is also available as an alternative to the oral contraceptive pill.[131] This ring typically contains estrogen and progesterone, and these hormones are released slowly into the vagina and local tissues following insertion. The ring is inserted vaginally for 3 weeks, and then removed for one week to allow menstruation (i.e., mimic the normal uterine cycle).[67] Transdermal patches and vaginal rings are similar to oral contraceptives in terms of effectiveness and side effects.[119] The primary advantages of the nonoral routes are increased convenience and adherence to the contraceptive regimen; that is, the use of patches or a vaginal ring can be very helpful in women who sometimes forget to take a pill every day.[49,76]

Other versions of oral contraceptives are available that contain only a progestin (norethindrone, norgestrel; see Table 30–6). These "minipills" were developed to avoid the adverse effects normally attributed to estrogen. Progestin-only minipills are somewhat less attractive as an oral contraceptive because these preparations are only about 97 to 98 percent effective and because they tend to cause irregular and unpredictable menstrual cycles. An implantable form of a progestin-only preparation (Norplant) has also been developed, whereby small, semipermeable tubes containing levonorgestrel are inserted subcutaneously in the arm.[56,143] The progestin is delivered in a slow, continuous fashion, allowing effective contraception for up to 5 years. These implants appear to have contraceptive efficacy that is better than progestin-only pills and is only slightly less effective than combined estrogen-progestin oral contraceptives. Progestin-only implants can be replaced at the end of 5 years to continue this method of contraception, or they can be removed at any time because of side effects or other reasons. There is likewise a form of progesterone (Depo Provera) that can be administered by

Table 30-6	HORMONAL CONTRACEPTIVES	

Estrogen Component	Progestin Component	Common Trade Name(s)
Oral Contraceptives		
Ethinyl estradiol	Desogestrel	Desogen, Mircette, others
Ethinyl estradiol	Ethynodiol diacetate	Demulen, Zovia
Ethinyl estradiol	Levonorgestrel	Levlen, Nordette, Triphasil, others
Ethinyl estradiol	Norethindrone acetate	Loestrin
Ethinyl estradiol	Norethindrone	Brevicon, Genora 1/35, Ortho-Novum 10/11, many others
Ethinyl estradiol	Norgestimate	Ortho-Cyclen, others
Ethinyl estradiol	Norgestrel	Lo/Ovral, Ovral
Mestranol	Norethindrone	Genora 1/50, Norinyl 1+50, Ortho-Novum 1/50, others
NA*	Norethindrone	Micronor, Nor-Q.D.
NA*	Norgestrel	Ovrette
Nonoral contraceptives		
Ethinyl estradiol	Norelgestromin	Ortho Evra (transdermal patch)
Ethinyl estradiol	Etonogestrel	NuvaRing (vaginal ring)
NA*	Levonorgestrel	Norplant (subcutaneous implants)
NA*	Medroxyprogesterone	Depo-Provera (intramuscular injection)

*NA = Not applicable; these products contain only progesterone.

deep intramuscular injection every 12 weeks.[137] Also, an intrauterine device has been developed that slowly releases a progestin within the uterus.[79,137] These implantable and injectable forms of progesterone therefore offer alternatives to women who cannot tolerate estrogen-progesterone pills or who have difficulty adhering to traditional oral contraceptive regimens.

Oral contraceptives that contain various hormones are sometimes used to prevent conception following sexual intercourse, especially in specific situations such as rape or unprotected sex. These post-coital interventions, or "morning-after pills," typically consist of a high dose of a natural or synthetic estrogen, a progestin such as levonorgestrel, or estrogen combined with a progestin (e.g., ethinyl estradiol combined with norgestrel). The exact mechanism of these morning-after pills is not known, but they appear to somehow interfere with ovulation or make the endometrium less favorable to implantation.[122] As indicated earlier, mifepristone can be used as a morning-after pill because this drug inhibits ovulation and blocks progesterone receptors in the uterus, thereby negating the effects of progesterone on the endometrium and developing placenta.[55] Hence, several options exist for preventing pregnancy after a specific incidence of sexual intercourse. Although these pills can be helpful in emergency situations, they are not meant to be an alternative to traditional birth control methods.

Mechanism of Contraceptive Action

Hormonal contraceptives exert their effects primarily by inhibiting ovulation and impairing the normal development of the uterine endometrium.[94,122] As discussed previously, the normal menstrual cycle is governed by the complex interaction between endogenous ovarian hormones and the pituitary gonadotropins. High levels of estrogen and progesterone in the bloodstream act as negative feedback and inhibit the release of LH and FSH from the anterior pituitary. Hormonal contraceptives maintain fairly high plasma levels of estrogen and progestin, thus limiting the release of LH and FSH through this negative feedback system. Because ovulation is normally caused by the midcycle LH surge (see Fig. 30–2), inhibition of LH release prevents ovulation. This event prevents an ovum from being made available for fertilization.

The estrogen and progestin supplied by the contraceptive also affect the development of the uterine lining. These hormones promote a certain amount of growth and proliferation of the uterine endometrium. The endometrium, however, does not develop to quite the same extent or in quite the same manner as it would if it were controlled by normal endogenous hormonal release. Consequently, the endometrial environment is less than optimal for implantation, even if ovulation and fertilization should take place. Also, there is an increase in the thickness and viscosity of the mucous secretions in the uterine cervix, thus impeding the passage of sperm through the cervical region, which adds to these preparations' contraceptive efficacy.

Through the effects on the endometrium, traditional contraceptive regimens can be used to mimic a normal menstrual flow. When the contraceptive hormones are withdrawn, the endometrium undergoes a sloughing similar to that in the normal cycle. Of course, the endometrium is being regulated by the exogenous hormones rather than the estrogen and progesterone normally produced by the ovaries. Still, this method of administration and withdrawal can produce a more or less normal pattern of uterine

activity, with the exception that chances of conception are dramatically reduced.

Adverse Effects of Hormonal Contraceptives

Although hormonal contraceptives provide an easy and effective means of birth control, their use has been limited somewhat by potentially serious side effects. In particular, contraceptive medications have been associated with cardiovascular problems such as thrombophlebitis, stroke, and myocardial infarction.[153] The incidence of these adverse effects, however, seems to depend to a large extent on whether the user has other risk factors associated with cardiovascular disease (smoking cigarettes, hyperlipidemia, hypertension, and so forth).[84,120,162] Likewise, cardiovascular risks may be diminished with the newer forms of hormonal contraceptives, which contain relatively less estrogen than their predecessors.

Over the years, the amount of estrogen contained in the combined estrogen-progesterone preparations has been reduced without sacrificing the contraceptive efficacy of these drugs.[164] The lower estrogen content theoretically reduces the risk of cardiovascular problems, although scientific studies have not been able to conclusively link the decreased risk of cardiovascular incidents with a decrease in estrogen content in contraceptive products.[52,153] Likewise, the newer hormonal contraceptives tend to contain progestins that have less androgenic properties; these newer progestins may help reduce the risk of cardiovascular complications.[9,14] This does not mean that hormonal contraceptives are devoid of cardiovascular side effects. These agents clearly have the potential to impair normal hemostasis and lead to venous thromboembolism, myocardial infarction, and stroke.[80,120] This risk is relatively modest, however, if modern estrogen-progesterone preparations are taken by relatively healthy young women.[120] Still, hormonal contraceptives should probably not be used by women with any preexisting cardiovascular problems (hypertension, recurrent thrombosis) or any conditions or situations that may lead to cardiovascular disease (e.g., cigarette smoking).[80,120,153]

There has been some indication that hormonal contraceptives may lead to certain forms of cancer. Some early versions of the pill were believed to cause tumors of the endometrium of the uterus. Early forms that were sequential in nature may have caused this effect; that is, they provided only estrogen for the first half of the menstrual cycle and estrogen combined with progesterone for the second half. However, the newer combined forms that supply both hormones throughout the cycle do not appear to increase the risk of uterine cancer. In fact, it appears that the form of oral contraceptive commonly used may actually *decrease* the risk of endometrial cancer, as well as prevent other forms of cancer, including ovarian cancer.[12,13,45] The carcinogenic properties of hormonal contraceptives have not been totally ruled out, however. The effects on breast cancer remain controversial, and the possibility exists that certain subgroups of women may have an increased risk of breast cancer, depending on factors such as how long they used the pill, their age, genetic predisposition, and so forth.[13,34,44] There is also considerable evidence that prolonged use of oral contraceptives (more than 8 years) may increase the risk of liver cancer.[91,163]

There are a number of other less serious but bothersome side effects associated with hormonal contraceptives. Problems such as nausea, loss of appetite, abdominal cramping, headache, dizziness, weight gain, and fatigue are fairly common. These symptoms are often transient and may diminish following continued use.

Consequently, the serious risks associated with hormonal contraceptives have diminished somewhat since their initial appearance on the market. These drugs are not without some hazards, however. In general, it is a good policy to reserve this form of birth control for relatively young, healthy women who do not smoke. Avoiding continuous, prolonged administration to diminish the risk of liver cancer may also be prudent. Finally, any increase in the other side effects associated with hormonal contraceptives, such as headache and abdominal discomfort, should be carefully evaluated to rule out a more serious underlying problem.

CASE STUDY

Male and Female Hormones

Brief History. S.K. is a 32-year-old woman who sustained a whiplash injury during a motor vehicle accident. She was being seen as an outpatient for physical therapy management of neck pain, decreased cervical range-of-motion, and cervicogenic headaches. The patient's neck pain was being managed pharmacologically by an oral muscle relaxant (carisoprodol), and she also took an over-the-counter acetaminophen product as needed. During the initial examination/evaluation, the therapist queried the patient about other medications, and the patient reported taking an oral contraceptive product containing an estrogen (ethinyl estradiol, 0.05 mg) and a progestin (norgestrel, 0.5 mg). This contraceptive facilitated traditional monthly cycles (3 weeks of the active pill, one week of placebo); she had been taking this product continuously for the past 11 years. The patient also smoked cigarettes, and she had recently increased cigarette use following the neck injury.

Problem/Influence of Medication. Approximately 2 weeks after beginning treatment, (i.e., during the fourth therapy session), the patient reported an increase in headache pain. This finding surprised the therapist because the patient's neck pain and cervical function had had been steadily improv-

ing. Upon further examination, the patient also reported a dull ache and tightness in the right calf, which was exacerbated by active and passive ankle dorsiflexion. Because the patient was taking an oral contraceptive and was also a cigarette smoker, the therapist was concerned that this patient might have a deep vein thrombosis (DVT). The therapist called the patient's physician, and the patient was referred immediately to the local hospital for further evaluation. Venous plethysmography revealed a large DVT that began in the calf but extended proximally into the popliteal vein. The patient was admitted to the hospital to begin anticoagulant therapy.

Decision/Solution. The patient was placed immediately on a low molecular weight heparin (enoxaparin), which was administered by subcutaneous injection (see Chapter 25). She also wore graduated compression stockings to reduce the risk of further thromboembolic disease. The oral contraceptive medication was discontinued, and she was counseled on strategies to quit smoking. The patient was eventually discharged to her home with instructions for continuing the subcutaneous heparin. After approximately 10 days, an oral anticoagulant (warfarin) was substituted for the heparin. She resumed physical therapy as an out-patient, where her neck problem was ultimately resolved without further incident.

Special Concerns of Sex Hormone Pharmacology in Rehabilitation Patients

■ ■ ■ Therapists should be cognizant of the adverse effects related to the estrogens, progesterones, and androgens so that they may help recognize problems related to these compounds. For instance, therapists should routinely monitor blood pressure during therapeutic administration of the sex hormones. These compounds tend to promote salt and water retention (mineralocorticoidlike properties), which may promote hypertension.

Therapists may also play an important role in educating patients about the dangers of androgen abuse. When dealing with an athletic population, physical therapists may serve as a source of information about anabolic steroids. Therapists should advise athletes about the potential side effects, such as liver, cardiovascular, and reproductive abnormalities. Therapists can also monitor blood pressure in athletes who appear to be using androgenic steroids. This interaction may help prevent a hypertensive crisis, as well as illustrate to the athlete the harmful effects of these drugs.

SUMMARY

The male hormones are the androgens, and the female hormones are the estrogens and progestins. These steroid hormones are primarily involved in the control of reproduction and sexual maturation. Male and female hormones also serve several important pharmacologic functions. These agents are often used as replacement therapy to resolve deficiencies in endogenous endocrine function. Androgens and estrogens and/or progestins are administered for a variety of other therapeutic reasons, including the control of some neoplastic diseases. Estrogens and progestins can also be administered to women as an effective means of birth control, and these hormones are used extensively as contraceptive agents. Finally, athletes sometimes use androgens in high doses in an attempt to increase muscle strength and performance. Although these drugs may produce increments in muscle strength in some individuals, the dangers of using high doses of anabolic steroids outweigh any potential ergogenic benefits.

References

1. Allan CM, Garcia A, Spaliviero J, et al. Complete Sertoli cell proliferation induced by follicle-stimulating hormone (FSH) independently of luteinizing hormone activity: evidence from genetic models of isolated FSH action. *Endocrinology.* 2004;145:1587–1593.
2. Anderson FD, Hait H. A multicenter, randomized study of an extended cycle oral contraceptive. *Contraception.* 2003;68:89–96.
3. Anderson GL, Limacher M, Assaf AR, et al. Effects of conjugated equine estrogen in postmenopausal women with hysterectomy: the Women's Health Initiative randomized controlled trial. *JAMA.* 2004;291:1701–1712.
4. Auranen A, Hietanen S, Salmi T, Grenman S. Hormonal treatments and epithelial ovarian cancer risk. *Int J Gynecol Cancer.* 2005;15:692–700.
5. Badimon L, Bayes-Genis A. Effects of progestins on thrombosis and atherosclerosis. *Hum Reprod Update.* 1999;5:191–199.
6. Bahrke MS, Yesalis CE. Abuse of anabolic androgenic steroids and related substances in sport and exercise. *Curr Opin Pharmacol.* 2004;4:614–620.
7. Barrett EJ. Organization of the endocrine system. In: Boron WF, Boulpaep EL, eds. *Medical Physiology: A Cellular and Molecular Approach.* New York: Saunders; 2003.
8. Beck JI, Boothroyd C, Proctor M, et al. Oral antioestrogens and medical adjuncts for subfertility associated with anovulation. *Cochrane Database Syst Rev.* 2005;CD002249.
9. Benagiano G, Primiero FM, Farris M. Clinical profile of contraceptive progestins. *Eur J Contracept Reprod Health Care.* 2004;9:182–193.
10. Berns JS, Mosenkis A. Pharmacologic adjuvants to epoetin in the treatment of anemia in patients on hemodialysis. *Hemodial Int.* 2005;9:7–22.
11. Bhavnani BR, Strickler RC. Menopausal hormone therapy. *J Obstet Gynaecol Can.* 2005;27:137–162.

12. Bose CK. Does hormone replacement therapy prevent epithelial ovarian cancer? *Reprod Biomed Online.* 2005;11:86–92.

13. Boyle P, Leon ME, Maisonneuve P, Autier P. Cancer control in women. Update 2003. *Int J Gynaecol Obstet.* 2003;83(suppl 1):179–202.

14. Burkman RT. Venous thromboembolism and oral contraceptives: current status and clinical implications. *Treat Endocrinol.* 2002;1:143–147.

15. Bushnell C. The cerebrovascular risks associated with tamoxifen use. *Expert Opin Drug Saf.* 2005;4:501–507.

16. Bushnell CD. Hormone replacement therapy and stroke: the current state of knowledge and directions for future research. *Semin Neurol.* 2006;26:123–130.

17. Cabasso A. Peliosis hepatis in a young adult bodybuilder. *Med Sci Sports Exerc.* 1994;26:2–4.

18. Cadepond F, Ulmann A, Baulieu EE. RU486 (mifepristone): mechanisms of action and clinical uses. *Annu Rev Med.* 1997;48:129–156.

19. Calfee R, Fadale P. Popular ergogenic drugs and supplements in young athletes. *Pediatrics.* 2006;117:e577–e589.

20. Cauley JA, Norton L, Lippman ME, et al. Continued breast cancer risk reduction in postmenopausal women treated with raloxifene: 4-year results from the MORE trial. Multiple outcomes of raloxifene evaluation. *Breast Cancer Res Treat.* 2001;65:125–134.

21. Chandrashekar V, Zaczek D, Bartke A. The consequences of altered somatotropic system on reproduction. *Biol Reprod.* 2004;71:17–27.

22. Christian CA, Mobley JL, Moenter SM. Diurnal and estradiol-dependent changes in gonadotropin-releasing hormone neuron firing activity. *Proc Natl Acad Sci USA.* 2005;102:15682–15687.

23. Cicinelli E, de Ziegler D, Alfonso R, et al. Endometrial effects, bleeding control, and compliance with a new postmenopausal hormone therapy regimen based on transdermal estradiol gel and every-other-day vaginal progesterone in capsules: a 3-year pilot study. *Fertil Steril.* 2005;83:1859–1863.

24. Cohen JC, Hickman R. Insulin resistance and diminished glucose tolerance in powerlifters ingesting anabolic steroids. *J Clin Endocrinol Metab.* 1987;64:960–963.

25. Col NF, Bowlby LA, McGarry K. The role of menopausal hormone therapy in preventing osteoporotic fractures: a critical review of the clinical evidence. *Minerva Med.* 2005;96:331–342.

26. Collins JA, Blake JM, Crosignani PG. Breast cancer risk with postmenopausal hormonal treatment. *Hum Reprod Update.* 2005;11:545–560.

27. Come SE, Borges VF. Role of fulvestrant in sequential hormonal therapy for advanced, hormone receptor-positive breast cancer in postmenopausal women. *Clin Breast Cancer.* 2005;6(suppl 1):S15–S22.

28. Compston J. How to manage osteoporosis after the menopause. *Best Pract Res Clin Rheumatol.* 2005;19:1007–1019.

29. Cosman F. Selective estrogen-receptor modulators. *Clin Geriatr Med.* 2003;19:371–379.

30. Cranney A, Adachi JD. Benefit-risk assessment of raloxifene in postmenopausal osteoporosis. *Drug Saf.* 2005;28:721–730.

31. Damber JE. Endocrine therapy for prostate cancer. *Acta Oncol.* 2005;44:605–609.

32. Darby E, Anawalt BD. Male hypogonadism: an update on diagnosis and treatment. *Treat Endocrinol.* 2005;4:293–309.

33. Davis JS, Rueda BR. The corpus luteum: an ovarian structure with maternal instincts and suicidal tendencies. *Front Biosci.* 2002;7:d1949–d1978.

34. Deligeoroglou E, Michailidis E, Creatsas G. Oral contraceptives and reproductive system cancer. *Ann N Y Acad Sci.* 2003;997:199–208.

35. Demling RH, DeSanti L. Oxandrolone induced lean mass gain during recovery from severe burns is maintained after discontinuation of the anabolic steroid. *Burns.* 2003;29:793–797.

36. Diamanti-Kandarakis E. Hormone replacement therapy and risk of malignancy. *Curr Opin Obstet Gynecol.* 2004;16:73–78.

37. Di Luigi L, Romanelli F, Lenzi A. Androgenic-anabolic steroids abuse in males. *J Endocrinol Invest.* 2005;28(suppl):81–84.

38. Dobs A. Role of testosterone in maintaining lean body mass and bone density in HIV-infected patients. *Int J Impot Res.* 2003;15(suppl 4):S21–S25.

39. Dohle GR, Smit M, Weber RF. Androgens and male fertility. *World J Urol.* 2003;21:341–345.

40. Donahue JL, Lowenthal DT. Androgens, anabolic-androgenic steroids, and inhibitors. *Am J Ther.* 2000;7:365–373.

41. Douketis J. Hormone replacement therapy and risk for venous thromboembolism: what's new and how do these findings influence clinical practice? *Curr Opin Hematol.* 2005;12:395–400.

42. Dowsett M, Nicholson RI, Pietras RJ. Biological characteristics of the pure antiestrogen fulvestrant: overcoming endocrine resistance. *Breast Cancer Res Treat.* 2005;93(suppl 1):S11–S18.

43. Edelman AB, Gallo MF, Jensen JT, et al. Continuous or extended cycle vs. cyclic use of combined oral contraceptives for contraception. *Cochrane Database Syst Rev.* 2005;CD004695.

44. ESHRE Capri Workshop Group. Hormones and breast cancer. *Hum Reprod Update.* 2004;10:281–293.

45. ESHRE Capri Workshop Group. Noncontraceptive health benefits of combined oral contraception. *Hum Reprod Update.* 2005;11:513–525.

46. Ettinger B. Vasomotor symptom relief versus unwanted effects: role of estrogen dosage. *Am J Med.* 2005;118(suppl 2):74–78.

47. Evans NA. Current concepts in anabolic-androgenic steroids. *Am J Sports Med.* 2004;32:534–542.

48. Fineschi V, Riezzo I, Centini F, et al. Sudden cardiac death during anabolic steroid abuse: morphologic and toxicologic findings in two fatal cases of bodybuilders. *Int J Legal Med.* 2005;121:48–53.

49. Forinash AB, Evans SL. New hormonal contraceptives: a comprehensive review of the literature. *Pharmacotherapy.* 2003;23:1573–1591.

50. Foster ZJ, Housner JA. Anabolic-androgenic steroids and testosterone precursors: ergogenic aids and sport. *Curr Sports Med Rep.* 2004;3:234–241.

51. Francucci CM, Camilletti A, Boscaro M. Raloxifene and cardiovascular health: its relationship to lipid and glucose metabolism, hemostatic and inflammation factors and cardiovascular function in postmenopausal women. *Curr Pharm Des.* 2005;11:4187–4206.

52. Gallo MF, Nanda K, Grimes DA, Schulz KF. Twenty micrograms vs. >20 microg estrogen oral contraceptives for contraception: systematic review of randomized controlled trials. *Contraception.* 2005; 71:162–169.

53. Gambacciani M, Vacca F. Postmenopausal osteoporosis and hormone replacement therapy. *Minerva Med.* 2004;95:507–520.

54. Gasco M, Argusti A, Bonanni B, Decensi A. SERMs in chemoprevention of breast cancer. *Eur J Cancer.* 2005; 41:1980–1989.

55. Gemzell-Danielsson K, Marions L. Mechanisms of action of mifepristone and levonorgestrel when used for emergency contraception. *Hum Reprod Update.* 2004;10:341–348.

56. Glasier A. Implantable contraceptives for women: effectiveness, discontinuation rates, return of fertility, and outcome of pregnancies. *Contraception.* 2002;65: 29–37.

57. Gluck O, Maricic M. Skeletal and nonskeletal effects of raloxifene. *Curr Osteoporos Rep.* 2003;1:123–128.

58. Gradishar W. Fulvestrant in the treatment of postmenopausal women with advanced breast cancer. *Expert Rev Anticancer Ther.* 2005;5:445–453.

59. Gradishar WJ. Tamoxifen—what next? *Oncologist.* 2004;9:378–384.

60. Grodstein F, Manson JE, Stampfer MJ. Hormone therapy and coronary heart disease: the role of time since menopause and age at hormone initiation. *J Womens Health.* 2006;15:35–44.

61. Haider SG. Cell biology of Leydig cells in the testis. *Int Rev Cytol.* 2004;233:181–241.

62. Hall RC, Hall RC. Abuse of supraphysiologic doses of anabolic steroids. *South Med J.* 2005;98:550–555.

63. Hall RC, Hall RC, Chapman MJ. Psychiatric complications of anabolic steroid abuse. *Psychosomatics.* 2005;46:285–290.

64. Hartgens F, Kuipers H. Effects of androgenic-anabolic steroids in athletes. *Sports Med.* 2004;34:513–554.

65. Henderson VW. Estrogen-containing hormone therapy and Alzheimer's disease risk: Understanding discrepant inferences from observational and experimental research. *Neuroscience.* 2006;138:1031–1039.

66. Henzl MR, Polan ML. Avoiding menstruation: a review of health and lifestyle issues. *J Reprod Med.* 2004;49:162–174.

67. Herndon EJ, Zieman M. New contraceptive options. *Am Fam Physician.* 2004;69:853–860.

68. Hijazi RA, Cunningham GR. Andropause: is androgen replacement therapy indicated for the aging male? *Annu Rev Med.* 2005;56:117–137.

69. Hiort O. Androgens and puberty. *Best Pract Res Clin Endocrinol Metab.* 2002;16:31–41.

70. Hitchcock CL, Prior JC. Evidence about extending the duration of oral contraceptive use to suppress menstruation. *Womens Health Issues.* 2004;14:201–211.

71. Holdcraft RW, Braun RE. Hormonal regulation of spermatogenesis. *Int J Androl.* 2004;27:335–342.

72. Homburg R. Clomiphene citrate—end of an era? A mini-review. *Hum Reprod.* 2005;20:2043–2051.

73. Honjo H, Iwasa K, Kawata M, et al. Progestins and estrogens and Alzheimer's disease. *J Steroid Biochem Mol Biol.* 2005;93:305–308.

74. Hulley S, Grady D, Bush T, et al. Randomized trial of estrogen plus progestin for secondary prevention of coronary heart disease in postmenopausal women. Heart and Estrogen/progestin Replacement Study (HERS) Research Group. *JAMA.* 1998;280:605–613.

75. Jarow JP, Lipshultz LI. Anabolic steroid-induced hypogonadotropic hypogonadism. *Am J Sports Med.* 1990;18:429–431.

76. Johansson ED. Future developments in hormonal contraception. *Am J Obstet Gynecol.* 2004;190(suppl): S69–S71.

77. Johnell O, Cauley JA, Kulkarni PM, et al. Raloxifene reduces risk of vertebral fractures in postmenopausal women regardless of prior hormone therapy. *J Fam Pract.* 2004;53:789–796.

78. Judge JO, Kleppinger A, Kenny A, et al. Home-based resistance training improves femoral bone mineral density in women on hormone therapy. *Osteoporos Int.* 2005;16:1096–1108.

79. Kaunitz AM. Beyond the pill: new data and options in hormonal and intrauterine contraception. *Am J Obstet Gynecol.* 2005;192:998–1004.

80. Keeling D. Combined oral contraceptives and the risk of myocardial infarction. *Ann Med.* 2003;35: 413–418.

81. Kelly MJ, Qiu J, Ronnekleiv OK. Estrogen signaling in the hypothalamus. *Vitam Horm.* 2005;71:123–145.

82. Kohen P, Castro O, Palomino A, et al. The steroidogenic response and corpus luteum expression of the steroidogenic acute regulatory protein after human chorionic gonadotropin administration at different times in the human luteal phase. *J Clin Endocrinol Metab.* 2003;88:3421–3430.

83. Kong A, Edmonds P. Testosterone therapy in HIV wasting syndrome: systematic review and meta-analysis. *Lancet Infect Dis.* 2002;2:692–699.

84. Kovacs L. Oral contraception over the age of 40. *Ann N Y Acad Sci.* 2003;997:194–198.

85. Krause W, Mueller U, Mazur A. Testosterone supplementation in the aging male: which questions have been answered? *Aging Male.* 2005;8:31–38.

86. Kuhl H. Pharmacology of estrogens and progestogens: influence of different routes of administration. *Climacteric.* 2005;8(suppl 1):3–63.

87. Kuhn CM. Anabolic steroids. *Recent Prog Horm Res.* 2002;57:411–434.

88. Kumar TR. What have we learned about gonadotropin function from gonadotropin subunit and receptor knockout mice? *Reproduction.* 2005;130:293–302.

89. Labrie F, Belanger A, Luu-The V, et al. Gonadotropin-releasing hormone agonists in the

treatment of prostate cancer. *Endocr Rev.* 2005;26: 361–379.

90. LaCroix AZ. Estrogen with and without progestin: benefits and risks of short-term use. *Am J Med.* 2005; 118(suppl 2):79–87.

91. La Vecchia C, Altieri A, Franceschi S, Tavani A. Oral contraceptives and cancer: an update. *Drug Saf.* 2001;24:741–754.

92. Lindsay R. Hormones and bone health in post-menopausal women. *Endocrine.* 2004;24:223–230.

93. Lombardo F, Sgro P, Salacone P, et al. Androgens and fertility. *J Endocrinol Invest.* 2005;28(suppl):51–55.

94. Loose DS, Stancel GM. Estrogens and progestins. In: Brunton LL, et al, eds. *The Pharmacological Basis of Therapeutics.* 11th ed. New York: McGraw-Hill; 2006.

95. Machado F, Rodriguez JR, Leon JP, et al. Tamoxifen and endometrial cancer. Is screening necessary? A review of the literature. *Eur J Gynaecol Oncol.* 2005; 26:257–265.

96. Maki PM. Hormone therapy and risk for dementia: where do we go from here? *Gynecol Endocrinol.* 2004; 19:354–359.

97. Malyala A, Kelly MJ, Ronnekleiv OK. Estrogen modulation of hypothalamic neurons: activation of multiple signaling pathways and gene expression changes. *Steroids.* 2005;70:397–406.

98. Maran RR. Thyroid hormones: their role in testicular steroidogenesis. *Arch Androl.* 2003;49:375–388.

99. Maravelias C, Dona A, Stefanidou M, Spiliopoulou C. Adverse effects of anabolic steroids in athletes. A constant threat. *Toxicol Lett.* 2005;158:167–175.

100. McLachlan RI. The endocrine control of spermatogenesis. *Baillieres Best Pract Res Clin Endocrinol Metab.* 2000;14:345–362.

101. Mechanick JI, Nierman DM. Gonadal steroids in critical illness. *Crit Care Clin.* 2006;22:87–103.

102. Miller VM, Jayachandran M, Heit JA, Owen WG. Estrogen therapy and thrombotic risk.*Pharmacol Ther.* 2006;111:792–807.

103. Millman RB, Ross EJ. Steroid and nutritional supplement use in professional athletes. *Am J Addict.* 2003; 12(suppl 2):S48–S54.

104. Mobasseri S, Liebson PR, Klein LW. Hormone therapy and selective estrogen receptor modulators for prevention of coronary heart disease in postmenopausal women estrogen replacement from the cardiologist's perspective. *Cardiol Rev.* 2004;12: 287–298.

105. Morales A. Testosterone treatment for the aging man: the controversy. *Curr Urol Rep.* 2004;5:472–477.

106. Morales A. Monitoring androgen replacement therapy: testosterone and prostate safety. *J Endocrinol Invest.* 2005;28(suppl):122–127

107. Moretti C, Frajese GV, Guccione L, et al. Androgens and body composition in the aging male. *J Endocrinol Invest.* 2005;28(suppl):56–64.

108. Morley JE, Haren MT, Kim MJ, et al. Testosterone, aging and quality of life. *J Endocrinol Invest.* 2005;28 (suppl):76–80.

109. Navarro JF, Mora C. Androgen therapy for anemia in elderly uremic patients. *Int Urol Nephrol.* 2001;32: 549–557.

110. Nelson AL. Extended-cycle oral contraception: a new option for routine use. *Treat Endocrinol.* 2005;4: 139–145.

111. Nicholson RI, Johnston SR. Endocrine therapy—current benefits and limitations. *Breast Cancer Res Treat.* 2005;93(suppl 1):S3–S10.

112. Nishiyama T, Suzuki K, Yamana K, et al. Stepping-stones to the further advancement of androgen-deprivation therapy for prostate cancer. *Expert Rev Anticancer Ther.* 2006;6:259–268.

113. Niswender GD, Juengel JL, Silva PJ, et al. Mechanisms controlling the function and life span of the corpus luteum. *Physiol Rev.* 2000;80:1–29.

114. Nzeako UC, Frigas E, Tremaine WJ. Hereditary angioedema: a broad review for clinicians. *Arch Intern Med.* 2001;161:2417–2429.

115. Orr R, Fiatarone Singh M. The anabolic androgenic steroid oxandrolone in the treatment of wasting and catabolic disorders: review of efficacy and safety. *Drugs.* 2004;64:725–750.

116. Pagonis TA, Angelopoulos NV, Koukoulis GN, Hadjichristodoulou CS. Psychiatric side effects induced by supraphysiological doses of combinations of anabolic steroids correlate to the severity of abuse. *Eur Psychiatry.* 2006;21:551–562.

117. Parssinen M, Seppala T. Steroid use and long-term health risks in former athletes. *Sports Med.* 2002;32:83–94.

118. Pettine KA. Association of anabolic steroids and avascular necrosis of femoral heads. *Am J Sports Med.* 1991;19:96–98.

119. Plourd DM, Rayburn WF. New contraceptive methods. *J Reprod Med.* 2003;48:665–671.

120. Pymar HC, Creinin MD. The risks of oral contraceptive pills. *Semin Reprod Med.* 2001;19:305–312.

121. Rackley CE. Hormones and coronary atherosclerosis in women. *Endocrine.* 2004;24:245–250.

122. Rivera R, Yacobson I, Grimes D. The mechanism of action of hormonal contraceptives and intrauterine contraceptive devices. *Am J Obstet Gynecol.* 1999;181(5 pt 1):1263–1269.

123. Robins DM. Androgen receptor and molecular mechanisms of male-specific gene expression. *Novartis Found Symp.* 2005;268:42–52; discussion 53–56, 96–99.

124. Rogol AD. New facets of androgen replacement therapy during childhood and adolescence. *Expert Opin Pharmacother.* 2005;6:1319–1336.

125. Rogol AD. Pubertal androgen therapy in boys. *Pediatr Endocrinol Rev.* 2005;2:383–390.

126. Rosenfield C. The use of ergogenic agents in high school athletes. *J Sch Nurs.* 2005;21:333–339.

127. Rossouw JE. Coronary heart disease in menopausal women: implications of primary and secondary prevention trials of hormones. *Maturitas.* 2005;51:51–63.

128. Roy AK, Tyagi RK, Song CS, et al. Androgen receptor: structural domains and functional dynamics after ligand-receptor interaction. *Ann N Y Acad Sci.* 2001; 949:44–57.

129. Sambrook P. Who will benefit from treatment with selective estrogen receptor modulators (SERMs)? *Best Pract Res Clin Rheumatol.* 2005;19:975–981.

130. Samsioe G. Transdermal hormone therapy: gels and patches. *Climacteric.* 2004;7:347–356.

131. Sarkar NN. The combined contraceptive vaginal device (NuvaRing): a comprehensive review. *Eur J Contracept Reprod Health Care.* 2005;10:73–78.

132. Sarkar NN. The potential of mifepristone (RU-486) as an emergency contraceptive drug. *Acta Obstet Gynecol Scand.* 2005;84:309–316.

133. Schindler AE. Endocrinology of pregnancy: consequences for the diagnosis and treatment of pregnancy disorders. *J Steroid Biochem Mol Biol.* 2005;97:386–388.

134. Schneider D, Hsia J. Coronary heart disease prevention in menopausal women. *Expert Opin Pharmacother.* 2005;6:695–705.

135. Schreiber C, Creinin M. Mifepristone in abortion care. *Semin Reprod Med.* 2005;23:82–91.

136. Shahidi NT. A review of the chemistry, biological action, and clinical applications of anabolic-androgenic steroids. *Clin Ther.* 2001;23:1355–1390.

137. Shulman LP. Advances in female hormonal contraception: current alternatives to oral regimens. *Treat Endocrinol.* 2003;2:247–256.

138. Shumaker SA, Legault C, Rapp SR, et al. Estrogen plus progestin and the incidence of dementia and mild cognitive impairment in postmenopausal women: the Women's Health Initiative Memory Study: a randomized controlled trial. *JAMA.* 2003;289:2651–2662.

139. Simon JA. Safety of estrogen/androgen regimens. *J Reprod Med.* 2001;46(suppl):281–290.

140. Simon T, Beau Yon de Jonage-Canonico M, Oger E, et al. Indicators of lifetime endogenous estrogen exposure and risk of venous thromboembolism. *J Thromb Haemost.* 2006;4:71–76.

141. Sitruk-Ware RL. Hormone therapy and the cardiovascular system: the critical role of progestins. *Climacteric.* 2003;6(suppl 3):21–28.

142. Sitruk-Ware R. New progestogens: a review of their effects in perimenopausal and postmenopausal women. *Drugs Aging.* 2004;21:865–883.

143. Sivin I. Risks and benefits, advantages and disadvantages of levonorgestrel-releasing contraceptive implants. *Drug Saf.* 2003;26:303–335.

144. Snyder PJ. In: Brunton LL, et al, eds. *The Pharmacological Basis of Therapeutics.* 11th ed. New York: McGraw-Hill; 2006.

145. Socas L, Zumbado M, Perez-Luzardo O, et al. Hepatocellular adenomas associated with anabolic androgenic steroid abuse in bodybuilders: a report of two cases and a review of the literature. *Br J Sports Med.* 2005;39:e27.

146. Sriraman V, Anbalagan M, Rao AJ. Hormonal regulation of Leydig cell proliferation and differentiation in rodent testis: a dynamic interplay between gonadotrophins and testicular factors. *Reprod Biomed Online.* 2005;11:507–518.

147. Sriraman V, Jagannadha Rao A. Evaluation of the role of FSH in regulation of Leydig cell function during different stages of its differentiation. *Mol Cell Endocrinol.* 2004;224:73–82.

148. Stevenson JC. Justification for the use of HRT in the long-term prevention of osteoporosis. *Maturitas.* 2005;51:113–126.

149. Strawford A, Barbieri T, Van Loan M, et al. Resistance exercise and supraphysiologic androgen therapy in eugonadal men with HIV-related weight loss: a randomized controlled trial. *JAMA.* 1999;281:1282–1290.

150. Taiwo BO. HIV-associated wasting: brief review and discussion of the impact of oxandrolone. *AIDS Patient Care STDS.* 2000;14:421–425.

151. Tan D, Haines CJ, Limpaphayom KK, et al. Relief of vasomotor symptoms and vaginal atrophy with three doses of conjugated estrogens and medroxyprogesterone acetate in postmenopausal Asian women from 11 countries: the Pan-Asia menopause (PAM) study. *Maturitas.* 2005;52:35–51.

152. Tan RS, Salazar JA. Risks of testosterone replacement therapy in ageing men. *Expert Opin Drug Saf.* 2004;3:599–606.

153. Tanis BC, Rosendaal FR. Venous and arterial thrombosis during oral contraceptive use: risks and risk factors. *Semin Vasc Med.* 2003;3:69–84.

154. Thein LA, Thein JM, Landry GL. Ergogenic aids. *Phys Ther.* 1995;75:426–439.

155. Tokish JM, Kocher MS, Hawkins RJ. Ergogenic aids: a review of basic science, performance, side effects, and status in sports. *Am J Sports Med.* 2004;32:1543–1553.

156. Trenton AJ, Currier GW. Behavioural manifestations of anabolic steroid use. *CNS Drugs.* 2005;19:571–595.

157. Urhausen A, Albers T, Kindermann W. Are the cardiac effects of anabolic steroid abuse in strength athletes reversible? *Heart.* 2004;90:496–501.

158. Verrijdt G, Haelens A, Claessens F. Selective DNA recognition by the androgen receptor as a mechanism for hormone-specific regulation of gene expression. *Mol Genet Metab.* 2003;78:175–185.

159. Walker WH, Cheng J. FSH and testosterone signaling in Sertoli cells. *Reproduction.* 2005;130:15–28.

160. Wenger NK. Menopausal hormone therapy and cardiovascular protection: state of the data 2003. *J Am Med Womens Assoc.* 2003;58:236–239.

161. Wiegratz I, Kuhl H. Long-cycle treatment with oral contraceptives. *Drugs.* 2004;64:2447–2462.

162. Wu O, Robertson L, Langhorne P, et al. Oral contraceptives, hormone replacement therapy, thrombophilias and risk of venous thromboembolism: a systematic review. The Thrombosis: Risk and Economic Assessment of Thrombophilia Screening (TREATS) Study. *Thromb Haemost.* 2005;94:17–25.

163. Yu MC, Yuan JM. Environmental factors and risk for hepatocellular carcinoma. *Gastroenterology.* 2004;127(suppl 1):S72–S78.

164. Yuzpe AA. Oral contraception: trends over time. *J Reprod Med.* 2002;47(suppl):967–973.

Chapter 31

Thyroid and Parathyroid Drugs: Agents Affecting Bone Mineralization

This chapter discusses the function and pharmacologic aspects of two important endocrine structures: the thyroid and parathyroid glands. Hormones secreted from the thyroid gland are involved in controlling metabolism; they also work synergistically with other hormones to promote normal growth and development. The parathyroid glands are essential in regulating calcium homeostasis and are important in maintaining proper bone mineralization.

Problems in the function of the thyroid or parathyroid glands are often treated by pharmacologic methods. Pharmacologic management of thyroid and parathyroid function should be of interest to rehabilitation specialists because physical therapists and occupational therapists treat patients with bone healing disorders and other endocrine problems related to these glands. This chapter first discusses normal physiologic function of the thyroid gland, followed by the types of drugs used to treat hyperthyroidism and hypothyroidism. The function of the parathyroid glands is covered next, discussing the role of the parathyroid glands and other hormones in maintaining bone mineral homeostasis. Finally, drugs used to regulate bone calcification are presented.

Function of the Thyroid Gland

The thyroid gland lies on either side of the trachea in the anterior neck region and consists of bilateral lobes that are connected by a central isthmus. The entire gland weighs approximately 15 to 20 g and receives a rich vascular supply as well as extensive innervation from the sympathetic nervous system.[55]

The thyroid gland synthesizes two primary hormones: thyroxine and triiodothyronine. A discussion of the synthesis and function of these hormones follows.

Synthesis of Thyroid Hormones

The chemical structures of thyroxine and triiodothyronine are shown in Figure 31–1. As shown in the figure, thyroid hormones are synthesized first by adding iodine to residues of the amino acid *tyrosine*. Addition of one iodine atom creates monoiodotyrosine, and the addition of a second iodine creates diiodotyrosine. Two of these iodinated tyrosines are then combined to complete the thyroid hormone. The combination of a monoiodotyrosine and a diiodotyrosine yields triiodothyronine, and the combination of two diiodotyrosines yields thyroxine.[55]

Because thyroxine contains four iodine residues, this compound is also referred to by the abbreviation T_4. Likewise, triiodothyronine contains three iodine residues, hence the abbreviation T_3. There has been considerable discussion about which hormone exerts the primary physiologic effects. Plasma levels of T_4 are much higher than T_3 levels, but T_3 may exert most of the physiologic effects on various tissues, which suggests that T_4 is a precursor to T_3 and that the conversion of T_4 to T_3 occurs in peripheral tissues.[23] Regardless of which hormone ultimately affects cellular metabolism, both T_4 and T_3 are needed for normal thyroid function.

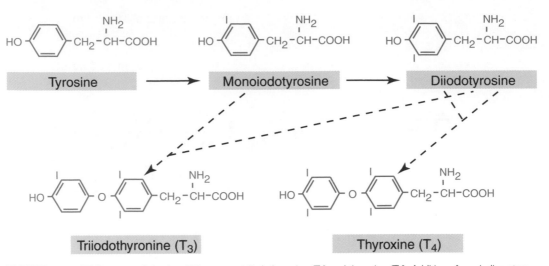

FIGURE 31–1 ▼ Structure of the thyroid hormones triiodothyronine (T₃) and thyroxine (T₄). Addition of one iodine atom (I) to tyrosine produces monoiodotyrosine; addition of a second iodine atom produces diiodotyrosine. A monoiodotyrosine and diiodotyrosine combine to form triiodothyronine (T₃). Coupling of two diiodotyrosines forms thyroxine (T₄).

The primary steps in thyroid hormone biosynthesis are shown schematically in Figure 31–2. Thyroid follicle cells take up and concentrate iodide from the bloodstream—this is significant because there must be a sufficient amount of iodine in the diet to provide what is needed for thyroid hormone production.[55] Thyroid cells also manufacture a protein known as thy-roglobulin (TGB), which contains tyrosine residues. The TGB molecule is manufactured within the follicle cell and stored in the central lumen of the thyroid follicle (see Fig. 31–2). During hormone synthesis, iodide is oxidized and covalently bonded to the tyrosine residues of the TGB molecule.[35] Two iodinated tyrosine residues combine within the TGB molecule to

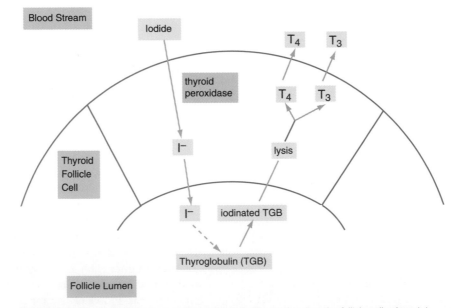

FIGURE 31–2 ▼ Thyroid hormone biosynthesis. Iodide is taken into the follicle cell, where it is converted by thyroid peroxidase to an oxidized form of iodine (I⁻). I⁻ is transported to the follicle lumen, where it is bonded to tyrosine residues of the thyroglobulin (TGB) molecule. Iodinated TGB is incorporated back into the cell, where it undergoes lysis to yield the thyroid hormones T₃ and T₄. See text for further discussion.

form T_4 (primarily), and smaller amounts of T_3 are also produced. At this point, the hormones are still incorporated within the large TGB molecule. The iodinated TGB molecule (TGB containing the iodinated tyrosines) is absorbed back into the follicle cell, where the large molecule is lysed to yield thyroid hormones. The hormones are then secreted into the systemic circulation, where they can reach various target tissues.

Regulation of Thyroid Hormone Release

Thyroid hormone production is controlled by the hypothalamic-pituitary system (see Chapter 28). Thyrotropin-releasing hormone (TRH) from the hypothalamus stimulates the release of thyroid-stimulating hormone (TSH) from the anterior pituitary.[17,63] TSH then travels via the systemic circulation to the thyroid gland to stimulate the production of thyroxine and triiodothyronine.

Thyroid hormone release is subject to the negative feedback strategy that is typical of endocrine systems controlled by the hypothalamic-pituitary axis. Increased circulating levels of the thyroid hormones (T_4, T_3) serve to limit their own production by inhibiting TRH release from the hypothalamus and TSH release from the anterior pituitary.[30,35] This negative feedback control prevents peripheral levels of thyroid hormones from becoming excessively high.

Physiologic Effects of Thyroid Hormones

Thyroid hormones affect a wide variety of peripheral tissues throughout the individual's life.[8,55] In some situations, these hormones exert a direct effect on cellular function (e.g., T_4 and T_3 appear to increase cellular metabolism by directly increasing oxidative enzyme activity). In other instances, thyroid hormones appear to play a permissive role in facilitating the function of other hormones. For instance, thyroid hormones must be present for growth hormone to function properly. The principal effects of the thyroid hormones are listed below.

Thermogenesis. **T_4 and T_3** increase the basal metabolic rate and subsequent heat production from the body, which are important in maintaining adequate body temperature during exposure to cold environments. Increased thermogenesis is achieved by thyroid hormone stimulation of cellular metabolism in various tissues, such as skeletal muscle, cardiac muscle, and liver and kidney cells.

Growth and Development. Thyroid hormones facilitate normal growth and development by stimulating the release of growth hormone and by enhancing the effects of growth hormone on peripheral tissues. Thyroid hormones also directly enhance the development of many physiologic systems, especially the skeletal system and central nervous system (CNS). If thyroid hormones are not present, severe growth restriction and mental retardation (cretinism) ensue.

Cardiovascular Effects. Thyroid hormones appear to increase heart rate and myocardial contractility, thus leading to an increase in cardiac output. It is unclear, however, if this occurrence is a direct effect of these hormones or if the thyroid hormones increase myocardial sensitivity to other hormones (norepinephrine and epinephrine).

Metabolic Effects. Thyroid hormones affect energy substrate utilization in a number of ways. For instance, these hormones increase intestinal glucose absorption and increase the activity of several enzymes involved in carbohydrate metabolism. Thyroid hormones enhance lipolysis by increasing the response of fat cells to other lipolytic hormones. In general, these and other metabolic effects help to increase the availability of glucose and lipids for increased cellular activity.

Mechanism of Action of Thyroid Hormones

The preponderance of evidence indicates that the thyroid hormones enter the cell and bind to specific receptors located within the cell's nucleus.[35,61] These thyroid hormone receptors act as DNA transcription factors that bind to specific DNA sequences regulating gene expression. When activated by the thyroid hormone, thyroid receptors induce transcription of specific DNA gene segments, which ultimately results in altered protein synthesis within the cell.[24,94] Most, if not all, of the physiologic effects of the thyroid hormones are related to this alteration in cellular protein production. For instance, thyroid hormones may act through nuclear DNA transcription to stimulate the synthesis of a particular enzymatic protein. Such a protein may increase the transport of specific substances (e.g., amino acids, glucose, sodium) across the cell membrane, or the newly synthesized protein may be directly involved in a metabolic pathway (e.g., glycolysis or lipid oxidation).

Table 31–1	PRIMARY TYPES OF HYPERTHYROIDISM AND HYPOTHYROIDISM

Hyperthyroidism (Thyrotoxicosis)	**Hypothyroidism (Hypothyroxinemia)**

Primary hyperthyroidism
  Graves disease
  Thyroid adenoma/carcinoma
Secondary hyperthyroidism
  Hyperthyroidism induced by excessive hypothalamic
    or pituitary stimulation
	Primary hypothyroidism
	  Genetic deficiency of enzymes that synthesize thyroid
	    hormones
	Secondary hypothyroidism
	  Hypothyroidism induced by hypothalamic or pituitary
	    deficiencies
	  Cretinism (childhood hypothyroidism)
	  Myxedema (adult hypothyroidism)
	Other forms of hypothyroidism
	  Hypothyroidism induced by peripheral insensitivity
	    to thyroid hormones, inadequate hormone transport,
	    other causes

Treatment of Thyroid Disorders

Thyroid disorders can be divided into two primary categories: conditions that increase thyroid function (hyperthyroidism) and conditions that decrease thyroid function (hypothyroidism).[8] There are several different types of hyperthyroidism and hypothyroidism, depending on the apparent etiology, symptoms, and age of onset of each type. The types of hyperthyroidism and hypothyroidism are listed in Table 31–1. Although we cannot review the causes and effects of all the various forms of thyroid dysfunction at this time, this topic is dealt with elsewhere extensively.[6,8,56,74]

The clinical manifestations of hyperthyroidism and hypothyroidism are listed in Table 31–2. From a pharmacotherapeutic standpoint, hyperthyroidism is treated with drugs that attenuate the synthesis and effects of thyroid hormones. Hypothyroidism is usually treated by thyroid hormone administration (replacement therapy). The general aspects and more common forms of hyperthyroidism and hypothyroidism are discussed here, along with the drugs used to resolve these primary forms of thyroid dysfunction.

Hyperthyroidism

Hyperthyroidism (thyrotoxicosis) results in the increased secretion of thyroid hormones. This condition may occur secondary to a number of conditions, including thyroid tumors and problems in the

endocrine regulation of thyroid secretion—for example, excess TSH secretion (see Table 31–1).[74] Hyperthyroidism is usually associated with enlargement of the thyroid gland, or goiter. One of the more common causes of hyperthyroidism is diffuse toxic goiter (Graves disease). Graves disease is thought to be caused by a problem in the immune system. Because of a genetic defect, antibodies are synthesized that directly stimulate the thyroid gland, resulting in exag-

Table 31–2	PRIMARY SYMPTOMS OF HYPERTHYROIDISM AND HYPOTHYROIDISM

Hyperthyroidism	**Hypothyroidism**
Nervousness	Lethargy/slow cerebration
Weight loss	Weight gain (in adult hypothyroidism)
Diarrhea	Constipation
Tachycardia	Bradycardia
Insomnia	Sleepiness
Increased appetite	Anorexia
Heat intolerance	Cold intolerance
Oligomenorrhea	Menorrhagia
Muscle wasting	Weakness
Goiter	Dry, coarse skin
Exophthalmos	Facial edema

Adapted from: Kuhn MA Thyroid and parathyroid agents. In: Kuhn MA ed. *Pharmacotherapeutics: A Nursing Process Approach.* 4th ed. Philadelphia: FA Davis; 1997.

gerated thyroid hormone production.[3,79] There are several other types of hyperthyroidism based on different causes and clinical features (see Table 31–1).[25,74]

The principal manifestations of hyperthyroidism are listed in Table 31–2. The treatment of this condition often consists of ablation of the thyroid gland, accomplished by surgically removing thyroid or by administering radioactive iodine. Several pharmacologic agents may also be used in the management of hyperthyroidism in various situations.[1,74] These drugs and their clinical applications are discussed in the following sections.

Antithyroid Agents. Antithyroid drugs directly inhibit thyroid hormone synthesis. The agents currently in use are propylthiouracil (Propyl-Thyracil) and methimazole (Tapazole).[19,45] These drugs inhibit the thyroid peroxidase enzyme necessary for preparing iodide for addition to tyrosine residues (see Fig. 31–2).[5] These agents also prevent the coupling of tyrosine residues within the thyroglobulin molecule.[19] Propylthiouracil also inhibits the effects of the thyroid hormones by blocking the conversion of T_4 to T_3 in peripheral tissues.[19] The most common adverse effects of antithyroid drugs are skin rash and itching, although this is usually mild and transient. Although serious problems involving formed blood elements (agranulocytosis and aplastic anemia) may occur, the incidence of such problems is relatively small. Finally, excessive inhibition of thyroid hormone synthesis from drug overdose may cause symptoms resembling hypothyroidism, such as coldness and lethargy.

Iodide. Relatively large dosages of iodide (exceeding 6 mg/d) cause a rapid and dramatic decrease in thyroid function.[35] In sufficient amounts, iodide inhibits virtually all the steps involved in thyroid hormone biosynthesis. For instance, high iodide levels limit the uptake of iodide into thyroid follicle cells, inhibit the formation of T_4 and T_3, and decrease the secretion of the completed hormones from the thyroid cell.

Although iodide is effective in treating hyperthyroidism for short periods, the effects of this drug begin to diminish after about 2 weeks of administration.[35] Consequently, iodide is used in limited situations, such as temporary control of hyperthyroidism prior to thyroidectomy. In addition, iodide may cause a severe hypersensitive reaction in susceptible individuals. Therefore, the use of iodide has been replaced somewhat by other agents such as antithyroid drugs and beta blockers.

Radioactive Iodine. A radioactive isotope of iodine(^{131}I) is often used to selectively destroy thyroid

tissues in certain forms of hyperthyroidism, such as in Graves disease.[67,74] A specific dose of radioactive iodine is administered orally and rapidly sequestered within the thyroid gland. The isotope then begins to emit beta radiation, which selectively destroys the thyroid follicle cells. Essentially no damage occurs to surrounding tissues because the radioactivity is contained within the thyroid gland. Thus, administration of radioactive iodine is a simple, relatively safe method of permanently ablating the thyroid gland and reducing excess thyroid hormone function.[35] Of course, patients who undergo radioactive destruction of the thyroid gland (or surgical thyroidectomy) must typically be given thyroid hormones as replacement therapy.[67]

Beta-Adrenergic Blockers. Beta-adrenergic blockers are usually associated with the treatment of cardiovascular problems such as hypertension and angina pectoris. Beta blockers may also be helpful as an adjunct in thyrotoxicosis.[65,84] Although these drugs do not directly lower plasma levels of thyroid hormones, they may help suppress symptoms such as tachycardia, palpitations, fever, and restlessness. Consequently, beta blockers are usually not the only drugs used in the long-term control of hyperthyroidism but serve as adjuncts to other medications such as antithyroid drugs. Beta blockers may be especially helpful in severe, acute exacerbations of thyrotoxicosis (thyroid storm). These drugs are also administered preoperatively to control symptoms until a more permanent means of treating thyrotoxicosis (thyroidectomy) can be implemented.[65] Some beta blockers that have been used effectively in thyrotoxicosis are acebutolol, atenolol, metoprolol, nadolol, oxprenolol, propranolol, sotalol, and timolol. The pharmacology and adverse effects of these compounds are described in Chapter 20.

Hypothyroidism

There are many forms of hypothyroidism, differing in their cause and age of onset (see Table 31–1). Severe adult hypothyroidism (myxedema) may occur idiopathically or may be caused by specific factors such as autoimmune lymphocytic destruction (Hashimoto disease). In the child, thyroid function may be congenitally impaired, and cretinism will result if this condition is untreated. Hypothyroidism may result at any age if the dietary intake of iodine is extremely low. Several other forms of hypothyroidism that have a genetic or familial basis also exist.[54]

The primary physiologic effects of decreased thyroid function are listed in Table 31–2. Although enlargement of the thyroid gland (*goiter*) is usually associated with hyperthyroidism, goiter may also be present in some forms of hypothyroidism (although for different reasons). For instance, thyroid enlargement occurs during hypothyroidism when there is a lack of dietary iodine (endemic goiter). Under the influence of TSH, the thyroid manufactures large quantities of thyroglobulin. Thyroid hormone synthesis is incomplete, however, because no iodine is available to add to the tyrosine residues. If no thyroid hormones are produced, there is no negative feedback to limit the secretion of TSH. Consequently, the thyroid gland increases in size because of the unabated production of thyroglobulin.

The primary method of treating hypothyroidism is to administer thyroid hormones as replacement therapy. Long-term administration of thyroid hormones is usually a safe, effective means of maintaining optimal patient health in hypothyroidism. Replacement therapy using thyroid hormone preparations is described below.

Thyroid Hormones. Replacement of deficient thyroid hormones with natural and synthetic analogs is necessary in most forms of hypothyroidism.[14,91] Preparations containing T_4 (levothyroxine), T_3 (liothyronine), or both hormones can be administered to mimic normal thyroid function whenever the endogenous production of these hormones is impaired. There has, however, been considerable debate about whether a replacement regimen should consist of T_4 only, or a combination of T_4 and T_3. It appears that combining both hormones does not provide additional benefits in certain physiologic responses (body weight, lipid metabolism) compared to replacement using only T_4.[15,33] Combining both hormones, however, may result in greater improvements in other responses, including mood, psychometric skills, and perceived quality-of-life.[23,91] Hence, the ideal replacement regimen may vary depending on each patient's needs, and efforts should be made to find the optimal type and dose of thyroid hormones for each patient.

Regardless of the exact regimen, thyroid hormone replacement is essential for maintaining optimal health in adults with various forms of hypothyroidism. Administration of thyroid hormones is likewise important in infants and children with hypothyroidism because adequate amounts of these hormones are needed for normal physical and mental development.[52] Thyroid hormone replacement is also necessary following thyroidectomy or pharmacologic ablation of the thyroid gland with radioactive iodine. Thyroid hormones may be used to prevent and treat cancer of the thyroid gland and to prevent enlargement of the thyroid gland (goiter) caused by other drugs such as lithium. Thyroid hormone maintenance may be beneficial in patients who are in the preliminary or sub- clinical phase of hypothyroidism. Some clinicians feel that administering these hormones in the early stages may prevent the disease from fully developing.[7]

Thyroid hormone preparations used clinically are listed in Table 31–3. The primary problems associated with these agents occur with overdosage. Symptoms of excess drug levels are similar to the symptoms of hyperthyroidism (see Table 31–2). Presence of these symptoms is resolved by decreasing the dosage or changing the medication.

Function of the Parathyroid Glands

In humans, there are usually four parathyroid glands that are embedded on the posterior surface of the thyroid gland. Each parathyroid gland is a pea-sized

Table 31–3	THYROID HORMONES USED TO TREAT HYPOTHYROIDISM		
Generic Name	**Trade Name(s)**	**Thyroid Hormone Content**	**Source**
Levothyroxine	Levothroid, Synthroid, others	T_4	Synthetic
Liothyronine	Cytomel	T_3	Synthetic
Liotrix	Thyrolar	T_3 and T_4	Synthetic
Thyroid	Armour Thyroid, others	T_3 and T_4	Natural

T_3 = triiodothyronine; T_4 = thyroxine.

structure weighing about 50 mg. Despite their diminutive size, parathyroids serve a vital role in controlling calcium homeostasis.[36,70] Because calcium is crucial in many physiologic processes—including synaptic transmission, muscle contraction, and bone mineralization—the importance of parathyroid function is obvious. In fact, removal of the parathyroid glands results in convulsions and death because of inadequate plasma calcium levels. The parathyroids control calcium homeostasis through the synthesis and secretion of parathyroid hormone (PTH), and the regulation and function of PTH is discussed below.

Parathyroid Hormone

PTH is a polypeptide hormone that is synthesized within the cells of the parathyroid glands. The primary factor controlling the release of PTH is the amount of calcium in the bloodstream.[36] A calcium-sensing receptor is located on the outer surface of the parathyroid cell membrane, and this receptor monitors plasma calcium levels.[11,88] A decrease in plasma calcium activates this receptor and causes increased release of PTH. As blood calcium levels increase, the receptor is inhibited, and PTH release is reduced.

The primary physiologic effect of PTH is to increase blood calcium levels by altering calcium metabolism in three primary tissues: bone, kidney, and the gastrointestinal tract.[47,88] PTH directly affects skeletal tissues by increasing bone turnover, thus liberating calcium from skeletal stores.[70] High levels of PTH appear to enhance the development and action of cells (osteoclasts) that break down skeletal tissues.[86] Increased osteoclast activity degrades the collagen matrix within the bone, thus releasing calcium into the bloodstream. PTH also increases plasma calcium levels by increasing renal reabsorption of calcium. As renal calcium reabsorption increases, PTH produces a simultaneous increase in phosphate excretion. Thus, PTH produces a rise in plasma calcium that is accompanied by a decrease in plasma phosphate levels.[36]

Finally, PTH helps increase the absorption of calcium from the gastrointestinal tract. This effect appears to be caused by the interaction between PTH and vitamin D metabolism. PTH increases the conversion of vitamin D to 1,25-dihydroxycholecalciferol (calcitriol).[36] Calcitriol directly stimulates calcium absorption from the intestine.

Consequently, PTH is crucial to maintaining adequate levels of calcium in the body. In addition,

PTH works with two other primary hormones—calcitonin and vitamin D—in regulating calcium homeostasis. These three hormones, as well as several other endocrine factors, are all involved in controlling calcium levels for various physiologic needs. How these hormones interact in controlling normal bone formation and resorption is of particular interest to rehabilitation specialists. Regulation of bone mineral homeostasis and the principal hormones involved in this process are presented in the following section.

Regulation of Bone Mineral Homeostasis

Bone serves two primary functions: to provide a rigid framework for the body and to provide a readily available and easily interchangeable calcium pool.[83] To serve both functions simultaneously, an appropriate balance must exist between bone formation and bone resorption.[72] As already discussed, bone resorption (breakdown) can supply calcium for various physiologic processes. Mineral resorption, however, occurs at the expense of bone formation. The primary minerals that enable bone to maintain its rigidity are calcium and phosphate. Excessive resorption of these minerals will result in bone demineralization, and the skeletal system will undergo failure (fracture). In addition, bone is continually undergoing specific changes in its internal architecture. This process of remodeling allows bone to adapt to changing stresses and optimally resist applied loads.[72]

Consequently, bone is a rather dynamic tissue that is constantly undergoing changes in mineral content and internal structure. The balance between bone resorption and formation is controlled by the complex interaction of local and systemic factors. In particular, several hormones regulate bone formation and help maintain adequate plasma calcium levels. The primary hormones involved in regulating bone mineral homeostasis are described below.

Parathyroid Hormone. The role of the parathyroid gland and PTH in controlling calcium metabolism was previously discussed. A prolonged or continuous increase in the secretion of PTH increases blood calcium levels by several methods, including increased resorption of calcium from bone. High levels of PTH accelerate bone breakdown (catabolic effect) to mobilize calcium for other physiologic needs.

However, normal or intermittent PTH release may actually enhance bone formation.[70,77] That is, intermittent release of moderate amounts of PTH can stimulate osteoblast activity and promote bone formation (anabolic effect). The anabolic effects of low or normal PTH levels seem limited to trabecular or cancellous bone; PTH does not seem to enhance formation of solid or cortical bone.[60] Nonetheless, the possibility that small intermittent doses of PTH may increase certain types of bone formation has sparked interest in using this hormone to prevent or reverse bone demineralization in certain conditions, including osteoporosis (see later).[71,77] Therefore, PTH plays an important and complex role in regulating bone metabolism. A prolonged, continuous increase in PTH secretion favors bone breakdown, whereas normal (intermittent) PTH release encourages bone synthesis and remodeling.

Vitamin D. Vitamin D is a steroidlike hormone that can be obtained from dietary sources or synthesized in the skin from cholesterol derivatives in the presence of ultraviolet light. Vitamin D produces several metabolites that are important in bone mineral homeostasis.[27,31] In general, vitamin D derivatives such as 1,25 dihydroxyvitamin D_3 increase serum calcium and phosphate levels by increasing intestinal calcium and phosphate absorption and by decreasing renal calcium and phosphate excretion.[27,46]

The effects of vitamin D metabolites on bone itself are somewhat unclear. Some metabolites seem to promote bone resorption and others seem to favor bone formation.[10] The overall influence of vitamin D, however, is to enhance bone formation by increasing the supply of the two primary minerals needed for bone formation (calcium and phosphate). Vitamin D also directly suppresses the synthesis and release of PTH from the parathyroid glands, an effect that tends to promote bone mineralization by limiting the catabolic effects of PTH.[46,92]

Calcitonin. Calcitonin is a hormone secreted by cells located in the thyroid gland. These calcitonin-secreting cells (also known as *parafollicular* or *C cells*) are interspersed between follicles that produce thyroid hormones. Calcitonin can be considered the physiologic antagonist of PTH.[36] Calcitonin lowers blood calcium by stimulating bone formation and increasing the incorporation of calcium into skeletal storage. The action of calcitonin also enhances the incorporation of phosphate into bone. Renal excretion of calcium and phosphate is increased by a direct effect of calcitonin on the kidneys, which further reduces the levels of these minerals in the bloodstream. The

effects of calcitonin on bone mineral metabolism, however, are relatively minor compared with PTH, and endogenous production of calcitonin is not essential for normal bone mineral homeostasis.[41] In contrast, PTH is a much more dominant hormone, and the absence of PTH produces acute disturbances in calcium metabolism that result in death. Calcitonin does have an important therapeutic function, and pharmacologic doses of calcitonin may be helpful in preventing bone loss in certain conditions (see "Pharmacologic Control of Bone Mineral Homeostasis," later).

Other Hormones. A number of other hormones influence bone mineral content.[10] Glucocorticoids produce a general catabolic effect on bone and other supporting tissues (see Chapter 29). Certain prostaglandins are also potent stimulators of bone resorption. A number of hormones, such as estrogens, androgens, growth hormone, insulin, and the thyroid hormones, generally enhance bone formation. In general, the effects of these other hormones are secondary to the more direct effects of PTH, vitamin D, and calcitonin. Nonetheless, all of the hormones that influence bone metabolism interact to some extent in the regulation of bone formation and breakdown. In addition, disturbances in any of these secondary endocrine systems may produce problems that are manifested in abnormal bone formation, including excess glucocorticoid activity and growth hormone deficiency.

Pharmacologic Control of Bone Mineral Homeostasis

Satisfactory control of the primary bone minerals is important in both acute and long-term situations. Blood calcium levels must be maintained within a limited range to ensure an adequate supply of free calcium for various physiologic purposes. The normal range of total calcium in the plasma is 8.6 to 10.6 mg/100 mL.[41] If plasma calcium levels fall to below 6 mg/100 mL, tetanic muscle convulsions quickly ensue. Excess plasma calcium (blood levels greater than 12 mg/100 mL) depresses nervous function, leading to sluggishness, lethargy, and possibly coma.

Chronic disturbances in calcium homeostasis can also produce problems in bone calcification. Likewise, various metabolic bone diseases can alter blood calcium levels, leading to hypocalcemia or **hypercalcemia**. Some of the more common metabolic diseases

Table 31–4	EXAMPLES OF METABOLIC BONE DISEASE	
Disease	**Pathophysiology**	**Primary Drug Treatment**
Hypoparathyroidism	Decreased parathyroid hormone secretion; leads to impaired bone resorption and hypocalcemia	Calcium supplements, vitamin D
Hyperparathyroidism	Increased parathyroid hormone secretion, usually caused by parathyroid tumors; leads to excessive bone resorption and hypercalcemia	Usually treated surgically by partial or complete resection of the parathyroid gland
Osteoporosis	Generalized bone demineralization; often associated with effects of aging and hormonal changes in post-menopausal women	Calcium supplements, vitamin D, calcitonin, bisphosphonates, intermittent parathyroid hormone, estrogen, or SERMs (raloxifene) (see Chapter 30)
Rickets	Impaired bone mineralization in children; caused by a deficiency of vitamin D	Calcium supplements, vitamin D
Osteomalacia	Adult form of rickets	Calcium supplements, vitamin D
Paget disease	Excessive bone formation and resorption (turnover); leads to ineffective remodeling and structural abnormalities within the bone	Calcitonin, bisphosphonates
Renal osteodystrophy	Chronic renal failure; induces complex metabolic changes resulting in excessive bone resorption	Vitamin D, calcium supplements
Gaucher disease	Excessive lipid storage in bone leads to impaired remodeling and excessive bone loss	No drugs are effective
Hypercalcemia of malignancy	Many forms of cancer accelerate bone resorption, leading to hypercalcemia	Calcitonin, bisphosphonates

SERMs = selective estrogen receptor modulators.

affecting bone mineralization are listed in Table 31–4. Various problems in bone metabolism may produce abnormal plasma calcium levels, thus leading to the aforementioned problems.

Consequently, pharmacologic methods must often be used to help control bone mineral levels in the bloodstream and maintain adequate bone mineralization. Specific drugs used to control bone mineralization and the clinical conditions in which they are used are discussed next.

Calcium Supplements

Calcium preparations are often administered to ensure that adequate calcium levels are available in the body for various physiologic needs, including bone formation. Specifically, calcium supplements can be used to help prevent bone loss in conditions such as osteoporosis, osteomalacia, rickets, and hypoparathyroidism. For instance, calcium supplements alone cannot prevent osteoporosis in postmenopausal women,[9] but these supplements are certainly helpful when combined with other treatments such as bisphosphonates (see "Bisphosphonates," later).[85] The use of oral calcium supplements appears to be especially important in individuals who do not receive sufficient amounts of calcium in their diet.[12,85]

Types of calcium supplements used clinically are listed in Table 31–5. The dose of a calcium supplement should make up the difference between dietary calcium intake and established daily guidelines for each patient. The exact dose for a patient therefore depends on factors such as the amount of dietary

Table 31–5	DRUGS USED TO CONTROL BONE MINERAL HOMEOSTASIS	
General Category	**Examples***	**Treatment Rationale and Principal Indications**
Bisphosphonates	Alendronate (Fosamax) Etidronate (Didronel) Ibandronate (Boniva) Pamidronate (Aredia) Risedronate (Actonel)	Appear to block excessive bone resorption and formation; is used to normalize bone turnover in conditions such as osteoporosis and Paget disease, and to prevent hypercalcemia resulting from excessive bone resorption in certain forms of cancer
Calcitonin	Human calcitonin (Cibacalcin) Salmon calcitonin (Calcimar, Miacalcin)	Mimic the effects of endogenous calcitonin and increase bone formation in conditions such as Paget disease and osteoporosis; also used to lower plasma calcium levels in hypercalcemic emergencies
Calcium supplements	Calcium carbonate (BioCal, Os-Cal 500, Tums, others) Calcium citrate (Citracal) Calcium glubionate (Calcionate, Neo-Calglucon) Calcium gluconate Calcium lactate Dibasic calcium phosphate Tribasic calcium phosphate (Posture)	Provide an additional source of calcium to prevent calcium depletion and encourage bone formation in conditions such as osteoporosis, osteomalacia, rickets, and hypoparathyroidism
Estrogens	Conjugated estrogens (Premarin) Esterified estrogen (Menest) Estradiol (Estrace, Climara, Estraderm, others) Estropipate (Ogen, Ortho-Est) Raloxifene** (Evista)	Stabilize bone turnover and promote bone mineralization in women that lack endogenous estrogen production (e.g., following menopause or ovariectomy)
Vitamin D analogs	Calcifediol (Calderol) Calcitriol (Rocaltrol) Dihydrotachysterol (DHT, Hytakerol) Ergocalciferol (Calciferol, Drisdol)	Generally enhance bone formation by increasing the absorption and retention of calcium and phosphate in the body; useful in treating disorders caused by vitamin D deficiency, including hypocalcemia, hypophosphatemia, rickets, and osteomalacia

*Common trade names are shown in parentheses.
**Selective estrogen receptor modulator; see text and Chapter 30 for details.

calcium, age, gender, and hormonal and reproductive status (e.g., women who are pregnant, premenopausal, or postmenopausal).[40,64] A woman, for example, who is postmenopausal and ingests 500 to 600 mg of dietary calcium per day would need a supplemental dosage of approximately 800 mg/d because the recommended dietary allowance (RDA) guideline for women after menopause is 1200 to 1500 mg/d.[13]

Clearly, the dosage of a calcium supplement must be determined by the specific needs of each individual. Excessive doses must also be avoided because they may produce symptoms of hypercalcemia, including constipation, drowsiness, fatigue, and headache. As hypercalcemia becomes more pronounced, confusion, irritability, cardiac arrhythmias, hypertension, nausea and vomiting, skin rashes, and pain in bones and muscle may occur. Hypercalcemia is a cause for concern because severe cardiac irregularities may prove fatal.

Vitamin D

Vitamin D is a precursor for a number of compounds that increase intestinal absorption and decrease renal excretion of calcium and phosphate. Metabolites of vitamin D and their pharmacologic analogs are typically used to increase blood calcium and phosphate levels and to enhance bone mineralization in conditions such as osteodystrophy, rickets, or other situations where people lack adequate amounts of vitamin D. Vitamin D analogs such as calcitriol have also been combined with calcium supplements to help treat postmenopausal osteoporosis,[4,9] and to treat bone loss caused by anti-inflammatory steroids (glucocorticoids; see Chapter 29).[28,76] Specific vitamin D–related compounds and their clinical applications are listed in Table 31–5.

Vitamin D is a fat-soluble vitamin, and excessive doses can accumulate in the body, leading to toxicity. Some early signs of vitamin D toxicity include headache, increased thirst, decreased appetite, metallic taste, fatigue, and gastrointestinal disturbances (nausea, vomiting, constipation, or diarrhea). Increased vitamin D toxicity is associated with hypercalcemia, high blood pressure, cardiac arrhythmias, renal failure, mood changes, and seizures. Vitamin D toxicity is a serious problem that can cause death because of cardiac and renal failure.

Bisphosphonates

The bisphosphonates (also called *diphosphonates*) are a group of inorganic compounds that include alendronate (Fosamax), pamidronate (Aredia), and several similar agents (see Table 31–5). Although their exact mechanism is unclear, these compounds appear to adsorb directly into calcium crystals in the bone and to reduce bone resorption by inhibiting osteoclast activity.[73,75] Thus, bisphosphonates are often used in Paget disease to help prevent exaggerated bone turnover and promote adequate mineralization.[53] These agents can also be used to inhibit abnormal bone formation in conditions such as heterotopic ossification and to prevent hypercalcemia resulting from increased bone resorption in neoplastic disease.[50,66] Bisphosphonates can also help prevent and treat bone loss during prolonged administration of anti-inflammatory steroids (glucocorticoids).[87]

Bisphosphonates have emerged as one of the primary treatments for osteoporosis, including osteoporosis associated with estrogen loss in women after menopause.[26,90] Use of these drugs can increase bone mineral density and reduce the risk of vertebral and nonvertebral fractures (e.g., hip fractures) in men and women with osteoporosis.[26,69,73] Bisphosphonates have become especially attractive in treating postmenopausal osteoporosis because they improve bone health in women without the risks associated with estrogen replacement (see "Estrogen Therapy," later). Hence, bisphosphonates have become a mainstay in treatment of osteoporosis, and researchers continue to investigate optimal dosing regimens that take advantage of the beneficial effects of these drugs.[22,32]

Bisphosphonates may produce some relatively minor side effects, including gastrointestinal disturbances such as nausea and diarrhea. In addition, patients should remain upright after taking a bisphosphonate so that the drug does not reflux into the esophagus and cause irritation (esophagitis). Specific agents may also be associated with certain side effects. Etidronate (Didronel), for example, can cause tenderness and pain over bony lesion sites in Paget disease, leading to fractures if excessive doses are taken for prolonged periods. Pamidronate (Aredia) may cause fever and localized pain and redness at the injection site, but these effects usually last for only a day or two.

Calcitonin

Calcitonin derived from synthetic sources can be administered to mimic the effects of the endogenous hormone. As described previously, endogenous calcitonin decreases blood calcium levels and promotes bone mineralization. Consequently, synthetically derived calcitonin is used to treat hypercalcemia and to decrease bone resorption in Paget disease.[53] Calcitonin has also been used to help prevent bone loss in a variety of other conditions, including rheumatoid arthritis,[81] postmenopausal osteoporosis,[44] and glucocorticoid-induced osteoporosis.[62] Administration of calcitonin can reduce the risk of vertebral fractures, but does not seem to be as effective as the bisphosphonates in reducing this risk.[82] On the other hand, calcitonin may have an analgesic effect on bone pain that compliments the drug's ability to promote bone healing.[59,81] Hence, calcitonin may be a suitable alternative for people with painful vertebral fractures who cannot tolerate other drugs such as bisphosphonates.[82,93]

In the past, calcitonin was administered by injection (intramuscular or subcutaneous), but aerosolized versions of calcitonin are now available that allow delivery in the form of nasal sprays.[51,68] Oral delivery of calcitonin is difficult because this hormone is absorbed poorly from the gastrointestinal (GI) tract and because calcitonin is degraded by proteolytic enzymes in the stomach.[57] Nonetheless, efforts are being made to overcome these limitations, and an oral form of calcitonin may be available someday.[62]

Hence, calcitonin has emerged as an effective and easy way to treat a variety of conditions that are characterized by increased bone resorption.[59,82] Calcitonin preparations used clinically are either identical to the human form of this hormone (Cibacalcin) or chemically identical to salmon calcitonin (Calcimar, Miacalcin). Redness and swelling may occur locally when these agents are administered by injection. Other side effects include gastrointestinal disturbances (stomach pain, nausea, vomiting, and diarrhea), loss of appetite, and flushing or redness in the head, hands, and feet.

Estrogen Therapy

The benefits and risks of estrogen replacement therapy were addressed in Chapter 30. There is little doubt that providing estrogen to women who lack endogenous estrogen production—that is, following menopause or ovariectomy—can help increase bone mineral content and reduce the risk of fractures.[16,18,38,58] Estrogen is critical in maintaining adequate bone mineralization in women, and low doses of estrogen alone or estrogen combined with a progestin can be administered in certain women when endogenous estrogen production is lost. Replacement of estrogen following menopause has been shown to be especially effective—this treatment can return the rate of bone formation and bone resorption to premenopausal levels.[38]

Recent studies, however, indicated that estrogen replacement is associated with substantial risks, including an increased incidence of cardiovascular disease and certain cancers (see Chapter 30).[2,89] Hence, estrogen replacement is no longer considered the cornerstone for the long-term management of women with postmenopausal osteoporosis.[34] Estrogen can be used on a limited basis to prevent osteoporosis in certain postmenopausal women with persistent vasomotor symptoms (i.e., hot flashes); that is, estrogen is used to improve bone health while simultaneously treating the vasomotor symptoms.[18] Candidates for this treatment, however, must be considered on a case-by-case basis to make sure they do not have an increased risk for cardiovascular disease or breast and uterine cancers.[43] Estrogen can also be combined with other treatments (calcium supplements, calcitonin, calcitriol, bisphosphonates) to promote optimal bone mineralization in suitable candidates.

Fortunately, concerns about estrogen led to the development of estrogenlike compounds that activate estrogen receptors on certain tissues such as bone while blocking the effects of estrogen on breast and uterine tissues. These agents are known as selective estrogen receptor modulators (SERMs) because of their ability to activate certain estrogen receptors on certain types of tissue preferentially.[20,78] The pharmacology of SERMs is addressed in more detail in Chapter 30

The primary SERM used to prevent osteoporosis is raloxifene (Evista).[21,42,48] This drug binds to and activates estrogen receptors in bone, thus preventing bone loss and demineralization. At the same time, raloxifene blocks estrogen receptors on breast and uterine tissues, thereby preventing the excessive stimulation of receptors that might lead to the development of cancer. Raloxifene also promotes positive effects on the cardiovascular system, including improvements in plasma lipid profiles. Hence, SERMs such as raloxifene provide an alternative to traditional estrogen therapy, and may be especially useful to women who are at risk for cardiovascular disease or have a history of breast or uterine cancer.[39] Efforts continue to develop other SERMs that will be effective in preventing osteoporosis while minimizing the risks associated with traditional estrogen replacement therapy.

Other Agents That Promote Bone Mineral Content

Several other innovative strategies have been developed recently to improve bone mineralization. Teriparatide (Forteo), for example, is a synthetic form of human parathyroid hormone (PTH) that was developed to treat severe cases of osteoporosis.[77,80] As indicated earlier, prolonged or continuous release of PTH increases bone resorption and breakdown, whereas intermittent doses of PTH may increase bone mineral density. Hence, small dosages of teriparatide (20 g) can be administered daily by subcutaneous injection to provide a burst of PTH activity.[37,71] This treatment can increase bone mineral density throughout the body, resulting in a reduced risk of vertebral and nonvertebral fractures.

Another new strategy involves drugs that stimulate calcium receptors on the parathyroid gland, thereby inhibiting the release of PTH.[49] As indicated earlier, plasma calcium ions regulate the release of PTH by affecting calcium receptors on the parathyroid gland. An increase in plasma calcium inhibits release of PTH, and a decrease in plasma calcium stimulates PTH release. Drugs mimicking the effects of endogenous calcium (i.e., calcimimetics) can therefore be used to reduce PTH release in people with parathyroid tumors or other conditions that cause prolonged, continuous release of PTH.[29,49] This effect will help prevent bone breakdown and the resulting increase in plasma calcium levels (hypercalcemia) that are associated with excessive PTH release. Cinacalcet (Sensipar) is the primary calcimimetic agent that is clinically used; other calcimimetics and strategies for controlling bone mineral content may be forthcoming.

Special Concerns in Rehabilitation Patients

■ ■ ■ Physical therapists and occupational therapists should generally be concerned about the potential side effects of the drugs discussed in this chapter. With regard to the treatment of thyroid disorders, excessive doses of drugs used to treat either hyperthyroidism or hypothyroidism tend to produce symptoms of the opposite disorder; that is, overdose of antithyroid drugs can produce signs of hypothyroidism, and vice versa. Therapists should be aware of the signs of thyroid dysfunction (see Table 31–2) and should be able to help detect signs of inappropriate drug dosage. Therapists should also avoid using rehabilitation techniques that may exacerbate any symptoms of thyroid dysfunction. For instance, care should be taken not to overstress the cardiovascular system of a patient with decreased cardiac output and hypotension caused by hypothyroidism (see Table 31–2).

Likewise, physical therapists and occupational therapists should be aware of the potential adverse effects of the drugs that regulate calcium homeostasis. For instance, excessive doses of calcium supplements may alter cardiovascular function, resulting in cardiac arrhythmias. Therapists may help detect these arrhythmias while monitoring pulses or electrocardiogram (ECG) recordings. Finally, therapists may enhance the effects of bone-mineralizing drugs by employing exercise and weight-bearing activities to stimulate bone formation. In addition, certain modalities may enhance the effects of bone-mineralizing agents. In particular, ultraviolet light increases endogenous vitamin D biosynthesis, thus facilitating calcium absorption and bone formation (see "Case Study").

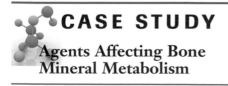

CASE STUDY

Agents Affecting Bone Mineral Metabolism

Brief History. R.D. is a 74-year-old woman with a history of generalized bone demineralization caused by osteomalacia that was primarily brought on by poor diet; that is, her total caloric intake and dietary levels of calcium and vitamin D have been very low. The patient is also rather reclusive, spending most of her time indoors. Consequently, she virtually lacks any exposure to natural sunlight. To treat her osteomalacia, she was placed on a regimen of oral calcium supplements and vitamin D. However, she has been reluctant to take these supplements because when she did, she occasionally experienced problems with diarrhea. Recently, she sustained a fracture of the femoral neck during a fall. She was admitted to the hospital, and the fracture was stabilized by open reduction and internal fixation. The patient was referred to physical therapy for strengthening and pre–weight-bearing activities.

Problem/Influence of Medication. During the postoperative period, calcium and vitamin D supplements were reinstituted to facilitate bone formation. The patient, however, soon began to experience bouts of diarrhea, apparently as a side effect of the vitamin D supplements. Consequently, the vitamin D supplements were withdrawn, and only the calcium supplement was continued. Because metabolic by-products of vitamin D accelerate the absorption of calcium from the gastrointestinal tract, both agents should be administered together. This patient, however, was apparently unable

to tolerate vitamin D (or its analogs), possibly because of hypersensitivity to these compounds.

Decision/Solution. The physical therapist working with this patient realized that ultraviolet radiation stimulates the production of endogenous vitamin D. Ultraviolet light catalyzes the conversion of a cholesterollike precursor (7-dehydrocholesterol) to vitamin D_3 within the skin. Vitamin D_3 then undergoes conversions in the liver and kidneys to form specific vitamin D metabolites (i.e., 1,25-dihydroxyvitamin D), which enhance intestinal calcium absorption. After conferring with the physician, the therapist incorporated a program of therapeutic ultraviolet radiation into the treatment regimen. The appropriate dose of ultraviolet exposure was first determined, followed by daily application of whole-body irradiation. Ultraviolet therapy was continued throughout the remainder of the patient's hospitalization, and callus formation at the fracture site was progressing well at the time of discharge.

SUMMARY

The thyroid and parathyroid glands serve a number of vital endocrine functions. The thyroid gland synthesizes and secretes the thyroid hormones T_3 and T_4. These hormones are important regulators of cellular metabolism and metabolic rate. Thyroid hormones also interact with other hormones to facilitate normal growth and development. The parathyroid glands control calcium homeostasis through the release of PTH. This hormone is crucial

in maintaining normal blood calcium levels and in regulating bone formation and resorption. PTH also interacts with other hormones such as vitamin D and calcitonin in the control of bone mineral metabolism. Acute and chronic problems in thyroid and parathyroid function are often successfully treated with various pharmacologic agents. Rehabilitation specialists should be aware of the general strategies for treating thyroid and parathyroid disorders and of the basic pharmacotherapeutic approach to these problems.

References

1. Abraham P, Avenell A, Park CM, et al. A systematic review of drug therapy for Graves' hyperthyroidism. *Eur J Endocrinol.* 2005;153:489–498.
2. Anderson GL, Limacher M, Assaf AR, et al. Effects of conjugated equine estrogen in postmenopausal women with hysterectomy: the Women's Health Initiative randomized controlled trial. *JAMA.* 2004; 291:1701–1712.
3. Ando T, Latif R, Davies TF. Thyrotropin receptor antibodies: new insights into their actions and clinical relevance. *Best Pract Res Clin Endocrinol Metab.* 2005;19: 33–52.
4. Avenell A, Gillespie WJ, Gillespie LD, O'Connell DL. Vitamin D and vitamin D analogues for preventing fractures associated with involutional and post-menopausal osteoporosis. *Cochrane Database Syst Rev.* 2005; CD000227.
5. Azizi F. The safety and efficacy of antithyroid drugs. *Expert Opin Drug Saf.* 2006;5:107–116.

6. Ban Y, Tomer Y. Genetic susceptibility in thyroid autoimmunity. *Pediatr Endocrinol Rev.* 2005;3: 20–32.
7. Biondi B, Palmieri EA, Klain M, et al. Subclinical hyperthyroidism: clinical features and treatment options. *Eur J Endocrinol.* 2005;152:1–9.
8. Boelaert K, Franklyn JA. Thyroid hormone in health and disease. *J Endocrinol.* 2005;187:1–15.
9. Boonen S, Rizzoli R, Meunier PJ, et al. The need for clinical guidance in the use of calcium and vitamin D in the management of osteoporosis: a consensus report. *Osteoporos Int.* 2004;15:511–519.
10. Bringhurst FR, Demay MB, Kronenberg HM. Hormones and disorders of mineral metabolism. In: Larsen PR, et al, eds. *Williams Textbook of Endocrinology.* 10th ed. Philadelphia: WB Saunders; 2003.
11. Brown EM. Calcium sensing by endocrine cells. *Endocr Pathol.* 2004;15:187–219.
12. Cashman KD. Calcium intake, calcium bioavailability and bone health. *Br J Nutr.* 2002;87(suppl 2): S169–S177.

13. Celotti F, Bignamini A. Dietary calcium and mineral/vitamin supplementation: a controversial problem. *J Int Med Res.* 1999;27:1.
14. Clarke N, Kabadi UM. Optimizing treatment of hypothyroidism. *Treat Endocrinol.* 2004;3:217–221.
15. Clyde PW, Harari AE, Getka EJ, Shakir KM. Combined levothyroxine plus liothyronine compared with levothyroxine alone in primary hypothyroidism: a randomized controlled trial. *JAMA.* 2003;290: 2952–2958.
16. Col NF, Bowlby LA, McGarry K. The role of menopausal hormone therapy in preventing osteoporotic fractures: a critical review of the clinical evidence. *Minerva Med.* 2005;96:331–342.
17. Colson AO, Gershengorn MC. Thyrotropin-releasing hormone analogs. *Mini Rev Med Chem.* 2006;6: 221–226.
18. Compston J. How to manage osteoporosis after the menopause. *Best Pract Res Clin Rheumatol.* 2005;19: 1007–1019.
19. Cooper DS. Antithyroid drugs. *N Engl J Med.* 2005; 352:905–917.
20. Cosman F. Selective estrogen-receptor modulators. *Clin Geriatr Med.* 2003;19:371–379.
21. Cranney A, Adachi JD. Benefit-risk assessment of raloxifene in postmenopausal osteoporosis. *Drug Saf.* 2005;28:721–730.
22. Cremers SC, Pillai G, Papapoulos SE. Pharmacokinetics/pharmacodynamics of bisphosphonates: use for optimisation of intermittent therapy for osteoporosis. *Clin Pharmacokinet.* 2005;44:551–570.
23. Danzi S, Klein I. Potential uses of T_3 in the treatment of human disease. *Clin Cornerstone.* 2005;7(suppl 2): S9–S15.
24. Danzi S, Klein I. Thyroid hormone and the cardiovascular system. *Minerva Endocrinol.* 2004;29:139–150.
25. Davies TF, Larsen PR. Thyrotoxicosis. In: Larsen PR, et al, eds. *Williams Textbook of Endocrinology.* 10th ed. Philadelphia: WB Saunders; 2003.
26. Delmas PD. The use of bisphosphonates in the treatment of osteoporosis. *Curr Opin Rheumatol.* 2005;17: 462–466.
27. DeLuca HF. Overview of general physiologic features and functions of vitamin D. *Am J Clin Nutr.* 2004;80 (Suppl):1689S–1696S.
28. de Nijs RN, Jacobs JW, Algra A, et al. Prevention and treatment of glucocorticoid-induced osteoporosis with active vitamin D_3 analogues: a review with meta-analysis of randomized controlled trials including organ transplantation studies. *Osteoporos Int.* 2004;15: 589–602.
29. Dong BJ. Cinacalcet: An oral calcimimetic agent for the management of hyperparathyroidism. *Clin Ther.* 2005;27:1725–1751.
30. Dupre SM, Guissouma H, Flamant F, et al. Both thyroid hormone receptor (TR) beta 1 and TR beta 2 isoforms contribute to the regulation of hypothalamic thyrotropin-releasing hormone. *Endocrinology.* 2004; 145:2337–2345.
31. Dusso AS, Brown AJ, Slatopolsky E. Vitamin D. *Am J Physiol Renal Physiol.* 2005;289:F8–F28.
32. Epstein S, Zaidi M. Biological properties and mechanism of action of ibandronate: application to the treatment of osteoporosis. *Bone.* 2005;37:433–440.
33. Escobar-Morreale HF, Botella-Carretero JI, Gomez-Bueno M, et al. Thyroid hormone replacement therapy in primary hypothyroidism: a randomized trial comparing L-thyroxine plus liothyronine with L-thyroxine alone. *Ann Intern Med.* 2005;142:412–424.
34. Farquhar CM, Marjoribanks J, Lethaby A, et al. Long term hormone therapy for perimenopausal and postmenopausal women. *Cochrane Database Syst Rev.* 2005; CD004143
35. Farwell AP, Braverman LE. Thyroid and antithyroid drugs. In: Brunton LL, et al, eds. *The Pharmacological Basis of Therapeutics.* 11th ed. New York: McGraw-Hill; 2006.
36. Friedman PA. Agents affecting ion mineral homeostasis and bone turnover. In: Brunton LL, et al, eds. *The Pharmacological Basis of Therapeutics.* 11th ed. New York: McGraw-Hill; 2006.
37. Frolik CA, Black EC, Cain RL, et al. Anabolic and catabolic bone effects of human parathyroid hormone (1–34) are predicted by duration of hormone exposure. *Bone.* 2003;33:372–379.
38. Gambacciani M, Vacca F. Postmenopausal osteoporosis and hormone replacement therapy. *Minerva Med.* 2004;95:507–520.
39. Gaudio A, Morabito N. Pharmacological management of severe postmenopausal osteoporosis. *Drugs Aging.* 2005;22:405–417.
40. Gennari C. Calcium and vitamin D nutrition and bone disease of the elderly. *Public Health Nutr.* 2001;4: 547–559.
41. Genuth SM. Endocrine regulation of the metabolism of calcium and phosphate. In: Berne RM, Levy MN, eds. *Physiology.* 3rd ed. St Louis: Mosby Year Book; 2000.
42. Gluck O, Maricic M. Skeletal and nonskeletal effects of raloxifene. *Curr Osteoporos Rep.* 2003;1:123–128.
43. Greenblatt D. Treatment of postmenopausal osteoporosis. *Pharmacotherapy.* 2005;25:574–584.
44. Hauselmann HJ, Rizzoli R. A comprehensive review of treatments for postmenopausal osteoporosis. *Osteoporos Int.* 2003;14:2–12.
45. He CT, Hsieh AT, Pei D, et al. Comparison of single daily dose of methimazole and propylthiouracil in the treatment of Graves' hyperthyroidism. *Clin Endocrinol.* 2004;60:676–681.
46. Hendy GN, Hruska KA, Mathew S, Goltzman D. New insights into mineral and skeletal regulation by active forms of vitamin D. *Kidney Int.* 2006;69: 218–223.
47. Hoenderop JG, Nilius B, Bindels RJ. Calcium absorption across epithelia. *Physiol Rev.* 2005;85:373–422.
48. Johnell O, Cauley JA, Kulkarni PM, et al. Raloxifene reduces risk of vertebral fractures in postmenopausal women regardless of prior hormone therapy. *J Fam Pract.* 2004;53:789–796.
49. Joy MS, Kshirsagar AV, Franceschini N. Calcimimetics and the treatment of primary and secondary hyperparathyroidism. *Ann Pharmacother.* 2004;38:1871–1880.

50. Kanakis I, Kousidou OCh, Karamanos NK. In vitro and in vivo antiresorptive effects of bisphosphonates in metastatic bone disease. *In Vivo.* 2005;19:311–318.

51. Kaskani E, Lyritis GP, Kosmidis C, et al. Effect of intermittent administration of 200 IU intranasal salmon calcitonin and low doses of 1alpha(OH) vitamin D3 on bone mineral density of the lumbar spine and hip region and biochemical bone markers in women with postmenopausal osteoporosis: a pilot study. *Clin Rheumatol.* 2005;24:232–238.

52. LaFranchi S. Congenital hypothyroidism: Etiologies, diagnosis, and management. *Thyroid.* 199; 9:735.

53. Langston AL, Ralston SH. Management of Paget's disease of bone. *Rheumatology.* 2004;43:955–959.

54. Larsen PR, Davies TF. Hypothyroidism and thyroiditis. In: Larsen PR, et al, eds. *Williams Textbook of Endocrinology.* 10th ed. Philadelphia: WB Saunders 2003.

55. Larsen PR, Davies TF, Schlumberger MJ, Hay ID. Thyroid physiology and diagnostic evaluation of patients with thyroid disorders. In: Larsen PR, et al, eds. *Williams Textbook of Endocrinology.* 10th ed. Philadelphia: WB Saunders 2003.

56. Lazarus JH. Thyroid disease in pregnancy and childhood. *Minerva Endocrinol.* 2005;30:71–87.

57. Lee YH, Sinko PJ. Oral delivery of salmon calcitonin. *Adv Drug Deliv Rev.* 2000;42:225–238.

58. Lindsay R. Hormones and bone health in postmenopausal women. *Endocrine.* 2004;24:223–230.

59. Mehta NM, Malootian A, Gilligan JP. Calcitonin for osteoporosis and bone pain. *Curr Pharm Des.* 2003;9:2659–2676.

60. Miyakoshi N. Effects of parathyroid hormone on cancellous bone mass and structure in osteoporosis. *Curr Pharm Des.* 2004;10:2615–2627.

61. Moore JM, Guy RK. Coregulator interactions with the thyroid hormone receptor. *Mol Cell Proteomics.* 2005;4: 475–482.

62. Munoz-Torres M, Alonso G, Raya MP. Calcitonin therapy in osteoporosis. *Treat Endocrinol.* 2004;3:117–132.

63. Nikrodhanond AA, Ortiga-Carvalho TM, Shibusawa N, et al. Dominant role of thyrotropin-releasing hormone in the hypothalamic-pituitary-thyroid axis. *J Biol Chem.* 2006;281:5000–5007.

64. North American Menopause Society. The role of calcium in peri- and postmenopausal women: consensus opinion of The North American Menopause Society. *Menopause.* 2001;8:84–95.

65. Panzer C, Beazley R, Braverman L. Rapid preoperative preparation for severe hyperthyroid Graves' disease. *J Clin Endocrinol Metab.* 2004;89:2142–2144.

66. Pavlakis N, Schmidt R, Stockler M. Bisphosphonates for breast cancer. *Cochrane Database Syst Rev.* 2005; CD003474.

67. Pearce EN, Braverman LE. Hyperthyroidism: advantages and disadvantages of medical therapy. *Surg Clin North Am.* 2004;84:833–847.

68. Peichl P, Griesmacher A, Kumpan W, et al. Clinical outcome of salmon calcitonin nasal spray treatment in postmenopausal women after total hip arthroplasty. *Gerontology.* 2005;51:242–252.

69. Perez-Lopez FR. Postmenopausal osteoporosis and alendronate. *Maturitas.* 2004;48:179–192.

70. Poole KE, Reeve J. Parathyroid hormone—a bone anabolic and catabolic agent. *Curr Opin Pharmacol.* 2005;5:612–617.

71. Qin L, Raggatt LJ, Partridge NC. Parathyroid hormone: a double-edged sword for bone metabolism. *Trends Endocrinol Metab.* 2004;15:60–65.

72. Raisz LG. Physiology and pathophysiology of bone remodeling. *Clin Chem.* 1999;45 (pt 2):1353–1358.

73. Recker RR, Barger-Lux J. Risedronate for prevention and treatment of osteoporosis in postmenopausal women. *Expert Opin Pharmacother.* 2005;6:465–477.

74. Reid JR, Wheeler SF. Hyperthyroidism: diagnosis and treatment. *Am Fam Physician.* 2005;72:623–630.

75. Reszka AA, Rodan GA. Nitrogen-containing bisphosphonate mechanism of action. *Mini Rev Med Chem.* 2004;4:711–719.

76. Richy F, Ethgen O, Bruyere O, Reginster JY. Efficacy of alphacalcidol and calcitriol in primary and corticosteroid-induced osteoporosis: a meta-analysis of their effects on bone mineral density and fracture rate. *Osteoporos Int.* 2004;15:301–310.

77. Rubin MR, Bilezikian JP. The potential of parathyroid hormone as a therapy for osteoporosis. *Int J Fertil Womens Med.* 2002;47:103–115.

78. Sambrook P. Who will benefit from treatment with selective estrogen receptor modulators (SERMs)? *Best Pract Res Clin Rheumatol.* 2005;19:975–981

79. Schott M, Scherbaum WA, Morgenthaler NG. Thyrotropin receptor autoantibodies in Graves' disease. *Trends Endocrinol Metab.* 2005;16:243–248.

80. Silver J, Bushinsky D. Harnessing the parathyroids to create stronger bones. *Curr Opin Nephrol Hypertens.* 2004;13:471–476.

81. Silverman SL. Calcitonin. *Rheum Dis Clin North Am.* 2001;27:187–196.

82. Silverman SL. Calcitonin. *Endocrinol Metab Clin North Am.* 2003;32:273–284.

83. Simon LS. Osteoporosis. *Clin Geriatr Med.* 2005;21: 603–629.

84. Streetman DD, Khanderia U. Diagnosis and treatment of Graves disease. *Ann Pharmacother.* 2003;37: 1100–1109.

85. Sunyecz JA, Weisman SM. The role of calcium in osteoporosis drug therapy. *J Womens Health.* 2005; 14:180–192.

86. Swarthout JT, D'Alonzo RC, Selvamurugan N, Partridge NC. Parathyroid hormone-dependent signaling pathways regulating genes in bone cells. *Gene.* 2002; 282:1–17.

87. Tamura Y, Okinaga H, Takami H. Glucocorticoid-induced osteoporosis. *Biomed Pharmacother.* 2004; 58:500–504.

88. Tfelt-Hansen J, Brown EM. The calcium-sensing receptor in normal physiology and pathophysiology: a review. *Crit Rev Clin Lab Sci.* 2005;42:35–70.

89. Warren MP, Halpert S. Hormone replacement therapy: controversies, pros and cons. *Best Pract Res Clin Endocrinol Metab.* 2004;18:317–332.

90. Watts NB. Bisphosphonate treatment of osteoporosis. *Clin Geriatr Med.* 2003;19:395–414.

91. Wiersinga WM. Thyroid hormone replacement therapy. *Horm Res.* 2001;56(suppl 1):74–81.

92. Willett AM. Vitamin D status and its relationship with parathyroid hormone and bone mineral status in older adolescents. *Proc Nutr Soc.* 2005;64:193–203.

93. Woo T, Adachi JD. Role of bisphosphonates and calcitonin in the prevention and treatment of osteoporosis. *Best Pract Res Clin Rheumatol.* 2001;15:469–481.

94. Yen PM, Chin WW. Genomic and nongenomic actions of thyroid hormone. In: Braverman LE, Utiger RD, eds. *Werner and Ingbar's The Thyroid.* 9th ed. New York: Lippincott Williams and Wilkins; 2005.

Chapter 32

Pancreatic Hormones and the Treatment of Diabetes Mellitus

The pancreas functions uniquely as both an endocrine and an exocrine gland. The gland's exocrine role consists of excretion of digestive enzymes into the duodenum via the pancreatic duct. Pancreatic endocrine function consists of the secretion of two principal hormones—insulin and glucagon—into the bloodstream. Insulin and glucagon are primarily involved with the regulation of blood glucose. Insulin also plays a role in protein and lipid metabolism and is important in several aspects of growth and development. Problems with the production and function of insulin cause a fairly common and clinically significant disease known as diabetes mellitus.

The purpose of this chapter is to review the normal physiologic roles of the pancreatic hormones and to describe the pathogenesis and treatment of diabetes mellitus. Diabetes mellitus has many sequelae that influence patients' neuromuscular and cardiovascular functioning. Patients with diabetes mellitus often undergo physical rehabilitation for problems related to the condition. Consequently, the nature of diabetes mellitus and the pharmacotherapeutic treatment of this disease are important to physical therapists and occupational therapists.

Structure and Function of the Endocrine Pancreas

The cellular composition of the pancreas has been described in great detail.[10,28,35] The bulk of the gland consists of acinar cells that synthesize and release pancreatic digestive enzymes (thereby providing the exocrine function). Interspersed within the acinar tissues are smaller clumps of tissue known as the *islets of Langerhans*. These islets contain cells that synthesize and secrete pancreatic hormones, thus constituting the endocrine portion of the gland.

The pancreatic islets consist of four primary cell types: alpha (A) cells, which produce glucagon; beta (B) cells, which produce insulin; delta (D) cells, which produce somatostatin; and (F) cells, which produce pancreatic polypeptide. As previously mentioned, this chapter focuses on the functions of insulin and glucagon. The exact physiologic roles of the other pancreatic hormones are not entirely clear. For example, the function of the pancreatic polypeptide released from pancreatic F cells remains to be determined.

Somatostatin, however, is a polypeptide hormone that appears to affect several physiologic systems, including the regulation of gastrointestinal (GI) absorption and motility. Although the exact role of pancreatic somatostatin is still somewhat unclear, this hormone may inhibit the release of glucagon and insulin.[93] Somatostatin is also produced in other tissues including the brain and GI tract, and this hormone may affect many other neuroendocrine responses.[92] Future studies may clarify the physiological effects of somatostatin and pancreatic polypeptide.

Insulin

Insulin is a large polypeptide of 51 amino acids arranged in a specific sequence and configuration. The primary effect of insulin is to lower blood glucose levels by facilitating the entry of glucose into peripheral tissues. The effects of insulin on energy metabolism, specific aspects of insulin release, and insulin's mechanism of action are discussed here.

Effects of Insulin on Carbohydrate Metabolism. Following a meal, blood glucose sharply increases. Insulin is responsible for facilitating the movement of glucose out of the bloodstream and into the liver and other tissues, where it can be stored for future needs.[35,122] Most tissues in the body (including skeletal muscle cells) are relatively impermeable to glucose and require the presence of some sort of transport system, or carrier, to help convey the glucose molecule across the cell membrane.[115,122] The carrier-mediated transport of glucose into muscle cells is believed to be a form of facilitated diffusion (see Chapter 2). Insulin appears to directly stimulate this facilitated diffusion, resulting in a 10-fold or greater increase in the rate of glucose influx.[60] The possible ways that insulin affects glucose transport on the cellular level are discussed later in "Cellular Mechanisms of Insulin Action."

Insulin affects the uptake and use of glucose in the liver somewhat differently than in skeletal muscle and other tissues. Hepatic cells are relatively permeable to glucose, and glucose enters these cells quite easily, even when insulin is not present. Glucose, however, is also free to leave liver cells just as easily, unless it is trapped in the cells in some manner. Insulin stimulates the activity of the glucokinase enzyme, which phosphorylates glucose and subsequently traps the glucose molecule in the hepatic cell. Insulin also increases the activity of enzymes that promote glycogen synthesis and inhibits the enzymes that promote glycogen breakdown. Thus, the primary effect of insulin on the liver is to promote the sequestration of the glucose molecule and to increase the storage of glucose in the form of hepatic glycogen.

Effects of Insulin on Protein and Lipid Metabolism. Although insulin is normally associated with regulating blood glucose, this hormone also exerts significant effects on proteins and lipids. In general, insulin promotes storage of protein and lipid in muscle and adipose tissue, respectively.[14,35,48] Insulin encourages protein synthesis in muscle cells by stimulating amino acid uptake, increasing DNA/RNA activity related to protein synthesis, and inhibiting protein breakdown. In fat cells, insulin stimulates the synthesis of triglycerides (the primary form of lipid storage in the body), and inhibits the enzyme that breaks down stored lipids (hormone-sensitive lipase). Consequently, insulin is involved in carbohydrate, protein, and lipid metabolism; disturbances in insulin function (diabetes mellitus) will affect the storage and use of all the primary energy substrates.

Cellular Mechanism of Insulin Action

Insulin exerts its effects first by binding to a receptor located on the surface membrane of target cells.[35,38] This receptor is a glycoprotein that is highly specific for insulin. The complete insulin receptor consists of two matching or paired units, with each unit consisting of an alpha and a beta subunit (Fig. 32–1). The alpha subunit is the binding site for insulin. The beta subunit appears to be an enzyme that functions as a tyrosine kinase, which means that the beta subunit catalyzes the addition of phosphate groups to tyrosine residues within the beta subunit.[35,93] Thus, binding insulin to the alpha subunit causes the beta subunit to undergo *autophosphorylation;* that is, the receptor adds phosphate groups to itself. This autophosphorylation of the insulin receptor then initiates a series of biochemical changes within the cell.

The way that the insulin-receptor interaction triggers subsequent changes in cellular activity has been the subject of extensive research. When activated, the insulin receptor begins to add phosphate molecules to other large intracellular proteins known as insulin receptor substrates (IRSs).[23,58] Although the exact details need to be elucidated, IRSs initiate changes in various metabolic pathways that ultimately result in increased glucose uptake, increased protein synthesis, and other changes in cell metabolism.[76,122] In particular, certain IRSs initiate the movement *(translocation)* of glucose transporters from intracellular storage sites to the cell membrane of skeletal muscle cells and other peripheral tissues (see Fig. 32–1). These glucose transporters are proteins that are synthesized and stored within the Golgi system of the cell. Glucose transporters are likewise often referred to as GLUT proteins or simply GLUTs; several different forms of GLUTs exist, depending on the specific cell that is affected by insulin. Perhaps the most important GLUT protein is the GLUT4 subtype, which is the glucose transporter in muscle and fat cells.[66,122] By binding to the insulin receptor on the cell membrane, insulin ultimately causes GLUT4 proteins to travel to the cell membrane, where they can then promote the facilitated diffusion of glucose into the cell (see Fig. 32–1).

Consequently, we now have a fairly clear idea of how insulin binds to a specific receptor and exerts its effects on target cells. Knowledge of exactly how insulin interacts with target tissues is important since defects in receptor binding and problems in the sub-

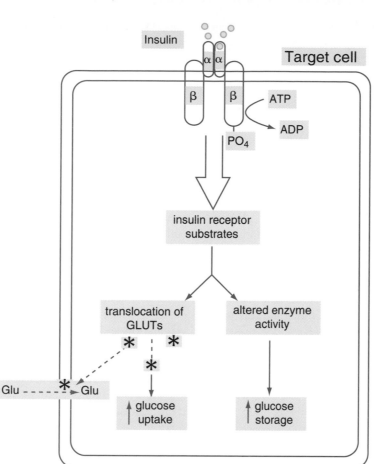

FIGURE 32–1 ▼ Possible mechanism of insulin action on glucose metabolism in skeletal muscle cells. An insulin receptor located on the cell's surface consists of 2 alpha (α) and 2 beta (β) subunits. Binding of insulin to the α subunits causes addition of phosphate groups (PO_4) to the β subunits. This receptor autophosphorylation causes the activation of one or more insulin receptor substrates (IRSs), which promote translocation of glucose carriers (GLUTs) to the cell membrane, where they increase facilitated diffusion of glucose (Glu) into the cell. Activated IRSs also increase the activity of enzymes that promote glucose storage.

sequent postreceptor events may be responsible for some of the changes seen in certain forms of diabetes mellitus. The possible role of these receptor-mediated problems in diabetes is discussed later in "Type 2 Diabetes."

Glucagon

Glucagon is considered to be the hormonal antagonist of insulin.[29,35] The primary effect of glucagon is to increase blood glucose to maintain normal blood glucose levels and to prevent hypoglycemia.[35,93] Glucagon pro-

duces a rapid increase in glycogen breakdown *(glycogenolysis)* in the liver, thus liberating glucose in the bloodstream from hepatic glycogen stores. Glucagon then stimulates a more prolonged increase in hepatic glucose production *(gluconeogenesis)*. This gluconeogenesis sustains blood glucose levels even after hepatic glycogen has been depleted.[93]

Glucagon appears to exert its effects on liver cells by a classic adenyl cyclase–cyclic adenosine monophosphate (cAMP) second messenger system (see Chapter 4).[93] Glucagon binds to a specific receptor located on the hepatic cell membrane. This stimulates the activity of the adenyl cyclase enzyme that transforms adenosine triphosphate (ATP) into cAMP. Then, cAMP acts as an intracellular second messenger that activates specific enzymes to increase glycogen breakdown and stimulate gluconeogenesis.

Control of Insulin and Glucagon Release

An adequate level of glucose in the bloodstream is necessary to provide a steady supply of energy for certain tissues, especially the brain. Normally, blood glucose is maintained between 80 and 90 mg of glucose per 100 mL of blood.[29] A severe drop in blood glucose (*hypoglycemia*) is a potentially serious problem that can result in coma and death. Chronic elevations in blood glucose (hyperglycemia) have been implicated in producing pathologic changes in neural and vascular structures. Consequently, insulin and glucagon play vital roles in controlling glucose levels, and the release of these hormones must be closely regulated.

The level of glucose in the bloodstream is the primary factor affecting pancreatic hormone release.[29] As blood glucose rises (e.g., following a meal), insulin secretion from pancreatic beta cells is increased. Insulin then promotes the movement of glucose out of the bloodstream and into various tissues, thus reducing plasma glucose back to normal levels. As blood glucose levels fall (e.g., during a sustained fast), glucagon is released from the alpha cells in the pancreas. Glucagon resolves this hypoglycemia by stimulating the synthesis and release of glucose from the liver.

The release of insulin and glucagon may also be governed by other energy substrates (lipids and amino acids), other hormones (thyroxine, cortisol), and autonomic neural control.[29,46] Nonetheless, the major factor influencing pancreatic hormone release is blood glucose. Cells located in the pancreatic islets are bathed directly by the blood supply reaching the pancreas. These cells act as glucose sensors, directly monitoring plasma glucose levels. In particular, the beta cells or insulin-secreting cells act as the primary glucose sensors, and adequate control of insulin release seems to be a somewhat higher priority than the control of glucagon function.[29]

An important interaction between insulin and glucagon may also take place directly within the pancreas, and insulin appears to be the dominant hormone controlling this interaction.[29,53] When the beta cells sense an increase in blood glucose, they release insulin, which in turn inhibits glucagon release from the alpha cells. When insulin release diminishes, the inhibition of glucagon production is removed, and glucagon secretion is free to increase. This intraislet regulation between insulin and glucagon is important during normal physiologic function as well as in pathologic conditions, such as diabetes mellitus.[53] A deficiency of insulin production permits an increase in glucagon release, and the effects of increased glucagon may contribute to some of the metabolic changes in diabetes mellitus (although the exact role of increased glucagon in diabetes mellitus remains controversial).[35]

Consequently, insulin and glucagon serve to maintain blood glucose within a finite range. If the endocrine portion of the pancreas is functioning normally, blood glucose levels remain remarkably constant, even in situations such as exercise and prolonged fasting. However, any abnormalities in pancreatic endocrine function can alter the regulation of blood glucose. In particular, problems associated with the production and effects of insulin can produce serious disturbances in glucose metabolism, as well as a number of other metabolic problems. Problems in insulin production and function are characteristic of a disease known as diabetes mellitus. The pathogenesis and treatment of this disease is presented in the following section.

Diabetes Mellitus

Diabetes mellitus is a disease caused by insufficient insulin secretion or a decrease in the peripheral effects of insulin. This disease is characterized by a primary defect in the metabolism of carbohydrates and other energy substrates. These metabolic defects can lead to serious acute and chronic pathologic changes. The term *diabetes mellitus* differentiates this disease from an unrelated disorder known as diabetes insipidus. Diabetes insipidus is caused by a lack of antidiuretic hormone (ADH) production or insensitivity to ADH. Consequently, the full terminology of "diabetes mellitus" should be used when referring to the insulin-related disease. Most clinicians, however, refer to diabetes mellitus as simply "diabetes."

Diabetes mellitus is a common disease that affects approximately 16 million people in the United States.[90] This disease is a serious problem in terms of increased morbidity and mortality. Diabetes mellitus is the leading cause of blindness in adults and is the primary factor responsible for 30 percent of the cases of end-stage renal failure.[90] It is also estimated that 67,000 lower-

Table 32–1	COMPARISON OF TYPE I AND TYPE II DIABETES MELLITUS	
Characteristic	**Type I**	**Type II**
Age at onset	Usually before 20	Usually after 30
Type of onset	Abrupt; often severe	Gradual; usually subtle
Usual body weight	Normal	Overweight
Blood insulin	Markedly reduced	Normal or increased
Peripheral response to insulin	Normal	Decreased
Clinical management	Insulin and diet	Diet; insulin or oral antidiabetics if diet control alone is ineffective

Adapted from: Craighead, p 1208.[28]

extremity amputations are performed annually because of complications related to diabetes mellitus.[90] Consequently, this disease is a serious problem affecting the lives of many individuals.

Diabetes mellitus is apparently not a single, homogeneous disease but rather a disease existing in at least two primary forms.[35,90] Patients with diabetes mellitus are usually classified as having either type 1 or type 2 diabetes, depending on the disease pathogenesis. The primary characteristics of type 1 and type 2 diabetes mellitus are summarized in Table 32–1. Specific aspects of these two primary forms of diabetes mellitus are discussed in more detail below.

Type 1 Diabetes

Type 1 diabetes accounts for approximately 5 to 10 percent of the individuals with diabetes mellitus.[31] Patients with type 1 diabetes are unable to synthesize any appreciable amounts of insulin. There appears to be an almost total destruction of pancreatic beta cells in these individuals. Because these patients are unable to produce insulin, type 1 diabetes has also been referred to as *insulin-dependent diabetes mellitus* (IDDM); that is, administration of exogenous insulin is necessary for survival. The onset of type 1 diabetes is usually during childhood, so this form of diabetes has also been referred to as *juvenile diabetes*. Classic type 1 diabetes, however, can develop in people of all ages.[35] Hence, terms such as *IDDM* and *juvenile diabetes* are no longer commonly used, and type 1 diabetes is generally the preferred term for this disease. Patients with type 1 diabetes are typically close to normal body weight or slightly underweight.

The exact cause of type 1 diabetes is unknown. There is considerable evidence, however, that the beta cell destruction characteristic of this disease may be caused in many patients by an autoimmune reaction.[40,126] Specifically, a virus or some other antigen may trigger an autoimmune reaction that selectively destroys the insulin-secreting beta cells in susceptible individuals.[71,126] Certain patients' susceptibility to such viral-initiated immunodestruction may be due to genetic predisposition, environmental factors, or other factors that remain to be determined.[31,71,80] The idea that type 1 diabetes may have an autoimmune basis has led to the use of immunosuppressant agents in the early stages of this disease (see "Immunosuppressants," later in this chapter).

Type 2 Diabetes

Type 2, also known previously as *non–insulin-dependent diabetes mellitus* (NIDDM), accounts for 90 to 95 percent of persons with diabetes mellitus.[19] This form of diabetes usually occurs in adults, especially in older individuals.[35,102] Type 2 diabetes, however, can also occur in young people, and there is concern that the incidence of this disease is increasing dramatically in children and adolescents.[9,83] Although the specific factors responsible for this disease are unknown, a genetic predisposition combined with poor diet, obesity, and lack of exercise all seem to contribute to the onset of type 2 diabetes.[50,81,83] Increased body weight is common in patients with type 2 diabetes.

Whereas insulin cannot be produced in type 1 diabetes, the problem in type 2 diabetes is somewhat more complex.[116] In most patients with type 2 diabetes, pancreatic beta cells remain intact and are capable of producing insulin. Therefore, the primary problem in type 2 diabetes is a decreased sensitivity of peripheral tissues to circulating insulin; this is referred to as *insulin resistance*.[19,105] For instance, tissues such as the liver and skeletal muscle fail to respond adequately to insulin in the bloodstream.[12] Thus, peripheral uptake and use of glucose are blunted, even when insulin is present.

The exact cellular mechanisms responsible for insulin resistance are unknown. The resistance may be caused by a primary (intrinsic) defect at the target cell that results in a decreased response of the cell to insulin. The decreased insulin response most likely occurs because of changes in the way the cell responds *after* insulin binds to the surface receptor. Problems in postreceptor signaling, such as decreased protein phosphorylation, impaired production of chemical mediators, and a lack of glucose transporters, have all been suggested as intracellular events that could help explain insulin resistance.[12,19] Therefore, even though insulin binds to the receptor, the cellular response is inadequate. Thus, insulin resistance appears to be a complex phenomenon that may involve a number of changes at the cellular level. The exact changes in receptor signaling or postreceptor function that cause this problem remain to be determined.

A defect in pancreatic beta cell function may also contribute to the manifestations of type 2 diabetes. As indicated, type 2 diabetes is often associated with plasma insulin levels that are normal or even slightly elevated. Insulin release, however, does not follow a normal pattern in people with type 2 diabetes. Normally, insulin is released from the beta cells following a meal, and release decreases substantially during fasting. In most people with type 2 diabetes, insulin is released continuously, even during fasting.[35] Following a meal, beta cells also fail to adequately increase insulin release in proportion to the increased glucose levels in the bloodstream. This abnormal pattern of insulin release suggests that beta cell function has been impaired in people with type 2 diabetes. Hence, the combination of peripheral tissue resistance and inappropriate beta cell response creates the fundamental metabolic abnormalities that underlie type 2 diabetes.

Finally, insulin resistance is present in disease states other than type 2 diabetes mellitus. Patients with conditions such as hypertension, obesity, and certain hyperlipidemias are also found to have decreased tissue sensitivity to circulating insulin.[19,72] As discussed in Chapter 21, a combination of these abnormalities is often described as metabolic syndrome, or syndrome X.[127,128] Metabolic syndrome occurs when insulin resistance, high blood pressure, abdominal obesity, and hyperlipidemia occur simultaneously in the patient.[61] Although the causes of insulin resistance in this syndrome are not completely understood, they probably involve a complex series of changes at the systemic, cellular, and subcellular levels.[19] There is consensus, however, that therapeutic strategies for resolving insulin resistance should be considered an important part of the management of various conditions that exhibit this phenomenon.[61,127]

Effects and Complications of Diabetes Mellitus

The most common symptom associated with diabetes mellitus is a chronic elevation of blood glucose (hyperglycemia). Hyperglycemia results from a relative lack of insulin-mediated glucose uptake and use by peripheral tissues. Hyperglycemia initiates a number of complex and potentially serious acute metabolic changes. For example, hyperglycemia is usually accompanied by increased glucose excretion by the kidneys (glycosuria). Glycosuria is caused by an inability of the kidneys to adequately reabsorb the excess amount of glucose reaching the nephron. Increased glucose excretion causes an osmotic force that promotes fluid and electrolyte excretion, thus leading to dehydration and electrolyte imbalance.[93] Also, the loss of glucose in the urine causes a metabolic shift toward the mobilization of fat and protein as an energy source. Increased use of fats and protein leads to the formation of acidic ketone bodies in the bloodstream. Excessive accumulation of ketones lowers plasma pH, producing acidosis (*ketoacidosis*), which can lead to coma and death.[24]

Diabetes mellitus is associated with several other long-term complications involving vascular and neural structures. Perhaps the most devastating complications associated with this disease result from the development of abnormalities in small blood vessels (*microangiopathy*).[35,103] Small vessels may undergo a thickening of the basement membrane, which can progress to the point of vessel occlusion.[125] The progressive ischemia caused by small-vessel disease is particularly damaging to certain structures such as the retina (leading to blindness) and the kidneys (leading to nephropathy and renal failure).[7,57,125] Damage to cutaneous vessels results in poor wound healing that can lead to ulcer formation.[85] Problems with large blood vessels (*macroangiopathy*) can also occur in diabetes because of defects in lipid metabolism that lead to atherosclerosis.[35,110] Macroangiopathy is a principal contributing factor in hypertension, myocardial infarction, and cerebral vascular accident in diabetic patients. Finally, peripheral neuropathies are quite common among patients with long-standing diabetes mellitus.[125]

The neurovascular complications described previously are directly related to the severity and duration of hyperglycemia in diabetic patients.[106,117] Although the details are somewhat unclear, prolonged elevations in blood glucose may promote structural and functional changes in vascular endothelial cells and peripheral neurons. These cellular changes are ultimately responsible for the gross pathologic abnormalities characteristic of poorly controlled diabetes mellitus.

Consequently, the primary goal in the treatment of both type 1 and type 2 diabetes mellitus is to control blood glucose levels. Maintenance of blood glucose at or close to normal levels—referred to as tight glycemic control—will prevent acute metabolic derangements and greatly reduce the risk of the chronic neurovascular complications associated with this disease.[100,117] The pharmacologic agents used to treat diabetes mellitus are described in the next sections.

Use of Insulin in Diabetes Mellitus

Therapeutic Effects and Rationale for Use

Exogenous insulin is administered to replace normal pancreatic hormone production in type 1 diabetes (IDDM). Exogenous insulin is crucial in maintaining normal glucose levels and proper metabolic function because beta cell function is essentially absent in patients with type 1 diabetes. Without exogenous insulin, the general health of type 1 patients is severely compromised, and they often succumb to the metabolic and neurovascular derangements associated with this disease.

Insulin may also be administered in some cases of type 2 diabetes to complement other drugs (oral antidiabetic agents) and to supplement endogenous insulin release.[64,70] In type 2 diabetes (NIDDM), exogenous insulin basically makes up the difference between the patient's endogenous hormone production and his or her specific insulin requirement. In addition, many patients with advanced cases of type 2 diabetes ultimately require supplemental insulin because other interventions (diet, exercise, other drugs) are not able to adequately control this disease.[35]

Insulin Preparations

There are many different forms of insulin, depending on the source of the hormones, chemical structure, and the length of pharmacologic effects. In the past, insulin used in the treatment of diabetes mellitus was often derived from animal sources; that is, beef and pork insulin. These sources were obtained by extracting the hormone from the pancreas of the host animal. The animal forms of insulin were effective in controlling glucose metabolism in humans, even though pork insulin has one amino acid that is different from the human insulin sequence, and beef insulin differs from human insulin by 3 amino acids.[35] Because of the development of human forms of insulin, animal sources are not used often, and the beef form is no longer available in the United States. Hence, most contemporary sources of insulin are manufactured chemically to mimic the structure and effects of human insulin.

Insulin that is identical to the human form of this hormone is produced through the use of cell cultures and recombinant DNA techniques.[69] Biosynthetically produced insulin that is identical to regular human insulin has advantages over the animal forms, including more rapid absorption after subcutaneous injection and a lower risk of immunologic (allergic) reactions.[35] Nonetheless, regular human insulin often takes effect more slowly than endogenous insulin released from pancreatic beta cells. That is, absorption of regular insulin from subcutaneous injection sites does not mimic the normal release of endogenous insulin occurring after a meal.[59]

Recently, biosynthetic techniques have been used to produce insulin analogs that are slightly different from human insulin. For example, insulin lispro (Humalog; see Table 32–2) is a synthetic insulin in which the sequence of two amino acids has been reversed.[35] This subtle change in insulin structure allows more rapid absorption than regular human insulin.[120] Insulin lispro can be administered immediately before or after a meal to more closely mimic the normal release of endogenous insulin.[89] Other rapidly acting insulin analogs such as insulin aspart and insulin glulisine are also available (see Table 32–2); these preparations can closely approximate the time course of insulin effects following the sudden increase in blood glucose occurring after a meal.[27,120]

On the other hand, it is sometimes advantageous to administer forms of insulin that are absorbed more slowly and have a more prolonged effect than regular human insulin (see Table 32–2). These intermediate-

Table 32–2	INSULIN PREPARATIONS				

Type of Insulin	Onset	Effects (hr) Peak	Duration	Common Trade Name(s) Human*	Animal**
Rapid-acting					
Regular insulin	0.5–1	2–4	5–7	Humulin R Novolin R	Regular Iletin II
Aspart	0.25	0.6–0.8	3–5	NovoLog	–
Lispro	<0.5	0.5–1.5	2–5	Humalog	–
Glulisine	–	0.5–1.5	1–2.5	Apidra	–
Intermediate-acting					
Isophane insulin	3–4	6–12	18–28	Humulin N Novolin N	NPH Insulin NPH Purified Insulin NPH Iletin II
Insulin zinc	1–3	8–12	18–28	Humulin L Novolin L	Lente Insulin Lente Insulin II
Long-acting					
Glargine	2–5	5–24	18–24	Lantus	–
Extended insulin zinc	4–6	18–24	36	Humulin U	–

*Human forms are derived from recombinant or biosynthetic human insulin.
**Animal sources are derived from purified pork insulin.

or long-acting forms provide a sustained background level of insulin effects throughout the day or night. Intermediate- and long-acting preparations can be created by adding acetate buffers and zinc (Lente insulins) or protamine and zinc (NPH insulins) to the insulin molecule.[35] These additions delay the absorption of the insulin molecule, thereby prolonging the effects and decreasing the need for frequent administration. In addition, insulin glargine is a long-acting insulin that has been produced biosynthetically.[120] Intermediate- and long-acting preparations are usually reserved for individuals who require less stringent control of blood glucose levels—for example, those who are helping to manage their condition through diet and weight control. Also, combinations of different preparations may be used to manage diabetes in specific situations.

For instance, a long-acting preparation may be supplemented by occasional administration of a rapid-acting agent to provide optimal glycemic control.

Finally, several commercial preparations are now available that combine two forms of insulin in the same product. Some common examples include preparations that contain a mixture of intermediate-acting insulin (e.g., isophane human insulin) and rapid-acting insulin (e.g., regular human insulin, aspart, or lispro). These insulins can be combined in specific amounts such as 50:50, 70:30, or 75:25 ratio of intermediate- to rapid-acting form, depending on the preparation. Products that combine two different forms of insulin can help provide optimal control of blood glucose levels while minimizing the number of injections needed to achieve this control.

Administration of Insulin

Insulin, a large polypeptide, is not suitable for oral administration. Even if the insulin molecule survived digestion by proteases in the stomach and small intestine, this compound is much too large to be absorbed through the gastrointestinal wall. Consequently, insulin is usually administered through subcutaneous injection. Insulin may also be administered by the intravenous route in emergency situations (e.g., diabetic coma).

Patients on long-term insulin therapy are usually trained to administer their own medication. In order to safely use insulin, it is important to provide adequate (refrigerated) storage of the preparation, to maintain sterile syringes, to accurately measure the dose and fill the syringe, and to use a proper injection technique. Patients should rotate the sites of administration (abdomen, upper thighs, upper arms, back, and buttocks) to avoid local damage from repeated injection.

The optimal dosage of insulin varies greatly from patient to patient, as well as within each patient. Factors such as exercise and dietary modification can change the insulin requirements for each individual. Consequently, the dosage of insulin is often adjusted periodically by monitoring the patient's blood glucose level. Adjustment of insulin dosage in poorly controlled diabetes mellitus is usually done under the close supervision of a physician. Advancements in glucose-monitoring devices that can be used in the home, however, now permit patients to routinely check their own blood glucose levels. Many patients can make their own insulin adjustments based on periodic blood glucose measurement. This process of glucose self-monitoring and insulin dosage adjustment permits optimal management of blood glucose levels on a day-to-day basis.

To avoid some of the problems of repeated subcutaneous injection, several alternative ways to administer insulin have been explored. Insulin pumps, for example, can be used to deliver a continuous (background) infusion of insulin that can also be supplemented at mealtime by manually activating the pump. These pumps can be worn outside the body, with insulin administered subcutaneously through a small catheter and needle that is held in place by skin tape.[42] Alternatively, small implantable pumps are being developed that can be placed surgically under the skin and programmed to release insulin as needed.[22] Insulin pumps are obviously much more convenient than using a hypodermic syringe to make multiple injections each day. These pumps may also provide better control over blood glucose levels while reducing the risk of side effects such as severe hypoglycemia.[95] The major drawback at present is that insulin pumps can malfunction, primarily because the catheter delivering insulin becomes occluded or obstructed.[42] Patients using insulin pumps must also monitor their glucose levels several times each day, and they must understand how to correctly use the pump to deliver the appropriate amount of insulin. Nonetheless, insulin pumps currently offer a convenient way to administer insulin, and technologic improvements in these devices may result in more extensive use in the future.[95]

Alternative routes for administering insulin are also being considered.[51] In particular, a form of insulin (Exubera) has been developed that can be administered by inhalation or nasal spray, thus precluding the need for subcutaneous injection.[88,104] Other modifications of the insulin molecule or use of chemical enhancers can increase the permeability of this hormone so that insulin can be administered through the skin (transcutaneously) or even via oral or buccal routes.[2,35] Technologic and practical advancements in insulin delivery continue to be explored, and methods for administering insulin may be safer and more convenient in the future.

Intensive Insulin Therapy

As indicated previously, the ultimate goal in the treatment of diabetes mellitus is to maintain blood glucose in the normal physiologic range as much as possible. To achieve this goal, an administration strategy known as intensive insulin therapy has been developed for persons who require exogenous insulin.[17] The idea of intensive insulin therapy is that the patient frequently monitors his or her blood glucose level and self-administers several (three or more) dosages of insulin per day, with each dose adjusted carefully to meet the patient's needs.[33] Basically, several relatively small doses of insulin are able to maintain blood glucose in the appropriate range much better than one or two relatively large doses. Likewise, different types of insulin can be combined to provide optimal results. For example, daily regimens can be designed that provide several doses of short-acting insulin (including the newer insulin analogs like insulin lispro, aspart, and glulisine), along with one or more doses of intermediate-acting insulin.[79,97] The short-acting doses can be administered at mealtimes or whenever immediate control of glucose levels is needed, and the intermediate-acting form can be administered once or twice a day to provide lower, background levels of insulin throughout the day or night.[34,79]

Of course, intensive insulin therapy requires more motivation and compliance on the part of the patient. Intensive therapy may also be associated with a somewhat greater risk of severe hypoglycemia if the insulin dosage does not carefully match the patient's needs throughout the day.[67] There is, nonetheless, considerable evidence that this strategy reduces the long-term complications associated with diabetes, including a lower incidence of neuropathies, renal disease, and other complications related to microangiopathy.[17,34,99] Hence, intensive insulin therapy may be worth the extra effort because this strategy can help prevent devastating complications that are typically associated with poorly controlled diabetes mellitus.

Adverse Effects of Insulin Therapy

The primary problem associated with insulin administration is *hypoglycemia*.[90,121] Exogenous insulin may produce a dramatic fall in blood glucose levels because insulin lowers blood glucose. Hypoglycemia may occur during insulin therapy if the dose of insulin is higher than the patient's needs. Missing a meal or receiving a delayed meal may also precipitate hypoglycemia. During insulin treatment, insulin is not released exclusively after a meal, as it would be during normal function. Insulin administered from an exogenous source may be present in the bloodstream even if the patient fails to provide glucose by eating. Hence, insulin may reduce blood glucose below normal levels because of the lack of a periodic replenishment of blood glucose from dietary sources.

Strenuous physical activity may promote hypoglycemia during insulin therapy. Exercise generally produces an insulinlike effect, meaning that exercise accelerates the movement of glucose out of the bloodstream and into the peripheral tissues (skeletal muscle) where it is needed. The combined effects of exercise and insulin may produce an exaggerated decrease in blood glucose, thus leading to hypoglycemia. To avoid exercise-induced hypoglycemia, the insulin dose should be decreased by 30 to 35 percent.[16] Careful measurement of blood glucose before and after exercise can help predict how much the insulin should be adjusted in each patient.

Initial symptoms of hypoglycemia include headache, fatigue, hunger, tachycardia, sweating, anxiety, and confusion. Symptoms progressively worsen as blood glucose continues to decrease, and severe hypoglycemia may lead to loss of consciousness, convulsions, and death. Consequently, early detection and resolution of hypoglycemia are imperative.[13,121] In the early stages, hypoglycemia can usually be reversed if the patient ingests foods containing glucose (soft drinks, fruit juice, glucose tablets, etc.). Typically, administration of the equivalent of 10 to 15 g of D-glucose is recommended to restore blood glucose in the early stages of hypoglycemia.[90]

Other problems that may be encountered are related to the immunologic effects of insulin use. Certain forms of insulin may evoke an immune reaction and stimulate antibody production. These anti-insulin antibodies may cause an allergic reaction in some individuals, as well as a resistance to the exogenous insulin molecule. As discussed previously, the incidence of these immunologic reactions seems to be greater when animal (i.e., pork) forms of insulin are used. Consequently, these problems are often resolved by switching the patient to another type of preparation, preferably biosynthetic human insulin.

Oral Antidiabetic Drugs

Several agents are now available that can be administered by mouth to help control blood glucose levels in people with type 2 (NIDDM) diabetes mellitus. These drugs tend to be most effective if some endogenous insulin production is present, but insulin secretion is relatively inadequate and the peripheral tissues are resistant to the effects of the endogenous insulin. These agents are therefore not effective for treating type 1 diabetes, but they can be used along with diet and exercise for the long-term management of type 2 diabetes.

Oral antidiabetic drugs do not offer a cure for type 2 diabetes, and their effectiveness varies considerably from patient to patient. Still, it appears that early and aggressive use of one or more of these agents can substantially reduce any complications associated with this disease. A brief description of currently available oral antidiabetic agents follows; agents that are categorized as sulfonylureas will be addressed first, followed by a diverse group of newer orally acting agents.

Sulfonylureas

The oldest and largest group of oral agents is classified chemically as *sulfonylureas*. These drugs act directly on pancreatic beta cells and stimulate the release of insulin,[3,18] which is released directly into the hepatic portal vein and subsequently travels to the liver, inhibiting hepatic glucose production.[36] Increased plasma levels of insulin also help facilitate glucose entry into muscle and other peripheral tissues. The combined effects of decreased hepatic glucose production and increased glucose uptake by muscle helps lower blood sugar in many people with type 2 diabetes. These drugs seem to be most effective in people who are in the early stages of type 2 diabetes and still have reasonable beta cell function.[30,96]

Specific sulfonylureas that are clinically used are listed in Table 32–3. These agents are all fairly similar in their pharmacologic efficacy and are primarily distinguished by individual potencies and pharmacokinetic properties (rate of absorption, duration of action, etc.).[35,74] The principal adverse effect of these drugs is hypoglycemia.[8,84] As with insulin therapy, hypoglycemia may be precipitated by sulfonylureas if the dose is excessive, if a meal is skipped, or if the patient increases his or her level of activity. Consequently, patients should be observed for any indications of low blood glucose, such as anxiety, confusion, headache, and sweating.[90] Other side effects that may occur include heartburn, gastrointestinal distress (nausea, vomiting, stomach pain, and diarrhea), headache, dizziness, skin rashes, and hematologic abnormalities

Table 32–3	**ORAL ANTIDIABETIC AGENTS**	
Classification and Examples*	**Mechanism of Action and Effects**	**Primary Adverse Effects**
Sulfonylureas Acetohexamide (Dymelor) Chlorpropamide (Diabinese) Glimepiride (Amaryl) Glipizide (Glucotrol) Glyburide (DiaBeta, Micronase) Tolazamide (Tolinase) Tolbutamide (Orinase)	Increase insulin secretion from pancreatic beta cells; increased insulin release helps reduce blood glucose by increasing glucose storage in muscle and by inhibiting hepatic glucose production	Hypoglycemia is the most common and potentially serious side effect of the sulfonylureas; other bothersome effects (gastrointestinal disturbances, headache, etc.) may occur depending on the specific agent
Biguanides Metformin (Glucophage)	Act directly on the liver to decrease hepatic glucose production; also increase sensitivity of peripheral tissues (muscle) to insulin	Gastrointestinal disturbances; lactic acidosis may also occur in rare cases, and this effect can be severe or fatal
Alpha-glucosidase inhibitors Acarbose (Precose) Miglitol (Glyset)	Inhibit sugar breakdown in the intestines and delay glucose absorption from the gastrointestinal tract	Gastrointestinal disturbances
Thiazolidinediones Pioglitazone (Actos) Rosiglitazone (Avandia)	Similar to the biguanides (metformin)	Headache; dizziness; fatigue/weakness; back pain; rare but potentially severe cases of hepatic toxicity
Benzoic acid derivatives Repaglinide (Prandin) Nateglinide (Starlix)	Similar to the sulfonylureas	Hypoglycemia; bronchitis; upper respiratory tract infections; joint and back pain; gastrointestinal disturbances; headache

*Examples include generic names with trade names listed in parentheses.

(e.g., leukopenia, agranulocytosis). These side effects are usually mild and transient, but may require attention if they are severe or prolonged.

Other Orally Active Drugs

In addition to the sulfonylureas, several other agents are currently available that can be administered orally to manage type 2 diabetes (Table 32–3).[49,75] These drugs differ in their chemical classification and mechanism of action, but they all attempt to normalize blood glucose levels in type 2 patients. Metformin (Glucophage), for example, is classified chemically as a biguanide agent that acts primarily on the liver to inhibit glucose production.[52,101] Metformin also increases the sensitivity of peripheral tissues to insulin, an effect that helps treat the fundamental problem in type 2 diabetes (i.e., decreased tissue sensitivity to insulin).[52] Acarbose (Precose) and miglitol (Glyset) are characterized as alpha-glucosidase inhibitors because they inhibit enzymes that break down sugars in the GI tract.[75] This effect helps delay glucose absorption from the intestines, thereby slowing the entry of glucose into the bloodstream and allowing time for the beta cells to respond to hyperglycemia after a meal.[118]

Rosiglitazone (Avandia) and pioglitazone (Actos) are members of a drug group called the thiazolidones.[37,123] These agents work like metformin; that is, they decrease hepatic glucose production and increase tissue sensitivity to insulin.[108,123] Repaglinide (Prandin) and nateglinide (Starlix) are classified as benzoic acid derivatives; these drugs act like the sulfonylureas because they directly increase the release of insulin from pancreatic beta cells.[21] Efforts continue to develop other thiazolidones and benzoic acid derivatives, and we may ultimately see additional drugs become available in the future.[32]

The adverse side effects of these orally acting drugs are summarized in Table 32–3. The drugs provide alternative treatments for patients who do not respond to sulfonylureas. These drugs can also be combined with one another, with a sulfonylurea, or with insulin therapy to provide optimal glucose control in certain patients.[54,96] That is, drugs from different classes can work together to provide more effective glycemic control in people with type 2 diabetes. Likewise, drug combinations can be tailored to the specific needs of each patient, thereby providing better long-term outcomes in type 2 diabetes.[25,49] Treatment of type 2 diabetes will undoubtedly contin-

ue to improve as more is learned about the best way to use existing oral drugs, and as other new oral antidiabetic agents become available.[32]

Other Drugs Used in the Management of Diabetes Mellitus

Glucagon

Glucagon is sometimes used to treat acute hypoglycemia induced by insulin or oral hypoglycemic agents.[35] As discussed previously, the initial effect of glucagon is to mobilize the release of glucose from hepatic glycogen stores. Consequently, the patient must have sufficient liver glycogen present for glucagon to be effective.

When used to treat hypoglycemia, glucagon is administered by injection (intravenous, intramuscular, or subcutaneous). Glucagon should reverse symptoms of hypoglycemia (including coma) within approximately 10 minutes after administration.[35] The primary adverse effects associated with glucagon are nausea and vomiting (although these effects may result from the hypoglycemia). Glucagon may also cause an allergic reaction (skin rash, difficulty in breathing) in some individuals.

Glucagon-like Peptide 1

Glucagon-like peptide 1 is a hormone that is normally released from the GI tract after eating a meal. This hormone increases the ability of blood glucose to stimulate insulin release from pancreatic beta cells.[56] Hence, a synthetic form of this hormone can be administered by injection to help provide better glycemic control following a sudden rise in blood glucose. Specifically, glucagon-like peptide 1 can exert effects similar to certain oral antidiabetic drugs (sulfonylureas, benzoic acids) that accentuate pancreatic insulin release, thereby helping to lower blood glucose following a meal. Glucagon-like peptide 1 can also decrease glucagon release from pancreatic alpha cells, delay absorption of food from the GI tract, and reduce appetite.[5,39] The combination of these effects may enable glucagon-like peptide 1 to be a novel way to improve glycemic control and decrease body weight in people with type 2 diabetes.[78] Exenatide (Byetta) is the first form of this hormone approved for clinical use; other biosynthetic hormones that mimic the effects of glucagon-like peptide 1 may be available in the future.

Immunosuppressants

As indicated earlier, most cases of type 1 diabetes are caused by an autoimmune response that selectively attacks and destroys pancreatic beta cells in susceptible individuals. Therefore, drugs that suppress this autoimmune response may be helpful in limiting beta cell destruction, thereby decreasing the severity of this disease.[4,41] Several immunosuppressants have been investigated as a way to potentially minimize beta cell loss from the autoimmune reactions underlying type 1 diabetes; some immunosuppressants that have been considered for this situation include cyclosporine, azathioprine, cyclophosphamide, methotrexate, and glucocorticoids.[11] The pharmacology of these immunosuppressants is discussed in more detail in Chapter 37.

Unfortunately, clinical trials using traditional immunosuppressive drugs have not been overwhelmingly successful in preventing the onset of type 1 diabetes. The lack of beneficial effects may be explained by the rather slow onset of autoimmune destruction that occurs prior to the onset of this disease; that is, these drugs might need to be used for several years prior to disease-onset in order to prevent beta cell destruction. Nonetheless, there is some evidence that certain immunosuppressants may blunt the severity of this disease in certain individuals.[11] Response to these agents, however, may vary greatly from patient to patient, and certain individuals may relapse when immunosuppressant therapy is discontinued.[11] Traditional immunosuppressant drugs are likewise notorious for producing severe side effects, especially when used at high dosages for prolonged periods (see Chapter 37). Hence, efforts continue to develop newer, less toxic immunosuppressants or immune system modulators that could be useful in preventing the onset of type 1 diabetes in genetically susceptible individuals.[1,41] The administration of effective immune system modulators that negate the autoimmune destruction of beta cells may be available some day, thereby preventing type 1 diabetes.[4]

Aldose Reductase Inhibitors

Drugs that selectively inhibit the aldose reductase enzyme represent a possible method for reducing peripheral neuropathies and other microvascular complications associated with poorly controlled type 1 or type 2 diabetes.[26,45] This enzyme, which is located in neurons and other cells, is responsible for converting glucose to another sugar known as sorbitol. The excessive accumulation of sorbitol within the cell may lead to structural and functional changes that are ultimately responsible for the complications associated with diabetes mellitus, especially peripheral neuropathies.[62,114] Consequently, aldose reductase inhibitors (ARIs) such as tolrestat, zenarestat, and epalrestat may be useful in preventing these complications by inhibiting the formation and accumulation of sorbitol within peripheral neurons. These agents may also have antioxidant effects that can help prevent inflammation and damage to various tissues.[112,114]

However, clinical trials using ARIs have been somewhat disappointing.[26,45] Although treatment with these drugs may slow the progression of diabetic neuropathy, ARIs do not appear to reverse any preexisting nerve damage.[94] Likewise, ARIs must be administered in a dose that is sufficient enough to inhibit more than 80 percent of the sorbitol production in the nerve cell.[55] That is, even relatively small amounts of sorbitol produced in the nerve can have a harmful effect. These drugs may also cause liver damage and hypersensitivity (allergic) reactions, thus further limiting their use in certain patients.[62] Because of these adverse effects and the relative lack of beneficial effects, ARIs are not currently available for clinical use in the United States. Safer and more effective agents are needed before these drugs can be used extensively in people with diabetes.[62]

Nonpharmacologic Intervention in Diabetes Mellitus

Dietary Management and Weight Reduction

Despite advancements in the pharmacologic treatment of diabetes mellitus, the most important and effective factor in controlling this disease is still proper nutrition.[82] In both type 1 and type 2 diabetes, total caloric intake, as well as the percentage of calories from specific sources (carbohydrates, fats, or proteins), is important in controlling blood glucose. Also, weight loss is a significant factor in decreasing the patient's need for drugs such as insulin and the oral hypoglycemics.[43] By losing weight, a patient may reduce the amount of tissue that requires insulin, thereby reducing the need for exogenous drugs. Because obesity is quite prevalent in patients with type 2 diabetes, weight loss seems to be especially effective in reducing drug requirements in these individuals.[44]

Exercise

Exercise appears to be beneficial in diabetes mellitus for several reasons. First, physical training may help facilitate weight loss, thus helping to decrease body mass and drug requirements.[6,107] Secondly, regular exercise appears to increase the sensitivity of peripheral tissues to insulin; that is, training helps overcome insulin resistance.[63,77] The exact reason for this effect is not clear. Finally, a program of physical training will improve general health and well being, making patients with diabetes less susceptible to various problems such as cardiovascular disease.[6,87] Of course, patients beginning a program of regular exercise should undergo a complete physical examination, and the frequency and intensity of the exercise should be closely monitored.

Tissue Transplants and Gene Therapy

A relatively new approach in treating diabetes mellitus is the transplantation of tissues containing pancreatic beta cells into patients with this disease.[73,109] For example, islet tissues containing functioning beta cells can be harvested from adult, neonatal, or fetal pancreatic tissues and surgically transplanted into the pancreas of patients with type 1 diabetes who lack adequate insulin production. Other strategies induce stem cells to develop into insulin-producing cells that can be transplanted into the pancreas.[91,98,111] Agents that induce differentiation and growth of endogenous beta cells may likewise help sustain or increase beta cell mass in certain patients with diabetes.[15,86,124] Alternatively, the entire pancreas can be transplanted from organ donors into patients with type 1 diabetes; this procedure may be done simultaneously with a kidney transplant in patients with diabetic nephropathy.[65,113] If successful, these tissue transplants can provide the patient with an endogenous source of insulin that will decrease or eliminate the need for insulin therapy. The success rates of these transplants are likewise improving steadily, primarily because newer immunosuppressant agents and gene-based strategies are available to prevent tissue rejection.[20,119]

New molecular strategies are also being investigated that could reestablish insulin production and insulin sensitivity by transplanting insulin-related genes into the cells of patients with diabetes mellitus.[47,68] These techniques basically attempt to either deliver insulin genes directly into patients' cells or focus on transplanting genetically altered cells that will produce or respond to insulin.[68] Although techniques such as tissue transplants and gene therapy are still relatively experimental, they may eventually be

Significance of Diabetes Mellitus in Rehabilitation

■ ■ ■ Patients often undergo rehabilitation for complications arising from diabetes mellitus. For instance, peripheral neuropathies may produce functional deficits that require physical therapy and occupational therapy. Small-vessel angiopathy may cause decreased peripheral blood flow, resulting in tissue ischemia, ulceration, and poor wound healing. This ischemia can lead to tissue necrosis and subsequent amputation, especially in the lower extremities. In advanced stages of diabetes, general debilitation combined with specific conditions (e.g., end-stage renal failure) creates multiple problems that challenge the health of the individual. Consequently, rehabilitation specialists will be involved in the treatment of various sequelae of diabetes mellitus throughout the course of this disease.

Physical therapists and occupational therapists should be aware of the possibility that acute metabolic derangements exist in their patients who have diabetes mellitus. Therapists should realize that patients on insulin and oral hypoglycemic medications could experience episodes of hypoglycemia due to these drugs' exaggerated lowering of blood glucose. Hypoglycemia may be precipitated if the patient has not eaten or is engaging in relatively strenuous physical activity. Therapists must ensure that patients are maintaining a regular dietary schedule and have not skipped a meal prior to the therapy session. Likewise, therapists should be especially alert for any signs of hypoglycemia during and after exercise.

Therapists should note any changes (confusion, fatigue, sweating, nausea) in the patient that may signal the onset of hypoglycemia. If these symptoms are observed, administration of a high-glucose snack is typically recommended. Therapists working with diabetic patients should have sources of glucose on hand to reverse these hypoglycemic symptoms. Some sources of glucose include soft drinks, fruit juices, and tablets containing D-glucose.[29]

Physical therapists and occupational therapists may help reinforce the importance of patient compliance during pharmacologic management of diabetes mellitus. Therapists can question whether patients have been taking their medications on a routine basis. Regular administration of insulin is essential in preventing a metabolic shift toward ketone body production and subsequent ketoacidosis, especially in patients with type 1 diabetes. In addition, therapists can help explain that adequate control of blood glucose not only prevents acute metabolic problems but also seems to decrease the incidence of the neurovascular complications.

Finally, rehabilitation specialists can encourage patient compliance in the nonpharmacologic management of their disease. Therapists can emphasize the importance of an appropriate diet and adequate physical activity in both type 1 and type 2 diabetes. Therapists may also play an important role in preventing the onset of diabetic foot ulcers and infection by educating the patient in proper skin care and footwear.

CASE STUDY

Diabetes Mellitus

Brief History. W.S. is an 18-year-old woman who began experiencing problems with glucose metabolism following a viral infection when she was 12. She was subsequently diagnosed as having type 1 diabetes mellitus. Since then, her condition has been successfully managed by insulin administration combined with dietary control. Once-daily administration of intermediate-acting insulin combined with periodic administration of short-acting insulin usually provides optimal therapeutic effects. She is also very active athletically and was a member of her high school soccer team. She is entering her first year of college and is beginning preseason practice with the college's soccer team. The physical therapist that serves as the team's athletic trainer was apprised of her condition.

Problem/Influence of Medication. Exercise produces an insulinlike effect; that is, it lowers blood glucose by facilitating the movement of glucose out of the bloodstream and into peripheral tissues. Because insulin also lowers blood glucose, the additive effects of insulin and exercise may produce profound hypoglycemia. As a result, a lower dosage of insulin is usually required on days that involve strenuous activ-

ity. The physical therapist was aware of this and other potential problems that could arise.

Decision/Solution. The therapist reminded the athlete to monitor her blood glucose levels before and after each practice session and to adjust her insulin dosage accordingly. During some of the initial practice sessions, blood glucose was also monitored during practice to ensure that insulin dosages were adequate. On practice days, insulin was injected into abdominal sites rather than around exercising muscles (thighs), in order to prevent the insulin from being absorbed too rapidly from the injection site. The therapist also reminded the athlete to eat a light meal before each practice and to be sure to eat again afterward. The therapist maintained a supply of glucose tablets and fruit juice on the practice field. The athlete was questioned periodically to look for early signs of hypoglycemia (confusion, nausea, etc.), and ingestion of carbohydrates was encouraged whenever appropriate. Finally, the therapist assigned a teammate to check on the athlete within an hour after practice ended to ensure that no delayed effects of hypoglycemia were apparent. With these precautions, the athlete successfully completed preseason training, as well as the entire soccer season without any serious incident.

developed to provide a more permanent means of treating diabetes mellitus.

SUMMARY

The islet cells of the pancreas synthesize and secrete insulin and glucagon. These hormones are important in regulating glucose uptake and use, as well as in other aspects of energy metabolism. Problems in the production and effects of insulin are typical of a disease known as diabetes mellitus. Diabetes mellitus can be categorized into two primary forms: type 1 diabetes, which is caused by an absolute deficiency of insulin, and type 2 diabetes, which is caused by a decrease in peripheral insulin effects, combined with abnormal insulin release.

Administration of exogenous insulin is required in the treatment of type 1 diabetes mellitus. Patients with type 2 diabetes may be treated with insulin or with oral antidiabetic drugs, depending on the severity of their disease. In both forms of diabetes mellitus, dietary control and adequate physical activity may help reduce the need for drug treatment, as well as improve the patient's general health and well-being. Physical therapists and occupational therapists play an important role in helping treat the complications of diabetes mellitus and in promoting good patient adherence to disease management. Therapists must be cognizant of the potential problems that may occur when working with these patients (hypoglycemia) and should be able to recognize and deal with any problems before a medical emergency arises.

References

1. Aly T, Devendra D, Eisenbarth GS. Immunotherapeutic approaches to prevent, ameliorate, and cure type 1 diabetes. *Am J Ther.* 2005;12:481–490.
2. Arbit E. The physiological rationale for oral insulin administration. *Diabetes Technol Ther.* 2004;6:510–517.
3. Ashcroft FM. ATP-sensitive potassium channelopathies: focus on insulin secretion. *J Clin Invest.* 2005;115:2047–2058.
4. Azam A, Eisenbarth GS. Immunopathogenesis and immunotherapeutic approaches to type 1A diabetes. *Expert Opin Biol Ther.* 2004;4:1569–1575.
5. Baggio LL, Drucker DJ. Clinical endocrinology and metabolism. Glucagon-like peptide-1 and glucagon-like peptide-2. *Best Pract Res Clin Endocrinol Metab.* 2004;18:531–554.
6. Bassuk SS, Manson JE. Epidemiological evidence for the role of physical activity in reducing risk of type 2 diabetes and cardiovascular disease. *J Appl Physiol.* 2005;99:1193–1204.
7. Bek T. Diabetic retinopathy: a review of the aarhus approach to studies on epidemiology, computerised grading, and the pathophysiology of the disease. *Horm Metab Res.* 2005;37(suppl 1):35–38.
8. Bell DS. Practical considerations and guidelines for dosing sulfonylureas as monotherapy or combination therapy. *Clin Ther.* 2004;26:1714–1727.
9. Berry D, Urban A, Grey M. Understanding the development and prevention of type 2 diabetes in youth (part 1). *J Pediatr Health Care.* 2006;20:3–10.
10. Bertelli E, Bendayan M. Association between endocrine pancreas and ductal system. More than an epiphenomenon of endocrine differentiation and development? *J Histochem Cytochem.* 2005;53:1071–1086.
11. Bertera S, Alexander A, Giannoukakis N, et al. Immunology of type 1 diabetes. Intervention and prevention strategies. *Endocrinol Metab Clin North Am.* 1999;28:841–864.
12. Bjornholm M, Zierath JR. Insulin signal transduction in human skeletal muscle: identifying the defects in type II diabetes. *Biochem Soc Trans.* 2005;33(Pt 2):354–357.
13. Bober E, Buyukgebiz A, Verrotti A, Chiarelli F. Hypoglycemia, hypoglycemia unawareness and counterregulation in children and adolescents with type 1 diabetes mellitus. *J Pediatr Endocrinol Metab.* 2005;18:831–841.
14. Bolster DR, Jefferson LS, Kimball SR. Regulation of protein synthesis associated with skeletal muscle hypertrophy by insulin-, amino acid- and exercise-induced signalling. *Proc Nutr Soc.* 2004;63:351–356.
15. Bouwens L, Rooman I. Regulation of pancreatic beta-cell mass. *Physiol Rev.* 2005;85:1255–1270.
16. Brannon FJ, Foley MW, Starr JA, Saul LM. *Cardiopulmonary Rehabilitation: Basic Theory and Application,* 3rd ed. FA Davis, Philadelphia, 1998.
17. Bretzel RG. Intensive insulin regimens: evidence for benefit. *Int J Obes Relat Metab Disord.* 2004;28(suppl 2):S8–S13.
18. Bryan J, Crane A, Vila-Carriles WH, et al. Insulin secretagogues, sulfonylurea receptors and K(ATP) channels. *Curr Pharm Des.* 2005;11:2699–2716.
19. Buse JB, Polonsky KS, Burant CF. Type 2 diabetes mellitus. In: Larsen PR, et al, eds. *Williams Textbook of Endocrinology.* 10th ed. Philadelphia: Saunders; 2003.
20. Calne R. Cell transplantation for diabetes. *Philos Trans R Soc Lond B Biol Sci.* 2005;360:1769–1774.
21. Campbell IW. Nateglinide—current and future role in the treatment of patients with type 2 diabetes mellitus. *Int J Clin Pract.* 2005;59:1218–1228.
22. Catargi B. Current status and future of implantable insulin pumps for the treatment of diabetes. *Expert Rev Med Devices.* 2004;1:181–185.
23. Chang L, Chiang SH, Saltiel AR. Insulin signaling and the regulation of glucose transport. *Mol Med.* 2004;10:65–71.
24. Charfen MA, Fernandez-Frackelton M. Diabetic ketoacidosis. *Emerg Med Clin North Am.* 2005;23:609–628.

25. Chipkin SR. How to select and combine oral agents for patients with type 2 diabetes mellitus. *Am J Med.* 2005;118(suppl 5A):4S–13S.

26. Chung SS, Chung SK. Aldose reductase in diabetic microvascular complications. *Curr Drug Targets.* 2005;6:475–486.

27. Cox SL. Insulin glulisine. *Drugs Today.* 2005;41: 433–440.

28. Craighead JE. Diabetes. In: Rubin E, Farber JL, eds. *Pathology.* 3rd ed. Philadelphia: Lippincott-Raven; 1999.

29. Cryer PE. Glucose homeostasis and hypoglycemia. In: Larsen PR, et al, eds. *Williams Textbook of Endocrinology.* 10th ed. Philadelphia: Saunders; 2003.

30. Dailey G. Insulin secretagogues: who, what, when, and how? *Curr Diab Rep.* 2005;5:329–332.

31. Daneman D. Type 1 diabetes. *Lancet.* 2006;367: 847–858.

32. Das SK, Chakrabarti R. Non-insulin dependent diabetes mellitus: present therapies and new drug targets. *Mini Rev Med Chem.* 2005;5:1019–1034.

33. Davidson J. Strategies for improving glycemic control: effective use of glucose monitoring. *Am J Med.* 2005; 118(suppl 9A):27S–32S.

34. Davidson JA. Treatment of the patient with diabetes: importance of maintaining target HbA(1c) levels. *Curr Med Res Opin.* 2004;20:1919–1927.

35. Davis SN. Insulin, oral hypoglycemic agents, and the pharmacology of the endocrine pancreas. In: Brunton LL, et Al, eds. *The Pharmacological Basis of Therapeutics.* 11th ed. New York: McGraw-Hill; 2006.

36. DeFronzo RA. Pharmacologic therapy for type 2 diabetes mellitus. *Ann Intern Med.* 1999;131:281–303.

37. Del Prato S, Marchetti P. Targeting insulin resistance and beta-cell dysfunction: the role of thiazolidinediones. *Diabetes Technol Ther.* 2004;6:719–731.

38. De Meyts P. Insulin and its receptor: structure, function and evolution. *Bioessays.* 2004;26:1351–1362.

39. Efendic S, Portwood N. Overview of incretin hormones. *Horm Metab Res.* 2004;36:742–746.

40. Eisenbarth GS, Polonsky KS, Buse JB. Type 1 diabetes mellitus. In: Larsen PR, et al, eds. *Williams Textbook of Endocrinology.* 10th ed. Philadelphia: Saunders; 2003.

41. Eldor R, Cohen IR, Raz I. Innovative immune-based therapeutic approaches for the treatment of type 1 diabetes mellitus. *Int Rev Immunol.* 2005;24:327–339.

42. Everett J. The role of insulin pumps in the management of diabetes. *Nurs Times.* 2004;100:48–49.

43. Foreyt JP, Poston WS, 2nd. The challenge of diet, exercise and lifestyle modification in the management of the obese diabetic patient. *Int J Obes Relat Metab Disord.* 1999;23(suppl 7):S5–S11.

44. Franz MJ. Prioritizing diabetes nutrition recommendations based on evidence. *Minerva Med.* 2004;95: 115–123.

45. Gabbay KH. Aldose reductase inhibition in the treatment of diabetic neuropathy: where are we in 2004? *Curr Diab Rep.* 2004;4:405–408.

46. Gagliardino JJ. Physiological endocrine control of energy homeostasis and postprandial blood glucose levels. *Eur Rev Med Pharmacol Sci.* 2005;9:75–92.

47. Giannoukakis N, Trucco M. Gene therapy for type 1 diabetes: a proposal to move to the next level. *Curr Opin Mol Ther.* 2005;7:467–475.

48. Giorgino F, Laviola L, Eriksson JW. Regional differences of insulin action in adipose tissue: insights from in vivo and in vitro studies. *Acta Physiol Scand.* 2005; 183:13–30.

49. Giorgino F, Laviola L, Leonardini A. Pathophysiology of type 2 diabetes: rationale for different oral antidiabetic treatment strategies. *Diabetes Res Clin Pract.* 2005; 68(suppl 11):S22–S29.

50. Golay A, Ybarra J. Link between obesity and type 2 diabetes. *Best Pract Res Clin Endocrinol Metab.* 2005; 19:649–663.

51. Gomez-Perez FJ, Rull JA. Insulin therapy: current alternatives. *Arch Med Res.* 2005;36:258–272.

52. Goodarzi MO, Bryer-Ash M. Metformin revisited: re-evaluation of its properties and role in the pharmacopoeia of modern antidiabetic agents. *Diabetes Obes Metab.* 2005;7:654–665.

53. Gosmanov NR, Szoke E, Israelian Z, et al. Role of the decrement in intraislet insulin for the glucagon response to hypoglycemia in humans. *Diabetes Care.* 2005;28:1124–1131.

54. Goudswaard AN, Furlong NJ, Rutten GE, et al. Insulin monotherapy versus combinations of insulin with oral hypoglycaemic agents in patients with type 2 diabetes mellitus. *Cochrane Database Syst Rev.* 2004; CD003418.

55. Greene DA, Arezzo JC, Brown MB. Effect of aldose reductase inhibition on nerve conduction and morphometry in diabetic neuropathy. *Zenarestat Study Group. Neurology.* 1999;53: 580–591.

56. Gromada J, Brock B, Schmitz O, Rorsman P. Glucagon-like peptide-1: regulation of insulin secretion and therapeutic potential. *Basic Clin Pharmacol Toxicol.* 2004;95:252–262.

57. Gross JL, de Azevedo MJ, Silveiro SP, et al. Diabetic nephropathy: diagnosis, prevention, and treatment. *Diabetes Care.* 2005;28:164–176.

58. Gual P, Le Marchand-Brustel Y, Tanti JF. Positive and negative regulation of insulin signaling through IRS-1 phosphorylation. *Biochimie.* 2005; 87:99–109.

59. Guerci B, Sauvanet JP. Subcutaneous insulin: pharmacokinetic variability and glycemic variability. *Diabetes Metab.* 2005;31:4S7–4S24.

60. Guyton AC, Hall JE. *Textbook of Medical Physiology.* 11th ed. Philadelphia: Elsevier Saunders; 2006.

61. Hafidh S, Senkottaiyan N, Villarreal D, Alpert MA. Management of the metabolic syndrome. *Am J Med Sci.* 2005;330:343–351.

62. Hamada Y, Nakamura J. Clinical potential of aldose reductase inhibitors in diabetic neuropathy. *Treat Endocrinol.* 2004;3:245–255.

63. Hawley JA. Exercise as a therapeutic intervention for the prevention and treatment of insulin resistance. *Diabetes Metab Res Rev.* 2004;20:383–393.

64. Hirsch IB. Intensifying insulin therapy in patients with type 2 diabetes mellitus. *Am J Med.* 2005;118(suppl 5A):21S–26S.

65. Hricik DE. Kidney-pancreas transplantation for diabetic nephropathy. *Semin Nephrol.* 2000;20:188–198.

66. Ishiki M, Klip A. Minireview: recent developments in the regulation of glucose transporter-4 traffic: new signals, locations, and partners. *Endocrinology.* 2005;146: 5071–5078.

67. Jacqueminet S, Masseboeuf N, Rolland M, et al. Limitations of the so-called "intensified" insulin therapy in type 1 diabetes mellitus. *Diabetes Metab.* 2005;31: 4S45–4S50.

68. Jun HS, Yoon JW. Approaches for the cure of type 1 diabetes by cellular and gene therapy. *Curr Gene Ther.* 2005;5:249–262.

69. Kamal AD, Dixon AN, Bain SC. Safety and side effects of the insulin analogues. *Expert Opin Drug Saf.* 2006; 5:131–143.

70. Karl DM. The use of bolus insulin and advancing insulin therapy in type 2 diabetes. *Curr Diab Rep.* 2004;4:352–357.

71. Kim MS, Polychronakos C. Immunogenetics of type 1 diabetes. *Horm Res.* 2005;64:180–188.

72. Kim SH, Reaven GM. The metabolic syndrome: one step forward, two steps back. *Diab Vasc Dis Res.* 2004;1:68–75.

73. Kizilel S, Garfinkel M, Opara E. The bioartificial pancreas: progress and challenges. *Diabetes Technol Ther.* 2005;7:968–985.

74. Korytkowski MT. Sulfonylurea treatment of type 2 diabetes mellitus: focus on glimepiride. *Pharmacotherapy.* 2004;24:606–620.

75. Krentz AJ, Bailey CJ. Oral antidiabetic agents: current role in type 2 diabetes mellitus. *Drugs.* 2005;65: 385–411.

76. Krook A, Wallberg-Henriksson H, Zierath JR. Sending the signal: molecular mechanisms regulating glucose uptake. *Med Sci Sports Exerc.* 2004;36: 1212–1217.

77. LaMonte MJ, Blair SN, Church TS. Physical activity and diabetes prevention. *J Appl Physiol.* 2005;99: 1205–1213.

78. Larsen PJ, Holst JJ. Glucagon-related peptide 1 (GLP-1): hormone and neurotransmitter. *Regul Pept.* 2005; 128:97–107.

79. Liebl A. Challenges in optimal metabolic control of diabetes. *Diabetes Metab Res Rev.* 2002;18(suppl 3):S36–S41.

80. Maier LM, Wicker LS. Genetic susceptibility to type 1 diabetes. *Curr Opin Immunol.* 2005;17:601–608.

81. Malecki MT. Genetics of type 2 diabetes mellitus. *Diabetes Res Clin Pract.* 2005;68(suppl ll):S10–S21.

82. Mann JI, De Leeuw I, Hermansen K, et al. Evidence-based nutritional approaches to the treatment and prevention of diabetes mellitus. *Nutr Metab Cardiovasc Dis.* 2004;14:373–394.

83. Marcovecchio M, Mohn A, Chiarelli F. Type 2 diabetes mellitus in children and adolescents. *J Endocrinol Invest.* 2005;28:853–863.

84. Melander A. Kinetics-effect relations of insulin-releasing drugs in patients with type 2 diabetes: brief overview. *Diabetes.* 2004;53(suppl 3):S151–S155.

85. Ngo BT, Hayes KD, DiMiao DJ, et al. Manifestations of cutaneous diabetic microangiopathy. *Am J Clin Dermatol.* 2005;6:225–237.

86. Nir T, Dor Y. How to make pancreatic beta cells—prospects for cell therapy in diabetes. *Curr Opin Biotechnol.* 2005;16:524–529.

87. Norris SL, Zhang X, Avenell A, et al. Long-term effectiveness of weight-loss interventions in adults with pre-diabetes: a review. *Am J Prev Med.* 2005; 28:126–139.

88. Odegard PS, Capoccia KL. Inhaled insulin: exubera. *Ann Pharmacother.* 2005;39:843–853.

89. Oiknine R, Bernbaum M, Mooradian AD. A critical appraisal of the role of insulin analogues in the management of diabetes mellitus. *Drugs.* 2005;65: 325–340.

90. Oki JC, Isley WL. Diabetes mellitus. In: DiPiro JT, et al, eds. *Pharmacotherapy: A Pathophysiologic Approach.* 5th ed. New York: McGraw-Hill; 2002.

91. Otonkoski T, Gao R, Lundin K. Stem cells in the treatment of diabetes. *Ann Med.* 2005;37:513–520.

92. Panteris V, Karamanolis DG. The puzzle of somatostatin: action, receptors, analogues and therapy. *Hepatogastroenterology.* 2005;52:1771–1781.

93. Peavey DE. The endocrine pancreas. In: Rhoades RA, Tanner GA, eds. *Medical Physiology.* 2nd ed. Philadelphia: Lippincott Williams and Wilkins; 2003.

94. Pfeifer MA, Schumer MP, Gelber DA. Aldose reductase inhibitors: the end of an era or the need for different trial designs? *Diabetes.* 1997;46(suppl 2): S82–S89.

95. Radermecker RP, Scheen AJ. Continuous subcutaneous insulin infusion with short-acting insulin analogues or human regular insulin: efficacy, safety, quality of life, and cost-effectiveness. *Diabetes Metab Res Rev.* 2004;20:178–188.

96. Riddle MC. Glycemic management of type 2 diabetes: an emerging strategy with oral agents, insulins, and combinations. *Endocrinol Metab Clin North Am.* 2005;34:77–98.

97. Ristic S, Bates PC. Effects of rapid-acting insulin analogs on overall glycemic control in type 1 and type 2 diabetes mellitus. *Diabetes Technol Ther.* 2003; 5:57–66.

98. Roche E, Enseat-Wase R, Reig JA, et al. Therapeutic potential of stem cells in diabetes. *Handb Exp Pharmacol.* 2006;174:147–167.

99. Rolla A. The pathophysiological basis for intensive insulin replacement. *Int J Obes Relat Metab Disord.* 2004;28(suppl 2):S3–S7.

100. Rosenberg DE, Jabbour SA, Goldstein BJ. Insulin resistance, diabetes and cardiovascular risk: approaches to treatment. *Diabetes Obes Metab.* 2005;7:642–653.

101. Saenz A, Fernandez-Esteban I, Mataix A, et al. Metformin monotherapy for type 2 diabetes mellitus. *Cochrane Database Syst Rev.* 2005;CD002966.

102. Sakharova OV, Inzucchi SE. Treatment of diabetes in the elderly. Addressing its complexities in this high-risk group. *Postgrad Med.* 2005;118: 19–26, 29.

103. Schalkwijk CG, Stehouwer CD. Vascular complications in diabetes mellitus: the role of endothelial dysfunction. *Clin Sci.* 2005;109:143–159.

104. Scherbaum WA. Unlocking the opportunity of tight glycaemic control. Inhaled insulin: clinical efficacy. *Diabetes Obes Metab.* 2005;7(suppl 1):S9–S13.

105. Schinner S, Scherbaum WA, Bornstein SR, Barthel A. Molecular mechanisms of insulin resistance. *Diabet Med.* 2005;22:674–682.

106. Schnell O. The links between diabetes and cardiovascular disease. *J Interv Cardiol.* 2005;18:413–416.

107. Schulze MB, Hu FB. Primary prevention of diabetes: what can be done and how much can be prevented? *Annu Rev Public Health.* 2005;26:445–467.

108. Seufert J, Lubben G, Dietrich K, Bates PC. A comparison of the effects of thiazolidinediones and metformin on metabolic control in patients with type 2 diabetes mellitus. *Clin Ther.* 2004;26: 805–818.

109. Shapiro AM, Lakey JR, Paty BW, et al. Strategic opportunities in clinical islet transplantation. *Transplantation.* 2005;79:1304–1307.

110. Sobel BE, Schneider DJ. Cardiovascular complications in diabetes mellitus. *Curr Opin Pharmacol.* 2005;5:143–148.

111. Soria B, Roche E, Reig JA, Martin F. Generation of insulin-producing cells from stem cells. *Novartis Found Symp.* 2005;265:158–167.

112. Srivastava SK, Ramana KV, Bhatnagar A. Role of aldose reductase and oxidative damage in diabetes and the consequent potential for therapeutic options. *Endocr Rev.* 2005;26:380–392.

113. Stegall MD, Larson TS, Kudva YC, et al. Pancreas transplantation for the prevention of diabetic nephropathy. *Mayo Clin Proc.* 2000;75:49–56.

114. Suzen S, Buyukbingol E. Recent studies of aldose reductase enzyme inhibition for diabetic complications. *Curr Med Chem.* 2003;10:1329–1352.

115. Thong FS, Dugani CB, Klip A. Turning signals on and off: GLUT4 traffic in the insulin-signaling highway. *Physiology.* 2005;20:271–284.

116. Tonelli J, Kishore P, Lee DE, Hawkins M. The regulation of glucose effectiveness: how glucose modulates its own production. *Curr Opin Clin Nutr Metab Care.* 2005;8:450–456.

117. Valeri C, Pozzilli P, Leslie D. Glucose control in diabetes. *Diabetes Metab Res Rev.* 2004;20(suppl 2):S1–S8.

118. Van de Laar FA, Lucassen PL, Akkermans RP, et al. Alpha-glucosidase inhibitors for type 2 diabetes mellitus. *Cochrane Database Syst Rev.* 2005;CD003639.

119. Van Linthout S, Madeddu P. Ex vivo gene transfer for improvement of transplanted pancreatic islet viability and function. *Curr Pharm Des.* 2005;11: 2927–2940.

120. Vazquez-Carrera M, Silvestre JS. Insulin analogues in the management of diabetes. *Methods Find Exp Clin Pharmacol.* 2004;26:445–461.

121. Vignesh JP, Mohan V. Hypoglycaemia unawareness. *J Assoc Physicians India.* 2004;52:727–732.

122. Watson RT, Pessin JE. Bridging the GAP between insulin signaling and GLUT4 translocation. *Trends Biochem Sci.* 2006;31:215–222.

123. Waugh J, Keating GM, Plosker GL, et al. Pioglitazone: a review of its use in type 2 diabetes mellitus. *Drugs.* 2006;66:85–109.

124. Yamada S, Kojima I. Regenerative medicine of the pancreatic beta cells. *J Hepatobiliary Pancreat Surg.* 2005;12:218–226.

125. Yamagishi S, Imaizumi T. Diabetic vascular complications: pathophysiology, biochemical basis and potential therapeutic strategy. *Curr Pharm Des.* 2005;11:2279–2299.

126. Yoon JW, Jun HS. Autoimmune destruction of pancreatic beta cells. *Am J Ther.* 2005;12:580–591.

127. Zarich SW. Cardiovascular risk factors in the metabolic syndrome: impact of insulin resistance on lipids, hypertension, and the development of diabetes and cardiac events. *Rev Cardiovasc Med.* 2005;6:194–205.

128. Zimmet P, Magliano D, Matsuzawa Y, et al. The metabolic syndrome: a global public health problem and a new definition. *J Atheroscler Thromb.* 2005; 12:295–300.

Chemotherapy of Infectious and Neoplastic Diseases

Chapter 33

Treatment of Infections I: Antibacterial Drugs

This chapter and the next two chapters in this text address drugs used to treat infections caused by pathogenic microorganisms and parasites. Microorganisms such as bacteria, viruses, and protozoa, as well as larger multicellular parasites, frequently invade human tissues and are responsible for various afflictions ranging from mild and annoying symptoms to life-threatening diseases. Often, the body's natural defense mechanisms are unable to deal with these pathogenic invaders, and pharmacologic treatment is essential in resolving infections and promoting recovery. Drugs used to treat infection represent one of the most significant advances in medical history, and these agents are among the most important and widely used pharmacologic agents throughout the world.

Drugs used to treat infectious diseases share a common goal of **selective toxicity,** meaning they must selectively kill or attenuate the growth of the pathogenic organism without causing excessive damage to the host (human) cells. In some cases, the pathogenic organism may have some distinctive structural or biochemical feature that allows the drug to selectively attack the invading cell. For instance, drugs that capitalize on certain differences in membrane structure, protein synthesis, or other unique aspects of cellular metabolism in the pathogenic organism will be effective and safe anti-infectious agents. Of course, selective toxicity is a relative term, because all of the drugs discussed in the following chapters exert some adverse effects on human tissues. However, drugs used to treat various infections generally impair function much more in the pathogenic organism than in human tissues.

Several other general terms are also used to describe the drugs used to treat infectious disease.

Agents used specifically against small, unicellular organisms (e.g., bacteria, viruses) are often referred to as *antimicrobial drugs*. Antimicrobial agents are also commonly referred to as *antibiotics*, indicating that these substances are used to kill other living organisms (i.e., anti-"bios," or life). To avoid confusion, drugs in this text are classified and identified according to the primary type of infectious organism they are used to treat—that is, whether they are antibacterial, antiviral, antifungal, and so on.

This chapter discusses drugs used to treat bacterial infections. Drugs used to treat and prevent viral infections are presented in Chapter 34, followed by the pharmacologic management of other parasitic infections (antifungal, antiprotozoal, and anthelmintic drugs) in Chapter 35. Because infectious disease represents one of the most common forms of illness, many patients undergoing therapists physical rehabilitation take one or more of these drugs. Physical therapists and occupational therapists will undoubtedly deal with patients undergoing chemotherapy for infectious disease on a routine basis. The pharmacotherapeutic management of infectious disease that is presented in Chapters 33 through 35 should be of interest to all rehabilitation specialists.

Bacteria: Basic Concepts

Bacterial Structure and Function

Bacteria are unicellular microorganisms, ranging in size from 0.8 to 15.0 μm in diameter.[45] Bacteria are distinguished from other microorganisms by several features, including a rigid cell wall that surrounds the bacterial cell and the lack of a true nuclear membrane (i.e., the genetic material within the bacterial cell is not confined by a distinct membrane).[50] Bacteria usually contain the basic subcellular organelles needed to synthesize proteins and maintain cellular metabolism, including ribosomes, enzymes, and cytoplasmic storage granules. Bacteria, however, must depend on some kind of nourishing medium to provide metabolic substrates to maintain function. Hence, these microorganisms often invade human tissues to gain access to a supply of amino acids, sugars, and other substances.

Pathogenic Effects of Bacteria

Bacterial infections can be harmful to host organisms in several ways.[32,45] First, bacteria multiply, competing with host (human) cells for essential nutrients. Bacteria also may directly harm human cells by releasing toxic substances. Moreover, bacteria may cause an immune response that will ultimately damage human tissues and the invading bacteria. Of course, not all bacteria in the human body are harmful. For example, certain bacteria in the gastrointestinal system inhibit the growth of other microorganisms and assist in the digestion of food and synthesis of certain nutrients. In addition, many bacteria that enter the body are adequately dealt with by normal immunologic responses. However, the invasion of pathogenic bacteria can lead to severe infections and death, especially if the patient's immune system is compromised or the body's endogenous defense mechanisms are unable to combat the infection. In some cases, bacteria may establish growth areas or colonies that remain innocuous for extended periods. However, this colonization may begin to proliferate and become a health threat when the patient succumbs to some other disorder or illness. Consequently, the chance of severe, life-threatening infections is especially high in individuals who are debilitated or have some immune system defect.

Bacterial Nomenclature and Classification

Bacteria are usually named according to their genus and species; these names are identified in italic typeface.[45] For instance, *Escherichia coli* refers to bacteria from the *Escherichia* genus, *coli* species. According to this nomenclature, the genus is capitalized and refers to bacteria with common genetic, morphologic, and biochemical characteristics. The species name is not capitalized and often refers to some physical, pathogenic, or other characteristic of the species. For example, *Streptococcus pyogenes* refers to bacteria from the

Streptococcus genus, which are commonly associated with pyogenic or pus-producing characteristics.

Because of diverse bacterial genera, bacteria are often categorized according to common characteristics, such as the shape and histologic staining of the bacterial cell.[50] For example, *gram-positive cocci* refers to spherical bacteria (cocci) that retain the discoloration of a particular staining technique (Gram's method of staining). However, development of a comprehensive taxonomy that neatly categorizes all bacteria is difficult because of the diverse morphologic and biochemical characteristics of the various bacterial families and genera.

For the purpose of this chapter, bacteria are categorized according to the criteria outlined in Table 33–1. This classification scheme does not fully identify all of the various characteristics of the many bacterial families. The classifications listed in Table 33–1 are used here only to categorize bacteria according to the use of antibacterial agents, which are discussed later in this chapter under "Specific Antibacterial Agents."

Treatment of Bacterial Infections: Basic Principles

Spectrum of Antibacterial Activity

Some drugs are effective against a variety of bacteria; these are usually referred to as *broad-spectrum agents*. For example, a drug such as tetracycline is considered to have a broad spectrum of activity because this drug is effective against many gram-negative, gram-positive, and other types of bacteria. In contrast, a drug such as isoniazid is specific for the bacillus that causes tuberculosis (i.e., *Mycobacterium tuberculosis*), and its spectrum of activity is relatively narrow. Hence, the antibacterial spectrum is one property of an antibacterial drug that determines the clinical applications of that agent. Other factors, including patient tolerance, bacterial resistance, and physician preference, also influence the selection of a particular drug for a particular condition. The clinical use of antibacterial drugs relative to specific bacterial pathogens is discussed in "Clinical Use of Antibacterial Drugs: Relationship to Specific Bacterial Infections."

Bactericidal Versus Bacteriostatic Activity

The term bactericidal refers to drugs that typically kill or destroy bacteria. In contrast, drugs that do not actu-

Table 33–1	TYPES OF BACTERIA	
Type	**Principal Features**	**Common Examples**
Gram-positive bacilli	Generally rod-shaped; retain color when treated by Gram's method of staining	*Bacillus anthracis, Clostridium tetani*
Gram-negative bacilli	Rod-shaped; do not retain color by Gram's method	*Escherichia coli, Klebsiella pneumoniae, Pseudomonas aeruginosa*
Gram-positive cocci	Generally spherical or ovoid in shape; retain color by Gram's method	*Staphylococcus aureus, Streptococcus pneumoniae*
Gram-negative cocci	Spherical or ovoid; do not retain color by Gram's method	*Neisseria gonorrhoeae* (gonococcus), *Neisseria meningitidis* (meningococcus)
Acid-fast bacilli	Rod-shaped; retains color of certain stains even when treated with acid	*Mycobacterium leprae, Mycobacterium tuberculosis*
Spirochetes	Slender; spiral shape; able to move about without flagella (intrinsic locomotor ability)	Lyme disease agent; *Treponema pallidum* (syphilis)
Actinomycetes	Thin filaments that stain positively by Gram's method	*Actinomyces israelii;* Nocardia
Others:		
Mycoplasmas	Spherical; lack the rigid, highly structured cell wall found in most bacteria	*Mycoplasma pneumoniae*
Rickettsiae	Small; gram-negative bacteria	*Rickettsia typhi, Rickettsia rickettsii*

ally kill bacteria but limit the growth and proliferation of bacterial invaders are referred to as bacteriostatic. Antibacterial drugs are usually classified as either bactericidal or bacteriostatic, depending on their mechanism of action. In addition, the classification of whether a drug is bactericidal or bacteriostatic may depend on the drug dosage. For instance, drugs such as erythromycin exhibit bacteriostatic activity at lower doses but are bactericidal at higher doses.

Basic Mechanisms of Antibacterial Drugs

As mentioned previously, antibacterial and other antimicrobial drugs must be selectively toxic to the infectious microorganism, without causing excessive damage to human cells. Drugs that exert selective toxicity against bacteria generally employ one of the mechanisms shown in Figure 33–1. These mecha-

nisms include (1) inhibition of bacterial cell wall synthesis and function, (2) inhibition of bacterial protein synthesis, and (3) inhibition of bacterial DNA/RNA function. The details of these mechanisms, along with the reasons why each mechanism is specific for bacterial (versus human) cells, are discussed next.

Inhibition of Bacterial Cell Wall Synthesis and Function

Penicillin, cephalosporins, and several other commonly used drugs exert antibacterial effects by inhibiting the synthesis of bacterial cell walls.[56] These drugs are selectively toxic because the bacterial cell walls differ considerably from those of their mammalian counterparts. The membrane surrounding most bacterial cells (with the exception of the *Mycoplasma* genus) is a relatively rigid, firm structure.[74] This rigidity appears to be essential in constraining the high osmotic pressure within the bacterial cell.[88] This behavior contrasts

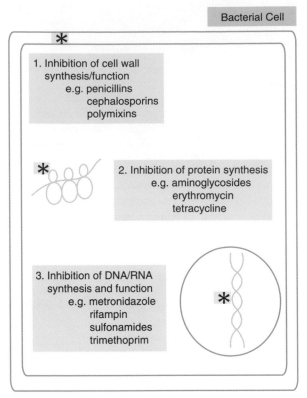

FIGURE 33–1 ▼ Primary sites of antibacterial drug action on bacterial cells. See text for discussion.

with the relatively supple, flexible membrane encompassing the mammalian cell.

The increased rigidity of bacterial cell walls is caused by the presence of protein-polysaccharide structures known as *peptidoglycans*.[74,88] Peptidoglycan units (also known as mureins) are cross-linked to one another within the cell wall in such a way as to provide a remarkable amount of rigidity and firmness to the cell. If these peptidoglycans are not present, the bacterial membrane will lack integrity and will cause altered function and impaired homeostasis within the bacterial cell. Also, the lack of adequate membrane cytoarchitecture appears to initiate a suicidal autolysis, whereby bacterial hydrolases released from lysosomes begin to break down the cell wall, thus further contributing to destruction of the microorganism.[50]

Consequently, drugs that cause inadequate production of peptidoglycans or other structural components within the cell wall may produce a selective bactericidal effect. Also, a limited number of antibacterial agents directly punch holes in the bacterial cell membrane, destroying the selective permeability and separation of internal from external environment,

which is crucial for the life of the microorganism.[31] These agents include the polymyxin antibiotics (polymyxin B, colistin). These drugs are cationic compounds that are attracted to negatively charged phospholipids in the bacterial cell membrane. The selectivity of these agents for bacterial cell membranes may be due to a greater attraction to certain bacterial phospholipids, as opposed to human cell membrane phospholipids. In any event, these drugs penetrate and disrupt the architecture and integrity of the surface membrane. In essence, these drugs act as detergents that break apart the phospholipid bilayer, creating gaps and leaks in the bacterial cell membrane.[31] The loss of cell membrane integrity leads to rapid death of the bacteria.

Inhibition of Bacterial Protein Synthesis

Bacteria, like most living organisms, must continually synthesize specific proteins to carry out various cellular functions, including enzymatic reactions and membrane transport. A fairly large and well-known group of antibacterial agents works by inhibiting or impairing the synthesis of these bacterial proteins. Drugs that exert their antibacterial effects in this manner include the aminoglycosides (e.g., gentamicin, streptomycin), erythromycin, the tetracyclines, and several other agents.[34,79] Generally, drugs that inhibit bacterial protein synthesis enter the bacterial cell and bind to specific ribosomal subunits.[5,59] Antibacterial drugs that work by this mechanism have a much greater affinity for bacterial ribosomes than for human ribosomes, hence their relative specificity in treating bacterial infections. Binding of the drug to the ribosome either blocks protein synthesis or causes the ribosome to misread the messenger RNA (mRNA) code, resulting in the production of meaningless or nonsense proteins.[34,87] The lack of appropriate protein production impairs bacterial cell membrane transport and metabolic function, resulting in retarded growth or death of the bacteria.

Inhibition of Bacterial DNA/RNA Synthesis and Function

As in any cell, bacteria must be able to replicate their genetic material to reproduce and function normally. An inability to produce normal DNA and RNA will prohibit the bacteria from mediating continued growth and reproduction. Drugs that exert their antibacterial activity by directly or indirectly interfering with the structure, synthesis, and function of DNA and RNA in susceptible bacteria include the fluoroquinolones, sulfonamides, and several other agents.[57] Apparently, these drugs are able to selectively impair bacterial DNA/RNA function because they have a greater affinity for bacterial genetic material and enzymes related to bacterial DNA/RNA synthesis.

Several antibacterial drugs inhibit bacterial nucleic acid synthesis by inhibiting the production of folic acid.[17] Folic acid serves as an enzymatic cofactor in a number of reactions, including synthesis of bacterial nucleic acids and certain essential amino acids. The pathway for synthesis of these folic acid cofactors is illustrated in Figure 33–2. Certain antibacterial drugs block specific steps in the folate pathway, thus impairing the production of this enzymatic cofactor and ultimately impairing the production of nucleic acids and

other essential metabolites. Examples of drugs that exert antibacterial effects by this mechanism are trimethoprim and the sulfonamide drugs (e.g., sulfadiazine, sulfamethoxazole).[33,82]

Specific Antibacterial Agents

Considering the vast number of antibacterial drugs, we cannot explore the pharmacokinetic and pharmacologic details of each individual agent. For the purposes of this chapter, the major groups of antibacterial drugs are categorized according to the basic modes of antibacterial action that were previously discussed (inhibition of cell wall synthesis, etc.). Pertinent aspects of each group's actions, uses, and potential side effects are briefly discussed. For a more detailed description of any specific agent, the reader is referred to one of the current drug indexes, such as the *Physician's Desk Reference (PDR)*.

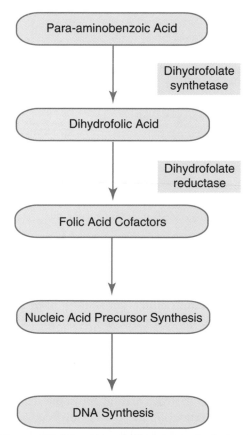

FIGURE 33–2 ▼ Folic acid metabolism in bacterial cells. Certain antibacterial drugs (e.g., sulfonamides and trimethoprim) inhibit the dihydrofolate synthetase and reductase enzymes, thus interfering with DNA biosynthesis.

Antibacterial Drugs That Inhibit Bacterial Cell Wall Synthesis and Function

Table 33–2 lists drugs that exert their primary antibacterial effects by impairing bacterial cell membrane synthesis and function. Clinical use and specific aspects of these drugs are presented below.

Penicillins

Penicillin, the first antibiotic, was originally derived from mold colonies of the *Penicillium* fungus during the early 1940s. Currently, there are several forms of natural and semisynthetic penicillins (see Table 33–2). These agents have a chemical structure and mode of action similar to the cephalosporin drugs and several other agents. Collectively, the penicillins and these other drugs are known as *beta-lactam antibiotics* because they share a common structure known as a *beta-lactam ring*.[56]

Penicillin and other beta-lactam agents exert their effects by binding to specific enzymatic proteins within the bacterial cell wall. These enzymatic proteins, known as penicillin-binding proteins (PBPs), are responsible for the normal synthesis and organization of the bacterial cell wall. In particular, PBPs help manufacture the peptidoglycans, which are essential for

| Table 33-2 | DRUGS THAT INHIBIT BACTERIAL CELL MEMBRANE SYNTHESIS |

Penicillins

Natural penicillins
    Penicillin G (Bicillin, Wycillin, many others)
    Penicillin V (Beepen-VK, V-Cillin K, others)
Penicillinase-resistant penicillins
    Cloxacillin (Cloxapen, Tegopen)
    Dicloxacillin (Dycill, Dynapen, Pathocil)
    Methicillin (Staphcillin)
    Nafcillin (Nafcil, Unipen, others)
    Oxacillin (Bactocill, Prostaphlin)
Aminopenicillins
    Amoxicillin (Amoxil, Polymox, others)
    Ampicillin (Omnipen, Polycillin, others)
    Bacampicillin (Spectrobid)
Extended-spectrum penicillins
    Carbenicillin (Geocillin, Geopen, Pyopen)
    Mezlocillin (Mezlan)
    Piperacillin (Pipracil)
    Ticarcillin (Ticar)

Cephalosporins

First-generation cephalosporins
    Cefadroxil (Duricef)
    Cefazolin (Ancef, Kefzol)
    Cephalexin (Keflex, others)
    Cephalothin (Keflin)
    Cephapirin (Cefadyl)
    Cephradine (Velosef)
Second-generation cephalosporins
    Cefaclor (Ceclor)
    Cefamandole (Mandol)
    Cefonicid (Monocid)

Cefotetan (Cefotan)
Cefoxitin (Mefoxin)
Cefprozil (Cefzil)
Cefuroxime (Ceftin, Kefurox, Zinacef)
Third-generation cephalosporins
    Cefdinir (Omnicef)
    Cefditoren (Spectracef)
    Cefoperazone (Cefobid)
    Cefotaxime (Claforan)
    Cefpodoxime (Vantin)
    Ceftazidime (Fortaz, Tazidime, others)
    Ceftibuten (Cedax)
    Ceftizoxime (Cefizox)
    Ceftriaxone (Rocephin)
Fourth-generation cephalosporins
    Cefepime (Maxipime)

Other Agents

Aztreonam (Azactam)
Bacitracin (Bacitracin ointment)
Colistin (Coly-Mycin S)
Cycloserine (Seromycin)
Imipenem/cilastatin (Primaxin)
Meropenem (Merrem I.V.)
Polymyxin B (generic)
Vancomycin (Vancocin)

Penicillin and Beta-lactamase Combinations

Ampicillin and clavulanate (Augmentin)
Ampicillin and sulbactam (Unasyn)
Piperacillin and tazobactam (Zosyn)
Ticarcillin and clavulanate (Timentin)

normal membrane structure and function.[47,78] Penicillins and other beta-lactam drugs attach to the PBPs and inhibit their function.[56,78] Thus, construction of the bacterial cell wall is impaired, and the cell dies from the membrane's inability to serve as a selective barrier and to contain the high internal osmotic pressure of the bacterial cell.

Classification and Use of Penicillins

As indicated in Table 33–2, penicillins can be classified according to their chemical background, spectrum of antibacterial activity, or pharmacokinetic features.[56] The naturally occurring penicillins (penicillin G and V) can be administered orally but have a relatively narrow antibacterial spectrum. Some semisynthetic penicillins (amoxicillin, ampicillin) have a broader antibacterial spectrum and may be administered either orally or parenterally, depending on the specific agent.

Penicillinase-resistant forms of penicillin were developed to overcome strains of bacteria that contain an enzyme known as a penicillinase or beta-lactamase. This enzyme destroys natural and some semisynthetic penicillins, rendering these drugs ineffective in bacteria containing this enzyme. For penicillinase-containing bacteria, the semisynthetic forms of penicillin that are resistant to destruction by the penicillinase must be used (see Table 33–2).

Discussing all the clinical applications of the penicillins goes well beyond the scope of this chapter. These agents are a mainstay in the treatment of infection and remain the drugs of choice in a diverse array of clinical disorders. Table 33–5 gives some indication of the clinical uses of the penicillins. Clearly, these agents continue to be one of the most important and effective antibacterial regimens currently available.

Adverse Effects

One of the primary problems with penicillin drugs is the potential for allergic reactions.[65] Hypersensitivity to penicillin is exhibited by skin rashes, hives, itching, and difficult breathing. In some individuals, these reactions may be minor and can often be resolved by changing the type of penicillin or the method of administration. In others, however, penicillin hypersensitivity may be severe and lead to an anaphylactic reaction (severe bronchoconstriction and cardiovascular collapse).

During prolonged administration, penicillin drugs may also cause central nervous system (CNS) problems (e.g., confusion, hallucinations), as well as certain blood disorders, such as hemolytic anemia and thrombocytopenia. Other relatively minor side effects of penicillin drugs include gastrointestinal problems such as nausea, vomiting, and diarrhea.

Cephalosporins

The cephalosporin drugs, which are also classified as beta-lactam antibiotics, exert their bactericidal effects in a manner similar to that of the penicillins (inhibition of PBPs, resulting in inadequate peptidoglycan production).[56] Generally, the cephalosporins serve as alternative agents to penicillins if the penicillin drugs are ineffective or poorly tolerated by the patient. Cephalosporins may also be the drugs of choice in certain types of urinary tract infections (see Tables 33–5).

Cephalosporins can be subdivided into first-, second-, third-, and fourth-generation groups, according to their spectrum of antibacterial activity (see Table 33–2). First-generation cephalosporins, which are generally effective against gram-positive cocci, may also be used against some gram-negative bacteria. Second-generation cephalosporins are also effective against gram-positive cocci, but they are somewhat more effective than first-generation agents against gram-negative bacteria. Third-generation cephalosporins have the broadest spectrum of effectiveness against gram-negative bacteria, but they have limited effects on gram-positive cocci. Fourth-generation agents have the broadest antibacterial spectrum of the cephalosporins, and they are effective against gram-positive and gram-negative organisms. Specific indications for cephalosporins are listed in Table 33–5.

Adverse Effects

In some patients, cephalosporins may cause an allergic reaction similar to the penicillin hypersensitivity described previously. A cross-sensitivity often exists: a patient who is allergic to penicillin drugs will also display hypersensitivity to cephalosporin agents. Other principal adverse effects of cephalosporins include gastrointestinal problems such as stomach cramps, diarrhea, nausea, and vomiting.

Other Agents That Inhibit Bacterial Cell Wall Synthesis

Aztreonam. Aztreonam (Azactam) is another type of beta-lactam antibiotic, but this drug is classified as a carbapenam agent rather than a penicillin or cephalosporin.[4] Nonetheless, aztreonam acts like the other beta-lactam agents and inhibits the synthesis and structure of the cell membrane in susceptible bacteria. Aztreonam has a limited spectrum, but it may be useful against serious infections caused by certain gram-negative bacilli (*Enterobacter aerogenes* and *Pseudomonas aeruginosa*). The principal problems associated with aztreonam include skin rashes, redness, and itching due to hypersensitivity in susceptible individuals.

Bacitracin. Bacitracin refers to a group of polypeptide antibiotics that have similar chemical and pharmacologic properties. These compounds inhibit bacterial cell wall synthesis by inhibiting the incorporation of amino acids and nucleic acid precursors into the bacterial cell wall. Bacitracin compounds, which have a broad range of antibacterial activity, are effective against many gram-positive bacilli and gram-positive cocci, as well as several other microorganisms. Bacitracin is usually applied topically to prevent and treat infection in superficial skin wounds and certain ophthalmic infections. Commercial preparations containing bacitracin may also contain other antibiotics, such as neomycin and polymyxin B. The primary problem associated with bacitracin is local hypersensitivity, as indicated by skin rashes and itching.

Colistin. Colistin (also known as *colistimethate* or *polymyxin E*) is similar to polymyxin B in terms of pharmacologic mechanism and antibacterial effects.[31] Colistin is used primarily in combination with other agents (neomycin and hydrocortisone) to treat local infections of the external auditory canal. Adverse effects are relatively rare during the local and topical use of this drug.

Cycloserine. Cycloserine inhibits bacterial wall synthesis by interfering with the final stage of peptidoglycan synthesis. Adding two units of the amino acid D-alanine completes the synthesis of peptidoglycans. Cycloserine, which is similar in structure to D-alanine, competitively inhibits the enzyme that adds the final D-alanine units onto the peptidoglycan structures. Cycloserine is considered a broad-spectrum antibiotic but is used primarily as an adjunct in the treatment of tuberculosis. The primary adverse effect of this drug is CNS toxicity, which may occur during prolonged use at relatively high dosages.

Ertapenem. Ertapenem (Invanz) is another carbapenam antibacterial agent that is similar to meropenem (see below).[11] Ertapenem is effective against gram-positive and gram-negative aerobic and anaerobic bacteria, and is often used to treat intra-abdominal and pelvic infections, as well as infections in the skin, urinary tract, and respiratory tract. Side effects include chest pain, gastrointestinal problems (nausea, diarrhea), headache, and fever.

Imipenem and Cilastatin. Imipenem is a beta-lactam drug that is classified as a carbapenam antibiotic.[10] Imipenem exerts bactericidal effects similar to the other beta-lactam agents (penicillins and cephalosporins); that is, imipenem inhibits PBP function and peptidoglycan synthesis. This drug is typically administered along with a second agent, cilastatin. Cilastatin enhances the bactericidal effects of imipenem by inhibiting metabolic inactivation of imipenem within the kidneys, even though cilastin does not exhibit any antibacterial activities by itself.[68]

Imipenem has one of the broadest antibacterial spectrums of the beta-lactam drugs and may be useful against a variety of aerobic gram-positive or gram-negative bacteria, as well as some anaerobic bacterial strains.[81] Side effects associated with imipenem include nausea, hypotension, and hypersensitivity (skin rashes, redness, itching). CNS abnormalities such as confusion, tremors, and seizures have also been reported in certain patients. The risk of imipenem-induced seizure is increased in patients who have a preexisting seizure disorder or if the drug dosage is too high, based on the patient's body weight.

Meropenem. Meropenem is a carbapenam antibacterial with effects and spectrum similar to imipen-

em.[81] Meropenem, however, does not need to be administered with cilastatin. This agent may likewise be effective against certain forms of gram-positive and gram-negative bacteria that are resistant to other beta-lactam drugs. Meropenem may cause CNS problems—including seizures—but the risk is relatively low when compared with the risk of seizures with imipenem.[23]

Polymyxin B. Polymyxin antibiotics are cationic compounds that are attracted to negatively charged phospholipids in the bacterial cell membrane. These drugs penetrate and disrupt the architecture and integrity of the surface membrane. Essentially, polymyxins act as detergents that break apart the phospholipid bilayer, which creates gaps in the bacterial cell wall, leading to the subsequent destruction of the bacteria.[31]

Polymyxin B is effective against many gram-negative bacteria, including *E. coli*, *Klebsiella*, and *Salmonella*. Systemic administration of this drug, however, is often associated with extreme nephrotoxicity. Hence, this agent is used primarily for the treatment of local, superficial infections of the skin, eyes, and mucous membranes. When applied topically for these conditions, adverse reactions are relatively rare. Polymyxin B is often combined with other antibiotics such as bacitracin and neomycin in commercial topical preparations.

Vancomycin. Vancomycin appears to bind directly to bacterial cell wall precursors such as D-alanine and to impair the incorporation of these precursors into the cell wall.[41] Vancomycin is effective against gram-positive bacilli and cocci and primarily serves as an alternative to the penicillins in a variety of infections (see Tables 33–5).[16] The emergence of bacteria that are resistant to vancomycin, however, has generated concern about the continued use of this drug (see "Resistance to Antibacterial Drugs" later in this chapter).[6] The primary adverse effects associated with vancomycin include hypersensitivity (e.g., skin rashes), a bitter or unpleasant taste in the mouth, and gastrointestinal disturbances (nausea and vomiting). Vancomycin also has the potential to cause nephrotoxicity and ototoxicity.

Use of Beta-Lactamase Inhibitors

A primary problem in using penicillins, cephalosporins, and other beta-lactam antibiotics is that certain bacteria produce enzymes known as beta-lactamases.[26,70] These beta-lactamase enzymes bind to the beta-lactam drug and destroy it before it can exert an antibacterial effect. Bacteria that produce these beta-lactamase enzymes are therefore resistant to penicillin and other beta-lactam antibacterial drugs (problems related to antibacterial drug resistance are discussed later in this chapter; see "Resistance to Antibacterial Drugs").[70] Fortunately, several drugs are available that inhibit these beta-lactamase enzymes.[13] These drugs include clavulanate, sulbactam, and tazobactam. These beta-lactamase inhibitors are typically combined with a specific type of penicillin in order to treat infections caused by bacteria that produce beta-lactamase enzymes.[14] The beta-lactamase inhibitor prevents the beta-lactamase enzyme from destroying the penicillin, thus allowing the penicillin to remain intact and effective against the bacterial infection.

Some common combinations of penicillins and specific beta-lactamase inhibitors are listed in Table 33–2. Administration of these drug combinations may produce side effects that are caused primarily by the penicillin component; that is, penicillin-related side effects such as headache, gastrointestinal problems, and allergic reactions. Nonetheless, combining a beta-lactamase inhibitor with a penicillin can be an effective way of treating bacterial infections that might otherwise be resistant to traditional antibacterial therapy.

Drugs That Inhibit Bacterial Protein Synthesis

Drugs that exert their primary antibacterial effects by inhibiting protein synthesis are listed in Table 33–3 and discussed below.

Aminoglycosides

The aminoglycosides are a group of antibacterial agents including streptomycin, gentamicin, neomycin, and similar agents (see Table 33–3). These agents bind irreversibly to certain parts of bacterial ribosomes and cause several changes in protein synthesis, including alterations in the ribosome's ability to read the mRNA genetic code.[15,39] This misreading results in the improper synthesis of proteins that control specific aspects of cell function, such as membrane structure and permeability.[15] The lack of normal cell proteins leads to the bacterial cell's death.

Antibacterial Spectrum and General Indications

Aminoglycosides have a very broad spectrum of antibacterial activity and are effective against many aerobic

Table 33–3	DRUGS THAT INHIBIT BACTERIAL PROTEIN SYNTHESIS		
Aminoglycosides	**Erythromycins**	**Tetracyclines**	**Other Agents**
Amikacin (Amikin)	Erythromycin (ERYC, E-Mycin, others)	Demeclocycline (Declomycin)	Chloramphenicol (Chloromycetin)
Gentamicin (Garamycin)	Erythromycin estolate (Ilosone)	Doxycycline (Monodox, Vibramycin, others)	Clindamycin (Cleocin)
Kanamycin (Kantrex)	Erythromycin ethylsuccinate (E.E.S., EryPed, others)	Minocycline (Minocin)	Ethionamide (Trecator-SC)
Neomycin (generic)	Erythromycin gluceptate (Ilotycin)	Oxytetracyline (Terramycin)	Lincomycin (Lincocin, Lincorex)
Netilmicin (Netromycin)	Erythromycin lactobionate (Erythrocin)	Tetracycline (Achromycin V, others)	Linezolid (Zyvox)
Streptomycin (generic)	Erythromycin stearate (Erythrocin, Erythrocot, others)		Quinupristin and Dalfopristin (Synercid)
Tobramycin (Nebcin)			Telithromycin (Ketek) Tigecycline (Tygacil)

gram-negative bacteria, including *E. coli*, *Pseudomonas*, and *Salmonella*.[15] Aminoglycosides are active against some aerobic gram-positive bacteria, such as certain species of *Staphylococcus*, and many anaerobic bacteria. Consequently, aminoglycosides are used to treat a variety of tissue and wound infections (see Table 33–5).

Adverse Effects

Aminoglycoside use is limited somewhat by problems with toxicity.[66] Nephrotoxicity, as indicated by bloody urine, acute renal tubular necrosis, and so on, is one of the more common and serious adverse effects.[49,66] Ototoxicity, as indicated by dizziness and ringing or fullness in the ears, may also occur. This effect can be irreversible in severe cases.[67] Toxicity may occur more frequently in certain individuals, such as patients with liver or kidney failure, or in elderly patients. To reduce the risk of toxicity, drug levels in the bloodstream must be periodically monitored so dosages can be adjusted for individual patients. Other adverse effects include hypersensitivity (e.g., skin rashes, itching) in susceptible individuals.

Erythromycin and Other Macrolides

Erythromycin and its chemical derivatives (azithromycin, clarithromycin, dirithromycin) comprise a group of agents known as macrolide antibiotics.[16] These drugs inhibit bacterial protein synthesis by binding to specific parts of the ribosomes in susceptible bacteria.[58] This binding impairs protein synthesis primarily by inhibiting the formation of peptide bonds between adjacent amino acids. In particular, erythromycin seems to encourage the dissociation of transfer RNA (tRNA) units from their binding site on the ribosome.[27] Normally, the tRNAs bring amino acids to the ribosome, where the amino acids are linked together to form proteins. By stimulating the detachment of tRNA, peptide bond formation is averted.

Antibacterial Spectrum and General Indications

Erythromycin and the other macrolides exhibit a very broad spectrum of antibacterial activities and are active against many gram-positive bacteria, as well as some gram-negative bacteria. These agents are often used as the primary or alternative drug in a variety of clinical conditions (see Table 33–5). Macrolides may be especially useful in patients who are allergic to penicillin.

Macrolides may produce other beneficial effects that compliment their antibacterial properties. These drugs, for example, seem to have anti-inflammatory effects, especially in diseases associated with airway inflammation.[80] Hence, these drugs may be particularly useful in treating certain airway infections in people with cystic fibrosis or other respiratory disorders associated with infection and inflammation in airway tissues.[8,75]

Adverse Effects

When given in high (bactericidal) dosages, gastrointestinal distress is a common problem with erythromycin administration; for example, stomach cramps, nausea, vomiting, and diarrhea may occur. Hence, erythromycin is usually given in doses that only impair the growth of bacteria (bacteriostatic doses). Some of the newer macrolides (clarithromycin, dirithromycin) may be somewhat safer and produce fewer side effects than erythromycin.[46] However, various degrees of allergic reactions—ranging from mild skin rashes to acute anaphylaxis—may occur when these drugs are used in susceptible individuals.

Tetracyclines

Tetracycline and tetracycline derivatives (see Table 33–3) inhibit protein synthesis by binding to several components of the ribosomal apparatus in susceptible bacteria.[3,12] Hence, these drugs may cause misreading of the mRNA code, as well as impair the formation of peptide bonds at the bacterial ribosome. Thus, tetracyclines are very effective in preventing bacterial protein synthesis.

Antibacterial Spectrum and General Indications

Tetracyclines are active against a variety of bacteria, including many gram-positive and gram-negative bacteria, as well as other bacterial microorganisms (*Rickettsia*, spirochetes).[16] Their use as a broad-spectrum antibiotic has diminished somewhat, however, because of the development of tetracycline-resistant bacterial strains. (The problem of drug-resistant bacteria is discussed in more detail in "Resistance to Antibacterial Drugs.")

Some of the newer tetracycline derivatives such as doxycycline may be used to overcome bacterial strains that are resistant to the traditional drugs.[16] Currently, tetracyclines are used to treat specific infections relating to such bacilli as *Chlamydia*, *Rickettsia*, and certain spirochetes (see Table 33–5). Tetracyclines may also be used as alternative agents in treating bacterial strains that are resistant to other drugs, such as chloramphenicol, streptomycin, and various penicillins.

Tetracyclines also seem to have anti-inflammatory and immunomodulating effects.[53,71] Although the exact reasons for these effects are unclear, tetracyclines have been used in a variety of noninfectious diseases with an inflammatory or autoimmune basis, including scleroderma and rheumatoid arthritis.[71] Clinical studies will continue to investigate how these drugs can be used effectively in the long-term management of chronic disease.

Adverse Effects

Gastrointestinal distress (nausea, vomiting, diarrhea) may be a problem with tetracycline use. Hypersensitivity reactions (such as rashes) may also occur, as well as an increase in skin sensitivity to ultraviolet light (photosensitivity).[16] Tetracyclines form chemical complexes with calcium that may impair the growth and development of calcified tissues such as bone and teeth, especially in children.[69] Tetracyclines also cause discoloration of teeth in children and pregnant women, apparently because of the tetracycline-calcium interaction.[69] As mentioned previously, development of tetracycline-resistant strains and resulting superinfections may be a serious problem during tetracycline therapy.

Other Agents That Inhibit Bacterial Protein Synthesis

Chloramphenicol. Chloramphenicol (Chloromycetin) is a synthetically produced agent that exerts antibacterial effects similar to those of erythromycin; that is, it binds to the 50S subunit of bacterial ribosomes and inhibits peptide bond formation. Chloramphenicol is a broad-spectrum antibiotic that is active against many gram-negative and gram-positive bacteria. This drug is administered systemically to treat serious infections such as typhoid fever, *Haemophilus* infections such as osteomyelitis, rickettsial infections such as Rocky Mountain spotted fever, and certain forms of meningitis. Chloramphenicol may also be administered topically to treat various skin, eye, and ear infections.

The most serious problem associated with chloramphenicol is the potential for bone marrow aplasia, which can lead to aplastic anemia and possibly death.[16,83] Chloramphenicol is also associated with other blood dyscrasias such as agranulocytosis and thrombocytopenia. Because of these risks, chloram-

phenicol is not typically used as a first-choice drug, but is reserved for severe infections that do not respond to other antibacterials, or situations where safer drugs are contraindicated (e.g., patients are allergic to other medications).[16]

Clindamycin. Clindamycin (Cleocin) is derived from lincomycin. Both drugs are similar in structure and function to erythromycin and inhibit protein synthesis by binding to the 50S ribosomal subunit of susceptible bacteria. These agents are effective against most gram-positive bacteria and some gram-negative microorganisms.[16] Typically, clindamycin and lincomycin are reserved as alternative drugs (rather than primary agents) in the treatment of local and systemic infections; these agents may be especially useful if patients are unable to tolerate either penicillin or erythromycin. The principal adverse effects associated with these drugs include gastrointestinal distress (nausea, diarrhea, colitis) and various allergic reactions, ranging from mild skin rashes to anaphylactic shock.

Ethionamide. Ethionamide (Trecator-SC) appears to inhibit bacterial protein synthesis, but the exact mechanism of action is unknown. This drug may act in a manner similar to that of some of the other drugs discussed previously in this section (binding to bacterial ribosomes), or it may mediate its effect by some other means. Ethionamide is effective against *M. tuberculosis* and is used primarily in the treatment of tuberculosis. This drug is usually used as a secondary agent when primary antituberculosis drugs are ineffective. Gastrointestinal distress (nausea, vomiting) is the most frequent problem encountered with ethionamide use. CNS disorders (drowsiness, mental depression, etc.), as well as severe postural hypotension, may also occur.

Lincomycin. Lincomycin (Lincocin, Lincorex) is similar in mechanism of action, clinical indications, and adverse side effects to clindamycin (see previously in this section).

Linezolid. Linezolid (Zyvox) binds to a specific site on the bacterial ribosome and inhibits protein synthesis in many gram-positive bacteria including staphlocci, streptococci, and enterococci. Hence, this drug is commonly used to treat pneumonia caused by *S. aureus* or *S. pneumoniae*, and other susceptible skin and soft tissue infections. Common side effects include gastrointestinal problems (nausea, diarrhea), with more serious blood dyscrasias (anemia, leukopenia, thrombocytopenia) occurring in some patients during prolonged drug administration.

Quinupristin and Dalfopristin. Quinupristin and Dalfopristin are combined in the same product (Synercid), which is used to treat certain gram-positive bacteria such as staphylococci and some enterococcal strains. These agents bind to the bacterial ribosome at slightly different sites, and work together to prevent the formation of bacterial polypeptide chains. Treatments are administered via intravenous infusion; primary side effects involve pain, irritation, and thrombophlebitis at the infusion site. Other side effects include muscle and joint pain and gastrointestinal disturbances (nausea, vomiting, diarrhea).

Telithromycin. Telithromycin (Ketek) is the first agent from a new class of drugs known as ketolide antibacterials.[77] This drug is derived from eryththromycin, but is altered structurally so that it is able to overcome certain forms of bacterial resistance. Telithromycin acts by binding to the bacterial ribosome and inhibiting protein synthesis. It has an antibacterial spectrum similar to eryththromycin, but is typically reserved for gram-negative strains that are resistant to other agents. Primary side effects include gastrointestinal disturbances (nausea, vomiting, diarrhea), liver toxicity, and cardiac arrhythmias in susceptible patients.

Tigecycline. Tigecycline (Tygacil) is a relatively new antibacterial drug that is classified chemically as a glycycline agent.[36] This drug is similar to tetracycline in structure and antibacterial spectrum, but tigecycline may be somewhat more effective in treating certain infections that are tetracycline-resistant.[25,89] This drug may also be useful against other resistant strains including methicillin-resistant *S. aureus*, and vancomycin-resistant *E. faecalis* and *E. faecium*.[89] The primary side effects of tigecycline include nausea, vomiting, headache, and dizziness.

Drugs That Inhibit Bacterial DNA/RNA Synthesis and Function

Table 33–4 lists drugs that exert their primary antibacterial effects by impairing the synthesis and replication of bacterial DNA and RNA. These agents are presented here.

Aminosalicylic Acid

Aminosalicylic acid (Paser, PAS) exerts its effects in a manner similar to the sulfonamide drugs; that is, aminosalicylic acid is structurally similar to para-aminobenzoic acid (PABA) and inhibits folic acid synthesis by competing with PABA in tuberculosis

Table 33–4	DRUGS THAT INHIBIT BACTERIAL DNA/RNA SYNTHESIS AND FUNCTION

Fluoroquinolones

Ciprofloxacin (Cipro)
Enoxacin (Penetrex)
Gatifloxacin (Tequin)
Levofloxacin (Levaquin)
Lomefloxacin (Maxaquin)
Moxifloxacin (Avelox)
Norfloxacin (Noroxin)
Ofloxacin (Floxin)
Sparfloxacin (Zagam)

Sulfonamides

Sulfadiazine (Silvadene)
Sulfamethizole (Thiosulfil Forte)
Sulfamethoxazole (Gantanol, Urobak)
Sulfisoxazole (Gantrisin)

Others

Aminosalicylic acid (Tubasal)
Clofazimine (Lamprene)
Dapsone (Avlosulfon)
Ethambutol (Myambutol)
Metronidazole (Flagyl, Protostat, others)
Mupirocin (Bactroban)
Rifabutin (Mycobutin)
Rifampin (Rifadin, Rimactane)
Rifapentine (Priftin)
Trimethoprim (Proloprim, Trimpex)

bacteria. This drug is used as an adjunct to the primary antitubercular agents, isoniazid and rifampin. Adverse effects are fairly common with aminosalicylic acid use and include gastrointestinal problems, hypersensitivity reactions, and blood dyscrasias (e.g., agranulocytosis, thrombocytopenia).

Clofazimine

Although the exact mechanism of clofazimine (Lamprene) is unclear, this drug appears to bind directly to bacterial DNA in susceptible microorganisms. Drug binding may prevent the double-stranded DNA helix from unraveling to allow replication of the DNA genetic code. An inability to replicate its genetic material will prevent the bacteria from undergoing mitosis.

Clofazimine is effective against *Mycobacterium leprae* and is used primarily as an adjunct in the treatment of leprosy. During clofazimine therapy, many patients experience problems with red to brownish-black discoloration of the skin. Although this discoloration is reversible, it may take several months to years before skin color returns to normal. Other adverse effects include abdominal pain, nausea, vomiting, and rough, scaly skin.

Dapsone

Dapsone (Avlosulfon) is a member of a class of chemical agents known as the sulfones. Dapsone is especially effective against *M. leprae* and is used with rifampin as the primary method of treating leprosy. Dapsone appears to exert its antibacterial effects in a manner similar to that of the sulfonamide drugs; that is, dapsone impairs folic acid synthesis by competing with PABA in bacterial cells. Primary adverse effects associated with dapsone include peripheral motor weakness, hypersensitivity reactions (skin rashes, itching), fever, and blood dyscrasias, such as hemolytic anemia.

Ethambutol

The mechanism of ethambutol (Myambutol) is not fully understood. This drug apparently suppresses RNA synthesis in susceptible bacteria, but it is not known how this occurs. Ethambutol is primarily effective against *M. tuberculosis* infections and is a secondary agent in the treatment of tuberculosis.[61] Adverse effects associated with this drug include joint pain, nausea, skin rash and itching, and CNS abnormalities (dizziness, confusion, hallucinations).

Fluoroquinolones

The fluoroquinolone antibiotics include ciprofloxacin (Cipro), enoxacin (Penetrex), gatifloxacin (Tequin), levofloxacin (Levaquin), lomefloxacin (Maxaquin), moxifloxacin (Avelox), norfloxacin (Noroxin), ofloxacin (Floxin), and sparfloxacin (Zagam). These drugs inhibit two specific enzymes—DNA-gyrase and topoisomerase IV—that affect DNA function in certain bacteria.[9,18] DNA-gyrase is responsible for controlling the amount of DNA winding (supercoiling) in bacterial cells. Topoisomerase IV enzymatically separates two new DNA strands that are formed during bacter-

ial cell division. Fluoroquinolones inhibit these enzymes, thereby impairing the normal DNA structure and function that is needed for cell growth and replication.[64]

Fluoroquinolones are effective against a wide range of gram-positive and gram-negative aerobic bacteria and are especially useful in urinary tract infections caused by *E. coli*, *Klebsiella*, *Proteus*, and *Enterobacter aerogenes*.[9,72] Other indications include the treatment of gastrointestinal infections, respiratory infections, osteomyelitis, and certain sexually transmitted diseases (gonorrhea).[18,20] A specific agent, ciprofloxacin (Cipro), is particularly effective against anthrax infections, and this drug received considerable attention as an intervention against bioterrorist activities that use anthrax.[21] Primary adverse effects include CNS toxicity, manifested by visual disturbances, headache, and dizziness. Gastrointestinal distress (nausea, vomiting, diarrhea) and allergic reactions (skin rashes, itching) may also occur.[57] These drugs produce photosensitivity and increase the skin's sensitivity to ultraviolet light.[2,57] Rare but potentially serious cases of nephrotoxicity may occur in certain patients.[43]

Finally, these drugs may cause tendon pain and inflammation (tendinopathy) that can be severe and can ultimately lead to tendon rupture in some patients.[37,48] Tendinopathy seems to occur most commonly in the Achilles tendon, but other tendons such as the patellar tendon and supraspinatus tendon may also be affected.[38,84] Although the overall incidence of tendinopathy is fairly low, patients may be more susceptible if they are older, have renal failure, are taking glucocorticoids, or have a history of fluoroquinolone-induced tendinopathy.[37] Although all of the fluoroquinolones can potentially cause tendinopathy, the risk of tendon damage seems highest with ofloxacin.[85] Hence, complaints of pain in any tendon should be carefully evaluated in patients taking fluoroquinolones, and the affected tendon(s) should not be exercised until the cause of tendinopathy can be determined. If it seems that fluoroquinolones are causing tendinopathy, these drugs should be discontinued, and efforts should be made to protect the tendon from excessive stress until the tendinopathy is resolved.

Metronidazole

The exact mechanism of metronidazole (Flagyl, Protostat, others) is not fully understood. This drug appears to be incorporated into bacterial cells, where it undergoes chemical reduction. Apparently, the reduced metabolite of metronidazole interacts with bacterial DNA and causes it to lose its characteristic double-helix structure. This leads to the disintegration of DNA molecules and loss of the ability to replicate and carry out normal genetic functions. Further details of this bactericidal effect remain to be determined.

Metronidazole is effective against most anaerobic bacteria and is useful in treating serious infections caused by *Bacteroides, Fusobacterium,* and other anaerobic bacteria. Metronidazole, is also effective against certain protozoa and is discussed in Chapter 35 with regard to its antiprotozoal effects. Common side effects associated with metronidazole include gastrointestinal distress (nausea, diarrhea), allergic reactions (such as rashes), and CNS symptoms (confusion, dizziness, mood changes). This drug may also cause peripheral neuropathies as indicated by numbness and tingling in the hands and feet.

Mupirocin

Mupirocin (Bactroban) inhibits a specific enzyme responsible for tRNA synthesis in susceptible bacteria. This drug is used topically to treat skin infections caused by *Staphylococcus aureus* or *Streptococcus pyogenes.* Likewise, mupirocin can be administered by nasal spray to treat local colonization of *S. aureus* in the nasal mucosa. This idea may be especially helpful in preventing systemic infection in individuals such as health care workers who are exposed to an outbreak of resistant strains of *S. aureus.* Local/topical administration of this drug is well tolerated, although some irritation of the skin may occur during topical use, and cough and respiratory irritation can occur when mupirocin is administered by nasal spray.

Rifampin

Rifampin (Rifadin, Rimactane), and similar agents such as rifabutin (Mycobutin) and rifapentine (Priftin), directly impair DNA replication by binding to and inhibiting the DNA-dependent RNA polymerase enzyme in susceptible bacteria. This enzyme initiates the replication of genetic material by generating the formation of RNA strands from the DNA template. By inhibiting this enzyme, rifampin blocks RNA chain synthesis and subsequent replication of the nucleic acid code in bacterial cells.

Rifampin is effective against many gram-negative and gram-positive bacteria and is one of the principal agents used to treat tuberculosis and leprosy. Typically, this drug is combined with another agent—for example, rifampin plus dapsone for leprosy, or rifampin plus isoniazid for tuberculosis—to increase effectiveness and to prevent the development of resistance to rifampin. Rifampin is also used in combination with erythromycin to treat Legionnaire disease and certain forms of meningitis (see Table 33–5).

Common adverse effects include gastrointestinal distress (nausea, vomiting, stomach cramps) and various hypersensitivity reactions (rashes and fever). Disturbances in liver function have also been noted, and serious hepatic abnormalities may occur in patients with preexisting liver disease.

Sulfonamides

The sulfonamides include sulfadiazine, sulfamethizole, and similar agents (see Table 33–4). Sulfonamides interfere with bacterial nucleic acid production by disrupting folic acid synthesis in susceptible bacteria. Sulfonamide drugs are structurally similar to PABA, which is the substance used in the first step of folic acid synthesis in certain types of bacteria (see Fig. 33–2). Sulfonamides either directly inhibit the enzyme responsible for PABA utilization or become a substitute for PABA, which results in the abnormal synthesis of folic acid. In either case, folic acid synthesis is reduced, and bacterial nucleic acid synthesis is impaired.

Sulfonamides have the potential to be used against a wide variety of bacteria, including gram-negative and gram-positive bacilli and cocci. The development of resistance in various bacteria, however, has limited the use of these drugs. Currently, sulfonamides are used systemically to treat certain urinary tract infections and infections caused by *Nocardia* bacteria. Sulfonamides may also be applied topically to treat vaginal infections, ophthalmic conditions, and other local infections. A specific agent, sulfadiazine, can also be combined with silver nitrate to form silver sulfadiazine, which is often applied topically to control bacterial infection in burns.[19,52]

The problems encountered most frequently with sulfonamide drugs include gastrointestinal distress, increased skin sensitivity to ultraviolet light, and allergic reactions. Serious disturbances in the formed blood elements, including blood dyscrasias such as agranulocytosis and hemolytic anemia, may also occur during systemic sulfonamide therapy.

Trimethoprim

Trimethoprim (Proloprim, Trimpex) interferes with the bacterial folic acid pathway by inhibiting the dihydrofolate reductase enzyme in susceptible bacteria (see Fig. 33–2). This enzyme converts dihydrofolic acid to tetrahydrofolic acid during the biosynthesis of folic acid cofactors. By inhibiting this enzyme, trimethoprim directly interferes with the production of folic acid cofactors, and subsequent production of vital bacterial nucleic acids is impaired.

Trimethoprim is effective against several gram-negative bacilli, including *E. coli*, *Enterobacter*, *Proteus mirabilis*, and *Klebsiella*. Trimethoprim is used primarily in the treatment of urinary tract infections caused by these and other susceptible bacteria (see Table 33–5). Trimethoprim is frequently used in combination with the sulfonamide drug sulfamethoxazole.[73] Primary adverse effects associated with trimethoprim include headache, skin rashes and itching, decreased appetite, an unusual taste in the mouth, and gastrointestinal problems (nausea, vomiting, diarrhea). Trimethoprim may also cause excessively high levels of potassium in the blood (hyperkalemia), especially in older adults.[55]

Other Antibacterial Drugs

Several other antibacterial drugs work by mechanisms that are either unknown or are different from the classical antibacterial mechanisms described previously. These drugs are discussed individually here.

Capreomycin

Capreomycin (Capastat) is used as an adjunct or alternative drug for the treatment of tuberculosis. The drug's mechanism of action is unknown. The primary problems associated with this drug include ototoxicity and nephrotoxicity.

Daptomycin

Daptomycin (Cubicin) is unique in that this drug binds to the cell membrane of susceptible bacteria and depolarizes the cell. Loss of membrane polarity results in a general inhibition of cell function and subsequent death of the bacterium. This drug is used primarily to treat skin infections caused by certain staphylococcal, streptococcal, and enterococcal bacteria. Because of its unique mechanism of action, daptomycin may also be

helpful in treating strains that are resistant to more traditional antibacterial drugs. Primary side effects of this drug include gastrointestinal problems (nausea, constipation, diarrhea), and higher doses may cause myopathy and neuropathy in some patients.

Isoniazid

Isoniazid (INH, Laniazid, Nydrazid, other names) is one of the primary drugs used to treat tuberculosis.[24,61] Although the exact mechanism of action is unknown, this drug appears to interfere with several enzymatic pathways involving protein, lipid, carbohydrate, and nucleic acid metabolism in susceptible bacteria. Adverse reactions to isoniazid are common, and patients may develop disorders such as hepatitis and peripheral neuropathies.

Methenamine

Methenamine (Hiprex, Mandelamine, Urex) exerts antibacterial properties in a unique fashion. In an acidic environment, this drug decomposes into formaldehyde and ammonia. Formaldehyde is bactericidal to almost all bacteria, and bacteria do not develop resistance to this toxin. This mechanism enables methenamine to be especially useful in treating urinary tract infections, because the presence of this drug in acidic urine facilitates the release of formaldehyde at the site of infection (i.e., within the urinary tract). Use of methenamine is safe, although high doses are associated with gastrointestinal upset and problems with urination (bloody urine, pain while urinating).

Nitrofurantoin

Bacterial enzymes reduce nitrofurantoin (Macrobid, Macrodantin, others) into a metabolite that is toxic to the bacterial cell. This toxic metabolite inhibits bacterial metabolic function by interfering with ribosomal function and other molecules involved in energy production and utilization in the bacterial cell. Nitrofurantoin is primarily used to treat urinary tract infections caused by a number of gram-negative and some gram-positive bacteria. Adverse effects associated with this drug include gastrointestinal distress (nausea, vomiting, and diarrhea) and neurotoxicity (as indicated by headache, numbness, and excessive fatigue). Acute pneumonitis (as indicated by coughing, chills, fever, and difficulty in breathing) may also occur soon after nitrofurantoin is initiated. This pneumonitis appears to be a direct chemical effect of the drug and usually disappears within hours after the drug is withdrawn.

Pyrazinamide

Pyrazinamide (generic) is used primarily as an adjunct to other drugs in treating tuberculosis. This drug's mechanism of action against *M. tuberculosis* is unknown. Problems associated with pyrazinamide include hepatotoxicity and lower-extremity joint pain.

Clinical Use of Antibacterial Drugs: Relationship to Specific Bacterial Infections

An incredible array of antibacterial agents is currently being used clinically. As mentioned previously, selection of a particular agent is based on the effectiveness of the drug against a range or spectrum of different bacteria. The clinical application of antibacterial drugs according to their effectiveness against specific bacteria is summarized in Table 33–5. As this table indicates, various antibacterial drugs can serve as either the primary or the alternative agents against specific bacterial infections. The actual selection of an antibacterial agent is often highly variable, depending on the particular patient, the type and location of the infection, the experience of the physician, and many other factors.

Resistance to Antibacterial Drugs

One of the most serious problems of antibacterial therapy is the potential for development of strains of bacteria that are resistant to one or more antibacterial agents.[1] Certain bacterial strains have a natural or acquired defense mechanism against specific antibacterial drugs. This enables the strain to survive the effects of the drug and continue to grow and reproduce similar resistant strains, thus representing a genetic selection process in which only the resistant strains survive the drug. As a result, bacteria that are invulnerable to the drug can breed. If other drugs are not effective against the resistant strain, or if cross-resistance to several antibacterial drugs occurs, the resistant bacteria become especially dangerous because of their immunity from antibacterial chemotherapy.[1]

Bacterial resistance can occur because of several mechanisms.[28,76] Certain bacterial strains may be able to enzymatically destroy the antibacterial drug. The best example is the beta-lactamase enzyme that is found in bacteria that are resistant to beta-lactam drugs (penicillins and cephalosporins).[54,86] As previously discussed, bacteria containing this enzyme can destroy certain penicillin and cephalosporin drugs, thus rendering the drug ineffective against these strains.

Resistance may also occur because the bacterial cell modifies or masks the site where the antibacterial drug typically binds on or within the cell. For instance, penicillins, aminoglycosides, vancomycin, and other drugs must bind to membrane proteins, intracellular proteins, ribosomes, and the like to exert their effect. Differences in the affinity of these binding sites may be acquired by bacterial mutation, thus decreasing the drug's effectiveness.[7,30] Bacteria may also develop resistance through genetic mutations that change the enzymes targeted by certain drugs. For example, fluoroquinolones, rifampin, and other drugs that normally inhibit enzymes responsible for bacterial DNA/RNA function will be ineffective if enzymes are modified within resistant bacteria.[7,35]

Resistance can likewise occur if the drug's ability to penetrate the bacterial cell is reduced. Most drugs must first penetrate the cell membrane and then enter the bacterial cell to exert their bactericidal effects. Specific bacteria that have a natural or acquired opposition to drug penetration render the drug useless, thus leading to the development of strains that are resistant to aminoglycosides and other agents.[28,76] Certain bacteria also develop drug efflux pumps that expel the drug from the bacterial cell, thus rendering the drug ineffective.[44] These pumps are a common way that bacteria develop resistance to tetracyclines and a number of other antimicrobial agents.[22,60]

Consequently, a number of factors may be responsible for mediating the formation of bacterial resistance to penicillins, cephalosporins, aminoglycosides, tetracyclines, and other antibacterial agents. Antibacterial resistance is typically categorized according to the name of the drug and the associated resistant bacterial strain. For example, some of the best known and most important types of resistance include vancomycin-resistant *Staphylococcus aureus (VRSA)*, methicillin-resistant *S. aureus (MRSA)*, vancomycin-resistant *Enterococcus (VRE)*, and penicillin-resistant *Streptococcus pneumoniae (PRSP)*.[1] Even though a resistant organism may be linked to a specific drug by name,

Text continued on page 517

Table 33–5	TREATMENT OF COMMON BACTERIAL INFECTIONS*		
Bacillus	**Common Disease(s)**	**Primary Agent(s)**	**Alternative Agent(s)**
Gram-positive bacilli			
Bacillus anthracis	Anthrax; pneumonia	Ciprofloxacin or doxycycline plus a penicillin ± another (alternative) agent	Clarithromycin; clindamycin; chloramphenicol; imipenem; rifampin; vancomycin
Clostridium difficile	Antibiotic-associated colitis	Metronidazole	Vancomycin
Clostridium perfringens	Gas gangrene	Penicillin G ± clindamycin	Cefazolin; clindamycin; doxycycline; metronidazole; imipenem
Clostridium tetani	Tetanus	Penicillin G; vancomycin	Clindamycin; doxycycline
Gram-negative bacilli			
Acinetobacter	Infections in various tissues; hospital-acquired infections	An aminoglycoside + ticarcillin	Imipenem or meropenem; ciprofloxacin; trimethoprim-sulfamethoxazole; ampicillin/sulbactam
Enterobacter species	Urinary tract and other infections	Aztreonam, imipenem, meropenem, or cefepime + an aminoglycoside	Ciprofloxacin; trimethoprim-sulfamethoxazole; 3rd generation cephalosporin
Escherichia coli	Meningitis	3rd-generation cephalosporin or meropenem	–
Escherichia coli	Bacteremia; urinary tract infections; other systemic infections	3rd-generation cephalosporin, ampicillin, amoxicillin/clavulanate, trimethoprim/sulfamethoxazole, or cephalexin	An aminoglycoside; ampicillin/sulbactam; imipenem; meropenem; a fluoroquinolone; 1st- or 2nd-generation cephalosporin
Haemophilus influenzae	Meningitis	Ceftriaxone or cefotaxime	Chloramphenicol; meropenem
Haemophilus influenzae	Otitis media; pneumonia; sinusitis	Amoxicillin, ampicillin, or amoxicillin-clavulanate	Azithromycin; clarithromycin; cefuroxime; ciprofloxacin; erythromycin; trimethoprim-sulfamethoxazole
Klebsiella pneumoniae	Pneumonia; urinary tract infection	3rd-generation cephalosporin ± an aminoglycoside	Cefuroxime; ciprofloxacin; ofloxacin; ampicillin/sulbactam; amoxicillin/clavulanate; imipenem; meropenem; trimethoprim-sulfamethoxazole

(Continued on following page)

Table 33-5 **TREATMENT OF COMMON BACTERIAL INFECTIONS*** *(Continued)*

Bacillus	Common Disease(s)	Primary Agent(s)	Alternative Agent(s)
Legionella pneumophila	Legionnaires' disease	Erythromycin ± rifampin or a fluoroquinolone	Azithromycin or clarithromycin; doxycycline; trimethoprim-sulfamethoxazole
Pasteurella multocida	Abscesses; bacteremia; meningitis; wound infections (animal bites)	Penicillin G	A cephalosporin; doxycycline; amoxicillin/clavulanate; trimethoprim-sulfamethoxazole
Proteus mirabilis	Urinary tract and other infections	Ampicillin or amoxicillin	An aminoglycoside; a cephalosporin; a fluoroquinolone
Pseudomonas aeruginosa	Bacteremia; pneumonia	Ceftazidime or piperacillin + an aminoglycoside	Aztreonam; cefepime; ciprofloxacin; imipenem; meropenem
Pseudomonas aeruginosa	Urinary tract infection	An aminoglycoside	Ciprofloxacin or ofloxacin
Salmonella typhi	Bacteremia; paratyphoid fever; typhoid fever	Ceftriaxone, ciprofloxacin, or cefotaxime	Trimethoprim-sulfamethoxazole
Serratia marcescens	Various opportunistic and hospital-acquired infections	3rd-generation cephalosporin ± gentamicin	Aztreonam; ciprofloxacin; imipenem; meropenem; trimethoprim-sulfamethoxazole
Gram-positive cocci			
Enterococcus faecalis	Endocarditis or other serious infection (bacteremia)	Ampicillin or penicillin G + gentamicin or streptomycin	Vancomycin + gentamicin or streptomycin
Enterococcus faecalis	Urinary tract infection	Ampicillin or amoxicillin	Ciprofloxacin; doxycycline; levofloxacin; fosfomycin
Staphylococcus aureus	Abscesses; bacteremia; cellulitis; endocarditis; osteomyelitis; pneumonia; others	If methicillin-sensitive: nafcillin or oxacillin. If methicillin-resistant: vancomycin ± gentamicin or rifampin	1st-generation cephalosporin; clindamycin; erythromycin; trimethoprim-sulfamethoxazole; a penicillin + a penicillinase inhibitor
Streptococcus pneumoniae	Arthritis; otitis; pneumonia; sinusitis	If penicillin sensitive: ampicillin or penicillin G or V. If penicillin resistant: vancomycin ± rifampin	A cephalosporin; erythromycin; azithromycin; clarithromycin; imipenem; meropenem; a fluoroquinolone; trimethoprim-sulfamethoxazole

Bacillus	Common Disease(s)	Primary Agent(s)	Alternative Agent(s)
Streptococcus (viridians group)	Bacteremia; endocarditis	Penicillin G ± gentamicin	1st-generation cephalosporin; erythromycin; azithromycin; clarithromycin; vancomycin ± gentamicin
Gram-negative cocci			
Moraxella catarrhalis	Otitis; pneumonia; sinusitis	Amoxicillin + clavulanate; ampicillin + sulbactam	A cephalosporin; azithromycin; clarithromycin; doxycycline; erythromycin; trimethoprim-sulfamethoxazole
Neisseria gonorrhoeae (gonococcus)	Arthritis-dermatitis syndrome; genital infections	Ceftriaxone, cefixime, cefotaxime, or cefpodoxime.	Ciprofloxacin or ofloxacin
Neisseria meningitidis (meningococcus)	Meningitis	Penicillin G	3rd-generation cephalosporin
Spirochetes			
Borrelia burgdorferi	Lyme disease	Amoxicillin; doxycycline; ceftriaxone; cefuroxime	Azithromycin; cefotaxime; clarithromycin; penicillin (high dose)
Treponema pallidum	Syphilis	Penicillin G, ceftriaxone	Doxycycline
Other Microorganisms			
Chlamydia pneumoniae	Pneumonia	Doxycycline	Azithromycin; clarithromycin; erythromycin; a fluoroquinolone
Chlamydia trachomatis	Blennorrhea; lymphogranuloma venereum; nonspecific urethritis; trachoma	Doxycycline or azithromycin	Levofloxacin or ofloxacin
Mycoplasma pneumoniae	"Atypical" pneumonia	Azithromycin, clarithromycin, or erythromycin	Doxycycline or a fluoroquinolone

*Selection of primary or alternative agents varies depending on the identification of specific bacterial strains and the presence or absence of resistance to each drug. Drug selection will also be influenced by other factors such as the patient's age, comorbidities, drug allergies, pregnancy, and its possible interactions with other medications.

the organism is typically resistant to other drugs as well (multidrug resistance).[1,51]

Development of resistant bacteria is understandably a very serious problem in contemporary drug therapy.[1] In addition, the number of resistant bacterial strains continues to progressively increase in certain institutions and in the community.[29,90] To limit the development of resistant strains, antibacterial drugs should be used judiciously and not overused.[62] For instance, it is often worthwhile to perform culture and sensitivity tests on sputum, blood, and other body fluids so that the pathogenic bacteria can be identified, leading to the use of more selective agents. Administering selective agents as opposed to broad-spectrum antibiotics may help attenuate and kill resistant strains more effectively, thus limiting the spread of bacterial resistance.[40,42] The selective use of current antibacterial drugs and the development of new bactericidal agents are needed to help control the problem of bacterial resistance.[63]

SUMMARY

Antibacterial drugs are used to prevent and treat infection in a variety of clinical situations. Some drugs are effective against a limited number of bacteria (narrow-spectrum), whereas other agents may be used against a relatively wide variety of bacterial pathogens (broad-spectrum). Specific agents may exert their antibacterial effects by preventing bacterial cell wall synthesis and function, or by inhibiting either bacterial protein syn-

Special Concerns in Rehabilitation Patients

■ ■ ■   Patients undergoing physical therapy and occupational therapy will be taking antibacterial drugs for any number of reasons. Antibacterial drugs may be administered to prevent or treat infection in conditions relating directly to the rehabilitation program. For instance, therapists are often involved in administering topical antibacterial agents (e.g., sulfadiazine) to patients with burns. Infection in other conditions related to rehabilitation, such as bone infections (osteomyelitis), infections sustained from trauma and various wounds, and infections following joint replacement and other types of surgery, will also require antibacterial therapy. Other types of infection that are not directly related to rehabilitation (e.g., urinary tract infection, pneumonia) are also very common, occurring frequently in hospitalized patients as well as those receiving outpatient physical therapy and occupational therapy. Consequently, therapists will be working routinely with patients who are receiving antibacterial treatment.

Therapists should generally be aware of the possible adverse effects of antibacterial drugs. Many of these agents have the potential to cause hypersensitivity reactions including skin rashes, itching, and respiratory difficulty (such as wheezing). Therapists may recognize the onset of such reactions when working with these patients. Other common side effects, including gastrointestinal problems (nausea, vomiting, diarrhea), are usually not serious but may be bothersome if they continually interrupt therapy. Therapists may have to alter the time of the rehabilitation session to work around these effects, especially if gastrointestinal and similar side effects tend to occur at a specific time of the day (e.g., early morning, late afternoon).

Certain agents may have adverse effects that directly interact with specific rehabilitation treatments. In particular, tetracyclines, sulfonamides, and fluoroquinolones (ciprofloxacin, norfloxacin, etc.) cause increased skin sensitivity to ultraviolet light. This problem is obvious if the therapist is administering ultraviolet treatments. Therapists must be especially careful to establish an accurate minimal erythemal dosage to ultraviolet light. Therapists should also be prepared to adjust the ultraviolet light treatments in accordance with changes in the dosage of the antibacterial drug.

Finally, therapists play a vital role in preventing the spread of bacterial and other infections. Therapists must maintain appropriate sterile technique when dealing with open wounds. Adequate sterilization of whirlpools with strong disinfectants is also critical in preventing the spread of infection from patient to patient in a rehabilitation setting. Therapists must also recognize the importance of hand washing in preventing the spread of infection and must not neglect to wash their own hands between patients.

CASE STUDY

Antibacterial Drugs

Brief History. J.B. is a 40-year-old former truck driver who was injured in a traffic accident 5 years ago, sustaining a spinal cord transection that resulted in complete paraplegia at the L1–2 level. He underwent extensive physical rehabilitation, including vocational retraining, and had recently been working as a computer programmer when he began to develop a pressure area in the region of the right ischial tuberosity. Despite conservative management, a pressure ulcer developed. Because the patient was in relatively good health otherwise, the ulcer was treated with local debridement and reconstructive surgery, using skin flaps. The patient was admitted to the hospital, and a routine preoperative culture of the ulcer revealed the presence of *E. coli*. The patient had a history of sensitivity to penicillin drugs and was therefore given a tetracycline antibiotic (Achromycin V, 250 mg orally every 6 hours) to resolve the infection prior to surgery. Physical therapy and

occupational therapy were also requested to help maintain the patient's upper body strength and functional activity while awaiting surgery. The physical therapist also suggested that ultraviolet radiation might be helpful in resolving the infection.

Problem/Influence of Medication. Tetracyclines and several other antibacterial agents increase the sensitivity of the skin to ultraviolet light.

Decision/Solution. The therapist carefully determined the minimal erythemal dosage for the patient prior to initiating ultraviolet treatments. In addition to using careful draping techniques, the therapist confined the treatment to the ulcer site, so that a minimum of the surrounding skin was exposed to the ultraviolet light. This approach ensured that the surrounding tissues would not be endangered if the patient's response to the ultraviolet treatment changed during the course of tetracycline treatment. The combination of drug therapy and ultraviolet radiation quickly resolved the infection, allowing the surgery to proceed as planned.

---

thesis or bacterial DNA/RNA synthesis and function. Although most bacterial infections can be effectively treated with one or more agents, the development of bacterial strains that are resistant to drug therapy continues to be a serious problem. Rehabilitation specialists will routinely treat patients receiving antibacterial

drugs for conditions that are directly or indirectly related to the need for physical therapy and occupational therapy. Therapists should be cognizant of the potential side effects of these drugs and should know how these drugs may interfere with specific physical therapy and occupational therapy procedures.

References

1. Alanis AJ. Resistance to antibiotics: are we in the postantibiotic era? *Arch Med Res.* 2005;36:697–705.
2. Albini A, Monti S. Photophysics and photochemistry of fluoroquinolones. *Chem Soc Rev.* 2003;32:238–250.
3. Anokhina MM, Barta A, Nierhaus KH, et al. Mapping of the second tetracycline binding site on the ribosomal small subunit of *E.coli. Nucleic Acids Res.* 2004;32:2594–2597.
4. Asbel LE, Levison ME. Cephalosporins, carbapenems, and monobactams. *Infect Dis Clin North Am.* 2000;14:435–447.
5. Auerbach T, Bashan A, Yonath A. Ribosomal antibiotics: structural basis for resistance, synergism and selectivity. *Trends Biotechnol.* 2004;22:570–576.
6. Barrett JF. Recent developments in glycopeptide antibacterials. *Curr Opin Investig Drugs.* 2005;6:781–790.
7. Bebear CM, Pereyre S. Mechanisms of drug resistance in *Mycoplasma pneumoniae. Curr Drug Targets Infect Disord.* 2005;5:263–271.
8. Bell SC, Senini SL, McCormack JG. Macrolides in cystic fibrosis. *Chron Respir Dis.* 2005;2:85–98.
9. Bhavnani SM, Andes DR. Gemifloxacin for the treatment of respiratory tract infections: in vitro susceptibility, pharmacokinetics and pharmacodynamics, clinical efficacy, and safety. *Pharmacotherapy.* 2005;25:717–740.
10. Bonfiglio G, Russo G, Nicoletti G. Recent developments in carbapenems. *Expert Opin Investig Drugs.* 2002;11:529–544.
11. Brink AJ, Feldman C, Grolman DC, et al. Appropriate use of the carbapenems. *S Afr Med J.* 2004;94:857–861.
12. Brodersen DE, Clemons WM, Jr, Carter AP, et al. The structural basis for the action of the antibiotics tetracycline, pactamycin, and hygromycin B on the 30S ribosomal subunit. *Cell.* 2000;103:1143–1154.
13. Buynak JD. The discovery and development of modified penicillin- and cephalosporin-derived beta-lactamase inhibitors. *Curr Med Chem.* 2004;11:1951–1964.
14. Buynak JD. Understanding the longevity of the beta-lactam antibiotics and of antibiotic/beta-lactamase

inhibitor combinations. *Biochem Pharmacol.* 2006;71: 930–940.

15. Chambers HF. Aminoglycosides. In: Brunton LL, et al, eds. *The Pharmacological Basis of Therapeutics.* 11th ed. New York: McGraw-Hill; 2006.

16. Chambers HF. Protein synthesis inhibitors and miscellaneous antibacterial agents. In: Brunton LL, et al, eds. *The Pharmacological Basis of Therapeutics.* 11th ed. New York: McGraw-Hill; 2006.

17. Chan DC, Anderson AC. Towards species-specific antifolates. *Curr Med Chem.* 2006;13:377–398.

18. Chen FJ, Lo HJ. Molecular mechanisms of fluoroquinolone resistance. *J Microbiol Immunol Infect.* 2003;36:1–9.

19. Costagliola M, Agrosi M. Second-degree burns: a comparative, multicenter, randomized trial of hyaluronic acid plus silver sulfadiazine vs. silver sulfadiazine alone. *Curr Med Res Opin.* 2005;21: 1235–1240.

20. Croom KF, Goa KL. Levofloxacin: a review of its use in the treatment of bacterial infections in the United States. *Drugs.* 2003;63:2769–2802.

21. Da Silva AD, De Almeida MV, De Souza MV, Couri MR. Biological activity and synthetic metodologies for the preparation of fluoroquinolones, a class of potent antibacterial agents. *Curr Med Chem.* 2003;10:21–39.

22. De Rossi E, Ainsa JA, Riccardi G. Role of mycobacterial efflux transporters in drug resistance: an unresolved question. *FEMS Microbiol Rev.* 2006;30:36–52.

23. Edwards SJ, Emmas CE, Campbell HE. Systematic review comparing meropenem with imipenem plus cilastatin in the treatment of severe infections. *Curr Med Res Opin.* 2005;21:785–794.

24. Enarson PM, Enarson DA, Gie R. Management of tuberculosis in children in low-income countries. *Int J Tuberc Lung Dis.* 2005;9:1299–1304.

25. Frampton JE, Curran MP. Tigecycline. *Drugs.* 2005; 65:2623–2637.

26. Georgopapadakou NH. Beta-lactamase inhibitors: evolving compounds for evolving resistance targets. *Expert Opin Investig Drugs.* 2004;13:1307–1318.

27. Goldman RC, Scaglione F. The macrolide-bacterium interaction and its biological basis. *Curr Drug Targets Infect Disord.* 2004;4:241–260.

28. Gootz TD. The forgotten Gram-negative bacilli: what genetic determinants are telling us about the spread of antibiotic resistance. *Biochem Pharmacol.* 2006;71: 1073–1084.

29. Gosbell IB. Epidemiology, clinical features and management of infections due to community methicillin-resistant Staphylococcus aureus (cMRSA). *Intern Med J.* 2005;35(suppl 2):S120–S35.

30. Guignard B, Entenza JM, Moreillon P. Beta-lactams against methicillin-resistant *Staphylococcus aureus. Curr Opin Pharmacol.* 2005;5:479–489.

31. Gump WC, Walsh JW. Intrathecal colistin for treatment of highly resistant Pseudomonas ventriculitis. Case report and review of the literature. *J Neurosurg.* 2005;102:915–917.

32. Harrington SM, Dudley EG, Nataro JP. Pathogenesis of enteroaggregative *Escherichia coli* infection. *FEMS Microbiol Lett.* 2006;254:12–18.

33. Hawser S, Lociuro S, Islam K. Dihydrofolate reductase inhibitors as antibacterial agents. *Biochem Pharmacol.* 2006;71:941–948.

34. Hermann T. Drugs targeting the ribosome. *Curr Opin Struct Biol.* 2005;15:355–366.

35. Hopkins KL, Davies RH, Threlfall EJ. Mechanisms of quinolone resistance in *Escherichia coli* and *Salmonella:* recent developments. *Int J Antimicrob Agents.* 2005; 25:358–373.

36. Jones CH, Petersen PJ. Tigecycline: a review of pre-clinical and clinical studies of the first-in-class glycylcycline antibiotic. *Drugs Today.* 2005;41:637–659.

37. Khaliq Y, Zhanel GG. Fluoroquinolone-associated tendinopathy: a critical review of the literature. *Clin Infect Dis.* 2003;36:1404–1410.

38. Khaliq Y, Zhanel GG. Musculoskeletal injury associated with fluoroquinolone antibiotics. *Clin Plast Surg.* 2005;32:495–502.

39. Kirsebom LA, Virtanen A, Mikkelsen NE. Aminoglycoside interactions with RNAs and nucleases. *Handb Exp Pharmacol.* 2006;173:73–96.

40. Kollef MH, Micek ST. Strategies to prevent antimicrobial resistance in the intensive care unit. *Crit Care Med.* 2005;33:1845–1853.

41. Li L, Xu B. Multivalent vancomycins and related antibiotics against infectious diseases. *Curr Pharm Des.* 2005;11:3111–3124.

42. Livermore DM. Minimising antibiotic resistance. *Lancet Infect Dis.* 2005;5:450–459.

43. Lomaestro BM. Fluoroquinolone-induced renal failure. *Drug Saf.* 2000;22:479–485.

44. Lynch AS. Efflux systems in bacterial pathogens: an opportunity for therapeutic intervention? An industry view. *Biochem Pharmacol.* 2006;71:949–956.

45. McAdam AJ, Sharpe AH. Infectious diseases. In: Kumar V, Abbas AK, Fausto N, eds. *Pathologic Basis of Disease.* 7th ed. New York: Elsevier Saunders; 2005.

46. McConnell SA, Amsden GW. Review and comparison of advanced-generation macrolides clarithromycin and dirithromycin. *Pharmacotherapy.* 1999;19:404–415.

47. McPherson DC, Popham DL. Peptidoglycan synthesis in the absence of class A penicillin-binding proteins in *Bacillus subtilis. J Bacteriol.* 2003;185:1423–1431.

48. Melhus A. Fluoroquinolones and tendon disorders. *Expert Opin Drug Saf.* 2005;4:299–309.

49. Nagai J, Takano M. Molecular aspects of renal handling of aminoglycosides and strategies for preventing the nephrotoxicity. *Drug Metab Pharmacokinet.* 2004; 19:159–170.

50. Neidhardt FC. Bacterial structures. In: Ryan KJ, Ray CG, eds. *Sherris Medical Microbiology.* 4th ed New York: McGraw-Hill; 2004.

51. Obritsch MD, Fish DN, MacLaren R, Jung R. Nosocomial infections due to multidrug-resistant *Pseudomonas aeruginosa:* epidemiology and treatment options. *Pharmacotherapy.* 2005;25:1353–1364.

52. Palmieri TL, Greenhalgh DG. Topical treatment of pediatric patients with burns: a practical guide. *Am J Clin Dermatol.* 2002;3:529–534.

53. Pasquale TR, Tan JS. Update on antimicrobial agents: new indications of older agents. *Expert Opin Pharmacother.* 2005;6:1681–1691.

54. Paterson DL, Bonomo RA. Extended-spectrum beta-lactamases: a clinical update. *Clin Microbiol Rev.* 2005;18:657–686.

55. Perazella MA. Trimethoprim-induced hyperkalemia: Clinical data, mechanism, prevention and management. *Drug Saf.* 2000;22:227–236.

56. Petri WA. Penicillins, cephalosporins, and other beta-lactam antibiotics. In: Brunton LL, et al, eds. *The Pharmacological Basis of Therapeutics.* 11th ed. New York: McGraw-Hill; 2006.

57. Petri WA. Sulfonamides, trimethoprim-sulfamethoxazole, quinolones, and agents for urinary tract infections. In: Brunton LL, et al, eds. *The Pharmacological Basis of Therapeutics.* 11th ed. New York: McGraw-Hill; 2006.

58. Poehlsgaard J, Douthwaite S. Macrolide antibiotic interaction and resistance on the bacterial ribosome. *Curr Opin Investig Drugs.* 2003;4:140–148.

59. Poehlsgaard J, Douthwaite S. The bacterial ribosome as a target for antibiotics. *Nat Rev Microbiol.* 2005;3:870–881.

60. Poole K. Efflux-mediated antimicrobial resistance. *J Antimicrob Chemother.* 2005;56:20–51.

61. Potter B, Rindfleisch K, Kraus CK. Management of active tuberculosis. *Am Fam Physician.* 2005;72:2225–2232.

62. Ramphal R. Importance of adequate initial antimicrobial therapy. *Chemotherapy.* 2005;51:171–176.

63. Rice LB. Unmet medical needs in antibacterial therapy. *Biochem Pharmacol.* 2006;71:991–995.

64. Richter S, Parolin C, Palumbo M, Palu G. Antiviral properties of quinolone-based drugs. *Curr Drug Targets Infect Disord.* 2004;4:111–116.

65. Rodriguez-Pena R, Antunez C, Martin E, et al. Allergic reactions to beta-lactams. *Expert Opin Drug Saf.* 2006;5:31–48.

66. Rougier F, Claude D, Maurin M, Maire P. Aminoglycoside nephrotoxicity. *Curr Drug Targets Infect Disord.* 2004;4:153–162.

67. Rybak LP, Whitworth CA. Ototoxicity: therapeutic opportunities. *Drug Discov Today.* 2005;10:1313–1321.

68. Sader HS, Gales AC. Emerging strategies in infectious diseases: new carbapenem and trinem antibacterial agents. *Drugs.* 2001;61:553–564.

69. Sanchez AR, Rogers RS, 3rd, Sheridan PJ. Tetracycline and other tetracycline-derivative staining of the teeth and oral cavity. *Int J Dermatol.* 2004;43:709–715.

70. Sandanayaka VP, Prashad AS. Resistance to beta-lactam antibiotics: structure and mechanism based design of beta-lactamase inhibitors. *Curr Med Chem.* 2002;9:1145–1165.

71. Sapadin AN, Fleischmajer R. Tetracyclines: nonantibiotic properties and their clinical implications. *J Am Acad Dermatol.* 2006;54:258–265.

72. Schaeffer AJ. The expanding role of fluoroquinolones. *Dis Mon.* 2003;49:129–147.

73. Schaeffer EM. Prophylactic use of antimicrobials in commonly performed outpatient urologic procedures. *Nat Clin Pract Urol.* 2006;3:24–31.

74. Scheffers DJ, Pinho MG. Bacterial cell wall synthesis: new insights from localization studies. *Microbiol Mol Biol Rev.* 2005;69:585–607.

75. Schultz MJ. Macrolide activities beyond their antimicrobial effects: macrolides in diffuse panbronchiolitis and cystic fibrosis. *J Antimicrob Chemother.* 2004;54:21–28.

76. Sheldon AT, Jr. Antibiotic resistance: a survival strategy. *Clin Lab Sci.* 2005;18:170–180.

77. Shi J, Montay G, Bhargava VO. Clinical pharmacokinetics of telithromycin, the first ketolide antibacterial. *Clin Pharmacokinet.* 2005;44:915–934.

78. Stewart GC. Taking shape: control of bacterial cell wall biosynthesis. *Mol Microbiol.* 2005;57:1177–1181.

79. Sutcliffe JA. Improving on nature: antibiotics that target the ribosome. *Curr Opin Microbiol.* 2005;8:534–542.

80. Tamaoki J, Kadota J, Takizawa H. Clinical implications of the immunomodulatory effects of macrolides. *Am J Med.* 2004;117(suppl 9A):5S–11S.

81. Tellado JM, Wilson SE. Empiric treatment of nosocomial intra-abdominal infections: a focus on the carbapenems. *Surg Infect.* 2005;6:329–343.

82. Then RL. Antimicrobial dihydrofolate reductase inhibitors—achievements and future options: review. *J Chemother.* 2004;16:3–12.

83. Turton JA, Andrews CM, Havard AC, Williams TC. Studies on the haemotoxicity of chloramphenicol succinate in the Dunkin Hartley guinea pig. *Int J Exp Pathol.* 2002;83:225–238.

84. van der Linden PD, Sturkenboom MC, Herings RM, et al. Fluoroquinolones and risk of Achilles tendon disorders: case-control study. *BMJ.* 2002;324:1306–1307.

85. van der Linden PD, van de Lei J, Nab HW, et al. Achilles tendinitis associated with fluoroquinolones. *Br J Clin Pharmacol.* 1999;48:433–437.

86. Wilke MS, Lovering AL, Strynadka NC. Beta-lactam antibiotic resistance: a current structural perspective. *Curr Opin Microbiol.* 2005;8:525–533.

87. Yonath A. Antibiotics targeting ribosomes: resistance, selectivity, synergism and cellular regulation. *Annu Rev Biochem.* 2005;74:649–679.

88. Young KD. Bacterial shape. *Mol Microbiol.* 2003;49:571–580.

89. Zhanel GG, Karlowsky JA, Rubinstein E, Hoban DJ. Tigecycline: a novel glycylcycline antibiotic. *Expert Rev Anti Infect Ther.* 2006;4:9–25.

90. Zirakzadeh A, Patel R. Epidemiology and mechanisms of glycopeptide resistance in enterococci. *Curr Opin Infect Dis.* 2005;18:507–512.

Treatment of Infections II: Antiviral Drugs

A virus is one of the smallest microorganisms, consisting of only a nucleic acid core that is surrounded by a protein shell.[18] Several types of viruses commonly infect human cells and are responsible for a diverse range of pathologies. Viral infections extend from relatively mild disorders such as the common cold to serious, life-threatening conditions such as acquired immunodeficiency syndrome (AIDS). Viruses are somewhat unique in that they must rely totally on the metabolic processes of the host (human) cell to function.[62] Hence, the pharmacologic treatment of viral infections is complex, because it is often difficult to selectively destroy the virus without also destroying human cells.

This chapter describes the basic characteristics of viruses and the relatively limited number of drugs that can act selectively as antiviral agents. Methods of preventing viral infections (antiviral vaccines) are also briefly discussed. Finally, the current methods of treating a specific viral-induced disease—AIDS—are presented. Rehabilitation specialists often treat patients who are in the active stages of a viral infection, as well as those suffering from the sequelae of viral disorders, such as gastroenteritis, encephalitis, and influenza. Hence, the pharmacotherapeutic treatment and prophylaxis of viral infections should concern physical therapists and occupational therapists.

Viral Structure and Function

Classification of Viruses

Viruses are classified according to several criteria, including physical, biochemical, and pathogenic characteristics.[18,62] The classifications of some of the more

common viruses affecting humans, and their associated diseases, are listed in Table 34–1. The table shows that viruses can be divided into two categories, depending on the type of genetic material contained in the virus (DNA or RNA viruses). Families within each major subdivision are classified according to physical characteristics (configuration of the genetic material, shape of the virus capsule) and other functional criteria.

Characteristics of Viruses

Viruses are somewhat unique in structure and function as compared with other microorganisms. The basic components of viral microorganisms are illustrated in Figure 34–1. A virus essentially consists of a core of viral DNA or RNA.[18,62] The genetic core is surrounded by a protein shell, or *capsid*. This structure—the capsid enclosing the nucleic acid core—is referred to as the *nucleocapsid*. In some viruses, the nucleocapsid is also surrounded by a viral membrane, or envelope, which is composed of glycoproteins extending outward from a lipid bilayer.

The virus, however, does not contain any of the cellular components necessary to replicate itself or synthesize proteins and other macromolecules; that is, the virus lacks ribosomes, endoplasmic reticulum, and so on.[18] The virus contains only the genetic code (viral genome) that will produce additional viruses. To replicate itself, the virus must rely on the biochemical machinery of the host cell.[95] In essence, the virus invades the host cell, takes control of the cell's metabolic function, and uses the host cell's macromolecular-synthesizing apparatus to crank out new viruses. Specific steps in the viral replication process are described in the next section.

Table 34-1	COMMON VIRUSES AFFECTING HUMANS	
DNA viruses		
Adenoviridae	Adenovirus, types 1–33	Respiratory tract and eye infections
Hepatitis B	Hepatitis B virus	Hepatitis B
Herpesviridae	Cytomegalovirus	Cytomegalic inclusion disease (i.e., widespread involvement of virtually any organ, especially the brain, liver, lung, kidney, intestine)
	Epstein-Barr virus	Infectious mononucleosis
	Herpes simplex, types 1 and 2	Local infections of oral, genital, and other mucocutaneous areas; systemic infections
	Varicella-zoster virus	Chickenpox; herpes zoster (shingles); other systemic infections
Poxviridae	Smallpox virus	Smallpox
RNA viruses		
Coronaviradae	Coronavirus	Upper respiratory tract infection
Flaviviridae	Hepatitis C virus	Hepatitis C
Orthomyxoviridae	Influenza virus, types A and B	Influenza
Paramyxoviridae	Measles virus	Measles virus
	Mumps virus	Mumps
	Respiratory syncytial virus	Respiratory tract infection in children
Picornaviridae	Hepatitis A virus	Hepatitis A
	Polioviruses	Poliomyelitis
	Rhinovirus, types 1–89	Common cold
Retroviridae	Human immunodeficiency virus (HIV)	AIDS
Rhabdoviridae	Rabies virus	Rabies
Togaviridae	Alphavirus	Encephalitis
	Rubella virus	Rubella

Viral Replication

Self-replication of a virus occurs in several distinct steps:[17,80] (1) adsorption, (2) penetration and uncoating, (3) biosynthesis, and (4) maturation and release. These steps are illustrated in Figure 34–2, and are briefly discussed below.

Adsorption. Initially, the virus attaches or adsorbs to the surface of the host cell. Most viruses are attracted to the host cell because of the interaction between proteins on the outer surface of the virus and receptorlike proteins on the host-cell membrane. The interaction of the virus with these surface proteins causes

the virus to adhere to the outer surface of the host-cell membrane.

Penetration and Uncoating. The virus enters the host cell either by passing directly through the cell membrane or by fusing with the host-cell membrane and releasing the viral genetic material into the host cell. Once inside the host cell, its proteolytic enzymes usually remove any coating that remains on the virus.

Biosynthesis. When viral genetic material is released within the host cell, the virus takes control of the cell's molecular synthesizing machinery to initiate the biosynthesis of new viral enzymes and proteins. Different viruses exert their effects on the host cell in

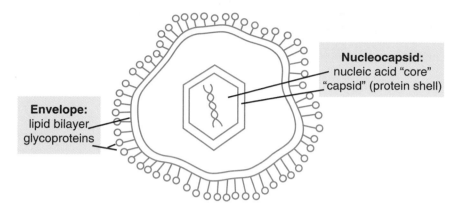

FIGURE 34–1 ▼ Basic components of a virus. Note the relative lack of most cellular organelles (ribosomes, endoplasmic reticulum, etc.).

different ways, but many viruses control the host cell through a direct effect on the cell's nucleus. Some viruses, including the virus that causes AIDS, actually insert their genetic material directly into the host cell's DNA, thereby becoming integrated within the genetic control of the infected cell.

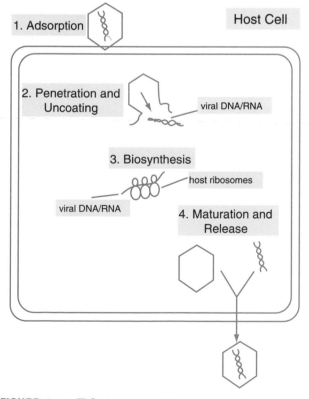

FIGURE 34–2 ▼ Basic sequence of viral replication. See text for details.

Regardless of the exact mechanism of infection, the virus essentially commands the cell to synthesize the enzymes that produce more copies of viral DNA or RNA and to synthesize structural proteins that will ultimately be used to form new viral shells or capsids. Thus, the virus uses the biosynthetic machinery as well as the structural components and nutrients of the cell (amino acids, nucleic acids, etc.) to replicate itself. Likewise, the virus often incapacitates the infected cell so that the infected cell cannot carry out its normal physiologic activities.

Maturation and Release. The component parts of the virus (the genetic core and surrounding shell) are assembled into mature viruses and released from the host cell. In some cases, the virus is released by a process of exocytosis, leaving the host cell relatively intact (although still infected with the original virus). Alternatively, the host cell may simply be destroyed (undergo lysis), thus releasing the viral offspring. Lysis of the host cell not only results in the release of the virus and the death of the cell, but also may stimulate the production of inflammatory mediators (prostaglandins, kinins, etc.), which create a hypersensitivity response.

The steps involved in viral replication are important pharmacologically because antiviral drugs may interrupt this process at one or more of the steps. Specific agents currently used as antiviral drugs and their pharmacodynamic aspects are discussed next.

Specific Antiviral Drugs

The primary agents that are approved for use as antiviral drugs are listed in Tables 34–2 and 34–3. Each agent is also briefly discussed below.

Table 34-2	ANTIVIRAL DRUGS	
Generic Name	**Trade Name(s)**	**Principal Indication(s)**
Acyclovir	Zovirax	Treatment of initial and recurrent herpesvirus infections (especially herpes simplex–related infections)
Amantadine	Symadine, Symmetrel	Prevention and treatment of influenza A infections (also used as an antiparkinsonism drug; see Chapter 10)
Cidofovir	Vistide	Treatment of cytomegalovirus (CMV) retinitis in immunocompromised patients
Docosanol	Abreva	Topical treatment of recurrent herpes simplex infections (cold sores)
Famciclovir	Famvir	Treatment and suppression of herpesvirus infections, including herpes simplex (genital herpes) and herpes zoster (shingles)
Fomivirsen	Vitravene	Injected into the eye to treat CMV retinitis
Foscarnet	Foscavir	Treatment of CMV infections in immunocompromised patients
Ganciclovir	Cytovene	Treatment of CMV retinitis in immunocompromised patients; also used to prevent CMV infection after organ transplants
Imiquimod	Aldara	Topical treatment for warts caused by condylomata acuminate
Oseltamivir	Tamiflu	Prevention and treatment of influenza A and B infections
Penciclovir	Denavir	Topical treatment of recurrent herpes simplex infections (cold sores)
Ribavirin	Virazole	Treatment of severe viral pneumonia caused by respiratory syncytial virus in infants and young children
Rimantadine	Flumadine	Prevention and treatment of influenza A infections
Trifluridine	Viroptic	Local (ophthalmic) administration for treatment of herpes simplex keratitis and keratoconjunctivitis
Valacyclovir	Valtrex	Treatment of initial and recurrent herpesvirus infections, including herpes simplex (genital herpes) and herpes zoster (shingles)
Valganciclovir	Valcyte	Treatment of cytomegalovirus (CMV) retinitis in immunocompromised patients; also used to prevent CMV infection after organ transplants
Vidarabine	Vira-A	Local (ophthalmic) administration for treatment of herpes simplex keratoconjunctivitis
Zanamivir	Relenza	Prevention and treatment of influenza A and B infections

Acyclovir and Valacyclovir

Antiviral Efficacy and Clinical Use. Acyclovir (Zovirax) is effective against herpesvirus infections, especially those involving herpes simplex types I and II.[24,97] Acyclovir is the principal drug used to treat genital herpes and herpes simplex–related infections in other mucosal and cutaneous areas (lips and face).[42] Acyclovir is also effective against other members of the herpesvirus family, including the varicella-zoster and Epstein-Barr virus.[24,89] This agent may be used to treat varicella-zoster–related infections such as herpes zoster and chickenpox. Epstein-Barr virus infections, including infectious mononucleosis, may also respond to acyclovir. This drug can also help decrease the risk of cytomegalovirus (CMV) infection in people receiving kidney transplants and transplants of other solid organs.[44,82]

Acyclovir can be applied topically as a cream to treat cutaneous and mucosal infections. This drug can also be administered systemically, either orally or intravenously in severe, acute infections.

Valacyclovir (Valtrex) is the precursor or "prodrug" of acyclovir.[89] When administered orally, valacyclovir is converted to acyclovir in the intestinal tract and liver. This conversion typically results in the eventual appearance of higher levels of acyclovir in the bloodstream, because valacyclovir is absorbed more readily from the gastrointestinal tract than acyclovir.[42] Thus, administration of valacyclovir is a more effective way to achieve the therapeutic effects of acyclovir when these drugs are orally administered.[42]

Mechanism of Action. Acyclovir inhibits viral DNA replication by inhibiting the function of the DNA polymerase enzyme.[42] This drug is taken into virus-infected cells and converted to acyclovir triphosphate by an enzyme known as viral thymidine kinase.[42] The phosphorylated drug directly inhibits the function of the viral DNA polymerase, thus impairing the replication of viral genetic material. The virus also incorporates the drug into viral DNA strands, which halts further production of DNA because of the presence of a false nucleic acid.[42]

The antiviral specificity of acyclovir is due to the drug's higher affinity for viral DNA polymerase rather than the analogous enzyme in human cells.[42] Also, the first step in the phosphorylation of acyclovir is greatly accelerated in virus-infected cells versus healthy cells. Hence, the amount of the activated (phosphorylated) form of acyclovir is much greater in the cells that really need it—that is, cells infected with the virus.

Adverse Effects. Topical application of acyclovir may produce local irritation of cutaneous and mucosal tissues. Prolonged systemic administration of acyclovir or valacyclovir may cause headaches, dizziness, skin rashes, and gastrointestinal problems (nausea, vomiting, diarrhea).

Amantadine and Rimantadine

Antiviral Efficacy and Clinical Use. Amantadine (Symmetrel) and rimantadine (Flumadine) are used in the prevention and treatment of infections caused by the influenza A virus.[24,28] When administered prophylactically, these drugs appear to be approximately 70 to 90 percent effective in preventing influenza A infections.[42] Also, these drugs usually decrease the severity and duration of flu symptoms in people infected with influenza A if drug therapy is initiated when symptoms first appear.[42,52] As discussed in Chapter 10, amantadine is also effective in alleviating some of the motor abnormalities of Parkinson disease. As an anti-Parkinson drug, amantadine may block the effects of excitatory neurotransmitters in the basal ganglia, thus exerting effects that are quite different from its antiviral effects (see Chapter 10).

Amantadine and rimantadine are administered to individuals already infected with influenza A to lessen the extent of the illness associated with the virus. These drugs are also given prophylactically to individuals who may have been exposed to influenza A and to high-risk patients such as the elderly or those with cardiopulmonary and other diseases. Amantadine may also be somewhat effective in treating certain cases of hepatitis C infection.[103] These drugs are typically administered orally, either in capsule form or in a syrup preparation.

Mechanism of Action. Amantadine and rimantadine appear to inhibit one of the early steps in influenza A replication by blocking the uncoating of the virus and preventing the release of viral nucleic acid within the host cell.[42] These drugs may also interfere with the assembly of viral components, thus inhibiting one of the final steps in the replication process.[42] This dual inhibitory effect on the early and late steps of viral replication accounts for these drugs' antiviral effectiveness.

Adverse Effects. These drugs may produce central nervous system (CNS) symptoms such as confusion, loss of concentration, mood changes, nervousness, dizziness, and light-headedness. These symptoms may be especially problematic in elderly patients. Excessive doses of amantadine and rimantadine may increase the severity of these CNS symptoms, and overdose may cause seizures.

Cidofovir

Antiviral Efficacy and Clinical Use. Cidofovir (Vistide) is used primarily to treat CMV retinitis in people with AIDS.[111] When used clinically, this drug is often combined with probenecid, an agent that inhibits renal excretion of cidofovir, thereby providing higher plasma levels of this antiviral agent.[112]

Mechanism of Action. Cidofovir works like acyclovir and ganciclovir; these drugs inhibit viral DNA replication by inhibiting DNA polymerase activity and by halting elongation of viral DNA chains.[42]

Adverse Effects. Cidofovir may cause nephrotoxicity, especially at higher doses. This drug may also decrease the number of neutrophilic leukocytes, resulting in neutropenia and related symptoms such as fever, chills, and sore throat. Other side effects include headache and gastrointestinal disturbances (anorexia, nausea, diarrhea).

Docosanol

Antiviral Efficacy and Clinical Use. Docosanol (Abreva) is applied topically to treat blisters and cold sores caused by herpes virus simplex.[42] This drug is available as an over-the-counter product, and is used primarily to treat recurrent outbreaks of orofacial herpes lesions.

Mechanism of Action. Docosanol does not inactivate the herpes virus, but appears to act on the host (human) cells so that the virus cannot adsorb to the surface of the cell. As such, it must be applied early in the course of outbreaks before the virus has a chance to cause substantial lesions.

Adverse Effects. Patients may experience headache and some local skin irritation during topical use of this drug.

Enfuvirtide

Antiviral Efficacy and Clinical Use. Enfuvirtide (Fuzeon) is the first approved drug that limits the ability of human immunodeficiency virus (HIV) to enter host cells.[77,86] As such, this drug is used as part of the antiviral regimen against HIV infection. Enfuvirtide is typically added to other agents (reverse transcriptase inhibitors, protease inhibitors) in patients who do not respond adequately to traditional anti-HIV treatment. This drug is effective against HIV type 1, but not against HIV type 2 (types of HIV are addressed later; see "HIV and the Treatment of AIDS").[77]

Enfuvirtide must be administered parenterally; it is associated with frequent and potentially serious side effects (see below). At the time of this writing, enfuvirtide is the only drug of its type, but other HIV entry inhibitors are currently in development, and the use of these drugs may be expanded in the future if newer, safer agents reach the market.[86]

Mechanism of Action. As indicated, enfuvirtide inhibits the ability of HIV to bind to, and enter, susceptible host cells such as CD4 lymphocytes. The drug actually binds to specific components on the outer glycoprotein envelop of the virus, thereby retarding the ability of the virus to change its shape in preparation for adsorbing to the surface of the host cell. If the virus cannot attach to host cells, the risk of infection is reduced.

Adverse Effects. Enfuvirtide must be administered by subcutaneous injection, and local pain and irritation occurs at the injection site in most patients. Other common side effects include peripheral neuropathy and immune complex reactions that can lead to serious problems including respiratory distress syndrome, kidney dysfunction, and possibly Guillain-Barré syndrome.

Famciclovir and Penciclovir

Antiviral Efficacy and Clinical Use. Penciclovir (Denavir) is similar to acyclovir in terms of its antiviral effects and clinical indications. However, penciclovir is absorbed poorly from the gastrointestinal tract. This drug is primarily administered topically to treat recurrent herpes simplex infections of the lips and face (cold sores).[58]

Famciclovir (Famvir) is the precursor (prodrug) to penciclovir; the drug is converted to penciclovir following oral administration.[91] This situation is analogous to the relationship between acyclovir and valacyclovir, where it is advantageous to administer the prodrug because it will be absorbed more completely and will ultimately result in higher plasma levels of the drug's active form. Hence, famciclovir is administered orally to treat infections related to herpes simplex (e.g., genital herpes) and varicella zoster (e.g., herpes zoster).[87,91,104] However, the actual antiviral effects of famciclovir occur because this drug is converted to penciclovir within the body.

Mechanism of Action. Penciclovir acts like acyclovir (see earlier); that is, the drug is activated (phosphorylated) within virus-infected cells, where it subsequently inhibits viral DNA synthesis and viral replication. As indicated, famciclovir exerts its antiviral effects after being converted to penciclovir in vivo.

Adverse Effects. Topical application of penciclovir may cause some skin reactions (rashes, irritation) at the application site, but the incidence of these reactions is fairly low. Systemic (oral) administration of famciclovir is generally well tolerated, with only minor side effects such as headache, dizziness, and gastrointestinal disturbances (nausea, diarrhea).

Fomivirsen

Antiviral Efficacy and Clinical Use. Fomivirsen (Vitravene) is injected into the vitreous humour to treat CMV infection in the eye.[42] This drug is often used to treat ocular CMV infections that are resistant to more traditional agents such as ganciclovir or foscarnet.

Mechanism of Action. Fomivirsen has a unique mechanism of antiviral action. This drug contains an amino acid sequence that is opposite or complimentary to the messenger RNA sequence controlling CMV replication. Because of this opposing or "antisense" sequence, fomivirsen inhibits several aspects of CMV replication, and also inhibits the viruses' ability to adsorb to the surface of host cells.

Adverse Effects. Injecting fomivirsen into the eye may cause localized pain, redness, or swelling, but serious side effects or vision disturbances are rare.

Foscarnet

Antiviral Efficacy and Clinical Use. Foscarnet (Foscavir) is primarily given to treat CMV retinitis in patients with AIDS.[6,24] This agent may also help control other infections in patients with a compromised immune system, including serious cytomegaloviral infections (pneumonia, gastrointestinal infections) and some herpesvirus infections (herpes simplex, varicella-zoster).

Mechanism of Action. Foscarnet works somewhat like acyclovir and ganciclovir; that is, foscarnet inhibits the DNA polymerase enzyme necessary for viral DNA replication. Foscarnet differs from these other antiviral drugs, however, in that it does not require phosphorylation (activation) by enzymes such as viral thymidine kinase. Certain strains of viruses are thymidine-kinase deficient, meaning that these viruses lack the enzyme needed to activate antiviral agents

such as acyclovir and ganciclovir. Hence, foscarnet is often used in patients with thymidine-kinase–resistant viruses who do not respond to acyclovir or ganciclovir.

Adverse Effects. The primary problem associated with foscarnet is impaired renal function, including acute tubular necrosis. Hematologic disorders (anemia, granulocytopenia, leukopenia), gastrointestinal disturbances (cramps, nausea, vomiting), and CNS toxicity (confusion, dizziness) may also occur during foscarnet treatment.

Ganciclovir and Valganciclovir

Antiviral Efficacy and Clinical Use. Ganciclovir (Cytovene) is given primarily to patients with AIDS to treat problems related to CMV infection, including CMV retinitis, polyradiculopathy, and other systemic CMV infections.[39,49] Valganciclovir (Valcyte) is the precursor (prodrug) form that is converted to ganciclovir within the body. Ganciclovir and similar agents (acyclovir and valacyclovir; see earlier) can also help reduce the risk of CMV infection in people receiving solid organ transplants such as kidney transplants.[44]

Mechanism of Action. Ganciclovir, like acyclovir, inhibits viral DNA replication by inhibiting DNA polymerase activity and by halting elongation of viral DNA chains.

Adverse Effects. The most serious problems associated with ganciclovir include anemia, granulocytopenia, thrombocytopenia, and related hematologic disorders. Ganciclovir may also cause gastrointestinal disturbances (nausea, loss of appetite) and CNS disturbances (mood changes, nervousness, tremor).

Imiquimod

Antiviral Efficacy and Clinical Use. Imiquimod (Aldara) is applied topically to treat condylomata acuminate infections that cause genital and perianal warts.[42] It can also be used to treat certain skin conditions such as actinic keratoses of the face and scalp.

Mechanism of Action. Although the details are unclear, imiquimod enhances the local production of interferons, tumour necrosis factor-alpha, and possibly other cytokines that produce antiviral responses. Hence, this drug does not act directly on the virus, but instead modulates the host (human) immune responses that have antiviral effects.

Adverse Effects. Some local skin irritation and blistering can occur when imiquimod is applied topically.

Trifluridine

Antiviral Efficacy and Clinical Use. Trifluridine (Viroptic) is administered by eye drops to treat local eye infections associated with herpes simplex virus; that is, herpes virus-related keratitis and keratoconjunctivitis.[42]

Mechanism of Action. This drug impairs viral DNA synthesis by inhibiting the enzymes that incorporate a specific nucleotide (thymidine) into viral DNA. The drug also substitutes itself for thymidine in the viral DNA sequence, thus creating a false DNA code that is ineffective in promoting viral replication.

Adverse Effects. Some local redness and irritation of the eye may develop during local/topical application of trifluridine, but serious adverse effects are rare.

Oseltamivir and Zanamivir

Antiviral Efficacy and Clinical Use. Oseltamivir (Tamiflu) and Zanamivir (Relenza) are effective against influenza virus types A and B. These drugs can reduce the duration and severity of flu symptoms if the drug is administered within 48 hours after symptoms first appear.[22,46] These drugs can also be taken prophylactically to reduce the risk of getting the flu, especially in people who are at high risk (older adults, people with respiratory disorders), or in cases where an individual is exposed to a family member or someone else with the flu.[3]

Mechanism of Action. Oseltamivir and zanamivir inhibit a specific enzyme (neuraminidase) that the influenza virus uses to complete its biosynthesis and release. By inhibiting this enzyme, these drugs impair a key step in viral replication, and reduce the ability of the virus to infect other respiratory cells.

Adverse Effects. Oral administration of oseltamivir can cause gastrointestinal disturbances such as nausea, vomiting, diarrhea, and abdominal cramps. Zanamivir, which is administered by inhalation, is associated with bronchospasm and reduced opening of the airway. The adverse effects of zanamivir can be quite severe in people with bronconstrictive disease (asthma, chronic obstructive pulmonary disease), and this drug should probably be avoided in these individuals.

Protease Inhibitors

Antiviral Efficacy and Clinical Use. These drugs inhibit an enzyme known as HIV protease. This enzyme is needed to manufacture specific HIV proteins, including enzymes such as the HIV reverse transcriptase enzyme and structural proteins that comprise the HIV molecule.[32] By inhibiting this enzyme, protease inhibitors prevent the synthesis and maturation of HIV, thus helping to prevent HIV replication and progression of HIV-related disease.[32,102] The protease inhibitors currently available include amprenavir (Agenerase), atazanavir (Reyataz), fosamprenavir (Lexiva), indinavir (Crixivan), lopinavir (Kaltetra; the trade name for lopinavir combined with ritonavir), nelfinavir (Viracept), ritonavir (Norvir), and saquinavir (Fortovase, Invirase) (see Table 34–3).

Protease inhibitors are often incorporated into the comprehensive treatment of people with HIV infection. Use of these drugs in combination with other anti-HIV agents is discussed in more detail later in this chapter (see "HIV and the Treatment of AIDS"). In addition, a specific protease inhibitor can be combined with a low dose of ritonavir—a process known as protease-inhibitor "boosting."[34,69] Ritonavir inhibits the hepatic breakdown of the other (primary) protease drug, thereby enabling the primary drug to exert better therapeutic effects at a lower dose.[34]

Mechanism of Action. Protease inhibitors bind to the HIV protease and prevent this enzyme from acting on HIV substrates.[32] This effect negates the ability of the protease enzyme to cleave polypeptide precursors from larger, polypeptide chains.[32] If these precursors are not available for the manufacture of HIV proteins, the virus cannot fully develop.[102] Treatment with protease inhibitors therefore results in the manufacture of incomplete and noninfectious fragments of HIV rather than the mature virus.[32]

Adverse Effects. Protease inhibitors may cause alterations in fat deposition in the body (lipodystrophy)—fat deposits atrophy in the limbs, but excess fat is deposited in the abdomen.[21,67] Blood lipids may also be adversely affected, resulting in increased plasma cholesterol, increased triglycerides, and decreased high-density lipoproteins.[55,56] These drugs may also cause other metabolic disturbances, including insulin resistance.[56,84] These drug-induced problems create a metabolic syndrome that can increase the risk of cardiovascular disease in people receiving protease inhibitors.[10] The extent of these metabolic problems depends on several factors, including the specific protease inhibitor, other anti-HIV medications that are also being administered, and the characteristics of each patient.[56,66] Other side effects include diarrhea, headache, and fatigue.[13,32]

Table 34-3	AGENTS USED TO INHIBIT HUMAN IMMUNODEFICIENCY VIRUS (HIV) REPLICATION

Generic Name	Trade Name(s)
Nucleoside reverse transcriptase inhibitors (NRTIs)	
Abacavir	Ziagen
Didanosine	Videx
Lamivudine	Epivir
Stavudine	Zerit
Tenofovir	Viread
Zalcitabine	Hivid
Zidovudine	Retrovir
Nonnucleoside reverse transcriptase inhibitors (NNRTIs)	
Delaviridine	Rescriptor
Efavirenz	Sustiva
Nevirapine	Viramune
Protease inhibitors	
Amprenavir	Agenerase
Atazanavir	Reyataz
Fosamprenavir	Lexiva
Indinavir	Crixivan
Lopinavir	Kaltetra*
Nelfinavir	Viracept
Ritonavir	Norvir
Saquinavir	Fortovase, Invirase
HIV entry inhibitors	
Enfuvirtide	Fuzeon

*Trade name for a combination of lopinavir and low-dose ritonavir.

Reverse Transcriptase Inhibitors

Antiviral Efficacy and Clinical Use. Reverse transcriptase inhibitors (RTIs) are used to inhibit the replication and proliferation of HIV type I (HIV-1). These agents act on a specific enzyme (HIV reverse transcriptase; see the section on "HIV and the Treatment of AIDS") and inhibit a key step in HIV replication.[16] Although these drugs do not eliminate the virus from infected cells, they are often effective in reducing HIV proliferation and the spread of HIV to noninfected cells.[107] These drugs are therefore beneficial in preventing or delaying the progression of HIV and AIDS. The use of RTIs in treating HIV infection is discussed in more detail later in this chapter.

Zidovudine (Retrovir), also known generically as azidothymidine or AZT, was the first RTI approved for treating people who are infected with HIV.[32] Other zidovudine-like drugs have also been developed; currently available agents include abacavir (Ziagen), didanosine (Videx), lamivudine (Epivir), stavudine (Zerit), tenofovir (Viread), and zalcitabine (HIVID).[32] These RTIs can also be subclassified as nucleoside reverse transcriptase inhibitors (NRTIs) because they share a common chemical background (see Table 34-3).

More recently, RTIs that are chemically distinct from zidovudine and other NRTIs have also been developed (see Table 34-3). These agents are known as nonnucleoside reverse transcriptase inhibitors (NNRTIs), and include drugs such as delavirdine (Rescriptor), efavirenz (Sustiva), and nevirapine (Viramune).[32] These drugs also inhibit the reverse transcriptase enzyme, but act at a different site on the enzyme than do their NRTI counterparts.

Therefore, several types of RTIs are available that can help prevent HIV replication and inhibit the proliferation and spread of this virus to noninfected cells. Although these drugs do not kill HIV, RTIs are the cornerstone of treatment for preventing the progression of HIV disease.[59] Use of the various RTIs in combination with each other and with other anti-HIV drugs is discussed in more detail in "HIV and the Treatment of AIDS," later in this chapter.

Mechanism of Action. RTIs impair HIV replication by inhibiting the reverse transcriptase enzyme that is needed to convert viral RNA to viral DNA (Fig. 34-3). With regard to zidovudine and the other NRTIs, these agents enter viral-infected cells, where they are progressively phosphorylated (activated) by

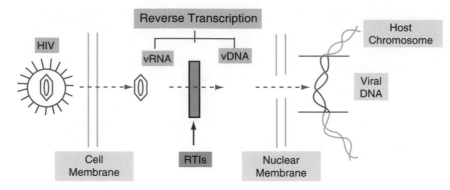

FIGURE 34–3 ▼ Schematic illustration of HIV replication and the site of action of the reverse transcriptase inhibitors (RTIs). These drugs interfere with the process of reverse transcription by inhibiting the enzyme that converts viral RNA (vRNA) to viral DNA (vDNA). See text for further discussion.

various intracellular enzymes.[32,37] The phosphorylated version of the drug then acts as a false nucleic acid, competing with the real nucleic acid (thymidine) for incorporation into growing viral DNA strands. This competition slows down the reverse transcriptase enzyme because the enzyme cannot handle the false nucleic acid (the drug) as easily as the real nucleic acid (thymidine). Even if the reverse transcriptase is successful in incorporating the drug into viral DNA strands, this action prematurely terminates DNA strand synthesis because a false nucleic acid has been added to the viral DNA instead of the real nucleic acid.

The newer agents (NNRTIs) such as delaviridine, efavirenz, and nevirapine directly inhibit the reverse transcriptase enzyme by binding to the enzyme's active (catalytic) site and preventing this enzyme from converting viral RNA to viral DNA.[37,94] Thus, these agents offer an alternative way to impair reverse transcriptase function and prevent viral replication.

Adverse Effects. RTIs are associated with a number of bothersome side effects, and certain agents can also cause potentially serious problems. The most common problems associated with zidovudine are blood dyscrasias, such as anemia and granulocytopenia. Other symptoms occurring during zidovudine administration may include fever, chills, nausea, diarrhea, dizziness, headache, and excessive fatigue. NRTI drugs may also cause myopathy, as indicated by skeletal muscle tenderness, weakness, and atrophy.[63] Likewise, peripheral neuropathies are common, especially when NRTIs such as didanosine, stavudine, and zacitabine are administered in higher doses.[63] These adverse neuromuscular effects are probably due to the toxic effects of these drugs on mitochondrial function in muscle and nerve tissues.[19,63] However, considering that these

drugs are often used in severely immunocompromised patients (such as patients with AIDS), adverse neuromuscular effects may be also be caused by other sequelae of AIDS in addition to the drug's effects. Hence, neuromuscular problems are seen frequently in patients with advanced cases of HIV infection and AIDS.

Other effects associated with NRTIs include pancreatitis, CNS toxicity (headache, irritability, insomnia), and gastrointestinal disturbances (nausea, diarrhea). Abacavir can cause an allergic (hypersensitivity) reaction that produces symptoms such as fever, joint and muscle pain, skin rashes, abdominal pain, nausea, diarrhea, and vomiting.[32] In severe cases, this reaction can progress to anaphylactic shock and possibly death.

Skin rashes are the most common side effect of the NNRTIs, and efavirenz may cause nervous system symptoms such as headache, dizziness, and insomnia.[41]

Ribavirin

Antiviral Efficacy and Clinical Use. Ribavirin (Virazole) is active against several RNA and DNA viruses, including respiratory syncytial virus (RSV).[106] Clinically, this drug is used to treat severe RSV pneumonia in infants and young children,[106] and RSV in certain adult populations, including the elderly, people with cardiopulmonary problems, and people with a compromised immune system.[29] Ribavirin may also be useful as a secondary agent in the treatment of influenza A and B in young adults. The combination of ribavirin and interferons (see section on "Interferons," later) is often the treatment of choice in chronic hepatitis C infection.[30,72]

Ribavirin is administered through oral inhalation. This drug is suspended in an aerosol form and administered to the patient by a mechanical aerosol generator and a ventilation mask, mouthpiece, or hood.

Mechanism of Action. The mechanism of action of this drug is not fully understood. Ribavirin appears to impair viral messenger RNA (mRNA) synthesis, probably by selectively inhibiting enzymes responsible for RNA replication.[35] Inadequate viral mRNA production leads to impaired viral protein synthesis, which ultimately curtails viral replication.

Adverse Effects. Ribavirin produces relatively few adverse effects when administered by inhalation. Most of the drug's action is confined to local pulmonary tissues, and severe systemic effects are rare. One adverse effect that may occur is local irritation of the eyes (conjunctivitis), due to the direct contact of aerosol with the eyes. This occurrence may be a problem if the drug is administered via some sort of hood or tent that encloses the patient's entire head.

Vidarabine

Antiviral Efficacy and Clinical Use. Vidarabine (Vira-A) was the first systemic agent used to treat herpesvirus infections, including CMV, herpes simplex virus, and varicella-zoster virus.[42] In the past, this drug was administered by continuous intravenous infusion to treat severe systemic infections caused by these viruses, but systemic use of vidarabine has been replaced by safer and less toxic agents. Vidarabine is currently used primarily to treat local viral infections of the eye (e.g., herpes simplex keratoconjunctivitis); it is applied topically by ophthalmic ointment to treat these infections.

Mechanism of Action. Vidarabine appears to exert its antiviral effects in a manner similar to acyclovir (see section on "Acyclovir"). Both drugs selectively inhibit viral enzymes that are responsible for viral DNA replication.[42]

Adverse Effects. The primary problems associated with systemic administration of vidarabine include gastrointestinal distress (nausea, vomiting, diarrhea) and CNS disturbances (dizziness, hallucinations, mood changes). Ophthalmic application may produce local irritation (itching, redness, swelling) in some individuals.

Viral Resistance

As discussed in the last chapter, certain bacteria can develop strategies that render them resistant to drug therapy. This fact is true for other microorganisms, including most types of virus. Viruses can mutate and alter their structural or functional characteristics so that previously effective drugs will be unable to control specific viral infections adequately. It is beyond the scope of this chapter to address all the resistant viral strains, and how these strains acquired resistance against antiviral drugs. Viral resistance, like bacterial resistance, is a growing concern. Efforts should be made to limit the indiscriminate or inappropriate use of antiviral drugs, and to contain the spread of resistant viruses. Developing methods to overcome viral resistance using new drugs or different drug combinations is also a critical area of laboratory and clinical research.

Interferons

Interferons are a group of proteins that produce a number of beneficial pharmacologic and physiologic effects.[40,71] These agents were first recognized as endogenous substances that exert nonspecific antiviral activity; that is, interferons enable healthy cells to resist infection from many viruses.[60] Interferons produce other beneficial effects, including the control of cell differentiation, the limiting of excessive cell proliferation, and the modification of certain immune processes.[17,40]

There are three primary classes of human interferons: alpha, beta, and gamma (Table 34–4). Certain cells and tissues produce each primary interferon class. Of these three types, alpha and beta interferons are often grouped together as type I interferons; these type I interferons seem more important in terms of antiviral activity.[40,96] Type II (gamma) interferons appear to be more important in regulating other aspects of the immune response and are responsible for promoting the growth of T lymphocytes and other responses promoting local inflammation.[42]

The possibility that interferons can be used as pharmacologic agents has aroused a great deal of interest. Recombinant DNA techniques and cell tissue cultures have been used to produce sufficient quantities of interferons for clinical drug trials. The rationale is that exogenously administered interferons will produce antiviral and other beneficial effects in healthy cells in a manner similar to their endogenously produced counterparts. Some of the pertinent aspects of interferon action and clinical applications are presented below.

Table 34-4	TYPES OF INTERFERONS	
Type and Subtype	**Specific Agents***	**Primary Indications**
Type I		
Alpha	Alphacon-1 (Infergen)	Chronic hepatitis C
	Alfa-2a (Roferon-A)	Hairy cell leukemia; Kaposi sarcoma (AIDS related)
	Alfa-2b (Intron A)	Hairy cell leukemia; Kaposi sarcoma (AIDS related); chronic hepatitis B; condyloma acuminatum; malignant melanoma
	Alfa-n3 (Alferon N)	Condyloma acuminatum
Beta	Beta-1A (Avonex)	Multiple sclerosis; condyloma acuminatum
	Beta-1B (Betaseron)	Multiple sclerosis
Type II		
Gamma	Gamma-1b (Actimmune)	Chronic granulomatous disease; osteopetrosis

*Specific agents are synthesized using recombinant DNA or other biosynthetic techniques to mimic the effects of naturally-occurring type I or type II interferons.

Synthesis and Cellular Effects of Interferons

The basic sequence of events in the cellular production and antiviral action of interferons is illustrated in Figure 34–4. Virtually all of the body's cells are capable of producing interferons, and these substances serve as an early step in preventing the virus from infecting healthy cells.[50] As illustrated in Figure 34–4, cells that have been infected by a virus produce interferons that are subsequently released from the infected cell. These interferons then travel to noninfected cells, where they bind to specific receptors located on the surface of the healthy cells. Binding of the interferon induces the healthy cell to synthesize its own antiviral proteins. Interferons apparently direct the healthy cell to synthesize the enzymes that inhibit viral messenger RNA and protein synthesis.[17,42] Thus, even if the virus does penetrate into the healthy cell, the virus cannot replicate because of an inability to synthesize viral proteins.

The manner in which interferons control cell growth and proliferation is not fully understood.

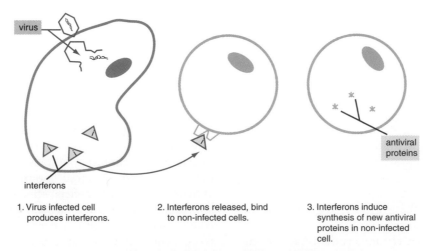

1. Virus infected cell produces interferons.

2. Interferons released, bind to non-infected cells.

3. Interferons induce synthesis of new antiviral proteins in non-infected cell.

FIGURE 34–4 ▼ Antiviral effects of interferons.

Interferons may limit excessive cell division by activating lymphocytes and other cytotoxic cells that combat the cancer, and by controlling specific gene segments in normal and cancerous cells.[71] In particular, interferons may inhibit specific gene-regulatory segments of tumor cells known as *oncogenes*. The inhibition of oncogenes would attenuate the excessive proliferation and lack of cell differentiation typifying neoplastic disease.[8] Interferons may also limit cancer growth by activating certain aspects of the immune system, including increased activity of natural killer cells and other cytotoxic cells that attack cancerous tissues.[8] Hence, interferons have proved effective in controlling several forms of cancer (see Table 34–4); the use of these agents as anticancer drugs is discussed in more detail in Chapter 36.

Pharmacologic Applications of Interferons

When interferons were first discovered, there was a great deal of optimism about their use as antiviral agents. Although early clinical trials with interferons were somewhat disappointing, their use as antiviral agents gained acceptance as more was learned about the three primary classes and subclasses of the interferons. We now realize that interferons cannot be used interchangeably as antiviral drugs, but that certain types of interferons can be administered to treat specific viruses (see Table 34–4). Currently, type I interferons (interferons alpha and beta) seem especially beneficial in treating hepatitis B and C infections.[42,70] These interferons can also be injected locally to treat certain forms of viral-induced warts such as condylomata acuminate infections (see Table 34–4). The clinical use of interferons as antiviral drugs should continue to increase as more is learned about various interferon subclasses and other factors influencing their effectiveness.[71]

As mentioned, interferons also help control abnormal cell proliferation, and these drugs have been approved for use in certain cancers. Interferons are often used as part of the treatment for certain leukemias, lymphomas, and several other forms of cancer (see Table 34–4). Interferon use in cancer chemotherapy is discussed in more detail in Chapter 36.

Finally, certain interferons may decrease exacerbations of multiple sclerosis (MS).[36,88] Specifically, interferon beta-1a (Avonex) and interferon beta-1b (Betaseron) may help reduce the incidence and severity of relapses in exacerbating-remitting MS.[36,64] This effect seems to occur because these beta interferons modulate several aspects of the autoimmune response that initiates the pathological changes associated with MS.[36,88] Although the details are unclear, it appears that type I interferons can reduce the activity of macrophages, lymphocytes, and other immune system components that are responsible for the autoimmune destruction of glial cells and neuronal structures in patients with MS.

Adverse Effects of Interferons

Interferons may cause flulike symptoms including fever, sweating, chills, muscle aches, and general malaise. Other side effects such as loss of appetite, nausea, vomiting, diarrhea, and unusual tiredness can also occur, depending on the type of interferon and the dosage. Interferons may also cause behavioral side effects such as depression, presumably because these drugs inhibit serotonin activity in the brain.[5,105] When interferons are administered by intramuscular or subcutaneous injection, some irritation may develop around the injection site. Finally, anti-interferon antibodies may be produced by the immune system, especially when interferons are administered for prolonged periods.[25] These antibodies can neutralize the interferons, thus decreasing their effectiveness in controlling viral infections and other conditions such as cancer and MS.

Control of Viral Infection with Vaccines

Vaccines prevent viral infection by stimulating the endogenous production of immune factors that will selectively destroy the invading virus. Hence, the vaccine can be administered to healthy individuals to provide them with immunity from certain viral infections. A vaccine acts as an antigen that induces the immune system to generate virus-specific antibodies. The vaccine, however, does not cause any appreciable viral infection because the vaccine contains a virus that has been modified in some way so that it retains its antigenic properties but lacks the ability to produce infection. Vaccines, for example, typically consist of a whole virus or part of the virus (viral particle or fragment) that has been completely inactivated (killed vaccines) or partially inactivated (live attenuated vaccines).[53] Thus, most antiviral vaccinations are accomplished by administering small amounts of the modified virus.

In general, it is somewhat easier to develop vaccines that prevent viral infection than to develop drugs that destroy the virus once it has infected human cells. This notion is reasonable when one considers that the virus is essentially coexisting with the host cell. As indicated previously, there are currently only a limited number of drugs that are able to selectively inhibit the virus without harming the host cell. A more practical strategy is to use vaccines to enable the body to destroy the virus before an infection is established.

At present, vaccines are available for several serious viral infections, including polio, smallpox, rabies, measles, mumps, rubella, hepatitis A and B, and influenza. In some situations, vaccination against certain viral infections is routine. For instance, schoolchildren must periodically show evidence of polio, measles, and other vaccinations according to state and local laws. In other cases, vaccines are administered prior to potential exposure to the virus or in high-risk groups. Influenza vaccinations, for example, are often administered to elderly and debilitated patients during seasonal influenza outbreaks.[75,109]

Although vaccines exist for many serious viral infections, some drawbacks still exist. Some vaccines are only partially effective, and viral infection still occurs in a significant percentage of vaccinated individuals. Other vaccines, especially killed vaccines, often require periodic readministration (boosters) to help maintain antiviral immunity. In addition, certain types of viruses still lack an effective vaccination. For example, no vaccine is currently approved for the HIV that causes AIDS.[51,98] Hence, the improvement of existing vaccines and the development of new vaccines remain two of the more important aspects of antiviral chemotherapy.[4]

HIV and the Treatment of AIDS

HIV is a member of the retrovirus family (see Table 34–1).[32] HIV impairs the function of certain cells in the immune system such as CD4+ (T-helper) lymphocytes.[11,26] Destruction of immune system components often leads to the severe immunocompromised state known as AIDS. This virus exists in at least two forms: HIV-1 and HIV-2. Both forms of the virus are capable of causing AIDS, but HIV-1 is more prevalent.[32] Hence, HIV-1 is also referred to informally as the "AIDS virus." Because there is currently no effective way to kill the AIDS virus in humans, there is no cure for AIDS.

AIDS is a life-threatening disorder because of the susceptibility of the immunocompromised patient to severe infections and certain forms of cancer.[65,73,76,101,113] In particular, patients with AIDS often suffer from severe viral infections (CMV, various herpesvirus infections), bacterial infections (*Mycobacterium tuberculosis*), fungal infections (*Pneumocystis jiroveci*), and infections caused by various other microbes and parasites. Patients with AIDS also develop relatively unusual neoplastic diseases, such as Kaposi sarcoma.

Considerable neuromuscular involvement also occurs in patients with AIDS.[47,100] Peripheral neuropathies, myopathies, and various CNS manifestations (dementia, other psychological manifestations) can occur directly from HIV infection or secondarily, due to some other opportunistic infection.[31,85,100] Likewise, peripheral neuropathies are a common side effect of certain anti-HIV drugs (didanosine, stavudine, zalcitabine), and myopathies are a side effect of zidovudine therapy.[63] Patients with HIV disease often have painful symptoms such as joint pain, back pain, and pain related to neuropathies and myopathies.[100] Hence, HIV disease can often be regarded as a degenerative neuromuscular disorder from the standpoint of a rehabilitation professional. Therapists can therefore help improve function and decrease pain in patients with HIV infection and AIDS.[1,33]

Individuals who are infected with HIV may remain very asymptomatic for several years before developing the full-blown clinical picture of AIDS. Even people exposed to HIV who do not initially develop AIDS carry the virus for the rest of their lives and are thus capable of transmitting the virus to others. Transmission of HIV from one individual to another occurs primarily through intimate sexual contact and through sharing intravenous needles. Transfusions of blood from HIV-infected donors are also a potential source of HIV transmission. Hence, practices such as safe sex, not sharing needles, and improved blood-screening techniques are crucial in preventing the transmission of HIV and the subsequent risk of developing AIDS.

The treatment of patients with AIDS and individuals infected by HIV is continually being modified as new drugs become available and more information is gained about the nature of the AIDS virus. Currently, the pharmacologic management of HIV-infected patients consists of two principal strategies: (1) controlling the proliferation and effects of HIV in individuals infected with this virus and (2) treatment and prevention of various opportunistic infections that attempt to take advantage of the compromised immune system in patients with AIDS. The pharmacologic methods used to accomplish these principal strategies are presented here.

Inhibition of HIV Proliferation in Infected Individuals

No drugs are currently available that selectively kill HIV in humans, hence the lack of a cure for this viral infection. Nonetheless, several antiviral drugs are given to inhibit the replication of this virus, thus decreasing the morbidity and mortality of HIV infection. These drugs are usually specific for the HIV-1 form of the virus, because HIV-1 is more prevalent in people infected by HIV. Several pharmacologic strategies for treating HIV infection are currently available, and these strategies are discussed briefly here.

Zidovudine (Retrovir, AZT) was the first drug approved as an anti-HIV agent.[32] Other agents that act like zidovudine were subsequently approved to prevent HIV replication. These drugs include abacavir (Ziagen), didanosine (Videx), lamivudine (Epivir), stavudine (Zerit), tenofovir (Viread), and zalcitabine (HIVID) (see Table 34–3). As discussed in "Specific Antiviral Drugs," zidovudine and similar drugs are classified as NRTIs because they share a common mechanism of action (illustrated in Figure 34–3); that is, these drugs inhibit the reverse transcriptase enzyme that HIV uses to synthesize viral DNA from viral RNA. This action impairs one of the early steps in viral replication, thus slowing the progression of HIV infection and the development of AIDS.

Protease inhibitors were the second major breakthrough in the pharmacologic treatment of HIV infection. Protease inhibitors are typically identified by generic names containing an "-avir" suffix. Protease inhibitors currently available include amprenavir (Agenerase), atazanavir (Reyataz), fosamprenavir (Lexiva), indinavir (Crixivan), lopinavir (Kaltetra; combination with Ritonavir), nelfinavir (Viracept), ritonavir (Norvir), and saquinavir (Fortovase, Invirase). As indicated earlier, these drugs impair the HIV protease enzyme that is responsible for several steps in HIV replication. Like the NRTIs, these drugs do not kill the virus but can slow its replication and prevent the spread of HIV to noninfected cells.

The third strategy developed to inhibit HIV replication is the NNRTIs. These drugs include delavirdine (Rescriptor), efavirenz (Sustiva), and nevirapine (Viramune). Like their nucleoside counterparts, NNR-TIs also inhibit the reverse transcriptase enzyme's ability to perform one of the initial steps in HIV replication. The NNRTIs, however, directly inhibit the active (catalytic) site on this enzyme, whereas zidovudine and other NRTIs serve as false substrates that take the place of the substance (thymidine) normally acted on by this enzyme (see "Reverse Transcriptase Inhibitors: Mechanism of Action"). Hence, NNRTIs provide another way to impair one of the key steps in HIV replication, and these drugs can be used along with other agents (NRTIs, protease inhibitors) to provide optimal benefits in preventing HIV replication and proliferation (see the next section).

Finally, a group of agents known as HIV entry inhibitors is beginning to reach the market. These drugs impair the ability of the virus to attach to the host cell's surface, thereby inhibiting HIV entry into susceptible lymphocytes. If the virus cannot enter the cell, it cannot infect that cell or begin the process of viral replication. Enfuviritide (Fuzeon) is the first HIV entry inhibitor to be approved, and other drugs of this type will hopefully be available in the near future.

The arsenal of anti-HIV agents has therefore grown steadily since the development of the first anti-HIV drug (zidovudine). In addition, other drugs and strategies that inhibit HIV infection continue to be explored.[32,61] As more is learned about the structure and function of this virus, drugs can be developed that impair specific steps in the absorption and replication of HIV in human cells. If clinical trials using these other drugs are favorable, they may also be approved for future use in individuals infected with HIV.

Anti-HIV Drug Combinations: Use of Highly Active Antiretroviral Therapy

Several anti-HIV drugs are often administered simultaneously to provide optimal inhibition of HIV replication and proliferation. The idea of combining several agents is referred to as highly active antiretroviral therapy, or HAART.[54] HAART often involves the simultaneous use of at least three anti-HIV agents.[114] A typical HAART strategy, for example, involves the use of two RTIs and one protease inhibitor.[54,90] There are, however, many variations of the specific drug combinations used during HAART. Moreover, HAART regimens are continually being revised as new drugs reach the market or problems arise with existing strategies. Hence, the exact number and types of drugs used during HAART are selected based on the specific needs of each patient.

Regardless of the exact drugs used, there is ample evidence that HAART can successfully delay the progression of HIV disease in people infected with the virus. In many cases, strict adherence to HAART regimens can reduce the viral load (that is, the amount of viral RNA present in the bloodstream) to levels that are undetectable with current testing procedures.[32] This fact does not mean that HAART has successfully eliminated the virus from the infected host or that the person infected with HIV has been cured. Even if HAART successfully reduces evidence of the virus in the plasma, the virus can be sequestered into T cells and other tissue "reservoirs" so that viral components cannot be detected in the bloodstream.[32,92] Still, HAART regimens can prevent the progression of HIV infection and help sustain immune function by allowing increases in the number of functioning CD4 lymphocytes.[54] The use of HAART is therefore associated with a substantial reduction in the incidence of AIDS and with improved clinical outcomes (fewer infections, decreased cancers, prolonged survival) in people who are infected with HIV.[54,81]

HAART regimens are, however, associated with several problems and limitations. A certain percentage of people with HIV do not respond adequately to HAART; that is, HAART may not be very successful in producing a sustained and complete reduction in viral load in anywhere from 30 to 50 percent of patients receiving these regimens.[32] The lack of effectiveness may be a consequence of poor adherence to the HAART regimen. Adherence to HAART is often difficult because of the potential for side effects with these drugs and because of difficulties in remembering the complicated dosage regimens associated with taking three or more agents.[32,54,90] Resistance to anti-HIV drugs can also develop,[20,74] especially if there is poor adherence to HAART regimens.[20,32] As mentioned earlier, HAART does not completely eliminate the virus from the infected host, because some of the viral components remain sequestered within tissues, where they remain hidden from HAART drugs.[92] Finally, the simultaneous use of several drugs during HAART increases the risk for drug-drug interactions, and likewise increases the chance for toxicity to the liver and other organs.[2,23]

Nonetheless, HAART can suppress HIV disease in many people who are infected with this virus. Drug combinations can be used successfully for the long-term management of HIV disease, and they offer hope that people with HIV do not have to progress inexorably toward AIDS and death. Research continues to find the best way to combine existing agents and to incorporate new agents into a comprehensive and successful regimen for people infected with HIV.

HIV Vaccines

An HIV vaccine has not yet been successfully developed and approved for use in the United States. As indicated earlier, vaccines are typically an altered form of the original virus that is administered to stimulate the immune system, so that the immune system can recognize and destroy the virus if a person is exposed to it. Creation of an HIV vaccine is understandably a complicated endeavor, given the complexity of this virus and its tendency to evolve and mutate into different types of HIV.[78,108] Nonetheless, the development of a safe, effective vaccine remains the best pharmacologic method for dealing with the spread of the virus, especially in underdeveloped nations that continue to experience a rise in the incidence of HIV and AIDS.[15,48]

Hence, efforts continue to develop an HIV vaccine that will produce adequate immunity from HIV infection without severe untoward side effects.[57] There is concern, however, that a successful vaccine may be very difficult to produce.[27,78] For example, development of an HIV vaccine that is not 100 percent effective might give recipients a false sense of security; that is, a vaccine that confers only partial immunity (e.g., a 50 to 75 percent reduction in the risk of contracting HIV) might encourage the recipient to forgo other precautions, such as safe sex, not sharing intravenous needles, and so forth. Likewise, the question arises about whether a single vaccine will be successful in providing immunity from all the various HIV strains and subtypes.[48,93] An HIV vaccine is urgently needed and would undoubtedly be received as one of the most important pharmacologic advancements of our time. The development of such a vaccine may be delayed, however, until we have a better understanding of HIV and how to best modify this virus into a successful vaccine.

We must therefore remember that zidovudine and other drugs currently available for treating HIV are not curative and may be helpful only in delaying or reducing AIDS-related deaths. A cure for AIDS, if possible, will take several years or even several decades before becoming a reality. As with many viruses, developing a vaccine against the AIDS virus is somewhat easier than making a drug that selectively destroys HIV. The development of an HIV vaccine, however, is probably still years away. Until a vaccine is developed, preventing transmission of HIV remains the best method of controlling the spread of AIDS.

Management of Opportunistic Infections

If HIV infection is not treated successfully, the body is open to infection from various other microorganisms. These infections are known commonly as opportunistic infections because microorganisms take advantage of the chance to infect people who lack normal immune defenses.[110] Fortunately, newer anti-HIV drugs and the use of HAART regimens have reduced the risk of opportunistic infections.[79,110] Hence, the best prevention against opportunistic infections is aggressive anti-HIV treatment that promotes T lymphocyte survival and helps maintain a functioning immune system.[12,99] Still, some patients are prone to opportunistic infections, including patients who are newly diagnosed with HIV infection, or patients that cannot tolerate, respond to, or adhere to HAART regimens.[45,110] Likewise, opportunistic infections are still a major cause of illness and death in areas of the world where HAART regimens are unavailable or unaffordable (i.e., developing countries).[14] When immune function deteriorates beyond a certain point (typically less than 200 CD4 lymphocytes per microliter), these patients are said to have AIDS.

Because of a virtual lack of immunologic defenses, patients with AIDS often succumb to a variety of opportunistic infections.[45] Essentially, these patients simply do not have the ability to fight off various viral, bacterial, and other microbial invaders.[12] Consequently, much of the pharmacologic approach to the treatment of AIDS is associated with trying to curtail various infections by using the respective antimicrobial drugs that are currently available.

It is beyond the scope of this chapter to give a detailed description of the pharmacologic treatment of all the possible opportunistic infections that occur in patients with AIDS. Nonetheless, some of the more common types of opportunistic infections and the drugs commonly used to treat them are listed in Table 34–5. Early recognition of infectious symptoms is crucial in helping initiate drug therapy before the infection becomes uncontrollable.[9] Because patients with AIDS essentially lack endogenous defense systems, drug therapy must often be continued indefinitely, or the infection will recur. On the other hand, successful implementation or reinstitution of HAART strategies can restore immune function in certain patients, and drugs for opportunistic infections can sometimes be discontinued.[38,43] Nonetheless, strategies for dealing with various infections are constantly changing, and drug therapy for HIV and opportunistic infections will surely be modified as new antimicrobial agents are developed and new evidence is provided about how these agents can be used in various infections.

Table 34–5 TREATMENT OF OPPORTUNISTIC INFECTIONS IN PATIENTS WITH AIDS

Organism	Type of Infection	Drug Treatment*
Viral infections		
Cytomegalovirus	Pneumonia; hepatitis; chorioretinitis; involvement of many other organs	Foscarnet or ganciclovir
Herpes simplex	Unusually severe vesicular and necrotizing lesions of mucocutaneous areas (mouth, pharynx) and gastrointestinal tract	Acyclovir, famciclovir, or valacyclovir
Varicella-zoster	Painful, vesicular eruption of skin according to dermatomal boundaries (shingles)	Acyclovir, famciclovir, or valacyclovir
Bacterial infections		
Mycobacterium avium complex	Involvement of bone marrow, reticuloendothelial tissues	Clarithromycin plus ethambutol; rifabutin
Mycobacterium tuberculosis	Tuberculosis	Isoniazid plus pyridoxine; rifampin (if isoniazid resistant)

(Continued on following page)

Table 34–5	TREATMENT OF OPPORTUNISTIC INFECTIONS IN PATIENTS WITH AIDS *(Continued)*	
Organism	**Type of Infection**	**Drug Treatment***
Salmonella	Enterocolitis and bacteremia	Ciprofloxacin or trimethoprim
Fungal infections		
Candida	Inflammatory lesions in oropharyngeal region and esophagitis	Oral infections: clotrimazole, fluconazole, or nystatin; Esophageal infections: fluconazole or ketoconazole
Coccidiodes	Primarily affects lungs but may disseminate to other tissues	Amphotericin B
Cryptococcus	Meningoencephalitis	Amphotericin B ± flucytosine, followed by fluconazole
Histoplasma capsulatum	Affects various tissues including lungs, lymphatics, and mucocutaneous tissues; also causes blood dyscrasias (anemias, leucopenia)	Amphotericin B or itraconazole
Pneumocystis jiroveci	Pneumonia	Trimethoprim-sulfamethoxazole, pentamidine, or atovaquone
Protozoal infections		
Toxoplasma	Central nervous system infections (cerebral degeneration, meningoencephalitis)	Pyrimethamine and sulfadiazine

*Choice of specific drugs varies according to disease status, presence of other infections, and so forth. Pharmacotherapeutic rationale is also constantly changing as new agents are developed and tested.

Relevance of Antiviral Chemotherapy in Rehabilitation Patients

■ ■ ■ The major significance of antiviral drugs to rehabilitation specialists and other health care professionals is the potential for controlling or eliminating infectious disease at present and in the future. As indicated in this chapter, only a few drugs can effectively resolve viral infections in humans at present. Nonetheless, the development of new antiviral agents and the improved use of existing compounds such as the interferons are exciting and important areas of pharmacology. In addition, viral prophylaxis through vaccination has virtually eliminated some types of serious infections, and the possibility of new and improved antiviral vaccines may enhance the health and welfare of patients throughout the world.

Consequently, physical therapists and occupational therapists should keep abreast of advances in treating and preventing viral infections. This notion is especially true for the AIDS crisis, which promises to be a major health issue for some time. By keeping informed of current developments in antiviral pharmacology, health care professionals will enrich their own knowledge while serving as a reliable source of information for their patients.

In addition, viral infections may produce pain and other symptoms that can be treated by physical rehabilitation. In particular, chronic HIV infection and the drug therapy for this disorder can both produce neuromuscular problems such as myopathy and peripheral neuropathy.[63,83] Neuromuscular impairments can occur at any stage in the disease process, but they become especially problematic in advanced cases of HIV infection, or when this disease progresses to AIDS.[7,63] Hence, therapists can use various physical agents to help decrease pain, and likewise implement aerobic and resistive exercise programs to help maintain muscle strength and function.[68] These interventions can be invaluable in helping maintain quality-of-life in people with HIV infection and AIDS.

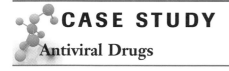

CASE STUDY

Antiviral Drugs

Brief History. R.K. is a 28-year-old man who was infected with HIV after sharing hypodermic syringes with a fellow drug abuser. He began a pharmacologic regimen of highly active antiretroviral therapy, consisting of two reverse transcriptase inhibitors (zidovudine [Retrovir], 600 mg/d and didanosine [Videx], 400 mg/d) and one protease inhibitor (indinavir [Crixivan], 2400 mg/d). This regimen was initially successful in controlling HIV replication and proliferation, but the patient began to lapse into periods of noncompliance and frequently failed to take his medications according to the proper dosing schedule. Hence, HIV proliferated and suppressed immune function to the point where he was considered to have developed AIDs. Recently, he developed a fever and respiratory infection due to *Pneumocystis jiroveci* pneumonia. He was admitted to the hospital and treated with a combination of pentamidine and trimethoprim-sulfamethoxazole. The patient also exhibited muscular weakness and began to develop burning pain in both lower extremities. The weakness and pain

were attributed to radiculopathy caused by infection of peripheral nerves by HIV or by some other opportunistic infection. The physical therapy department was consulted to determine what could be done to alleviate the neuropathic pain and dysfunction.

Decision/Solution. The therapist initiated a program of transcutaneous electrical nerve stimulation (TENS) along the affected nerve pathways. The patient was instructed in the use of the TENS unit, and intensity and other stimulation parameters were adjusted to tolerance by the patient. The therapist also found that cold neon laser treatment helped decrease pain and increase function along the more severely affected nerves, and daily laser treatments were instituted. The combination of TENS and laser therapy helped to decrease the pain in this viral-related disorder, thus improving the patient's well being without the use of additional pharmacologic agents (pain medications). Progressive involvement of other peripheral neurons occurred over the course of the next few weeks, however, and the patient eventually died of respiratory failure.

SUMMARY

Viruses present a unique problem in terms of the pharmacologic treatment of infectious disease. These microorganisms rely totally on the metabolic function of host (human) cells to function and replicate more viruses. Hence, there are currently only a limited number of effective antiviral agents that selectively kill or attenuate the virus without seriously harming the human cells. Developing and administering antiviral vaccines that stimulate the immunity of the host to specific viral infections is often more practical. In the future, the development of new antiviral agents and vaccines may help treat and eliminate viral infections that currently pose a serious health threat.

References

1. Abbaticola MM. A team approach to the treatment of AIDS wasting. *J Assoc Nurses AIDS Care.* 2000;11: 45–53.

2. Abrescia N, D'Abraccio M, Figoni M, et al. Hepatotoxicity of antiretroviral drugs. *Curr Pharm Des.* 2005; 11:3697–3710.

3. Alymova IV, Taylor G, Portner A. Neuraminidase inhibitors as antiviral agents. *Curr Drug Targets Infect Disord.* 2005;5:401–409.

4. Arvin AM, Greenberg HB. New viral vaccines. *Virology.* 2006;344:240–249.

5. Asnis GM, De La Garza R. Interferon-induced depression: strategies in treatment. *Prog Neuropsychopharmacol Biol Psychiatry.* 2005;29:808–818.

6. Ausayakhun S, Watananikorn S, Ngamtiphakorn S, Prasitsilp J. Intravitreal foscarnet for cytomegalovirus retinitis in patients with AIDS. *J Med Assoc Thai.* 2005; 88:103–107.

7. Authier FJ, Chariot P, Gherardi RK. Skeletal muscle involvement in human immunodeficiency virus (HIV)-infected patients in the era of highly active antiretroviral therapy (HAART). *Muscle Nerve.* 2005;32:247–260.

8. Balmer CM, Valley AW. Cancer treatment and chemotherapy. In: DiPiro JT, et al, eds. *Pharmacotherapy: A Pathophysiologic Approach.* 5th ed. New York: McGraw-Hill; 2002.

9. Banerjee U. Progress in diagnosis of opportunistic infections in HIV/AIDS. *Indian J Med Res.* 2005;121: 395–406.

10. Barbaro G. Metabolic and cardiovascular complications of highly active antiretroviral therapy for HIV infection. *Curr HIV Res.* 2006;4:79–85.

11. Beck JM. The immunocompromised host: HIV infection. *Proc Am Thorac Soc.* 2005;2:423–427.

12. Berenguer J, Laguna F, Lopez-Aldeguer J, et al. Prevention of opportunistic infections in adult and adolescent patients with HIV infection. GESIDA/National AIDS Plan guidelines, 2004. *Enferm Infecc Microbiol Clin.* 2004;22:160–176.

13. Boyle BA, Elion RA, Moyle GJ, Cohen CJ. Considerations in selecting protease inhibitor therapy. *AIDS Rev.* 2004;6:218–225.

14. Boyton RJ. Infectious lung complications in patients with HIV/AIDS. *Curr Opin Pulm Med.* 2005;11: 203–207.

15. Burgers WA, Williamson C. The challenges of HIV vaccine development and testing. *Best Pract Res Clin Obstet Gynaecol.* 2005;19:277–291.

16. Castro HC, Loureiro NI, Pujol-Luz M, et al. HIV-1 reverse transcriptase: a therapeutical target in the spotlight. *Curr Med Chem.* 2006;13:313–324.

17. Champoux JJ. Viral multiplication. In: Ryan KJ, Ray CG, eds. *Sherris Medical Microbiology.* 4th ed. New York: McGraw-Hill; 2004.

18. Champoux JJ. Viral structure. In: Ryan KJ, Ray CG, eds. *Sherris Medical Microbiology.* 4th ed. New York: McGraw-Hill; 2004.

19. Cherry CL, Lala L, Wesselingh SL. Mitochondrial toxicity of nucleoside analogues: mechanism, monitoring and management. *Sex Health.* 2005;2:1–11.

20. Clotet B. Strategies for overcoming resistance in HIV-1 infected patients receiving HAART. *AIDS Rev.* 2004; 6:123–130.

21. Cohen CJ. Ritonavir-boosted protease inhibitors, part 2: cardiac implications of lipid alterations. *AIDS Read.* 2005;15:528–532, 537–538.

22. Colman PM. Zanamivir: an influenza virus neuraminidase inhibitor. *Expert Rev Anti Infect Ther.* 2005;3: 191–199.

23. Daugas E, Rougier JP, Hill G. HAART-related nephropathies in HIV-infected patients. *Kidney Int.* 2005;67:393–403.

24. De Clercq E. Antiviral drugs in current clinical use. *J Clin Virol.* 2004;30:115–133.

25. Deisenhammer F, Schellekens H, Bertolotto A. Measurement of neutralizing antibodies to interferon beta in patients with multiple sclerosis. *J Neurol.* 2004; 251(suppl 2):II31–II39.

26. Eger KA, Unutmaz D. The innate immune system and HIV pathogenesis. *Curr HIV/AIDS Rep.* 2005; 2:10–15.

27. Esparza J. The global HIV vaccine enterprise. *Int Microbiol.* 2005;8:93–101.

28. Evans CT, Lavela SL, Smith B, et al. Influenza diagnosis and treatment in veterans with spinal cord injury. *Arch Phys Med Rehabil.* 2006;87:291–293.

29. Falsey AR, Walsh EE. Respiratory syncytial virus infection in adults. *Clin Microbiol Rev.* 2000;13: 371–384.

30. Feld JJ, Hoofnagle JH. Mechanism of action of interferon and ribavirin in treatment of hepatitis C. *Nature.* 2005;436:967–972.

31. Ferrari S, Vento S, Monaco S, et al. Human immunodeficiency virus-associated peripheral neuropathies. *Mayo Clin Proc.* 2006;81:213–219.

32. Flexner C. Antiretroviral agents and treatment of HIV infection. In: Brunton LL, et al, eds. *The Pharmacological Basis of Therapeutics.* 11th ed. New York: McGraw-Hill; 2006.

33. Galantino ML, Jermyn RT, Tursi FJ, Eke-Okoro S. Physical therapy management for the patient with HIV. Lower extremity challenges. *Clin Podiatr Med Surg.* 1998;15:329–346.

34. Gallant JE. Protease-inhibitor boosting in the treatment-experienced patient. *AIDS Rev.* 2004;6:226–233.

35. Gish RG. Treating HCV with ribavirin analogues and ribavirin-like molecules. *J Antimicrob Chemother.* 2006; 57:8–13.

36. Goodin DS. Treatment of multiple sclerosis with human beta interferon. *Int MS J.* 2005;12:96–108.

37. Gotte M. Inhibition of HIV-1 reverse transcription: basic principles of drug action and resistance. *Expert Rev Anti Infect Ther.* 2004;2:707–716.

38. Green H, Hay P, Dunn DT, et al. A prospective multicentre study of discontinuing prophylaxis for opportunistic infections after effective antiretroviral therapy. *HIV Med.* 2004;5:278–283.

39. Griffiths P. Cytomegalovirus infection of the central nervous system. *Herpes.* 2004;11(suppl 2):95A–104A.

40. Haller O, Kochs G, Weber F. The interferon response circuit: induction and suppression by pathogenic viruses. *Virology.* 2006;344:119–130.

41. Harris M, Montaner JS. Clinical uses of non-nucleoside reverse transcriptase inhibitors. *Rev Med Virol.* 2000;10: 217–229.
42. Hayden FG. Antiviral agents (nonretroviral). In: Brunton LL, et al, eds. *The Pharmacological Basis of Therapeutics.* 11th ed. New York: McGraw-Hill; 2006.
43. Hermsen ED, Wynn HE, McNabb J. Discontinuation of prophylaxis for HIV-associated opportunistic infections in the era of highly active antiretroviral therapy. *Am J Health Syst Pharm.* 2004;61:245–256.
44. Hodson EM, Jones CA, Webster AC, et al. Antiviral medications to prevent cytomegalovirus disease and early death in recipients of solid-organ transplants: a systematic review of randomized controlled trials. *Lancet.* 2005;365:2105–2115.
45. Hung CC, Chang SC. Impact of highly active anti-retroviral therapy on incidence and management of human immunodeficiency virus-related opportunistic infections. *J Antimicrob Chemother.* 2004;54:849–853.
46. Jefferson T, Demicheli V, Rivetti D, et al. Antivirals for influenza in healthy adults: systematic review. *Lancet.* 2006;367:303–313.
47. Jones G, Power C. Regulation of neural cell survival by HIV-1 infection. *Neurobiol Dis.* 2006;21:1–17.
48. Joseph J, Etcheverry F, Alcami J, Maria GJ. A safe, effective and affordable HIV vaccine—an urgent global need. *AIDS Rev.* 2005;7:131–138.
49. Kappel PJ, Charonis AC, Holland GN, et al. Outcomes associated with ganciclovir implants in patients with AIDS-related cytomegalovirus retinitis. *Ophthalmology.* 2006;113:683.e1-8.
50. Kawai T, Akira S. Innate immune recognition of viral infection. *Nat Immunol.* 2006;7:131–137.
51. Koff WC, Johnson PR, Watkins DI, et al. HIV vaccine design: insights from live attenuated SIV vaccines. *Nat Immunol.* 2006;7:19–23.
52. Kolbe F, Sitar DS, Papaioannou A, Campbell G. An amantadine hydrochloride dosing program adjusted for renal function during an influenza outbreak in elderly institutionalized patients. *Can J Clin Pharmacol.* 2003; 10:119–122.
53. Krensky AM, Vincenti F, Bennett WM. Immunosuppressants, tolerogens, and immunostimulants. In: Brunton LL, et al, eds. *The Pharmacological Basis of Therapeutics.* 11th ed. New York: McGraw-Hill; 2006.
54. Kress KD. HIV update: emerging clinical evidence and a review of recommendations for the use of highly active antiretroviral therapy. *Am J Health Syst Pharm.* 2004;61(suppl 3):S3–S14.
55. Kulasekaram R, Peters BS, Wierzbicki AS. Dyslipidaemia and cardiovascular risk in HIV infection. *Curr Med Res Opin.* 2005;21:1717–1725.
56. Lee GA, Rao MN, Grunfeld C. The effects of HIV protease inhibitors on carbohydrate and lipid metabolism. *Curr Infect Dis Rep.* 2004;6:471–482.
57. Levy Y. Therapeutic HIV vaccines: an update. *Curr HIV/AIDS Rep.* 2005;2:5–9.
58. Lin L, Chen XS, Cui PG, et al. Topical application of penciclovir cream for the treatment of herpes simplex facialis/labialis: a randomized, double-blind, multicentre, aciclovir-controlled trial. *J Dermatolog Treat.* 2002; 13:67–72.
59. Locatelli GA, Cancio R, Spadari S, Maga G. HIV-1 reverse transcriptase inhibitors: current issues and future perspectives. *Curr Drug Metab.* 2004;5:283–290.
60. Malmgaard L. Induction and regulation of IFNs during viral infections. *J Interferon Cytokine Res.* 2004; 24:439–454.
61. Marks K, Gulick RM. New antiretroviral agents for the treatment of HIV infection. *Curr HIV/AIDS Rep.* 2004;1:82–88.
62. McAdam AJ, Sharpe AH. Infectious diseases. In: Kumar V, Abbas AK, Fausto N, eds. *Pathologic Basis of Disease.* 7th ed. New York: Elsevier Saunders; 2005.
63. Moyle G. Mechanisms of HIV and nucleoside reverse transcriptase inhibitor injury to mitochondria. *Antivir Ther.* 2005;10(suppl 2):M47–M52.
64. Murdoch D, Lyseng-Williamson KA. Subcutaneous recombinant interferon-beta-1a (Rebif): a review of its use in relapsing-remitting multiple sclerosis. *Drugs.* 2005;65:1295–1312.
65. Nagappan V, Kazanjian P. Bacterial infections in adult HIV-infected patients. *HIV Clin Trials.* 2005; 6:213–228.
66. Nolan D, Mallal S. Antiretroviral-therapy–associated lipoatrophy: current status and future directions. *Sex Health.* 2005;2:153–163.
67. Nolan D, Reiss P, Mallal S. Adverse effects of antiretroviral therapy for HIV infection: a review of selected topics. *Expert Opin Drug Saf.* 2005;4: 201–218.
68. O'Brien K, Nixon S, Glazier RH, Tynan AM. Progressive resistive exercise interventions for adults living with HIV/AIDS. *Cochrane Database Syst Rev.* 2004; CD004248.
69. O'Brien WA, 3rd. Saquinavir/Ritonavir: its evolution and current treatment role. *AIDS Read.* 2006;16:38–44.
70. Ocama P, Opio CK, Lee WM. Hepatitis B virus infection: current status. *Am J Med.* 2005;118:1413.
71. Pang KR, Wu JJ, Huang DB, et al. Biological and clinical basis for molecular studies of interferons. *Methods Mol Med.* 2005;116:1–23.
72. Pawlotsky JM. Therapy of hepatitis C: from empiricism to eradication. *Hepatology.* 2006;43(suppl 1): S207–S220.
73. Petrosillo N, Nicastri E, Viale P. Nosocomial pulmonary infections in HIV-positive patients. *Curr Opin Pulm Med.* 2005;11:231–235.
74. Pillay D, Taylor S, Richman DD. Incidence and impact of resistance against approved antiviral drugs. *Rev Med Virol.* 2000;10:231–253.
75. Poole PJ, Chacko E, Wood-Baker RW, Cates CJ. Influenza vaccine for patients with chronic obstructive pulmonary disease. *Cochrane Database Syst Rev.* 2006; CD002733.
76. Pop SM, Kolls JK, Steele C. Pneumocystis: immune recognition and evasion. *Int J Biochem Cell Biol.* 2006; 38:17–22.
77. Poveda E, Briz V, Soriano V. Enfuvirtide, the first fusion inhibitor to treat HIV infection. *AIDS Rev.* 2005;7:139–147.
78. Puls RL, Emery S. Therapeutic vaccination against HIV: current progress and future possibilities. *Clin Sci (Lond).* 2006;110:59–71.

79. Pulvirenti JJ. Inpatient care of the HIV infected patient in the highly active antiretroviral therapy (HAART) era. *Curr HIV Res.* 2005;3:133–145.

80. Radtke K, Dohner K, Sodeik B. Viral interactions with the cytoskeleton: a hitchhiker's guide to the cell. *Cell Microbiol.* 2006;8:387–400.

81. Rathbun RC, Lockhart SM, Stephens JR. Current HIV treatment guidelines—an overview. *Curr Pharm Des.* 2006;12:1045–1063.

82. Reischig T, Opatrny K, Jr, Treska V, et al. Prospective comparison of valacyclovir and oral ganciclovir for prevention of cytomegalovirus disease in high-risk renal transplant recipients. *Kidney Blood Press Res.* 2005;28:218–225.

83. Roedling S, Pearl D, Manji H, et al. Unusual muscle disease in HIV infected patients. *Sex Transm Infect.* 2004;80:315–317.

84. Rudich A, Ben-Romano R, Etzion S, Bashan N. Cellular mechanisms of insulin resistance, lipodystrophy and atherosclerosis induced by HIV protease inhibitors. *Acta Physiol Scand.* 2005;183:75–88.

85. Rumbaugh JA, Nath A. Developments in HIV neuropathogenesis. *Curr Pharm Des.* 2006;12:1023–1044.

86. Rusconi S, Scozzafava A, Mastrolorenzo A, Supuran CT. New advances in HIV entry inhibitors development. *Curr Drug Targets Infect Disord.* 2004;4:339–355.

87. Sacks SL. Famciclovir suppression of asymptomatic and symptomatic recurrent anogenital herpes simplex virus shedding in women: a randomized, double-blind, double-dummy, placebo-controlled, parallel-group, single-center trial. *J Infect Dis.* 2004;189:1341–1347.

88. Sandberg-Wollheim M. Interferon-beta1a treatment for multiple sclerosis. *Expert Rev Neurother.* 2005;5: 25–34.

89. Sandy MC. Herpes zoster: medical and nursing management. *Clin J Oncol Nurs.* 2005;9:443–446.

90. Sax PE, Gathe JC, Jr. Beyond efficacy: the impact of combination antiretroviral therapy on quality of life. *AIDS Patient Care STDS.* 2005;19:563–576.

91. Shafran SD, Tyring SK, Ashton R, et al. Once, twice, or three times daily famciclovir compared with aciclovir for the oral treatment of herpes zoster in immunocompetent adults: a randomized, multicenter, double-blind clinical trial. *J Clin Virol.* 2004;29:248–253.

92. Shehu-Xhilaga M, Tachedjian G, Crowe SM, Kedzierska K. Antiretroviral compounds: mechanisms underlying failure of HAART to eradicate HIV-1. *Curr Med Chem.* 2005;12:1705–1719.

93. Slobod KS, Coleclough C, Bonsignori M, et al. HIV vaccine rationale, design and testing. *Curr HIV Res.* 2005;3:107–112.

94. Sluis-Cremer N, Temiz NA, Bahar I. Conformational changes in HIV-1 reverse transcriptase induced by nonnucleoside reverse transcriptase inhibitor binding. *Curr HIV Res.* 2004;2:323–332.

95. Smith AE, Helenius A. How viruses enter animal cells. *Science.* 2004;304:237–242.

96. Smith PL, Lombardi G, Foster GR. Type I interferons and the innate immune response—more than just antiviral cytokines. *Mol Immunol.* 2005;42: 869–877.

97. Sozen E, Avunduk AM, Akyol N. Comparison of efficacy of oral valacyclovir and topical acyclovir in the treatment of herpes simplex keratitis: a randomized clinical trial. *Chemotherapy.* 2006;52:29–31.

98. Spearman P. Current progress in the development of HIV vaccines. *Curr Pharm Des.* 2006;12:1147–1167.

99. Tantisiriwat W, Powderly WG. Prophylaxis of opportunistic infections. *Infect Dis Clin North Am.* 2000; 14:929–944.

100. Tehranzadeh J, Ter-Oganesyan RR, Steinbach LS. Musculoskeletal disorders associated with HIV infection and AIDS. Part II: non-infectious musculoskeletal conditions. *Skeletal Radiol.* 2004;33:311–320.

101. Thom K, Forrest G. Gastrointestinal infections in immunocompromised hosts. *Curr Opin Gastroenterol.* 2006;22:18–23.

102. Tomasselli AG, Heinrikson RL. Targeting the HIV-protease in AIDS therapy: A current clinical perspective. *Biochem Biophys Acta.* 2000;1477:189–214.

103. Torre F, Campo N, Giusto R, et al. Antiviral activity of amantadine in elderly patients with chronic hepatitis C. *Gerontology.* 2001;47:330–333.

104. Tyring SK, Diaz-Mitoma F, Shafran SD, et al. Oral famciclovir for the suppression of recurrent genital herpes: the combined data from two randomized controlled trials. *J Cutan Med Surg.* 2003;7:449–454.

105. Valentine AD, Meyers CA. Neurobehavioral effects of interferon therapy. *Curr Psychiatry Rep.* 2005; 7:391–395.

106. Ventre K, Randolph A. Ribavirin for respiratory syncytial virus infection of the lower respiratory tract in infants and young children. *Cochrane Database Syst Rev.* 2004;CD000181.

107. Vivet-Boudou V, Didierjean J, Isel C, Marquet R. Nucleoside and nucleotide inhibitors of HIV-1 replication. *Cell Mol Life Sci.* 2006;63:163–186.

108. Wang LX. Toward oligosaccharide- and glycopeptide-based HIV vaccines. *Curr Opin Drug Discov Devel.* 2006;9:194–206.

109. While A, George C, Murgatroyd B. Promoting influenza vaccination in older people: rationale and reality. *Br J Community Nurs.* 2005;10:427–430.

110. Willemot P, Klein MB. Prevention of HIV-associated opportunistic infections and diseases in the age of highly active antiretroviral therapy. *Expert Rev Anti Infect Ther.* 2004;2:521–532.

111. Williams-Aziz SL, Hartline CB, Harden EA, et al. Comparative activities of lipid esters of cidofovir and cyclic cidofovir against replication of herpesviruses in vitro. *Antimicrob Agents Chemother.* 2005; 49:3724–3733.

112. Wolf DL, Rodriguez CA, Mucci M, et al. Pharmacokinetics and renal effects of cidofovir with a reduced dose of probenecid in HIV-infected patients with cytomegalovirus retinitis. *J Clin Pharmacol.* 2003;43: 43–51.

113. Wood C, Harrington W, Jr. AIDS and associated malignancies. *Cell Res.* 2005;15:947–952.

114. Young B. Review: mixing new cocktails: drug interactions in antiretroviral regimens. *AIDS Patient Care STDS.* 2005;19:286–297.

Treatment of Infections III: Antifungal and Antiparasitic Drugs

In addition to bacteria and viruses, several parasitic microorganisms may produce infections in humans. In particular, certain species of fungi, protozoa, and helminths (worms) frequently cause infections in humans. Although some types of parasitic infections are limited or unknown in developed nations such as the United States, parasitic infections generally represent the most common form of disease worldwide. These infections are especially prevalent in tropical and subtropical environments and in impoverished areas of the world where sanitation and hygiene are inadequate. In addition, the incidence of serious fungal and other parasitic infections has been increasing in industrialized nations because of the increased susceptibility of immunocompromised patients, such as patients with acquired immunodeficiency syndrome (AIDS), to these infections.[2,16,70] Hence, the effective pharmacologic treatment of these infections remains an important topic in the global management of disease.

The pharmacologic treatment of parasitic infections is a complex and extensive topic. In this limited space, it is difficult to describe the many species of each parasite, all the diseases caused by parasites, and the chemical methods currently available to selectively destroy various fungi, protozoa, and helminths in humans. Consequently, the general aspects of each type of parasitic infection are reviewed briefly, followed by the primary drugs used to treat specific fungal, protozoal, and helminthic infections. This discussion will acquaint physical therapists and occupational therapists with the nature of these types of infections and the basic chemotherapeutic techniques and agents that are used to treat these problems.

Antifungal Agents

Fungi are plantlike microorganisms that exist ubiquitously throughout the soil and air and in plants and animals. Although abundant in nature (about 100,000 species exist), only a few species produce serious infections in humans.[25,67] A disease caused by fungal infection is also referred to as a *mycosis*. Some fungal infections are relatively local or superficial, affecting cutaneous and mucocutaneous tissue. Examples of common superficial fungal infections include the tinea (ringworm) infections that cause problems such as athlete's foot. Common mucocutaneous fungal infections include candidiasis and yeast infections of vaginal tissues. Other fungal infections are deeper or more systemic. For instance, fungal infections may affect the lungs, central nervous system (CNS), or other tissues and organs throughout the body.[43,44,54]

Often, fungal infections are relatively innocuous because they can be destroyed by the body's normal immune defense mechanisms. However, some infections require pharmacologic treatment, especially if the patient's endogenous defense mechanisms are compromised in some way. For instance, patients undergoing immunosuppressive drug treatment with glucocorticoids or certain antibiotics may develop systemic fungal infections. In addition, diseases that attack the immune system, such as AIDS, leave the patient vulnerable to severe fungal infections (see Chapter 34). Fungal infections that are relatively easy to treat in the immunocompetent person may become invasive and life threatening in those who lack adequate immune function.[11,42] Hence, there is a significant need for effective systemic antifungal agents in certain high-risk patients.

Agents used to treat common fungal infections are listed in Tables 35–1 and 35–2. As indicated in Table 35–1, certain drugs can be administered systemically to treat infections in various tissues. Other agents are more toxic; their use is limited to local or topical application for fungal infections in the skin and mucous membranes (Table 35–2). The use of systemic and topical antifungal agents is addressed in more detail below.

Systemic Antifungal Agents

The antifungal agents that can be administered systemically by oral or intravenous routes are listed here. These agents are often used to treat invasive (deep) fungal infections in the body, or they can be administered systemically to treat more superficial infections that have disseminated over a large area of the skin or subcutaneous tissues. The clinical use, mechanism of action, and potential adverse effects of these drugs are addressed here.

Amphotericin B

Clinical Use. Amphotericin B (Amphocin, Fungizone Intravenous) is one of the primary drugs used to treat severe systemic fungal infections.[26,39] This drug is often chosen to treat systemic infections and meningitis caused by *Candida*, *Cryptococcus*, and several other

Table 35–1	USE OF SYSTEMIC ANTIFUNGAL AGENTS IN INVASIVE AND DISSEMINATED MYCOSES*		
Type of Infection	**Principal Sites of Infection**	**Principal Agent(s)**	**Secondary/Alternative Agent(s)**
Aspergillosis	Lungs, other organs, body orifices	Amphotericin B	Itraconazole, voriconazole
Blastomycosis	Lungs, skin; may disseminate to other tissues	Amphotericin B	Itraconazole
Candidiasis	Intestinal tract, skin, mucous membranes (mouth, pharynx, vagina)	Amphotericin B, fluconazole	Caspofungin, flucytosine, itraconazole
Coccidioidomycosis	Lungs, skin, subcutaneous tissues; may form disseminated lesions throughout the body	Amphotericin B	Fluconazole, itraconazole
Cryptococcosis	Lungs, meninges, other tissues	Amphotericin B, fluconazole	Flucytosine, itraconazole
Histoplasmosis	Lungs, spleen	Amphotericin B	Itraconazole
Tinea (ringworm) infections	Skin, subcutaneous tissues	Griseofulvin	Itraconazole, terbinafine

*Drugs indicated here are administered systemically (orally, intravenously) to treat widespread or invasive fungal infections. Some of these agents are also available in topical preparations, especially in the treatment of candidiasis and tinea infections in the skin and mucocutaneous tissues (see text). Selection of a specific drug or preparation will also depend on patient-specific factors, such as immune function, age, pregnancy, and identification of resistant fungal species.

Table 35–2	TOPICAL ANTIFUNGALS		
Generic Name	**Trade Name**	**Type of Preparation**	**Primary Indication(s)**
Azoles			
Butoconazole	Femstat 3	Vaginal cream; vaginal suppositories	Vulvovaginal candidiasis
Clotrimazole	Gyne-Lotrimin; Fem-Care; others	Vaginal cream; vaginal tablets	Vulvovaginal candidiasis
	Mycelex Troches	Lozenges	Oropharyngeal candidiasis
	Mycelex Creme; Lotrim-in; others	Cream; lotion; solution	Cutaneous candidiasis, tinea (ringworm) infections
Econazole	Spectazole	Cream	Cutaneous candidiasis, tinea (ringworm) infections
Miconazole	Femizol-M; Monistat; others	Vaginal cream; vaginal suppositories; vaginal tampons	Vulvovaginal candidiasis
Oxiconazole	Oxistat	Cream; lotion	Tinea (ringworm) infections
Sulconazole	Exelderm	Cream; solution	Tinea (ringworm) infections
Terconazole	Terazol	Vaginal cream; vaginal suppositories	Vulvovaginal candidiasis
Tioconazole	Monistat 1; Vagistat-1	Vaginal ointment; vaginal suppositories	Vulvovaginal candidiasis
Other Topical Agents			
Butenafine	Mentax	Cream	Tinea (ringworm) infections
Naftifine	Naftin	Cream; gel	Tinea (ringworm) infections
Nystatin	Mycostatin; Nilstat; others	Lozenges; oral suspension; tablets	Oropharyngeal candidiasis
	Mycostatin; Nilstat; Nystex	Cream; ointment; powder	Cutaneous and mucocutaneous candidiasis
	Generic	Vaginal cream; vaginal tablets	Vulvovaginal candidiasis
Tolnaftate	Aftate; Tinactin; many others	Aerosol powder; aerosol solution; powder; solution	Tinea (ringworm) infections

Note: Drugs listed here are only available in topical or local preparations. Certain systemic agents listed in Table 35–1 can also be applied locally to treat various superficial fungal infections.

species of pathogenic fungi (see Table 35–1). Amphotericin is also effective against certain protozoal infection such as leishmaniasis.[5] Typically, this drug is administered by slow intravenous infusion. Local and topical administration may also be used to treat limited infections caused by susceptible fungi.

Several newer forms of amphotericin B (Abelcet, AmBisome, Amphotec) have also been developed. These drugs are encapsulated in small lipid spheres (liposomes) and then injected slowly by intravenous infusion.[26,57] The lipid-based preparations appear to deliver higher doses of amphotericin B to the site of fungal infections more directly, thereby reducing the risk of adverse effects such as renal toxicity.[20,29] Clinical studies suggest that these lipid forms can therefore be used to treat serious fungal infections while reducing the risk of nephrotoxicity and other side effects.[39]

Mechanism of Action. Amphotericin B appears to work by binding to specific steroidlike lipids (sterols) located in the cell membrane of susceptible fungi.[7] This binding causes increased permeability in the cell membrane, leading to a leaky membrane and loss of cellular components.

Adverse Effects. The effectiveness of amphotericin B against serious systemic fungal infections is tempered somewhat by a high incidence of side effects.[39] Most patients experience problems such as headache, fever, muscle and joint pain, muscle weakness, and gastrointestinal distress (nausea, vomiting, stomach pain or cramping). As indicated, nephrotoxicity may also occur in some patients, but the use of the lipid-based formulations of this drug may reduce this risk. Considering the life-threatening nature of some fungal infections such as meningitis, certain side effects of amphotericin B must often be tolerated while the drug exerts its antifungal actions.

Fluconazole

Clinical Use. Fluconazole (Diflucan) can be administered orally to treat serious systemic fungal infections.[15] This drug is often the primary treatment for urinary tract infections, pneumonia, and infections of the mouth and esophagus caused by the *Candida* species of fungus.[19,63] This agent may also be used to treat cryptococcal meningitis and may help prevent recurrence of cryptococcal infections in patients with AIDS. Fluconazole is somewhat less toxic than more traditional agents such as amphotericin B, and can be administered orally, which is an advantage over amphotericin B.

There is some concern, however, about fluconazole's effectiveness in treating deep, systemic fungal infections in severely ill patients.[35] Hence, this drug can be combined with other antifungals such as amphotericin B to provide optimal treatment for certain cases of candidiasis and other severe fungal infections.[4]

Mechanism of Action. Fluconazole and similar agents (itraconazole, ketoconazole) inhibit certain enzymes in fungal cells that are responsible for the synthesis of important sterols.[9,15] A deficiency of these sterols results in impaired membrane function and other metabolic abnormalities within the fungal cell. Fluconazole also directly damages the fungal membrane by destroying certain membrane components such as triglycerides and phospholipids. Loss of normal membrane structure and function results in the destruction of the fungus.

Adverse Effects. Hepatotoxicity is the most serious adverse effect of fluconazole; this drug should be used cautiously in patients with impaired liver function. Other common side effects include headache and gastrointestinal disturbances (abdominal pain, nausea, vomiting).

Flucytosine

Clinical Use. The antifungal spectrum of flucytosine (Ancobon) is limited primarily to the *Candida* and *Cryptococcus* species.[7] This drug is used systemically to treat endocarditis, urinary tract infections, and the presence of fungi in the bloodstream (fungemia) during candidiasis. Flucytosine is also used to treat meningitis and severe pulmonary infections caused by cryptococcosis. This drug is often combined with amphotericin B to provide optimal effects and to decrease the chance of fungal resistance.[4,8]

Mechanism of Action. Flucytosine is incorporated into susceptible fungi, where it undergoes enzymatic conversion to fluorouracil,[7] which acts as an antimetabolite during RNA synthesis in the fungus. Fluorouracil is incorporated into RNA chains but acts as a false nucleic acid. This event ultimately impairs protein synthesis, thus disrupting the normal function of the fungus.

Adverse Effects. Flucytosine may cause hepatotoxicity and may also impair bone marrow function, resulting in anemia, leukopenia, and several other blood dyscrasias.[69] This drug may also produce severe gastrointestinal disturbances, including nausea, vomiting, diarrhea, and loss of appetite.

Griseofulvin

Clinical Use. Griseofulvin (Fulvicin, Grisactin, other names) is used primarily in the treatment of common fungal infections of the skin known as tinea, or ringworm.[33,56] For example, this drug is administered to treat fungal infections of the feet (tinea pedis, or "athlete's foot"), infections in the groin area (tinea cruris, or "jock rash"), and similar infections of the skin, nails, and scalp. Griseofulvin is administered orally.

Mechanism of Action. Griseofulvin enters susceptible fungal cells and binds to the mitotic spindle during cell division.[9] This binding impairs the mitotic process, thus directly inhibiting the ability of the cell to replicate itself.

Adverse Effects. Common side effects of griseofulvin administration include headaches—which may be severe—and gastrointestinal disturbances (nausea, vomiting, diarrhea). Some individuals may exhibit hypersensitivity to this drug as evidenced by skin rashes. Skin photosensitivity (increased reaction to ultraviolet light) may also occur.

Itraconazole

Clinical Use. Itraconazole (Sporanox) is an azole antifungal agent that is effective against many systemic fungal infections.[64] For example, this drug is used to treat blastomycosis and histoplasmosis infections in the lungs and other tissues, especially in patients with a compromised immune system.[10,37] Itraconazole may also be used as the primary or alternative treatment for other fungal infections, such as aspergillosis, chromomycosis, coccidioidomycosis, and various infections caused by the *Candida* species. Like fluconazole, itraconazole can be administered orally and can be given intravenously in severe systemic infections.[64]

Mechanism of Action. Itraconazole works like fluconazole and similar azoles. These drugs disrupt membrane function of the fungal cell by inhibiting the synthesis of key membrane components such as sterols, and by directly damaging other membrane components such as phospholipids. Impaired membrane function leads to metabolic abnormalities and subsequent death of the fungal cell.

Adverse Effects. Side effects associated with itraconazole include headache, gastrointestinal disturbances (nausea, vomiting), and skin rash.

Ketoconazole

Clinical Use. Ketoconazole (Nizoral) is used to treat a variety of superficial and deep fungal infections.[9,35,72] This drug can be administered orally to treat pulmonary and systemic infections in candidiasis, coccidioidomycosis, histoplasmosis, and several other types of deep fungal infections. Oral administration is also used to treat tinea infections of the skin, scalp, and other body areas. Ketoconazole is available in topical preparations for the treatment of tinea infections and other relatively localized infections, including certain vaginal infections.

Mechanism of Action. Ketoconazole selectively inhibits certain enzymes that are responsible for the synthesis of important sterols in fungal cells.[9] A deficiency of sterols results in impaired membrane function and other metabolic abnormalities within the fungal cell. At higher concentrations, ketoconazole may also directly disrupt the cell membrane, resulting in the destruction of the fungus.

Adverse Effects. Gastrointestinal disturbances (nausea, vomiting, stomach pain) are the most common adverse effects when ketoconazole is administered systemically. Some degree of hepatotoxicity may occur, and severe or even fatal hepatitis has been reported on rare occasions. In large, prolonged dosages, this drug may also impair testosterone and adrenocorticosteroid synthesis, resulting in breast tenderness and enlargement (gynecomastia) and decreased sex drive in some men. Because of these side effects, other drugs such as itraconazole have largely replaced systemic use of ketoconazole.

Echinocandins

Clinical Use. Echinocandins comprise a relatively new group of antifungals that includes drugs such as caspofungin (Cancidas) and micafungin (Mycamine).[7] These drugs are administered intravenously to treat severe esophageal infections caused by *Candida*. Caspofungin is also used to treat systemic aspergillosis infections in patients who cannot tolerate other drugs such as amphotericin B or fluconazole.[45] Other echinocandin drugs are currently being developed, and their use may expand in the future if newer agents reach the market.

Mechanism of Action. These drugs inhibit the glucan synthase enzyme that is responsible for the biosynthesis of beta-D-glucan—a component of the fungal cell membrane.[45] Loss of this membrane component disrupts the integrity of the fungal cell wall, resulting in death of the fungus.

Adverse Effects. Primary side effects of caspofungin and micafungin include gastrointestinal disturbances (nausea, vomiting) and headache. Some local irritation may also occur at the injection site when these drugs are administered intravenously.

Terbinafine

Clinical Use. Terbinafine (Lamisil) is effective against a broad spectrum of fungi and can be administered systemically to treat infections in the toenails and fingernails (onychomycosis) that are caused by various fungi.[17,30] Oral administration of this drug may also be useful in treating ringworm infections such as tinea corporis, tinea capitis (ringworm of the scalp), and tinea cruris, especially if these infections do not respond to topical treatment. Terbinafine is likewise available in creams and solutions for topical treatment of various tinea infections, including tinea pedis and tinea versicolor.

Mechanism of Action. Terbinafine inhibits a specific enzyme (squalene epoxidase) that is responsible for sterol synthesis in the fungal cell membrane. This action impairs cell wall synthesis, with subsequent loss of cell membrane function and integrity. Inhibition of this enzyme causes squalene to accumulate in the fungal cell, which can also impair cell function and lead to death of the fungus.

Adverse Effects. Systemic administration of terbinafine may cause a hypersensitivity reaction (skin rashes, itching) and gastrointestinal problems such as nausea, vomiting, and diarrhea. This drug may also cause a change or loss of taste, an effect that may last several weeks after the drug is discontinued. Topical administration is generally well tolerated, although signs of local irritation (itching, redness, peeling skin) may indicate a need to discontinue this drug.

Voriconazole

Clinical Use. Voriconazole (Vfend) is similar chemically to other azole antifungals such as fluconazole. Voriconazole has a broad antifungal spectrum, and is administered systemically to treat aspergillosis and other serious fungal infections caused by *Scedosporium apiospermum* and *Fusarium*.[31]

Mechanism of Action. Voriconazole inhibits sterol biosynthesis in fungal cell membranes.[53] That is, this drug acts like fluconazole and similar agents to impair membrane synthesis, which results in membrane integrity loss and death of the fungal cell.

Adverse Effects. Skin rashes and vision disturbances (blurred vision, seeing bright spots) are common during voriconazole administration, but these side effects are usually transient and fairly uneventful. Serious problems, such as liver toxicity and cardiac arrhythmias, may occur in susceptible patients.

Topical Antifungal Agents

As mentioned earlier, certain antifungals are too toxic to be administered systemically, but these drugs can be applied topically to treat fungal infections in the skin and mucous membranes. These drugs are therefore commonly used to treat various fungal infections in the skin (dermatophytosis), including tinea infections such as tinea pedis and tinea cruris.[38] These drugs can also be applied locally to treat *Candida* infections in the mucous membranes of the mouth, pharynx, and vagina. The primary topical antifungals are listed in Table 35–2, and are addressed briefly below.

Topical Azole Antifungals

Clinical Use. Azole antifungals that are administered topically include clotrimazole, miconazole, and other topical agents listed in Table 35–2. These drugs are related to the systemic azoles (fluconazole, itraconazole, ketoconazole; see earlier) and share a common chemical background, mechanism of action, and antifungal spectrum. The topical azoles, however, are too toxic for systemic use and are therefore restricted to local application. Nonetheless, these drugs are valuable in controlling fungal infections in the skin and mucocutaneous tissues (see Table 35–2). For example, azoles such as butoconazole, clotrimazole, miconazole, terconazole, and tioconazole can be applied via creams, ointments, and suppositories to treat vaginal *Candida* infections. Other agents such as econazole, oxiconazole, and sulconazole can be applied via creams, solutions, or powders to treat tinea infections that cause athlete's foot (tinea pedis) and jock rash (tinea cruris). Certain azoles can also be applied locally via lozenges or elixirs (syrups) to treat oral candidiasis infections that occur in patients with a compromised immune system (see Table 35–2). Hence, these agents are used to treat local mycoses that occur in a variety of clinical situations.

Mechanism of Action. Like the systemic azoles, clotrimazole and other topical antifungal azoles work by inhibiting the synthesis of key components of the fungal cell membrane; that is, these drugs impair production of membrane sterols, triglycerides, and phospholipids.[9] Loss of these components results in the membrane's inability to maintain intracellular homeostasis, leading to death of the fungus.

Adverse Effects. There are relatively few side effects when these drugs are applied locally. Gastrointestinal distress (cramps, diarrhea, vomiting) can occur if azole lozenges are swallowed. Other problems associated with topical use include local burning or irritation of the skin or mucous membranes.

Other Topical Agents

Clinical Use. Other topical antifungals include nystatin (Mycostatin, Nilstat, others), naftifine (Naftin), butenafine (Mentax), and tolnaftate (Aftate, Tinactin, other names) (see Table 35–2).

Nystatin has a wide spectrum of activity against various fungi, but is not used to treat systemic infections because it is not absorbed from the gastrointestinal tract. Therefore, nystatin is administered via several topical preparations to treat cutaneous, oropharyngeal, or vaginal candidiasis. Topical and local (oropharyngeal) use of nystatin is especially important in treating candidiasis in immunocompromised patients, including patients with AIDS.[1]

Naftifine, tolnaftate, and butenafine are used primarily to treat local and superficial cases of tinea infection. These agents are found in several over-the-counter products that are administered topically to treat tinea infections such as tinea pedis and tinea cruris.

Mechanism of Action. Nystatin exerts its antifungal effects in a manner similar to that of amphotericin B; that is, this drug binds to sterols in the cell membrane, which causes an increase in membrane permeability and a loss of cellular homeostasis. Naftifine and butenafine inhibit a fungal enzyme (squalene epoxidase) that is responsible for the synthesis of a key membrane component (ergosterol), resulting in the loss of membrane integrity and death of the fungus. Tolnaftate appears to stunt the growth of fungal cell bodies, but the exact mechanism of this drug is unknown.

Adverse Effects. Nystatin is generally well tolerated when applied locally. Systemic absorption through mucous membranes may cause some gastrointestinal disturbances (nausea, vomiting, diarrhea), but these side effects are generally mild and transient. Topical use of butenafine, naftifine, and tolnaftate is likewise safe, although local burning and irritation of the skin may occur in some individuals.

Antiprotozoal Agents

Protozoa are single-celled organisms that represent the lowest division of the animal kingdom. Of the several thousand species of protozoa, approximately 35 represent a threat of parasitic infection in humans.[25]

One relatively common disease caused by protozoal infection is malaria. Malaria is caused by several species of a protozoan parasite known as plasmodia. Although this disease has been virtually eliminated in North America and Europe, malaria continues to be a primary health problem throughout many other parts of the world.[44] Individuals who live in these areas, as well as those traveling to parts of the world where malaria is prevalent, must often undergo antimalarial chemotherapy. Hence, drugs that prevent and treat malaria are extremely important.

In addition to malaria, several other serious infections may occur in humans due to parasitic invasion by protozoa.[2,44] Severe intestinal infections (dysentery) produced by various protozoa occur quite frequently, especially in areas where contaminated food and drinking water are prevalent. Infections in tissues such as the liver, heart, lungs, brain, and other organs may also occur because of protozoal infestation. As mentioned in this chapter's introduction, individuals with a compromised immune system may be especially susceptible to these intestinal and extraintestinal infections.[2,70]

The primary agents used to treat protozoal infections are listed in Tables 35–3 and 35–4, and each agent is described subsequently. Drugs that are primarily used to treat and prevent malaria are grouped together, followed by drugs that are used to treat other types of protozoal infections (intestinal and extraintestinal infections).

Antimalarial Agents

Chloroquine

Clinical Use. Historically, chloroquine (Aralen) has been one of the primary antimalarial drugs.[27] This drug provides a safe, effective, and relatively inexpensive method for treating malaria, and is also administered routinely to individuals who are traveling to areas of the world where they may be exposed to malaria infection.[49] Resistance to this drug, however, has emerged in many areas of the world where malaria is prevalent.[55] That is, the parasite that causes this disease (the *Plasmodium* amoeba) has developed mechanisms that render this drug ineffective. If these chloroquine-resistant strains are encountered, other antimalarial drugs such as quinine or artemisinin derivatives must be used (see Table 35–3).[21]

Table 35–3	TREATMENT OF MALARIA	
Type of Malaria	**Primary Agent(s)**	**Adjunctive/Alternative Agent(s)**
Chloroquine-sensitive	Chloroquine	Primaquine
Chloroquine-resistant	Quinine	Artemisinin derivatives Atovaquone-proguanil Mefloquine Pyrimethamine-sulfadoxine Antibacterials (e.g., clindamycin, doxycycline, sulfamethoxazole, or tetracycline)

Chloroquine is also used for the treatment of conditions other than malaria. This drug is effective against other types of protozoal infections such as amebiasis and may be used with iodoquinol or emetine to treat infections in the liver and pericardium. As discussed in Chapter 16, chloroquine is effective in rheumatoid disease and is used in the treatment of conditions such as rheumatoid arthritis and systemic lupus erythe-

Table 35–4	TREATMENT OF OTHER PROTOZOAL INFECTIONS		
Type of Infection	**Principal Site(s) of Infection**	**Primary Agent(s)**	**Alternative/Secondary Agent(s)**
Amebiasis	Intestinal tract; liver; lungs	Metronidazole	Dehydroemetine, iodoquinol, tinidazole, antibacterials (paromomycin, tetracylcine)
Balantidiasis	Lower gastrointestinal tract	Iodoquinol (tetracycline antibiotics are also effective)	Metronidazole
Giardiasis	Small intestine	Metronidazole	Albendazole, paromomycin, nitazoxanide, tinidazole
Leishmaniasis	Skin; mucocutaneous tissues; viscera	Amphotericin B	Itraconazole, ketoconazole pentamidine, sodium stibogluconate
Trichomoniasis	Vagina; genitourinary tract	Metronidazole	Tinidazole
Toxoplasmosis	Lymph nodes; many organs and tissues	Pyrimethamine-sulfadiazine (see antimalarial drugs); other antibacterials (clindamycin)	Trimethoprim-sulfamethoxazole ± another agent (azithromycin, clarithromycin, atovaquone, or dapsone)
Trypanosomiasis (Chagas disease; African sleeping sickness)	Heart; brain; many other organs	Early stages: pentamidine, suramin Later stages: melarsoprol	Nifurtimox

matosus. However, the reasons why this antiprotozoal agent is also effective against rheumatoid disease are unclear. Chloroquine is administered orally.

Mechanism of Action. Although the exact mechanism is unknown, chloroquine may impair metabolic and digestive function in the protozoa by becoming concentrated within subcellular vacuoles and raising the pH of these vacuoles.[65] This effect may inhibit the ability of the parasite to digest hemoglobin from the blood of the host erythrocytes. Impaired hemoglobin digestion leads to the accumulation of toxic heme by-products in the protozoa, which subsequently leads to death of this parasite.[28] Chloroquine may also bind directly to DNA within susceptible parasites and inhibit DNA/RNA function and subsequent protein synthesis. The ability to impair protein synthesis may contribute to the antiprotozoal actions of this drug.

Adverse Effects. The most serious problem associated with chloroquine is the possibility of toxicity to the retina and subsequent visual disturbances. This issue is usually insignificant, however, when this drug is used for short periods in relatively low doses (see Chapter 16). Other relatively mild side effects may occur, including gastrointestinal distress (nausea, vomiting, stomach cramps, diarrhea), behavior and mood changes (irritability, confusion, nervousness, depression), and skin disorders (rashes, itching, discoloration).

Hydroxychloroquine

Hydroxychloroquine (Plaquenil) is derived chemically from chloroquine and is similar to it in clinical use, mechanism of action, and adverse effects. Hydroxychloroquine does not have any distinct therapeutic advantages over chloroquine, but it may be substituted in certain individuals who do not respond well to chloroquine.

Mefloquine

Clinical Use. Mefloquine (Lariam) has emerged as one of the most important antimalarial agents.[61] This drug is especially important in the prevention and treatment of malaria that is resistant to traditional antimalarial drugs such as chloroquine and quinine.[50] Mefloquine is often the drug of choice for antimalarial prophylaxis, especially in areas of the world where chloroquine-resistant strains of malaria are common.[23] Mefloquine can be used alone, but combining this

drug with other antimalarials such as an artemisinin derivative may provide more effective treatment against malaria.[14]

Mechanism of Action. Although the drug's exact mechanism of action is unknown, mefloquine may exert antimalarial effects similar to chloroquine; that is, these drugs inhibit hemoglobin digestion in malarial parasites, thus causing heme by-products to accumulate within the protozoa and cause toxicity and death of this parasite.[65]

Adverse Effects. Mefloquine is safe and well tolerated when used at moderate doses to prevent malarial infection. At higher doses, such as those used to treat infection, mefloquine may cause dizziness, headache, fever, joint and muscle pain, and gastrointestinal problems (abdominal pain, nausea, vomiting, diarrhea). These side effects, however, may be difficult to distinguish from the symptoms associated with malaria. Although rare, neuropsychiatric symptoms such as confusion, psychosis, and seizures may occur, especially when this drug is used at higher dosages for prolonged periods.[60]

Primaquine

Clinical Use. Primaquine is typically used to treat the relapses of specific forms of malaria,[12] and is generally administered in acute or severe exacerbations, or when other drugs (chloroquine, mefloquine) are ineffective in suppressing malarial attacks. Primaquine may also be used to prevent the onset of malaria in individuals who are especially at risk because of prolonged exposure to the disease.[50] This drug is administered orally.

Mechanism of Action. Primaquine appears to impair DNA function in susceptible parasites. The exact manner in which this occurs is unknown.

Adverse Effects. Gastrointestinal disturbances (nausea, vomiting, abdominal pain), headache, and visual disturbances may occur during primaquine therapy. A more serious side effect, acute hemolytic anemia, may occur in patients who have a specific deficiency in the enzyme glucose-6-phosphate dehydrogenase. This enzymatic deficiency is genetic, and is more common in certain individuals of African, Mediterranean, and Asian descent; hence there is an increased risk of hemolytic anemia in these groups.[61] People with specific cases of this enzyme deficiency should be identified so that alternative antimalarial drugs can be used.[34]

Pyrimethamine

Clinical Use. When used alone, pyrimethamine (Daraprim) is only of minor use in treating and preventing malaria. However, the antimalarial effectiveness of pyrimethamine is increased dramatically by combining it with the antibacterial drug sulfadoxine.[61] The combination of these two drugs (known commercially as Fansidar) has been used to prevent or treat certain forms of chloroquine-resistant malaria (see Table 35–3).[61] Regrettably, resistance to pyrimethamine/sulfadoxine treatment has also increased in many areas to the point where this drug combination is no longer effective.[62]

Pyrimethamine may also be combined with other antimalarials such as artemisinin derivatives, but these regimens should only be used if the malarial parasites are not resistant to the specific drugs in the regimen.[13] Pyrimethamine can also be combined with a sulfonamide drug such as dapsone, sulfadiazine, or sulfamethoxazole to treat protozoal infections that cause toxoplasmosis, or fungal infections that cause *Pneumocystis* pneumonia. These agents are administered orally.

Mechanism of Action. Pyrimethamine blocks the production of folic acid in susceptible protozoa by inhibiting the function of the dihydrofolate reductase enzyme. Folic acid helps catalyze the production of nucleic and amino acids in these parasites. Therefore, this drug ultimately impairs nucleic acid and protein synthesis by interfering with folic acid production. The action of sulfadoxine and other sulfonamide antibacterial agents was discussed in Chapter 33. These agents also inhibit folic acid synthesis in certain bacterial and protozoal cells.

Adverse Effects. The incidence and severity of side effects from pyrimethamine-sulfadoxine are related to the dosage and duration of therapy. Toxicity is fairly common when these drugs are given in high dosages for prolonged periods, and adverse effects include gastrointestinal disturbances (vomiting, stomach cramps, loss of appetite), blood dyscrasias (agranulocytosis, leukopenia, thrombocytopenia), CNS abnormalities (tremors, ataxia, seizures), and hypersensitivity reactions (skin rashes, anaphylaxis, liver dysfunction). As indicated above, resistance may also occur during repeated use, and this drug strategy may be ineffective in certain strains of malaria that have already developed resistant mechanisms. Hence, pyrimethamine-sulfadoxine is usually administered on a very limited basis, such as a single dose at the onset of malarial symptoms.

Quinine

Clinical Use. Quinine is one of the oldest forms of antimalarial chemotherapy, having been obtained from the bark of certain South American trees as early as the 1600s.[61] Although quinine was the principal method of preventing and treating malaria for many years, the use of this drug has diminished somewhat because it is relatively toxic and expensive to produce.[61] Hence, the routine use of this drug has largely been replaced by newer, safer agents such as mefloquine and artemisinin derivatives. Quinine, however, remains one of the most effective antimalarial drugs and is currently used to treat severe malaria that is resistant to other drugs.[40,68] Quinine sulfate is administered orally, and quinine dihydrochloride is administered by slow intravenous infusion.

Mechanism of Action. The exact mechanism of quinine is not known. This drug probably exerts antimalarial effects similar to those of chloroquine—that is, inhibition of hemoglobin digestion and subsequent accumulation of toxic heme by-products that lead to death in susceptible protozoa.[22]

Adverse Effects. Quinine is associated with many adverse effects involving several primary organ systems. This drug may produce disturbances in the CNS (headache, visual disturbances, ringing in the ears), gastrointestinal system (nausea, vomiting, abdominal pain), and cardiovascular system (cardiac arrhythmias). Problems with hypersensitivity, blood disorders, liver dysfunction, and hypoglycemia may also occur in some individuals.

Other Antimalarials: Use of Artemisinin Derivatives

Clinical Use. Artemisinin derivatives are naturally occurring compounds that appear to be effective against many forms of the protozoa that cause malaria.[71] These drugs consist of the parent compound (artemisinin) and several products that can be synthesized from artemisinin such as artesunate, artemether, and dihydroartemisinin.[61] It does not appear that any one derivative is superior to another in treating malaria, hence the term artemisinin derivative can be used to collectively describe this group.[71] These agents act rapidly and appear to be effective against all malarial parasites that infect humans.[55] Moreover, resistance to artemisinin derivatives has not yet emerged, so these drugs have moved to the forefront as primary antimalarial agents, especially in parts of the world where resistance to traditional drugs is problematic.[71] Artemisinin derivatives can likewise be used alone or combined with other antimalarials (e.g., mefloquine or piperaquine) to improve efficacy and reduce the chance of drug resistance.[3,18]

Mechanism of Action. Artemisinin derivatives appear to work by a two-step process occurring within the malarial parasite.[46] In the first step, the drug is activated when it is cleaved by the heme-iron component within the protozoa. This cleavage forms a highly reactive free radical that, in the second step, reacts with and destroys essential protozoal proteins.[46] Destruction of these proteins results in the loss of cellular function and subsequent death of the protozoa.

Adverse Effects. Because these drugs are fairly new, the potential for side effects remains to be determined fully. Studies on animals suggested that these drugs may be neurotoxic, but this effect has not been proven conclusively in humans.[46] Future research should help determine the relative risks and benefits of these agents, as well as how artemisinin derivatives can complement other drugs in the antimalarial armamentarium.

Drugs Used to Treat Protozoal Infections in the Intestines and Other Tissues

Atovaquone

Clinical Use. Atovaquone (Mepron) is used primarily to treat the protozoon that causes toxoplasmosis and the fungus that causes pneumocystis pneumonia in immunocompromised patients.[6] This drug is not typically the primary treatment for pneumocystis, but is often reserved for patients who cannot tolerate more traditional treatments using sulfamethoxazole and trimethoprim (see Chapter 34) or pentamidine (see later). Atovaquone can also be used to prevent and treat resistant cases of malaria, and the antimalarial effects of this drug seem especially useful when combined with proguanil.[48]

Mechanism of Action. Atovaquone appears to selectively inhibit electron transport in susceptible microorganisms.[6] This inhibition directly decreases production of ATP in the microorganism and may interfere with nucleic acid synthesis, ultimately resulting in death of the parasite.

Adverse Effects. Atovaquone may cause side effects such as fever, skin rash, cough, headache, and gastrointestinal problems (nausea, vomiting, diarrhea).

Emetine and Dehydroemetine

Clinical Use. Emetine and dehydroemetine (Mebadin) are used primarily to treat protozoal infections in the intestinal tract and extraintestinal sites such as the lungs and liver. These drugs are powerful amebicides and are generally reserved for severe, acute cases of intestinal amebiasis (dysentery).[51] Because of the potential for adverse effects, these drugs are no longer marketed in the United States, and safer agents like metronidazole are often used in their place. Emetine and dehydroemetine are typically administered by deep subcutaneous injection or intramuscular injection.

Mechanism of Action. These drugs exert a direct effect on susceptible protozoa by causing degeneration of subcellular components such as the nucleus and reticular system within the parasite.

Adverse Effects. As indicated earlier, the effectiveness of emetine and dehydroemetine is limited by a number of potentially serious side effects. In particular, problems with cardiotoxicity may occur, as reflected by arrhythmias, palpitations, and other changes in cardiac conduction and excitability. Gastrointestinal disturbances such as diarrhea, nausea, and vomiting are also quite common. Generalized muscular aches and weakness may occur, as well as localized myositis near the site of administration. Hence, these drugs are administered under close medical supervision and are withdrawn as soon as the amebicidal effects are apparent.

Iodoquinol

Clinical Use. Iodoquinol (Diquinol, Yodoxin, other names) is used primarily to treat protozoal infections within the intestinal tract,[51] and it is often combined with a second tissue amebicide, which kills protozoa at extraintestinal sites. For instance, iodoquinol may be combined with metronidazole to ensure the destruction of parasites throughout the body. Iodoquinol is usually administered orally. Because iodoquinol is relatively toxic, the routine use of this drug has been replaced somewhat by other agents such as paromomycin, which may be somewhat safer.

Mechanism of Action. The mechanism of action of iodoquinol as an amebicide is unknown.

Adverse Effects. Iodoquinol is neurotoxic and may produce optic and peripheral neuropathies when administered in large dosages for prolonged periods. Problems with muscle weakness and ataxia may also occur because of the neurotoxic effects of this drug.

Other adverse effects include gastrointestinal distress (nausea, vomiting, cramps) and various skin reactions (rashes, itching, discoloration), but these effects are relatively mild and transient.

Metronidazole

Clinical Use. Metronidazole (Flagyl, Protostat, other names) is effective against a broad spectrum of protozoa and is often the primary agent used against protozoal infections in intestinal and extraintestinal tissues.[51] Metronidazole is often the drug of choice for treating several intestinal infections (amebiasis, giardiasis) and amebic abscesses in other tissues such as the liver. Metronidazole is also the primary drug used to treat trichomoniasis, a sexually transmitted protozoal disease affecting the vagina and male genitourinary tract.[59]

As indicated in Chapter 33, metronidazole has bactericidal effects and is used in certain gram-negative bacterial infections. This drug may be administered orally or intravenously. Other agents have also been developed that are structurally and functionally similar to metronidazole. Tinidazole (Tindamax), for example, can be used in cases where metronidazole is not tolerated or is ineffective.[24]

Mechanism of Action. The exact mechanism of action of metronidazole is not known. It is believed that this drug is reduced chemically within the parasitic cell to a metabolite that impairs nucleic acid and DNA synthesis.[32] The exact nature of this metabolite, however, and other features of the cytotoxic effects of this drug remain to be determined.

Adverse Effects. Gastrointestinal disturbances including nausea, vomiting, diarrhea, stomach pain, and an unpleasant taste in the mouth are relatively common with metronidazole. Other adverse effects such as hypersensitivity reactions, peripheral neuropathy, hematologic abnormalities, and genitourinary problems have been reported, but their incidence is relatively low.

Nitazoxanide

Clinical Use. Nitazoxanide (Alinia) is a relatively new agent that is used primarily to treat diarrhea caused by intestinal cryptosporidia and giardia infections.[51] This drug is approved for use in children aged 1 to 11, and is administered orally.

Mechanism of Action. Nitazoxanide appears to inhibit electron transport in susceptible protozoa, thus inhibiting energy metabolism in these parasites. This drug may have other antiprotozoal effects that remain to be determined.

Adverse Effects. This drug is generally well tolerated. Gastrointestinal disturbances (vomiting, diarrhea) and headache have been reported, but these effects may be due to the intestinal infection rather than the drug.

Paromomycin

Clinical Use. Paromomycin (Humatin) is an aminoglycoside antibacterial (see Chapter 33) that is used primarily to treat mild to moderate intestinal infections (amebiasis).[51] This drug may also be used as an adjunct to other amebicides during the treatment of more severe protozoal infections. Paromomycin is also effective against some bacteria and tapeworms, and may be used as a secondary agent in certain bacterial or helminthic infections. This drug is administered orally.

Mechanism of Action. Paromomycin acts selectively on protozoa within the intestinal lumen and destroys these parasites by a direct toxic effect.

Adverse Effects. Paromomycin is not absorbed from the intestine to any great extent, so adverse effects are fairly limited. Nonetheless, problems with gastrointestinal distress (nausea, vomiting, abdominal pain) may occur as this drug exerts amebicidal effects within the intestine.

Pentamidine

Clinical Use. Pentamidine (Nebupent, Pentam, other names) is effective against several types of extraintestinal protozoal infections, including certain forms of trypanosomiasis (African sleeping sickness) and visceral infections caused by Leishmania protozoa. Typically, pentamidine is reserved as a secondary agent in treating these infections and is used when the principal drug in each case is not available or is tolerated poorly (see Table 35–4). Use of this drug as a primary agent has increased, however, in the treatment of pneumocystis infections in patients with AIDS.[51] This drug is usually administered by parenteral routes such as deep intramuscular injection or slow intravenous infusion. Pentamidine may also be administered by oral inhalation to treat lung infections, and this strategy is now commonly used as prophylaxis and treatment of pneumocystis pneumonia in patients with AIDS.[47]

Mechanism of Action. The exact mechanism of this drug is not clear, and pentamidine may affect different parasites in different ways. Some possible antiprotozoal actions of this drug include the inhibition of protein and nucleic acid synthesis, cellular metabolism, and oxidative phosphorylation in susceptible parasites.

Adverse Effects. The primary adverse effect of systemic pentamidine administration is renal toxicity. Renal function may be markedly impaired in some patients, but kidney function usually returns to normal when the drug is withdrawn. Other adverse effects include hypotension, hypoglycemia, gastrointestinal distress, blood dyscrasias (leukopenia, thrombocytopenia), and local pain and tenderness at the site of injection. Adverse effects are reduced substantially when the drug is given by inhalation, and this method of administration is desirable when pentamidine is used to prevent pneumocystis pneumonia in patients with human immunodeficiency virus (HIV) disease.

Other Antiprotozoal Drugs

Several additional agents have been developed to treat intestinal and extraintestinal infections caused by various protozoa. These agents include melarsoprol, nifurtimox, sodium stibogluconate, and suramin. The use and distribution of these drugs, however, is quite different from the agents described previously. In the United States, these additional drugs are usually available only from the Centers for Disease Control (CDC), in Atlanta, Georgia. At the request of the physician, the CDC dispenses the drug to the physician, who then provides the agent to the patient.

Clinical applications of individual drugs in this category are indicated in Table 35–4. In general, these drugs are reserved for some of the more serious or rare types of protozoal infections. As might be expected, adverse side effects of these drugs are quite common. However, these drugs may be lifesaving in some of the more severe infections, which is why the CDC controls their distribution. For more information about specific agents in this group, the reader is referred to other sources.[51]

Anthelmintics

Infection from helminths, or parasitic worms, is the most common form of disease in the world.[41,44] There are several types of worms that may invade and subsist from human tissues.[44,52] Common examples include tapeworms (cestodes), roundworms (nematodes), and flukes (trematodes).[52] Worms can enter the body by various routes but often are ingested as eggs in contaminated food and water. Once in the body, the eggs hatch, and adult worms ultimately lodge in various tissues, especially the digestive tract. Some types (flukes) may also lodge in blood vessels such as the hepatic portal vein. Depending on the species, adult worms may range from a few millimeters to several meters in length. The adult worms begin to steal nutrients from their human host and may begin to obstruct the intestinal lumen or other ducts if they reproduce in sufficient numbers.

Some of the common **anthelmintics** used to kill the basic types of worms in humans are listed in Table 35–5. These agents are often very effective; a single oral dose is usually sufficient to selectively destroy the parasite. Brief descriptions of the basic pharmacologic effects and possible adverse effects of the primary anthelmintic agents are presented below. Several authors have also extensively reviewed the pharmacologic treatment of helminthic infections.[36,41,52,58,66]

Albendazole

Albendazole (Albenza) is primarily used to treat infections caused by the larval form of certain cestodes (tapeworms). These infections often cause cysts (hydatid disease) in the liver, lungs, and other tissues; albendazole is used as an adjunct to the surgical removal of these cysts or as the primary treatment if these cysts are inoperable. This drug is also effective against many gastrointestinal roundworms and hookworms, and is typically used as a secondary agent if other anthelmintics are not effective in treating these infections.

Albendazole exerts its anthelmintic effects by acting on the intestinal cells of parasitic worms and by inhibiting glucose uptake and glycogen storage by these parasites. This effect ultimately leads to lack of energy production, degeneration of intracellular components, and subsequent death of the parasite. Albendazole is usually well tolerated when used for short-term treatment of infections in gastrointestinal or other tissues. Long-term treatment for conditions such as hydatid disease may result in abnormal liver function tests (e.g., increased serum aminotransferase activity), and liver function should therefore be monitored periodically to prevent hepatotoxicity if this drug is used for extended periods.

Table 35–5	TREATMENT OF COMMON HELMINTHIC INFECTIONS	
Parasite	**Primary Agent(s)**	**Secondary Agent(s)**
Roundworms (nematodes)		
Ascariasis (roundworm)	Albendazole, mebendazole, pyrantel pamoate	Piperazine citrate
Filariasis	Albendazole, diethylcarbamazine, ivermectin	–
Hookworm	Albendazole, mebendazole	Ivermectin, pyrantel pamoate, thiabendazole
Pinworm	Albendazole, mebendazole, pyrantel pamoate	Piperazine citrate
Trichinosis	Albendazole, mebendazole	Thiabendazole
Tapeworms (cestodes)		
Beef tapeworm	Niclosamide, praziquantel	–
Pork tapeworm	Albendazole, praziquantel	Niclosamide
Fish tapeworm	Niclosamide, praziquantel	–
Flukes (trematodes)		
Blood flukes	Praziquantel	Oxamniquine
Fluke infections in other organs	Praziquantel	–

Diethylcarbamazine

Diethylcarbamazine (Hetrazan) is used to treat certain roundworm infections of the lymphatics and connective tissues, including loiasis, onchocerciasis, and *Bancroft filariasis*. This agent immobilizes immature roundworms (microfilariae) and facilitates the destruction of these microfilariae by the body's immune system. Diethylcarbamazine is also effective against the adult forms of certain roundworms, but the mechanism of this anthelmintic action against mature nematodes is not known.

Side effects associated with diethylcarbamazine include headache, malaise, weakness, and loss of appetite. More severe reactions (fever, acute inflammatory response) may also occur following diethylcarbamazine use, but these reactions may be caused by the release of antigenic substances from the dying roundworms rather than from the drug itself.

Ivermectin

Ivermectin (Mectizan, Stromectol) is the primary treatment for filarial nematode infections (onchocerciasis) that invade ocular tissues and cause loss of vision (river blindness). Ivermectin may also be used in filarial infections in other tissues (lymphatics, skin). This drug is a secondary agent for treating intestinal nematodes such as strongyloidosis.

Ivermectin binds to chloride ion channels in parasitic nerve and muscle cells, thereby increasing membrane permeability to chloride. Increased intracellular chloride results in hyperpolarization of nerve and muscle tissues, which results in paralysis and death of the parasite. Ivermectin is well tolerated during short-term use in mild-to-moderate infections. Administration in more severe infections may cause swollen or tender lymph glands, fever, skin rash, itching, and joint and muscle pain, but these reactions may be caused by the death of the infectious parasites rather than by the drug itself.

Mebendazole

Mebendazole (Vermox) is effective against many types of roundworms and a few tapeworms that parasitize humans. Like albendazole, this drug selectively damages intestinal cells in these worms, thus inhibiting the uptake and intracellular transport of glucose and other nutrients into these parasites. This activity leads to the destruction of the epithelial lining and subsequent death of the parasite. Mebendazole is a relatively safe drug, although some mild, transient gastrointestinal problems may occur.

Niclosamide

Niclosamide (Niclocide) is effective against several types of tapeworm (see Table 35–5). This drug inhibits certain mitochondrial enzymes in these parasites, which ultimately results in the breakdown of the protective integument of the worm, thus allowing the digestive enzymes in the host (human) intestine to attack the parasite. Ultimately, the worm is digested and expelled from the gastrointestinal tract. There are relatively few adverse effects of niclosamide treatment, probably because the drug is not absorbed to any great extent from the human intestine. Thus, this drug remains in the intestinal lumen, where it can act directly on the tapeworm.

Oxamniquine

Oxamniquine (Vansil) is effective against a genus of parasitic worms known as blood flukes (schistosomes). These parasites typically adhere to the wall of blood vessels such as the hepatic portal vein. Oxamniquine inhibits muscular contraction of the sucker that holds the fluke to the vessel wall, thus allowing the worm to dislodge and travel to the liver. In the liver, the parasite is engulfed and destroyed by hepatic phagocytes. Common side effects associated with this drug include headache, dizziness, and drowsiness. However, these adverse effects are generally mild and transient.

Piperazine Citrate

Piperazine citrate is typically used as a secondary agent in ascariasis (roundworm) and enterobiasis (pinworm) infections (see Table 35–5). This drug appears to paralyze the worm by blocking the effect of acetylcholine at the parasite's neuromuscular junction. The paralyzed worm can then be dislodged and expelled from the host (human) intestine during normal bowel movements. Side effects such as headache, dizziness, and gastrointestinal disturbance may occur during piperazine citrate administration, but these effects are generally mild and transient.

Praziquantel

Praziquantel (Biltricide) is one of the most versatile and important anthelmintic agents, and is the drug of choice in treating all major trematode (fluke) infections and several common types of tapeworm infections (see Table 35–5). This drug's exact mechanism of action is unknown. Praziquantel may stimulate muscular contraction of the parasite, resulting in a type of spastic paralysis, which causes the worm to lose its hold on intestinal or vascular tissue. At higher concentrations, this drug may initiate destructive changes in the integument of the worm, allowing the host defense mechanisms (e.g., enzymes, phagocytes) to destroy the parasite. Praziquantel is associated with a number of frequent side effects, including gastrointestinal problems (abdominal pain, nausea, vomiting), CNS effects (headache, dizziness), and mild hepatotoxicity. These effects can usually be tolerated, however, for the relatively short time that the drug is in effect.

Pyrantel Pamoate

Pyrantel pamoate (Antiminth, other names) is one of the primary agents used in several types of roundworm and pinworm infections (see Table 35–5). This drug stimulates acetylcholine release and inhibits acetylcholine breakdown at the neuromuscular junction, thus producing a prolonged state of excitation and muscular contraction that causes spastic paralysis of the worm. The worm is unable to retain its hold on the intestinal tissue and can be expelled from the digestive tract by normal bowel movements. This drug is generally well tolerated, with only occasional problems of mild gastrointestinal disturbances.

Thiabendazole

Thiabendazole (Mintezol) is often used in trichinosis and several other types of roundworm infections (see Table 35–5). The anthelmintic mechanism of this drug is not fully understood, but selective inhibition of certain key metabolic enzymes in susceptible parasites is probable. Although thiabendazole is quite effective, the use of this drug has declined somewhat in favor of less toxic agents such as mebendazole. The most common side effects associated with this drug involve gastrointestinal distress (nausea, vomiting, loss of appetite). Allergic reactions (skin rash, itching, chills) may also occur in some individuals.

Significance of Antifungal and Antiparasitic Drugs in Rehabilitation

■ ■ ■ The drugs discussed in this chapter are relevant because they relate largely to specific groups of patients seen in a rehabilitation setting. Therapists working in sports physical therapy may deal frequently with topical antifungal agents in the treatment of cutaneous ringworm infections. For instance, physical therapists and athletic trainers may be responsible for recognizing and helping treat tinea pedis, tinea cruris, and similar infections. Therapists and trainers can make sure the drugs are being applied in the proper fashion and as directed by the physician. Therapists may also play a crucial role in preventing the spread of these infections by educating athletes about how to prevent transmission among team members (e.g., not sharing towels and combs).

Physical therapists and occupational therapists working with patients who have AIDS will frequently encounter patients taking systemic antifungal and antiprotozoal drugs. The use of these agents is critical in controlling parasitic infections in patients with AIDS and other individuals with a compromised or deficient immune system.

Finally, the drugs discussed in this chapter will have particular importance to therapists working in or traveling to parts of the world where parasitic infections remain a primary health problem and source of human suffering. Therapists involved in the Peace Corps or similar organizations will routinely treat patients taking these drugs. Also, therapists working in these areas may be taking some of the drugs themselves, such as the prophylactic antimalarial agents chloroquine and mefloquine. Hence, therapists should be aware of the pharmacology and potential side effects of these agents, both in their patients and in themselves. Of course, therapists working in North America should know that individuals who have returned from or have immigrated from certain geographic areas may carry various fungal and parasitic infections and that these patients will also require chemotherapy using the drugs discussed in this chapter.

CASE STUDY

Antifungal Drugs

Brief History. A physical therapist working with a college football team was taping a team member's ankle when he noticed redness and inflammation between the athlete's toes. The athlete reported that the redness and itching had developed within the last few days and was becoming progressively worse. The therapist suspected a cutaneous fungal infection (probably tinea pedis) and reported this information to the team physician.

Decision/Solution. The physician prescribed a topical antifungal preparation containing miconazole (Monistat-Derm). The athlete was instructed to apply this preparation twice daily. The physical therapist also instructed the athlete in proper skin hygiene (such as thoroughly washing and drying the feet, wearing clean socks). In addition, the physical therapist had the locker room floors and shower areas thoroughly disinfected to prevent transmission of the fungus to other team members. This isolated case of tinea pedis was resolved without further incident.

SUMMARY

This chapter presented three general groups of drugs that are used to treat infection caused by specific microorganisms in humans. Antifungal drugs are used against local or systemic infections caused by pathogenic fungi. Antiprotozoal agents are used to prevent and treat protozoal infections such as malaria, severe intestinal infection (dysentery), and infections in other tissues and organs. Anthelmintic drugs are used against parasitic worms (tapeworm, roundworm, etc.), which may infect the human intestinal tract and other tissues. Although the use of some of these agents is relatively limited in the United States, these drugs tend to be some of the most important agents in controlling infection and improving health on a worldwide basis. In addition, the use of some of these agents has increased lately in treating opportunistic fungal and protozoal infections in patients who have AIDS and others with compromised immune systems. Physical and occupational therapists may be involved with treating specific groups of patients taking these drugs, including patients with AIDS and patients located in geographic areas where these types of infections are prevalent.

References

1. Albougy HA, Naidoo S. A systematic review of the management of oral candidiasis associated with HIV/AIDS. *SADJ.* 2002;57:457–466.
2. Allen JE, Liu LX. Immunity to parasitic and fungal infections. In: Pier GB, et al, eds. *Immunology, Infection, and Immunity.* Washington, DC: ASM Press; 2004.
3. Ashley EA, White NJ. Artemisinin-based combinations. *Curr Opin Infect Dis.* 2005;18:531–536.
4. Baddley JW, Pappas PG. Antifungal combination therapy: clinical potential. *Drugs.* 2005;65:1461–1480.
5. Barratt G, Legrand P. Comparison of the efficacy and pharmacology of formulations of amphotericin B used in treatment of leishmaniasis. *Curr Opin Infect Dis.* 2005;18:527–530.
6. Basselin M, Hunt SM, Abdala-Valencia H, Kaneshiro ES. Ubiquinone synthesis in mitochondrial and microsomal subcellular fractions of *Pneumocystis spp*: differential sensitivities to atovaquone. *Eukaryot Cell.* 2005;4: 1483–1492.
7. Bennett JE. Antifungal agents. In: Brunton LL, et al, eds. *The Pharmacological Basis of Therapeutics.* 11th ed. New York: McGraw-Hill; 2006.
8. Bicanic T, Harrison TS. Cryptococcal meningitis. *Br Med Bull.* 2005;72:99–118.
9. Borgers M, Degreef H, Cauwenbergh G. Fungal infections of the skin: infection process and antimycotic therapy. *Curr Drug Targets.* 2005;6:849–862.
10. Bradsher RW, Chapman SW, Pappas PG. Blastomycosis. *Infect Dis Clin North Am.* 2003;17:21–40.
11. Brakhage AA. Systemic fungal infections caused by Aspergillus species: epidemiology, infection process and virulence determinants. *Curr Drug Targets.* 2005; 6:875–886.
12. Buchachart K, Krudsood S, Singhasivanon P, et al. Effect of primaquine standard dose (15 mg/day for 14 days) in the treatment of vivax malaria patients in Thailand. *Southeast Asian J Trop Med Public Health.* 2001;32:720–726.
13. Bukirwa H, Critchley J. Sulfadoxine-pyrimethamine plus artesunate versus sulfadoxine-pyrimethamine plus amodiaquine for treating uncomplicated malaria. *Cochrane Database Syst Rev.* 2006;CD004966.
14. Bukirwa H, Orton L. Artesunate plus mefloquine versus mefloquine for treating uncomplicated malaria. *Cochrane Database Syst Rev.* 2005;CD004531.
15. Cha R, Sobel JD. Fluconazole for the treatment of candidiasis: 15 years experience. *Expert Rev Anti Infect Ther.* 2004;2:357–366.
16. Chakrabarti A. Microbiology of systemic fungal infections. *J Postgrad Med.* 2005;51(suppl 1):S16–S20.
17. Darkes MJ, Scott LJ, Goa KL. Terbinafine: a review of its use in onychomycosis in adults. *Am J Clin Dermatol.* 2003;4:39–65.
18. Davis TM, Karunajeewa HA, Ilett KF. Artemisinin-based combination therapies for uncomplicated malaria. *Med J Aust.* 2005;182:181–185.
19. Deck DH, Guglielmo BJ. Pharmacological advances in the treatment of invasive candidiasis. *Expert Rev Anti Infect Ther.* 2006;4:137–149.
20. Deray G. Amphotericin B nephrotoxicity. *J Antimicrob Chemother.* 2002;49(suppl 1):37–41.
21. Farooq U, Mahajan RC. Drug resistance in malaria. *J Vector Borne Dis.* 2004;41:45–53.
22. Fitch CD. Ferriprotoporphyrin IX, phospholipids, and the antimalarial actions of quinoline drugs. *Life Sci.* 2004;74:1957–1972.
23. Franco-Paredes C, Santos-Preciado JI. Problem pathogens: prevention of malaria in travellers. *Lancet Infect Dis.* 2006;6:139–149.
24. Fung HB, Doan TL. Tinidazole: a nitroimidazole antiprotozoal agent. *Clin Ther.* 2005;27:1859–1884.
25. Genta RM, Connor DH. Infectious and parasitic diseases. In: Rubin E, Farber JL, eds. *Pathology.* 3rd ed. Philadelphia: Lippincott-Raven; 1999.
26. Gibbs WJ, Drew RH, Perfect JR. Liposomal amphotericin B: clinical experience and perspectives. *Expert Rev Anti Infect Ther.* 2005;3:167–181.
27. Ginsburg H. Should chloroquine be laid to rest? *Acta Trop.* 2005;96:16–23.
28. Ginsburg H, Golenser J. Glutathione is involved in the antimalarial action of chloroquine and its modulation affects drug sensitivity of human and murine species of Plasmodium. *Redox Rep.* 2003;8:276–279.

29. Goldman RD, Koren G. Amphotericin B nephrotoxicity in children. *J Pediatr Hematol Oncol.* 2004;26: 421–426.

30. Gupta AK, Ryder JE, Lynch LE, Tavakkol A. The use of terbinafine in the treatment of onychomycosis in adults and special populations: a review of the evidence. *J Drugs Dermatol.* 2005;4:302–308.

31. Herbrecht R. Voriconazole: therapeutic review of a new azole antifungal. *Expert Rev Anti Infect Ther.* 2004; 2:485–497.

32. Hrdy I, Cammack R, Stopka P, et al. Alternative pathway of metronidazole activation in Trichomonas vaginalis hydrogenosomes. *Antimicrob Agents Chemother.* 2005;49:5033–5036.

33. Huang DB, Ostrosky-Zeichner L, Wu JJ, et al. Therapy of common superficial fungal infections. *Dermatol Ther.* 2004;17:517–522.

34. Jalloh A, Tantular IS, Pusarawati S, et al. Rapid epidemiologic assessment of glucose-6-phosphate dehydrogenase deficiency in malaria-endemic areas in Southeast Asia using a novel diagnostic kit. *Trop Med Int Health.* 2004;9:615–623.

35. Kam LW, Lin JD. Management of systemic candidal infections in the intensive care unit. *Am J Health Syst Pharm.* 2002;59:33–41.

36. Keiser J, Utzinger J. Chemotherapy for major foodborne trematodes: a review. *Expert Opin Pharmacother.* 2004;5:1711–1726.

37. Kurowski R, Ostapchuk M. Overview of histoplasmosis. *Am Fam Physician.* 2002;66:2247–2252.

38. Kyle AA, Dahl MV. Topical therapy for fungal infections. *Am J Clin Dermatol.* 2004;5:443–451.

39. Lemke A, Kiderlen AF, Kayser O. Amphotericin B. *Appl Microbiol Biotechnol.* 2005;68:151–162.

40. Lesi A, Meremikwu M. High first dose quinine regimen for treating severe malaria. *Cochrane Database Syst Rev.* 2004;CD003341.

41. Loukas A, Hotez PJ. Chemotherapy of helminth infections. In: Brunton LL, et al, eds. *The Pharmacological Basis of Therapeutics.* 11th ed. New York: McGraw-Hill; 2006.

42. Marty F, Mylonakis E. Antifungal use in HIV infection. *Expert Opin Pharmacother.* 2002;3:91–102.

43. Mavor AL, Thewes S, Hube B. Systemic fungal infections caused by Candida species: epidemiology, infection process and virulence attributes. *Curr Drug Targets.* 2005;6:863–874.

44. McAdam AJ, Sharpe AH. Infectious diseases. In: Kumar V, Abbas AK, Fausto N, eds. *Pathologic Basis of Disease.* 7th ed. New York: Elsevier Saunders; 2005.

45. McCormack PL, Perry CM. Caspofungin: a review of its use in the treatment of fungal infections. *Drugs.* 2005;65:2049–2068.

46. Meshnick SR. Artemisinin: mechanisms of action, resistance and toxicity. *Int J Parasitol.* 2002;32: 1655–1660.

47. Obaji J, Lee-Pack LR, Gutierrez C, Chan CK. The pulmonary effects of long-term exposure to aerosol pentamidine: a 5-year surveillance study in HIV-infected patients. *Chest.* 2003;123:1983–1987.

48. Patel SN, Kain KC. Atovaquone/proguanil for the prophylaxis and treatment of malaria. *Expert Rev Anti Infect Ther.* 2005;3:849–861.

49. Pellegrini M, Ruff TA. Malaria. The latest in advice for travelers. *Aust Fam Physician.* 1999;28:683–688.

50. Petersen E. Malaria chemoprophylaxis: when should we use it and what are the options? *Expert Rev Anti Infect Ther.* 2004;2:119–132.

51. Phillips MA. Stanley SL. Chemotherapy of protozoal infections: amebiasis, giardiasis, trichomoniasis, trypanosomiasis, leishmaniasis, and other protozoal infections. In: Brunton LL, et al, eds. *The Pharmacological Basis of Therapeutics.* 11th ed. New York: McGraw-Hill; 2006.

52. Plorde JJ. Introduction to pathogenic parasites: pathogenesis and chemotherapy of parasitic diseases. In: Ryan KJ, Ray CG, eds. *Sherris Medical Microbiology.* 4th ed. New York: McGraw-Hill; 2004.

53. Polak A. Antifungal therapy—state of the art at the beginning of the 21st century. *Prog Drug Res.* 2003; Spec No:59–190.

54. Rao S, Ali U. Systemic fungal infections in neonates. *J Postgrad Med.* 2005;51(suppl 1):S27–S29.

55. Rathore D, McCutchan TF, Sullivan M, Kumar S. Antimalarial drugs: current status and new developments. *Expert Opin Investig Drugs.* 2005;14:871–883.

56. Roberts BJ, Friedlander SF. Tinea capitis: a treatment update. *Pediatr Ann.* 2005;34:191–200.

57. Sastry PS, Parikh PM, Kulkarni PS, et al. Use of liposomal amphotericin B in bone marrow transplant. *J Postgrad Med.* 2005;51(suppl 1):S49–S52.

58. Schantz PM. Progress in diagnosis, treatment and elimination of echinococcosis and cysticercosis. *Parasitol Int.* 2006;55(suppl):S7–S13.

59. Schwebke JR, Burgess D. Trichomoniasis. *Clin Microbiol Rev.* 2004;17:794–803.

60. Shanks GD, Edstein MD. Modern malaria chemoprophylaxis. *Drugs.* 2005;65:2091–2110.

61. Shapiro TA, Goldberg DE. Chemotherapy of protozoal infections: malaria. In: Brunton LL, et al, eds. *The Pharmacological Basis of Therapeutics.* 11th ed. New York: McGraw-Hill;2006.

62. Sibley CH, Hyde JE, Sims PF, et al. Pyrimethamine-sulfadoxine resistance in Plasmodium falciparum: what next? *Trends Parasitol.* 2001;17:582–588.

63. Sims CR, Ostrosky-Zeichner L, Rex JH. Invasive candidiasis in immunocompromised hospitalized patients. *Arch Med Res.* 2005;36:660–671.

64. Slain D, Rogers PD, Cleary JD, Chapman SW. Intravenous itraconazole. *Ann Pharmacother.* 2001;35: 720–729.

65. Spiller DG, Bray PG, Hughes RH, et al. The pH of the Plasmodium falciparum digestive vacuole: holy grail or dead-end trail? *Trends Parasitol.* 2002;18: 441–444.

66. Tisch DJ, Michael E, Kazura JW. Mass chemotherapy options to control lymphatic filariasis: a systematic review. *Lancet Infect Dis.* 2005;5:514–523.

67. Tournu H, Serneels J, Van Dijck P. Fungal pathogens research: novel and improved molecular approaches for

the discovery of antifungal drug targets. *Curr Drug Targets.* 2005;6:909–922.

68. Trampuz A, Jereb M, Muzlovic I, Prabhu RM. Clinical review: severe malaria. *Crit Care.* 2003;7:315–323.

69. Vermes A, Guchelaar HJ, Dankert J. Flucytosine: a review of its pharmacology, clinical indications, pharmacokinetics, toxicity, and drug interactions. *J Antimicrob Chemother.* 2000;46:171–179.

70. Wiwanitkit V. Intestinal parasite infestation in HIV infected patients. *Curr HIV Res.* 2006;4:87–96.

71. Woodrow CJ, Haynes RK, Krishna S. Artemisinins. *Postgrad Med J.* 2005;81:71–78.

72. Yamada H, Kotaki H, Takahashi T. Recommendations for the treatment of fungal pneumonias. *Expert Opin Pharmacother.* 2003;4:1241–1258.

Chapter 36

Cancer Chemotherapy

Cancer encompasses a group of diseases that are marked by rapid, uncontrolled cell proliferation and a conversion of normal cells to a more primitive and undifferentiated state.[11,41] Large tumors, or *neoplasms*, may form from excessive cell proliferation. Although some types of tumors are well contained (benign), malignant tumors continue to proliferate within local tissues and can possibly spread (metastasize) to other tissues in the body. The term *cancer* specifically refers to the malignant forms of neoplastic disease, which can often be fatal as tumors invade and destroy tissues throughout the body. However, benign tumors can also be life threatening; for example, a large benign tumor may produce morbidity and mortality by obstructing the intestinal tract or by pressing on crucial central nervous system (CNS) structures. Cancer cells, however, are unique in their progressive invasion of local tissues and their ability to metastasize to other tissues.[41]

Cancer ranks second to cardiovascular disease as the leading cause of death in the United States.[31] There are many different types of cancer, and malignancies are classified by the location and the type of tissue from which the cancer originated.[41] For instance, cancers arising from epithelial tissues (e.g., skin, gastrointestinal lining) are labeled as *carcinomas;* cancers arising from mesenchymal tissues (e.g., bone, striated muscle) are labeled as *sarcomas*. In addition, cancers associated with the formed blood elements are connoted by the suffix "-emia" (e.g., "leukemia" is the cancerous proliferation of leukocytes). Many other descriptive terms are used to describe various malignancies, and certain forms of cancer are often named after a specific person (e.g., Hodgkin disease, Wilms tumor). We cannot, however, describe all the various types of malignancies. The reader may want to consult a pathology text or similar reference for more infor-

mation about the location and morphology of particular forms of cancer.[41,76]

The exact cause of many cases of neoplastic disease is unknown. However, a great deal has been learned about possible environmental, viral, genetic, and other elements, or **carcinogens,** that may cause or increase a person's susceptibility to various types of cancer. Conversely, certain positive lifestyles, including adequate exercise, a high-fiber diet, and the avoidance of tobacco products, may be crucial in preventing certain forms of cancer. Of course, routine checkups and early detection play a vital role in reducing cancer mortality.

When cancer is diagnosed, three primary treatment modalities are available: surgery, radiation treatment, and cancer chemotherapy. The purpose of this chapter is to describe the basic rationale of cancer **chemotherapy** and to provide an overview of the drugs that are currently available to treat specific forms of cancer. Rehabilitation specialists will routinely work with patients undergoing cancer chemotherapy. For reasons that will become apparent in this chapter, these drugs tend to produce toxic effects that directly influence physical therapy and occupational therapy procedures. Therefore, this chapter should provide therapists with a better understanding of the pharmacodynamic principles and beneficial effects, as well as the reasons for the potential adverse effects of these important drugs.

General Principles

Cytotoxic Strategy

The basic strategy of anticancer drugs is to limit cell proliferation by killing or attenuating the growth of the cancerous cells. However, the pharmacologic treatment of cancer represents a unique and perplexing problem. Although cancer cells have become more primitive and have lost much of their normal appearance, they are still human cells that have simply gone wild. In addition, they cannot be easily destroyed without also causing some harm to healthy human tissue. The concept of selective toxicity becomes more difficult to achieve when using anticancer drugs versus drugs that attack foreign invaders and parasites such as antibacterial drugs or antifungal drugs (see Chapters 33– 35).

Hence, most anticancer drugs rely on the basic strategy of inhibiting DNA/RNA synthesis and function, or on directly inhibiting cell division (mitosis). Cancerous cells have a greater need to replicate their genetic material and undergo mitosis than noncancerous cells. Healthy cells will, of course, also suffer to some extent because traditional anticancer drugs typically lack specificity and impair function in noncancerous tissues as well as cancerous cells.[20,35] The cancerous cells, however, will be affected to a greater extent because of their need to undergo mitosis at a much higher rate than most healthy cells.

Cell-Cycle–Specific Versus Cell-Cycle–Nonspecific Drugs

Antineoplastic drugs are sometimes classified by whether they act at a specific phase of cell division.[14] Cancer cells and most normal cells typically undergo a life cycle that can be divided into several distinct phases: a resting phase (G_0), a pre-DNA synthesis phase (also the phase of normal cell metabolism; G_1), a period of DNA synthesis (S), a post-DNA synthesis phase (G_2), and the period of actual cell division or mitosis (M) (Fig. 36–1).[11,41] Certain antineoplastic drugs are referred to as cell-cycle–specific because they exert their effects only when the cancer cell is in a certain phase. For instance, most antimetabolites (cytarabine, methotrexate, others) act when the cell is in the S phase (Fig. 36–1). Other drugs are classified as cell-cycle–nonspecific because they exert antineoplastic effects on the cell regardless of the cell cycle's phase. Examples of cell-cycle–nonspecific agents include most alkylating agents and antineoplastic antibiotics.

The significance of cell-cycle–specificity or nonspecificity is obvious. Cell-cycle–specific drugs will be effective only in cells that are progressing through the cell cycle—that is, cells that are not remaining in the resting (G_0) phase. Cell-cycle–nonspecific agents have a more general effect and should inhibit replication in all the cells that the drug reaches.

Concepts of Growth Fraction and Total Cell Kill

Cancer cells are not all uniform in their rate of replication and proliferation. In any given tumor or type of disseminated cancer, certain cells do not proliferate, while other cells reproduce at variable rates. The term *growth fraction* refers to the percentage of proliferating cells relative to total neoplastic cell population.[6] The cells included in the growth fraction are more susceptible to antineoplastic drugs because these cells must synthesize and replicate their genetic material. Fortunately, these cells also must be killed to prevent the cancer from spreading.

The concept of *total cell kill* refers to the fact that virtually every tumor cell capable of replicating must be killed in order to eliminate the cancer completely.[6] Theoretically, even a single surviving malignant cell could eventually replicate in sufficient numbers and cause death. The difficulty of achieving total cell kill is illustrated by the following example. The number of malignant cells in a patient with acute lymphocytic leukemia could be as high as 10^{12}. If an anticancer drug kills 99.99 percent of these cells, one might think that the drug was successful in resolving the cancer. However, 10^8—or approximately 1 billion—cells would remain alive and capable of advancing the leukemia. Obviously, total cell kill is always a chemotherapeutic goal but may be sometimes difficult to achieve. In reality, chemotherapy regimens often reduce the number of cancer cells to the point where the body's endogenous defense mechanisms (i.e., cytotoxic immune responses) can deal with the remaining cancerous tissues, and the disease is considered to be in remission.[6]

Prevalence and Management of Adverse Effects

Because antineoplastic agents often impair replication of normal tissues, these drugs are generally associated with a number of common and relatively severe adverse effects. Normal human cells must often undergo controlled mitosis to sustain normal function. This fact is especially true for certain tissues such as hair follicles, bone marrow, immune system cells, and epithelial cells in the skin and gastrointestinal tract. Obviously, most chemotherapy agents for cancer will also affect these tissues to some extent. In fact, the primary reason for most of the common adverse effects (e.g., hair loss, anemia, nausea) is that normal cells are also experiencing the same toxic changes as the tumor cells. The can-

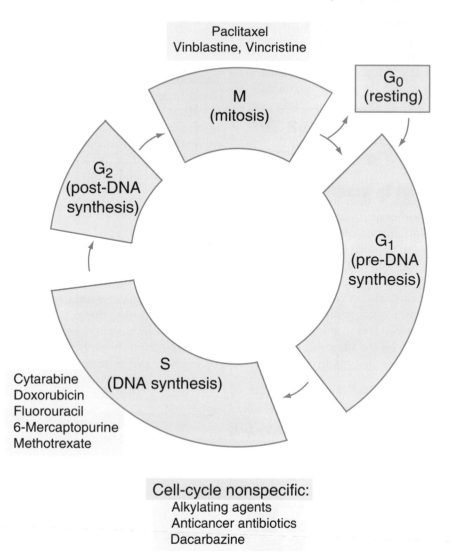

FIGURE 36–1 ▼ Phases of the cell cycle. Examples of cell-cycle–specific drugs are listed next to the phase of the cycle they act on. Examples of cell-cycle–nonspecific drugs are listed below the figure. See text for more details.

cer cells, however, tend to suffer these toxic effects to a greater extent because of their increased rate of replication and cell division. Still, healthy cells often exhibit some toxic effects, even at the minimum effective doses of the chemotherapeutic agents.

Consequently, antineoplastic drugs typically have a very low therapeutic index compared with drugs that are used to treat less serious disorders (see Chapter 1). Considering that cancer is usually life threatening, these toxic effects must be expected and tolerated during chemotherapeutic treatments. Some side effects, however, can be treated with other drugs. In particular, gastrointestinal disturbances (e.g., nausea,

vomiting, loss of appetite) may be relieved to some extent by administering traditional antiemetic agents such as glucocorticoids (dexamethasone) or drugs that block dopamine receptors (metoclopramide).[4,30] In addition, newer antiemetic and antinausea agents such as dolasetron (Anzemet), granisetron (Kytril), ondansetron (Zofran), and palonosetron (Aloxi) have been developed to treat chemotherapy-induced nausea and vomiting. These newer agents, which block a specific type of CNS serotonin receptor known as the 5-hydroxytryptamine type 3 (5-HT$_3$) receptor, reduce the nausea and vomiting caused when serotonin binds to that receptor.[1,4] Likewise, a new agent known as aprepitant (Emend) is available that blocks the neurokinin-1 receptor in the CNS, thereby inhibiting the nausea and vomiting mediated by other neuropeptides such as substance P.[4,68] Hence, several drugs are now available that can be used alone or in combinations to reduce the severity of gastrointestinal distress commonly associated with cancer chemotherapy agents.[2,68]

Other forms of supportive care can also be helpful in improving the quality-of-life for patients with cancer. Analgesics (see Chapters 14 and 15) are often needed to help patients cope with cancer pain and to make the rigors of chemotherapy treatment more tolerable.[59,70] A variety of other medications can also be used to treat specific symptoms such as anemia, cough, weight loss, and constipation.[45,78,85] Support from medical, nursing, and other health care providers (including physical therapists and occupational therapists) can likewise help immeasurably in reassuring the patient that chemotherapy-induced side effects are normal—and even necessary—for the cancer chemotherapy drugs to exert their antineoplastic effects.

Specific Drugs

Drugs used against cancer can be classified by their chemical structure, source, or mechanism of action. The primary groups of antineoplastic drugs are the alkylating agents, antimetabolites, antineoplastic antibiotics, plant alkaloids, antineoplastic hormones, and several other miscellaneous drug groups and individual agents. The principal antineoplastic medications are presented below.

Alkylating Agents

Alkylating agents exert cytotoxic effects by inducing binding within DNA strands and by preventing DNA function and replication.[22,56] Essentially, the drug causes cross-links to be formed between the strands of the DNA double helix or within a single DNA strand (Fig. 36–2). In either case, these cross-links effectively tie up the DNA molecule, eliminating the ability of the DNA double helix to untwist. If the DNA double helix cannot unravel, the genetic code of the cell cannot be

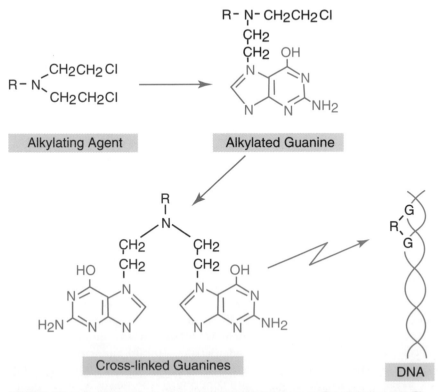

FIGURE 36–2 ▼ Mechanism of action of anticancer alkylating agents. The alkylating agent (R) causes alkylation of guanine nucleotides located in the DNA strand. Cross-links are then formed between two alkylated guanines, thus creating strong bonds between or within the DNA strands that inhibit DNA function and replication.

reproduced, and cell reproduction is arrested. In addition, cross-linking within the double helix impairs cellular protein synthesis because the DNA double helix cannot unwind to allow formation of messenger RNA strands. The cell therefore cannot synthesize vital cellular proteins (enzymes, transport proteins, etc.). Alkylating agents likewise initiate a process of cell death (apoptosis) by disrupting DNA function, in which several degradative enzymes (nucleases, proteases) are released and begin to destroy the cell.[11]

Alkylating agents are so named because they typically generate a chemical alkyl group on one of the bases, such as guanine in the DNA chain. This alkyl group acts as the bridge that ultimately links two bases in the DNA molecule (see Fig. 36–2). The bonds formed by this cross-linking are strong and resistant to breakage. Thus, the DNA double helix remains tied up for the cell's life.

Anticancer drugs that work primarily as alkylating agents are listed in Table 36–1. As indicated, these agents represent the largest category of anticancer drugs and are used to treat a variety of leukemias, carcinomas, and other neoplasms. Common side effects of alkylating agents are also listed in Table 36–1. As previously discussed, most of these adverse effects are caused by the effect of the alkylating agent on DNA replication in normal, healthy tissues.

Antimetabolites

Cells are able to synthesize genetic material (DNA, RNA) from endogenous metabolites known as purine and pyrimidine nucleotides (Fig. 36–3). Certain anticancer drugs are structurally similar to these endogenous metabolites and compete with these compounds during DNA/RNA biosynthesis. These drugs are therefore called antimetabolites because they interfere with the normal metabolites during cellular biosynthesis.[16,80]

Antimetabolites can impair the biosynthesis of genetic material in two primary ways.[11] First, the drug may be incorporated directly into the genetic material, thus forming a fake and nonfunctional genetic product. This effect would be like baking a cake but substituting an inappropriate ingredient (salt) for a normal ingredient (sugar). Obviously, the product would not work (or taste) very well. The second manner in which antimetabolites may impair DNA/RNA biosynthesis is by occupying the enzymes that synthesize various components of the genetic material. These enzymes do not recognize the difference between the antimetabolite

drug and the normal metabolite and waste their time trying to convert the antimetabolite into a normal metabolic product. The enzyme, however, cannot effectively act on the drug, so the normal metabolic products are not formed. In either case, the cell's ability to synthesize normal DNA and RNA is impaired, and the cell cannot replicate its genetic material or carry out normal protein synthesis because of a lack of functional DNA and RNA.

Cancer chemotherapeutic agents that act as antimetabolites and the principal neoplastic diseases for which they are indicated are listed in Table 36–2. As stated previously, these drugs interrupt cellular pathways that synthesize DNA and RNA; the primary sites where specific antimetabolites interrupt these pathways are indicated in Figure 36–3. As with most anticancer drugs, these agents are especially toxic to cells that have a large growth fraction and undergo extensive replication. These cells have a great need to synthesize nucleic acids—hence the preferential effect of antimetabolites on these cells.

Antibiotics

Several anticancer drugs are chemically classified as antibiotics but are usually reserved for neoplastic diseases because of their relatively high toxicity. The exact mechanism of action for these antibiotics to exert antineoplastic effects is still being investigated. These drugs may act directly on DNA by becoming intercalated (inserted) between base pairs in the DNA strand. This insertion would cause a general disruption or even lysis of the DNA strand, thus preventing DNA replication and RNA synthesis.[25] Alternatively, these antibiotics may act in other ways, including having direct effects on the cancerous cell membrane, inhibiting DNA-related enzymes, and forming highly reactive free radicals that directly damage the DNA molecule.[51,83] Regardless of their exact mechanism, these agents play a role in the treatment of several neoplastic diseases. Antibiotic agents used for cancer chemotherapy are listed in Table 36–3.

Plant Alkaloids

Alkaloids are nitrogen-based compounds frequently found in plants. Plant alkaloids that are used in treating cancer in humans include traditional agents, such as vincristine and vinblastine, and newer agents, such as vinorelbine, paclitaxel, and docetaxel (Table 36–4). These agents are also known as antimitotic drugs be-

Text continued on page 573

Table 36–1	ALKYLATING AGENTS		
Generic Name	**Trade Name**	**Primary Antineoplastic Indication(s)***	**Common Adverse Effects**
Altretamine	Hexalen	Ovarian cancer	GI distress (nausea, vomiting, loss of appetite); blood disorders (leukopenia, thrombocytopenia); CNS neurotoxicity (unusual tiredness, dizziness, confusion, depression, anxiety); peripheral neuropathies
Busulfan	Myleran	Chronic myelocytic leukemia	Blood disorders (anemia, leukopenia, thrombocytopenia); metabolic disorders (hyperuricemia, fatigue, weight loss, other symptoms)
Carmustine	BCNU, BiCNU	Primary brain tumors; Hodgkin disease; non-Hodgkin lymphomas; multiple myeloma	Blood disorders (thrombocytopenia, leukopenia); GI distress (nausea, vomiting); hepatotoxicity; pulmonary toxicity
Chlorambucil	Leukeran	Chronic lymphocytic leukemia; Hodgkin disease; non-Hodgkin lymphomas	Blood disorders (leukopenia, thrombocytopenia, anemia,); skin rashes/itching; pulmonary toxicity; seizures
Cyclophosphamide	Cytoxan, Neosar	Acute and chronic lymphocytic leukemia; acute and chronic myelocytic leukemia; carcinoma of ovary, breast; Hodgkin disease; non-Hodgkin lymphomas; multiple myeloma	Blood disorders (anemia, leukopenia, thrombocytopenia); GI distress (nausea, vomiting, loss of appetite); bladder irritation; hair loss; cardiotoxicity; pulmonary toxicity
Dacarbazine	DTIC-Dome	Malignant melanoma; refractory Hodgkin's lymphomas	GI distress (nausea, vomiting, loss of appetite); blood disorders (leukopenia, thrombocytopenia)
Ifosfamide	IFEX	Testicular cancer	Blood disorders (leukopenia, thrombocytopenia); CNS effects (agitation, confusion, dizziness); urotoxicity; GI distress (nausea, vomiting)
Lomustine	CeeNU	Brain tumors; Hodgkin disease	Blood disorders (anemia, leukopenia); GI disorders (nausea, vomiting)
Mechlorethamine	Mustargen, nitrogen mustard	Bronchogenic carcinoma; chronic leukemia; Hodgkin disease; non-Hodgkin lymphomas; blood disorders (leukopenia, thrombocytopenia); skin rashes/itching	Blood disorders (anemia, leukopenia, thrombocytopenia); GI distress (nausea, vomiting); CNS effects (headache, dizziness, convulsions); local irritation at injection site

Generic Name	Trade Name	Primary Antineoplastic Indication(s)*	Common Adverse Effects
Melphalan	Alkeran	Ovarian carcinoma; multiple myeloma	Blood disorders (leukopenia, thrombocytopenia); skin rashes/itching
Procarbazine	Matulane	Hodgkin disease	Blood disorders (leukopenia, thrombocytopenia); GI distress (nausea, vomiting); CNS toxicity (mood changes, incoordination, motor problems)
Streptozocin	Zanosar	Pancreatic carcinoma	Nephrotoxicity; GI distress (nausea, vomiting); blood disorders (anemia, leukopenia, thrombocytopenia); local irritation at injection site
Thiotepa	Thioplex	Carcinoma of breast, ovary, and bladder; Hodgkin disease	Blood disorders (anemia, leukopenia, thrombocytopenia, pancytopenia)
Uracil mustard	Generic	Chronic lymphocytic leukemia; chronic myelocytic leukemia; non-Hodgkin lymphomas	Blood disorders (anemia, leukopenia, thrombocytopenia); GI distress (nausea, vomiting, diarrhea, loss of appetite)

*Only the indications listed in the U.S. product labeling are included here. Many anticancer drugs are used for additional types of neoplastic disease.
GI = gastrointestinal; CNS = central nervous system.

Table 36–2   ANTIMETABOLITES

Generic Name	Trade Name	Primary Antineoplastic Indication(s)*	Common Adverse Effects
Capecitabine	Xeloda	Breast cancer	Blood disorders (anemia, neutropenia, thrombocytopenia); GI distress (abdominal pain, nausea, vomiting); dermatitis; stomatitis; unusual tiredness
Cladribine	Leustatin	Hairy cell leukemia	Blood disorders (anemia, neutropenia, thrombocytopenia); fever; infection; GI distress (loss of appetite, nausea, vomiting); skin rash; headache; unusual tiredness
Cytarabine	Cytosar-U, Depocyt	Several forms of acute and chronic leukemia; non-Hodgkin lymphomas	Blood disorders (anemia, megaloblastosis, reticulocytopenia, others); GI distress (nausea, vomiting); skin rash; hair loss
Floxuridine	FUDR	Carcinoma of the GI tract and liver	GI disorders (nausea, vomiting, loss of appetite); skin disorders (discoloration, rash, hair loss)

(Continued on following page)

Table 36–2	ANTIMETABOLITES *(Continued)*		
Generic Name	**Trade Name**	**Primary Antineoplastic Indication(s)***	**Common Adverse Effects**
Fludarabine	Fludara	Chronic lymphocytic leukemia	Blood disorders (anemia, leukopenia, thrombocytopenia); infection; pneumonia; GI distress (nausea, vomiting, diarrhea); skin rash; unusual tiredness; hair loss
Fluorouracil	Adrucil	Carcinoma of colon, rectum, stomach, and pancreas	GI distress (loss of appetite, nausea); blood disorders (anemia, leukopenia, thrombocytopenia); skin disorders (rash, hair loss)
Gemcitabine	Gemzar	Carcinoma of the pancreas; nonsmall cell lung cancer	Blood disorders (anemia, leukopenia, neutropenia, thrombocytopenia); dyspnea; edema; fever; skin rash; hematuria; GI distress (nausea, vomiting, constipation, diarrhea)
Mercaptopurine	Purinethol	Acute lymphocytic and myelocytic leukemia; chronic myelocytic leukemia	Blood disorders (anemia, leukopenia, thrombocytopenia); GI distress (nausea, loss of appetite); hepatotoxicity
Methotrexate	Generic (when used for cancer)	Acute lymphocytic leukemia; meningeal leukemia; carcinoma of head and neck region, lung; non-Hodgkin lymphomas	Blood disorders (anemia, leukopenia, thrombocytopenia); GI distress (including ulceration of GI tract); skin disorders (rashes, photosensitivity, hair loss); hepatotoxicity; CNS effects (headaches, drowsiness, fatigue)
Pemetrexed	Alimta	Mesothelioma	Blood disorders (anemia, leukopenia, thrombocytopenia); allergic reaction
Pentostatin	Nipent	Hairy cell leukemia	Blood disorders (anemia, leukopenia, thrombocytopenia); allergic reaction; CNS toxicity (unusual tiredness, anxiety, confusion); headache; muscle pain; GI distress (nausea, vomiting, diarrhea)
Thioguanine	Generic	Acute lymphocytic leukemia; acute and chronic myelocytic leukemia	Blood disorders (anemia, leukopenia, thrombocytopenia); GI distress (nausea, vomiting); hepatotoxicity

*Only the indications listed in the U.S. product labeling are included here. Many anticancer drugs are used for additional types of neoplastic disease.
GI = gastrointestinal; CNS = central nervous system.

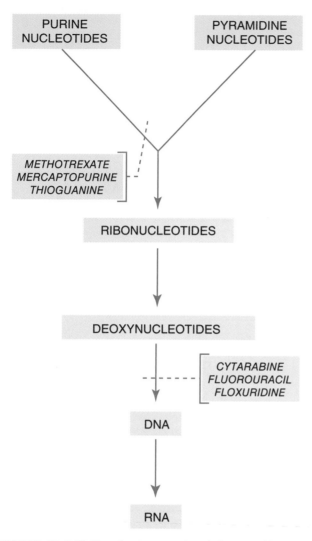

FIGURE 36–3 ▼ Sites of anticancer antimetabolite action. Various drugs interfere with DNA/RNA production by inhibiting nucleic acid biosynthesis at specific sites indicated by the dashed lines.

the nuclear material becomes disrupted and dispersed throughout the cytosol. This effect causes direct damage to the chromosomes, leading to subsequent cell dysfunction and death.

Other drugs classified as plant alkaloids include etoposide, irinotecan, teniposide, and topotecan (see Table 36–4). These drugs inhibit specific enzymes known as topoisomerase enzymes, which are necessary for DNA replication.[11] Inhibition of these enzymes causes a break in both strands of the DNA double helix, which leads to DNA destruction and cell death. Etoposide and teniposide inhibit the topoisomerase I form of this enzyme, and irinotecan and topotecan inhibit the topoisomerase II form of this enzyme. These drugs are therefore used to limit cell division and cancer growth in various types of neoplastic disease (see Table 36–4).

Hormones

Several forms of cancer are referred to as hormone sensitive because they tend to be exacerbated by certain hormones and attenuated by others. In particular, adrenocorticosteroids (see Chapter 29) and the sex hormones (androgens, estrogens, progesterone; see Chapter 30) may influence the proliferation of certain tumors. Hence, drugs that either mimic or block (antagonize) the effects of these hormones may be useful in treating certain hormone-sensitive forms of cancer.[29] Hormonal anticancer drugs are typically used as adjuvant therapy; that is, they are used in conjunction with surgery, radiation treatment, and other anticancer drugs.

The primary drugs that inhibit neoplasms via hormonal mechanisms are listed in Table 36–5. In some cases, these drugs work by direct inhibitory effects on cancerous cells (e.g., adrenocorticoid suppression of lymphocyte function) or by negative feedback mechanisms that decrease the endogenous hormonal stimulation of the tumor (e.g., gonadotropin-releasing hormones). In other cases, drugs can directly block the effects of the endogenous hormone and prevent that hormone from stimulating specific tumors. In particular, androgen receptor blockers (flutamide, others) can treat prostate cancer by blocking the effects of testosterone on the prostate gland.[28]

Estrogen receptor blockers (fulvestrant, tamoxifen) can likewise help prevent and treat breast and uterine cancers that are stimulated by estrogen.[37] Fulvestrant (Faslodex) is classified as a "pure" antiestrogen

cause they directly impair cell division. These drugs exert their antimitotic effects by binding to cellular microtubules and altering the function of these microtubules.[38,92] In particular, these drugs disrupt the function of the microtubules that are involved in the mitotic apparatus of the cell (the mitotic spindle). Certain agents (vincristine, vinblastine, vinorelbine) inhibit the formation of the mitotic apparatus, whereas others (paclitaxel, docetaxel) inhibit breakdown of these microtubules, thereby creating a stable but nonfunctional mitotic apparatus.[38,58] In either situation, these drugs disrupt the normal function of the mitotic apparatus and prevent the cell from dividing and proliferating. In fact, when the cell attempts to divide,

Text continued on page 577

Table 36–3 **ANTINEOPLASTIC ANTIBIOTICS**

Generic Name	Trade Name	Primary Antineoplastic Indication(s)*	Common Adverse Effects
Bleomycin	Blenoxane	Carcinoma of head, neck, cervical region, skin, penis, vulva, and testicle; Hodgkin disease; non-Hodgkin lymphomas	Pulmonary toxicity (interstitial pneumonitis); skin disorders (rash, discoloration); mucosal lesions; fever; GI distress; general weakness and malaise
Dactinomycin	Cosmegen	Carcinoma of testicle and endometrium; carcinosarcoma of kidney (Wilms tumor); Ewing sarcoma; rhabdomyosarcoma	Blood disorders (leukopenia, thrombocytopenia, others); GI distress (nausea, vomiting, loss of appetite); mucocutaneous lesions; skin disorders (rash, hair loss); local irritation at injection site
Daunorubicin	Cerubidine, DaunoXome	Several forms of acute leukemia	Blood disorders (anemia, leukopenia, thrombocytopenia); cardiotoxicity (arrhythmias, congestive heart failure); GI distress (nausea, vomiting, GI tract ulceration); hair loss
Doxorubicin	Adriamycin RDF, Rubex, others	Acute leukemias; carcinoma of bladder, breast, ovary, thyroid, and other tissues; Hodgkin disease; non-Hodgkin lymphomas; several sarcomas	Similar to daunorubicin
Idarubicin	Idamycin	Acute myelocytic leukemia	Similar to daunorubicin
Mitomycin	Mutamycin	Carcinoma of stomach and pancreas; chronic myelocytic leukemia	Blood disorders (leukopenia, thrombocytopenia); GI distress (nausea, vomiting, GI irritation and ulceration); nephrotoxicity; pulmonary toxicity
Mitoxantrone	Novantrone	Carcinoma of the prostate; acute nonlymphocytic leukemia	Cough, shortness of breath; leukopenia or infection; stomatitis/mucositis; GI problems (stomach pain, nausea, vomiting, diarrhea, GI bleeding)
Plicamycin	Mithracin	Testicular carcinoma	Blood disorders (leukopenia, thrombocytopenia); GI distress (nausea, vomiting, diarrhea, GI tract irritation); general weakness and malaise

*Only the indications listed in the U.S. product labeling are included here. Many anticancer drugs are used for additional types of neoplastic disease.
GI = gastrointestinal.

Table 36–4	PLANT ALKALOIDS		
Generic Name	**Trade Name**	**Primary Antineoplastic Indication(s)***	**Common Adverse Effects**
Docetaxel	Taxotere	Breast cancer	Blood disorders (anemia, leukopenia, neutropenia); fever; fluid retention; paresthesias/dysthesias; skin rashes/itching; stomatitis; GI distress (nausea, diarrhea);
Etoposide	Etopophos, VePesid	Carcinoma of lung, testes	Blood disorders (anemia, leukopenia, thrombocytopenia); GI distress (nausea, vomiting); hypotension, allergic reactions; hair loss; neurotoxicity (peripheral neuropathies, CNS effects)
Irinotecan	Camptosar	Colorectal cancer	Blood disorders (anemia, leukopenia, neutropenia); dyspnea; GI distress (nausea, vomiting, diarrhea, constipation, loss of appetite, abdominal cramps)
Paclitaxel	Taxol	Carcinoma of the breast, ovaries; Kaposi sarcoma; nonsmall cell lung cancer	Blood disorders (anemia, leukopenia, neutropenia, thrombocytopenia); hypersensitivity reaction (skin rash/itching, shortness of breath); joint/muscle pain; peripheral neuropathies; GI distress (nausea, vomiting, diarrhea)
Teniposide	Vumon	Acute lymphocytic leukemia	Blood disorders (anemia, leukopenia, neutropenia, thrombocytopenia); hypersensitivity reaction; mucositis; GI distress (nausea, vomiting, diarrhea)
Topotecan	Hycamtin	Ovarian cancer; small lung cell carcinoma	Blood disorders (anemia, leukopenia, neutropenia, thrombocytopenia); dyspnea; fever; neurological effects (muscle weakness, paresthesias); stomatitis; GI distress (abdominal pain, loss of appetite, nausea, vomiting, diarrhea, constipation)
Vinblastine	Velban, Velsar	Carcinoma of breast, testes, other tissues; Hodgkin disease; non-Hodgkin lymphomas; Kaposi sarcoma	Blood disorders (primarily leukopenia); GI distress (nausea, vomiting); hair loss; central and peripheral neuropathies; local irritation at injection site

(Continued on following page)

Table 36–4	PLANT ALKALOIDS *(Continued)*		
Generic Name	**Trade Name**	**Primary Antineoplastic Indication(s)***	**Common Adverse Effects**
Vincristine	Oncovin, Vincasar	Acute lymphocytic leukemia; neuroblastoma; Wilms tumor; Hodgkin disease; non-Hodgkin lymphomas; Ewing sarcoma	Neurotoxicity (peripheral neuropathies, CNS disorders); hair loss; local irritation at injection site
Vinorelbine	Navelbine	Nonsmall cell lung cancer	Blood disorders (anemia, granulocytopenia, leukopenia); unusual weakness/fatigue; GI distress (loss of appetite, nausea, vomiting, constipation); hair loss

*Only the indications listed in the U.S. product labeling are included here. Many anticancer drugs are used for additional types of neoplastic disease.
GI = gastrointestinal; CNS = central nervous system.

Table 36–5	ANTINEOPLASTIC HORMONES		
Types of Hormones	**Primary Antineoplastic Indications(s)***	**Common Adverse Effects**
Adrenocorticosteroids Prednisone Prednisolone Others	Acute lymphoblastic leukemia; chronic lymphocytic leukemia; Hodgkin disease	Adrenocortical suppression; general catabolic effect on supporting tissues (see Chapter 29)
Androgens Fluoxymesterone Methyltestosterone Testosterone	Advanced, inoperable breast cancer in postmenopausal women	Masculinization in women (see Chapter 30)
Antiandrogens Bicalutamide Flutamide Nilutamide	Inhibits the cellular uptake and effects of androgens in advanced, metastatic prostate cancer	Nausea; vomiting; diarrhea; decreased sex drive
Aromatase inhibitors Anastrozole Exemestane Letrozole	Inhibits estrogen biosynthesis to reduce the effects of estrogen in estrogen-sensitive breast cancer	Nausea; vomiting; dizziness; hot flashes; joint and muscle pain; dyspnea; (generally well-tolerated relative to other antineoplastic hormones; side effects vary depending on the specific drug)
Estrogens Diethylstilbestrol Estradiol Others	Advanced, inoperable breast cancer in selected men and postmenopausal women; advanced, inoperable prostate cancer in men	Cardiovascular complications (including stroke and heart attack—especially in men); many other adverse effects (see Chapter 30)

Types of Hormones	Primary Antineoplastic Indications(s)*	Common Adverse Effects
Antiestrogens Fulvestrant Tamoxifen	Acts as an estrogen antagonist to decrease the recurrence of cancer following mastectomy or to reduce tumor growth in advanced stages of breast cancer	Nausea; vomiting; hot flashes (generally well-tolerated relative to other antineoplastic hormones)
Progestins Hydroxyprogesterone Medroxyprogesterone Megestrol	Carcinoma of the breast and endometrium; advanced prostate cancer; advanced renal cancer	Menstrual irregularities; hyperglycemia; edema; mood changes; unusual tiredness; abdominal pain/cramps
Gonadotropin-releasing hormone drugs Abarelix Leuprolide Goserelin Triptorelin	Works by negative feedback mechanisms to inhibit testosterone or estrogen production; used primarily in advanced prostate cancer or breast cancer	Hot flashes; bone pain; CNS effects (headache, dizziness); GI disturbances (nausea, vomiting)

*Only the indications listed in the U.S. product labeling are included here. Many anticancer drugs are used for additional types of neoplastic disease.

GI = gastrointestinal; CNS = central nervous system.

because this drug binds to all estrogen receptors without activating them; that is, fulvestrant is a true estrogen receptor antagonist or blocker. As indicated in Chapter 30, tamoxifen is actually classified as a selective estrogen receptor modulator (SERM), meaning that this drug blocks estrogen receptors on certain tissues (breast, uterus), while stimulating other estrogen receptors in bone, cardiovascular tissues, skin, and so forth.[23,37]

In contrast to estrogen blockers, **aromatase inhibitors** such as anastrozole (Arimidex), letrozole (Femara), and exemestane (Aromasin) can decrease estrogen production in breast and other tissues by inhibiting the aromatase enzyme that is responsible for estrogen biosynthesis.[8,24] That is, these aromatase inhibitors do not block estrogen receptors, but instead reduce estrogen production, thereby decreasing the influence of estrogen on breast tumors.[17] Hence, several options are now available for controlling hormone-sensitive cancers that are responsive to estrogen and androgens in women and men, respectively. Refer to Chapter 30 for more details about the effects of androgens, estrogens, and their respective receptor blocking agents.

Biologic Response Modifiers

Agents such as the interferons, interleuklin-2, and **monoclonal antibodies** are classified as biologic re-

sponse modifiers because they enhance the body's ability to respond to neoplasms; that is, these drugs are not necessarily cytotoxic, but they affect the mechanisms that regulate cell division or influence specific aspects of immune function that help inhibit or destroy the cancerous tissues. These drugs are listed in Table 36–6, and are addressed briefly below.

The chemistry and pharmacology of the interferons were discussed in Chapter 34. These peptide compounds exert a number of beneficial effects, including antiviral and antineoplastic activity. However, the exact mechanism of action for interferons to impair cancerous cell growth is not clear. It is possible that interferons affect several aspects of tumor growth, including the inhibition of cancerous genes (oncogenes), the activation of cytotoxic immune cells (natural killer cells), and the inhibition of other aspects of cell metabolism and proliferation in cancerous tissues.[6] These agents are currently used to treat certain types of leukemias, lymphomas, Kaposi sarcoma, and cancer in other organs and tissues (Table 36–6).[11,33]

Interleukin-2 (IL-2) is an endogenous cytokine that normally exerts a number of beneficial immunologic responses. In particular, IL-2 stimulates the growth and differentiation of T-cell lymphocytes that are selectively toxic for tumor cells.[11,33] Hence, recombinant DNA techniques are now used to synthesize IL-2 so that this agent can be used to treat cancers such as renal cancer and malignant melanoma (see

Table 36–6	OTHER ANTINEOPLASTIC DRUG CATEGORIES	
Drug(s)	**Primary Antineoplastic Indication(s)***	**Common Adverse Effects**
Biologic response modifiers		

Interferons
  Interferon alfa-2a
    (Roferon-A)
  Interferon alfa-2b
    (Intron-A)
	Hairy-cell leukemia; Kaposi sarcoma; chronic myelocytic leukemia; renal and bladder cancers	Flulike syndrome (mild fever, chills, malaise)

Interleukin-2 Aldesleukin (Proleukin)	Renal carcinoma	Blood disorders (anemia, eosinophilia, leukopenia, thrombocytopenia); cardiac arrhythmias; hypotension; pulmonary toxicity; renal toxicity; neuropsychiatric effects; hypothyroidism
Monoclonal antibodies		
Alemtuzumab (Campath)	Chronic lymphocytic leukemia	Blood disorders (anemia, leukopenia, neutropenia, thrombocytopenia); chest pain, dyspnea; infection; nausea
Bevacizumab (Avastin)	Colorectal carcinoma	Hemorrhage; hypertension; GI distress (nausea, vomiting, diarrhea); blood disorders (leukopenia, neutropenia); others
Cetuximab (Erbitux)	Colorectal carcinoma	Rash; fever; infection; dyspnea; GI distress (nausea, vomiting, diarrhea)
Gemtuzumab (Mylotarg)	Acute myeloid leukemia	Hemorrhage; liver toxicity; infection; joint pain; lung toxicity; GI distress (nausea, vomiting, diarrhea); others
Rituximab (Rituxan)	Non-Hodgkin lymphoma	Blood disorders (anemia, leukopenia, neutropenia, thrombocytopenia); hypertension; hyperglycemia; joint and muscle pain; fatigue; rash; GI distress (nausea, vomiting, diarrhea); others
Heavy metal compounds		
Carboplatin (Paraplatin)	Carcinoma of the ovaries	Blood disorders (anemia, leukopenia, neutropenia, thrombocytopenia); unusual tiredness; GI distress (nausea, vomiting)
Cisplatin (Platinol)	Carcinoma of bladder, ovaries, testicles, and other tissues	Nephrotoxicity; GI distress (nausea, vomiting); neurotoxicity (cranial and peripheral nerves); hypersensitive reactions (e.g., flushing, respiratory problems, tachycardia)

Drug(s)	Primary Antineoplastic Indication(s)[*]	Common Adverse Effects
Oxaliplatin	Colorectal cancer	Blood disorders (anemia, leukopenia, neutropenia, thrombocytopenia); joint pain, chest pain
Tyrosine kinase inhibitors		
Erlotinib	Nonsmall cell lung cancer; carcinoma of the pancreas	GI distress (nausea, diarrhea); rash; lung toxicity
Geftinib	Nonsmall cell lung cancer	Blurred vision; dyspnea; rash; GI distress (nausea, vomiting, diarrhea)
Imatinib	Chronic myeloid leukemia	GI distress (nausea, vomiting); blood disorders (anemia, neutropenia, thrombocytopenia); joint and muscle pain; chest pain

[*]Only the indications listed in the U.S. product labeling are included here. Many anticancer drugs are used for additional types of neoplastic disease.
GI = gastrointestinal.

Table 36–6). Research continues to identify the antineoplastic role of interleukins, interferons, and other cytokines, as well as to define how these agents can be used alone or in combination to treat various forms of cancer.[33,77]

Monoclonal antibodies represent a method for targeting an anticancer drug against cancerous tissues.[53,75] These drugs are manufactured using cell cloning techniques that produce an antibody that is specific for an antigen on the surface of a particular type of cancer cell. When administered, the monoclonal antibody is attracted directly to the cancer cell, without any appreciable affect on healthy tissues. That is, healthy cells lack the antigen that is present on the cancerous cell, and should therefore remain unaffected by the drug. Once it has reached the cancerous cell, monoclonal antibodies exert several complex effects that limit cell function, inhibit mitosis, and can possibly result in the cell's death.[34] Some newer monoclonal agents known as bispecific antibodies may also contain a second antibody that produces an additional beneficial effect such as stimulating production of cytotoxic T lymphocytes or other immune system components that attack the tumor.[47] Although the use of monoclonal antibodies is still relatively new, several agents are currently available (Table 36–6). Likewise, development of anticancer antibodies continues to be an important area of research, and other antibodies

that selectively inhibit or kill cancer cells with minimal or no effects on healthy tissues may be available in the future.[34,75]

Certain monoclonal antibodies such as bevacizumab (Avastin) can also be used as **angiogenesis** inhibitors; that is, these agents inhibit the formation of new blood vessels in growing tumors.[65,88] Because tumors often need a rich vascular supply to grow and proliferate, angiogenesis inhibitors can literally starve the tumor of oxygen and nutrients.[87,91] Bevacizumab binds specifically to vascular endothelial growth factor (VEGF), and prevents it from stimulating the formation of blood vessels in the tumor.[62,88] Hence, this intervention can be used along with other more traditional anticancer drugs to treat specific cancers such as advanced colorectal cancer. Other strategies to prevent angiogenesis are currently being developed, and various types of angiogenesis inhibitors may be forthcoming.[21,65]

Heavy Metal Compounds

Heavy metal compounds used to treat cancer include cisplatin, carboplatin, and oxaliplatin (see Table 36–6). These drugs, which contain platinum, are also known as platinum coordination complexes.[10,27] Heavy metal drugs act like the alkylating agents; that is, they form strong cross-links between and within DNA strands, thereby preventing DNA translation and replication. The chemical nature of these cross-links, however, involves the platinum component of the drug rather than actual formation of an alkyl side group. Heavy metal compounds are especially important in treating certain epithelial cancers, including testicular cancer, ovarian cancer, bladder cancer, and others (see Table 36–6).[11,89]

Aspirin and Other NSAIDs

Considerable evidence exists that aspirin and similar nonsteroidal anti-inflammatory drugs (NSAIDs) can prevent colorectal cancer, and that these drugs might also decrease malignancies in other tissues such as the stomach, esophagus, breast, bladder, and lungs.[79,82] This effect seems to be dose-related, with increased protection occurring in people who use aspirin on a regular basis.[82] Although the exact reason for this anti-cancer effect is unknown, certain prostaglandins such as prostaglandin E2 may promote the growth and proliferation of certain tumors.[12,82] As indicated in Chapter 15, aspirin and similar drugs inhibit the cyclo-oxygenase enzyme that synthesizes prostaglandins in various cells in the body. Hence, aspirin and other NSAIDs may reduce the risk of colorectal cancer and other cancers by inhibiting the synthesis of certain prostaglandins. In addition, the COX-2 form of the cyclooxygenase enzyme seems to be prevalent in certain tumors, and inhibition of this enzyme using COX-2 selective drugs may ultimately provide optimal results in certain cancers.[13] More information will surely be forthcoming about how aspirin and other NSAIDs can help prevent specific types of cancer.

Tyrosine Kinase Inhibitors

As discussed in Chapter 4, tyrosine kinase is an enzyme found in many cells and is responsible for transmitting signals from the cell membrane to other functional components throughout the cell. In certain types of cancer, defective function of tyrosine kinases leads to abnormal cell function and proliferation. Hence, drugs that inhibit tyrosine kinase activity will be especially useful in some cancers.[11] Several tyrosine kinase drugs are currently available including erlotinib (Tarceva), geftinib (Iressa), and imatinib (Glivec). These drugs are gaining acceptance as a part of the treatment of certain leukemias, as well as cancers affecting other tissues such as the lungs, stomach, and pancreas. Use of these drugs is fairly new, however, and more informa-tion about optimal use of tyrosine kinase inhibitors will surely be forthcoming.

Miscellaneous Agents

Certain chemotherapy agents do not fall into one of the categories addressed above. These miscellaneous drugs are listed in Table 36–7, and are described briefly below.

Arsenic trioxide. Arsenic is a heavy metal that can exert toxic, poisonous effects. Therapeutic dosages of arsenic trioxide (Trisenox), however, may limit the growth of certain leukemias such as acute promyelo-cytic leukemia.[11] However, because of its potential toxicity, arsenic trioxide is not usually an initial treat-ment, but is reserved for patients who relapse or who are resistant to other treatments. Although the exact mechanism of action is unclear, this drug apparently induces several cytotoxic effects by directly damaging DNA and proteins that regulate DNA synthesis and replication.

Asparaginase. Asparaginase (Elspar) is an enzyme that converts the amino acid asparagine into aspartic acid and ammonia. Most normal cells are able to syn-thesize sufficient amounts of asparagine to function properly. Some tumor cells (especially certain leukemic cells) must rely on extracellular sources for a supply of asparagine, however. By breaking down asparagine in the bloodstream and extracellular fluid, asparaginase deprives tumor cells of their source of asparagine, thus selectively impairing cell metabolism in these cells.[36] Asparaginase is used primarily in the treatment of acute lymphocytic leukemia (see Table 36–7).

Bortezomib. Bortezomib (Velcade) inhibits pro-teasome activity in mammalian cells.[11] Mammalian proteasome is responsible for degrading certain cellu-lar proteins affecting cell function and division. By prolonging the activity of these proteins, bortezomib brings about complex changes in cell function that lead to cell dysfunction and death. Certain types of cancer, such as multiple myeloma, are more sensitive to impaired proteasome regulation, hence the use of this drug in these cancers.

Denileukin Diftitox. Denileukin Diftitox (Ontak) is formulated by combining interleukin-2 with diph-theria toxin.[11] Certain leukemia and lymphoma cells have a surface receptor that has a high affinity for interleukin-2, thus attracting this drug directly to these cells. Upon binding with the receptor, the diphtheria toxin component of the drug inhibits cellular protein synthesis, which ultimately results in cell death. This

| **Table 36–7** | **MISCELLANEOUS ANTINEOPLASTIC DRUGS** |

Drug	Primary Antineoplastic Indication(s)*	Common Adverse Effects
Arsenic trioxide (Trisenox)	Acute promyelocytic leukemia	Dyspnea; GI distress (nausea, vomiting, diarrhea); headache; fatigue; others
Asparaginase (Elspar)	Acute lymphocytic leukemia	Allergic reactions; renal toxicity; hepatic toxicity; delayed hemostasis; CNS toxicity (fatigue, mood changes); GI distress (nausea, vomiting); pancreatitis
Bortezomib (Velcade)	Multiple myeloma	Blood disorders (anemia, neutropenia, thrombocytopenia); dyspnea; joint and muscle pain; peripheral neuropathies
Denileukin Diftitox (Ontak)	Cutaneous T-cell lymphomas	Acute allergic reactions; joint and muscle pain; flulike symptoms; infection; GI distress (nausea, vomiting, diarrhea)
Estramustine (Emcyt)	Prostate cancer	Sodium and fluid retention; blood disorders (leukopenia, thrombocytopenia); thrombosis; GI distress (nausea, diarrhea)
Hydroxyurea (Hydrea)	Carcinoma of the ovaries, head/neck region, other tissues; chronic myelocytic leukemia; melanomas	Blood disorders (primarily leukopenia); GI distress (nausea, vomiting, loss of appetite, GI tract irritation and ulceration); skin rash
Mitotane (Lysodren)	Suppresses adrenal gland; used primarily to treat adrenocortical carcinoma	GI distress (nausea, vomiting, diarrhea, loss of appetite); CNS toxicity (lethargy, fatigue, mood changes); skin rashes
Thalidomide (Thalomid)	Multiple myeloma	Peripheral neuropathy; dizziness; drowsiness; GI distress (nausea, diarrhea, stomach pain); contraindicated in pregnant women because of teratogenic potential
Tretinoin (Vesanoid)	Acute promyelocytic leukemia	Cardiac arrhythmias; edema; blood pressure abnormalities (hypotension, hypertension); phlebitis; respiratory tract problems; muscle pain; paresthesias; CNS toxicity (depression, anxiety, confusion); skin rash; GI distress (abdominal distension; nausea, vomiting)

*Only the indications listed in the U.S. product labeling are included here. Many anticancer drugs are used for additional types of neoplastic disease.

GI = gastrointestinal; CNS = central nervous system.

drug is used primarily to treat recurrent cutaneous T-cell lymphoma.

Estramustine. Estramustine (Emcyt) is a chemical combination of mechlorethamine (an alkylating agent) and estrogen. It is not clear, however, how this drug exerts antineoplastic effects. The beneficial effects of this drug are probably not related to any alkylating effects. Rather, they may be the direct result of its estrogenic component, or its inhibitory effect on the microtubules that comprise the mitotic apparatus.[11] This drug is typically used for the palliative treatment of advanced prostate cancer.[60]

Hydroxyurea. It is believed that hydroxyurea (Hydrea) impairs DNA synthesis by inhibiting a specific enzyme (ribonucleoside reductase) involved in synthesizing nucleic acid precursors.[11] The uses of hydroxyurea are listed in Table 36–7.

Mitotane. Although the exact mechanism of this drug is unknown, mitotane (Lysodren) selectively inhibits adrenocortical function. This agent is used exclusively to treat carcinoma of the adrenal cortex.

Thalidomide. Thalidomide (Thalomid) was originally developed as a sedative and antinausea drug, but was withdrawn from the market because it caused severe birth defects when administered to pregnant women. This drug, however, has reemerged as a potential treatment for cancers such as multiple myeloma.[39,73] Although the exact reasons for its anticancer effects are not clear, thalidomide exerts a number of complex effects on immune function, including the suppression of tumor necrosis factor alpha.[40] This drug also inhibits angiogenesis, and may therefore limit the growth of solid tumors by inhibiting vascularization and nutrient supply.[63]

Tretinoin. Tretinoin (Vesanoid), also known as all-*trans*-retinoic acid, is derived from vitamin A (retinol).[86] This drug is not cytotoxic, but it may help cells differentiate and replicate at a more normal rate. However, the exact way that this agent affects cell differentiation is not known. Tretinoin is used primarily to treat certain forms of leukemia.[7]

Combination Chemotherapy

Frequently, several different anticancer drugs are administered simultaneously. This process of combination chemotherapy increases the chance of successfully treating the cancer because of the additive and synergistic effect of each agent. Often, different types of anticancer drugs are combined in the same regimen to provide optimal results.[11] For instance, a particular drug regimen may include an alkylating agent, an antineoplastic antibiotic, a hormonal agent, or some other combination of anticancer drugs.

Some common anticancer drug combinations and the types of cancer in which they are used are listed in Table 36–8. These drug combinations are often indicated by an acronym of the drug names. For instance, "FAC" indicates a regimen of fluorouracil, doxorubicin (Adriamycin), and cyclophosphamide. These abbreviations are used to summarize drug therapy in a patient's medical chart, so therapists should be aware of the more common chemotherapy combinations.

Use of Anticancer Drugs with Other Treatments

Cancer chemotherapy is only one method of treating neoplastic disease. The other primary weapons in the anticancer arsenal are surgery and radiation treatment.[18,61] The choice of one or more of these techniques depends primarily on the patient, the type of cancer, and the tumor location. In many situations, chemotherapy may be the primary or sole form of treatment in neoplastic disease, especially for certain advanced or inoperable tumors, or in widely disseminated forms of cancer, such as leukemia or lymphoma.[6] In other situations, chemotherapy is used in combination with other techniques, such as an adjuvant to surgery and radiation treatment.[18,27] Primary examples of adjuvant cancer chemotherapy include using anticancer drugs following a mastectomy or surgical removal of other carcinomas.[19,54,43,61]

Whether anticancer drugs are used as the primary treatment or as adjuvant therapy, a common general strategy is upheld. To achieve a total cell kill, all reasonable means of dealing with the cancer must be employed as early as possible. Cancer is not the type of disease in which a wait-and-see approach can be used. The general strategy is more aligned with the idea that a barrage of anticancer modalities (i.e., surgery, radiation, and a combination of several different antineoplastic drugs) may be necessary to achieve a successful outcome. In addition, a multimodal approach (combining chemotherapy with radiation or using several drugs simultaneously) may produce a synergistic effect between these modalities. For instance, certain drugs may sensitize cancer cells to radiation treatment.[71,90]

Table 36–8	FREQUENTLY USED COMBINATION CHEMOTHERAPY REGIMENS	
Chemotherapeutic Regimen[*]	Components of Regimen	Primary Indication
ABVD	Doxorubicin (Adriamycin), bleomycin (Blenoxane), vinblastine (Velban), dacarbazine (DTIC)	Hodgkin Disease
BEP	Bleomycin, etoposide, cisplatin (Platinol)	Germ cell tumors
CHOP	Cyclophosphamide (Cytoxan), doxorubicin,[**] vincristine (Oncovin), prednisone	Non-Hodgkin lymphoma
CMF	Cyclophosphamide (Cytoxan), methotrexate, 5-fluorouracil	Breast cancer
COP	Cyclophosphamide (Cytoxan), vincristine (Oncovin), prednisone	Non-Hodgkin lymphoma
FAC	5-Fluorouracil, doxorubicin (Adriamycin), cyclophosphamide (Cytoxan)	Breast cancer
ICE	Ifosfamide, carboplatin, etoposide	Nonsmall cell lung cancer
MOPP	Mechlorethamine (Mustargen), vincristine (Oncovin), procarbazine, prednisone	Hodgkin Disease
VAD	Vincristine, doxorubicin (Adriamycin), dexamethasone	Multiple myeloma
VIP	Vincristine, ifosfamide, cisplatin (Platinol)	Germ cell tumors

[*]A few examples of commonly used regimens are listed here. Many other combinations are used clinically, and regimens are often tailored for the needs of each patient.
[**]The H in this regimen refers to hydroxydaunorubicin, the chemical synonym for doxorubicin.

Likewise, several drugs working together may increase the antineoplastic effects of one another through a synergistic cytotoxic effect.[11]

Success of Anticancer Drugs

Various forms of cancer exhibit a broad spectrum of response to antineoplastic medications. Some forms of cancer (choriocarcinoma, Wilms tumor) can be cured in more than 90 percent of affected patients. In other neoplastic disorders, chemotherapy may not cure the disease but may succeed in mediating remission and prolonging survival in a large patient percentage. Of course, other factors such as early detection and the concomitant use of other interventions (surgery, radiation) will greatly influence the success of chemotherapy drugs.

However, several types of cancer do not respond well to treatment. For example, the majority of metastatic cancers cannot be cured by current chemotherapeutic methods or by any other type of treatment.[11] In addition, some of the most common forms of adult neoplastic disease are difficult to treat by using anticancer drugs. As indicated in Table 36–9, the number of deaths associated with colorectal, prostate, and breast cancer is unacceptably high, and the mortality rate for lung cancer and pancreatic cancer is well over 90 percent in both men and women.

Exactly why some forms of cancer are more difficult to treat pharmacologically than others remains unclear. Differences in the biochemistry, genetics, and location of certain cancer cells may make them less sensitive to the toxic effects of anticancer drugs.[6] Resistance to anticancer drugs

Table 36–9	INCIDENCE AND MORTALITY OF THE LEADING FORMS OF CANCER IN WOMEN AND MEN*	
Type/Site of Cancer	Number of New Cases	Number of Deaths
Women		
Breast	212,920	40,970
Colon and rectum	57,460	27,300
Leukemia	15,070	9,810
Lung and bronchus	81,770	72,130
Lymphoma	31,800	9,560
Ovary	20,180	15,310
Pancreas	16,580	16,210
Uterine cervix	9,710	3,700
Uterine corpus	41,200	7,350
Men		
Colon and rectum	49,220	27,870
Esophagus	11,260	10,730
Leukemia	20,000	12,470
Liver and bile duct	12,600	10,840
Lung and bronchus	92,700	90,330
Lymphoma	34,870	10,770
Pancreas	17,150	16,090
Prostate	234,460	27,350
Urinary system	70,940	17,530

*Source: The American Cancer Society Department of Epidemiology and Surveillance Research, estimates for 2006.

(see the next section, "Resistance to Cancer Chemotherapy Drugs") may also explain why certain cancers respond poorly to chemotherapy. Consequently, investigations of how to improve the efficacy of existing agents and the development of new anticancer drugs remain major foci in pharmacologic research. Some of the primary strategies in improving cancer chemotherapy are discussed later in "Future Perspectives."

Resistance to Cancer Chemotherapy Drugs

As indicated previously, certain cancers do not respond well to cancer chemotherapy. A primary reason is that cancers may develop resistance to a broad range of chemotherapeutic agents (multiple drug resistance), thus rendering these drugs ineffective in treating the cancer.[9,74]

Cancers can become resistant to drugs through several different mechanisms. One common mechanism occurs when the cancer cell synthesizes a glycoprotein that acts as a drug efflux pump.[15,74] The glycoprotein pump is inserted into the cancer cell's membrane and effectively expels different types of anticancer drugs from the cancer cell. Thus, cancer chemotherapeutic agents are ineffective because they are removed from the cell before they have a chance to exert cytotoxic effects.

Cancer cells also use other mechanisms to induce drug resistance, including the production of specific substances (glutathione, glutathione-*S*-transferases) that inactivate anticancer drugs within the cancer cell, or the development of mechanisms that repair DNA that is damaged by anticancer drugs.[22,48] Likewise, many anticancer drugs must bind to a specific receptor on or within the cancer cell; these cells can develop drug resistance by modifying the structure or function of these receptors so that the drug is unable to bind to the receptor.[28,50] Cancer cells are therefore capable of developing several methods for self-preservation against a broad range of cytotoxic drugs. Hence, various strategies are being explored to prevent or overcome multiple-drug resistance during cancer chemotherapy. These strategies include altering the dosage, timing, and sequence of administration of different medications and using different combinations of medications to combat resistance.[49,52,84] Use of these strategies, along with the development of new anticancer agents that do not cause resistance (see the next section, "Future Perspectives"), should help increase the effectiveness of chemotherapy in certain types of cancer.

Future Perspectives

Several new strategies are being explored to increase the effectiveness and decrease the toxicity of anticancer drugs.[57,64] As discussed previously, most of the traditional drugs are toxic not only to tumor cells but also to normal cells. Nonetheless, if the drug can be delivered or targeted specifically for tumor cells, it will produce a more selective effect. One way to accomplish this targeting is by attaching the drug to another substance that is attracted specifically to tumor cells. An example of this strategy is the use of monoclonal antibodies (see the section on "Biological Response Modifiers"). By joining the drug with an antibody that recognizes receptors only on cancerous cells, the drug is delivered directly to the neoplastic tissues. Although the use of antibodies in treating cancer is still relatively new, these and other vehicles that specifically target the tumor will almost certainly expand in the future.[35,69]

Drugs may likewise be delivered more effectively to cancerous cells by encapsulating the drug in a microsphere or liposome that becomes lodged in the tumor.[3,66] Drug microspheres or other drug formulations can also be implanted surgically so that the drug remains fairly localized at the tumor site, thereby reducing its systemic effects.[26] Variations on these techniques and other delivery methods continue to be explored and may someday be used on a widespread basis to increase effectiveness, while decreasing the toxicity of anticancer drugs.

Other unique strategies are being developed to selectively impair the chemistry or metabolism of cancerous tissues. As indicated earlier, drugs such as bevacizumab act as angiogenesis inhibitors that restrict the formation of new blood vessels in developing tumors. This effect can limit tumor growth and promote the death of cancerous cells by starving the tumor of oxygen and nutrients. This idea is especially attractive because agents that inhibit angiogenesis can have a fairly selective effect on the tumor without producing excessive effects on the vascularization of normal tissues.[21,91] Although the number of angiogenesis inhibitors is currently limited, clinical

trials of other angiogenesis inhibitors are ongoing, and these agents will hopefully become a more common component in the treatment of various neoplasms.[87,91]

A number of other experimental strategies that limit the metabolism and proliferation of cancerous cells are likewise being explored. These strategies typically capitalize on some enzymatic process or other unique aspect of cancer cell metabolism so that normal tissues remain largely unaffected by the drug.[11] An example is the use of drugs such as imatinib and geftinib that inhibit abnormal tyrosine kinase activity in certain cancerous cells (see "Tyrosine Kinase Inhibitors" above). As more is learned about the unique aspects of cancer cell metabolism, other agents will be developed that selectively impair the biochemistry of the cancer cell with minimal effects on the metabolism and function of normal cells.

Additionally, strategies are being explored to administer drugs that can protect healthy cells from the more traditional anticancer agents.[32,44] An example is the possible use of antioxidants or free-radical scavengers that reduce chemotherapy-induced damage to healthy cells.[55,67] Hence, several preliminary strategies have been developed to provide more selective and less toxic chemotherapeutic regimens. Future research will almost certainly expand these ideas to provide effective and safer treatments for cancer.

Finally, important advances have been made in understanding how the body's immune system can be recruited to help prevent and treat certain cancers. If the body's immune system recognizes the cancer cell as an invader, then various endogenous immune responses can be initiated to combat the cancerous cells. Hence, various strategies are being explored to help stimulate this immunologic response, including genetic modification of the cancer cells to increase their antigenic properties and expose these cells to immune attack.[5,81] The most promising efforts center around the development of anticancer vaccines, whereby the immune system can be sensitized to search out and destroy cancerous cells before they can develop into serious cancers.[42,46,72] Increased knowledge about the nature of cancer, combined with a better understanding of the endogenous control of cell replication, may ultimately provide drugs that are safe and effective in curing all forms of cancer.

Implications of Cancer Chemotherapy in Rehabilitation Patients

■ ■ ■ The major way in which antineoplastic drugs will affect physical therapy and occupational therapy is through the adverse side effects of these agents. These drugs are routinely associated with a number of severe toxic effects, including gastrointestinal problems, blood disorders, and profound fatigue. In addition, neurotoxic effects, including CNS abnormalities (such as convulsions and ataxia) and peripheral neuropathies, may be a problem, especially with plant alkaloids (vinblastine, vincristine). In terms of physical rehabilitation, these side effects are typically a source of frustration to both the patient and therapist. On some days, the patient undergoing cancer chemotherapy will simply not be able to tolerate even a relatively mild rehabilitation session. This reality can be especially demoralizing to patients who want to try to overcome the disease and actively participate in therapy as much as possible. Physical therapists and occupational therapists must take into account the debilitating nature of these drugs and be sensitive to the needs of the patient on a day-to-day basis. At certain times, the therapist must simply back off in trying to encourage active participation from the patient. Therapists, however, can often be particularly helpful in providing psychological support to patients undergoing antineoplastic drug treatment. Therapists can reassure the patient that the side effects of these drugs are usually transient and that there will be better days when rehabilitation can be resumed.

Therapists may also be helpful in treating other problems associated with neoplastic disease. In particular, therapists may be involved in reducing the severe pain typically associated with many forms of cancer. Therapists can use transcutaneous electric nerve stimulation (TENS) or other physical agents as a nonpharmacologic means to attenuate pain. Other physical interventions such as massage can also be invaluable in helping decrease the pain and anxiety that often occur in people receiving cancer chemotherapy. These approaches may reduce the need for pain medications, thus reducing the chance that these drugs will cause additional adverse effects and drug interactions with anticancer drugs.

As previously mentioned, physical therapists and occupational therapists also play a vital role in providing encouragement and support to the patient with cancer. This support can often help immeasurably in improving the patient's quality-of-life.

CASE STUDY

Cancer Chemotherapy

Brief History. R.J. is a 57-year-old woman who was diagnosed with metastatic breast cancer 1 year ago, at which time she underwent a modified radical mastectomy followed by antineoplastic drugs. The cancer, however, had evidently metastasized to other tissues, including bone. She recently developed pain in the lumbosacral region, which was attributed to metastatic skeletal lesions in the lower lumbar vertebrae. She was admitted to the hospital to pursue a course of radiation treatment to control pain and minimize bony

destruction at the site of the skeletal lesion. Her current pharmacologic regimen consists of an antineoplastic antimetabolite (doxorubicin) and an antiestrogen (tamoxifen). She was also given a combination of narcotic and non-narcotic analgesics (codeine and aspirin) to help control pain. Physical therapy was initiated to help control pain and maintain function in this patient.

Problem/Influence of Medication. The patient began to experience an increase in gastrointestinal side effects, including nausea, vomiting, loss of appetite, and epigastric pain. These problems may have been caused by the analgesic drugs or by the combination of the analgesics and the antimetabolite. However, the patient, experienced adequate pain relief from the aspirin-codeine combination and was reluctant to consider alternative medications. The persistent nausea and loss of appetite had a general debilitating effect on the patient, and the physical therapist was having difficulty engaging the patient in an active general conditioning program.

Decision/Solution. The therapist instituted a program of local heat (hot packs) and TENS to help control pain in the lumbosacral region. This approach provided a nonpharmacologic means of alleviating pain, thereby decreasing the patient's analgesic drug requirements and related gastrointestinal problems. The patient was able to participate actively in a rehabilitation program throughout the course of her hospitalization, thus maintaining her overall strength and physical condition.

SUMMARY

Antineoplastic drugs typically limit excessive growth and proliferation of cancer cells by impairing DNA synthesis and function or by directly limiting cell division (mitosis). To replicate at a rapid rate, cancer cells must synthesize rather large quantities of DNA and RNA and continually undergo mitosis. Hence, cancer cells tend to be affected by antineoplastic drugs to a somewhat greater extent than normal cells. Normal cells, however, are also frequently affected by these drugs, resulting in a high incidence of side effects. Currently, cancer chemotherapy is effective in reducing and even curing many neoplastic diseases. However, other forms of cancer are much more difficult to treat pharmacologically. Several strategies have been developed to target the antineoplastic drug directly for cancer cells. Increased use of these targeted strategies may improve the efficacy and safety of anticancer agents. Rehabilitation specialists should be aware of the general debilitating nature of traditional chemotherapy regimens, and therapists must be prepared to adjust their treatment based on the ability of the patient to tolerate the adverse effects of cancer chemotherapy.

References

1. Aapro M. 5-HT(3)-receptor antagonists in the management of nausea and vomiting in cancer and cancer treatment. *Oncology.* 2005;69:97–109.
2. Aapro M. Optimising antiemetic therapy: what are the problems and how can they be overcome? *Curr Med Res Opin.* 2005;21:885–897.
3. Andresen TL, Jensen SS, Kaasgaard T, Jorgensen K. Triggered activation and release of liposomal prodrugs and drugs in cancer tissue by secretory phospholipase A2. *Curr Drug Deliv.* 2005;2:353–362.
4. Aranda Aguilar E, Constenla Figueiras M, Cortes-Funes H, et al. Clinical practice guidelines on antiemetics in oncology. *Expert Rev Anticancer Ther.* 2005;5:963–972.
5. Baecher-Allan C, Anderson DE. Immune regulation in tumor-bearing hosts. *Curr Opin Immunol.* 2006;18:214–219.
6. Balmer CM, Valley AW. Cancer treatment and chemotherapy. In: DiPiro JT, et al, eds. *Pharmacotherapy: A Pathophysiologic Approach.* 5th ed. New York: McGraw-Hill; 2002.
7. Bastie JN, Balitrand N, Guillemot I, et al. Cooperative action of 1alpha,25-dihydroxyvitamin D3 and retinoic acid in NB4 acute promyelocytic leukemia cell differentiation is transcriptionally controlled. *Exp Cell Res.* 2005;310:319–330.
8. Berry J. Are all aromatase inhibitors the same? A review of controlled clinical trials in breast cancer. *Clin Ther.* 2005;27:1671–1684.
9. Bosch TM, Meijerman I, Beijnen JH, Schellens JH. Genetic polymorphisms of drug-metabolising enzymes and drug transporters in the chemotherapeutic treatment of cancer. *Clin Pharmacokinet.* 2006;45:253–285.
10. Brabec V, Kasparkova J. Modifications of DNA by platinum complexes. Relation to resistance of tumors to platinum antitumor drugs. *Drug Resist Update.* 2005; 8:131–146.
11. Chabner BA, Amrein PC, Druker BJ, et al: Antineoplastic agents. In: Brunton LL, et al, eds. *The Pharmacological Basis of Therapeutics.* 11th ed. New York: McGraw-Hill 2006.
12. Chell S, Patsos HA, Qualtrough D, et al. Prospects in NSAID-derived chemoprevention of colorectal cancer. *Biochem Soc Trans.* 2005;33:667–671.
13. Chow LW, Loo WT, Toi M. Current directions for COX-2 inhibition in breast cancer. *Biomed Pharmacother.* 2005;59(suppl 2):S281–S284.
14. Chu E, Sartorelli AC. Cancer chemotherapy. In: Katzung BG, ed. *Basic and Clinical Pharmacology.* 9th ed. New York: Lange Medical Books/McGraw-Hill; 2004.
15. Clarke R, Leonessa F, Trock B. Multidrug resistance/P-glycoprotein and breast cancer: review and meta-analysis. *Semin Oncol.* 2005;32(suppl 7):S9–S15.
16. Coulthard S, Hogarth L. The thiopurines: an update. *Invest New Drugs.* 2005;23:523–532.
17. Cuzick J, Sasieni P, Howell A. Should aromatase inhibitors be used as initial adjuvant treatment or sequenced after tamoxifen? *Br J Cancer.* 2006; 94:460–464.

18. Elshaikh M, Ljungman M, Ten Haken R, Lichter AS. Advances in radiation oncology. *Annu Rev Med.* 2006; 57:19–31.

19. Evans DB. Preoperative chemoradiation for pancreatic cancer. *Semin Oncol.* 2005;32(suppl 9):S25–S29.

20. Floyd JD, Nguyen DT, Lobins RL, et al. Cardiotoxicity of cancer therapy. *J Clin Oncol.* 2005;23:7685–7696.

21. Folkman J. Angiogenesis. *Annu Rev Med.* 2006;57:1–18.

22. Francia G, Green SK, Bocci G, et al. Down-regulation of DNA mismatch repair proteins in human and murine tumor spheroids: implications for multicellular resistance to alkylating agents. *Mol Cancer Ther.* 2005; 4:1484–1494.

23. Gasco M, Argusti A, Bonanni B, Decensi A. SERMs in chemoprevention of breast cancer. *Eur J Cancer.* 2005; 41:1980–1989.

24. Geisler J, Lonning PE. Aromatase inhibitors as adjuvant treatment of breast cancer. *Crit Rev Oncol Hematol.* 2006;57:53–61.

25. Gruber BM, Anuszewska EL, Bubko I, et al. Relationship between topoisomerase II-DNA cleavable complexes, apoptosis and cytotoxic activity of anthracyclines in human cervix carcinoma cells. *Anticancer Res.* 2005; 25(3B):2193–2198.

26. Hamstra DA, Moffat BA, Hall DE, et al. Intratumoral injection of BCNU in ethanol (DTI-015) results in enhanced delivery to tumor—a pharmacokinetic study. *J Neurooncol.* 2005;73:225–238.

27. Hao D, Ritter MA, Oliver T, Browman GP. Platinum-based concurrent hemoradiotherapy for tumors of the head and neck and the esophagus. *Semin Radiat Oncol.* 2006;16:10–19.

28. Hirawat S, Budman DR, Kreis W. The androgen receptor: structure, mutations, and antiandrogens. *Cancer Invest.* 2003;21:400–417.

29. Hoffmann J, Sommer A. Steroid hormone receptors as targets for the therapy of breast and prostate cancer—recent advances, mechanisms of resistance, and new approaches. *J Steroid Biochem Mol Biol.* 2005;93: 191–200.

30. Horiot JC. Antiemetic therapy in cancer: an update. *Expert Opin Pharmacother.* 2005;6:1713–1723.

31. Hoyert DL, Heron MP, Murphy SL, Kung HC. Deaths: final data for 2003. *Natl Vital Stat Rep.* 2006;54:1–120.

32. Hussain AE, Blakley BW, Nicolas M, Balderston J. Assessment of the protective effects of amifostine against cisplatin-induced toxicity. *J Otolaryngol.* 2003;32:294–297.

33. Hutson TE, Quinn DI. Cytokine therapy: a standard of care for metastatic renal cell carcinoma? *Clin Genitourin Cancer.* 2005;4:181–186.

34. Iannello A, Ahmad A. Role of antibody-dependent cell-mediated cytotoxicity in the efficacy of therapeutic anti-cancer monoclonal antibodies. *Cancer Metastasis Rev.* 2005;24:487–499.

35. Jaracz S, Chen J, Kuznetsova LV, Ojima I. Recent advances in tumor-targeting anticancer drug conjugates. *Bioorg Med Chem.* 2005;13:5043–5054.

36. Jarrar M, Gaynon PS, Periclou AP, et al. Asparagine depletion after pegylated *E. coli* asparaginase treatment and induction outcome in children with acute lymphoblastic leukemia in first bone marrow relapse: A Children's Oncology Group study (CCG-1941). *Pediatr Blood Cancer.* 2006;47:141–146.

37. Johansen AM. Breast cancer chemoprevention: a review of selective estrogen receptor modulators. *Clin J Oncol Nurs.* 2005;9:317–320.

38. Jordan MA. Mechanism of action of antitumor drugs that interact with microtubules and tubulin. *Curr Med Chem Anticancer Agents.* 2002;2:1–17.

39. Kumar S, Anderson KC. Drug insight: thalidomide as a treatment for multiple myeloma. *Nat Clin Pract Oncol.* 2005;2:262–270.

40. Kumar S, Witzig TE, Rajkumar SV. Thalidomide as an anti-cancer agent. *J Cell Mol Med.* 2002;6:160–174.

41. Kumar V, Abbas AK, Fausto N. Neoplasia. In: Kumar V, Abbas AK, Fausto N, eds. *Pathologic Basis of Disease.* 7th ed. New York: Elsevier Saunders; 2005.

42. Lage A, Perez R, Fernandez LE. Therapeutic cancer vaccines: at midway between immunology and pharmacology. *Curr Cancer Drug Targets.* 2005;5:611–627.

43. Laskar SG, Agarwal JP, Srinivas C, Dinshaw KA. Radiotherapeutic management of locally advanced head and neck cancer. *Expert Rev Anticancer Ther.* 2006;6:405–417.

44. Links M, Lewis C. Chemoprotectants: a review of their clinical pharmacology and therapeutic efficacy. *Drugs.* 1999;57:293–308.

45. Littlewood T, Collins G. Epoetin alfa: basic biology and clinical utility in cancer patients. *Expert Rev Anticancer Ther.* 2005;5:947–956.

46. Lollini PL, Cavallo F, Nanni P, Forni G. Vaccines for tumour prevention. *Nat Rev Cancer.* 2006;6: 204–216.

47. Lum LG, Davol PA, Lee RJ. The new face of bispecific antibodies: targeting cancer and much more. *Exp Hematol.* 2006;34:1–6.

48. Madhusudan S, Middleton MR. The emerging role of DNA repair proteins as predictive, prognostic and therapeutic targets in cancer. *Cancer Treat Rev.* 2005; 31:603–617.

49. Mahadevan D, Shirahatti N. Strategies for targeting the multidrug resistance-1 (MDR1)/P-gp transporter in human malignancies. *Curr Cancer Drug Targets.* 2005;5:445–455.

50. Michor F, Nowak MA, Iwasa Y. Evolution of resistance to cancer therapy. *Curr Pharm Des.* 2006;12: 261–271.

51. Mizutani H, Tada-Oikawa S, Hiraku Y, et al. Mechanism of apoptosis induced by doxorubicin through the generation of hydrogen peroxide. *Life Sci.* 2005;76: 1439–1453.

52. Molnar J, Gyemant N, Tanaka M, et al. Inhibition of multidrug resistance of cancer cells by natural diterpenes, triterpenes and carotenoids. *Curr Pharm Des.* 2006;12:287–311.

53. O'Brien S, Albitar M, Giles FJ. Monoclonal antibodies in the treatment of leukemia. *Curr Mol Med.* 2005;5: 663–675.

54. Oehler C, Ciernik IF. Radiation therapy and combined modality treatment of gastrointestinal carcinomas. *Cancer Treat Rev.* 2006;32:119–138.

55. Ozcan A, Korkmaz A, Oter S, Coskun O. Contribution of flavonoid antioxidants to the preventive effect

of mesna in cyclophosphamide-induced cystitis in rats. *Arch Toxicol.* 2005;79:461–465.

56. Paik J, Duncan T, Lindahl T, Sedgwick B. Sensitization of human carcinoma cells to alkylating agents by small interfering RNA suppression of 3-alkyladenine-DNA glycosylase. *Cancer Res.* 2005; 65:10472–10477.

57. Parvez T. Cancer treatment: what's ahead? *J Coll Physicians Surg Pak.* 2005;15:738–745.

58. Pellegrini F, Budman DR. Review: tubulin function, action of antitubulin drugs, and new drug development. *Cancer Invest.* 2005;23:264–273.

59. Pharo GH, Zhou L. Pharmacologic management of cancer pain. *J Am Osteopath Assoc.* 2005;105(suppl 5):S21–S28.

60. Pinter O, Molnar J, Toth C, et al. Administration of estramustine in response to changes in the prostate-specific antigen and Karnofsky index in the treatment of prostate cancer. *In Vivo.* 2005;19: 787–792.

61. Podnos YD, Wagman LD. Surgical management of hepatic breast cancer metastases. *Oncology.* 2005;19:1583–1588.

62. Pradeep CR, Sunila ES, Kuttan G. Expression of vascular endothelial growth factor (VEGF) and VEGF receptors in tumor angiogenesis and malignancies. *Integr Cancer Ther.* 2005;4:315–321.

63. Raje N, Anderson KC. Thalidomide and immunomodulatory drugs as cancer therapy. *Curr Opin Oncol.* 2002;14:635–640.

64. Reddy LH. Drug delivery to tumours: recent strategies. *J Pharm Pharmacol.* 2005;57:1231–1242.

65. Ryan CJ, Lin AM, Small EJ. Angiogenesis inhibition plus chemotherapy for metastatic hormone refractory prostate cancer: history and rationale. *Urol Oncol.* 2006;24:250–253.

66. Sapra P, Tyagi P, Allen TM. Ligand-targeted liposomes for cancer treatment. *Curr Drug Deliv.* 2005; 2:369–381.

67. Schimmel KJ, Richel DJ, van den Brink RB, Guchelaar HJ. Cardiotoxicity of cytotoxic drugs. *Cancer Treat Rev.* 2004;30:181–191.

68. Schwartzberg L. Chemotherapy-induced nausea and vomiting: state of the art in 2006. *J Support Oncol.* 2006;4(suppl 1):3–8.

69. Shukla GS, Krag DN. Selective delivery of therapeutic agents for the diagnosis and treatment of cancer. *Expert Opin Biol Ther.* 2006;6:39–54.

70. Slatkin N. Cancer-related pain and its pharmacologic management in the patient with bone metastasis. *J Support Oncol.* 2006;4(suppl 1):15–21.

71. Soffietti R, Costanza A, Laguzzi E, et al. Radiotherapy and chemotherapy of brain metastases. *J Neurooncol.* 2005;75:31–42.

72. Srivastava PK. Therapeutic cancer vaccines. *Curr Opin Immunol.* 2006;18:201–205.

73. Suppiah R, Srkalovic JG, Hussein MA. Immunomodulatory analogues of thalidomide in the treatment of multiple myeloma. *Clin Lymphoma Myeloma.* 2006; 6:301–305.

74. Szakacs G, Paterson JK, Ludwig JA, et al. Targeting multidrug resistance in cancer. *Nat Rev Drug Discov.* 2006;5:219–234.

75. Tanner JE. Designing antibodies for oncology. *Cancer Metastasis Rev.* 2005;24:585–598.

76. Tannock IF, Hill RP, Bristow RG, Harrington L, eds. *The Basic Science of Oncology.* 4th ed. New York: McGraw-Hill; 2005.

77. Tarhini AA, Agarwala SS. Novel agents in development for the treatment of melanoma. *Expert Opin Investig Drugs.* 2005;14:885–892.

78. Temel JS, Pirl WF, Lynch TJ. Comprehensive symptom management in patients with advanced-stage non-small-cell lung cancer. *Clin Lung Cancer.* 2006;7:241–249.

79. Ulrich CM, Bigler J, Potter JD. Non-steroidal anti-inflammatory drugs for cancer prevention: promise, perils and pharmacogenetics. *Nat Rev Cancer.* 2006;6: 130–140.

80. Van den Neste E, Cardoen S, Offner F, Bontemps F. Old and new insights into the mechanisms of action of two nucleoside analogs active in lymphoid malignancies: fludarabine and cladribine (review). *Int J Oncol.* 2005;27:1113–1124.

81. Waldmann TA. Effective cancer therapy through immunomodulation. *Annu Rev Med.* 2006;57:65–81.

82. Wang D, Dubois RN. Prostaglandins and cancer. *Gut.* 2006;55:115–122.

83. Wang S, Konorev EA, Kotamraju S, et al. Doxorubicin induces apoptosis in normal and tumor cells via distinctly different mechanisms. intermediacy of H(2) O(2)- and p53-dependent pathways. *J Biol Chem.* 2004; 279:25535–25543.

84. Weinberg OK, Marquez-Garban DC, Pietras RJ. New approaches to reverse resistance to hormonal therapy in human breast cancer. *Drug Resist Update.* 2005;8: 219–233.

85. Yavuzsen T, Davis MP, Walsh D, et al. Systematic review of the treatment of cancer-associated anorexia and weight loss. *J Clin Oncol.* 2005; 23:8500–8511.

86. Yen A, Varvayanis S, Smith JL, Lamkin TJ. Retinoic acid induces expression of SLP-76: expression with c-FMS enhances ERK activation and retinoic acid-induced differentiation/G0 arrest of HL-60 cells. *Eur J Cell Biol.* 2006;85:117–132.

87. Younes A. Angiogenesis in lymphoma: a short review. *Curr Mol Med.* 2005;5:609–613.

88. Zakarija A, Soff G. Update on angiogenesis inhibitors. *Curr Opin Oncol.* 2005;17:578–583.

89. Zaniboni A, Meriggi F. The emerging role of oxaliplatin in the treatment of gastric cancer. *J Chemother.* 2005;17:656–662.

90. Zhang M, Chakravarti A. Novel radiation-enhancing agents in malignant gliomas. *Semin Radiat Oncol.* 2006; 16:29–37.

91. Zhong H, Bowen JP. Antiangiogenesis drug design: multiple pathways targeting tumor vasculature. *Curr Med Chem.* 2006;13:849–862.

92. Zhou J, Giannakakou P. Targeting microtubules for cancer chemotherapy. *Curr Med Chem Anticancer Agents.* 2005;5:65–71.

Chapter 37

Immunomodulating Agents

The immune system is responsible for controlling the body's response to various types of injury and for defending the body from invading pathogens, including bacteria, viruses, and other parasites.[16,18] The importance of this system in maintaining health is illustrated by the devastating effects that can occur in people who lack adequate immune function, such as patients with acquired immunodeficiency syndrome (AIDS). The use of drugs to modify immune responses, or immunomodulating agents, is therefore an important area of pharmacology. For example, it may be helpful to augment immune function if a person's immune system is not functioning adequately. By contrast, it is sometimes necessary to suppress immune function pharmacologically to prevent immune-mediated injury to certain tissues or organs. Following organ transplants and tissue grafts, the immune system may cause the rejection of tissues transplanted from other donors (*allografts*) or from other sites in the patient's body (*autografts*).[60,72] Likewise, immunosuppression may be helpful when the immune system causes damage to the body's tissues. Such conditions are often referred to as *autoimmune diseases*. Clinical disorders such as rheumatoid arthritis, myasthenia gravis, and systemic lupus erythematosus are now recognized as having an autoimmune basis.[25,44,68]

This chapter addresses immunosuppressive drugs, or **immunosuppressants,** that are currently available to prevent the rejection of transplants or to treat specific diseases caused by an autoimmune response. Clearly, these drugs must be used very cautiously because too much suppression of the immune system will increase a patient's susceptibility to infection from foreign pathogens. Likewise, these drugs are rather toxic and often cause a number of adverse effects to the kidneys, lungs, musculoskeletal system, and other tissues. Nonetheless, immunosuppressive agents are often life-saving because of their ability to prevent and treat organ rejection and to decrease immune-mediated tissue damage in other diseases.

Drugs that increase immune function, or immunostimulants, are also addressed in this chapter. This group of agents is rather small, and the clinical use of immunostimulants is limited when compared with the indications for immunosuppressive drugs. Nonetheless, the development and use of immunostimulants is an exciting area of pharmacology, and some insight into the therapeutic use of these drugs is provided.

This chapter begins with a brief overview of the immune response, followed by the drugs that are currently available to suppress or stimulate this response. Physical therapists and occupational therapists may be involved in the rehabilitation of patients who have received organ transplants, skin grafts, or similar procedures that necessitate the use of immunosuppressant drugs. Rehabilitation specialists also treat patients with autoimmune disorders or immunodeficiency syndromes that affect the musculoskeletal system; these patients are also likely to be taking immunomodulating drugs. Hence, this chapter will provide therapists with knowledge about the pharmacology of these drugs and how the drugs' effects and side effects can affect physical rehabilitation.

Overview of the Immune Response

As indicated, one of the primary responsibilities of the immune system is to protect the body from bacteria, viruses, and other foreign pathogens. The immune response consists of two primary components: innate and adaptive (acquired) immunity.[18,23] Innate immunity involves specific cells (leukocytes) that are present at birth and provide a relatively rapid and nonselective defense against foreign invaders and pathogens throughout the individual's lifetime.[67] Adaptive immunity primarily involves certain lymphocytes (T and B) that develop slowly but retain the ability to recognize specific invading microorganisms and to initiate specific steps to attack and destroy the invading cell.[18]

The innate and adaptive branches of the immune response are both needed for optimal immune function, and the two interact extensively.[18,23] The adaptive response's ability to recognize and deal with foreign pathogens likewise involves an incredibly complex interaction between various cellular and chemical (humoral) components.[23,48,51] A detailed description of the intricacies of how these components work together is beyond the scope of this chapter. Many aspects of the immune response are still being investigated. An overview of key cellular and humoral elements that mediate acquired immunity is illustrated in Figure 37–1, and these elements are described briefly below.

1. *Antigen ingestion, processing, and presentation.* An invading substance (*antigen*) is engulfed by phagocytes such as macrophages and other antigen-presenting cells (APCs).[41,51] The APCs process the antigen by forming a complex between the antigen and specific membrane proteins known as major histocompatibility complex (MHC) proteins. The antigen-MHC complex is placed on the surface of the APC, where it can be presented to other lymphocytes such as the T cells. The APCs also synthesize and release chemical mediators such as interleukin-1 (IL-1) and other cytokines, which act on other immune cells (T cells) to amplify these cells' response to immune mediators.

2. *Antigen recognition and T-cell activation.* Lymphocytes derived from thymic tissues (hence the term *T cell*) recognize the antigen-MHC complex that is presented to the T cell on the macrophage surface. This recognition activates certain T cells (T-helper cells), which begin to synthesize and release a number of chemical mediators known as **lymphokines**.[28,48] Lymphokines are cytokines and chemokines derived from activated T lymphocytes and include mediators such as interleukin-2 (IL-2), other interleukins, gamma interferon, B-cell growth and differentiation factors, and other chemicals that stimulate the immune system.[10] Certain T cells

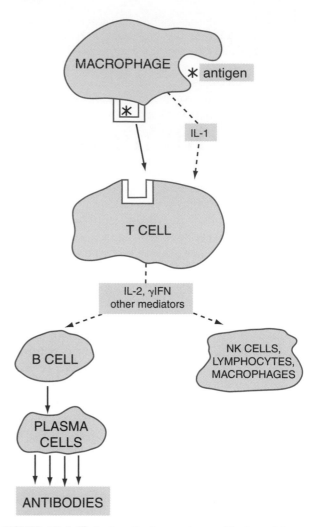

FIGURE 37–1 ▼ A schematic diagram of some of the key cellular and humoral elements involved in the acquired immune response. Macrophages engulf and process antigens and present these antigens to T lymphocytes (T cells). Macrophages also stimulate T-cell function by releasing interleukin-1 (IL-1). T cells synthesize and release humoral factors, including interleukin-2 (IL-2), gamma interferon (γ IFN), and other mediators. These mediators activate other lymphocytes (B cells) and cause these cells to differentiate into plasma cells, which produce various antibodies. T-cell–derived mediators also stimulate the activity of other immune system cells, such as natural killer (NK) cells, other cytotoxic lymphocytes, and other macrophages. See text for further explanation.

(T-killer cells) are also activated by APC presentation, and directly destroy targeted antigens.

3. *Proliferation, amplification, and recruitment.* T cells continue to replicate and proliferate, thus producing more lymphokines, which further amplifies the T-cell effects. These lymphokines also recruit lymphocytes derived from bone marrow—that is, B cells.[74] Under the direction

of IL-1 and other lymphokines, B cells proliferate and differentiate into plasma cells. Plasma cells ultimately release specific antibodies known as *immunoglobulins* (IgG, IgA, IgM, and the like). Likewise, T-cell and macrophage-derived lymphokines recruit additional cellular components, including other macrophages, cytotoxic lymphocytes (natural killer, or NK, cells), and various cells that can participate in the destruction of the foreign antigen.

Clearly, the immune response is an intricate sequence of events that involves a complex interaction between a number of cellular and humoral components. The overview provided here is just a brief summary of how some of the primary components participate in mediating acquired immunity. Readers are referred to additional sources for more information on this topic.[16,18,49]

Pharmacologic Suppression of the Immune Response

Drugs are used to suppress the immune system for two basic reasons (Table 37–1). First, the immune response is often attenuated pharmacologically following the transplantation of organs or tissues to prevent the rejection of these tissues.[5,72] Sometimes, organs and other tissues can be attacked by the recipient's immune system, even if these tissues appear to be cross-matched between donor and recipient. This rejection is often caused by membrane proteins on the donor tissue that are recognized as antigens by the host's immune system.[60] Hence, drugs that suppress the cellular and chemical response to these membrane proteins can help prevent them from destroying the transplanted tissues and causing additional injury to the host's tissues.

Often, several different types of immunosuppressants are used together in fairly high doses to prevent or treat transplant rejection.[5,72] For instance, a glucocorticoid such as betamethasone is often administered with nonsteroidal drugs such as cyclosporine and azathioprine to provide optimal success and viability of the transplant. Of course, giving several powerful drugs at high doses often causes unpleasant or even toxic side effects. These effects must often be tolerated, however, considering the limited number of organs available for transplantation and the need to ensure the survival of the transplant as much as possible.

A second major indication for these drugs is to limit immune-mediated damage to the body's tissues—that is, suppression of an autoimmune response.[11,25] Autoimmune responses occur when the immune system loses the ability to differentiate the body's own tissues from foreign or pathogenic tissues.[67] Exactly what causes this defect in immune recognition is often unclear, but prior exposure to some pathogen such as a virus may activate the immune response in a way that causes the immune system to mistakenly attack normal tissues while trying to destroy the virus. This autoimmune activation may remain in effect even after the original pathogen has been destroyed, thus leading to chronic immune–mediated injury to the body's tissues.

Autoimmune responses seem to be the underlying basis for a number of diseases, including rheumatoid arthritis, diabetes mellitus, myasthenia gravis, systemic lupus erythematosus, scleroderma, polymyositis/dermatomyositis, and several other disorders.[25,27,44] As indicated previously, it is not exactly clear what factors cause autoimmune responses, as well as why certain individuals are more prone to autoimmune-related diseases. Nonetheless, drugs that suppress the immune system can limit damage to various other tissues, and these drugs may produce dramatic improvements in patients with diseases that are caused by an autoimmune response.

Specific Immunosuppressive Agents

Drugs commonly used to suppress the immune system are listed in Table 37–1; the pharmacology of specific agents follows.

Azathioprine

Clinical Use. Azathioprine (Imuran) is a cytotoxic agent that is structurally and functionally similar to certain anticancer drugs, such as mercaptopurine.[22,30] Azathioprine is primarily used to prevent the rejection of transplanted organs, especially in patients with kidney transplants. Azathioprine may also be used to suppress immune responses in a wide range of other conditions, such as systemic lupus erythematosus, dermatomyositis, inflammatory myopathy, hepatic disease, myasthenia gravis, and ulcerative colitis. As presented in Chapter 16, azathioprine is also used as an antiarthritic disease–modifying agent.

| Table 37-1 | COMMON IMMUNOSUPPRESSIVE AGENTS | | |

| | | Primary Indications* | |
Generic Name	Trade Name(s)	Prevention or Treatment of Transplant Rejection	Diseases That Have an Autoimmune Response
Antibodies	Names vary according to specific lymphocyte targets; see Table 37–2	Bone marrow, other organ transplants (see Table 37–2)	Idiopathic thrombocytic purpura, other hemolytic disorders
Azathioprine	Imuran	Kidney, heart, liver, pancreas	Rheumatoid arthritis, inflammatory bowel disease, myasthenia gravis, systemic lupus erythematosus (SLE), others
Cyclophosphamide	Cytoxan, Neosar	Bone marrow, other organ transplants	Rheumatoid arthritis, multiple sclerosis, SLE, dermatomyositis, glomerulonephritis, hematologic disorders
Cyclosporine	Neoral, Sandimmune	Kidney, liver, heart, lung, pancreas, bone marrow	Psoriasis, rheumatoid arthritis, nephrotic syndrome
Glucocorticoids	See text for listing	Heart, kidney, liver, bone marrow	Multiple sclerosis, rheumatoid arthritis, SLE, inflammatory bowel disease, hemolytic disorders, others.
Methotrexate	Folex, Rheumatrex	–	Rheumatoid arthritis, psoriasis
Mycophenolate mofetil	CellCept	Heart, kidney	–
Sirolimus	Rapamune	Kidney, heart, liver	Rheumatoid arthritis, psoriasis, SLE
Sulfasalazine	Azulfidine, others	–	Rheumatoid arthritis, inflammatory bowel disease
Tacrolimus	Prograf	Liver, kidney, heart, lung, pancreas	Uveitis

*Indications vary considerably and many indications listed here are not in the U.S. product labeling for each drug; optimal use of these drugs alone or in combination with each other continues to be investigated.

Mechanism of Action. Although the exact mechanism of azathioprine is unknown, this drug probably interferes with DNA synthesis in cells mediating the immune response. Azathioprine appears to act like the antimetabolite drugs used in cancer chemotherapy (see Chapter 36). The cell normally uses various endogenous substances such as purines as ingredients during DNA synthesis. Azathioprine is structurally similar to these purines, and this drug acts as a false ingredient that competes with the naturally occurring substances to slow down and disrupt DNA synthesis. Impaired nucleic acid synthesis slows down the replication of lymphocytes and other key cellular components that direct the immune response. Thus, azathioprine directly limits cellular proliferation through this inhibitory effect on DNA synthesis and ultimately limits the production of humoral components (antibodies) produced by these cells.

Adverse Effects. The primary side effects of azathioprine are related to suppression of bone marrow function, including leukopenia, megaloblastic anemia, and similar blood dyscrasias. Other side effects include skin rash and gastrointestinal distress (appetite loss, nausea, vomiting); hepatic dysfunction can also occur when higher doses are used.

Cyclophosphamide

Clinical Use. Cyclophosphamide (Cytoxan, Neosar) is an anticancer alkylating agent that is commonly used in a variety of neoplastic disorders (see Chapter 36). This drug may also be helpful in suppressing the immune response in certain autoimmune diseases, such as multiple sclerosis, systemic lupus erythematosus, and rheumatoid arthritis.[12,43] High doses of cyclophosphamide are also used to prevent tissue rejection in patients receiving bone marrow transplants and other organ transplants.

Mechanism of Action. The mechanism of cyclophosphamide as an anticancer alkylating agent is described in Chapter 36. This drug causes the formation of strong cross-links between strands of DNA and RNA, thus inhibiting DNA/RNA replication and function. Cyclophosphamide probably exerts immunosuppressant effects in a similar manner; that is, this drug inhibits DNA and RNA function in lymphocytes and other key cells, thus limiting the rapid proliferation of these cells during the immune response.

Adverse Effects. Cyclophosphamide is used very cautiously as an immunosuppressant because of the possibility of severe side effects, including carcinogenic effects during long-term use. Other side effects include hematologic disorders (leukopenia, thrombocytopenia), cardiotoxicity, nephrotoxicity, and pulmonary toxicity.

Cyclosporine

Clinical Use. Cyclosporine (Neoral, Sandimmune) is one of the primary medications used to suppress immune function following organ transplantation.[14,21,69] This medication can be used alone or combined with glucocorticoids, azathioprine, and other immunosuppressants to prevent the rejection of a kidney, lung, liver, heart, pancreas, and other organ transplants.

Cyclosporine is used to a somewhat lesser extent in treating autoimmune diseases, but it may be helpful in conditions such as psoriasis, rheumatoid arthritis, inflammatory bowel disease, and glomerulonephritis.[15,32,63] As discussed in Chapter 32, cyclosporine has also been used in the early stages of type 1 diabetes mellitus to help control immune-mediated destruction of pancreatic beta cells, thus decreasing the severity of this disease in some patients.[9]

Although cyclosporine is one of the most effective immunosuppressants, the traditional form of this drug is associated with unpredictable absorption from the gastrointestinal (GI) tract and potentially severe side effects, such as nephrotoxicity and neurotoxicity.[33,58] In a newer form of cyclosporine (Neoral), the drug is modified into microemulsion capsules that disperse more easily within the GI tract, thereby enabling the drug to be absorbed in a more predictable fashion.[26] The microemulsion form of cyclosporine appears to be safer because it is not as toxic to the kidneys and other tissues as is the regular formulation.[8] Hence, this microemulsion formulation is often the optimal way to administer cyclosporine following organ transplantation or other situations requiring immunosuppression.[26,36]

Mechanism of Action. Cyclosporine and tacrolimus (see below) are known as calcineurin inhibitors because they inhibit a specific protein (calcineurin) in lymphoid tissues. This inhibition ultimately suppresses the production of IL-2, a cytokine that plays a critical role in immune response by promoting the growth and proliferation of activated T lymphocytes and other immune cells, such as NK cells (see Fig. 37–1).[5,52] Thus, cyclosporine is one of the premier immunosuppressants because of its relative selectivity for T cells and its inhibition of a key mediator of the immune response (IL-2).[41] This relatively specific inhibition is often advantageous when compared with other nonselective drugs such as azathioprine, cyclophosphamide, and glucocorticoids that inhibit virtually all the cells and chemical mediators involved in the immune response.

Adverse Effects. The primary problem associated with cyclosporine is nephrotoxicity, which can range from mild, asymptomatic cases to severe kidney dysfunction, which requires discontinuation of the drug.[33,46] Hypertension is also a common adverse effect, especially when cyclosporine is used for prolonged periods.[58] Other problems include neurotoxicity, gingival hyperplasia, hair growth (hirsutism), and increased infections. These problems, however, tend to be less severe with cyclosporine than with other less-selective immunosuppressants.

Glucocorticoids

Clinical Use. As described in Chapter 29, glucocorticoids are powerful anti-inflammatory and immunosuppressive drugs. Glucocorticoids exert a rather nonspecific inhibition of virtually all aspects of cell- and chemical-mediated immunity, thus enabling these drugs to be used in a variety of situations when it is necessary to suppress immune function. Hence, these drugs are a mainstay in preventing transplant rejection and in treating various diseases associated with an autoimmune response.[29,72]

Glucocorticoids commonly used as immunosuppressants include the following:

- betamethasone (Celestone)
- cortisone (Cortone)
- dexamethasone (Decadron, others)
- hydrocortisone (Cortef)
- methylprednisolone (Medrol)
- prednisolone (Pediapred, Prelone, others)
- prednisone (Deltasone, others)
- triamcinolone (Aristocort, others)

Mechanism of Action. Although their exact mechanism of immunosuppression is unclear, glucocorticoids probably interrupt the immune response by a complex effect at the genomic level of various immune cells.[5,57] These drugs enter immune system cells, where they bind to a cytoplasmic receptor. The drug-receptor complex then migrates to the cell's nucleus, where it acts directly on specific immunoregulatory genes. In particular, glucocorticoids influence the expression of cytokines and other chemicals that orchestrate the immune response; that is, glucocorticoids inhibit the transcription of messenger RNA units that are normally translated into immunostimulatory signals such as interleukin-1, gamma interferon, and other substances that activate the cells responsible for mediating the immune response. Hence, these drugs disrupt the production of chemical signals that activate and control various immune system cellular components. For more details about how glucocorticoids exert their effects on various cells and tissues, see Chapter 29.

Adverse Effects. The immunosuppressive effects of glucocorticoids are balanced by several side effects. As described in Chapter 29, glucocorticoids typically produce a catabolic effect on collagenous tissues, and breakdown of muscle, bone, skin, and various other tissues is a common adverse effect. Glucocorticoids also produce other side effects, including hypertension, adrenocortical suppression, growth retardation in children, an increased chance of infection, glaucoma, decreased glucose tolerance, and gastric ulcer. These side effects can be especially problematic when glucocorticoids are used to prevent transplant rejection because these drugs are often given in high dosages for extended periods.

Therefore, glucocorticoids are typically combined with other nonsteroidal immunosuppressants such as cyclosporine, azathioprine, or immunosuppressive antibodies so that synergistic effects can be obtained and immunosuppression can be achieved with relatively low doses of each drug.[54] In addition, efforts are often made to progressively decrease the glucocorticoid dose so that immunosuppression is achieved by using the lowest possible dose. In some cases, the glucocorticoid may even be withdrawn during maintenance immunosuppressive therapy, and nonsteroidal drugs (cyclosporine, tacrolimus, mycophenolate mofetil) are used to provide long-term immunosuppression following organ transplantation.[39]

Methotrexate

Clinical Use. Methotrexate (Folex, Rheumatrex) was originally developed as an anticancer agent (see Chapter 36), but this drug is also used occasionally in certain noncancerous conditions that have an autoimmune component.[15,78] As indicated in Chapter 16, methotrexate is commonly used as a disease-modifying drug in rheumatoid arthritis. Methotrexate is also approved for use in psoriasis. This agent has only mild immunosuppressive effects, however, and is not typically used to treat organ transplants or other conditions that require more extensive immunosuppression.

Mechanism of Action. The pharmacology of methotrexate is described in Chapter 36. This drug acts as an antimetabolite that interferes with the production of DNA and RNA precursors in rapidly proliferating cells. This interference produces a general inhibition of the replication of lymphocytes inherent in the immune response.

Adverse Effects. The major problems associated with methotrexate include hepatic and pulmonary toxicity. These problems are dose-related, however, and serious adverse effects tend to occur less frequently at doses used for immunosuppression than at those for anticancer treatment.

Mycophenolate Mofetil

Clinical Use. Mycophenolate mofetil (CellCept) is primarily used to prevent or treat organ rejection following cardiac and renal transplantation. This drug is typically combined with other immunosuppressants (cyclosporine, glucocorticoids) to provide optimal immunosuppression in patients receiving these transplant types.[39,40,70] Mycophenolate mofetil may also be useful in suppressing the immune response associated with autoimmune conditions such as systemic lupus erythematosus.[2]

Mechanism of Action. Mycophenolate mofetil inhibits a specific enzyme (inosine monophosphate dehydrogenase) that is responsible for the synthesis of DNA precursors in T and B lymphocytes.[39,50] Because these lymphocytes cannot synthesize adequate amounts of DNA, their ability to replicate and proliferate is impaired, thus blunting the immune response. This drug may also inhibit lymphocyte attraction and adhesion to the vascular endothelium, thereby impairing the lymphocytes' ability to migrate to the site of the foreign (transplanted) tissues and to infiltrate from the bloodstream into these tissues.[50]

Adverse Effects. The primary adverse effects associated with mycophenolate mofetil are blood disorders (anemia, leukopenia, neutropenia) and gastrointestinal problems (abdominal pain, nausea, vomiting, heartburn, diarrhea, constipation).[50] Other side effects include chest pain, cough, dyspnea, muscle pain, weakness, and cardiovascular problems (hypertension, arrhythmias).

Sulfasalazine

Clinical Use. Sulfasalazine (Azulfidine, other names) has unique properties, with some antibacterial characteristics similar to sulfonamide drugs (see Chapter 33) and some of anti-inflammatory characteristics similar to the salicylates (see Chapter 15). This drug is primarily used to suppress the immune response associated with rheumatoid arthritis and inflammatory bowel disease.[38,61]

Mechanism of Action. The exact mechanism of this drug in immune-related disorders is not fully understood. Sulfasalazine may affect key components in the immune system, including suppression of NK cells. Other effects may be related to the drug's breakdown into active metabolites, including sulfapyridine and mesalamine, which exert antibiotic and anti-inflammatory effects, respectively.

Adverse Effects. Primary side effects include headache, blood dyscrasias (agranulocytosis, anemia, thrombocytopenia), increased sensitivity to ultraviolet light, and hypersensitivity reactions (fever, skin rash, itching). Hypersensitivity can be severe or even fatal in susceptible individuals.

Sirolimus

Clinical Use. Sirolimus (rapamycin, Rapamune) is one of the newest immunosuppressants and is an antibiotic that also has substantial immunosuppressant effects. This drug is used primarily to prevent organ rejection in people with solid organ transplants (kidney, heart, and so forth).[42,55] Sirolimus is especially helpful following kidney transplants because it helps prevent organ rejection without adversely affecting glomerular filtration and other aspects of the kidney function.[45] Likewise, this drug is often used preferentially in patients with renal dysfunction instead of more nephrotoxic drugs (cyclosporine, tacrolimus).[45,55]

To provide optimal immunosuppressant effects, sirolimus is typically combined with glucocorticoids or other immunosuppressants. Sirolimus exerts a number of other beneficial effects, including the ability to inhibit smooth muscle proliferation in blood vessel walls. For this reason, sirolimus is sometimes incorporated into drug-eluting stents; that is, a supportive tubular structure (stent) is placed in the lumen of a partially occluded artery, and the drug is released slowly from the stent to help reduce vessel occlusion.[64]

Mechanism of Action. Unlike other immunosuppressants (cyclosporine, tacrolimus), sirolimus does not interfere directly with cytokine production. Instead, sirolimus inhibits the function of a specific enzyme commonly known as the mammalian target of rapamycin (mTOR).[37,42] This enzyme plays a key role in signaling pathways that promote the growth and proliferation of T and B cells.[37,45] By inhibiting this enzyme, sirolimus causes cell division to stop at a specific stage (G1), thereby limiting the ability of these cells to mount an attack on transplanted tissues.[65]

Adverse Effects. Sirolimus may cause blood lipid disorders, including hypercholesterolemia and hypertriglyceridemia.[42] Other side effects include blood disorders (anemia, leukopenia, thrombocytopenia), diarrhea, skin rash, joint and muscle pain, and hypertension.[42]

Tacrolimus

Clinical Use. Tacrolimus (Prograf) is similar to cyclosporine in structure and in immunosuppressive effects, but tacrolimus is approximately 10 to 100 times more potent than cyclosporine.[41] Tacrolimus may be somewhat less toxic than cyclosporine and other immunosuppressants, although serious side effects may still occur at higher doses (see "Adverse Effects" in this section). Tacrolimus is used primarily to prevent rejection of kidney and liver transplants.[76,77] This drug may also be useful in preventing or treating the rejection of other organs and tissues including heart, lung, pancreas, and bone marrow transplants.[36,41] Topical preparations of tacrolimus or an analogous drug known as pimecrolimus (Elidel) can also be used to treat skin disorders such as atopic dermatitis.[7,31]

Mechanism of Action. Tacrolimus acts like cyclosporine by binding to a specific protein (calcineurin) in lymphoid tissues and inhibiting the production of key immune mediators such as IL-2.[5] IL-2 plays a critical role in the immune response because this substance promotes the growth and proliferation of activated T lymphocytes and other immune cells, such as NK cells (see Fig. 37–1). This binding provides a somewhat more selective inhibition of immune function than other drugs that exert a general or nonselective inhibition of the immune response.

Adverse Effects. Common side effects of tacrolimus include gastrointestinal disturbances (cramps, nausea, diarrhea, constipation), weakness, fever, and skin rashes and itching. More serious problems include renal and central nervous system (CNS) toxicity (headache, anxiety, nervousness, seizures).[41] Tacrolimus is also associated with problems with glucose metabolism (hyperglycemia, glucose intolerance), and can cause diabetes mellitus in certain individuals.[73]

Other Methods of Immunosuppression

Immunosuppressant Antibodies

Immune function can also be suppressed by using antibodies that interact with specific immune system cells and interfere with the cell's function (Table 37–2).[13,47] These antibodies can be obtained from animal sources and cell culture techniques (monoclonal antibodies) to provide a rather selective method of suppressing

Table 37–2	ANTIBODY REAGENTS USED AS IMMUNOSUPPRESSANTS	
Generic Name	**Trade Name**	**Primary Indication(s)**
Antithymocyte globulin	–	Treatment of rejection of kidney, heart, liver, lung, pancreas, and bone marrow transplants
Muromonab-CD3 monoclonal antibody	Orthoclone OKT3	Acute rejection of heart, liver, and kidney transplants
$Rh_0(D)$ immune globulin	BayRho-D, RhoGAM, others	Prevention of Rh hemolytic disease of the newborn
Interleukin-1 receptor antagonists		
Basiliximab	Simulect	Prevention of acute rejection of kidney transplants
Daclizumab	Zenapax	Prevention of acute rejection of kidney transplants
Tumor necrosis factor-alpha inhibitors		
Adalimumab	Humira	Rheumatoid arthritis
Infliximab	Remicade	Rheumatoid arthritis; ulcerative colitis

immune function. For example, antibodies such as Rho(D) immunoglobulin are used routinely to suppress immune response in mothers who have been exposed to a fetus's incompatible blood type. This immunosuppression prevents the mother from developing antibodies that will be passed on to the fetus or to a fetus in a subsequent pregnancy, thus blocking the production of maternal antibodies that can attack the fetus's blood and cause a potentially fatal condition known as hemolytic anemia of the newborn.[41]

Antibodies have also been developed that are very selective for antigens located on the surface of specific T cells and other lymphocytes; these antibodies inhibit cell function or cause destruction of the cell.[20] Anti–T-cell antibodies are primarily used to help prevent or treat rejection of organ and bone marrow transplants (see Table 37–2).[13,75]

Antibodies that block the interleukin-2 receptor, thus preventing interleukin-2 from activating T lymphocytes, have also been developed.[24,62] These anti–interleukin-2 receptor agents, such as basiliximab (Simulect) and daclizumab (Zenapax), may be helpful in reducing the incidence of acute transplant rejection.[13] Antibodies seem to be especially useful in the initial (induction) phase of antirejection treatment because these drugs can delay or supplant the use of more toxic immunosuppressants such as the glucocorticoids and calcineurin inhibitors (cyclosporine and tacrolimus).[3,56]

Finally, antibodies such as adalimumab (Humira) and infliximab (Remicade) have been developed that bind directly to tumor necrosis factor alpha (TNF-alpha), thereby preventing this cytokine from causing damage to joints and other tissues. These anti-TNF–alpha drugs are therefore helpful in autoimmune diseases such as rheumatoid arthritis; their pharmacology is addressed in more detail in Chapter 16.

Immunosuppressant antibodies continue to gain acceptance as a method for preventing rejection of transplanted tissues and for treating various autoimmune diseases.[17,47] For more information on the use of specific antibodies in specific disorders, please refer to other sources on this topic.[17,41,47,56]

Miscellaneous Immunosuppressants

A variety of other agents with cytotoxic effects has been used to suppress the immune system. These drugs include chlorambucil (Leukeran), dactinomycin (Cosmegen), mercaptopurine (Purinethol), vinblastine (Velban), and vincristine (Oncovin, Vincasar).[41] These agents are similar to methotrexate; they exert cytotoxic effects that interfere with the proliferation of immune system cellular components. These drugs are used primarily as anticancer agents; the pharmacology of these drugs is described in more detail in Chapter 36. The use of these agents as immunosuppressants, however, has generally declined in favor of drugs that have a more selective and strategic effect on immune function. Nonetheless, these drugs may be helpful in certain autoimmune disorders, or in preventing the rejection of tissue and organ transplants in specific situations.

Finally, thalidomide can be used as an immunosuppressant in conditions such as systemic lupus erythematosus (SLE)[53] and in preventing graft-versus-host disease following bone marrow transplant.[35,71] This drug was originally developed as a sedative, but was later discovered to produce severe birth defects when administered to women during pregnancy. Nonetheless, thalidomide may help blunt immunologic responses by regulating the genes that express tumor necrosis factor-alpha.[53] Decreased production of this factor results in diminished activation of neutrophils and other immune components, thereby reducing the severity of immunologic reactions. The effects of thalidomide on immune function appear to be very complex, however, and this drug may actually increase the production of tumor necrosis factor alpha in certain conditions such as human immunodeficiency virus (HIV) infection.[41] Hence, thalidomide's immunomodulatory effects continue to be investigated, and use of this drug in specific diseases may be modified in the future.

Immunostimulants

A number of agents can suppress the immune system. However, there has been considerable interest in developing pharmacologic methods to modify or even stimulate immune function in specific situations. In particular, agents that have a positive immunomodulating effect could be beneficial to patients with compromised immune function (such as AIDS or certain cancers) or chronic infections.[19,41] Development of immunostimulants, however, is understandably a complex and potentially dangerous proposition. Excessive or incorrect immune activation could trigger myriad problems that resemble autoimmune diseases. Likewise, it may be difficult to selectively stimulate certain aspects of the immune system to treat a specific problem without also causing a more widespread and systemic immunologic response. Nonetheless, a few strategies are currently available to modify or stimulate immune function in a limited number of situations.

Bacille Calmette-Guérin

Clinical Use. Bacille Calmette-Guérin (BCG, TheraCys, others) is an active bacterial strain that can be administered systemically as a vaccine against tuberculosis. This agent may also stimulate immune function and can be administered locally within the bladder (intravesicularly) to treat certain forms of superficial bladder cancer.[66]

Mechanism of Action. The exact reason that this agent is effective in treating cancer is unknown. Some evidence suggests that it may activate macrophages locally at the site of the cancer and that these macrophages engulf and destroy tumor cells.[79]

Adverse Effects. When administered directly into the bladder, common side effects include bladder irritation and infection. Systemic administration (immunization) may also cause dermatologic reactions (peeling or scaling of the skin), allergic reactions, inflammation of lymph nodes, and local irritation or ulceration at the injection site.

Immune Globulin

Clinical Use. Immune globulin (Gamimune, Gammagard, other names) is prepared by extracting immunoglobulins from donated human blood.[41] These preparations contain all subclasses of immunoglobulin (Ig) but consist primarily of IgG. Immune globulin is administered intravenously to boost immune function in several conditions, including primary immunodeficiency syndromes (congenital agammaglobulinemia, common variable immunodeficiency, and severe combined immunodeficiency), idiopathic thrombocytopenic purpura, Kawasaki disease, chronic lymphocytic leukemia, and HIV infection in children.[4,59] Other potential indications for immune globulin include dermatomyositis, Guillain-Barré syndrome, demyelinating polyneuropathies, Lambert-Eaton myasthenia syndrome, and relapsing-remitting multiple sclerosis.

Mechanism of Action. Commercial preparations of immune globulin mimic the normal role of endogenous immunoglobulins. These preparations therefore directly act as antibodies against infectious agents. They can also help modulate the activity of T lymphocytes, macrophages, and other immune system cells to maintain immune system competence.[6,59]

Adverse Effects. Immune globulin may cause several side effects, such as joint and muscle pain, headache, general malaise, and gastrointestinal disturbances (nausea, vomiting).[34] Although rare, allergic reactions, including anaphylaxis, can occur in some individuals. Because immune globulin is obtained from human blood, care must also be taken to prevent transmission of hepatitis and HIV from infected donors.

Levamisole

Clinical Use. Levamisole (Ergamisol) is primarily used to treat colorectal carcinoma. Specifically, this drug is administered with fluorouracil (see Chapter 36) to prevent recurrence of colorectal cancer after surgical removal of the primary tumor.[1]

Mechanism of Action. Although the exact effects are not known, levamisole may augment immune function by activating macrophages and immune cells that selectively engulf and destroy any residual cancerous cells.[41]

Adverse Effects. Levamisole may cause blood disorders such as agranulocytosis, leukopenia, or thrombocytopenia. Other side effects include nausea, diarrhea, and a metallic taste in the mouth.

Other Immunomodulators

Cytokines are a potential way to modify the immune system in several situations because of their ability to act as immunoregulatory chemicals. For example, cytokines such as interferon-alpha and interleukin-2 can be administered to treat certain forms of cancer (see Chapter 36). Likewise, certain interferons can help control viral infections, and interferon-beta may be helpful in autoimmune diseases such as multiple sclerosis (see Chapter 34). Researchers continue to investigate how immune function can be manipulated to treat various diseases, and additional immune system modulators will almost certainly be forthcoming.

Significance of Immunomodulating Agents in Rehabilitation

■ ■ ■ Physical therapists and occupational therapists are often involved in the rehabilitation of patients who have received heart, liver, kidney, and other organ transplants. Therapists also frequently deal with patients who have received autologous grafts, such as skin grafts for treating burns, and bone marrow transplants during the treatment of certain cancers. Hence, therapists frequently deal with patients taking drugs to prevent tissue rejection.

Therapists also deal with the rehabilitation of musculoskeletal disorders that are caused by an autoimmune response. Many of these diseases attack connective tissues, and autoimmune diseases such as rheumatoid arthritis, dermatomyositis, and systemic lupus erythematosus are often the primary reason that patients undergo rehabilitation. Patients with a compromised immune system may develop musculoskeletal problems related to their immunodeficient state. Hence, immunomodulating drugs are frequently used in many patients receiving physical therapy and occupational therapy.

The most significant impact of these drugs on rehabilitation is related to their side effects, especially those of the immunosuppressants. These drugs are typically used in high doses to produce immunosuppressive effects, which are often achieved at the expense of serious and toxic side effects. Many immunosuppressants, especially the glucocorticoids, exert catabolic effects on bone, muscle, and other tissues. Other immunosuppressants, such as cyclosporine and tacrolimus, are neurotoxic and may cause peripheral neuropathies and CNS-related problems in balance and posture.

Hence, rehabilitation specialists can play a critical role in offsetting some of these adverse effects. Therapists can institute strengthening and general conditioning exercises to prevent breakdown of muscle, bone, and other tissues, as well as to maintain cardiovascular function. Problems associated with peripheral neuropathies, such as pain and weakness, may respond to TENS and other electrotherapeutic treatments. Balance and gait training may help patients overcome problems caused by CNS toxicity and vestibular problems. Thus, therapists can implement specific strategies as required to help patients cope with the adverse drug effects associated with immunomodulating agents.

CASE STUDY

Immunomodulating Agents

Brief History. A.S. is a 47-year-old concert musician who experienced a progressive decline in renal function that ultimately led to renal failure. Kidney function was maintained artificially through renal dialysis until a suitable kidney transplant became available from a donor who died in an automobile accident. The kidney was transplanted successfully, and A.S. was placed on a prophylactic regimen of three different immunosuppressive drugs to prevent the rejection of the transplanted kidney. At the time of the transplant, cyclosporine was initiated at a dosage of 10 mg/kg of body weight

each day. After 15 days, the dosage was decreased to 8 mg/kg per day, and was progressively decreased over the next 2 months until a maintenance dosage of 2 mg/kg per day was achieved. On the day of surgery, he also received an intravenous dose of 0.5 g of methylprednisolone. Oral doses of methylprednisolone were then administered in dosages of 16 mg/d for the first 3 months, 12 mg/d for the next 3 months, and 8 mg/d thereafter. Azathioprine was administered at a dosage of 1 mg/kg per day throughout the posttransplant period. Physical therapy was initiated in the intensive care unit (ICU) 1 day after the transplant to increase strength and to facilitate recovery from the surgery.

Problem/Influence of Medication. The therapist noted that several drugs were being used to prevent rejection, including rather high doses of methylprednisolone, a glucocorticoid agent. Glucocorticoids are notorious for their catabolic effects, and the therapist was aware that a program of strengthening and weight-bearing exercise would help offset the breakdown of muscle and bone that can often occur with prolonged glucocorticoid administration.

Decision/Solution. Gentle resistance exercises were initiated in the ICU as soon as the patient was alert and could follow basic instructions. Strengthening exercises were progressively increased using manual resistance, and various weights and exercise machines were incorporated into the strengthening regimen as tolerated by the patient. The thera-

pist also initiated weight-bearing activities as soon as the patient was able to tolerate standing. Weight-bearing activities were progressively increased, and the patient was able to walk independently for distances up to 1000 feet and climb two flights of stairs at the time of discharge. The therapist also worked closely with the patient and the patient's family to make sure that strengthening exercises and a progressive ambulation program were continued at home. The patient did not experience any problems related to tissue rejection, and he was able to resume his musical career and maintain an active lifestyle that included daily walks and regular visits to a health club, where he participated in a supervised program of strength training.

SUMMARY

Our knowledge of how the immune system functions in both normal and disease states has increased dramatically over the last several decades, and we now have drugs that can moderate the effects of the immune response in certain clinical situations. Immunosuppressants are a mainstay in preventing tissue rejection, and much of the current success of organ transplants is due to the judicious use of immunosuppressive drugs. These drugs are also beneficial in a number of diseases that have an autoimmune basis, and immunosuppressants can help alleviate symptoms or possibly even reverse the sequelae of certain diseases

such as rheumatoid arthritis. A few agents are also available that can augment or stimulate immune function in certain situations. The use of these immunostimulants will continue to expand as more is learned about how we can enhance the immune response in conditions such as cancer and certain immunocompromised states. However, immunomodulating drugs are not without problems because many agents cause a rather nonspecific effect on immune function, which leads to serious side effects. As more is learned about the details of immune function, new drugs will be developed that are more selective in their ability to modify immune responses without causing a generalized suppression or activation of the immune system.

References

1. Andre T, de Gramont A, Study Group of Clinical Research in Radiotherapies Oncology, Oncology Multidiciplinary Research Group. An overview of adjuvant systemic chemotherapy for colon cancer. *Clin Colorectal Cancer.* 2004;4(suppl 1):S22–S28.
2. Appel GB, Radhakrishnan J, Ginzler EM. Use of mycophenolate mofetil in autoimmune and renal diseases. *Transplantation.* 2005;80(suppl): S265–S271.
3. Bakr MA. Induction therapy. *Exp Clin Transplant.* 2005;3:320–328.
4. Ballow M. Clinical and investigational considerations for the use of IGIV therapy. *Am J Health Syst Pharm.* 2005;62(suppl 3):S12–S18.
5. Barshes NR, Goodpastor SE, Goss JA. Pharmacologic immunosuppression. *Front Biosci.* 2004;9:411–420.
6. Bayary J, Dasgupta S, Misra N, et al. Intravenous immunoglobulin in autoimmune disorders: an insight

into the immunoregulatory mechanisms. *Int Immunopharmacol.* 2006;6:528–534.
7. Beck LA. The efficacy and safety of tacrolimus ointment: a clinical review. *J Am Acad Dermatol.* 2005;53 (suppl 2):S165–S170.
8. Belitsky P. Neoral use in the renal transplant recipient. *Transplant Proc.* 2000;32(suppl 3A):10S.
9. Bertera S, Alexander A, Giannoukakis N, et al. Immunology of type 1 diabetes. Intervention and prevention strategies. *Endocrinol Metab Clin North Am.* 1999;28:841–864.
10. Blach-Olszewska Z. Innate immunity: cells, receptors, and signaling pathways. *Arch Immunol Ther Exp (Warsz).* 2005;53:245–253.
11. Braun F, Behrend M. Basic immunosuppressive drugs outside solid organ transplantation. *Expert Opin Investig Drugs.* 2006;15:267–291.
12. Brodsky RA. High dose cyclophosphamide treatment for autoimmune disorders. *Scientific World Journal.* 2002; 2:1808–1815.

13. Buhaescu I, Segall L, Goldsmith D, Covic A. New immunosuppressive therapies in renal transplantation: monoclonal antibodies. *J Nephrol.* 2005;18:529–536.

14. Calne R. Cyclosporine as a milestone in immunosuppression. *Transplant Proc.* 2004;36(suppl):13S–15S.

15. Cather J, Menter A. Novel therapies for psoriasis. *Am J Clin Dermatol.* 2002;3:159–173.

16. Chaplin DD. Overview of the human immune response. *J Allergy Clin Immunol.* 2006;117(suppl mini-primer):S430–S435.

17. Cianci R, Cammarota G, Raducci F, Pandolfi F. The impact of biological agents interfering with receptor/ligand binding in the immune system. *Eur Rev Med Pharmacol Sci.* 2005;9:305–314.

18. Clark R, Kupper T. Old meets new: the interaction between innate and adaptive immunity. *J Invest Dermatol.* 2005;125:629–637.

19. Clerici M. Immunomodulants for the treatment of HIV infection: the search goes on. *Expert Opin Investig Drugs.* 2006;15:197–200.

20. Cobbold SP. T cell tolerance induced by therapeutic antibodies. *Philos Trans R Soc Lond B Biol Sci.* 2005; 360:1695–1705.

21. Cortesini R. Cyclosporine—lessons from the first 20 years. *Transplant Proc.* 2004;36(suppl):158S–162S.

22. Coulthard S, Hogarth L. The thiopurines: an update. *Invest New Drugs.* 2005;23:523–532.

23. Dempsey PW, Vaidya SA, Cheng G. The art of war: innate and adaptive immune responses. *Cell Mol Life Sci.* 2003;60:2604–2621.

24. Di Filippo S. Anti-IL-2 receptor antibody vs. polyclonal anti-lymphocyte antibody as induction therapy in pediatric transplantation. *Pediatr Transplant.* 2005; 9:373–380.

25. Drachman DB, Brodsky RA. High-dose therapy for autoimmune neurologic diseases. *Curr Opin Oncol.* 2005;17:83–88.

26. Dunn CJ, Wagstaff AJ, Perry CM, Plosker GL, Goa KL. Cyclosporin: an updated review of the pharmacokinetic properties, clinical efficacy and tolerability of a microemulsion-based formulation (neoral)1 in organ transplantation. *Drugs.* 2001;61: 1957–2016.

27. Eldor R, Cohen IR, Raz I. Innovative immune-based therapeutic approaches for the treatment of type 1 diabetes mellitus. *Int Rev Immunol.* 2005;24:327–339.

28. Esche C, Stellato C, Beck LA. Chemokines: key players in innate and adaptive immunity. *J Invest Dermatol.* 2005;125:615–628.

29. Franchimont D. Overview of the actions of glucocorticoids on the immune response: a good model to characterize new pathways of immunosuppression for new treatment strategies. *Ann N Y Acad Sci.* 2004;1024: 124–137.

30. Gearry RB, Barclay ML. Azathioprine and 6-mercaptopurine pharmacogenetics and metabolite monitoring in inflammatory bowel disease. *J Gastroenterol Hepatol.* 2005;20:1149–1157.

31. Gisondi P, Ellis CN, Girolomoni G. Pimecrolimus in dermatology: atopic dermatitis and beyond. *Int J Clin Pract.* 2005;59:969–974.

32. Gremese E, Ferraccioli GF. Benefit/risk of cyclosporine in rheumatoid arthritis. *Clin Exp Rheumatol.* 2004; 22(suppl 35):S101–S107.

33. Grinyo JM, Cruzado JM. Cyclosporine nephrotoxicity. *Transplant Proc.* 2004;36(suppl):240S–242S.

34. Hamrock DJ. Adverse events associated with intravenous immunoglobulin therapy. *Int Immunopharmacol.* 2006;6:535–542.

35. Joglekar S, Levin M. The promise of thalidomide: evolving indications. *Drugs Today.* 2004;40:197–204.

36. Keogh A. Calcineurin inhibitors in heart transplantation. *J Heart Lung Transplant.* 2004;23(suppl):S202–S206.

37. Kirken RA, Wang YL. Molecular actions of sirolimus: sirolimus and mTor. *Transplant Proc.* 2003;35(suppl): 227S–230S.

38. Klotz U. Colonic targeting of aminosalicylates for the treatment of ulcerative colitis. *Dig Liver Dis.* 2005;37: 381–388.

39. Klupp J, Pfitzmann R, Langrehr JM, Neuhaus P. Indications of mycophenolate mofetil in liver transplantation. *Transplantation.* 2005;80(suppl):S142–S146.

40. Kobashigawa JA, Meiser BM. Review of major clinical trials with mycophenolate mofetil in cardiac transplantation. *Transplantation.* 2005;80(suppl): S235–S243.

41. Krensky AM, Vincenti F, Bennett WM. Immunosuppressants, tolerogens, and immunostimulants. In: Brunton LL, et al, eds. *The Pharmacologic Basis of Therapeutics.* 11th ed. New York: McGraw-Hill; 2006.

42. Kuypers DR. Benefit-risk assessment of sirolimus in renal transplantation. *Drug Saf.* 2005;28:153–181.

43. La Mantia L, Milanese C, Mascoli N, et al. Cyclophosphamide for multiple sclerosis. *Cochrane Database Syst Rev.* 2002;CD002819.

44. Lee SJ, Kavanaugh A. Autoimmunity, vasculitis, and autoantibodies. *J Allergy Clin Immunol.* 2006;117(suppl mini-primer):S445–S450.

45. Lee VW, Chapman JR. Sirolimus: its role in nephrology. *Nephrology (Carlton).* 2005;10:606–614.

46. Li C, Lim SW, Sun BK, Yang CW. Chronic cyclosporine nephrotoxicity: new insights and preventive strategies. *Yonsei Med J.* 2004;45:1004–1016.

47. Liossis SN, Tsokos GC. Monoclonal antibodies and fusion proteins in medicine. *J Allergy Clin Immunol.* 2005;116:721–729.

48. Luster AD. The role of chemokines in linking innate and adaptive immunity. *Curr Opin Immunol.* 2002;14: 129–135.

49. McCullough KC, Summerfield A. Basic concepts of immune response and defense development. *ILAR J.* 2005;46:230–240.

50. Mele TA, Halloran PF. The use of mycophenolate mofetil in transplant recipients. *Immunopharmacology.* 2000;47:215.

51. Munz C, Steinman RM, Fujii S. Dendritic cell maturation by innate lymphocytes: coordinated stimulation of innate and adaptive immunity. *J Exp Med.* 2005;202: 203–207.

52. Parekh K, Trulock E, Patterson GA. Use of cyclosporine in lung transplantation. *Transplant Proc.* 2004; 36(suppl):318S–322S.

53. Pelle MT, Werth VP. Thalidomide in cutaneous lupus erythematosus. *Am J Clin Dermatol.* 2003;4:379–387.

54. Ponticelli C, Tarantino A, Campise M, Montagnino G, Aroldi A, Passerini P. From cyclosporine to the future. *Transplant Proc.* 2004;36(suppl):557S–560S.

55. Radovancevic B, Vrtovec B. Sirolimus therapy in cardiac transplantation. *Transplant Proc.* 2003;35(suppl): 171S–176S.

56. Regazzi MB, Alessiani M, Rinaldi M. New strategies in immunosuppression. *Transplant Proc.* 2005;37: 2675–2678.

57. Reichardt HM. Immunomodulatory activities of glucocorticoids: insights from transgenesis and gene targeting. *Curr Pharm Des.* 2004;10:2797–2805.

58. Rezzani R. Cyclosporine A and adverse effects on organs: histochemical studies. *Prog Histochem Cytochem.* 2004;39:85–128.

59. Rhoades CJ, Williams MA, Kelsey SM, Newland AC. Monocyte-macrophage system and targets for immunomodulation by intravenous immunoglobulin. *Blood Rev.* 2000;14:14–30.

60. Sacks SH, Zhou W. Allograft rejection: effect of local synthesis of complement. *Springer Semin Immunopathol.* 2005;27:332–344.

61. Sandborn WJ, Feagan BG. Review article: mild to moderate Crohn's disease—defining the basis for a new treatment algorithm. *Aliment Pharmacol Ther.* 2003;18: 263–277.

62. Sandrini S. Use of IL-2 receptor antagonists to reduce delayed graft function following renal transplantation: a review. *Clin Transplant.* 2005;19:705–710.

63. Sands BE. Immunosuppressive drugs in ulcerative colitis: twisting facts to suit theories? *Gut.* 2006;55: 437–441.

64. Schluter M, Schofer J. Direct stenting with sirolimus-eluting stents. *Am Heart Hosp J.* 2005;3: 182–186, 192.

65. Sehgal SN. Sirolimus: its discovery, biological properties, and mechanism of action. *Transplant Proc.* 2003;35 (suppl):7S–14S.

66. Sengupta S, Blute ML. The management of superficial transitional cell carcinoma of the bladder. *Urology.* 2006;67(suppl 1):48–55.

67. Shi F, Ljunggren HG, Sarvetnick N. Innate immunity and autoimmunity: from self-protection to self-destruction. *Trends Immunol.* 2001;22:97–101.

68. Sieb JP. Myasthenia gravis: emerging new therapy options. *Curr Opin Pharmacol.* 2005;5:303–307.

69. Sivathasan C. Experience with cyclosporine in heart transplantation. *Transplant Proc.* 2004;36(suppl): 346S–348S.

70. Srinivas TR, Kaplan B, Schold JD, Meier-Kriesche HU. The impact of mycophenolate mofetil on long-term outcomes in kidney transplantation. *Transplantation.* 2005;80(suppl):S211–S220.

71. Svennilson J. Novel approaches in GVHD therapy. *Bone Marrow Transplant.* 2005;35(suppl 1):S65–S67.

72. Taylor AL, Watson CJ, Bradley JA. Immunosuppressive agents in solid organ transplantation: mechanisms of action and therapeutic efficacy. *Crit Rev Oncol Hematol.* 2005;56:23–46.

73. van Hooff JP, Christiaans MH, van Duijnhoven EM. Tacrolimus and posttransplant diabetes mellitus in renal transplantation. *Transplantation.* 2005;79: 1465–1469.

74. Viau M, Zouali M. B-lymphocytes, innate immunity, and autoimmunity. *Clin Immunol.* 2005;114: 17–26.

75. Webster A, Pankhurst T, Rinaldi F, et al. Polyclonal and monoclonal antibodies for treating acute rejection episodes in kidney transplant recipients. *Cochrane Database Syst Rev.* 2006;CD004756.

76. Webster AC, Woodroffe RC, Taylor RS, et al. Tacrolimus versus ciclosporin as primary immunosuppression for kidney transplant recipients: meta-analysis and meta-regression of randomised trial data. *BMJ.* 2005;331:810.

77. Wong W, Venetz JP, Tolkoff-Rubin N, Pascual M. 2005 immunosuppressive strategies in kidney transplantation: which role for the calcineurin inhibitors? *Transplantation.* 2005;80:289–296.

78. Zeiser R, Marks R, Bertz H, Finke J. Immunopathogenesis of acute graft-versus-host disease: implications for novel preventive and therapeutic strategies. *Ann Hematol.* 2004;83:551–565.

79. Zlotta AR, Schulman CC. Biological response modifiers for the treatment of superficial bladder tumors. *Eur Urol.* 2000;37(suppl 3):10.

Chapter 38

Complementary and Alternative Medications

In addition to traditional medications, consumers have access to many substances that are not considered a part of conventional or mainstream pharmacotherapeutics. These substances often consist of natural products such as herbal preparations, vitamins, minerals, and other nutritional substances that are taken to promote optimal health or to treat various conditions. These products are usually classified as dietary supplements by the Food and Drug Administration (FDA), and are therefore not subjected to the rigorous testing and scrutiny required for prescription drugs and many over-the-counter medications.

These nontraditional products are often described as complementary or alternative medications (CAMs), to differentiate them from the more conventional medications that are classified as drugs by the FDA. To be specific, a complementary medication is a substance that is used in addition to a conventional treatment, whereas an alternative medication is used as a substitute for a more traditional or mainstream treatment.[44] Other terms are applied to specific interventions, such as herbal remedies, naturopathic treatments, phytomedicines, and so forth. However, for the purpose of this chapter the term CAM will be used to encompass the array of substances that fall outside conventional pharmacotherapeutic regimens.

CAMs and other nontraditional healing philosophies (meditation, yoga, acupuncture, and so forth) have been a mainstay in certain cultures and societies. Western cultures, however, have generally been more aligned with conventional treatments and medications. Nonetheless, the interest and use of CAMs in persons living in the United States has increased dramatically over the past several years. Although it is dif-

ficult to determine the exact prevalence of CAM use, it is estimated that over 38 million adults in the United States use some form of CAM.[41,75] Interest in CAMs will almost certainly continue to increase as the popular media, the Internet, and other resources promote the potential benefits of CAMs.

Because CAMs represent such a broad range of substances and interventions, it is difficult to address this topic in a single chapter. This chapter will, however, present a general overview of the topic and will then describe some of the common CAMs that are taken by persons undergoing physical rehabilitation. This chapter aims to alert readers to some of the more pertinent and unique aspects of CAM use, and to help clinicians understand how these substances can affect how patients respond to rehabilitation interventions.

Unique Aspects of CAMs

Misconceptions about CAM Safety

Many CAMs are derived from natural sources such as herbs and other plants. Therefore, some consumers assume that a "natural" product is inherently safer than a synthetic or manufactured chemical.[57] These individuals may likewise believe that they can take an unlimited amount of a CAM; that is, they may exceed dose limits with the idea that the product can do no harm. These misconceptions can lead to tragic consequences, as was the case with ephedra. Ephedra, derived from an evergreen shrub, also contains epinephrine (adrenaline). As discussed in Chapter 20, epinephrine is a powerful agonist (stimulant) of alpha and beta receptors on various tissues throughout the body. People took ephedra to capitalize on these effects, especially its adrenalinelike effects in promoting weight loss and enhancing athletic performance.[1,19] Unfortunately, ephedra is also a powerful cardiovascular stimulant of beta-1 receptors on the heart and alpha-1 receptors on the peripheral vasculature. Hence, some well-documented cases of heart attack and stroke were attributed to ephedra, especially when it was taken in high doses to promote weight loss.[1] Concerns about the safety of ephedra prompted the FDA to ban dietary supplements containing ephedra in 2004.[66]

Patients should be reminded that CAMs are subject to all the same restrictions and potential problems as conventional medications. The case of ephedra serves as a primary example of how a product can produce powerful physiologic effects regardless of whether it is derived from natural or synthetic sources. It might also help to remind patients that some very important and powerful traditional medications such as opioids (Chapter 14), digoxin (Chapter 24), and certain anticancer drugs (Chapter 36) were originally derived from plant sources. Hence, patients should adhere to proper dosages even if the CAM originated from a natural source.

Failure to Report CAM Use

Patients are sometimes reluctant to tell their physician, nurse, pharmacist, or therapist that they are using CAMs.[41] These patients are often afraid that health care providers will criticize the use of these products as being unscientific and not consistent with conventional health care. This lack of reporting may result in an adverse interaction if a specific traditional medication is administered with a CAM. Likewise, CAMs can alter the metabolism of other medications (see "Potential Adverse Effects of CAMs," below), necessitating a change in the dose of the traditional medication to maintain efficacy or avoid an adverse drug reaction. Hence, patients should be encouraged to disclose CAM use as well as the use of any other nontraditional interventions, and clinicians should maintain a constructive, nonjudgmental dialogue with patients about the potential benefits and adverse effects of CAMs.[25]

Lack of Standards for Quality and Purity of CAMs

Because many CAMs are classified as food or dietary supplements, these substances are not subject to the same standards for quality and purity as traditional

medications.[7] As a result, the active ingredients in certain products may vary considerably or may be inadequate to exert a therapeutic effect.[49,64] This fact seems especially true for CAMs that are derived from plant sources. Plants that grow under different environmental or soil conditions will invariably contain different amounts of the active ingredients. In addition, some CAMs may inadvertently contain toxins that are sequestered by the plant when it is growing in its natural environment. There is also the possibility that the wrong plants will be harvested and subsequently marketed as a specific type of CAM. Hence, consumers should be aware that the quality of CAMs may vary from product to product, and that poor quality can result in a lack of therapeutic effects or an increased risk of toxic effects.

Delayed Use of Conventional Medications

A major concern among health care providers is that the use of ineffective alternative medications can delay or postpone the use of effective conventional interventions.[12] Consumers may begin to self-treat various conditions with alternative medications, hoping that these treatments will provide relief and that they can forego conventional or mainstream treatments. If the alternative treatment is not effective, however, the condition can worsen to the point where conventional treatment is no longer effective or takes much longer to achieve beneficial effects. Consumers should be counseled to avoid over-reliance on these alternative medications, and to seek conventional medical treatment if symptoms fail to resolve quickly or if they worsen during alternative medication use.

Potential Adverse Effects of CAMs

CAMs are often safe and are not typically associated with severe adverse effects when taken as recommended by reasonably healthy persons.[20] CAMs, however, can interact with conventional medications, and directly increase or decrease these medications' effects.[35] Moreover, CAMs often influence the absorption, distribution, metabolism, and excretion of conventional medications.[11,37] In particular, CAMs can stimulate the liver to synthesize more drug-metabolizing enzymes, a process known as enzyme induction (the phenomenon of enzyme induction is addressed in Chapter 3).[80] During enzyme induction, the liver is capable of metabolizing conventional drugs faster than normal, and the drugs fail to reach therapeutic levels because they are broken down too quickly.[37] Hence, conventional medications may fail to exert beneficial effects, and the disease can continue to progress even though the patient is taking the conventional medication as directed. Once again, physicians must be aware of whether patients are consuming CAMs so that doses of conventional medications can be adjusted to maintain therapeutic effects.

Excessive or prolonged dosages of CAMs can likewise produce toxic effects on various tissues and organs. In particular, the liver may be damaged, and cases of acute liver failure have been documented during inappropriate CAM use or in patients with preexisting liver disease.[45,70] This fact makes sense considering that the liver often metabolizes CAMs in the same way that it deals with other drugs and toxins.[22] Other organs, including the heart, kidneys, and lungs, can also be subjected to toxic effects by high doses of CAMs much in the same way that these organs are vulnerable to untoward effects of conventional medications.

Finally, CAMs can produce side effects and adverse reactions similar to conventional medications.[61] Gastrointestinal disturbances (nausea, vomiting, diarrhea), headache, allergic responses, and various other reactions are possible even when CAMs are taken at appropriate doses. The type and severity of these reactions depends on many factors including the type of CAM and the individual characteristics of each patient (genetic factors, diseases, other medications, and so forth). Clearly, CAMs can produce the same types of problems as conventional medications, and consumers must be reminded that these products are actual drugs even though they may be derived from natural or nontraditional sources.

 ## Specific CAMs

The array of CAMs is so vast that even a partial listing is difficult. Some of the more common CAMs are listed in Table 38–1, and are addressed briefly below to provide some indication of their source, primary indications, and potential adverse effects. These discussions are not intended to advocate the use of these substances or to provide a detailed evaluation of the evidence supporting or refuting their use. For more information about these or other CAMs, please refer to several sources listed at the end of the chapter.[53,67,73]

Bee Venom

Bee venom, administered in the form of actual bee stings, has been used to treat people with multiple sclerosis, rheumatoid arthritis, and other disease that have an autoimmune basis.[48,78] This treatment is supposed to modulate the immune response and suppress the damage caused by the activation and attack of immune cells on specific tissues.[30] There is little evidence, however, that bee sting therapy can produce beneficial effects in humans.[78] Additional research is needed to determine whether these treatments can promote short- or long-term benefits in persons with various autoimmune diseases.

Echinacea

Echinacea is derived from the root and seeds of the Echinacea plant that grows in parts of the Midwestern United States. This herb is used primarily to stimulate or support the immune system, and is often used to treat cold symptoms and other relatively minor respiratory tract infections.[8,38] Although the exact reasons for beneficial effects are unclear, there is considerable evidence that echinacea preparations can reduce symptoms of the common cold when taken soon after symptoms appear.[5,71] The ability of echinacea to prevent colds and other infections, however, is less well defined.[49] Echinacea can also be administered topically to treat burns and other localized wounds. The most common side effects associated with echinacea are gastrointestinal (GI) upset, skin rash, and other allergic or hypersensitivity reactions.[36]

Garlic

Garlic is a bulb that grows throughout the world; its potential health benefits have been extolled for ages. Evidence suggests that garlic extract may reduce the risk of cardiovascular disease by reducing plasma lipids, lowering blood pressure, and inhibiting platelet aggregation.[10,69] Other purported benefits include antineoplastic, antimicrobial, anti-inflammatory, antihyperglycemic, and antioxidant effects.[15,60,74] The exact reasons for these effects are not clear, but are usually attributed to allicin, a chemical that is considered to be the active component of garlic. Side effects are generally mild, consisting primarily of garlic breath odor and GI upset. Serious bleeding problems could occur, however, if patients experience antiplatelet effects from the garlic and are taking other anticoagulants such as heparin, warfarin, or aspirin.

Table 38–1 **COMPLEMENTARY AND ALTERNATIVE MEDICATIONS**

Common Name	Scientific Name	Original Source	Primary Indications/Effects
Bee venom	—	Live bees	Multiple sclerosis; rheumatoid arthritis; other diseases with an autoimmune basis
Chondroitin	*Chondroitin sulfate*	Bovine tracheal cartilage	Osteoarthritis (combined with glucosamine)
Echinacea	Echinacea species *(E. angustifolia; E. pallida; E. purpurea)*	Roots and seeds from the echinacea plant	Immune stimulant; treatment of colds and upper respiratory tract infections; applied topically to promote wound healing
Garlic	*Allium sativum L*	Bulb of the garlic plant	Decrease cholesterol and other plasma lipids; anti-inflammatory; antimicrobial; antioxidant; other effects
Ginger	*Zingiber officinale*	Root of the ginger plant	Antiemetic; anti-inflammatory; antioxidant; migraine headaches; indigestion; infection; fever; other effects
Ginkgo	*Ginkgo biloba*	Leaf of the gingko tree	Improve memory and cognition; increase vascular perfusion of brain and other tissues; antioxidant; anti-inflammatory
Ginseng	*Panax ginseng*	Root of the ginseng plant	Increase well-being; reduce fatigue; used in the treatment of cancer, diabetes, cardiovascular dysfunction, and various other diseases
Glucosamine	2-amino-2-deoxyglucose; glucosamine sulfate	Manufactured synthetically from sugar-protein precursors	Osteoarthritis (combined with chondroitin)
Kava	*Piper methysticum*	Root of the kava plant	Sedative-hypnotic and antianxiety effects
Melatonin	N-acetyl-5-methoxytryptamine	Manufactured synthetically to mimic the endogenous hormone	Sedative-hypnotic; regulate sleep-wake cycles; used in various other conditions because of antioxidant and immunomodulating effects
Saw palmetto	*Serenoa repens*	Fruit of the saw palmetto palm	Benign prostatic hypertrophy
St. John's wort	*Hypericum perforatum L*	Flowers of the St. John's wort plant	Antidepressant
Valerian	*Valeriana officinalis*	Root of the valerian plant	Sedative-hypnotic and antianxiety effects

Ginger

Ginger is extracted from the root of the ginger plant; the plant originated in Asia but now grows throughout other parts of the world. Ginger is noted for its substantial antiemetic effects, and can be used to control the nausea and vomiting that occurs during pregnancy or after surgery.[9,14] It also produces anti-inflammatory effects by inhibiting prostaglandin synthesis in a manner similar to aspirin and other NSAIDs (see Chapter 15).[28] Ginger may likewise inhibit leukotriene production (see Chapter 26), and it may affect specific genes to reduce the production of other pro-inflammatory products.[28] Ginger has been used for other conditions, including the treatment of sore throats, migraine headaches, indigestion, infection, and fever. Side effects of ginger are usually minor, consisting primarily of GI problems (nausea, vomiting) and allergic reactions.

Ginkgo biloba

Ginkgo biloba is extracted from the leaves of the gingko tree that originated in Japan and China. This herb has become synonymous with attempts to increase memory and cognition. Hence, gingko products are used extensively by many older adults, especially as a complementary or alternative treatment of Alzheimer disease.[52] Gingko is reported to improve circulation, and some of its effects on cognitive function have been attributed to increased cerebral perfusion. Gingko may also exert antioxidant effects, and some of its therapeutic benefits have been attributed to its ability to limit free-radical damage on vascular and other tissues.[23] The primary problem associated with *Gingko biloba* is an increased risk of hemorrhage,[6] and gingko products should be avoided in people at risk for bleeding events or who are taking anticoagulants (heparin, warfarin, aspirin and other NSAIDs).

Ginseng

Ginseng, derived from the root of the Panax plant, is renowned as an herbal remedy for various conditions. It is often administered to increase general well-being, reduce fatigue, improve mental acuity, and promote optimal health.[18,40] Ginseng has likewise been advocated in the prevention and treatment of many diseases including cancer, diabetes, neurodegenerative disorders, and cardiovascular disease.[13,33,68,83] The potential benefits of ginseng products are typically attributed to its antioxidant properties and ability to support the immune system.[40,85] The exact effects of ginseng, however, are not well understood. Ginseng is well tolerated when taken in moderate amounts, but it can reduce the effectiveness of anticoagulant medications such as warfarin, and it can exaggerate the effects of antihyperglycemic medications such as insulin and oral antidiabetic drugs.[42]

Glucosamine and Chondroitin

As discussed in Chapter 16, glucosamine and chondroitin are dietary supplements that have been advocated for the treatment of osteoarthritis. These compounds can be obtained from natural sources, or they can be manufactured synthetically. The primary rationale for taking glucosamine and chondroitin is to supply the body with the ingredients needed to build healthy articular cartilage and to maintain synovial fluid viscosity.[64] That is, these supplements can provide glycosaminoglycans, proteoglycans, and hyaluronic acid, which comprise the fundamental constituents needed to repair damaged cartilage and to increase synovial viscosity, thus limiting the joint damage associated with osteoarthritis.[34,64]

The potential benefits of glucosamine and chondroitin have been studied extensively in several clinical trials.[17] It appears that these supplements may not be helpful in reducing pain or in improving function in all patients with osteoarthritis, but certain patients with more severe pain or an increased rate of cartilage turnover may experience some beneficial effects.[17] These substances are generally well tolerated, although headache and GI problems (nausea, cramping, heartburn) may occur. Researchers continue to study the long-term effects of glucosamine and chondroitin, and future studies may provide better insight into how this CAM treatment can benefit certain subpopulations of people with osteoarthritis.

Kava

Kava originates from the root of the *Piper methysticum* (kava) plant that grows predominately in the South Pacific islands. This drug has been used for centuries by various local cultures because of its sedative and antianxiety effects. Kava has likewise gained popularity in western societies, and studies suggest that kava extracts can be used as an alternative to traditional sedative-hypnotic and anxiolytic drugs, such as benzodiazepines (see Chapter 6).[21,39] Kava may also produce analgesic and muscle relaxant effects, and some patients may use this product for self-treatment of back pain and other musculoskeletal injuries. Although the exact mechanism of action is unclear, kava extracts probably affect receptors within the limbic system, and enhance the inhibitory effects of GABA and other neurotransmitters. Liver toxicity is the most serious effect associated with kava, and the risk of liver damage is especially problematic when higher dosages are taken for prolonged periods.[77] Because of the potential for liver toxicity, kava products are banned in many countries throughout Europe.[2]

Melatonin

Melatonin is an endogenous neurohormone that is produced primarily by the pineal gland. In humans, melatonin is normally released at night, with plasma levels tending to peak between 2 and 4 AM.[47] Melatonin is associated with the ability to regulate sleep-wake cycles, and perhaps other circadian rhythms.[3,31] Because of this effect, synthetic melatonin supplements have been used primarily to treat insomnia, especially in individuals with disturbed sleep cycles or persons who are blind and cannot regulate melatonin release because they are unable to respond visually to normal light-dark cycles.[3]

Melatonin is also associated with antioxidant effects; these effects may be beneficial in several situations, such as preventing the neurodegenerative changes in Parkinson disease,[54,81] reducing migraine headaches,[65] and improving insulin responses in type 2 diabetes mellitus.[62] Melatonin may also stimulate and support the immune system, and may therefore be helpful in treating certain forms of cancer.[58,59] Clearly, melatonin has the ability to regulate a number of important physiologic functions, and researchers continue to investigate the potential benefits of melatonin supplements in a number of conditions. Side effects of melatonin are usually minor, consisting primarily of headache, change in sleep cycles, vivid dreams, GI disturbances, and allergic reactions (skin rashes and itching).

Saw Palmetto

Saw palmetto is a palm that grows in the southern United States, and extracts from the fruit of this palm are used primarily to treat benign prostatic hypertrophy (BPH).[27] Evidence suggests that saw palmetto extracts can reduce urinary restriction and increase urine flow in mild to moderate cases of BPH.[24,82] This effect is apparently due to a reduction in swelling and inflammation of the prostate, but the exact mechanism of saw palmetto on BPH is not clear.[26] Possible side effects include headache, GI upset, and allergic reactions. Saw palmetto treatments, however, are generally well tolerated, especially when compared to conventional medications such as finasteride (Proscar) (see Chapter 30).[27,82]

St. John's Wort

St. John's wort is derived from the flowers of the *Hypericum perforatum* plant that grows throughout England, Europe, Asia, and parts of the United States. This herbal supplement has been used extensively to treat symptoms of depression and anxiety. Although the details are unclear, St. John's wort probably contains several chemicals that alter the balance of central nervous system (CNS) neurotransmitters affecting mood and behavior.[46,84] As discussed in Chapter 7, depression seems to be associated with a fundamental defect in amine neurotransmitters such as serotonin, norepinephrine, and dopamine. St. John's wort may promote changes in these neurotransmitters in a manner similar to conventional prescription antidepressants.[56,84] Many people have therefore used St. John's wort as an alternative medication to help improve mood and resolve the symptoms of depression.[46,72]

Several studies have suggested that products containing adequate amounts of the active chemicals from St. John's wort may be successful in treating mild-to-moderate depression.[46,72] The success of this product in more severe or resistant forms of depression remains unclear.[50] St. John's wort is generally well tolerated,[43,51] but use of this product can accelerate the metabolism of other therapeutic medications such as warfarin (Chapter 25), reverse transcriptase inhibitors (Chapter 34), cyclosporine (Chapter 37), and certain anticancer agents (Chapter 36).[16,72] Hence, St. John's wort can prevent these other medications from reaching therapeutic levels, and dosages of other medications may have to be adjusted to maintain their efficacy when administered with St. John's wort.[46]

Valerian

Valerian is derived from the root of the valerian plant that grows throughout many parts of the world. It is generally used to treat mild cases of anxiety and to promote normal sleep. As a sleep aid, valerian may need to be taken for a week or so before beneficial effects become apparent.[29] Nonetheless, this product can be an alternative long-term treatment for people with mild-to-moderate cases of insomnia and restlessness.[79] Valerian appears to exert sedative and antianxiety effects in a manner similar to benzodiazepines; that is, enhancement of GABA inhibition in specific parts of the brain that control sleep (see Chapter 6).[63] Side effects of valerian are generally mild, and consist of headache and GI problems (nausea, vomiting).

Vitamins and Minerals

Vitamins and minerals are not considered medications, but these substances are essential for maintaining physiologic function and homeostasis throughout the body. Many individuals consume these substances to compliment other medications and to help promote optimal health. It is beyond the scope of this chapter to address all the pertinent issues related to vitamin and mineral metabolism. Nonetheless, a brief overview of these substances and their use as dietary supplements is provided here and summarized in Tables 38–2 and 38–3. Readers are also referred to other sources for a more detailed discussion of vitamins and minerals.[4,55,76]

Vitamins

Vitamins comprise a diverse group of organic chemicals that the body needs to facilitate specific metabolic and biosynthetic processes.[4] In many cases, vitamins act as enzymatic cofactors; that is, the vitamin works directly with the enzyme to catalyze a specific chemical reaction. In other situations, the vitamin forms an essential component of a chemical structure or species that is needed for a specific chemical reaction. The body typically needs small amounts of vitamins to promote normal growth and development, and to maintain optimal health throughout adulthood.[32]

Table 38–2 summarizes the key aspects of vitamins needed throughout the body. Most of these vitamins cannot be synthesized within the body and must be ingested from an outside source.[76] Eating certain foods on a regular basis will provide the body with an adequate supply of the specific vitamins it needs. Fruits and vegetables, for example, often serve as a source of dietary vitamins. Alternatively, there are myriad vitamin supplements that consumers can purchase and self-administer to insure adequate daily vitamin intake.

Vitamin supplements are usually required if the dietary supply of vitamins is inadequate to meet the body's daily requirements.[4] In most cases, a relatively balanced diet will provide adequate amounts of all the

Text continued on page 614

Table 38–2   VITAMINS

Vitamin	RDA/AI*	Physiological Function	Adverse Effects of Excessive Consumption
Biotin	Men & women: 30 µg/d	Coenzyme in the synthesis of fat, glycogen, and amino acids	No adverse effects have been reported**
Folic acid	Men & women: 400 µg/d	Coenzyme in the metabolism of nucleic acids and amino acids; prevents megaloblastic anemia	Adverse effects have not been documented, but high doses may mask neurological complications in people with Vitamin B_{12} deficiency
Niacin	Men: 16 mg/d Women: 14 mg/d	Coenzyme or cosubstrate in many biological reactions required for energy metabolism	Gastrointestinal distress; vasomotor reactions (flushing)
Pantothenic acid	Men & women: 5 mg/d	Coenzyme in fatty acid metabolism	No adverse effects have been reported**

(Continued on following page)

Table 38–2	VITAMINS *(Continued)*		
Vitamin	**RDA/AI***	**Physiological function**	**Adverse Effects of Excessive Consumption**
Vitamin A (retinol)	Men: 900 µg/d Women: 700 µg/d	Required for normal vision, gene expression, reproduction, embryonic development, and immune function	Teratological effects; liver toxicity
Vitamin B_1 (thiamin)	Men: 1.2 mg/d Women: 1.1 mg/d	Coenzyme in the metabolism of carbohydrates and certain amino acids; prevents beriberi	No adverse effects have been reported**
Vitamin B_2 (riboflavin)	Men: 1.3 mg/d Women: 1.1 mg/d	Coenzyme in numerous oxidative metabolic reactions	No adverse effects have been reported**
Vitamin B_6 (pyridoxine)	Men: 1.3–1.7 mg/d Women: 1.3–1.5 mg/d	Coenzyme in the metabolism of amino acids and glycogen	No adverse effects have been reported**
Vitamin B_{12} (cobalamin)	Men & women: 2.4 µg/d	Coenzyme in nucleic acid metabolism; prevents megaloblastic/pernicious anemia	No adverse effects have been reported**
Vitamin C (ascorbic acid)	Men: 90 mg/d Women: 75 mg/d	Cofactor for reactions requiring reduced copper or iron metalloenzyme and as a protective antioxidant; prevents scurvy	Gastrointestinal disturbances, kidney stones, excess iron absorption
Vitamin D (calciferol)	Men & women: 5–15 µg/d	Maintain serum calcium and phosphorus concentrations; prevents rickets	Hypercalcemia secondary to elevated vitamin D metabolites in plasma
Vitamin E (α-tocopherol)	Men & women: 15 mg/d	Antioxidant effects	Hemorrhagic toxicity
Vitamin K	Men: 120 µg/d Women: 90 µg/d	Coenzyme during the synthesis of many proteins involved in blood clotting and bone metabolism	No adverse effects have been reported**

*Recommended daily requirement (RDA) or adequate intake (AI) for men and nonpregnant women over 20 years old. Recommended values for certain vitamins (e.g., folic acid) may be higher in women who are pregnant. Values for children are typically lower, and are adjusted according to the child's age.

**Absence of reported adverse effects does not mean that there is no potential for adverse effects from high intake. Caution should still be used when taking doses well in excess of the recommended daily amounts.

Adapted from: Institute of Medicine of the National Academies (www.iom.edu): Food & Nutrition > Dietary Reference Intakes > DRI Tables > Vitamins.

Table 38–3	MINERALS	

Major minerals (> 0.005% body weight)

Mineral	**Primary Physiologic Function(s)**	**RDA/AI***
Calcium	Mineralization of bone and teeth; synaptic transmission; muscle contraction; blood clotting	Men & women: 1000 mg/d
Chloride	With sodium and potassium, helps maintain electrochemical and water balance across cell membrane	Men & women: 2.3 g/d
Magnesium	Cofactor for enzyme systems	Men: 420 mg/d Women: 320 mg/d
Phosphate	Facilitates energy storage and release, nucleotide synthesis, and maintenance of acid-base balance in body fluids	Men & women: 700 mg/d
Potassium	With sodium and chloride, helps maintain electrochemical and water balance across cell membrane; promotes repolarization of nerve and muscle tissues	Men & women: 4.7 g/d
Sodium	With potassium and chloride, helps maintain electrochemical and water balance across cell membrane; initiates depolarization of nerve and muscle tissues	Men & women: 1.5 g/d
Inorganic Sulfate	Provides precursors for sulfur-containing compounds	Unknown

Trace minerals (< 0.005% body weight)

Mineral	**Primary Physiologic Function(s)**	**RDA/AI***
Chromium	Helps maintain normal blood glucose levels	Men: 35 μg/d Women: 25 μg/d
Copper	Component of enzymes in iron metabolism	Men & women: 900 μg/d
Fluoride	Stimulates new bone formation; prevents formation of dental cavities	Men: 4 mg/d Women: 3 mg/d
Iodine	Component of the thyroid hormones; prevents goiter and cretinism	Men & women: 150 μg/d
Iron	Component of hemoglobin and numerous enzymes; prevents certain anemias	Men: 8 mg/d Women: 18 mg/d
Manganese	Involved in bone formation and in enzymes involved in amino acid, cholesterol, and carbohydrate metabolism	Men: 2.3 mg/d Women: 1.8 mg/d
Molybdenum	Cofactor for enzymes involved in catabolism of certain amino acids and nucleic acids	Men & women: 45 μg/d
Selenium	Defense against oxidative stress; regulates thyroid hormone action and metabolism of vitamin C and other molecules	Men & women: 55 μg/d
Zinc	Component of many enzymes and proteins; involved in the regulation of gene expression	Men: 11 mg/d Women: 8 mg/d

*Recommended daily requirement (RDA) or adequate intake (AI) for men and nonpregnant women 30–50 years old. Values may differ for children, older adults, and pregnant women.
Adapted from: Institute of Medicine of the National Academies (www.iom.edu): Food & Nutrition > Dietary Reference Intakes > DRI Tables > Electrolytes and Water; Elements.

vitamins needed. People with diets that are extremely poor in nutrients or lacking in certain foods may benefit from vitamin supplements. Certain metabolic disorders may likewise impair the absorption or utilization of specific vitamins, and supplements can help resolve a potential vitamin imbalance in these situations.[32] In other situations, the body's demand for certain vitamins may increase, and dietary sources may be unable to provide enough of a specific vitamin. During pregnancy, for example, a supplement with folic acid is helpful in supplying an adequate source of this vitamin for the mother and developing fetus.

Hence, vitamin supplements should be administered to make up any differences between the dietary supply and the body's demand for specific vitamins. Some individuals, however, self-administer large dosages of vitamins on a regular basis with the misconception that these supplements will promote better health and offer protection from disease. Excessive dosages of vitamins are unnecessary and can be harmful if they begin to accumulate in certain tissues and organs. This fact is especially true for the fat soluble vitamins A, D, E, and K.[4,55] Water soluble vitamins (B complex, vitamin C) are generally less problematic because excess doses of these vitamins are excreted in the urine. Fat-soluble vitamins, however, can accumulate in adipose tissue, the liver, and various other sites throughout the body. Excess vitamin administration can result in various signs of toxicity, including drowsiness, headache, fatigue, nausea, muscle weakness, and enlargement of the liver and spleen (see Table 38–2).[4]

Clinicians should therefore advise patients about the need for adequate dietary vitamin intake, but should also caution patients about the indiscriminate or excessive use of vitamin supplements. Patients with specific questions can also be referred to a registered dietician who can analyze the person's vitamin needs, and suggest whether supplements may be helpful.

Minerals

Minerals are small chemical substances that play key roles in various physiologic processes.[55] Consider, for example, the ways that minerals such as sodium, potassium, chloride, and calcium influence the function and homeostasis of virtually every cell in the body. These minerals and several other major minerals (see Table 38–3) are essential for life. Other minerals, known commonly as trace minerals, are not as abundant in the body, but are still needed to promote the function of specific cells and tissues.

The primary roles and the recommended daily intake of major and trace minerals are listed in Table 38–3. Similar to vitamins, these minerals are typically obtained from dietary sources. Specific minerals may likewise be included in various multivitamins and other dietary supplements, with the intent that these minerals will promote good health and prevent disease. Again, there is generally no need for mineral supplements for most people eating a reasonably balanced diet. On the other hand, mineral supplements can be helpful in specific situations where the body's need for a mineral may exceed dietary supply. Some examples of appropriate supplementation include calcium supplements for people with osteoporosis (see Chapter 31), potassium supplements for people on diuretics (see Chapter 21), and iron supplements for people with certain anemias. Hence, mineral supplements may be helpful in certain individuals, but the dose and type of supplement should be adjusted carefully.

Special Concerns in Rehabilitation Patients

■ ■ ■ Considering the extensive use of CAMs, many patients receiving physical therapy or occupational therapy will be taking these products to promote health and to prevent disease. Patients may also feel empowered to take a more active role in controlling their health and well-being, especially if they experience beneficial effects from exercise and other rehabilitation interventions. Hence, these patients may be interested in how nutritional and dietary supplements can be used in a safe and effective manner. CAMs are likewise used as part of the treatment for many conditions seen in patients receiving rehabilitation, including back pain, fibromyalgia, rheumatoid and osteoarthritis, and myriad other systemic diseases and conditions.

Rehabilitation specialists will therefore be in an optimal position to serve as health care educators in discussing the appropriate uses of CAMs, and dispelling myths about unproven or improbable claims about these products' benefits. Therapists should query their patients about CAM use as part of the evaluation process. In fact, patients may be more willing to divulge their use of CAMs to therapists as opposed to physicians and other health care practitioners. Therapists may identify potential problems in patients taking excessive or inappropriate CAMs, and can refer such patients to a physician, nurse practitioner, or registered dietician for further evaluation of the risks of using CAMs. However, therapists should not advise patients to take specific CAMs because ingestion of any chemical may cause untoward effects that are simply not apparent given our knowledge of the patient's medical background, comorbidities, diet, other medications, and so forth. Patients who are interested in taking CAMs should always be referred to other practitioners who are experts in the use of these products.

Finally, therapists should look for signs that might indicate excessive use of CAMs such as muscle weakness, incoordination, excessive fatigue, balance problems, skin rashes or bruising, neuropathic changes, and cardiovascular impairments (increased blood pressure, arrhythmias, and so forth). These signs or any unexplained change in function should be brought to the attention of the physician so that the potential risks of CAMs can be evaluated and dealt with accordingly.

CASE STUDY
Complementary and Alternative Medications

Brief History. S.G. is a 75-year-old man who began experiencing osteoarthritic changes in his right knee when he was in his 50s. This condition worsened progressively, necessitating a total knee arthroplasty, which was performed two years ago. The initial knee replacement, however, became unstable, and was recently revised surgically to decrease pain and to promote better function. While in the hospital for this revision, the patient developed a deep vein thrombosis, and was placed on heparin followed by warfarin (Coumadin) to control excessive coagulation. He continued taking the warfarin when he was discharged, and a physical therapist began providing home care on a regular basis. During the initial visit, the therapist asked the patient if he was taking any additional medications. He replied that he had recently started taking St. John's wort on the advice of a friend. Apparently, this patient had become very discouraged and despondent because of problems with his knee replacement and his inability to resume his hobbies and social activities (playing golf, gardening, and so forth). He hoped

that the St. John's wort would provide an alternative way to improve his mood while recovering from the most recent knee surgery.

Problem/Influence of Medication. St. John's wort can cause enzyme induction, which results in an increase in the liver's ability to metabolize other medications, including warfarin. This process could result in the warfarin being metabolized too rapidly and therefore failing to reach therapeutic levels. Lack of adequate anticoagulant effects would place the patient at increased risk for subsequent thrombosis and pulmonary embolism.

Decision/Solution. The therapist called the physician and related the fact that the patient had recently started taking St. John's wort. To get an indication of warfarin efficacy, the physician ordered blood tests to assess the patient's clotting times. These tests revealed that clotting times were indeed slightly decreased, indicating that the blood was clotting too rapidly and that the dose of warfarin needed to be increased. The dose of warfarin was adjusted accordingly, and clotting time was monitored periodically to ensure that the new dose was appropriate. The patient recovered from the surgery without any further thrombotic events.

SUMMARY

CAMs represent a diverse array of nutritional supplements and other products that are used to promote health and prevent disease. Because CAMs are often derived from natural sources, patients may have certain misconceptions about the safety and efficacy of these products. CAMs are likewise not subjected to the scrutiny and control of traditional medications, and patient responses may be influenced by problems with the product's purity and quality. Many patients undergoing physical rehabilitation will self-administer CAMs to help treat various conditions or to maintain optimal health. Therapists should query their patients about CAM use, serve as a source of information about the potential benefits and detriments of these products, and remain alert for any untoward reactions that might indicate toxic effects of CAMs.

References

1. Andraws R, Chawla P, Brown DL. Cardiovascular effects of ephedra alkaloids: a comprehensive review. *Prog Cardiovasc Dis.* 2005;47:217–225.
2. Anke J, Ramzan I. Pharmacokinetic and pharmacodynamic drug interactions with Kava (Piper methysticum Forst. f.). *J Ethnopharmacol.* 2004;93:153–160.
3. Arendt J. Melatonin: characteristics, concerns, and prospects. *J Biol Rhythms.* 2005;20:291–303.
4. Barone S. Vitamins. In: Craig CR, Stitzel RE, eds. *Modern Pharmacology with Clinical Applications.* 5th ed. Boston: Little, Brown and Company; 1997.
5. Barnes J, Anderson LA, Gibbons S, Phillipson JD. Echinacea species (*Echinacea angustifolia (DC.) Hell., Echinacea pallida (Nutt.) Nutt., Echinacea purpurea (L.) Moench)*: a review of their chemistry, pharmacology and clinical properties. *J Pharm Pharmacol.* 2005;57:929–954.
6. Bent S, Goldberg H, Padula A, Avins AL. Spontaneous bleeding associated with *ginkgo biloba*: a case report and systematic review of the literature: a case report and systematic review of the literature. *J Gen Intern Med.* 2005;20:657–661.
7. Bircher AJ, Surber C. Unregulated alternative medicine. *J Drugs Dermatol.* 2003;2:58–61.
8. Block KI, Mead MN. Immune system effects of echinacea, ginseng, and astragalus: a review. *Integr Cancer Ther.* 2003;2:247–267.
9. Boone SA, Shields KM. Treating pregnancy-related nausea and vomiting with ginger. *Ann Pharmacother.* 2005;39:1710–1713.
10. Borek C. Garlic reduces dementia and heart-disease risk. *J Nutr.* 2006;136(suppl):810S–812S.
11. Brazier NC, Levine MA. Drug-herb interaction among commonly used conventional medicines: a compendium for health care professionals. *Am J Ther.* 2003;10:163–169.
12. Brienza RS, Stein MD, Fagan MJ. Delay in obtaining conventional healthcare by female internal medicine patients who use herbal therapies. *J Womens Health Gend Based Med.* 2002;11:79–87.
13. Buettner C, Yeh GY, Phillips RS, et al. Systematic review of the effects of ginseng on cardiovascular risk factors. *Ann Pharmacother.* 2006;40:83–95.
14. Chaiyakunapruk N, Kitikannakorn N, Nathisuwan S, et al. The efficacy of ginger for the prevention of postoperative nausea and vomiting: a meta-analysis. *Am J Obstet Gynecol.* 2006;194:95–99.
15. Chauhan NB. Multiplicity of garlic health effects and Alzheimer's disease. *J Nutr Health Aging.* 2005;9:421–432.
16. Choudhuri S, Valerio LG, Jr. Usefulness of studies on the molecular mechanism of action of herbals/botanicals: the case of St. John's wort. *J Biochem Mol Toxicol.* 2005;19:1–11.
17. Clegg DO, Reda DJ, Harris CL, et al. Glucosamine, chondroitin sulfate, and the two in combination for painful knee osteoarthritis. *N Engl J Med.* 2006;354:795–808.
18. Coleman CI, Hebert JH, Reddy P. The effects of *Panax ginseng* on quality of life. *J Clin Pharm Ther.* 2003;28:5–15.
19. Dwyer JT, Allison DB, Coates PM. Dietary supplements in weight reduction. *J Am Diet Assoc.* 2005;105(suppl 1):S80–S86.
20. Ernst E. The risk-benefit profile of commonly used herbal therapies: Ginkgo, St. John's wort, ginseng, echinacea, saw palmetto, and kava. *Ann Intern Med.* 2002;136:42–53.
21. Ernst E. Herbal remedies for anxiety—a systematic review of controlled clinical trials. *Phytomedicine.* 2006;13:205–208.
22. Fogden E, Neuberger J. Alternative medicines and the liver. *Liver Int.* 2003;23:213–220.
23. Frank B, Gupta S. A review of antioxidants and Alzheimer's disease. *Ann Clin Psychiatry.* 2005;17:269–286.
24. Gerber GS, Fitzpatrick JM. The role of a lipidosterolic extract of *Serenoa repens* in the management of lower urinary tract symptoms associated with benign prostatic hyperplasia. *BJU Int.* 2004;94:338–344.
25. Giveon SM, Liberman N, Klang S, Kahan E. A survey of primary care physicians' perceptions of their patients' use of complementary medicine. *Complement Ther Med.* 2003;11:254–260.
26. Gong EM, Gerber GS. Saw palmetto and benign prostatic hyperplasia. *Am J Chin Med.* 2004;32:331–338.
27. Gordon AE, Shaughnessy AF. Saw palmetto for prostate disorders. *Am Fam Physician.* 2003;67:1281–1283.
28. Grzanna R, Lindmark L, Frondoza CG. Ginger—an herbal medicinal product with broad anti-inflammatory actions. *J Med Food.* 2005;8:125–132.

29. Hadley S, Petry JJ. Valerian. *Am Fam Physician.* 2003;67:1755–1758.

30. Hamedani M, Vatanpour H, Saadat F, et al. Bee venom, immunostimulant or immunosuppressor? Insight into the effect on matrix metalloproteinases and interferons. *Immunopharmacol Immunotoxicol.* 2005;27:671–681.

31. Hardeland R, Pandi-Perumal SR, Cardinali DP. Melatonin. *Int J Biochem Cell Biol.* 2006;38:313–316.

32. Heimburger DC, McLaren DS, Shils ME. Clinical manifestations of nutrient deficiencies and toxicities: a resume. In: Shils ME, et al, eds. *Modern Nutrition in Health and Disease.*10th ed. Philadelphia: Lippincott Williams and Wilkins; 2006.

33. Helms S. Cancer prevention and therapeutics: *Panax ginseng. Altern Med Rev.* 2004;9:259–274.

34. Homandberg GA, Guo D, Ray LM, Ding L. Mixtures of glucosamine and chondroitin sulfate reverse fibronectin fragment mediated damage to cartilage more effectively than either agent alone. *Osteoarthritis Cartilage.* 2006;14:793–806.

35. Hu Z, Yang X, Ho PC, et al. Herb-drug interactions: a literature review. *Drugs.* 2005;65:1239–1282.

36. Huntley AL, Thompson Coon J, Ernst E. The safety of herbal medicinal products derived from Echinacea species: a systematic review. *Drug Saf.* 2005;28:387–400.

37. Ioannides C. Pharmacokinetic interactions between herbal remedies and medicinal drugs. *Xenobiotica.* 2002;32:451–478.

38. Islam J, Carter R. Use of Echinacea in upper respiratory tract infection. *South Med J.* 2005;98: 311–318.

39. Jorm AF, Christensen H, Griffiths KM, et al. Effectiveness of complementary and self-help treatments for anxiety disorders. *Med J Aust.* 2004;181(suppl): S29–S46.

40. Kaneko H, Nakanishi K. Proof of the mysterious efficacy of ginseng: basic and clinical trials: clinical effects of medical ginseng, Korean red ginseng: specifically, its anti-stress action for prevention of disease. *J Pharmacol Sci.* 2004;95:158–162.

41. Kennedy J. Herb and supplement use in the US adult population. *Clin Ther.* 2005;27:1847–1858.

42. Kiefer D, Pantuso T. *Panax ginseng. Am Fam Physician.* 2003;68:1539–1542.

43. Knuppel L, Linde K. Adverse effects of St. John's Wort: a systematic review. *J Clin Psychiatry.* 2004; 65:1470–1479.

44. Kronenberg F, Mindes J, Jacobson JS. The future of complementary and alternative medicine for cancer. *Cancer Invest.* 2005;23:420–426.

45. Krueger KJ, McClain CJ, McClave SA, Dryden GW. Nutritional supplements and alternative medicine. *Curr Opin Gastroenterol.* 2004;20: 130–138.

46. Lawvere S, Mahoney MC. St. John's wort. *Am Fam Physician.* 2005;72:2249–2254.

47. Lee CO. Complementary and alternative medicines patients are talking about: melatonin. *Clin J Oncol Nurs.* 2006;10:105–107.

48. Lee JY, Kang SS, Kim JH, et al. Inhibitory effect of whole bee venom in adjuvant-induced arthritis. *In Vivo.* 2005;19:801–805.

49. Linde K, Barrett B, Wolkart K, et al. Echinacea for preventing and treating the common cold. *Cochrane Database Syst Rev.* 2006;CD000530.

50. Linde K, Berner M, Egger M, Mulrow C. St John's wort for depression: meta-analysis of randomised controlled trials. *Br J Psychiatry.* 2005;186:99–107.

51. Linde K, Knuppel L. Large-scale observational studies of hypericum extracts in patients with depressive disorders—a systematic review. *Phytomedicine.* 2005;12: 148–157.

52. Luo Y. Alzheimer's disease, the nematode *Caenorhabditis elegans,* and *Ginkgo biloba* leaf extract. *Life Sci.* 2006; 78:2066–2072.

53. Massey PB. Dietary supplements. *Med Clin North Am.* 2002;86:127–147.

54. Mayo JC, Sainz RM, Tan DX, et al. Melatonin and Parkinson's disease. *Endocrine.* 2005;27:169–178.

55. McArdle WD, Katch FI, Katch VL. The micronutrients and water. In: *Sports and Exercise Nutrition.* 2nd ed. Philadelphia: Lippincott Williams and Wilkins; 2005.

56. Mennini T, Gobbi M. The antidepressant mechanism of *Hypericum perforatum. Life Sci.* 2004;75:1021–1027.

57. Mevorah B, Orion E, Matz H, Wolf R. Cutaneous side effects of alternative therapy. *Dermatol Ther.* 2003;16: 141–149.

58. Miller SC, Pandi-Perumal SR, Esquifino AI, et al. The role of melatonin in immuno-enhancement: potential application in cancer. *Int J Exp Pathol.* 2006;87:81–88.

59. Mills E, Wu P, Seely D, Guyatt G. Melatonin in the treatment of cancer: a systematic review of randomized controlled trials and meta-analysis. *J Pineal Res.* 2005; 39:360–366.

60. Milner JA. Preclinical perspectives on garlic and cancer. *J Nutr.* 2006;136(suppl):827S–831S.

61. Niggemann B, Gruber C. Side-effects of complementary and alternative medicine. *Allergy.* 2003;58:707–716.

62. Nishida S. Metabolic effects of melatonin on oxidative stress and diabetes mellitus. *Endocrine.* 2005;27: 131–136.

63. Ortiz JG, Nieves-Natal J, Chavez P. Effects of Valeriana officinalis extracts on [3H]flunitrazepam binding, synaptosomal [3H]GABA uptake, and hippocampal [3H]GABA release. *Neurochem Res.* 1999;24:1373–1378.

64. Owens S, Wagner P, Vangsness CT, Jr. Recent advances in glucosamine and chondroitin supplementation. *J Knee Surg.* 2004;17:185–193.

65. Peres MF, Masruha MR, Zukerman E, et al. Potential therapeutic use of melatonin in migraine and other headache disorders. *Expert Opin Investig Drugs.* 2006; 15:367–375.

66. Phillips GC. Medicolegal issues and ergogenic aids: trade, tragedy, and public safety, the example of ephedra and the Dietary Supplement Health and Education Act. *Curr Sports Med Rep.* 2004;3:224–228.

67. *Physician's Desk Reference (PDR) for Nonprescription Drugs, Dietary Supplements, and Herbs: The Definitive Guide to OTC Medications.* Montvale, NJ: Thompson PDR; 2006.

68. Radad K, Gille G, Liu L, Rausch WD. Use of ginseng in medicine with emphasis on neurodegenerative disorders. *J Pharmacol Sci.* 2006;100:175–186.

69. Rahman K, Lowe GM. Garlic and cardiovascular disease: a critical review. *J Nutr.* 2006;136(suppl): 736S–740S.

70. Schiano TD. Hepatotoxicity and complementary and alternative medicines. *Clin Liver Dis.* 2003;7: 453–473.

71. Schoop R, Klein P, Suter A, Johnston SL. Echinacea in the prevention of induced rhinovirus colds: a meta-analysis. *Clin Ther.* 2006;28:174–183.

72. Schulz V. Safety of St. John's Wort extract compared to synthetic antidepressants. *Phytomedicine.* 2006;13: 199–204.

73. Skidmore-Roth L. *Mosby's Handbook of Herbal and Natural Supplements.* 3rd ed. St Louis: Mosby; 2006.

74. Tattelman E. Health effects of garlic. *Am Fam Physician.* 2005;72:103–106.

75. Tindle HA, Davis RB, Phillips RS, Eisenberg DM. Trends in use of complementary and alternative medicine by US adults: 1997–2002. *Altern Ther Health Med.* 2005;11:42–49.

76. Tso P. Gastrointestinal secretion, digestion, and absorption. In: Rhoades RA, Tanner GA, eds. *Medical Physiology.* 2nd ed. Philadelphia: Lippincott Williams and Wilkins; 2003.

77. Ulbricht C, Basch E, Boon H, et al. Safety review of kava *(Piper methysticum)* by the Natural Standard Research Collaboration. *Expert Opin Drug Saf.* 2005;4:779–794.

78. Wesselius T, Heersema DJ, Mostert JP, et al. A randomized crossover study of bee sting therapy for multiple sclerosis. *Neurology.* 2005;65:1764–1768.

79. Wheatley D. Medicinal plants for insomnia: a review of their pharmacology, efficacy and tolerability. *J Psychopharmacol.* 2005;19:414–421.

80. Williamson EM. Drug interactions between herbal and prescription medicines. *Drug Saf.* 2003;26:1075–1092.

81. Willis GL. The role of ML-23 and other melatonin analogues in the treatment and management of Parkinson's disease. *Drug News Perspect.* 2005;18:437–444.

82. Wilt T, Ishani A, Mac Donald R. Serenoa repens for benign prostatic hyperplasia. *Cochrane Database Syst Rev.* 2002;CD001423.

83. Xie JT, Mchendale S, Yuan CS. Ginseng and diabetes. *Am J Chin Med.* 2005;33:397–404.

84. Zanoli P. Role of hyperforin in the pharmacological activities of St. John's Wort. *CNS Drug Rev.* 2004;10: 203–218.

85. Zhou W, Chai H, Lin PH, et al. Molecular mechanisms and clinical applications of ginseng root for cardiovascular disease. *Med Sci Monit.* 2004;10:RA187–RA192.

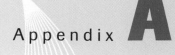

Drugs Administered by Iontophoresis and Phonophoresis

Drugs that may be administered by iontophoresis and phonophoresis are listed here. Administration of these agents by these techniques is largely empirical. The use of these substances in the conditions listed is based primarily on clinical observation and anecdotal reports in the literature. Likewise, the preparation strengths given here are merely suggestions based on currently available information.

Drug	Principal Indication(s)	Treatment Rationale	Iontophoresis	Phonophoresis
Acetic acid	Calcific tendinitis	Acetate is believed to increase solubility of calcium deposits in tendons and other soft tissues	2%–5% aqueous solution from negative pole	–
Calcium chloride	Skeletal muscle spasms	Calcium stabilizes excitable membranes; appears to decrease excitability threshold in peripheral nerves and skeletal muscle	2% aqueous solution from positive pole	–
Dexamethasone	Inflammation	Synthetic steroidal anti-inflammatory agent (see Chapter 29)	4 mg/mL in aqueous solution from negative pole	0.4% ointment
Hydrocortisone	Inflammation	Anti-inflammatory steroid (see Chapter 29)	0.5% ointment from positive pole	0.5%–1.0% ointment
Hyaluronidase	Local edema (subacute and chronic stage)	Appears to increase permeability in connective tissue by hydrolyzing hyaluronic acid, thus decreasing encapsulation and allowing disbursement of local edema	Reconstitute with 0.9% sodium chloride to provide a 150 mg/mL solution from positive pole	–

(Continued on following page)

Drug	Principal Indication(s)	Treatment Rationale	Iontophoresis	Phonophoresis
Iodine	Adhesive capsulitis and other soft-tissue adhesions; microbial infections	Iodine is a broad-spectrum antibiotic, hence its use in infections, etc.; the sclerolytic actions of iodine are not fully understood	5%–10% solution or ointment from negative pole	10% ointment
Lidocaine	Soft-tissue pain and inflammation (e.g., bursitis, tenosynovitis)	Local anesthetic effects (see Chapter 12)	4%–5% solution or ointment from positive pole	5% ointment
Magnesium sulfate	Skeletal muscle spasms; myositis	Muscle relaxant effect may be caused by decreased excitability of the skeletal muscle membrane and decreased transmission at the neuromuscular junction	2% aqueous solution or ointment from positive pole	2% ointment
Salicylates	Muscle and joint pain in acute and chronic conditions (e.g., overuse injuries, rheumatoid arthritis)	Aspirinlike drugs with analgesic and anti-inflammatory effects (see Chapter 15)	10% trolamine salicylate ointment or 2%–3% sodium salicylate solution from negative pole	10% trolamine salicylate ointment or 3% sodium salicylate ointment
Tolazoline hydrochloride	Indolent cutaneous ulcers	Increases local blood flow and tissue healing by inhibiting vascular smooth muscle contraction	2% aqueous solution or ointment from positive pole	–
Zinc oxide	Skin ulcers; other dermatologic disorders	Zinc acts as a general antiseptic; may increase tissue healing	20% ointment from positive pole	20% ointment

Use of the *Physicians' Desk Reference*

Several drug indexes are available that can supplement this text by serving as a detailed source of information about individual drugs. One of the most readily available and frequently used indexes is the *Physicians' Desk Reference*, or *PDR*. The *PDR* is published annually by Thomson PDR, Montvale, NJ 07645-1742.

Drug manufacturers submit information about the indications, dosages, adverse effects, and so on, of individual agents for inclusion in the *PDR*. The *PDR* is then published annually, providing a relatively current source of information. The *PDR* is also updated within a given year through periodic supplements.

The *PDR* begins by listing all the manufacturers who submitted information to the *PDR* in the "Manufacturers' Index." Immediately following the "Manufacturers' Index," drugs are listed according to the "Brand and Generic Name Index" and the "Product Category Index." These listings are followed by detailed descriptions of the drugs in the "Product Information Section," which constitutes the bulk of the *PDR*.

Using the *PDR* for the first time can be somewhat confusing because drugs are listed in several different ways. This brief outline may help individuals use the *PDR* more effectively to obtain information about specific agents.

1. **If the Trade Name or Brand Name of the Drug Is Known.** Begin by looking in the "Brand and Generic Name Index" in the front of the *PDR*, easily found by locating the PINK pages. Drugs are listed alphabetically according to the name given by the drug manufacturer (trade, or brand name) as well as by the generic name (see section 2, below). Each trade name is followed by the name of the manufacturer (in parentheses) and by a page number, which indicates where the drug is described in the "Product Information" section. Some trade names are preceded by a small diamond and will usually have two page numbers following the name. This diamond indicates that a color photograph of the actual medication is provided in the special section of the *PDR* known as the "Product Identification Guide." The first page number following the drug name is the page that illustrates a picture of the drug, and the second page number identifies where the written information can be found.

Many drugs listed in the "Brand and Generic Name Index" have several variations on the trade name, depending on different forms of the drug and routes of administration. For example, a drug that is available in tablets, capsules, and injectable forms may have slight variations on the trade name that reflect these different preparations.

2. **If the Generic or Chemical Name Is Known.** If you are using an edition of the *PDR* published in 1994 or later, begin by looking in the "Brand and Generic Name Index" (PINK pages). This section integrates generic names into the alphabetical listing of trade names. The generic name of each drug is followed by the trade name, manufacturer (in parentheses), and pages where the drug is illustrated and described. Often, the generic heading in this section is followed by several different trade names, indicating that several different manufacturers market the drug.

Older editions of the *PDR* (1993 and earlier) list generic and chemical names in a separate section called the "Generic and Chemical Name Index," marked by YELLOW pages. If you are using an older edition, consult this section if you know only the generic name.

3. **To Find Out What Drugs Are Available to Treat a Given Disorder.** The best place to begin is the "Product Category Index" located in the BLUE pages. Here, drugs are listed according to the principal pharmacologic classifications, such as anesthetics, laxatives, and sedatives. Major categories in this section are often subdivided into subcategories that are more specific. For example, cardiovascular preparations are subdivided into antiarrhythmics, beta-adrenergic blocking agents, vasodilators, and others. Drugs in each category (or subcategory) are listed according to their trade name, followed by the manufacturer (in parentheses) and the pages on which the drug is illustrated and described.

4. **If You Want to Contact the Manufacturer for More Information about the Drug.** Look in the "Manufacturers' Index" located in the WHITE pages at the very beginning of the *PDR*. Manufacturers who have contributed to the *PDR* are listed alphabetically, with an address and phone number that serve as a source for inquiries. In addition, a partial listing of the products available from each manufacturer is included following the manufacturer's name and address.

5. **If You Want to Identify the Name of a Specific Pill, Capsule, or Tablet.** Locate the "Product Identification Guide," which contains glossy color photographs of many of the drugs. Drugs are categorized alphabetically according to their manufacturer. Often, individual pills, tablets, and other forms have the name of the manufacturer scored or printed directly on the medication. An unknown medication can be identified by matching the drug to the pictures listed under that manufacturer.

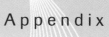

Drugs of Abuse

Some of the more frequently abused drugs are listed here. Agents such as cocaine and the psychedelics are illicit drugs with no major pharmacotherapeutic value. Other drugs such as barbiturates, benzodiazepines, and opioids are routinely used for therapeutic reasons but have a strong potential for abuse when taken indiscriminately. Finally, drugs such as alcohol, caffeine, and nicotine are readily available in various commercial products but may also be considered drugs of abuse when consumed in large quantities for prolonged periods.

Drug(s)	Classification/ Action	Route/Method of Administration	Effect Desired by User	Principal Adverse Effects	Additional Information
Alcohol	Sedative-hypnotic	Oral, from various beverages (wine, beer, other alcoholic drinks)	Euphoria; relaxed inhibitions; decreased anxiety; sense of escape	Physical dependence; impaired motor skills; chronic degenerative changes in the brain, liver, and other organs	See Chapter 6
Barbiturates Nembutal Seconal Others	Sedative-hypnotic	Oral or injected (IM, IV)	Relaxation and a sense of calmness; drowsiness	Physical dependence; possible death from overdose; behavior changes (irritability, psychosis) following prolonged use	See Chapter 6
Benzodiazepines Valium Librium Others	Similar to barbiturates	Similar to barbiturates	Similar to barbiturates	Similar to barbiturates	Similar to barbiturates
Caffeine	CNS stimulant	Oral; from coffee, tea, other beverages	Increased alertness; decreased fatigue; improved work capacity	Sleep disturbances; irritability; nervousness; cardiac arrhythmias	See Chapter 26

(Continued on following page)

Drug(s)	Classification/ Action	Route/Method of Administration	Effect Desired by User	Principal Adverse Effects	Additional Information
Cannabinoids Hashish Marijuana	Psychoactive drugs with mixed (stimulant and depressant) activity	Smoked; possible oral ingestion	Initial response: euphoria, excitement, increased perception; later response: relaxation, stupor, dreamlike state	Endocrine changes (decreased testosterone in males) and changes in respiratory function similar to chronic cigarette smoking are associated with heavy use	—
Cocaine	CNS stimulant (when taken systemically)	"Snorted" (absorbed via nasal mucosa); smoked (in crystalline form)	Euphoria; excitement; feelings of intense pleasure and well-being	Physical dependence; acute CNS and cardiac toxicity; profound mood swings	See Chapter 12
Narcotics Demerol Morphine Heroin Others	Natural and synthetic opioids; analgesics	Oral or injected (IM, IV)	Relaxation; euphoria; feelings of tranquility; prevent onset of opiate withdrawal	Physical dependence; respiratory depression; high potential for death due to overdose	See Chapter 14
Nicotine	CNS toxin; produces variable effects via somatic and autonomic nervous system interaction	Smoked or absorbed from tobacco products (cigarettes, cigars, chewing tobacco)	Relaxation; calming effect; decreased irritability	Physical dependence; possible carcinogen; associated with pathologic changes in respiratory function during long-term tobacco use	—
Psychedelics LSD Mescaline Phencyclidine (PCP) Psilocybin	Hallucinogens	Oral; may also be smoked or inhaled	Altered perception and insight; distorted senses; disinhibition	Severe hallucinations; panic reaction; acute psychotic reactions	—

Glossary

Common terms related to pharmacology and a brief definition of each term are listed here. Synonyms (SYN), antonyms (ANT), and common abbreviations (ABBR) are also included, whenever applicable.

Acetylcholine: A neurotransmitter in the somatic and autonomic nervous systems; principal synapses using acetylcholine include the skeletal neuromuscular junction, autonomic ganglia, and certain pathways in the brain.

Adenylate cyclase: An enzyme located on the inner surface of many cell membranes; it is important in mediating biochemical changes in the cell in response to drug and hormone stimulation (SYN: adenyl cyclase).

Adrenergic: Refers to synapses or physiologic responses involving epinephrine and norepinephrine.

Adrenocorticosteroids: The group of steroid hormones produced by the adrenal cortex. These drugs include the glucocorticoids (cortisol, cortisone), mineralocorticoids (aldosterone), and sex hormones (androgens, estrogens, progestins).

Affinity: The mutual attraction between a drug and a specific cellular receptor.

Agonist: A drug that binds to a receptor and causes some change in cell function (ANT: antagonist).

Akathisia: A feeling of extreme motor restlessness and an inability to sit still; may occur because of antipsychotic drug therapy.

Allergy: A state of hypersensitivity to foreign substances (e.g., environmental antigens and certain drugs), manifested by an exaggerated response of the immune system.

Alpha receptors: A primary class of receptors that are responsive to epinephrine and norepinephrine. Alpha receptors are subclassified into alpha-1 and alpha-2 receptors based on their sensitivity to various drugs.

Anabolic steroids: Natural and synthetic male hormones that may be misused in an attempt to increase muscle size and improve athletic performance (SYN: androgens).

Analgesia: To lessen or relieve pain. Drugs with this ability are known as *analgesics*.

Androgen: A male steroid such as testosterone.

Angina pectoris: Severe pain and constriction in the chest region, usually associated with myocardial ischemia.

Angiogenesis: The development of new blood vessels. Drugs that inhibit this effect can be useful in limiting the growth and proliferation of certain tumors.

Antagonist: A drug that binds to a receptor but does not cause a change in cell activity (SYN: blocker).

Anthelmintic: A drug that destroys parasitic worms (e.g., tapeworms, roundworms) in the gastrointestinal tract and elsewhere in the body.

Anticholinergic: Drugs that decrease activity at acetylcholine synapses. These agents are often used to diminish activity in the parasympathetic nervous system (SYN: parasympatholytic).

Anticoagulation: A decrease in the blood's capacity to coagulate (clot). Drugs with the ability to decrease coagulation are known as *anticoagulants*.

Antimetabolite: The general term for drugs that impair function in harmful cells and microorganisms by antagonizing or replacing normal metabolic substrates in those cells. Certain anti-infectious and antineoplastic agents function as antimetabolites.

Antineoplastic: A drug that prevents or attenuates the growth and proliferation of cancerous cells.

Antipyresis: The reduction of fever. Drugs with the ability to reduce fevers are known as *antipyretics.*

Antitussive: A drug that reduces coughing.

Aromatase: An enzyme responsible for estrogen biosynthesis.

Asthma: A chronic disease of the respiratory system characterized by bronchoconstriction, airway inflammation, and the formation of mucous plugs in the airway.

Bactericidal: An agent that kills or destroys bacteria.

Bacteriostatic: An agent that inhibits the growth and proliferation of bacteria.

Beta receptor: A primary class of the receptors that are responsive to epinephrine and (to a lesser extent) norepinephrine. Beta receptors are subclassified into beta-1 and beta-2 receptors based on their sensitivity to various drugs.

Bioavailability: The extent to which a drug reaches the systemic circulation following administration by various routes.

Biotransformation: Biochemical changes that occur to the drug within the body, usually resulting in the breakdown and inactivation of the drug (SYN: drug metabolism).

Bipolar disorder: A psychological disorder characterized by mood swings ranging from excitable (manic) periods to periods of depression (SYN: manic-depression).

Blood-brain barrier: The specialized anatomic arrangement of cerebral capillary walls that serves to restrict the passage of some drugs into the brain.

Blood dyscrasia: A pathologic condition of the blood, usually referring to a defect in one or more of the blood's cellular elements.

Carcinogen: Any substance that produces cancer or increases the risk of developing cancer.

Catecholamine: A group of chemically similar compounds that are important in the modulation of cardiovascular activity and many other physiologic functions. Common catecholamines include epinephrine, norepinephrine, and dopamine.

Cathartic: An agent that causes a relatively rapid evacuation of the bowels.

Ceiling effect: The point at which no further increase in response occurs as a drug dose is progressively increased; this effect is represented by a plateau on the drug's dose-response curve (SYN: maximal efficacy).

Chemical name: A drug name that is derived from the specific chemical structure of the compound. Chemical names are not used clinically but are shortened in some way to form the drug's generic name.

Chemotherapy: The use of chemical agents to treat infectious or neoplastic disease.

Cholinergic: Refers to synapses or physiologic responses involving acetylcholine.

Cholinesterase: The enzyme that breaks down acetylcholine (SYN: acetylcholinesterase).

Clearance: The process by which the active form of the drug is removed from the bloodstream by either metabolism or excretion.

Congestive heart failure: A clinical syndrome of cardiac disease that is marked by decreased myocardial contractility, peripheral edema, shortness of breath, and decreased tolerance for physical exertion.

Cretinism: A congenital syndrome of mental retardation, decreased metabolism, and impaired physical development secondary to insufficient production of thyroid hormones.

Cyclic adenosine monophosphate (ABBR: cAMP): The ring-shaped conformation of adenosine monophosphate, which is important in acting as a second messenger in mediating the intracellular response to drug stimulation.

Cyclooxygenase (ABBR: COX): The key enzyme involved in prostaglandin biosynthesis. This enzyme converts arachidonic acid into prostaglandin G_2, thereby providing the precursor for the cell to synthesize additional prostaglandins.

Cytokine: The general term used to describe proteins produced by various immune and inflammatory cells. These proteins act as intercellular chemical signals that help orchestrate immune and inflammatory responses. Common cytokines include the interferons, interleukins, and certain growth factors.

Demand dose: Amount of drug administered when a patient activates certain drug delivery systems, such as those used during patient-controlled analgesia.

Desensitization: A brief and transient decrease in the responsiveness of cellular receptors to drug effects.

Diabetes insipidus: A disease marked by increased urination (polyuria) and excessive thirst (polydipsia) due to inadequate production of antidiuretic hormone (ADH) and/or a decrease in the renal response to ADH.

Diabetes mellitus: A disease marked by abnormal metabolism of glucose and other energy substrates caused by a defect in the production of insulin and/or a decrease in the peripheral response to insulin.

Diuretic: A drug that increases the formation and excretion of urine.

Dopa decarboxylase: The enzyme that converts dihydroxyphenylalanine (dopa) into dopamine.

Dopamine: A neurotransmitter located in the central nervous system (CNS) that is important in motor control as well as in certain aspects of behavior. The presence of endogenous or exogenous dopamine in the periphery also affects cardiovascular function.

Dosage: The amount of medication that is appropriate for treating a given condition or illness.

Dose: The amount of medication that is administered at one time.

Dose-response curve: The relationship between incremental doses of a drug and the magnitude of the reaction that those doses will cause.

Down-regulation: A prolonged decrease in the number and/or sensitivity of drug receptors, usually occurring as a compensatory response to overstimulation of the receptor.

Drug holiday: A period of several days to several weeks in which medications are withdrawn from the patient to allow recovery from drug tolerance or tox-icity; sometimes used in patients with advanced cases of Parkinson disease.

Drug microsomal metabolizing system (ABBR: DMMS): A series of enzymes located on the smooth endoplasmic reticulum that are important in catalyzing drug biotransformation.

Dysentery: The general term for severe gastrointestinal distress (diarrhea, cramps, bloody stools) that is usually associated with the presence of infectious microorganisms in the intestines.

Eicosanoids: The general term for the group of 20-carbon fatty acids that includes the prostaglandins, thromboxanes, and leukotrienes. These substances are involved in mediating inflammation and other pathologic responses.

Emetic: A drug that initiates or facilitates vomiting.

End-of-dose akinesia: A phenomenon in Parkinson disease in which the effectiveness of the medication wears off toward the end of the dosing interval, resulting in a virtual lack of volitional movement from the patient.

Enteral administration: Administration of drugs by way of the alimentary canal.

Enzyme induction: The process wherein some drugs provoke cells to synthesize more drug-metabolizing enzymes, thus leading to accelerated drug biotransformation.

Epidural nerve block: Administration of local anesthesia into the spinal canal between the bony vertebral column and the dura mater (i.e., the injection does not penetrate the spinal membranes but remains above the dura).

Epilepsy: A chronic neurologic disorder characterized by recurrent seizures that are manifested as brief periods of altered consciousness, involuntary motor activity, or vivid sensory phenomena.

Epinephrine: A hormone synthesized primarily in the adrenal medulla, mimicking the peripheral effects of norepinephrine. Epinephrine is involved in the sympathetic nervous system response to stress and is especially effective in stimulating cardiovascular function (SYN: adrenaline).

Estrogens: The general term for natural and synthetic female hormones such as estradiol and estrone.

Expectorant: A drug that facilitates the production and discharge of mucous secretions from the respiratory tract.

First-pass effect: The phenomenon in which drugs absorbed from the stomach and small intestine must pass through the liver before reaching the systemic circulation. Certain drugs undergo extensive hepatic metabolism because of this first pass through the liver.

Food and Drug Administration (ABBR: FDA): The official government agency involved in regulating the pharmaceutical industry in the United States.

Gamma-aminobutyric acid (ABBR: GABA): An inhibitory neurotransmitter in the brain and spinal cord.

Generic name: The name applied to a drug, which is not protected by a trademark; usually a shortened version of the drug's chemical name (SYN: nonproprietary name).

Glucocorticoid: The general class of steroid agents that affect glucose metabolism and are used pharmacologically to decrease inflammation and suppress the immune system. Principle examples include cortisol and corticosterone.

Glycosuria: The presence of glucose in the urine.

Gonadotropin: A hormone that produces a stimulatory effect on the gonads (ovaries and testes); primary gonadotropins include luteinizing hormone (LH) and follicle-stimulating hormone (FSH).

G proteins: Proteins that bind with guanine nucleotides and regulate cell activity. G proteins often serve as a link between surface receptors and intracellular enzymes such as adenylate cyclase.

Half-life: The time required to eliminate 50 percent of the drug existing in the body.

Histamine: A chemical produced by various cells in the body that is involved in the modulation of certain physiologic responses (e.g., secretion of gastric acid), as well as in the mediation of hypersensitivity (allergic) responses.

Hypercalcemia: An excessive concentration of calcium in the bloodstream (ANT: hypocalcemia).

Hyperglycemia: An excessive concentration of glucose in the bloodstream (ANT: hypoglycemia).

Hypersensitivity: An exaggerated response of the immune system to a foreign substance (SYN: allergic response).

Hypertension: A pathologic condition characterized by a sustained, reproducible increase in blood pressure.

Hypnotic: A drug that initiates or maintains a relatively normal state of sleep.

Hypokalemia: An abnormally low concentration of potassium in the bloodstream (ANT: hyperkalemia).

Hyponatremia: An abnormally low concentration of sodium in the bloodstream (ANT: hypernatremia).

Immunosuppressant: A drug used to attenuate the body's immune response. These agents are often used to prevent rejection of organ transplants or to treat diseases caused by overactivity in the immune system (ANT: immunostimulant).

Interferon: A member of the group of proteins that exert a number of physiologic and pharmacologic effects, including antiviral and antineoplastic activity.

Intrathecal: Administration of substances within a sheath; typically refers to injection into the subarachnoid space surrounding the spinal cord.

Laxative: An agent that promotes peristalsis and evacuation of the bowel in a relatively slow manner (as opposed to a cathartic).

Leukotriene: One of the 20-carbon fatty acid compounds (eicosanoids) formed from arachidonic acid by the lipoxygenase enzyme. Leukotrienes are important in mediating certain allergic and inflammatory responses, especially in respiratory tissues.

Lipoxygenase (ABBR: LOX): The enzyme that initiates leukotriene biosynthesis. This enzyme converts arachidonic acid into precursors that the cell uses to synthesize specific leukotrienes.

Loading dose: Amount of drug administered at the onset of treatment to rapidly bring the amount of drug in the body to therapeutic levels.

Lockout interval: The minimum amount of time that must expire between each dose of medication that is administered by patient-controlled analgesia (PCA). The PCA pump is inactivated during the lockout interval so that the patient cannot self-administer excessive amounts of drugs.

Lymphokines: Chemicals released from activated lymphocytes that help mediate various aspects of the immune response. Common lymphokines include the interleukins and gamma interferon.

Malignancy: A term usually applied to cancerous tumors that tend to become progressively worse.

Maximal efficacy: The maximum response a drug can produce; the point at which the response does not increase even if the dosage continues to increase (SYN: ceiling effect).

Median effective dose (ABBR: ED_{50}): The drug dose that produces a specific therapeutic response in 50 percent of the patients in whom it is tested.

Median lethal dose (ABBR: LD_{50}): The drug dose that causes death in 50 percent of the experimental animals in which it is tested.

Median toxic dose (ABBR: TD_{50}): The drug dose that produces a specific adverse (toxic) response in 50 percent of the patients in whom it is tested.

Metabolite: The compound that is formed when the drug undergoes biotransformation and is chemically altered by some metabolic process.

Metastasize: The transfer or spread of diseased (i.e., cancerous) cells from a primary location to other sites in the body.

Mineralocorticoid: A steroid hormone (e.g., aldosterone) that is important in regulating fluid and electrolyte balance by increasing the reabsorption of sodium from the kidneys.

Monoamine oxidase (ABBR: MAO): An enzyme that breaks down monoamine neurotransmitters such as dopamine, norepinephrine, and serotonin.

Monoclonal antibody: An antibody created by fusing a mouse myeloma cell with a human B lymphocyte. These antibodies recognize specific cell-surface antigens on cancer cells or other tissues to target the drug directly to that tissue.

Mucolytic: A drug that decreases the viscosity and increases the fluidity of mucous secretions in the respiratory tract, thus making it easier for the patient to cough up secretions.

Muscarinic receptor: A primary class of cholinergic receptors that are named according to their affinity for the muscarine toxin. Certain cholinergic agonists and antagonists also have a relatively selective affinity for muscarinic receptors.

Myxedema: The adult or acquired form of hypothyroidism characterized by decreased metabolic rate, lethargy, decreased mental alertness, weight gain, and other somatic changes.

Neuroleptic: A term frequently used to describe antipsychotic drugs, referring to the tendency of these drugs to produce a behavioral syndrome of apathy, sedation, decreased initiative, and decreased responsiveness (SYN: antipsychotic).

Nicotinic receptor: A primary class of cholinergic receptors, named according to their affinity for nicotine, as well as certain other cholinergic agonists and antagonists.

Norepinephrine: A neurotransmitter that is important in certain brain pathways and in the terminal synapses of the sympathetic nervous system (SYN: noradrenaline).

On-off phenomenon: The fluctuation in response seen in certain patients with Parkinson disease, in which the effectiveness of medications may suddenly diminish at some point between dosages.

Opioid: An analgesic drug with morphinelike effects; commonly refers to the synthetic forms of these analgesics (SYN: narcotic).

Orthostatic hypotension: A sudden fall in blood pressure that occurs when the patient stands erect; this is a frequent side effect of many medications.

Ototoxicity: The harmful side effect of some drugs and toxins influencing the ear's hearing and balance functions.

Over-the-counter drugs (ABBR: OTC): Drugs that can be purchased directly by the consumer without a prescription (SYN: nonprescription drugs).

Parenteral administration: Administration of drugs by routes other than via the alimentary canal: by injection, transdermally, topically, and so on.

Parkinson disease or **parkinsonism:** The clinical syndrome of bradykinesia, rigidity, resting tremor, and postural instability associated with neurotransmitter abnormalities within the basal ganglia.

Pharmacodynamics: The study of how drugs affect the body; that is, the physiologic and biochemical mechanisms of drug action.

Pharmacokinetics: The study of how the body handles drugs; that is, the manner in which drugs are absorbed, distributed, metabolized, and excreted.

Pharmacologic dose: An amount of drug given that is much greater than the amount of a similar substance produced within the body; this increased dose is used to exaggerate the beneficial effects normally provided by the endogenous compound.

Pharmacotherapeutics: The study of how drugs are used in the prevention and treatment of disease.

Pharmacy: The professional discipline dealing with the preparation and dispensing of medications.

Physical dependence: A phenomenon that develops during prolonged use of addictive substances, signified by the onset of withdrawal symptoms when the drug is discontinued.

Physiologic dose: The amount of drug given that is roughly equivalent to the amount of a similar substance normally produced within the body; this dose is typically used to replace the endogenous substance when the body is no longer able to produce the substance.

Placebo: A medication that contains inert or inactive ingredients; used to pacify a patient or test a patient's psychophysiologic response to treatment.

Potency: The dose of a drug that produces a given response in a specific amplitude. When two drugs are compared, the more potent drug will produce a given response at a lower dose.

Progestins: The general term for the natural and synthetic female hormones such as progesterone.

Prostaglandin: A member of the family of 20-carbon fatty acid compounds (eicosanoids) formed from arachidonic acid by the cyclooxygenase enzyme. Prostaglandins help regulate normal cell activity, and may help mediate certain pathologic responses, including pain, inflammation, fever, and abnormal blood coagulation.

Psychosis: A relatively severe form of mental illness characterized by marked thought disturbances and an impaired perception of reality.

Receptor: The component of the cell (usually a protein) to which the drug binds, thus initiating a change in cell function.

Salicylate: The chemical term commonly used to denote compounds such as aspirin that have anti-inflammatory, analgesic, antipyretic, and anticoagulant properties.

Second messenger: The term applied to compounds formed within the cell, such as cyclic AMP. The second messenger initiates a series of biochemical changes within the cell following stimulation of a receptor on the cell's outer surface by drugs, hormones, and so on.

Sedative: A drug that produces a calming effect and serves to pacify the patient. These agents are sometimes referred to as *minor tranquilizers.*

Seizure: A sudden attack of symptoms usually associated with diseases such as epilepsy. Epileptic seizures are due to the random, uncontrolled firing of a group of cerebral neurons, which results in a variety of sensory and motor manifestations.

Selective toxicity: A desired effect of antineoplastic and anti-infectious agents, wherein the drug kills the pathogenic organism or cells without damaging healthy tissues.

Serotonin: A neurotransmitter located in the central nervous system (CNS) that is important in many functions, including mood, arousal, and inhibition of painful stimuli (SYN: 5-hydroxytryptamine).

Side effect: Any effect produced by a drug that occurs in addition to the principal therapeutic response.

Spinal nerve block: Administration of local anesthesia into the spinal canal between the arachnoid membrane and the pia mater (i.e., the subarachnoid space).

Status epilepticus: An emergency characterized by a rapid series of epileptic seizures that occur without any appreciable recovery between seizures.

Steroid: The general term used to describe a group of hormones and their analogs that have a common chemical configuration but are divided into several categories depending on their primary physiologic effects. Common types of steroids include the glucocorticoids (cortisone, prednisone, many others), mineralocorticoids (aldosterone), androgens/anabolic steroids (testosterone), and steroids related to female physiologic function (estrogen, progesterone).

Supersensitivity: An increased response to drugs and endogenous compounds caused by an increase in the number and/or sensitivity of receptors for that drug.

Sympatholytics: Drugs that inhibit or antagonize function within the sympathetic nervous system.

Sympathomimetics: Drugs that facilitate or increase activity within the sympathetic nervous system.

Tardive dyskinesia: A movement disorder characterized by involuntary, fragmented movements of the mouth, face, and jaw (i.e., chewing, sucking, tongue protrusion, and the like). This disorder may occur during the prolonged administration of antipsychotic drugs.

Therapeutic index (ABBR: TI): A ratio used to represent the relative safety of a particular drug; the larger the therapeutic index, the safer the drug. It is calculated as the median toxic dose divided by the median effective dose. (In animal trials, the median lethal dose is often substituted for the median toxic dose.)

Therapeutic window: The range of drug concentrations in the body that will promote optimal beneficial effects. Drug concentrations less than the lower end of this range will be ineffective, and concentrations greater than the upper end of this range will create excessive side effects.

Thyrotoxicosis: Abnormally high production of thyroid hormones resulting in symptoms such as nervousness, weight loss, and tachycardia (SYN: hyperthyroidism).

Tolerance: The acquired phenomenon associated with some drugs, in which larger dosages of the drug are needed to achieve a given effect when the drug is used for prolonged periods.

Toxicology: The study of the harmful effects of drugs and other chemicals.

Trade name: The name given to a drug by the pharmaceutical company; it is protected by a trademark and used by the company for marketing the drug (SYN: proprietary name).

Vaccine: A substance typically consisting of a modified infectious microorganism that is administered to help prevent disease by stimulating the endogenous immune defense mechanisms against infection.

Viscosupplementation: Injection of a polysaccharide (hyaluronin) into osteoarthritic joints to help restore the viscosity of synovial fluid.

Volume of distribution (ABBR: V_d): A ratio used to estimate the distribution of a drug within the body relative to the total amount of fluid in the body. It is calculated as the amount of drug administered divided by the plasma concentration of the drug.

Withdrawal syndrome: The clinical syndrome of somatic and psychologic manifestations that occur when a drug is removed from a patient who has become physically dependent on a drug (SYN: abstinence syndrome).

Index